Fundamentals of Operative Dentistry: A Contemporary Approach

Third Edition

Fundamentals of
Operative Dentistry

A Contemporary Approach

Third Edition

Edited by

James B. Summitt, DDS, MS
Professor and Chairman
Department of Restorative Dentistry
University of Texas Health Science Center at San Antonio
San Antonio, Texas

J. William Robbins, DDS, MA
Private Practice, General Dentistry
Clinical Professor
Department of General Dentistry
University of Texas Health Science Center at San Antonio
San Antonio, Texas

Thomas J. Hilton, DMD, MS
Alumni Centennial Professor in Operative Dentistry
Department of Restorative Dentistry
Oregon Health & Science University
School of Dentistry
Portland, Oregon

Richard S. Schwartz, DDS
Private Practice, Endodontics
San Antonio, Texas

Illustrations by
Jose dos Santos, Jr, DDS, PhD
Adjunct Professor
Department of Restorative Dentistry
University of Texas Health Science Center at San Antonio
San Antonio, Texas

Quintessence Publishing Co, Inc

Chicago, Berlin, Tokyo, London, Paris, Milan, Barcelona, Istanbul,
São Paulo, New Delhi, Moscow, Prague, and Warsaw

To my wife and one love, Joanne, my loving children, Carrie and J.B., J.B.'s wife, Minna, and our grandson, Will.
—JBS

To my favorite kids, Alyssa, Sarah, and Andrew, and my wife and best friend, Brenda.
—JWR

To my wife, DeaDea, for her constant love, support and encouragement; to my parents for instilling in me the qualities that have served me throughout my life; and to my mentors, three of whom are my fellow editors for this book, for inspiring me to strive for excellence.
—TJH

To my wife Jeannette, who puts up with me, takes care of me, and loves me.
She is the perfect partner in life.
—RSS

Library of Congress Cataloging-in-Publication Data

Fundamentals of operative dentistry : a contemporary approach / edited
    by James B. Summitt ... [et al.] ; illustrations by Jose dos Santos Jr.
    -- 3rd ed.
        p. ; cm.
    Includes bibliographical references and index.
    ISBN 0-86715-452-7
    1. Dentistry, Operative.   I. Summitt, James B.
    [DNLM: 1. Dentistry, Operative--instrumentation. 2. Dentistry,
Operative--methods. 3. Dental Caries--prevention & control.
4. Dental Materials--therapeutic use. 5. Dental Prosthesis.
6. Esthetics, Dental.   WU 300 F981 2006]
RK501.S436 2006
617.6'05--dc22

                                        2005028570

© 2006 Quintessence Publishing Co, Inc

Quintessence Publishing Co, Inc
4350 Chandler Drive
Hanover Park, Illinois 60133
www.quintpub.com

Editor: Lindsay Harmon
Production: Sue Robinson
Design: Dawn Hartman

Printed in India

Table of Contents

Preface

Dental educators and practicing dentists have, at times, been slow to respond to advances in dental materials and techniques. Operative dentistry, in particular, has often been influenced more by history and tradition than by science. Until recently, many restorative procedures taught in dental schools and practiced by dentists were based primarily on Dr G. V. Black's classic textbook, *A Work on Operative Dentistry*, published in 1908. The many advances in materials and instrumentation, linked with the development of reliable dental adhesives, have allowed us to modify many of Black's original concepts to more conservative, tooth-preserving procedures and to offer a much wider range of restorative options. Black was, indeed, one of dentistry's greatest innovators and original thinkers. Were he alive today, he would be leading the advance of new technology and innovation. We best honor his memory not by clinging to concepts of the past but rather by looking to recent scientific innovations and incorporating them into our practices and dental school curricula.

This textbook is about contemporary operative dentistry. It is a blend of traditional, time-proven methods and recent scientific developments. Whereas preparations for cast-gold restorations have changed relatively little over the years, preparations for amalgam and resin composite restorations are smaller and require removal of less sound tooth structure because of the development of adhesive technologies. While we still use many luting agents in the traditional manner, adhesive cements provide greater retention for cast restorations and allow expanded use of ceramic and resin composite materials. Many concepts of caries management and pulpal protection have changed drastically as well. It is our hope that this textbook, which represents an ardent effort to present current concepts and the latest scientific evidence in restorative and preventive dentistry, will be helpful to students, educators, and practicing dentists during this time of rapidly developing technologies.

Several themes echo throughout this textbook. The first is the attempt to provide a scientific basis for the concepts described. The authors are clinically active, and many are engaged in clinical and laboratory research in the areas of cariology, restorative dentistry, and/or dental materials. Whenever possible, the diagnosis and treatment options described are based on current research findings. When convincing evidence is not available, we have attempted to present a consensus founded on a significant depth of experience and informed thought.

A second theme reflected in the book is our commitment to conservative dentistry. The treatment modalities described involve the preservation of as much sound tooth structure as possible within the framework of the existing destruction and the patient's expectations for esthetic results. When disease necessitates a restoration, it should be kept as small as possible. However, it must be kept in mind that a conservative philosophy is also based on predictability. The treatment that is most predictable in terms of functional and esthetic longevity, based as much as possible on scientific evidence, must also be considered the most conservative. Therefore, when an extensive amount of tooth structure has been destroyed and remaining cusps are significantly weakened, occlusal coverage with a restoration may be the most predictable, and therefore most conservative treatment. When portions of axial tooth surfaces are healthy, their preservation is desirable. In the conservative philosophy on which this book is based, a complete-coverage restoration (complete crown) is generally considered the least desirable treatment alternative, unless the tooth condition is such that a complete-coverage restoration will provide the most predictable clinical outcome.

The book describes techniques for the restoration of health, function, and esthetics of individual teeth and the dentition as a whole. Included are descriptions of direct conservative restorations fabricated from dental amalgam, resin composite, and resin-ionomer materials. Also detailed are techniques for partial- and complete-coverage indirect restorations of gold alloy, porcelain, metal-ceramic, and resin composite.

The second edition brought greater depth to the subjects that were a part of the first edition and was expanded to include more information related to esthetic dentistry. The third edition has been updated with new information based on evidence reported since the second edition. Because of this new evidence, reference lists have been expanded. New authors were added to 9 chapters. There are only 20 chapters in the third edition instead of the 21 in the second edition because the publisher and editors wanted only a single chapter on cast-gold restorations.

This edition has also undergone a change in editorship with the addition of Tom Hilton, who contributed chapters for the first two editions, as an editor. He participated in the planning, editing, and revision of this textbook as a whole.

As in the previous editions, the primary objective in producing this book is to provide students and practitioners with current and practical concepts of prevention and management of caries as a disease and of restoration of individual teeth. It is our hope that the changes made in this edition will make it of greater benefit to those who use it.

Contributors

Thomas G. Berry, DDS, MA
Professor
Department of Restorative Dentistry
University of Colorado
School of Dentistry
Denver, Colorado

James C. Broome, DDS, MS
Associate Dean for Clinical Affairs
The University of Alabama at Birmingham
School of Dentistry
Birmingham, Alabama

John O. Burgess, DDS, MS
Assistant Dean for Clinical Research
Louisiana State University Health Science Center
School of Dentistry
New Orleans, Louisiana

Daniel C. N. Chan, DDS, MS, DDS
Professor and Director
Division of Operative Dentistry
Department of Oral Rehabilitation
Medical College of Georgia
Augusta, Georgia

Michael A. Cochran, DDS, MSD
Professor and Director
Graduate Operative Dentistry Program
Department of Restorative Dentistry
Indiana University
School of Dentistry
Indianapolis, Indiana

Richard D. Davis, DDS
Private Practice, Endodontics
San Antonio, Texas

Jan De Munck, DDS, PhD
Postdoctoral Researcher
Leuven BIOMAT Research Cluster
Department of Conservative Dentistry
School of Dentistry, Oral Pathology, and Maxillofacial
  Surgery
Catholic University of Leuven
Leuven, Belgium

Patrice P. Fan, DDS, MSD, FRCD (C)
Affiliate Assistant Professor
Department of Restorative Dentistry
University of Washington
Seattle, Washington

Dennis J. Fasbinder, DDS
Clinical Professor
Director of Graduate Education
Director of Advanced Education in
  General Dentistry Program
Department of Cariology, Endodontics,
  and Restorative Sciences
University of Michigan
School of Dentistry
Ann Arbor, Michigan

Carl W. Haveman, DDS, MS
Associate Professor
Department of General Dentistry
University of Texas Health Science Center at San Antonio
San Antonio, Texas

Van B. Haywood, DMD
Professor
Department of Oral Rehabilitation
Medical College of Georgia
Augusta, Georgia

Thomas J. Hilton, DMD, MS
Alumni Centennial Professor in Operative Dentistry
Department of Restorative Dentistry
Oregon Health & Science University
School of Dentistry
Portland, Oregon

Satoshi Inoue, DDS, PhD
Assistant Professor
Division of General Dentistry
Center for Dental Clinics
Hokkaido University Hospital
Sapporo, Japan

Edwina A. M. Kidd, BDS, FDSRCS, PhD
Professor of Cariology
Division of Conservative Dentistry
The Dental School of Guy's, King's, and St Thomas' Hospital
London, United Kingdom

Paul Lambrechts, DDS, PhD
Professor and Program Director
Leuven BIOMAT Research Cluster
Department of Conservative Dentistry
School of Dentistry, Oral Pathology, and Maxillofacial
  Surgery
Catholic University of Leuven
Leuven, Belgium

Mark L. LittleStar, DDS
Clinical Associate Professor
Department of Restorative Dentistry
University of Texas Health Science Center at San Antonio
San Antonio, Texas

Bruce A. Matis, DDS, MSD
Professor and Director
Clinical Research Section
Department of Restorative Dentistry
Indiana University
School of Dentistry
Indianapolis, Indiana

David F. Murchison, DDS, MMS
Program Director, General Dentistry Residency
Department of General Dentistry
Wilford Hall USAF Medical Center
Lackland Air Force Base
San Antonio, Texas

Jerry W. Nicholson, MA, DDS
Assistant Professor
Department of Restorative Dentistry
University of Texas Health Science Center at San Antonio
San Antonio, Texas

John W. Osborne, DDS, MSD
Professor and Director of Clinical Research
Department of Restorative Dentistry
University of Colorado Health Science Center
Denver, Colorado

J. D. Overton, DDS
Head, Division of Operative Dentistry
Department of Restorative Dentistry
University of Texas Health Science Center at San Antonio
San Antonio, Texas

Jorge Perdigão, DDS, MS, PhD
Associate Professor and Head
Division of Operative Dentistry
University of Minnesota
School of Dentistry
Minneapolis, Minnesota

Marleen Peumans, DDS, PhD
Assistant Professor
Leuven BIOMAT Research Cluster
Department of Conservative Dentistry
School of Dentistry, Oral Pathology, and Maxillofacial
  Surgery
Catholic University of Leuven
Leuven, Belgium

J. William Robbins, DDS, MA
Private Practice, General Dentistry
Clinical Professor
Department of General Dentistry
University of Texas Health Science Center at San Antonio
San Antonio, Texas

Joost Roeters, DDS, PhD
Associate Professor
Department of Cariology and Endodontology
Radboud University Medical Center
Nijmegen, The Netherlands

William F. Rose, Jr, DDS
Assistant Professor
Department of General Dentistry
University of Texas Health Science Center at San Antonio
San Antonio, Texas

Jeffrey S. Rouse, DDS
Clinical Associate Professor
Department of Prosthodontics
University of Texas Health Science Center at San Antonio
San Antonio, Texas

Clifford B. Starr, DMD
Clinical Associate Professor
Director, Advanced Education in General Dentistry Residency
Department of Operative Dentistry
University of Florida
College of Dentistry
Jacksonville, Florida

James B. Summitt, DDS, MS
Professor and Chairman
Department of Restorative Dentistry
University of Texas Health Science Center at San Antonio
San Antonio, Texas

J. Peter van Amerongen, DDS, PhD
Associate Professor
Department of Cariology, Endodontology, and
  Pedodontology
Academic Center for Dentistry Amsterdam (ACTA)
Amsterdam, The Netherlands

Cor van Loveren, DDS, PhD
Associate Professor
Department of Cariology, Endodontology, and
  Pedodontology
Academic Center for Dentistry Amsterdam (ACTA)
Amsterdam, The Netherlands

Kirsten Van Landuyt, DDS
Doctoral Student
Leuven BIOMAT Research Cluster
Department of Conservative Dentistry
School of Dentistry, Oral Pathology, and Maxillofacial
  Surgery
Catholic University of Leuven
Leuven, Belgium

Bart Van Meerbeek, DDS, PhD
Professor
Department of Conservative Dentistry
School of Dentistry, Oral Pathology, and Maxillofacial
  Surgery
Catholic University of Leuven
Leuven, Belgium

Marcos A. Vargas, DDS, MS
Associate Professor and Graduate Program Director
Department of Operative Dentistry
University of Iowa
Iowa City, Iowa

Xiaoming Xu, PhD
Assistant Professor
Department of Operative Dentistry and Biomaterials
Louisiana State University Health Science Center
School of Dentistry
New Orleans, Louisiana

Yasuhiro Yoshida, DDS, PhD
Department of Biomaterials
Okayama University
Graduate School of Medicine and Dentistry
Okayama, Japan

Biologic Considerations

Jerry W. Nicholson

Success in clinical dentistry requires a thorough understanding of the anatomic and biologic nature of the tooth, with its components of enamel, dentin, pulp, and cementum, as well as the supporting tissues of bone and gingiva (Fig 1-1; see also Fig 1-9a). Dentistry that violates the physical, chemical, and biologic parameters of tooth tissues can lead to premature restoration failure, compromised coronal integrity, recurrent caries, patient discomfort, or even pulpal necrosis. It is only within a biologic framework that the principles, materials, and techniques that constitute operative dentistry are validated. This chapter presents a morphologic and histologic review of tooth tissues with emphasis on their clinical significance for the practice of restorative dentistry.

Enamel

Enamel provides shape and a hard, durable surface for teeth and a protective cap for the dentin and pulp (see Fig 1-9a). Both color and form contribute to the esthetic appearance of enamel. Much of the art of restorative dentistry comes from efforts to simulate the color, texture, translucency, and contours of enamel with synthetic dental materials such as resin composite or porcelain. Nevertheless, the lifelong preservation of the patient's own enamel is one of the defining goals of operative dentistry. Although enamel is capable of lifelong service, its crystalline mineral makeup and rigidity, exposed to an oral environment of occlusal, chemical, and bacterial challenges, make it vulnerable to acid demineralization, attrition (wear),

and fracture (Fig 1-2). Compared to other tissues, mature enamel is unique in that, except for alterations in the dynamics of mineralization, repair or replacement can only be accomplished through dental therapy.

Permeability

At maturity, enamel is 96% inorganic hydroxyapatite mineral by weight and more than 86% by volume. Enamel also contains a small volume of organic matrix, as well as 4% to 12% water, which is contained in the intercrystalline spaces and in a network of micropores opening to the external surface.[1] These microchannels form a dynamic connection between the oral cavity and the pulpal interstitial and dentinal tubule fluids.[2,3] Various fluids, ions, and low-molecular-weight substances, whether deleterious, physiologic, or therapeutic, can diffuse through the semipermeable enamel. Therefore, the dynamics of acid demineralization, reprecipitation or remineralization, fluoride uptake, and vital bleaching therapy are not limited to the surface but are active in three dimensions.[4-9] When teeth become dehydrated, as from nocturnal mouth breathing or rubber dam isolation for dental treatment, the empty micropores make the enamel appear chalky and lighter in color (Fig 1-3). The condition is reversible with return to the "wet" oral environment.

Lifelong exposure of semipermeable enamel to the ingress of elements from the oral environment into the mineral structure of the tooth results in coloration intensity and resistance to demineralization. The yellowing of older teeth may be attributed to

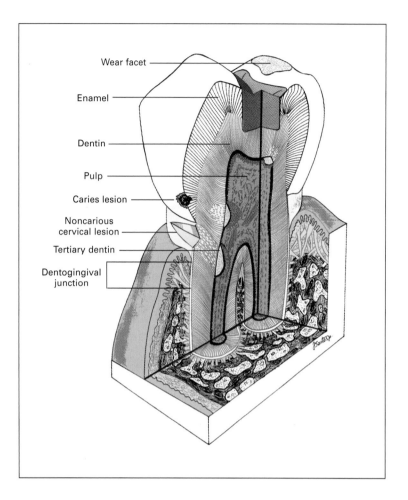

Fig 1-1 Component tissues and supporting structures of the tooth.

Wear facet

Enamel

Dentin

Pulp

Caries lesion

Noncarious
cervical lesion

Tertiary dentin

Dentogingival
junction

thinning or increased translucency of enamel, accumulation of trace elements in the enamel structure, and perhaps the sclerosis of mature dentin. The yellowing may be treated conservatively with at-home or in-office bleaching. The enamel remineralization process benefits from the incorporation of fluoride from water sources or toothpaste and from the fluoride concentrated in the biofilm that adheres to enamel surfaces. Fluoride enhances the remineralization repair of enamel damaged by plaque-acids to increase the ratio or conversion of hydroxyapatite to more stable and less acid-soluble crystals of fluorohydroxyapatite or fluoroapatite.[10] Therefore, with aging, color (hue) is intensified, but acid solubility of enamel, pore volume, water content, and permeability are reduced.[11]

Clinical Appearance and Defects

The dentist must pay close attention to the surface characteristics of enamel for evidence of pathologic or traumatic conditions. Key diagnostic signs include color changes associated with demineralization, cavitation, excessive wear, morphologic faults or fissures, and cracks (see Fig 1-2).

Color

Enamel translucency is directly related to the degree of mineralization, and its color is primarily a function of its thickness and the color of the underlying dentin. From a thickness of approximately 2.5 mm at cusp tips and 2.0 mm at incisal edges, enamel thickness decreases significantly below deep occlusal fissures and tapers to become very thin in the cervical area near the cementoenamel junction (CEJ). Therefore, the young anterior tooth has a translucent gray or slightly bluish enamel tint near the incisal edge. A more chromatic yellow-orange shade predominates cervically, where dentin shows through thinner enamel. Coincidentally, in about 10% of teeth, a gap between enamel and cementum in the cervical area leaves vital, potentially sensitive dentin completely exposed.[12]

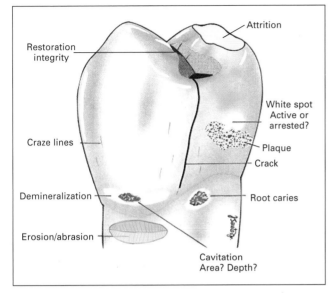

Fig 1-2 Observations of clinical importance on the tooth surface.

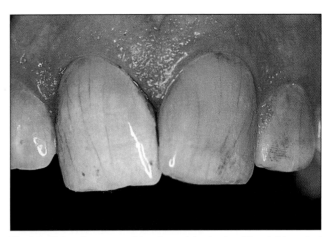

Fig 1-3 Color change resulting from dehydration. The right central incisor was isolated by rubber dam for approximately 5 minutes. Shade matching of restorative materials should be determined with full-spectrum lighting before isolation.

Anomalies of development and mineralization, extrinsic stains, antibiotic therapy, and excessive fluoride can alter the natural color of the teeth.[13] However, because caries is the primary disease threat to the dentition, enamel discoloration related to demineralization caused by acid from a few organisms, primarily mutans streptococci, within plaque[14] is a critical diagnostic observation. Subsurface enamel porosity from demineralization is manifested clinically by a milky white opacity termed a *white spot lesion* (Figs 1-2, 1-4a, and 1-4b). Early enamel fissure-caries lesions are difficult to detect on bitewing radiographs. However, diagnostic accuracy can be improved by a systematic visual ranking of the enamel discoloration adjacent to pits and fissures, which, in turn, is correlated with the histologic depth of demineralization.[15,16] In the later stages of enamel demineralization extending to near the dentinoenamel junction (DEJ), the white-spot opacity is evident not only when the tooth is air dried, but also when it is wet with saliva.[17] It may take 4 to 5 years for demineralization to progress through the enamel,[18,19] but with improved plaque removal and remineralization, the lesion may arrest and, with time, again appear normal. In one study, 182 white spot lesions in 8-year-old children were reevaluated at age 15: 9% had cavitated, 26% appeared unchanged, and 51% appeared clinically sound.[20] A longstanding chalky and roughened white-spot appearance of the facial or lingual enamel surface (see Fig 1-4a) generally indicates that the patient practices inadequate oral hygiene, has a cariogenic diet, and

is at a higher risk for caries. If the caries process continues, a blue or gray tint to the overlying enamel is a sign of advanced dentin involvement. With the advent of effective remineralization, dentin bonding techniques, and fissure sealants, several authorities have suggested that invasive restorative procedures or replacement restorations should be considered only if caries lesion extension to dentin can be confirmed by visual signs of deep discoloration, enamel cavitation to dentin, or radiographic evidence.[21]

Cavitation

In the early stages of an enamel caries lesion, the acid from the surface plaque biomass penetrates through the eroded crystal spaces to form a subsurface lesion of demineralized and porous mineral structure that appears clinically as a white spot. The acid protons follow the direction of the widened intercrystalline spaces of the affected enamel rods toward the DEJ. If the etiology of the lesion, the dentopathic plaque, is not regularly removed through preventive measures, the lesion will progress in depth to the DEJ and into the dentin. Smooth-surface enamel lesions are triangular in two dimensions, with the base of the triangle at the enamel surface; but in three dimensions, the proximal enamel lesion is a cone with its base equivalent in location and area to the demineralized enamel surface and its apex closest to the DEJ. The deepest demineralized enamel rods, those at the apex of the cone, are the rods most exposed in time and acid concentration to the

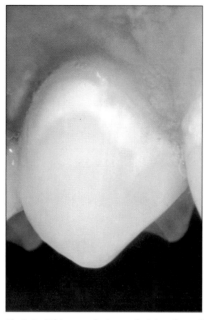

Fig 1-4a White spot lesion on facial surface of maxillary premolar.

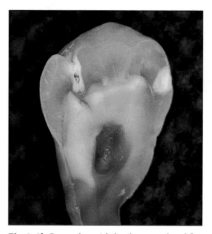

Fig 1-4b Premolar with both an occlusal fissure caries lesion (Class 1), extending into the dentin, and a proximal smooth-surface caries lesion (Class 2).

surface biomass and are first to be demineralized to the depth of the DEJ. The nature of enamel caries lesions in occlusal fissures is similar, but the shape is more complex as it occurs simultaneously at the confluence of two or more cuspal lobes, each with divergent rod directions (see Fig 1-4b). In two dimensions, a fissure-caries lesion presents with the apex of the triangular lesion at the sides of the occlusal fissure and with the divergent rods of both lobes forming a broad base parallel to the DEJ.

Along with regular plaque removal, topical fluoride applications help to limit or even reverse enamel demineralization.[22] New preventive materials attempt to replace minerals in the subsurface enamel lesion using home applications of amorphous and reactive calcium phosphate complexes.[23] A newly developed product employing synthetic hydroxyapatite in an acid paste is said to repair defects and replace crystals within a matter of minutes.[24]

Unless prevention or remineralization can abort or reverse the carious demineralization, dentin structure is compromised and can no longer support the enamel, which eventually breaks away to create a "cavity" (Fig 1-5). A restoration must then be placed. Untreated, the cavitation expands to compromise the structural strength of the crown, and microorganisms proliferate and infiltrate deep into dentin to jeopardize the vitality of the pulp. When the caries lesion extends past the CEJ, as in root caries (see Fig 1-2), isolation, access, and gingival tissue response complicate the restorative procedure.

Wear

Enamel is as hard as steel,[25] with a Knoop Hardness Number of 343 (compared with 68 for dentin). However, enamel will wear because of attrition or frictional contact against opposing enamel or harder restorative materials such as porcelain. The normal physiologic contact wear rate for enamel is as much as 29 µm per year.[26] Restorative materials that replace or function against enamel should have compatible wear, smoothness, and strength characteristics. Heavy occlusal wear is demonstrated when rounded occlusal cuspal contours are ground to flat facets (see Fig 1-1). Depending on factors such as bruxism, other parafunctional habits, malocclusion, age, and diet, cusps may be lost completely and enamel abraded away so that dentin is exposed and occlusal function compromised (Fig 1-6). In preparing a tooth for restoration, cavity outline form should be designed so that the margins of restorative materials avoid critical, high-stress areas of occlusal contact.[27] The effects of lost vertical dimension from tooth wear are offset by apical cementogenesis and passive tooth eruption.

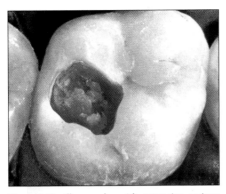

Fig 1-5 Maxillary molar with extensive carious dentin. This is only the initial entry through unsupported enamel into the carious dentin; the final preparation of the tooth will likely remove at least the distolingual cusp and marginal ridge to eliminate unsupported enamel.

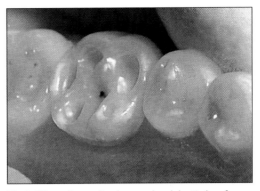

Fig 1-6 Excessive occlusal enamel and dentin loss from a combination of bruxism, attrition, and erosion. (Courtesy of Dr Van B. Haywood.)

Faults and Fissures

Various defects of the enamel surface may contribute to the accumulation and retention of plaque. Perikymata (parallel ridges formed by cyclic deposition of enamel), pitting defects formed by termination of enamel rods, and other hypoplastic flaws are common, especially in the cervical area.[1] Limited linear defects or craze lines result from a combination of occlusal loading and age-related loss of resiliency but are not clinically significant. Organic films of surface pellicle and dendritic cuticles extending 1 to 3 μm into the enamel may play key roles in ion exchange and in adhesion and colonization of bacterial plaque on the enamel surface.[28]

Of greater concern are the fissure systems on the occlusal surfaces and, to a lesser extent, on buccal and lingual surfaces of posterior teeth. A deep fissure is formed by incomplete fusion of lobes of cuspal enamel in the developing tooth. The resulting narrow clefts provide a protected niche for acidogenic bacteria and the nutrients they require (Figs 1-4b and 1-7). It is estimated that caries lesions are five times more likely to occur in occlusal fissures, and two and a half times more likely to occur in buccal and lingual fissures than are caries lesions in proximal smooth surfaces.[29] The 2000 US Surgeon General's report,[30] which was based on a national survey of dental health, confirms that overall caries experience, especially smooth-surfaces lesions, is declining. However, the fissured surfaces of the teeth are relatively inaccessible for plaque-control measures and account for nearly 90% of total decayed, missing, and filled surfaces (DMFS) in US schoolchildren. The Surgeon General's report concludes that the physical barrier provided by an enamel-bonded resin fissure sealant is an effective preventive treatment for high-caries-risk patients and for individual teeth with incipient enamel pit and fissure lesions.[31,32]

Cracks

Although craze lines in the surface enamel are of little consequence, pronounced cracks that extend from developmental grooves across marginal ridges to axial surfaces, or from the margins of large restorations, may portend coronal or cuspal fracture. A crack defect is especially critical when the crack, viewed within a cavity preparation, extends through dentin, or when the patient has pain when chewing (Fig 1-8). A cracked tooth that is symptomatic or involves dentin requires a restoration that provides complete occlusal coverage or at least adhesive splinting.[33,34]

Rod and Interrod Crystal Structure

Enamel is a mineralized epidermal tissue. Ameloblast cells of the developing tooth secrete the organic matrix gel to define the enamel contours and initiate its mineralization. Calcium ions are transported both extra- and intracellularly to form "seeds" of hydroxyapatite throughout the developing matrix. These hydroxyapatite seeds form nidi for crystallization, and the crystals enlarge and supplant the organic matrix. The repeating molecular units of hydroxyapatite, $Ca^{10}(PO_4)^6(OH)^2$, make up the building blocks of the enamel crystal. However, the majority of apatite units exist in an impure form in which

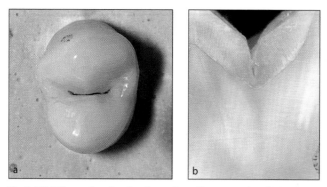

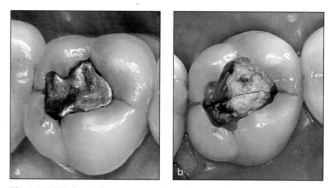

Fig 1-7 *(a)* Fissured occlusal surface of maxillary premolar. *(b)* Cross section of fissure shown in Fig 1-7a.

Fig 1-8 *(a)* Molar with pronounced cracks extending across mesial and distal marginal ridges. *(b)* Same molar with occlusal restoration removed, exposing a mesiodistal incomplete fracture across pulpal floor. (Courtesy of Dr Van Haywood.)

carbonate is substituted in the lattice, with a destabilizing effect on the crystal. When exposed to plaque acids, the carbonated components of the crystal are the most susceptible to demineralization and the first to be solubilized. Both the therapeutic substitution of fluoride into the enamel apatite crystal and the facilitatory role of fluoride to enhance remineralization following cycles of acid dissolution are key to the dynamics of remineralization. Enamel crystals in the incipient caries lesion, in the presence of fluorides, are replaced or repaired with fluoroapatite or fluorohydroxyapatite, which are relatively insoluble. Therefore, the best outcome of repeated cycles of demineralization-remineralization, when accompanied by plaque control and availability of fluoride, is a more caries-resistant enamel.[35,36]

The maturing ameloblast cell develops a cytoplasmic extension, the Tomes' process, that simultaneously secretes enamel protein matrix and initiates the mineralization and orientation of enamel crystals. The divergent directions of the crystals generated from the central and peripheral surfaces of Tomes' processes, repeated in a symmetric pattern, form the two basic structural units of enamel, cylindrical enamel rods and the surrounding interrod enamel. Figures 1-9a to 1-9f are electron microscope photomicrographs of enamel, progressing from a macrostructural image to ultrastructural images showing individual enamel crystals. The crystals in the enamel rods and interrod enamel differ only in the orientation of the crystals: interrod crystals are almost perpendicular to rod crystals. In mature enamel, the closely packed, hexagonal crystals have cross-sectional dimensions of approximately 30 × 60 nm (Fig 1-9f). The matrix proteins, enamelins, and water of hydration form a shell, or envelope, around each crystal. With the exception of the amorphous inner and outer

enamel surface, the rod and interrod enamel are thought to be continuous throughout the thickness of the enamel. The multitude of crystals that form these two entities may also span the width of the enamel structure. The crystals within the cylinders of rod enamel run parallel to the long axis of the rods, which are, in turn, approximately perpendicular to the enamel surface. A narrow space filled with organic material around three fourths of each rod, called the *rod sheath*, separates the two enamel units. However, the two separate enamel components are connected at the portion of the rod circumference that is not bounded by the rod sheath, to form an isthmus of confluent crystals (see Fig 1-9d). In cross section, the rod core and connecting isthmus of interrod enamel together have traditionally been described as keyhole-shaped and as the basic repeating structural unit of enamel. However, recent studies show the interrod enamel to be continuous within the enamel mass and to be a step ahead of the rod in development. Therefore, the current interpretation of the structure of enamel is that of cylindrical enamel rods embedded in the surrounding interrod enamel.[11]

Enamel and Acid Etching

The spacing and divergent orientation of the crystals in the rod and in the interrod enamel make the enamel rod differentially soluble when exposed for a brief time to weak acids. Depending on the acid, contact time, and plane of cavity preparation, either the ends or the sides of the crystals may be preferentially exposed. Different etch patterns have been described depending on type and contact time of the etchant and whether the primary dissolution affects the rod or the interrod structure.[37,38]

Fig 1-9a to 1-9f Enamel composition. (From Nanci.[11] Reprinted with permission from Elsevier.)

Fig 1-9a Scanning electron photomicrograph of a cross-section of a tooth crown showing enamel as the outer protective covering for the tooth. (Bar = 1 μm.)

Fig 1-9b Scanning electron photomicrograph showing the complex of enamel rods and the DEJ. (Bar = 100 μm.)

Fig 1-9c Scanning electron photomicrograph showing enamel rods (R) and interrod enamel (IR). (Bar = 6 μm.)

Fig 1-9d Scanning electron photomicrograph of a cross-section of enamel rods (R) and interrod enamel (IR). Note the connecting isthmus between the two enamel components and the gap (sheath) around the rods. (Bar = 10 μm.)

Fig 1-9e Transmission electron photomicrograph showing divergent crystal orientation in rodent enamel rod and interrod enamel. (Bar = 0.1 μm.)

Fig 1-9f Transmission electron photomicrograph showing the elongated hexagonal shape of hydroxyapatite crystals in enamel. The dimensions of each crystal are in the range of 30 × 60 nm. (Bar = 20 nm.)

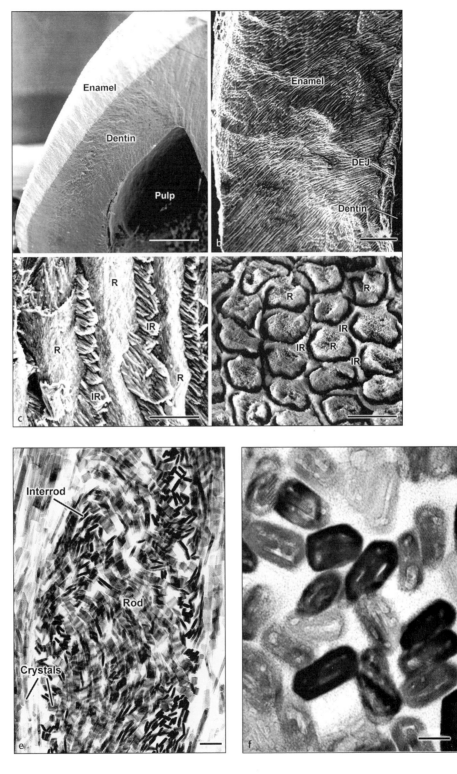

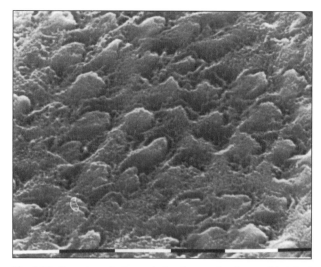

Fig 1-10 Scanning electron photomicrograph of an acid-etched enamel surface. Note the keyhole-shaped rods and uneven surface formed by the disparity in depth of rod heads and rod peripheries. (Bar = 10 µm.)

The initial effect of acid contact in etching enamel for bonding to restorative materials is to remove about 10 µm of surface enamel, which typically contains no rod structure. Then, with rod and interrod structure exposed, the differential dissolution of enamel rod and interrod structure forms a three-dimensional macroporosity (Fig 1-10, see also Fig 8-3). The acid-treated enamel surface has a high surface energy so that resin monomer flows into, intimately adheres to, and polymerizes within the pores to form retentive resin tags that are up to 20 µm deep. At the same time, the internal cores of all the exposed individual crystals are solubilized to create a multitude of microporosities. It is these countless numbers of minitags, formed within the individual crystal cores, that contribute the most to the enamel-resin bond.[39] Because there are 30,000 to 40,000 enamel rods per square millimeter of a surface of cut enamel and the etch penetration increases the bondable surface area 10- to 20-fold, the attachment of resin adhesives to enamel through micromechanical interlocking is extremely strong.[40–42]

As stated, the crystals within the enamel rod cylinders run parallel to the length of the enamel rods, which are, in turn, approximately perpendicular to the external surface. A cavity wall preparation that is perpendicular to the surface will expose predominantly the sides of both the enamel rods and their crystals. This configuration is recommended for amalgam preparations because it preserves the dentinal support of the enamel, but it does not present the optimum bondable enamel substrate. When the transverse section or face of the crystal, rather than its side, is exposed to acid, the central core

of the crystal is most susceptible to acid dissolution. Resin bond strengths are twice as high when adhering to the acid-etched ends of the crystals as compared to the sides of the crystals.[43] Thus, a tangential cut or bevel of approximately 45 degrees across a 90-degree cavosurface angle of a prepared cavity will expose the ends of the rods and their rod crystals. Beveling enamel cavosurface angles of cavity preparations for resin composite is generally recommended to expose the ends of the rods and to maximize the integrity of the restoration at its margins.[44,45] An exception is on occlusal surfaces, where beveling would extend tapering resin margins into areas of increased stress. Regardless of the variation in etch pattern, the orientation of the enamel crystals, or the selected tooth surface, the acid-etch modification of enamel for micromechanical retention provides a conservative, reliable alternative to macromechanical undercuts traditionally used for retention of restorations.[46]

Strength and Resilience

Enamel is hard and durable, but the rod sheaths, where the crystals of the interrod enamel abut three fourths of each enamel rod cylinder, form natural cleavage lines through which longitudinal fracture may occur. The tensile-bond strength of enamel rods is as low as 11.4 MPa.[47] The fracture resistance between enamel rods is weakened if the underlying dentinal support is pathologically destroyed or mechanically removed (Figs 1-11a and 1-11b). Fracture dislodgment of the enamel rods that form the cavity wall or cavomargin of a dental restoration creates a gap defect. Leakage or ingress of bacteria and their by-products may lead to secondary caries lesions.[48] When resin composite is etch-bonded to approximately parallel opposing walls of a cavity preparation, strain relief due to polymerization shrinkage has led to reports of enamel microcracks and crazing at margins.[49] Therefore, beveling acute or right-angle enamel cavosurface margins so that the bond near margins is primarily to cross-sectioned rods and not to the sides of rods is believed to be beneficial in preventing these fractures.[50] Considering the variation in direction of enamel rods and interrod enamel and the structural damage caused by high-speed eccentric bur rotation, planing the cavosurface margin with hand instruments or low-speed rotary instruments to remove any friable or fragile enamel structure is recommended as a finishing step.

Although enamel is incapable of self-repair, its protective and functional adaptation is noteworthy. Carious demineralization to the point of cavitation generally takes several years. Demineralization is impeded because the apatite crystals in enamel are 10 times larger than those in dentin[51] and offer less surface-to-volume exposure to acids. The crystals are

Fig 1-11a Coronal section through interproximal box in a cavity preparation. Use of a rotary instrument (bur), which may leave the proximal wall with an acute enamel angle and undermined enamel, requires careful planing.

Fig 1-11b Marginal defect, resulting from improper cavity wall preparation, leads to eventual loss of enamel at the restoration interface.

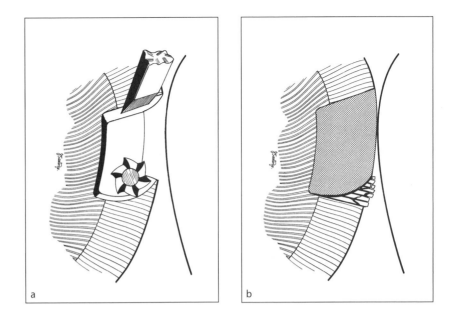

pressed so tightly together that their hexagonal shape is distorted,[11] but this tight adaptation makes for little or no space for acid penetration between the crystals. With preventive measures and exogenous or salivary renewal of calcium, phosphates, and especially fluorides, the dynamics of demineralization can be stopped or therapeutically reversed. Additionally, the crystals are separated by a thin organic matrix that provides some additional strain relief to help prevent fracture.[52]

Enamel thickness and its degree of mineralization are greatest in occlusal and incisal areas of enamel where masticatory contact occurs.[53] The enamel rods are grouped in bundles that undulate in an offset pattern as they course to the surface. As a functional adaptation to occlusal stress, the spiraling weave of rod direction is so pronounced at the cusp tips of posterior teeth that it is referred to as *gnarled* enamel. If enamel were uniformly crystalline, it would shatter with occlusal function. An enamel structure with divergent crystal orientations organized into two interwoven substructures, enamel rods and interrod enamel, yet bound at a connecting area by continuous crystals, provides a strong latticework. The enamel rods, which are parallel to each other and perpendicular to the surface structurally, limit the lateral propagation of occlusal stress and transfer it unidirectionally to the resilient dentinal foundation.[54]

Dentin

Dentin provides both color and an elastic foundation for the enamel. The radicular (root) dentin covered with cementum and the coronal (crown) dentin supporting the enamel form the bulk structure of the tooth. The strength and durability of the coronal structures are related to dentin integrity. To the extent that open dentinal tubules can become closed and impermeable, dentin is a protective barrier and chamber for the vital pulp tissues. As a tissue without substantive vascular supply or innervation, it is nevertheless able to respond to external thermal, chemical, or mechanical stimuli.

Support

Tooth strength, rigidity, and integrity rely on an intact dentinal substrate. To appreciate the magnitude of occlusal loading, a mean maximum bite force of 738 N (166 lb)[55,56] applied to an average contact area of 4 mm² distributed over 20 occlusal contacts[57] yields more than 26,000 psi. Several investigators have reported that resistance to tooth fracture is compromised with increasing depth and/or width of cavity preparation.[58–60] A posterior tooth with an endodontic access preparation retains only a third of the fracture resistance of an intact tooth.[61] In vitro studies report that large mesio-occlusodistal (MOD) preparations increase the strain or deflection of facial cusps threefold compared to that of intact control teeth, and coronal stiffness decreases more than 60%.[61] Elastic deformation of the crown and cuspal flexure are factors that can contribute to noncarious cervical lesions,[62] cervical debonding of restorations,[63] marginal breakdown,[64,65] fatigue failure, crack propagation, and fracture.[66,67] Removal and replacement of dental restorations over a patient's lifetime generally result in successively larger or deeper prepara-

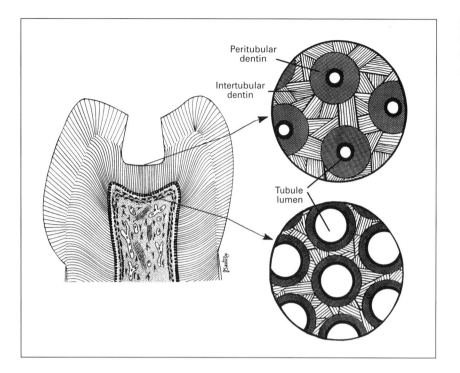

Fig 1-12 Dentin near the DEJ *(outer)* and near the pulp *(inner)* are compared to show relative differences in intertubular and peritubular dentin and in lumen spacing and volume.

Peritubular dentin

Intertubular dentin

Tubule lumen

tions.[68,69] Therefore, to preserve coronal integrity, a conservative approach that combines localized removal of carious tooth structure with preservation of sound tooth structure, placement of sealants, and placement of bonded restorations is recommended.[70] If a large preparation is required, the dentist should consider complete coverage of the occlusal surface with an onlay or a crown.

Dentin Morphology

Dentin is primarily composed of small, thin apatite crystal flakes embedded in a protein matrix of cross-linked collagen fibrils. The odontoblast, with its cell body at the pulp periphery and its extended process within the dentinal tubule, secretes the organic dentin matrix and regulates mineralization. The converging paths of the odontoblastic processes form channels or tubules averaging about 1 µm in diameter and traverse the full 3.0- to 3.5-mm (3,000- to 3,500-µm) thickness of the dentin from the DEJ to the pulp. The tubules comprise about 10% of dentin volume.[71] From near the axial coronal DEJs, the tubule paths form a double curve or S shape, whereas tubules from near the DEJs in occlusal areas and from root surfaces form a relatively straight path to the pulp interface. In mature dentin, the odontoblastic process extends within the dentinal tubule to about one third the dentin thickness.[72,73] Unlike enamel, which is acellular and predominantly mineralized, dentin is, by volume, 45% to 50% inorganic apatite crystals, about 30% organic matrix,

and about 25% water. Dentin is typically pale yellow in color and is slightly harder than bone. Two main types of dentin are present: (1) *intertubular dentin*, the structural component of the hydroxyapatite-embedded collagen matrix forming the bulk of dentin structure, and (2) *peritubular dentin*, limited to the lining of the tubule walls (Fig 1-12). Peritubular dentin has little organic matrix but is densely packed with miniscule apatite crystals. Though primary intertubular dentin remains dimensionally stable, the hypermineralized peritubular lining gradually increases in width over time.[74] The relative and changing proportions of mineralized crystals, organic collagen matrix, and cellular and fluid-filled tubular volume determine the clinical and biologic responses of dentin. These component ratios vary according to location (depth) in dentin, age, and trauma history of the tooth.

Dentin Permeability

Although functional in forming and maintaining dentin, the open tubular channels of dentin compromise its function as a protective barrier. When the external covering of enamel or cementum is removed from dentin through cavity preparation, root planing, caries, trauma, or abrasion and erosion, the exposed tubules, if patent, become conduits between the pulp and the external oral environment. The exposure of the tubules with cavity preparation is somewhat offset by a layer of tenacious grinding debris, the *smear layer*, which adheres to the surface and plugs the tubular orifices.[75] For optimum

Fig 1-13 Leaking restoration interface *(left)*; sealed restoration interface *(right)*. Microleakage is exacerbated by polymerization shrinkage, condensation gaps around the restorative material, and/or differences in thermal expansion. When microleakage is present, the tubule openings in dentin form a potential pathway between the oral environment and the pulp. Various restorative materials, together with the tooth's defenses of tubule sclerosis and reparative dentin, restrict the noxious infiltration.

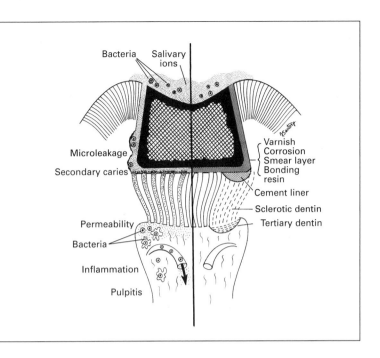

success, dentin bonding systems must remove or penetrate this organic-inorganic barrier to facilitate resin diffusion and micromechanical bonding with the demineralized dentinal substrate.[76]

When injury or active caries affect dentin, the immediate inflammatory response is pulpal vasodilation, increased blood flow, and increased interstitial fluid pressure, which results in an increased outward flow rate of tubular fluid.[77] In vitro studies have shown the fluid outflow may partially counteract the inward diffusion of toxic solutes through the tubules by 50% to 60%.[78] In addition, vasodilation and temporary gaps between the junctional complexes of adjacent odontoblast cells accommodate the passage of plasma proteins, such as albumin and immunoglobulins, into the dentinal fluid. These components agglutinate within the tubules to limit the diffusion to the pulp of exogenous stimuli and possibly to provide a direct immune response to bacteria.[79–81] Thus, with exposure of the tubules, a vascular response and accelerated outward flow of the tubular fluid constitutes an immediate protective response. Nonetheless, tubules that are blocked or constricted provide the pulp with better protection from the permeation of noxious substances.

The diffusion gradient is reduced by both smaller tubular diameters and greater tubular lengths, ie, greater remaining dentinal thickness (RDT). Indeed, the functional diameter of the tubule is only a fraction of the anatomic lumen because intratubular cellular, collagenous, and mineral inclusions restrict flow through the tubular channels.[82] Furthermore, the long 3,000+-µm length of tubules and inherent buffering capacity of a full thickness of dentin create an effective biofilter of diffusion products.[83,84] There are also regional differences in dentin permeability. The coronal occlusal dentin (pulpal floor of a cavity preparation) is inherently less permeable than is the dentin around the pulp horns or axial surfaces.[85–87] As a result, although the fissured occlusal surfaces of posterior teeth often require cavity preparation, only about 30% of the subjacent dentinal tubules are patent over their entire length. However, gingival areas of preparations, such as prepared proximal boxes or crown margins, which are relatively more susceptible to microleakage and development of recurrent caries lesions, are located where the dentin is most permeable.[88–90]

The presence of bacteria or their by-products in deep dentin causes an acute histopathologic and inflammatory response within the pulp.[91–93] Even restored teeth are at risk of continued toxic diffusion through the phenomenon of *microleakage*, the temperature-mediated flux of substances between the oral environment and the restoration-tooth interface due to the differing coefficients of thermal expansion of tooth structure and restorative materials[92] (Fig 1-13). No restorative material or technique can ensure a complete hermetic seal of the restoration-tooth interface, and leakage at the gingival (cementum or dentin) margins of resin-bonded restorations is commonly reported.[94] Through marginal defects, differential thermal expansion, and capillary action, various cytotoxic components or bacterial endotoxins may diffuse through the

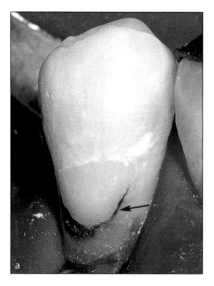

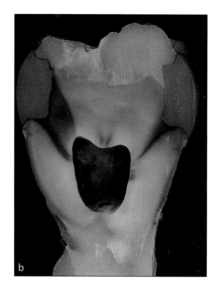

Fig 1-14a Failed resin composite restoration. Polymerization shrinkage and cervical debonding created a restoration-wall gap defect, leading to microleakage and secondary caries. (*Arrow*, cervical margin.)

Fig 1-14b In vitro dye penetration reveals microleakage and diffusion through dentinal tubules.

dentinal substrate to reach the pulp. Clinically, an open margin or leaking restoration contributes to a wide range of problems from marginal stains to sensitivity and chronic pulpitis and is, therefore, frequently cited as the reason for replacement of an existing restoration[95] (Figs 1-14a and 1-14b).

Tubule conduits connecting the pulp to the external oral environment create a virtual micropulpal exposure. Newly erupted teeth with relatively open tubules are particularly vulnerable to pulpal effects from active caries and rapid penetration of bacteria.[96] Without treatment, loss of tooth structure due to carious demineralization or excessive wear results in a diminished thickness of dentin separating the pulp from the oral environment. If the threatening stimuli are moderate and slow in developing, the dentin-pulp complex may have time to hypermineralize or sclerose the tubule channels or to add new tertiary dentin at the pulp-dentin junction (PDJ). Blockage of the tubules and dentin repair are the most important defensive reactions of the dentin. However, with trauma, rapid advance of a caries lesion, or deep cavity preparation, a minimal RDT with numerous open tubules renders the pulp vulnerable to the influx of noxious substances. Without intervention, bacteria eventually reach the level of the PDJ, and pulpal necrosis is the probable outcome.[97]

Dentinal Substrates

Primary and Secondary Physiologic Dentin

Bioactive signaling molecules and growth factors in the inner dental epithelium differentiate ectomesenchymal cells of the dental papilla into mature odontoblast cells. They synthesize and secrete extracellular organic matrix, which, following

mineralization, forms the primary and secondary physiologic dentin[74,98] (Fig 1-15). The first-formed, 150-µm-thick layer of primary dentin subjacent to the enamel is termed *mantle dentin*. It differs from other primary dentin in that it is 4% less mineralized and the collagen fiber orientation is perpendicular rather than parallel to the DEJ. Following mantle deposition, odontoblasts begin to form odontoblastic processes and create tubules as the cell bodies converge pulpally. When mature, as long as the root apex remains undeveloped and open, the odontoblasts produce primary dentin, mainly intertubular dentin, at a rate of 4 to 8 µm/day. Approximately 2 to 3 years following tooth eruption, and coincident with root apexification, the bulk of dentin surrounding the pulp chamber and canal systems, termed *circumpulpal dentin*, is completely formed. The synthesis of dentin then slows to 1 to 2 µm/day, decreasing in rate with age but continuing as long as the tooth is vital. The tubules remain regularly spaced and continuous with tubules within the primary dentin. As the tooth matures, this secondary dentin is distributed gradually and asymmetrically to create pulp-chamber volume reduction with a relatively constricted occlusogingival dimension. The pulp horns and root canals are also gradually reduced in volume. Before starting a cavity preparation or crown preparation, the dentist should radiographically assess the size and location of the pulpal tissues in relation to the size and location of the caries lesion in order to anticipate the need for an indirect pulp capping procedure and to avoid a pulpal exposure.

Outer Dentin

In the first-formed dentin near the DEJ, the tubules of the outer dentin (Figs 1-12 and 1-16) are relatively far apart and, with time, mineral supplementation of peritubular walls pro-

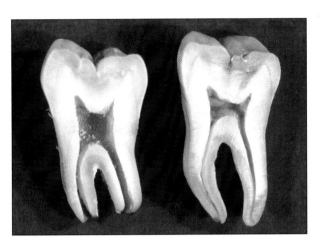

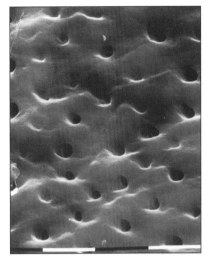

Fig 1-15 Primary and secondary dentin. *(left)* Primary dentin and large pulp chamber and root canals of a mandibular molar after eruption but before completion of root formation when accelerated primary dentin formation ceases and secondary dentinogenesis begins. *(right)* Mature molar that has had gradual and continued deposition of secondary dentin. Note the large mesiobuccal pulp horn that is susceptible to exposure with deep cavity preparation. There is asymmetric deposition of secondary dentin on the pulp chamber roof and floor to narrow the vertical dimension. (Courtesy of Dr James A. Gillis.)

Fig 1-16 Scanning electron photomicrograph of tubules in outer dentin. All highly mineralized peritubular dentin has been removed in the specimen preparation. (Bar = 10 μm.)

gressively narrows the lumen. With relatively fewer tubules at the periphery, around 20,000 tubules/mm², and small tubule diameters of approximately 0.8 μm, the tubule lumens only constitute about 4% of the surface area of cut outer dentin[99] (see Fig 1-16). However, there is extensive terminal branching of the tubules in the outer 250 μm of dentin and regularly spaced connecting branches between tubules. Smaller fine canaliculi and even microfine 0.1-μm pores extend from the tubule walls to permeate the intertubular dentin (Figs 1-17 and 1-18). Similar to the vascular system, this highly interconnected and fluid-filled tubular system acts as a transporting medium for mineral exchange and for bioactive molecules released from the dentin matrix.[71,100] This networking of tubules may account for the paradox that pressure as localized as an explorer tip moving across a surface of cut dentin may indirectly stimulate a plexus of neurons to cause a sensation of pain. Also, when the prepared dentin surface is acid etched for resin bonding, the highly mineralized peritubular walls are the first to be solubilized to create wide funnel-shaped tubules and expose connecting branches. Resin penetration into tubules and branches, together with the micro-mechanical bond of the resin-dentin hybrid layer, form a mechanical interlocking of resin tags to create the best possible bond to the etched-dentin substrate.[101]

Since the processes of the odontoblastic cells extend no farther than the inner third of adult dentin (approximately 1.0 mm), cavity preparations or caries lesions confined to the outer dentin do not directly sever or degrade the vital cellular component of the dentin-pulp complex. Peripheral preparations or lesions with a substantial remaining dentin thickness of 2.0 mm or more provide a sufficient physiologic barrier to safeguard pulpal health from routine restorative techniques.[102] One important exception is an extensive crown preparation without water coolant and with constant, as opposed to intermittent, cutting, which may generate a level of heat or rate of temperature increase capable of creating histopathologically evident pulpal injury.[103,104]

Inner Dentin

The dentinal substrate near the predentin and PDJ is quite different from that near the DEJ. The 20-μm-thick predentin layer consists of newly secreted organic matrix awaiting mineralization. The converging tubules at the predentin, the portion of the dentin closest to the pulp, number up to 58,000 per square millimeter in cross section and contain the processes of the odontoblast cells[105] (Figs 1-19 and 1-20). Careful cavity preparation and proper restorative technique are required to limit surgical trauma to the odontoblast cell bodies

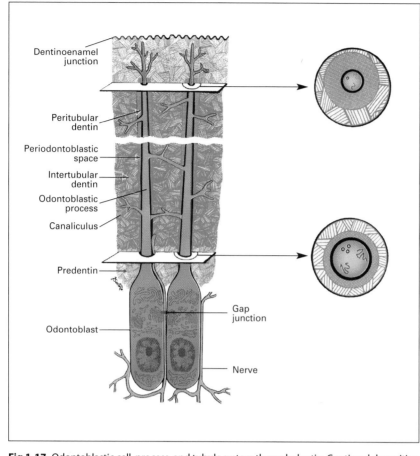

Fig 1-17 Odontoblastic cell, process, and tubule system through dentin. Continual deposition of peritubular dentin and minerals, accelerated by a chronic, noxious stimulus, gradually occludes the tubules peripherally. Note terminal branching and interconnections between odontoblastic cell processes and between cellular walls. Direct neural penetration of dentin is limited to less than 20% of the tubules, and then, rarely beyond the predentin.

Fig 1-18 Scanning electron photomicrograph of resin penetration into a dentinal tubule system after etching with phosphoric acid. The acid etching caused the tapered appearance of the tubules near their exit on the cut surface *(top)*. The dentin was then demineralized with hydrochloric acid and the organic component removed with sodium hypochlorite, leaving the resin to illustrate tubule configuration. Note the cross branching of tubules; this illustrates the complexity of the dentinal tubule. (Courtesy of Dr Jorge Perdigao.)

and prevent their injurious displacement into the tubules,[106] but with good technique and a healthy pulp prior to tooth preparation, the likely outcome of a deep preparation is pulpal healing without clinical symptoms. The tubule diameters near the PDJ are larger (2.5 to 3.0 µm), the distance between tubule centers is half that between tubule centers at the DEJ, and the peritubular dentin is diminished in thickness or absent.[107] At the PDJ, the area of the intertubular dentin is as little as 12% of the surface and the volume of the fluid-filled tubule lumens approaches 80%.[71,108,109] Therefore, at this level, the dentin is more permeable and about 22 times wetter than the dentin at the DEJ.[110] The fluid in the dentinal

tubules is an extension of the interstitial fluid within the pulp, which has a positive pressure of 5 to 20 mm Hg. Therefore, the deeper the cavity preparation, the greater the outward flow of dentinal fluid from the exposed tubules to "wet" the cut surface. Some moisture has been shown to facilitate dentin bonding.[111] However, studies of various bonding systems incorporating simulated pulpal pressure in deep dentin have demonstrated "overwet" conditions and lower bond strengths.[112–114] Also, deep cavity preparation extending near to the pulp may injure the cellular tissues, and a minimal RDT, whether from preparation, trauma, or a caries lesion, places the pulp in close proximity to toxic or immunologic stimuli.

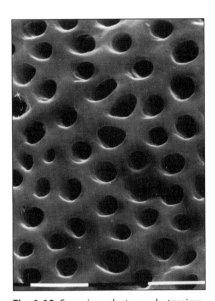

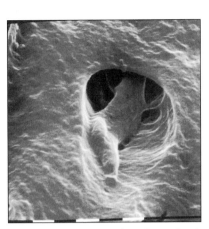

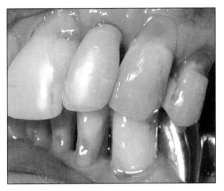

Fig 1-19 Scanning electron photomicrograph of tubules in inner dentin of tooth in Fig 1-16. The section was approximately parallel to the walls of the pulp chamber. All highly mineralized peritubular dentin has been removed in the specimen preparation. (Bar = 10 μm.)

Fig 1-20 Magnified tubule orifice with collagen matrix and odontoblastic process. (Bar = 1.0 μm.)

Fig 1-21 Large NCCLs in the central incisor, canine, and first premolar that illustrate the appearance of sclerotic dentin.

Sclerotic Dentin

A combination of abrasion, attrition, erosion from dietary sources or gastric acid, or occlusal stress may lead to the loss of enamel, cementum, and dentin. The progressive loss of tooth structure at the CEJ typically presents as a wedge-shaped defect. Although the etiology of the lesion is multifactorial, it is not primarily a result of demineralization from bacteria-produced acids and is termed a *noncarious cervical lesion* (NCCL). The exposed root-surface dentin of an advanced NCCL differs in appearance from cut coronal dentin in that it is generally deep yellow in color and has a transparent, glossy surface (Fig 1-21).[115] These lesions may be episodically and acutely sensitive to touch or to changes in temperature, so that the dentin is termed *hypersensitive*. The condition is directly related to the percentage of open or patent tubules between the exposed root surface and the pulp; nearly 75% are present in sensitive dentin vs about 24% in insensitive root dentin.[116] Sclerotic dentin is characterized by hypermineralization or blockage of the tubules with Whitlockite crystals and by a denatured collagen network. Recent studies have demonstrated acid-resistant, bacteria-embedded, hypermineralized, layered plaques on the surface of the sclerotic dentin of NCCLs.[117] The altered surface and substrate limit the formation of both the hybrid layer and the resin tags, so that the bond strengths to sclerotic dentin in a NCCL is 20%

to 40% less than the bond strengths to dentin in artificially created wedge-shaped lesions in the cervical area.[118] The optimum mechanical or chemical preparation of the hypermineralized surface, types of bonding systems, and techniques to bond restorations to sclerotic dentin are currently being investigated.[115,119]

Carious Dentin

The caries process is driven by the presence on the tooth surface of a plaque biomass containing acid-producing bacteria. Without intervention, a progression of destructive changes occurs, prompting pulpal and dentinal responses. This begins with the subsurface enamel lesion and is followed by dentin demineralization, cavitation, infection of demineralized dentin, dentin-matrix dissolution, and ultimately, pulpal necrosis.[120] The degree and type of response is related to the caries activity, which may be active and rapidly progressive, chronic and slowly progressive, or arrested. Over time, with the changing interplay of the oral environment, lesion development, host response, and preventive practices, the same lesion may assume any of these forms.

The earliest dentinal response occurs adjacent to the center or apex of the enamel lesion, where deepest demineralization of enamel rods approaches the DEJ. Even before the enamel lesion reaches the DEJ histologically, acid protons, sol-

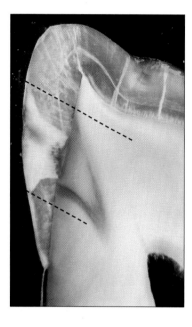

1-22 Precavitated smooth-surface caries lesion with demineralization of enamel rods in center of enamel lesion extending to the DEJ; dentin demineralization is guided by direction of dentinal tubules. Note that the affected dentin area at the DEJ is adjacent to the enamel rods that have suffered demineralization at the outer surface *(dotted lines)* as well as those that have been demineralized to the DEJ. (From Bjørndal and Mjör.[121] Used with permission.)

ubilized matrix components, and released bioactive molecules diffuse through the tubules contiguous with the affected enamel rods to stimulate morphologic changes and metabolic activity in the affected primary odontoblasts. Mineralizing components are released into the tubular fluid of the periodontoblastic space to augment the existing peritubular walls and form a localized zone of hypermineralized dentin subjacent to the enamel lesion of permeable enamel rods.[121,122]

When the enamel-rod dissolution and enamel porosity reaches the DEJ, the hypermineralized zone then becomes subject to accelerated acid dissolution. In contrast to enamel, dentin demineralization is more rapid because of the tubular network and the high surface-to-volume ratio of the small hydroxyapatite crystallites embedded in the collagen.[123] Clinically, the affected dentin is often distinguished from normal dentin by decreased hardness and by a yellow-brown discoloration due to acid effect on the organic dentin matrix or possibly from exogenous staining.[124] Unchecked, demineralization of the soft and discolored dentin progresses toward the pulp (Fig 1-22). It is a misconception that the precavitation caries lesion spreads laterally along the DEJ beyond the area of the affected enamel rods of the white spot lesion.[125,126] Also, as long as the enamel surface remains intact, the dentin lesion is relatively sterile and devoid of viable bacteria.[127] Incipient, noncavitated lesions may be arrested with plaque control or with other noninvasive preventive therapies.[128]

A pivotal point of caries lesion progression occurs if the 20- to 50-μm surface layer of enamel over the internal enamel lesion fractures so that the surface becomes cavitated. With-

in the defect, which is generally inaccessible to brushing or flossing, the facultative dentopathic bacteria multiply to generate a destructive acidic environment. A pathologic cycle of tooth destruction, infection, and tubular invasion of the dentin structure ensues (Figs 1-5 and 1-23). Following the demineralization of the peritubular walls and the intertubular crystals, proteolytic enzymes from the bacteria disrupt the cross-linked collagen framework of intertubular dentin. Clinically, advanced or acutely infected dentin differs from normal dentin or dentin of an arrested caries lesion in that it is soft, readily excavated, wet, and generally light yellow to orange in color.[129] This amorphous lesion is referred to as *infected dentin* and histologically as the *zone of destruction*. Beneath this zone, where the dentin matrix is still intact and limited bacterial penetration is confined to the tubules, the dentin is termed *affected dentin*.[130] Only select microorganisms invade the tubules. In the outer superficial or cavitated lesion, strains of gram-positive streptococcus prevail, whereas anaerobic rods are the bacteria primarily found in deep dentinal tubules and infected pulps and root canals.[131] If the caries lesion progress is gradual, the pH gradient in the deeper tubules below the affected dentin promotes recrystallization of the solubilized minerals. The precipitated crystals, called the *zone of sclerosis*, occlude the tubule lumens to restrict diffusion of toxins to the pulp. However, without operative intervention, the acidic and bacterial front eventually breaches the hard tissue defenses that protect the pulp. The infusion of endotoxins and bacterial antigens into the pulp evokes severe immunologic, inflammatory, and cellular responses, with the

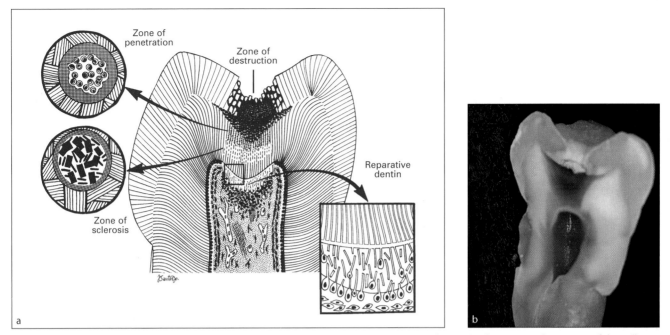

Figs 1-23a and 1-23b Tooth response to carious destruction of tooth structure. Acid demineralization and enzymatic destruction of the collagen matrix lead to cavitation, an irreversible change. *(a)* Bacteria fill and demineralize the lumens of the tubules peripherally, but dissolved minerals reprecipitate deeper to augment sclerosis and hypermineralization of subcarious dentin. Reparative dentin with irregular and noncontinuous tubules forms a final barricade against bacterial metabolites. *(b)* Note the lateral spread of the caries lesion at the DEJ and a hypermineralized sclerotic zone around the pulp.

probable outcome of irreversible pulpitis. However, several clinical studies of sealants, sealed restorations, and indirect pulp-capping procedures in vital teeth suggest that even advanced or infected dentin caries lesions may be arrested in situ if the bonded materials successfully seal the lesion and entomb the bacteria.[132–134]

In the event of cavitation and dentinal infection, restorative treatment is necessary to remove the infected dentin and restore the integrity of the coronal surface. Discoloration is an unreliable guide to excavation of carious dentin, but the degree of dentin hardness, as determined by tactile feedback from excavating burs and hand instruments, is the most reliable guide to differentiation between infected, affected, and normal dentin.[135] As with dentin of different depths, some types of bonding systems are better suited to dentin altered by caries. Total-etch systems have bonded well to moist, caries-affected dentin,[136] and extended etching times have helped.[137] However, self-etching systems provide significantly reduced bond strengths when applied to affected and infected dentin.[138]

Both RDT and a moderate-to-slow rate of caries lesion progression are key to marshalling hard and soft tissue defensive and reparative responses of the pulpodentin complex. The degree of hard tissue alterations reflects the progress and intensity of the pathologic conditions.

Altered Dentin

Altered dentin describes morphologic changes in the dentin matrix with age and from localized defensive and repair responses to injury caused by caries or wear. The mechanisms of biologic control and coordination of pulpal and dentinal responses are beginning to be understood. The hard tissue responses to injury include tubular hypermineralization and sclerosis, which restrict the tubular diffusion of noxious agents. Also, tertiary dentinogenesis adds new barrier dentin at the pulpal interface. At the same time, a pulpal response is underway, including activation of odontoblastic and subodontoblastic cells, proliferation of vascular and neural tissues that support these cells, a heightened immune response, and inflammation.

Hypermineralized Dentin

Following root formation and for as long as the tooth is vital, the odontoblasts slowly produce extracellular dentin matrix and concentrate minerals for the production of physiologic secondary dentin. It is theorized that a portion of the mineralizing components released into the tubules gradually augments the thickness of the mineralized peritubular walls. As the tooth matures, beginning at the periphery of the dentin, the tubules become progressively hypermineralized and, with constriction of the lumen, less permeable. Just as secondary

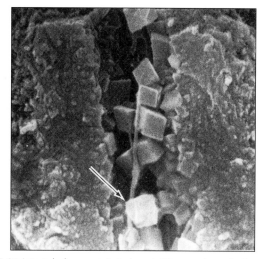

Fig 1-24 Intertubular precipitated crystallites nearly occluding dentin tubule. (Original magnification ×27,000. From Yoshiyama et al.[116] Used with permission.)

dentin deposition is primarily physiologic, tubular hypermineralization or sclerosis is an age-related process of the coronal dentin and, especially, of the root dentin.[139] However, with an external stimulus or irritation, such as a slowly progressing caries lesion, attrition, or restorative procedures, the rate of mineral augmentation to the tubular walls can be accelerated.

Mineral crystallization within the tubules, as in sclerotic dentin in the walls of NCCLs, is also an important defensive response to attrition and to an active caries process in dentin. The apatite minerals of the inorganic dentin are dissolved in the acidic environment of the peripheral cavitated lesion. The supersaturated acidic solution is diluted and buffered by diffusion through and contact with the tubular walls, and the pH kinetics reverse to favor reprecipitation of calcium and phosphates. Platelike, cuboidal, or rhomboid mineral crystals form to barricade the open lumen[140] (Fig 1-24). Similar crystals are observed within tubules of coronal or root dentin exposed to the oral environment through attrition or abrasion.[141]

The combination of peritubular wall thickness and intratubular crystals creates a zone of hypermineralized dentin beneath exposed or carious dentin, the *zone of sclerosis* or *translucent zone* (see Fig 1-23a). Sclerotic dentin is frequently found beneath both active caries lesions and restorations and is an important defense reaction of the hard tissues because it limits the permeability of dentin.[142] Rate of caries lesion progression and patient age are important factors. Rapidly progressive caries lesions in newly erupted teeth can lead to *dead tracts,* empty tubules in which the odontoblast and its process are destroyed before any defensive restriction of the tubules can occur.[143] In one study, the sclerotic zones

beneath caries lesions in young adults limited the dentin permeability to only 14% of the permeability of noncarious controls. With subjects age 45 to 69 years, the dentin beneath caries lesions was completely impermeable.[144] However, as with the sclerotic dentin of NCCLs, the altered sclerosed dentinal substrate may limit bond strengths of restorative systems. It is not clear to what extent the genesis of the sclerotic dentin is purely physicochemical or is biologically controlled. However, hard tissue responses to external noxious stimuli generally occur in conjunction with an active biologic cellular response of tertiary dentinogenesis.

Tertiary Dentin

Newly formed dentin at the dentin-pulp interface compensates for the loss of peripheral dentin from caries or injury and may provide a superior pulpal seal against noxious diffusion through the tubules (Fig 1-25). If the stimulus is relatively low-grade, such as from an incipient enamel caries lesion, the primary odontoblasts are metabolically reactivated to produce a localized tertiary dentin termed *reactionary dentin* (Fig 1-26a). At the same time, complex biochemical signaling systems promote proliferation of supportive vascular and neural tissues among the affected odontoblast cells. Paradoxically, despite being reactivated, the odontoblasts do not assume the increased size and complexity observed during secretion of the primary dentin matrix.[98] The affected odontoblasts are smaller and have a decreased cytoplasm-to-nucleus ratio.[147,148] The rate of reactionary dentin formation, the inclusion of tubular and cellular components, and the continuity of tubules in reactionary dentin with tubules in the overlying dentin vary according to the severity of the stimulus. Reactionary dentin resulting from a mild, slowly progressing caries lesion may resemble secondary dentin with connecting tubules between the two tissues. An active noncavitated lesion may result in atubular reactionary dentin.[149] With a rapidly progressing caries lesion, neither tubular hypermineralization nor reactionary dentin has an opportunity to form.[150]

When cavity preparation reduces the RDT to less than 0.25 mm, the trauma to the odontoblastic cell bodies and their processes reduces their numbers by up to 41%.[151] Even before restorative tooth preparation, an advancing caries lesion generates hydrogen ions and endotoxins that have the potential to critically injure the primary odontoblasts. With a mechanical pulpal exposure, 100% of the primary odontoblasts are destroyed. Yet, with vital pulp tissue surrounding the area of destroyed cells, the pulp-dentin complex can recruit other pulpal cells, including stem cells, to become odontoblast-like cells.[152] The cascade of biologic signals to other pulp cells is complex because recruitment, migration to

Fig 1-25 Reparative dentin forming a localized defense barrier and replacement for lost carious dentin at periphery. The effectiveness of the diffusion barrier is shown by the absence of pulpal inflammation. (From Trowbridge.[145] Used with permission.)

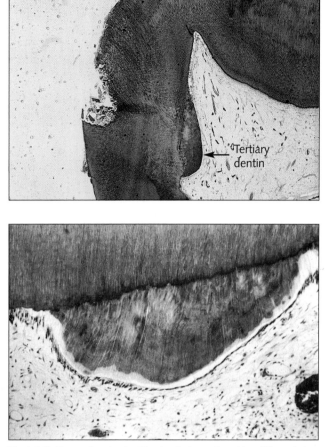

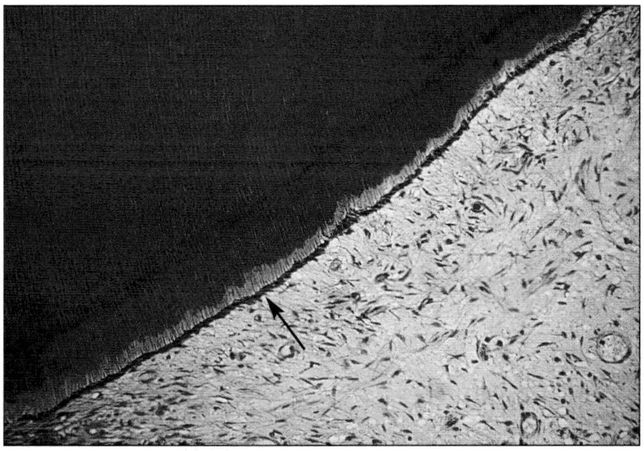

Fig 1-26a Reactionary dentin. Note the layer of intact primary odontoblast cells and the regular pattern of tubules continuous with those of the physiological secondary dentin. (H&E stain, original magnification ×56. From Trowbridge.[145] Used with permission.)

Fig 1-26b Reparative dentin. The dentin is produced by differentiation of subodontoblastic cells that replace the primary odontoblasts killed from the effects of caries. The tubules are less regular and not continuous with those of the overlying dentin. (From Trowbridge.[146] Used with permission.)

the odontoblastic layer, differentiation, and a change in form and function must precede the secretion of new dentin matrix. The process takes 20 to 40 days before dentinogenesis begins.[153] With a mechanical pulp exposure, the formation of a tertiary dentin "bridge" is expedited by direct pulp-capping procedures that limit bacterial contamination and seal the exposure site.[154] Tertiary dentin produced by odontoblast-like replacement cells is termed *reparative dentin* (Figs 1-25 and 1-26b). The layer of reparative matrix formed at the dentin-pulp interface, termed *interface dentin*, is atubular and is, therefore, a superior barrier because it seals and terminates the tubular pathways of the overlying dentin.[155,156] Depending on the nature and rate of progression of the caries lesion, subsequent layers of tertiary dentin, equivalent to wound healing or scar formation, may vary in their tubular content.[149] Both reactionary and reparative dentin can form

beneath the same caries lesion because the periphery of a dentin lesion may be less advanced than the center.[148] To the extent that bacterial antigens and cytotoxins begin to breach the hard tissue barriers, the pulp defenses must rely on increased vascular clearance, activated immune response, and inflammation.

Molecular signals link caries-inflicted or other injury to the tooth with the hard and soft tissue responses of the dentin-pulp complex. Until recently, mature dentin was considered inert and tertiary dentin a type of irritation response.[157] Recent research has identified molecules trapped within the mineralized dentin matrix that are equivalent to the signaling molecules responsible for the differentiation and activation of the embryonic preodontoblast cells. During primary dentinogenesis, they are synthesized and secreted by the odontoblasts into the extracellular dentin matrix. These bioactive

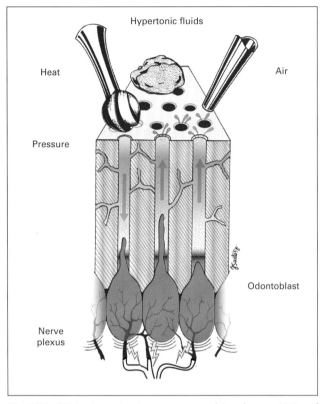

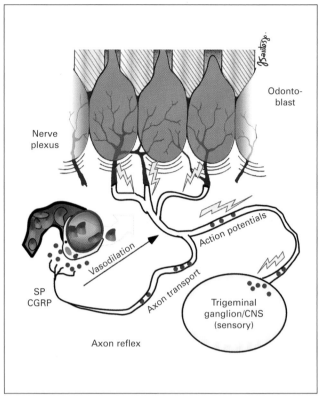

Fig 1-27a Hydrodynamic phenomenon explains the sensitivity of dentin, which is without significant innervation. Fluid dynamics of the tubules move the odontoblastic cell bodies and mechanically depolarize approximating sensory afferent nerve endings.

Fig 1-27b Axon loops from activated sensory nerves provide reflex efferent functions to pulpal, immunologic, and vascular cells by release of neuropeptides from terminal nerve endings. Whereas the sensory action potentials along nerve membranes are nearly instantaneous, the axonal transport of chemical factors and neuropeptide replacements may take hours or days.[174]

molecules are embedded in both the soluble mineral and the insoluble collagen components of the dentin. Cells that have receptors for these growth factors, including odontoblasts and subodontoblastic cells,[158] are directed to various activities, including migration, metabolic functions, proliferation, and differentiation.[146] Some of the active growth factors in dentin, such as bone morphogenic protein-2 (BMP-2) are also present and instrumental in bone regeneration.[159] The foremost and most abundant of the numerous dentin growth factors is transforming growth factor-β_1 (TGF-β_1), one of a group of transforming growth factors.[160] With injury or caries, TGF-β_1 is a pivotal molecule that initiates tertiary repair and modulates the inflammatory reaction.[161] Experimental extracts of solubilized dentin matrix contain the released growth factors. When placed in deep, atraumatically prepared cavities with a minimum RDT, the growth factors diffuse across the dentin to stimulate both reactionary and reparative tertiary dentin.[162] With caries, growth factors are released by demineralization, caused by either bacterial or restorative etching acids, and

then diffuse pulpally through the dentinal tubules to interact with the odontoblasts and pulpal cells.[163] Also relevant to pulp therapy, dentin extracts or chips of dentin experimentally placed on vital pulp tissue expedite reparative dentinogenesis.[164] The therapeutic application of growth factors incorporated into restorative materials to induce dentin impermeability and repair is an exciting prospect for future research.

Dentin Sensitivity

Dentin can be painfully sensitive, but there is no direct anatomic explanation. Although sensitive to thermal, tactile, chemical, and osmotic agents, dentin is neither vascularized nor innervated, except in about 20% of tubules that have nerve fibers penetrating inner dentin by no more than a few microns. The possibility of the odontoblastic cell body and process having a role in direct transmission of sensation is doubtful.[74] The odontoblastic process does not extend beyond the inner third of mature dentin.[165] In addition, the cell membranes of odontoblasts are nonconductive, and there is no synaptic connection between the odontoblastic cell and the contiguous terminal branches of the pulpal nerve plexus. Finally, pain sensation remains even when concentrated anesthetic solutions are placed on the dentin surface or when the odontoblastic layer is disrupted.[166]

Brännström et al[167] proposed a theory based on the capillary flow dynamics of the fluid-filled dentinal tubules (Fig 1-27a). Tubular fluid flow of 4 to 6 mm/sec is produced by the application of a stimulus that expands or contracts the tubular fluid volume and/or creates rapid shifts in the rate and/or direction of the fluid flow. An outward flow apparently causes more sensation than does flow in a pulpal direction.[168] Common clinical procedures associated with tooth preparation, such as air drying, cold water rinses, or pressure from probing and cutting dentin, generate outward fluid displacement. The "current," or hydrostatic pressure, displaces the odontoblastic cell bodies and stretches the intertwined terminal branches of the nerve plexus to allow the entry of sodium to initiate depolarization and the perception of pain.[169] Adenosine triphosphate (ATP), released from damaged cells or by stimulation of endothelial cells, may provide a chemical rather than mechanical explanation for depolarization, because ATP receptors have been identified on terminal branches of the pulpal sensory neurons.[170] Ahlquist et al[171] correlated intensity of pain with rapid changes of hydrostatic pressure applied to smear-free dentin in axial walls of cavity preparations. Other evidence supporting the hydrodynamic theory is the in vivo correlation of tubule patency with hypersensitivity of root dentin. With hypersensitive root dentin, the degree of tubule closure from intratubular crystals was directly correlated with decreased sensitivity to touch, air, or temperature stimuli.[117,172] Chemical compounds that promote intratubular crystallization, such as oxalates or strontium chloride, are active ingredients in some toothpastes and professional desensitizing compounds.[173]

A painful stimulus-reflex response is protective as an alarm to avoid trauma or injury. However, the advantages of painful and sensitive dentin to foods and fluids are less clear, and pain is not a reliable indicator of histopathologic changes or of dentin demineralization caused by caries. It is possible that the major protective benefit of stimulating the sensory pulpal nerves is not the registering of pain in the central nervous system. Branches of these afferent nerves loop back via an axon reflex to stimulate the contractile components of the vascular complex (Fig 1-27b). When triggered, they release potent neuropeptides to activate vasodilation, increase blood flow, and elevate interstitial pressure.[74,175] Thus, rather than discomfort, homeostasis and pulpal defense may be the critical protective outcomes of the hydrodynamic response.

Conclusion

The elastic nature of dentin provides stress relief for brittle enamel. The integrity of dentin is related to coronal strength and durability and can be compromised by carious demineralization, traumatic injury, wear, or poor restorative techniques. Unlike the relatively homogenous nature of enamel, the dentinal substrate varies considerably with location, age, and response to external stimuli. Differences in dentin permeability, wetness and dryness, hypermineralization, and pathologic events complicate comparative research studies on dentin and on dentin bonding systems. The dentin matrix can no longer be considered biologically inert. Signaling molecules and growth factors are released in dentin injury or demineralization to activate tertiary dentin repair and to initiate mobilization of pulp defenses. The barrier protection of the pulp tissue is directly related to the impermeability of the dentinal tubules. When carious metabolites, toxins, and bacterial by-products access the pulpal tissues through these portals, both hard (dentinal) tissue and soft (pulpal) tissue defensive reactions are activated to seal the tubules and repair the damage. Because of the numerous interactions between tissues of the dentin and pulp, the two are often discussed together as one complex.

Pulp

Dental pulp,[74,176] composed of 75% water and 25% organic material, is a viscous connective tissue of collagen fibers and organic ground substance supporting the vital cellular, vascular, and nerve structures of the tooth. It is a unique connective tissue in that its vascularization is essentially channeled through one opening, the apical foramen at the root apex, and it is completely encased within relatively rigid dentinal walls. Therefore, it is without the advantage of an unlimited collateral blood supply or an expansion space for the swelling that accompanies the typical inflammatory response of tissue to injury. However, the protected and isolated position of the pulp belies the fact that it is a sensitive and resilient tissue with great potential for healing.

The dental pulp fulfills several functions:

1. *Formative:* Generates primary, secondary, and tertiary dentin (dentinogenesis)
2. *Nutritive:* Provides the vascular supply and ground substance transfer medium for metabolic functions and maintenance of cells and organic matrix
3. *Sensory:* Transmits afferent pain sensation (nociception)
4. *Protective:* Coordinates inflammatory, antigenic, neurogenic, and dentinogenic responses to injury and noxious stimuli

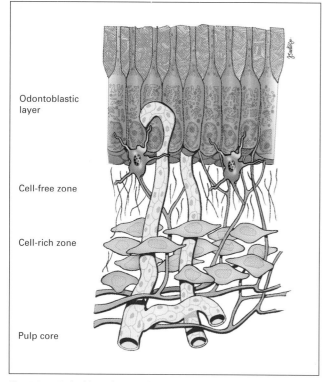

Fig 1-28a Pulpal histology. Odontoblast cell layer with immunocompetent dendritic cells, cell-free zone filled with both nerve and capillary plexuses, cell-rich zone of fibroblasts and undifferentiated cells, and pulp core.

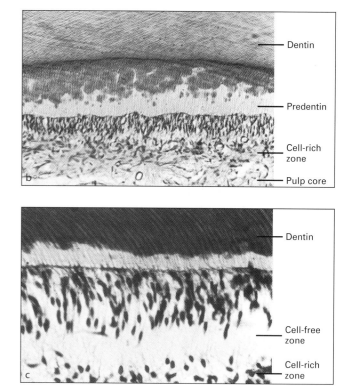

Figs 1-28b and 1-28c Photomicrographs of dentin and underlying pulpal tissues. The multilayered appearance of odontoblast cells is an artifact. (Courtesy of Dr Charles Cox.)

Additional protective functions include homeostasis and clearance of noxious and antigenic substances through the vascular and lymphatic systems and through defense cells such as macrophages and leukocytes.

Morphology

The pulpal tissue is traditionally described in histologically distinct, concentric zones: the peripheral odontoblastic layer, the cell-free zone, the cell-rich zone, and the innermost pulp core (Figs 1-28a to 1-28c).

The radicular and coronal pulp core is largely ground substance, an amorphous hydrated matrix gel that, with collagen fibrils, surrounds and supports the pulpal cells and the vascular and sensory elements. The matrix gel, like interstitial fluid, serves as a transfer medium for transport of nutrients and by-products between widely separated cells of the pulp core and the vasculature. Arterioles and venules, myelinated and unmyelinated nerves, and lymphatic channels, bundled into trunks, pass into and out of the pulp core through the apical foramen or foramina. Collagen is a component of all connec-

tive tissues, but in the pulp, the discreet bundles of fibers are dispersed rather than organized into a supportive framework as in dentin. The proportion of collagen increases with age and is concentrated in the radicular pulp; this facilitates its removal with a barbed broach if a pulpectomy is required. The cell-rich zone consists of fibroblasts and undifferentiated cells. The cells of the stratified odontoblastic layer and of the cell-rich zone are separated and supported by a plexus of capillaries and axons that forms the cell-free zone. Cells of the pulp function for matrix production, immune reactions, defense, vascular control, and inflammatory response.

Pulpal Cells

Odontoblast cell bodies form the outer periphery of the pulp tissue. These specialized, postmitotic cells, each with a process extending into a dentinal tubule, form a single layer at the predentin-pulp interface. As long as the tooth remains vital, they produce and adapt the dentin matrix, including collagen, and they may provide an active transport of calcium ions.[177] The odontoblasts synthesize and secrete various noncollagenous proteins that affect the structure and mineralization of the dentin. Also synthesized are bioactive growth and signaling molecules that supplement neuropeptides within the pulp to coordinate pulpal-dentinal responses for healing and repair. The cellular morphology reflects the stage of activity: large, complex and columnar when active, small and flattened when quiescent, injured, or aged. Each cell body forms a loose "plug" at the pulpal terminus of the dentinal tubule and is therefore subject to the hydrostatic shear currents of the tubular fluid. The hydrodynamic effects range from "aspiration" of the cell bodies into the tubules and autolysis of the cells to minor displacement and depolarization of nerve terminals in close contact with the cells. The cell membranes are bound together through a variety of membrane junctions characterized as tight and permanent or gapped and adhesive.[178] Prominent fibers interconnect the cells to form a terminal web, which may orchestrate their secretory functions and stimulus responses as a unified zone. The membrane junctions may modulate either a physiologic barrier or a molecular sieve to regulate transfer of ions and plasma molecules between the interstitial fluid of the pulp and the tubular fluid.[179] Either injury or routine operative procedures can temporarily disrupt the odontoblastic barrier to permit infusion of plasma proteins and to increase outward tubular flow.[180,181]

Fibroblasts, the most numerous pulpal cells, form a dispersed but interconnecting network through their cytoplasmic extensions. They produce, maintain, and remodel pulp matrix and collagen. They are concentrated in the cell-rich zone supporting the odontoblastic cells. Fibroblasts, undifferentiated mesenchymal cells, stem cells, pericytes, and smooth muscle cells supporting the capillary walls are all prime candidates as progenitor cells capable of differentiation and phenotype conversion into matrix-secreting replacements for destroyed primary odontoblasts.[182]

Immunocompetent cells include macrophages, lymphocytes, and dendritic cells that function as a host defense system against foreign bodies and antigens.[98,176] *Macrophages* are large cells that are scavengers, able to phagocytize microorganisms, cellular debris, and damaged extracellular matrix. *Dendritic cells* are highly motile cells with branched extensions up to 50 μm long; they have great capacity for encoding antigens on their membrane surfaces. With early caries lesions or injury, they congregate among layers of injured or destroyed odontoblasts and even extend their branches into the affected tubules for surveillance of protein antigens.[183,184] Once antigens are captured, they migrate to nearby lymph nodes to present their encoded antigens to *T-lymphocytes*. This initial phase is the primary immune response in which memory T-cells carrying the antigen "blueprint" are cloned and released back into the pulp tissue. After 3 to 5 days, following another antigen exposure, encoded dendritic cells or macrophages directly interface with the preprogrammed memory T-cells in the pulp tissue to release proinflammatory cytokines.[185] With dental caries, this secondary phase of the cell-mediated immune response typically produces chronic inflammation because bacterial by-products diffuse into the pulp long before the organisms themselves directly reach and infect the tissue.[145] Tubular sclerosis, tertiary dentin, and restorative treatment limit or eliminate the antigen stimulus so that an area in which there is chronic inflammation should revert to a healthy histologic state. However, if microorganisms penetrate the tertiary dentin that forms beneath the caries lesion, the host responds with a prompt and massive influx of neutrophilic and mononuclear leukocytes typical of an acute inflammatory response.[186]

Vascular System

The microvascular system of the pulp[187] contains vessels no larger than arterioles and venules. The primary function is maintenance of tissue homeostasis. Also, thin-walled lymphatic vessels return tissue fluid and high-molecular-weight plasma proteins back to the vascular system. Capillaries supply oxygen and nutrients that dissolve in and diffuse through the viscous ground substance of the pulp to reach the cells. In turn, the circulation removes waste products, such as carbon dioxide, by-products of inflammation,[143] and diffusion products that have permeated through the dentin so that they do not accumulate to toxic levels[188] (see Fig 1-13). The equilibrium between diffusion and clearance may be temporarily threatened by use of long-acting anesthetic agents that contain vasoconstrictors such as epinephrine. An intraligamental injection of a canine tooth with 2% lidocaine with 1:100,000 epinephrine will cause pulpal blood flow to cease for 20 minutes or more.[189] Fortunately, the respiratory requirements of mature pulp cells are so low that no permanent cellular damage ensues.

Inflammation, the normal tissue response to injury and the first stage of repair, is somewhat modified by the pulp's unique location within the noncompliant walls of the pulp chamber. A stimulus that produces cellular damage initiates neural and chemical signals that increase blood flow and capillary permeability. Plasma proteins, fluids, and leukocytes spill into the confined extracellular space and elevate interstitial fluid pressure.[190] The smooth muscle sphincters that regulate capillary blood flow are under the control of both neurons and local cellular conditions so that a localized vascular response to stimuli may occur independent of the overall system. Theoretically, elevated extravascular tissue pressure could collapse the thin venule walls and start a destructive cycle of restricted circulation and expanding ischemia. However, the pulpal circulation is unique because it contains numerous arteriole "U-turns," or reverse flow loops, and arteriole-venule anastomoses, or shunts, to bypass the affected capillary bed.[191] Many of these capillaries are normally nonfunctional but facilitate instantaneous localized hyperemia in response to injury. Also, at the periphery of the affected area, where high tissue pressure is attenuated, capillary recapture and lymphatic adsorption of edematous fluids are expedited.[192] These processes confine the edema and elevated tissue pressure to the immediate inflamed area. Animal studies indicate that tissue pressure in an area of pulpal inflammation is two to three times higher than normal but is diminished to nearly normal levels approximately 1.0 mm from the affected area.[193]

Another protective effect of elevated but localized pulpal tissue pressure is a vigorous outward flow of tubular fluid to counteract the pulpal diffusion of noxious solutes through permeable dentin.[194,195] However, an inflammatory condition and higher tissue pressure may also induce *hyperalgesia*, a lowered threshold of sensitivity of pulpal nerves. Thus, an afflicted tooth exposed to the added stress of cavity preparation and restoration may become hypersensitive to cold or other stimuli.[196]

Innervation

Some patients seek dental services because their teeth, through caries lesion(s), injury, or exposed cervical dentin, are painful. Various noxious, thermal, electrical, and mechanical stimuli may all be interpreted to some degree as pain. However, pain perception, termed *nociception*, is less important to preservation of pulp vitality than is the role of neuromediation of vascular, inflammatory, immune, and defense functions.[174]

Nociception

Innervation of the pulp[197] is primarily from sensory (afferent) axons with their cell bodies located a great distance away in the trigeminal ganglion. There are also sympathetic (efferent) axons, with nuclei in the cervical sympathetic ganglia, that produce vasoconstriction when activated. Nerves are classified according to purpose, myelin sheathing, diameter, and conduction velocity. Although a few large and very high-conduction-velocity A-β nerves with a proprioceptive or touch pressure function have been identified, most sensory interdental nerves are either A-δ nerves or smaller, unmyelinated C fibers. About 13% of the nerves innervating premolars are myelinated A nerves,[198] but they gradually lose their myelin coating as they form the sensory plexus of the cell-free zone and branch into multiple free-end terminals.[199] Up to 40% of the tubules at the pulp horns contain neural filaments extending up to 200 μm into inner dentin,[200] but their role in nociception is unclear. The A-δ nerves have conduction velocities of 13.0 m/sec and low sensitization thresholds to react to hydrodynamic phenomena.[201,202] Activation of the A-δ system results in pain characterized as a sharp, intense jolt.[203]

About 87% of axons innervating premolars are smaller, unmyelinated C fibers, which are more uniformly distributed through the pulp.[204] The conduction velocities of C fibers are slower, 0.5 to 1.0 m/sec, and C fibers are only activated by a level of stimuli capable of creating tissue destruction, such as prolonged high temperatures or pulpitis. The C fibers are also resistant to tissue hypoxia and are not affected by reduction of blood flow or high tissue pressure. Therefore, pain may persist in anesthetized, infected, or even nonvital teeth.[205,206] The sensation resulting from activation of the C fibers is a diffuse burning or throbbing pain, and the patient may have difficulty locating the affected tooth.[203]

Neuromediation of Pulp Functions

The close proximity of terminal sensory fibers to odontoblast cells responding to hydrodynamic fluid movement accounts for dentin sensitivity, but the central nervous system is not the sole terminus. As with the odontoblast cells, multiple branches from the axon form the same close apposition with fibroblast cells, perivascular cells, and immunocompetent cells. The terminal nerve ends contain receptors for released or generated bioactive factors caused by injury to the dentin, pulpal cells, or interstitial environment (see Fig 1-27b). Examples include released dentin growth factors for tertiary dentinogenesis or nerve growth factor (NGF) from fibroblasts to activate sprouting and new growth of additional neurons.[207] Appropriate signals from nearby cells (paracrine), through the blood supply (endocrine), or even from the same cell (autocrine) trigger the release of potent neuropeptides stored within the terminal neurons. Two potent neuropeptides having receptor sites on vascular cells are calcitonin gene–related peptide (CGRP) and substance P; these induce vasodilation and increased blood flow to commence inflammation.[208,209] The importance of the neurogenic link was demonstrated when teeth that were experimentally denervated and exposed to trauma showed significantly greater pulpal damage because they lacked sufficient inflammatory response.[210] The neuropeptides are so potent that the experimental stimulation of a single C fiber resulted in a detectable increase in blood flow.[211] The exchanges of factors and neuropeptides regulate the inflammatory, dentinogenic, and immunologic functions and other defenses of the pulpodentin complex. The responses are dynamic, increasing or decreasing with the severity of the external stimulus and with the phase of response: acute, chronic, or healed. These effector functions of the sensory neurons are critical to the function and vitality of the pulpo-dentin complex.

Restorative Dentistry and Pulpal Health

Mechanically cutting tooth structure, especially dentin, during restorative treatments generate considerable physical, chemical, and thermal irritation of the pulp. However, if the dentist uses an acceptable and conservative technique and achieves bacterial control, even a mechanical pulp exposure or use of acidic restorative materials poses few problems for pulpal health.[212–215] Although microleakage around restorations is ubiquitous, the fact that almost all pulps remain healthy is related to diminished virulence of the bacteria, relative imper-meability of the dentin, and the healing potential of the pulp. An animal study reported 15% pulpal necrosis after a 5.5°C increase in intrapulpal temperature and up to 60% necrosis after an 11°C increase.[216] In vitro crown preparation studies without water coolant record increased intrapulpal tempera-tures of this degree.[217,218] Although a retrospective radio-graphic study of teeth prepared for crowns using only air coolant reported good success,[219] many authorities state that water coolant and intermittent rotary instrument contact with tooth structure during crown preparations is essential to avoid histopathologic damage.[220,221]

The aged tooth is less able to respond to noxious stimuli and injury. Age-related changes include reduced blood sup-ply, a smaller pulp chamber, 50% reduction of pulp cells with a lower ratio of pulp cells to collagen fiber, loss and degener-ation of myelinated and unmyelinated nerves, decreased neu-ropeptides, loss of water from the ground substance, and increased intrapulpal mineralizations (denticles).[74,222] Howev-er, the aged tooth is generally less sensitive and is protected by sclerotic and tertiary dentin that make it impermeable to diffusion of injurious agents. The pulpodentin complex is nei-ther static nor noncompliant but is dynamic and adaptive to environmental stresses. Advances in clinical dentistry such as effective preventive measures, sensitive diagnostic tools, improved bonding systems and restorative materials, and conservative surgical preparations should extend the durabil-ity and biocompatibility of dental services to preserve the teeth for a lifetime.

Gingiva

The gingiva[223,224] is that component of the periodontal tissues that covers the alveolar bone, seals the cervical areas of teeth and the periodontal structures from the external environ-ment, and defines the cervical contours of the clinical crown.

Just as durable enamel protects the vulnerable tooth tissues it overlays, the keratinized surface of the attached gingiva safe-guards the deeper supporting structures of the periodontium. The keratinized epithelial surface protects against the friction of tooth brushing and mastication; against the chemical effects of food, drink, and plaque; and, most critically, against the destructive effects of oral pathogens. Color, contour, and symmetry of the oral tissues define esthetic form, but high or low gingival levels and red, swollen gingival tissues subvert biologic and esthetic norms. Periodontal disease affects up to 70% of the population. Gingivitis, the most prevalent form, is characterized as a chronic but reversible inflammatory response of the gingiva to bacterial plaque. In 20% to 30% of the affected population who have a genetically susceptible profile (host factor), the gingival inflammatory response to plaque progresses to periodontitis. This is a more severe and destructive disease, associated with specific subgingival path-ogenic microorganisms and characterized by a loss of connec-tive tissue attachment and bone support.[225,226] In general, the initial stages of gingivitis and periodontitis are prevented or controlled by access to and the timely removal of supragingi-val and accessible plaque or by establishment of an oral biota that excludes periodontal pathogens.[227,228] To this end, the oral hygiene of the patient is essential.[229–231] When restora-tions are required, the clinician can contribute to a healthy gingival response by ensuring that restorations precisely mimic contours and surface smoothness of the tooth struc-ture they are replacing.

Anatomic Description

A normal, healthy gingiva (Fig 1-29) presents a scalloped marginal outline, firm texture, coral-pink or normally pig-mented coloration (depending on ethnicity), and, in about 40% of the population, a stippled surface. Coronally, free gin-giva includes the scalloped cuff of tissue forming the margin-al crest, which curves internally to form a narrow internal crevice or sulcus around the tooth. The external free gingiva extends apically 1.0 to 2.0 mm to the free gingival groove located at the level of the CEJ in a healthy situation. The main component of the gingiva, the attached gingiva, is firmly affixed to the periosteum of the alveolar bone and hard palate and to the supra-alveolar cementum of the root of each tooth. The free and attached gingiva extends interprox-imally to form the interdental papilla that fills the gingival embrasure below the interproximal contacts. Figure 1-30 shows the various collagen fiber bundles that attach the tooth and gingival tissue to the bone and to each other. The inter-dental papilla does not completely fill the gingival embrasure. In a healthy periodontium in which the gingival tissue and

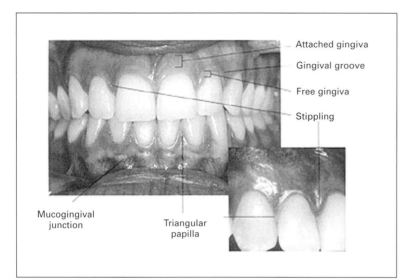

Fig 1-29 Clinically healthy, normal gingiva. (From Chapple and Gilbert.[232] Used with permission.)

Attached gingiva

Gingival groove

Free gingiva

Stippling

Mucogingival junction

Triangular papilla

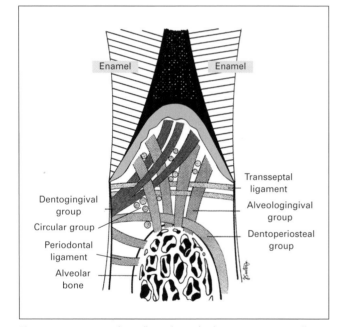

Enamel   Enamel

Transseptal ligament

Alveologingival group

Dentoperiosteal group

Dentogingival group

Circular group

Periodontal ligament

Alveolar bone

Fig 1-30 Interproximal papilla and attached gingiva. Various collagen fiber bundles continuous with the connective tissue attachment circle the teeth or attach the gingiva to the cementum and bone. The gingival embrasure or interdental space below the contact is prone to plaque accumulation, which is responsible for both caries lesion development and gingivitis.

bone have not receded apically, the interdental papilla completely fills the gingival embrasure. Unlike attached gingiva, the epithelial lining of the sulcus and of the papillary col between the facial and lingual papilla is not keratinized. Therefore, in a mouth that harbors periodontal pathogens,

without effective oral hygiene procedures, both the sulcus and papilla are susceptible to inflammatory reactions to the plaque biomass that accumulates there. The *vertical width*, or *zone*, of keratinized gingiva refers to the distance from the free gingival margin to the mucogingival junction. The mucogingival junction is the junction of the keratinized gingiva with the alveolar mucosa, which is mobile, darker red, and nonkeratinized. The usual width of keratinized gingiva varies by location on both the facial and lingual aspects of the teeth. Facially, it is normally widest in the incisor areas and narrowest in the canine and first premolar regions. Lingually, it varies from less than 2.0 mm in the area of the mandibular incisors to 9.0 mm on the lingual aspects of mandibular molars.[233]

The significance of the width (zone) of keratinized gingiva in restorative dentistry is somewhat controversial. Lang and Löe[233] evaluated sites without restorations in adults with effective oral hygiene and concluded that a minimum width of 2.0 mm of keratinized gingiva is required to prevent chronic gingival inflammation. Maynard and Wilson[234] recommended 5 mm of keratinized gingiva (2 mm of free and 3 mm of attached gingiva) to achieve predictability of gingival response to restorations with margins placed within the gingival crevice or sulcus. These same authors also advised that the thickness of the gingiva be evaluated. In clinical situations in which the tissue is thin enough to see the periodontal probe through the free gingival margin, the soft tissues may be unable to support intracrevicular restorative procedures.[234] In a human clinical study, Stetler and Bissada[235] compared areas of a narrow (less than 2 mm) zone of keratinized gingiva to wide (greater than 2 mm) areas. In sites with no restorations present, there was no clinical difference in gingival inflammation between narrow and wide areas. Teeth in narrow keratinized areas with subgingival restorations had greater inflammation.[235] In a similar study,[236] restored teeth with margins placed within the gingival sulcus adjacent to narrow areas of keratinized gingiva suffered increased recession and attachment loss. In summary, both the width (zone) and thickness of the gingival tissues should be evaluated prior to the placement of restorations that will extend subgingivally. In compromised areas, mucogingival therapy (soft tissue grafting) prior to placing restorations should be considered.

Dentogingival Complex and Biologic Width

The junctional epithelium and the subjacent connective tissue between the base of the gingival sulcus and the alveolar crest stabilize and seal the gingiva around the cervical enamel and supra-alveolar cementum surfaces. The combination of these two tissues (junctional epithelium and connective tissue attachment) is termed the *dentogingival junction*, and their combined vertical dimension is the *biologic width* (Fig 1-31). The junctional epithelium (or epithelial attachment) is nonkeratinized and provides intimate adhesion against the cervical enamel or, with gingival recession or attachment loss, against the cementum. With inflammation, a periodontal probe used to measure pocket depth may easily penetrate the junctional epithelium to the level of the connective tissue attachment. The clinical attachment level is the distance from the CEJ to the tip of the probe. As a defensive mechanism against pathogenic bacterial penetration, the junctional epithelial cells have a high mitotic rate and are rapidly exfoliated and replaced. The cellular spacing and narrow, tapering width of the junctional epithelium layer facilitates the movement of serum exudates containing defensive cells, complement, and antibodies into the sulcus as gingival crevicular fluid. The inflammatory response may become exaggerated and result in gingival edema, color changes, and bleeding, classic signs of gingivitis. The amount of crevicular fluid exudate and of bleeding with probing are two quantitative indices of gingival inflammation.[232,237] The protective body defenses can be overcome by the chronic accumulation of pathogenic bacteria in the plaque biomass or at local plaque-retaining sites such as calculus or imperfect restoration margins. With unfavorable genetic host factors, the inflammatory response can become destructive. Proliferation and apical migration of the junctional epithelial cells create greater pocket depths and a loss of attachment with resorption of alveolar bone, both manifestations of periodontitis. The internal and external epithelium layers are supported by a network of collagen fiber bands coursing around and between the teeth and affixing the gingiva to alveolar bone and cementum of the roots (see Fig 1-30). From periodontally healthy adult cadaver dissec-

tions, Vacek et al[238] reported that the mean vertical dimension of the junctional epithelium was 1.14 mm. The subjacent connective tissue attachment measured a relatively consistent 0.77 mm. Together, the mean biologic width dimension was 1.91 mm (1.75 mm for anterior teeth and 2.08 mm for posterior teeth). The results affirm an earlier dissection study by Gargiulo et al[239] in which the biologic width averaged 2.04 mm. Based on these dissections and on clinical experience, clinicians have generally accepted a 1.0-mm depth guideline for a healthy gingival sulcus. Thus, at a midfacial location, 3.0 mm (2.0 mm biologic width plus an additional 1.0-mm sulcus depth) is a simplified working construct termed the *dentogingival complex* (see Fig 1-31). Interproximally, with adjacent teeth present, the dentogingival complex dimension is reported to be in a range of 3.0 to 4.5 mm.[240,241]

Several clinical studies have demonstrated that the closer a crown margin is to the dentogingival attachment, ie, the deeper into the gingival sulcus the margin is placed, the greater the probability of an inflammatory response, as evidenced by increased gingival plaque, increased bleeding indices, and, with time, the loss of attachment.[242–245] A prospective clinical study[246] evaluating 480 ceramometal crowns found that the risk of gingival bleeding was related to the baseline oral hygiene index and was twice as high for intrasulcular margins as for supragingival margins. Thus, it is generally accepted that a supragingival crown margin is beneficial for periodontal health. However, an intrasulcular or even subgingival preparation margin is often necessary because of a short clinical crown, cervical or root caries lesions, a coronal fracture, or the need to hide the margin. Maintenance of the 2.0-mm dimension of the dentogingival junction is generally deemed a high-priority condition for biologic health. The assumption is that a violation of the biologic width, especially into the connective tissue attachment, will lead to chronic inflammation and perhaps the loss of attachment, bone resorption, and gingival recession.[247]

It is difficult to clinically measure the separate tissue components of the biologic width. Kois[240,241] advocates the diagnostic use of a periodontal probe to confirm the level of the bone support to validate a biologically safe placement of the gingival margin. With anesthesia, the probe penetrates the midfacial sulcus to contact the osseous crest, a process called *bone sounding* (see Fig 1-31). The distance from the free gingival margin to the osseous crest defines the dentogingival complex, ie, the biologic width plus the sulcus depth. In 85% of subjects, a 3.0-mm reading confirms existence of an optimum biologic width, and the preparation margin may be safely placed 0.5 mm below the existing gingival margin. In addition, the preparation must follow the contours of the gingival margin, which parallels the CEJ, to avoid violation of the

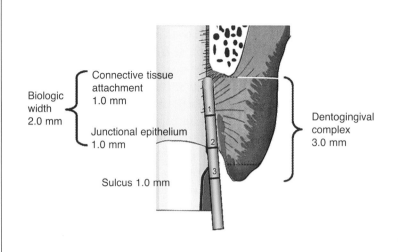

Fig 1-31 Biologic width and dentogingival complex. Note that the gingival crown cavosurface margin is ideally no more than ½ mm into the sulcus. The tip of the periodontal probe has been pushed through the DEJ (junctional epithelium and connective tissue attachment) to the osseous crest (bone sounding).

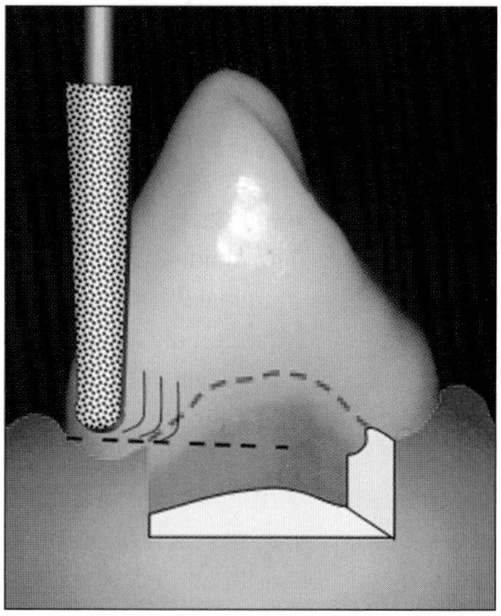

Fig 1-32 The dentist should carefully parallel and duplicate the pronounced curve of the interproximal gingiva (and CEJ) during crown preparation, as shown by the pink dotted line, in order to prevent violation of the biologic width.

biologic width (or biologic zone), especially in the interproximal areas. With maxillary incisors, the proximal CEJ and junctional attachment may be scalloped as much as 3.5 mm incisal to the level of the facial CEJ (Fig 1-32). A midfacial reading greater than 3.0 mm confirms distant osseous support for the gingiva so that recession of the gingiva or interdental papilla may result following restorative procedures. A supporting anatomic probing study reported a relationship between a healthy gingival papilla and the distance from the alveolar crest to the base of the proximal contact. At a distance of 5.0 mm, 98% of the dental papillae completely filled the restored gingival embrasure; but at 6.0 mm, only 56% did so.[248] The dentist might be able to adjust the incisal/occlusal-gingival level of restored proximal contacts accordingly. If the dimension of the dentogingival complex is less than 3.0 mm, which suggests a compromised biologic width, a mucogingival flap and osseous resection (a crown lengthening procedure) is generally recommended to achieve the necessary dentogingival complex dimension in the area.[249]

The clinical imperative of 2.0 mm biologic width is based on the averages of dimensions determined in the autopsy studies cited above; however, much variation was found in the individual dimensions of the sulcus, junctional epithelium, and connective tissue attachment.[238,250] Fifteen percent of teeth in the study by Vacek et al[238] had restoration margins less than 2.0 mm from the osseous crest with no related loss of attachment. In an animal study, Class 5 restorations were

placed directly at the osseous crest. At 1 year, a functional biologic width reformed apically with one fifth the linear dimensions of the preoperative nonrestored controls.[251] A 2-year prospective clinical study evaluated the periodontal effects of subgingival crown margins within the dentogingival complex in three groups of patients: Group 1 consisted of patients with subgingival crown margins 1.0 mm or less from the alveolar crest (within the connective tissue attachment); Group 2, patients with margins from 1.0 mm to less than or equal to 2.0 mm from the alveolar crest (within the junctional epithelium); and Group 3, patients with margins 2.0 mm or greater from the alveolar crest (within the sulcus). A marked increase in papillary bleeding for Group 1 was the most significant sign that the health of the periodontium was compromised. Even though gingival inflammation resulted from the violation of the connective tissue attachment, there were no signs of either gingival recession or bone resorption.[252] Excepting this clinical study, a review[253] of the literature on placement of the gingival margin based on traditional concepts of biologic width concluded that the evidence is primarily based on opinion and anecdotal cases. Nevertheless, the authors suggest that "clinical experience and prudence" favor a 3.0-mm space between the alveolar crest and the restoration margin.[253] For additional discussion of evaluation and management of tissue during crown preparation, see chapter 17.

Defective Restorations and Periodontal Health

In addition to the subgingival placement of the restoration margin, poor quality of the restoration margin, including marginal openings, roughness, and overhangs, may impair periodontal health. With an ideal preparation, it is technically possible to obtain a marginal discrepancy of less than 10 μm with a cast metallic restoration and less than 50 μm with a ceramic restoration.[254] However, with additive effects of luting cement thickness, preparation design deficiencies, and technique errors, the interface discrepancy can be much greater. In a retrospective study of 42 crowns with intrasulcular margins and more than 4 years service, the mean marginal discrepancy was 160 μm, and 15 crowns (36%) had discrepancies greater than 200 μm. The investigators reported a direct quantitative correlation between increased marginal discrepancy and an increased gingival index and crevicular fluid-flow volume.[255] Another study reported that, in addition to increased inflammation, radiographically determined bone loss was associated with crown margin discrepancies greater than 50 μm.[256] With a marginal discrepancy of 200 μm completely surrounding a restored tooth, the total computed area of exposed cement surface amounts to several square millimeters. This interface is rough, porous, and retentive to plaque.[257]

Another concern with restoration margins, especially with Class 2 direct restorations, is *overhang*, the extension of the restorative material beyond the cavity preparation. The morphologic variation in the cervical aspect of teeth, including furcations, fluting, and concavities, makes it difficult to consistently place a wedge and matrix band to fully adapt to the gingival cavomargin. Lervik et al[258] magnified bite-wing radiographs and found that 25% of proximal-surface restorations presented overhangs. Of these, 29% were greater than 0.2 mm and 4% were greater than 0.5 mm. Jeffcoat and Howell[259] grouped 100 restorations with overhangs by the percentage of intrusion or invasion into the interproximal space and compared adjacent bone loss with the 100 contralateral nonrestored controls. They concluded that gingival displacement caused by large overhangs intruding 51% or more into the interproximal space is directly related to alveolar bone loss. In a literature review of overhanging dental restorations (ODRs) and their effects on the periodontium, Brunsvold and Lane[260] reported a prevalence range of interproximal overhangs from 25% to 76%. The authors attributed the wide range to differences in classification criteria and diagnostic methods. Their conclusions, which follow, are validated by recent studies and reviews:[261,262]

- Prevalence of ODR is high, involving at least 25% of restored teeth.
- Radiographic and tactile exploration must be combined to improve ODR detection.
- Increased bone loss, attachment loss, pocket depth, and inflammation occur adjacent to teeth with ODR; the periodontal destruction is related to the size of the ODR.

Restoration overhangs have been described as "permanent calculus." As with poor marginal fit of crowns, iatrogenic defects in restorations contribute to the retention and concentration of plaque biomass. Lang et al[263] found that an ODR also alters the pathologic nature of the plaque bacteria. Two sets of MOD onlays were made for each subject, one with normal contours and one with a 0.5- to 1.0-mm overhang. One of the restorations was temporarily cemented, and after 19 to 27 weeks, that restoration was removed and the other was placed in a crossover study design. With the overhanging restorations, a normally healthy sulcus microflora changed to a gram-negative, anaerobic culture typical of chronic periodontitis. It is important to note that when the onlays with overhangs were exchanged for the properly fitted restorations, equivalent to the clinical removal of an overhang, the gingival index and microflora returned to a healthy state. However, in a study in which amalgam overhangs were removed with an ultrasonic scaler and followed for 3 months, baseline gingival inflammation and early bone loss were not significantly reversed except in the group with meticulous plaque control.[264] Thus, in addition to encouraging patients' oral hygiene, the clinician should carefully plan the location of restoration margins and strive for excellent fit and contour of the restoration. When overhangs are detected, their removal should be part of the treatment plan.[265]

Other parameters of restorations that have a less directly detrimental effect on the health of the periodontium are overcontoured axial surfaces, traumatic occlusion, and defective interproximal contacts. Undercontoured or "flat" facial and lingual profiles have been advocated to benefit periodontal health, while overcontoured restorations have been associated with plaque retention.[266] Crowns are commonly overcontoured, from 0.7 to 1.28 mm wider than the dimension of the teeth before restoration.[267] It appears that some latitude in facial and lingual contours is acceptable, but it is important to incorporate "fluting" in areas where the restoration abuts furcations to facilitate plaque removal.[268] A common clinical sign of traumatic occlusion on a specific tooth or group of teeth, especially with a loss of periodontal support, is hypermobility. A clinical study of patients with periodontitis found a relationship between tooth mobility and increased loss of both attachment and bone.[269] In their review, the authors concluded that in patients with preexisting plaque-induced periodontitis, concomitant occlusal trauma may increase the rate of destruction, but "trauma from occlusion cannot induce periodontal tissue breakdown."[270]

Another aspect of restorations that relates to the health and comfort of the periodontium is deficient or open interproximal contacts. Acceptable interproximal contacts should contribute to tooth stability, deflect food to the vestibular or oral embrasures to protect the nonkeratinized gingival col, and prevent food impaction. However, when the level of oral hygiene is good and there is no food impaction, there is no clear relationship between deficient interproximal contacts and periodontal problems.[271] Indeed, the majority of healthy teeth, unless in heavy occlusion, have a slight interproximal gap that will often allow shimstock to pass through the contact.[272] Nevertheless, if the teeth are in contact preoperatively, authorities agree that the new restoration should restore the contact to prevent possible gingival irritation and patient discomfort from food impaction.

Conclusion

Just like the dentition, the periodontium is at risk from specific plaque organisms and therefore benefits from routine effective plaque removal. Errors in diagnosis and treatment planning and iatrogenic problems associated with restoration of teeth can exacerbate plaque retention, inflammation, loss of connective tissue attachment, and loss of bone support. A healthy periodontium is essential for the well-being, comfort, and esthetics of the oral structures.

Acknowledgment

The author wishes to thank Dr David Lasho, clinical assistant professor, Department of Periodontics, University of Texas Health Science Center Dental School at San Antonio, for his review of and assistance with the section on the gingiva.

References

1. Fejerskov O, Thylstrup A. Dental enamel. In: Mjör IA, Fejerskov O (eds). Human Oral Embryology and Histology. Copenhagen: Munksgaard, 1986:5–89.

2. Bartelstone HJ, Mandel ID, Oshry E, Seidlin SM. Use of radioactive iodine as a tracer in the study of the physiology of the teeth. Science 1947;106:132–133.

3. Wainwright WW, Lemoine FA. Rapid diffuse penetration of intact enamel and dentin by carbon 14 labeled urea. J Am Dent Assoc 1950;41: 135–145.

4. Featherstone JDB, Ten Cate JM. Physicochemical aspects of fluoride enamel interactions. In: Ekstrand J, Fejerskov O, Silverstone LM (eds). Fluoride in Dentistry. Copenhagen: Munksgaard, 1988:125–149.

5. Murray JJ, Rugg-Gunn AJ, Jenkins GN. Fluorides in Caries Prevention, ed 3. Boston: Wright, 1991.

6. Kirkham J, Robinson C, Strong M, Shore RC. Effects of frequency of acid exposure on demineralization/remineralization behavior of human enamel in vitro. Caries Res 1994;28:9–13.

7. Yanagisawa T, Miake Y. High-resolution electron microscopy of enamel-crystal demineralization and remineralization in carious lesions. J Electron Microscopy 2003;52:605–613.

8. De Freitas PM, Turssi CP, Hara AT. Serra MC. Dentin microhardness during and after whitening treatments. Quintessence Int 2004;35:411–417.

9. Robinson C, Shore RC, Brookes SJ, Strafford S, Wood SR, Kirkam J. The chemistry of enamel caries. Crit Rev Oral Biol Med 2000;11:481–495.

10. Donly KJ, Stookey GK. Topical fluoride therapy. In: Harris NO, Garcia-Godoy F (eds). Primary Preventive Dentistry, ed 6. Upper Saddle River, NJ: Pearson Prentice Hall, 2004:241–284.

11. Nanci A. Enamel: Composition, formation, and structure. In: Nanci A (ed). Ten Cate's Oral Histology: Development, Structure, and Function, ed 6. St Louis: Mosby, 2003:145–191.

12. Muller CFJ, van Wyk CW. The amelo-cemental junction. J Dent Assoc South Afr 1984;39:799–803.

13. Frysh H. The chemistry of bleaching. In: Goldstein RE, Garber DA (eds). Complete Dental Bleaching. Chicago: Quintessence, 1995:25–33.

14. Shklair I, Keene H, Cullen P. The distribution of Streptococcus mutans on the teeth of two groups of naval recruits. Arch Oral Biol 1974;19: 199–202.

15. Ricketts DN, Ekstrand KR, Kidd EA, Larsen T. Relating visual and radiographic ranked scoring systems for occlusal caries detection to histological and microbiological evidence. Oper Dent 2002;27:231–237.

16. Heinrich-Weltzien R, Weerheijm KL, Kuhnisch J, Oehme T, Stosser L. Clinical evaluation of visual, radiographic, and laser fluorescence methods for detection of occlusal caries. J Dent Child 2002;69:127–132.

17. Ekstrand KR, Ricketts DN, Kidd EAM. Reproducibility and accuracy of three methods for assessment of demineralization depth on the occlusal surface: An in-vitro examination. Caries Res 1997;31:224–232.

18. Pitts NG, Kidd EAM. Some of the factors to be considered in the prescription and timing of bitewing radiographs in the diagnosis and management of dental caries: Contemporary recommendations. Br Dent J 1992;172:225–227.

19. Mejare I, Kallest IC, Stenlund H. Incidence and progression of approximal caries from 11 to 22 years of age in Sweden: A prospective radiographic study. Caries Res 1999;33:93–100.

20. Backer Diirks O. Posteruptive changes in dental enamel. J Dent Res 1966;45:503–511.

21. Van Amerongen JP, Davidson CL, Opdam NJM, Roeters FJM, Kidd EAM (eds). Restoring the tooth: "The seal is the deal." In: Fejerskov O, Kidd EAM (eds). Dental Caries: The Disease and Its Clinical Management. Oxford: Blackwell Munksgaard, 2003:275–292.

22. Hausen H. Benefits of topical fluorides firmly established. Evid Based Dent 2004;5:36–37.

23. Cai F, Shen P, Morgan MV, Reynolds EC. Remineralization of enamel subsurface lesions in situ by sugar-free lozenges containing casein phosphopeptide-amorphous calcium phosphate. Aust Dent J 2003;48: 240–243.

24. Yamagishi K, Onuma K, Suzuki T, et al. Materials chemistry: A synthetic enamel for rapid tooth repair. Nature 2005;433:819.

25. Caldwell RC, Muntz ML, Gilmore RW, Pigman W. Microhardness studies of intact surface enamel. J Dent Res 1957;36:732–738.

26. Lambrechts P, Braem M, Vuylsteke-Wauters M, Vanherle G. Quantitative in vivo wear of human enamel. J Dent Res 1989;68:1752–1754.

27. Christensen GT. Alternatives for Class 2 restorations. Clin Res Assoc Newsletter 1994;18(5):1–3.

28. Listgarten MA, Korostoff J. The development and structure of dental plaque (a bacterial biofilm), calculus, and other tooth-adherent organic materials. In: Harris NO, Garcia-Godoy F (eds). Primary Preventive Dentistry, ed 6. Upper Saddle River, NJ: Pearson Prentice Hall, 2004:23–44.

29. Kaste LM, Selwitz RH, Oldakowski RJ, Brunelle JA, Winn DM, Brown LJ. Coronal caries in the primary and permanent dentition of children and adolescents 1–17 years of age: United States, 1988–1991. J Dent Res 1996;75(special issue):631–641.

30. US Department of Health and Human Services. Oral Health in America: A Report of the Surgeon General. Rockville, MD: US Department of Health and Human Services, National Institute of Dental and Craniofacial Research, National Institutes of Health, 2000.

31. Llodra JC, Bravo M, Delgado-Rodriguez M, Baca P, Galvey R. Factors influencing the effectiveness of sealants—A meta-analysis. Community Dent Oral Epidemiol 1993;21:261–268.

32. Heller KE, Reed SG, Bruner FW, Eklund SA, Burt BA. Longitudinal evaluation of sealing molars with and without incipient dental caries in a public health program. J Public Health Dent 1995;55:148–153.

33. Ailor JE Jr. Managing incomplete tooth fractures. J Am Dent Assoc 2000;131:1168–1174.

34. Geurtsen W, Schwarze T, Gunay H. Diagnosis, therapy, and prevention of the cracked tooth syndrome. Quintessence Int 2003;34:409–417.

35. Robinson C, Shore RC, Brookes SJ, Strafford S, Wood SR, Kirkam J. The chemistry of enamel caries. Crit Rev Oral Biol Med 2000;11:481–495.

36. Featherstone JDB. Prevention and reversal of dental caries: Role of low level fluoride. Community Dent Oral Epidemiol 1999;27:31–40.

37. Silverstone LM, Saxton CA, Dogon IL, Fejerskov O. Variation in the pattern of acid etching of human dental enamel examined by scanning electron microscopy. Caries Res 1975;9:373–387.

38. Hewlett ER. Resin adhesion to enamel and dentin: A review. J Calif Dent Assoc 2003;31:469–476.

39. Van Meerbeek B, De Munck J, Yoshida Y, et al. Buonocore memorial lecture. Adhesion to enamel and dentin: Current status and future challenges. Oper Dent 2003;28:215–235.

40. Buonocore MG. A simple method of increasing the adhesion of acrylic filling materials to enamel surfaces. J Dent Res 1955;34:849–853.

41. Gwinnett AJ, Matsui A. A study of enamel adhesives. The physical relationship between enamel and adhesive. Arch Oral Biol 1967;12:1615–1620.

42. Buonocore MG. The Use of Adhesives in Dentistry. Springfield, IL: Thomas, 1975:75.

43. Munechika T, Suzuki K, Nishiyama M, Ohashi M, Horie K. A comparison of the tensile bond strengths of composite resins to longitudinal and transverse sections of enamel prisms in human teeth. J Dent Res 1984;63:1079–1082.

44. Opdam NJ, Roeters JJ, Kuijs R, Burgersdijk RC. Necessity of bevels for box only Class II composite restorations. Am J Dent 1993;6:85–87.

45. Hilton TJ, Ferracane JL. Cavity preparation factors and microleakage of Class II composite restorations filled at intraoral temperatures. Quintessence Int 2002;33:337–346.

46. Hobson RS, McCabe JF. Relationship between enamel etch characteristics and resin-enamel bond strength. Br Dent J 2002;192:463–468.

47. Giannini M, Soares CJ, de Carvalho RM. Ultimate tensile strength of tooth structures. Dent Mater 2004;20:322–329.

48. Kidd EAM, Toffenetti F, Mjör IA. Secondary caries. Int Dent J 1992;42:127–138.

49. Christensen RP, Palmer TM, Ploeger BJ, Yost MP. Resin polymerization problems—Are they caused by resin curing lights, resin formulations, or both? Compend Contin Educ Dent Suppl 1999; Nov(25):S42–S54.

50. Marzouk MA, Simonton AL, Grpss RD. Operative Dentistry—Modern Theory and Practice. St Louis: Ishiyaku EuroAmerica, 1985:33–37.

51. Simmelink JW. Histology of enamel. In: Avery JK (ed). Oral Development and Histology. Baltimore: Williams & Wilkins, 1987:140–150.

52. Boyde A. Enamel structure and cavity margins. Oper Dent 1976;1:13–28.

53. Crabb HS, Darling AI. The gradient of mineralization in developing enamel. Arch Oral Biol 1960;52:118–122.

54. Spears IR, van Noort R, Crompton RH, Cardew GE, Howard IC. The effects of enamel anisotrophy on the distribution of stress in a tooth. J Dent Res 1993;72:1526–1531.

55. Anderson DJ. Measurement of stress in mastication. J Dent Res 1956;35:671–673.

56. Braun S, Bantleon HP, Hnat WP, Freudenthaler JW, Marcotte MR, Johnson BE. A study of bite force, part I: Relationship to various physical characteristics. Angle Orthod 1995;65:367–372.

57. Hoffmann F, Eismann D. The total surface and number of occlusal contacts in static and dynamic occlusion. Bilt Udrux Ortodonata Jugosl 1991;24:71–78.

58. Vale WA. Cavity preparations. Ir Dent Rev 1956;2:33–41.

59. Mondelli J, Steagall L, Ishikiriama A, de Lima Navarro MF, Soares FB. Fracture strength of human teeth with cavity preparations. J Prosthet Dent 1980;43:419–422.

60. Blaser PK, Lund MR, Cochran MA. Effects of designs of Class 2 preparations on resistance of teeth to fracture. Oper Dent 1983;8:6–10.

61. Reeh ES, Douglas WH, Messer HH. Stiffness of endodontically treated teeth related to restoration technique. J Dent Res 1989;68:1540–1544.

62. Rees JS, Jagger DC. Abfraction lesions: Myth or reality? J Esthet Restor Dent 2003;15:263–271.

63. Heymann HO, Sturdevant JR, Bayne S, Wilder AD, Sluder TB, Brunson WD. Examining tooth flexure effects on cervical restorations: A two-year clinical study. J Am Dent Assoc 1991;122:41–47.

64. Palamara D, Palamara JE, Tyas ML, Messer HH. Strain patterns in cervical enamel of teeth subjected to occlusal loading. Dent Mater 2000;16;412–419.

65. Rees JS, Hammadeh M. Undermining of enamel as a mechanism of abfracture lesion formation: A finite element study. Eur J Oral Sci 2004;112:342–352.

66. el-Mowafy OM. Fracture strength and fracture patterns of maxillary premolars with approximal slot cavities. Oper Dent 1993;18:160–166.

67. Zidan O, Abdel-Keriem U. The effect of amalgam bonding on the stiffness of teeth weakened by cavity preparation. Dent Mater 2003;19:680–685.

68. Elderton RJ. Clinical studies concerning re-restoration of teeth. Adv Dent Res 1990;4:4–9.

69. Brantley CF, Bader JD, Shugars DA, Nesbit SP. Does the cycle of rerestoration lead to larger restorations? J Am Dent Assoc 1995;126:1407–1413.

70. Burke FJ. From extension for prevention to prevention of extension: (minimal intervention dentistry). Dent Update 2003;30:492–498, 500, 502.

71. Garberoglio R, Brännström M. Scanning electron microscopic investigation of human dentinal tubules. Arch Oral Biol 1976;21:355–362.

72. Mjör IA, Sveen OB, Heyeraas KJ. Normal structure and physiology. In: Mjör IA. Pulp-Dentin Biology in Restorative Dentistry. Chicago: Quintessence, 2002:1–22.

73. Goracci G, Mori G, Baldi M. Terminal end of the human odontoblast process: A study using SEM and confocal microscopy. Clin Oral Investig 1999;3:126–132.

74. Nanci A. Dentin-pulp complex. In: Nanci A (ed). Ten Cate's Oral Histology: Development, Structure, and Function, ed 6. St Louis: Mosby, 2003:192–239.

75. Pashley DH, Depew DD. Effects of the smear layer, Copalite, and oxalate on microleakage. Oper Dent 1986;11:95–102.

76. Ayad MF. Effects of rotary instrumentation and different enchants on removal of smear layer on human dentin. J Prosthet Dent 2001;85:67–72.

77. Vongsavan N, Matthews RW, Matthews B. The permeability of human dentine in vitro and in vivo. Arch Oral Biol 2000;45:931–935.

78. Pashley DH, Matthews WG. The effects of outward forced convective flow on inward diffusion in human dentine, in vitro. Arch Oral Biol 1993;38:577–582.

79. Pashley DH, Kepler EE, Williams, EC, Okabe A. Progressive decrease in dentine permeability following cavity preparation. Arch Oral Biol 1983;28:853–858.

80. Hahn CL, Overton B. The effects of immunoglobulins on the convective permeability of human dentine in vitro. Arch Oral Biol 1997;42:835–843.

81. Love RM. The effect of tissue molecules on bacterial invasion of dentine. Oral Microbiol Immunol 2002;117:32–37.

82. Dai X-F, Ten Cate AR, Limeback H. The extent and distribution of intratubular collagen fibrils in human dentin. Arch Oral Biol 1991;36:775–778.

83. Michelich V, Pashley DH, Whitford GM. Dentin permeability: A comparison of functional versus anatomical tubular radii. J Dent Res 1978;57:1019–1024.

84. Pashley DH. Dentine permeability and its role in the pathobiology of dentine sensitivity. Arch Oral Biol 1994;39(suppl):73S–80S.

85. Maroli S, Khea SC, Krell KV. Regional variation in permeability of young dentin. Oper Dent 1992;17:93–100.

86. Rauchenberger CR. Dentin permeability: The clinical ramifications. Dent Clin North Am 1992;36:527–542.

87. Richardson DW, Tao L, Pashley DH. Dentin permeability: Effects of crown preparation. Int J Prosthodont 1991;4:219–225.

88. Mjör IA. Frequency of secondary caries at various anatomical locations. Oper Dent 1985;10:88–92.

89. Pashley DH, Andringa HJ, Derkson GD, Derkson ME, Kalathoor SR. Regional variability in the permeability of human dentine. Arch Oral Biol 1987;32:519–523.

90. Hughes NP, Littlewood D, Macpherson JV, Beeston MA, Unwin PR. Direct measurements of fluid flow rate in dentinal tubules using scanning electro-chemical microscopy. In: Shimono M, Takahashi K (eds). Dentin/Pulp Complex. Tokyo: Quintessence, 1996:333–335.

91. Brännström M, Vojinovic O, Nordenvall KJ. Bacteria and pulpal reactions under silicate cement restorations. J Prosthet Dent 1979;41:290–295.

92. Bergenholtz G, Cox CF, Loesche WJ, Syed SA. Bacterial leakage around dental restorations: Its effect on the dental pulp. J Oral Pathol 1982;11:439–450.

93. Bergenholtz G. Evidence for bacterial causation of adverse pulpal responses in resin-based dental restorations. Crit Rev Oral Biol Med 2000;11:467–480.

94. Hilton TJ. Can modern restorative procedures and materials reliably seal cavities? In vitro investigations: Part 1. Am J Dent 2002;15:198–210.

95. Mjör IA, Moorhead JE, Dahl JF. Reasons for replacement of restorations in permanent teeth in general dental practice. Int Dent J 2000;50:361–366.

96. Piesco NP. Histology of dentin. In: Avery JK, Steele PF (eds). Oral Development and Histology, ed 3. New York: Thieme, 2002:172–189.

97. Langeland K. Tissue response to dental caries. Endod Dent Traumatol 1987;3:149–171.

98. Garant PR. Oral Cells and Tissues. Chicago: Quintessence, 2003.

99. Pashley DH. Dentin: A dynamic substrate—A review. Scanning Microsc 1989;3:161–176.

100. Smith AJ, Matthews JB, Hall RC. Transforming growth factor-β1 (TGB-β1) in dentine matrix. Ligand activation and receptor expression. Eur J Oral Sci 1998;106(suppl 1):179–184.

101. Chappell RP, Cobb CM, Spencer P, Eick JD. Dentine tubule anastomosis: A potential factor in adhesive bonding. J Prosthet Dent 1994;72:183–188.

102. Stanley HR. Design of a human pulp study 1. Oral Surg 1968;25:633–647.

103. Zach L, Cohen G. Thermogenesis in operative techniques: Comparison of four methods. J Prosthet Dent 1962;12:977–984.

104. Goodis HE, Pashley D, Staabholtz A. Pulpal effects of thermal and mechanical irritants. In: Hargreaves KM, Goodis HE (eds). Selzer and Bender's Dental Pulp. Chicago: Quintessence, 2002:371–388.

105. Mjör IA, Nordahl I. The density and branching of dentinal tubules in human teeth. Arch Oral Biol 1996;41:401–412.

106. Mjör IA. Initial reactions to tooth preparation. In: Mjör IA. Pulp-Dentin Biology in Restorative Dentistry. Chicago: Quintessence, 2002:23–37.

107. Fosse F, Saele PK, Eide R. Numerical density and distribution pattern of dentin tubules. Acta Odontol Scand 1992;50:201–210.

108. Outhwaite WC, Livingston MJ, Pashley DH. Effects of changes in surface area, thickness, temperature, and post-extraction time on human dentine permeability. Arch Oral Biol 1976;21:599–603.

109. Pashley DH, Pashley EL, Carvalho RM, Tay FR. The effects of dentin permeability on restorative dentistry. Dent Clin North Am 2002;46:211–245.

110. Pashley DH. Dynamics of the pulpo-dentin complex. Crit Rev Oral Biol Med 1996;7:104–133.

111. Gwinnett AJ. Dentin bond strength after drying and rewetting. Am J Dent 1994;7:144–148.

112. Prati C, Pashley DH, Montanari G. Hydrostatic intrapulpal pressure and bond strength of bonding systems. Dent Mater 1991;7:54–58.

113. Tay F, Gwinnett A, Wei S. The overwet phenomenon: A scanning electron microscopic study of surface moisture in the acid-conditioned, resin-dentin interface. Am J Dent 1996;9:109–114.

114. Moll K, Haller B. Effect of intrinsic and extrinsic moisture on bond strength to dentin. J Oral Rehab 2000;27:150–165.

115. El-din AK, Miller BH, Griggs JA. Resin bonding to sclerotic, noncarious, cervical lesions. Quintessence Int 2004;35:529–540.

116. Yoshiyama M, Masada J, Uchida A, Ishida H. Scanning electron microscopic characterization of sensitive vs. insensitive human radicular dentin. J Dent Res 1989;68:1498–1502.

117. Tay FR, Pashley DH. Resin bonding to cervical sclerotic dentin: A review. J Dent 2004;32:173–196.

118. Kwong SM, Cheung GS, Kei LH, et al. Micro-tensile bond strengths to sclerotic dentin using a self-etching and a total-etching technique. Dent Mater 2002;18:359–369.

119. Lopes GC, Baratieri CM, Baratieri LN, Monteiro S Jr, Carkoso Vieira LC. Bonding to cervical sclerotic dentin: Effect of acid etching time. J Adhes Dent 2004;6:19–23.

120. Bjørndal L, Mjör IA. Dental caries: Characteristics of lesions and pulpal reactions. In: Mjör IA. Pulp-Dentin Biology in Restorative Dentistry. Chicago: Quintessence, 2002:55–75.

121. Bjørndal L, Thylstrup A. A structural analysis of approximal enamel caries lesions and subjacent dentin reactions. Eur J Oral Sci 1995;103:25–31.

122. Bjørndal L, DarvannT, Thylstrup A. A quantitative light microscopic study of the odontoblast and subodontoblastic reactions to active and arrested enamel caries without cavitation. Caries Res 1998;31:59–69.

123. ten Cate JM, Larsen MJ, Pearch IEF, Fejerskov O. Chemical interactions between the tooth and oral fluids. In: Fejerskov O, Kidd EAM (eds). Dental Caries: The Disease and Its Clinical Management. Oxford, UK: Blackwell Munksgaard, 2003:49–70.

124. Fejerskov O, Nyvad B, Kidd EAM. Clinical and histological manifestations of dental caries. In: Fejerskov O, Kidd EAM (eds). Dental Caries: The Disease and Its Clinical Management. Oxford, UK: Blackwell Munksgaard, 2003:71–98.

125. Bjørndal L, Darvann T, Lussi A. A computerized analysis of the relation between the occlusal enamel caries lesion and the demineralized dentin. Eur J Oral Sci 1999;107:176–182.

126. Bjørndal L. Dentin caries: Progression and clinical management. Oper Dent 2002;27:211–217.

127. Ricketts DN, Ekstrand KR, Kidd EA, Larsen T. Relating visual and radiographic ranked scoring systems for occlusal caries detection to histological and microbiological evidence. Oper Dent 2002;27:231–237.

128. Helfenstein U, Steiner J. Fluoride varnishes (Duraphat): A meta-analysis. Community Dent Oral Epidemiol 1994;22:1–5.

129. Maltz M, de Oliveira D, Fontanella V, Bianchi R. A clinical, microbiologic, and radiographic study of deep caries lesions after incomplete caries removal. Quintessence Int 2002;33:151–159.

130. Fusayama T. Two layers of carious dentin; diagnosis and treatment. Oper Dent 1979;4:63–70.

131. Love RM, Jenkinson HF. Invasion of dentinal tubules by oral bacteria. Crit Rev Oral Biol Med 2002;3:171–183.

132. Mertz-Fairhurst EJ, Curtis JW Jr, Ergle JW, Rueggeberg FA, Adair SM. Ultraconservative and cariostatic sealed restorations: Results at year 10. J Am Dent Assoc 1998;129:55–66.

133. Ricketts DN, Kidd EA, Beignton D. Operative and microbiological validation of visual, radiographic, and electronic diagnosis of occlusal caries in non-cavitated teeth judged to be in need of operative care. Br Dent J 1995;179:214–220.

134. Kidd EAM. How 'clean' must a cavity be before restoration? Caries Res 2004;38:306–313.

135. Bonecker M, Grossman G, Cleaton-Jones PE, Parak R. Clinical, histological and microbiological study of hand-excavated carious dentine in extracted permanent teeth. SADJ 2003;58:273–278.

136. Nakajima M, Sano H, Zhang L, Tagami J, Pashley DH. Effect of moist vs dry bonding to normal vs caries-affected dentin with Scotchbond Multi-Purpose Plus. J Dent Res 1999;78:1298–1303.

137. Arrais CA, Giannini M, Nakajima M, Tagami J. Effects of additional and extended acid etching on bonding to caries-affected dentine. Eur J Oral Sci 2004;112:458–464.

138. Yoshiyama Y, Tay FR, Toru Y, et al. Resin adhesion to carious dentin. Am J Dent 2003;16:47–52.

139. Torneck CD. Dentin-pulp complex. In: Ten Cate AR (ed). Oral Histology: Development, Structure, and Function, ed 4. St Louis: Mosby Year-Book, 1994:169–217.

140. Shimizu C, Yamashita Y, Ichigo T, Fusayama T. Carious change of dentin observed on longspan ultrathin sections. J Dent Res 1981;60:1826–1831.

141. Yagi T, Suga S. SEM investigations on the human sclerosed dentinal tubules [in Japanese]. Shigaku 1990;78:313–337.

142. Stanley HR, Pereira JC, Spiegel E, Broom C, Schultz M. The detection and prevalence of reactive and physiologic sclerotic dentin, reparative dentin and dead tracts beneath various types of dental lesions according to tooth surface and age. J Oral Pathol 1983;12:257–289.

143. Kim S, Trowbridge HO. Pulpal reaction to caries and dental procedures. In: Cohen S, Burns RC (eds). Pathways of the Pulp, ed 7. St Louis: Mosby, 1998:532–551.

144. Tagami J, Hosoda H, Burrow MF, Nakajima M. Effect of aging and caries on dentin permeability. Proc Finn Dent Soc 1992;88(suppl 1):149–154.

145. Trowbridge HO. Histology of pulpal inflammation. In: Hargreaves KM, Goodis H (eds). Seltzer and Bender's Dental Pulp. Chicago: Quintessence, 2002:227–246.

146. Trowbridge HO. Pulp biology: Progress during the past 25 years. Aust Endod J 2003;29:5–12.

147. Magloire H, Joffre A, Couble ML, Chavrier C, Dumont J. Ultrastructural alterations of human odontoblasts and collagen fibres in the pulpal border zone beneath early caries lesions. Cell Mol Biol Incl Cyto Enzymol 1981;27:437–443.

148. Bjørndal L, Darvann T. A light microscopic study of odontoblastic and non-odontoblastic cells involved in tertiary dentinogenesis in well-defined cavitated carious lesions. Caries Res 1999;33:500–560.

149. Bjørndal L. Presence or absence of tertiary dentinogenesis in relation to caries progression. Adv Dent Res 2001;15:80–83.

150. Bjørndal L, Mjör IA. Pulp-dentin biology in restorative dentistry. Part 4. Dental caries—Characteristics of lesions and pulpal reactions. Quintessence Int 2001;32:717–736.

151. Murray PE, About I, Lumley PJ, Franquin JC, Remusat M, Smith AJ. Cavity remaining dentin thickness and pulpal activity. Am J Dent 2002;15:41–48.

152. Tecles O, Laurent P, Zygouritsas S, et al. Activation of human dental pulp progenitor/stem cells in response to odontoblast injury. Arch Oral Biol 2005;50:103–108.

153. Stanley HR. White CL, McCray L. The rate of tertiary (reparative) dentine formation in the human tooth. Oral Surg 1966;21:180–189.

154. Cox CF, Bogen G, Koper HM, Ruby JD. Repair of pulpal injury by dental materials. In: Hargreaves, KM, Goodis, HE (eds). Seltzer and Bender's Dental Pulp. Chicago: Quintessence, 2002:325–344.

155. Mjör IA, Ferrari M. Reactions to restorative materials, tooth-restoration interfaces, and adhesive techniques. In: Mjör IA (ed). Pulp-Dentin Biology in Restorative Dentistry. Chicago: Quintessence, 2002:101–103.

156. Izumi T, Inoue H, Matsuura H, et al. Changes in the pattern of horseradish peroxidase diffusion into predentin and dentin after cavity preparation in rat molars. Oral Surg Oral Med Oral Path Oral Radiol Endod 2001;92:675–681.

157. Tziafas D, Smith AJ, Lesot H. Designing new treatment strategies in vital pulp therapy. J Dent 2000;28:77–92.

158. Sloan AJ, Matthews JB, Smith AJ. TGF-beta receptor expression in human odontoblasts and pulpal cells. Histochem J 1999;31:565–569.

159. Iohara K, Nakashima M, Ito M, Ishikawa M, Nakasima A, Akamine A. Dentin regeneration by dental pulp stem cell therapy with recombinant human bone morphogenetic protein 2. J Dent Res 2004;83:590–595.

160. Cassidy N, Fahey M, Prime SS, Smith AJ. Comparative analysis of transforming growth factor-beta (TGF-β) isoforms 1–3 in human and rabbit dentine matrices. Arch Oral Biol 1997;42:219–223.

161. D'Souza RN, Cavender A, Dickinson D, Roberts A, Letterio J. TGF-β$_1$ is essential for the homeostasis of the dentin-pulp complex. Eur J Oral Sci 1998;106:185–191.

162. Smith AJ, Tobias RS, Cassidy N, et al. Odontoblast stimulation in ferrets by dentine matrix components. Arch Oral Biol 1994;39:13–22.

163. Smith AJ. Pulpal responses to caries and dental repair. Caries Res 2002;36:223–232.

164. Tziafas D, Alvanou A, Panagiotakopoulos N, et al. Induction of odontoblast-like cell differentiation in dog dental pulps after in vivo implantation of dentine matrix components. Arch Oral Biol 1995;40:883–893.

165. Goracci G, Mori G, Baldi M. Terminal end of the human odontoblast process: A study using SEM and confocal microscopy. Clin Oral Investig 1999;3:126–132.

166. Brännström M, Aström A. The hydrodynamics of the dentine: The possible relationship to dental pain. Int Dent J 1972;22:219–227.

167. Brännström M, Johnson G, Linden LA. Fluid flow and pain response in the dentin produced by hydrostatic pressure. Odontol Rev 1969;20:15–16.

168. Andrew D, Matthews B. Displacement of the contents of dentinal tubules and sensory transduction in intradental nerves of the cat. J Physiol 2000;529(part 3):791–802.

169. Trowbridge HO. Intradental sensory units: Physiological and clinical aspects. J Endod 1985;11:489–498.

170. Alavi AM, Dubyak GR, Burnstock G. Immunohistochemical evidence for ATP receptors in human dental pulp. J Dent Res 2001;80:476–483.

171. Ahlquist M, Franzein O, Coffey J, Pashley D. Dental pain evoked by hydrostatic pressures applied to exposed dentin in man: A test of the hydrodynamic theory of dental sensitivity. J Endod 1994;20:130–137.

172. Cuenin MF, Scheidt MJ, O'Neal RB, et al. An in vivo study of dentin sensitivity: The relation of dentin sensitivity and the patency of dentin tubules. J Periodontol 1991;62:668–673.

173. Kolker JL, Vargas MA, Armstrong SR, Dawson DV. Effect of desensitizing agents on dentin permeability and dentin tubule occlusion. J Adhes Dent 2002;4:211–221.

174. Byers MR, Närhi MV. Nerve supply of the pulpodentin complex and responses to injury. In: Hargreaves KM, Goodis H (eds). Seltzer and Bender's Dental Pulp. Chicago: Quintessence, 2002:151–179.

175. Heyeraas KJ, Sveen OB, Mjör IA. Pulpal inflammation and its sequelae. In: Mjör IA. Pulp-Dentin Biology in Restorative Dentistry. Chicago: Quintessence, 2002:39–54.

176. Okiji T. Pulp as a connective tissue. In: Hargreaves KM, Goodis H (eds). Seltzer and Bender's Dental Pulp. Chicago: Quintessence, 2002:95–122.

177. Linde A. Dentin mineralization and the role of odontoblasts in calcium transport. Connect Tissue Res 1995;33:169–179.

178. Sasaki T, Nakagawa K, Higashi S. Ultrastructure of odontoblasts in kitten tooth germs as revealed by freeze-fracture. Arch Oral Biol 1982;27:897–904.

179. Bishop MA. Yoshida S. A permeability barrier to lanthanum and the presence of collagen between odontoblasts in pig molars. J Anat 1992;181:29–38.

180. Brännström M. Communication between the oral cavity and the dental pulp associated with restorative treatment. Oper Dent 1984;9:57–68.

181. Turner DF, Marfurt CF, Sattleberg C. Demonstration of physiological barrier between pulpal odontoblasts and its perturbation following routine restorative procedures: Horseradish peroxidase tracing study in the rat. J Dent Res 1989;68:1262–1268.

182. Smith AJ. Questions and controversies. In: Nanci A, Ten Cate AR (eds). Ten Cate's Oral Histology: Development, Structure, and Function, ed 6. St. Louis: Mosby, 2003:192–239.

183. Sakurai K, Okiji T, Suda H. Co-increase of nerve fibers and HLA-DR and/or factor-XIIIa-expressing dendritic cells in dentinal caries-affected regions of the human dental pulp: An immunohistochemical study. J Dent Res 1999;78:1596–1608.

184. Ohshima H, Nakakura-Ohshima K, Takeuchi K, Hoshino M, Takano Y, Maeda T. Pulpal regeneration after cavity preparation, with special reference to close spatio-relationships between odontoblasts and immunocompetent cells. Microsc Res Tech 2003;60:483–490.

185. Jontell M, Okiji T, Dahlgren U, Bergenholtz G. Immune defense mechanisms of the dental pulp. Crit Rev Oral Biol Med 1998;9:179–200.

186. Reeves R, Stanley HR. The relationship of bacterial penetration and pulpal pathosis in carious teeth. Oral Surg Oral Med Oral Pathol 1966;22:59–65.

187. Suda H, Ikeda H. The circulation of the pulp. In: Hargreaves KM, Goodis HE (eds). Seltzer and Bender's Dental Pulp. Chicago: Quintessence, 2003:123–150.

188. Pashley DH. The influence of dentin permeability and pulpal blood flow on pulpal solute concentrations. J Endod 1979;5:355–361.

189. Kim S. Ligamental injection: A physiological explanation of its efficacy. J Endod 1986;12:486–491.

190. Stenvik A, Iverson J, Mjör IA. Tissue pressure and histology of normal and inflamed tooth pulps in Macaque monkeys. Arch Oral Biol 1972;17:1501–1511.

191. Takahashi K, Kishi Y, Kim S. A scanning electron microscope study of the blood vessels of dog pulp using corrosion resin casts. J Endod 1982;8:131–135.

192. Heyeraas KJ. Interstitial fluid pressure and transmicrovascular fluid flow. In: Inoki R, Judo T, Olgart L (eds). Dynamic Aspects of Dental Pulp. London: Chapman and Hall, 1990:189–198.

193. Tonder KJ, Kvinnsland I. Micropuncture measurement of interstitial tissue pressure in normal and inflamed dental pulp in cats. J Endod 1983;9:105–109.

194. Gerzina TMO, Hume WR. Effect of hydrostatic pressure on the diffusion of monomers through dentin in vitro. J Dent Res 1995;74:369–373.

195. Pashley DH, Matthews WG. The effect of outward forced convective flow on inward diffusion in human dentine in vitro. Arch Oral Biol 1993;38:577–582.

196. Trowbridge HO. Intradental sensory units: Physiological and clinical aspects. J Endod 1985;11:489–498.

197. Nair PN. Neural elements in dental pulp and dentin. Oral Surg Oral Med Oral Pathol Oral Radiol Endod 1995;80:710–719.

198. Nair PNR, Luder HU, Schroeder HE. The number and size spectra of myelinated nerves in human premolars. Anat Embryol 1992;92:123–128.

199. Johnsen DC, Harshabarger J, Rymer HD. Quantitative assessment of neural development in human premolars. Anat Rec 1983;205:431–439.

200. Byers MR. Dental sensory receptors. Int Rev Neurobiol 1984;25:39–94.

201. Narhi M, Hirvonen TK, Hakamura M. Responses of intradental nerve fibers to stimulation of dentin and pulp. Acta Physiol Scand 1982;115:173–178.

202. Narhi M, Virtanen A, Huopaniemi T, Hirvonen T. Conduction velocities of single pulp nerve fiber units in the cat. Acta Physiol Scand 1982;116:209–213.

203. Figdor D. Aspects of dentinal and pulpal pain. Pain of dentinal and pulpal origin—A review for the clinician. Ann R Australas Coll Dent Surg 1994;12:131–142.

204. Nair PNR, Schroeder HE. Number and size-spectra of non-myelinated axons of human premolars. Anat Embryol 1995;192:35–41.

205. Edwall L, Scott D Jr. Influence of changes in microcirculation on the excitability of the sensory unit in the tooth of the cat. Acta Physiol Scand 1971;82:555–566.

206. Torebjork HE, Hallin RG. Perceptual changes accompanying controlled preferential blocking of A and C fiber responses in intact human skin nerves. Exp Brain Res 1973;16:321–332.

207. Byers MR, Wheeler EF, Bothwell M. Altered expression of NGF and P75 NGF-receptor by fibroblasts of injured teeth precedes sensory nerve sprouting. Growth Factors 1992;6:41–52.

208. Gazelius B, Edwall B, Olgart L, Lundberg JM, Hokfelt T, Fischer JA. Vasodilatory effects and coexistence of calcitonin gene-related peptide (CGRP) and substance P in sensory nerves of cat dental pulp. Acta Physiol Scand 1987;130:33–40.

209. Olgart L. Neural control of pulpal blood flow. Crit Rev Oral Biol 1996;7:159–171.

210. Byers MO, Taylor PE. Effect of sensory denervation on the response of rat molar pulp to exposure injury. J Dent Res 1993;72:613–618.

211. Andrew D, Matthews B. Some properties of vasodilatory nerves innervating tooth pulp in the cat. In: Shimono M, Maeda T, Suda H, Takahashi K (eds). Dentin/Pulp Complex. Tokyo: Quintessence, 1996:254–257.

212. Cox CF. Biocompatibility of dental materials in the absence of bacterial infection. Oper Dent 1987;12:146–152.

213. Mjör IA. Pulp-dentin biology in restorative dentistry. Part 7: The exposed pulp. Quintessence Int 2002;33:113–135.

214. Mjör IA, Ferrari M. Pulp-dentin biology in restorative dentistry. Part 6: Reactions to restorative materials, tooth restoration interfaces, and adhesive techniques. Quintessence Int 2002;33:35–63.

215. Murray PE, Lumley PJ, Smith AJ. Preserving the vital pulp in operative dentistry: 2. Guidelines for successful restoration of unexposed dentinal lesions. Dent Update 2002;29:127–134.

216. Zach L, Cohen G. Pulp response to externally applied heat. Oral Surg Oral Med Oral Pathol 1965;19:515–530.

217. Cavalcanti BN, Otani C, Rode SM. High-speed cavity preparation techniques with different water flows. J Prosthet Dent. 2002;87:158–161.

218. Ozturk B, Usumez A, Ozturk AN, Ozer F. In vitro assessment of temperature change in the pulp chamber during cavity preparation. J Prosthet Dent 2004;9:436–440.

219. Lockard MW. A retrospective study of pulpal response in vital adult teeth prepared for complete coverage restorations at ultrahigh speed using only air coolant. J Prosthet Dent 2002;88:473–478.

220. Seltzer S, Bender IB. Early human pulp reactions to full crown preparations. J Am Dent Assoc 1959;59:915–930.

221. Swerdlow H, Stanley H Jr. Reaction of human dental pulp to cavity preparation. 2. At 150,000 rpm with air-water spray. J Prosthet Dent 1959;9:121–131.

222. Freid K. Changes in pulpal nerves with aging. Proc Finn Dent Soc 1992;88(suppl 1):517–528.

223. Lindhe H, Karring T, Araújo M. Anatomy of the periodontium. In: Lindhe J, Karring T, Lang N (eds). Clinical Periodontology and Implant Dentistry, ed 4. Oxford: Blackwell, 2003:327.

224. Holmstrup P. Anatomy of the periodontium. In: Wilson TG, Kornman KS (eds). Fundamentals of Periodontics, ed 2. Chicago: Quintessence, 2003:21–38.

225. Brown LJ, Oliver RC, Löe H. Periodontal diseases in the U.S. in 1981: Prevalence, severity, extent and role in tooth mortality. J Periodontol 1989;60:363–370.

226. Kornman KS. The pathogenesis of periodontitis. In: Wilson TG, Kornman KS (eds). Fundamentals of Periodontics, ed 2. Chicago: Quintessence, 2003:3–12.

227. Hillman JD, Brooks TA, Michalek SM, Harmon CC, Snoep JL, van Der Weijden CC. Construction and characterization of an effector strain of Streptococcus mutans for replacement therapy of dental caries. Infect Immun 2000;68:543–549.

228. Tagg JR, Dierksen KP. Bacterial replacement therapy: Adapting "germ warfare" to infection prevention. Trends Biotechnol 2003;21:217–223.

229. Petersilka GJ, Ehmke B, Flemmig TF. Antimicrobial effects of mechanical debridement. Periodontol 2000 2002;28:56–71.

230. Ower P. The role of self-administered plaque control in the management of periodontal diseases: I. A review of the evidence. Dent Update 2003;30:60–68.

231. Trombelli L, Scapoli C, Orlandini E, Tosi M, Bottega S, Tatakis DN. Modulation of clinical expression of plaque-induced gingivitis. III. Response of "high responders" and "low responders" to therapy. J Clin Periodontol 2004;31:253–259.

232. Chapple ILC, Gilbert AD. Understanding Periodontal Diseases: Assessment and Diagnostic Procedures in Practice. London: Quintessence, 2002:4–5.

233. Lang NP, Löe H. The relationship between the width of keratinized gingiva and gingival health. J Periodontol 1972;43:623–627.

234. Maynard JG Jr, Wilson RDK. Physiologic dimensions of the periodontium significant to the restorative dentist. Periodontol 1979;50:170–174.

235. Stetler KJ, Bissada NF. Significance of the width of keratinized gingiva on the periodontal status of teeth with submarginal restorations. J Periodontol 1987;58:696–700.

236. Koke U, Sander C, Heinecke A, Müller H. A possible influence of gingival dimensions on attachment loss and gingival recession following placement of artificial crowns. Int J Periodont Restorative Dent 2003;23:439–445.

237. Wilson TG, Magnusson I. Examination of patients to detect periodontal diseases. In: Wilson TG, Kornman KS (eds). Fundamentals of Periodontics, ed 2. Chicago: Quintessence, 2003:255–257.

238. Vacek JS, Gher ME, Assad DA, Richardson AC, Giambarresi LI. The dimensions of the human dentogingival junction. J Periodont Restorative Dent 1994;14:155–165.

239. Gargiulo AW, Wentz FM, Orban B. Dimensions and relations of the dentogingival junction in humans. J Periodontol 1961;32:261–267.

240. Kois JC. Altering gingival levels: The restorative connection. Part 1: Biologic variables. J Esthet Dent 1994;6:3–9.

241. Kois JC. New paradigms for anterior tooth preparation. Rationale and technique. Oral Health 1998;88:19–22, 25–27, 29–30.

242. Löe H. Reactions of marginal periodontal tissues to restorative procedures. Int Dent J 1968;18:759–778.

243. Silness J. Periodontal conditions in patients treated with dental bridges. 2. The influence of full and partial crowns on plaque accumulation, development of gingivitis, and pocket formation. J Periodontal Res 1970;5:219–224.

244. Newcomb GM. The relationship between the location of subgingival crown margins and gingival inflammation. J Periodontol 1974;45:151–154.

245. Flores-de-Jacoby L, Zafiropoulos GG, Ciancis S. The effect of crown margin location on plaque and periodontal health. Int J Periodont Restorative Dent 1989;9:197–205.

246. Reitemeier B, Hansel K, Walter MH, Kastner C, Toutenburg H. Effect of posterior crown margin placement on gingival health. J Prosthet Dent 2002;87:167–172.

247. Kois JC. The restorative-periodontal interface: Biological parameters. Periodontol 2000 1996;11:29–38.

248. Tarnow DP, Magner AW, Fletcher P. The effect of the distance from the contact point to the crest of bone on the presence or absence of the interproximal dental papilla. J Periodontol 1992;63:995–996.

249. Loughlin DM, Glover ME, Loughlin RM. Clinical crown lengthening. In: Wilson GW, Kornman KS (eds). Fundamentals of Periodontics, ed 2. Chicago: Quintessence, 2003:406–427.

250. Gargiulo AW, Wentz FM, Orban B. Dimensions and relations of the dentogingival junction in humans. J Periodontol 1961;32:261–267.

251. Tal H, Soldinger M, Dreiangel A, Pitaru S. Periodontal response to long-term abuse of the gingival attachment by supracrestal amalgam restorations. J Clin Periodontol 1989;16:654–659.

252. Günay H, Seeger A, Tschernitschek H, Geutsen W. Placement of the preparation line and periodontal health—A prospective 2-year clinical study. Int J Periodont Restorative Dent 2000;20:173–181.

253. Padbury A Jr, Eber R, Wang H-L. Interactions between the gingiva and the margin of restorations. J Clin Periodontol 2003;30:379–385.

254. Rosenstiel SF, Land MF, Jujimoto J. Contemporary Fixed Prosthodontics, ed 3. St Louis: Mosby, 2001:174.

255. Felton DA, Kanoy BE, Bayne MS, Wirthman GP. Effect of in vivo crown margin discrepancies on periodontal health. J Prosthet Dent 1991;65:357–364.

256. Sorensen SE, Larsen IM, Jörgensen KD. Gingival and alveolar bone reaction to marginal fit of subgingival crown margins. Scand J Dent Res 1986;94:109–114.

257. Silness J, Hegdahl T. Area of the exposed zinc phosphate cement surfaces in fixed restorations. Scand J Dent Res 1970;78:163–177.

258. Lervik T, Riodan PJ, Haugejorden O. Periodontal disease and approximal overhangs on amalgam restorations in Norwegian 21-year-olds. Community Dent Oral Epidemiol 1984;12:264–268.

259. Jeffcoat MK, Howell TH. Alveolar bone destruction due to overhanging amalgam in periodontal disease. J Periodontol 1980;51:599–602.

260. Brunsvold MA, Lane JJ. The prevalence of overhanging dental restorations and their relationship to periodontal disease. J Clin Periodontol 1990;17:67–72.

261. Matthews DC, Tabesh M. Detection of localized tooth-related factors that predispose to periodontal infections. Periodontol 2000 2004;34:136–150.

262. Parsell DE, Streckfus CF, Stewart BM, Buchanan WT. The effect of amalgam overhangs on alveolar bone height as a function of patient age and overhang width. Oper Dent 1998;23:94–99.

263. Lang NP, Kiel RA, Anderhalden K. Clinical and microbiological effects of subgingival restorations with overhanging or clinically perfect margins. J Clin Periodontol 1983;10:563–578.

264. Highfield JE, Powell RN. Effects of removal of posterior overhanging metallic margins of restorations upon the periodontal tissues. J Clin Periodontol 1987;5:169–181.

265. Axelsson P. Diagnosis and Risk Prediction of Periodontal Diseases, vol 3. Chicago: Quintessence, 2002:181–186.

266. Youdelis RA, Weaver JD, Sapkos S. Facial and lingual contours of artificial complete crown restoration and their effects on the periodontium. J Prosthet Dent 1973;29:61–66.

267. Ehrlich J, Yaffe A, Weisgold AS. Faciolingual width before and after tooth restoration: A comparative study. J Prosthet Dent 1981;46:153–156.

268. Becker CM, Kaldahl WB. Current theories of crown contour, margin placement, and pontic design. J Prosthet Dent 1981;37:163–179.

269. Pihlstrom BE, Anderson KA, Aeppli D, Schaffer EM. Association between signs of trauma from occlusion and periodontitis. J Periodontol 1986;57:1–6.

270. Lindhe J, Nyman S, Ericsson I. Trauma from occlusion. In: Lindhe J, Karring T, Lang N (eds). Clinical Periodontology and Implant Dentistry, ed 4. Oxford: Blackwell Munksgaard, 2003:354–365.

271. Hancock EB, Mayo CV, Schwab RR, Wirthlin MR. Influence of interdental contacts on periodontal status. J Periodontol 1980;51:445–449.

272. DuBois LM, Niles SM, Boice PA. The magnitude of interproximal spaces between adjacent teeth. Am J Dent 1993;6:315–317.

Patient Evaluation and Problem-Oriented Treatment Planning

William F. Rose, Jr
Carl W. Haveman
Richard D. Davis

Excellence in dental care is achieved through the dentist's ability to assess the patient, determine his or her needs, design an appropriate plan of treatment, and execute the plan with proficiency. Inadequately planned treatment, even when well executed, will result in less-than-ideal care. The process of identifying problems and designing the treatment for those problems is the essence of treatment planning and the focus of this chapter.

As an integral part of comprehensive dental care, treatment planning for the restoration of individual teeth must be done in concert with the diagnosis of problems and treatment planning for the entire masticatory system. The objective of this chapter is to present a problem-oriented approach to treatment planning for restorative dentistry. This approach begins with a comprehensive patient evaluation and gradually narrows its focus to the restoration of individual teeth. Emphasis is placed on the decision-making processes involved in identifying problems related to restorative dentistry; assessing the demands of the oral environment; and selecting the materials, operative modalities, and sequence best suited to the treatment of these problems.

The Problem-Oriented Treatment Planning Model

Treatment planning is generally accomplished with either a treatment-oriented model or a problem-oriented model. In the *treatment-oriented model*, the dentist examining the patient finds certain intraoral conditions and mentally equates those problems to the need for certain forms of treatment. The examination findings are summarized in the form of a list of needed treatments, which then becomes the treatment plan. The *problem-oriented model* requires that the examination lead to the formulation of a list of problems. Each problem on the list is then considered in terms of treatment options, each of which has different advantages and disadvantages. The optimal solution for each problem is then chosen, and, after sequencing, this list of solutions becomes the treatment plan.

For patients with only a few, uncomplicated problems, the outcomes are similar whether the treatment plan is problem based or treatment based. In more complex cases, problems are often interrelated, and the solution to one problem may affect the treatment needed to resolve other problems. In these instances, the process of identifying and listing the individual problems enables the dentist to think through each one and the various options for treating it without getting lost in the magnitude of the overall task.

The problem-oriented approach directs the dentist to perform a systematic evaluation of the patient, so that no problems are overlooked, either in diagnosis or in treatment planning. It is designed to prevent tunnel vision of obvious pathoses at the expense of less obvious but equally important problems.

The problem-oriented treatment planning process includes the following steps: a thorough evaluation of the patient's general health and the stomatognathic system; identification of the problems requiring treatment; and development of an integrated treatment plan. Armed with knowledge of all the problems, the clinician envisions the state of the dentition after the seriously compromised and nonrestorable teeth have been removed. Based on this vision of the remaining sound dentition, the dentist visualizes the optimal state to which the patient's dentition can be restored and maintained. Treatment needed to achieve this optimal result can then be documented. This process of retrograde planning, or planning in reverse, starting with the desired end result, often enables the clinician to identify previously unrecognized or unforeseen problems and add them to the problem list. The orthograde approach to treatment planning, which is based on identification of existing problems, can be combined and coordinated with a retrograde approach so that treatment of each problem on the problem list is consistent with the desired optimal treatment goal. A list of integrated treatment steps can then be generated.

Problem List Formulation

The dentist initially evaluates the patient from a subjective standpoint, ascertaining the chief complaint and the patient's goals of treatment. A medical history and a dental history are then elicited. The objective portion of the assessment consists of a categorical evaluation of the patient, beginning with vital signs and an extraoral head and neck examination and progressing through a thorough intraoral evaluation. The examination procedures are standardized and routinely completed in the same order and fashion to simplify the procedure and to ensure that crucial steps are not omitted. Related nonclinical portions of the evaluation include examinations of radiographs, diagnostic casts (usually mounted in an articulator), and photographs.

The objectives of the examination are to distinguish normal from abnormal findings and to determine which of the abnormal findings constitute problems that require treatment or will influence treatment. From the findings of the initial examination, a problem list is established. If the problems are listed under categorical headings (eg, periodontal problems, endodontic problems), the dentist is unlikely to omit problems. This list is dynamic and can be modified as new problems arise.

Problem-Oriented Planning

In the next phase of treatment planning, the dentist considers the various problems with which the patient presents and uses clinical judgment to estimate which teeth have a sufficiently favorable prognosis to justify being retained and which

teeth, if any, should be removed. Mental imaging is used to visualize the state of the dentition after the removal of nonsalvageable teeth. The dentist then formulates a mental image of the optimal condition to which the patient can be rehabilitated. This visualization requires the dentist to decide which teeth need to be replaced and which form of prosthodontic replacement and restorative treatment is most appropriate. Once this optimal condition has been visualized, a treatment solution is proposed for each problem on the problem list, with each individual solution planned to coincide with the final visualized optimal treatment objective.

If the treatment plan for any of the individual problems conflicts with the optimal treatment plan, either the treatment for the individual problem or the optimal treatment goal must be altered until they are coincident. When the clinician believes that, in consideration of all the problems and proposed treatments, the optimal treatment objective is feasible and maintainable, this list of individual treatments becomes the unsequenced treatment plan.

Treatment Sequencing

The final step in treatment planning, sequencing the treatment, is completed by arranging the solutions to the various problems in a set order (see box).

Chief complaint
Medical/systemic care
Emergency care
Treatment plan presentation
Disease control
Reevaluation
Definitive care
Maintenance care

The proposed treatment sequencing follows the logic of the medical model, so disease is treated in the priority of importance to the patient's overall health. This method of sequencing ignores the common technique of treating by specialty, where, for example, all the periodontal care is provided, followed by the endodontic care, which is followed by the restorative care.

Chief Complaint

The patient's *chief complaint* should be addressed at the outset of treatment, even if only via discussion, and even if definitive treatment of this problem will be deferred.

Medical/Systemic Care

The *medical/systemic care* phase includes aspects of treatment that affect the patient's systemic health. These take precedence over the treatment of dental problems and must be considered before dental problems are addressed. This most commonly includes medically related diagnostic tests and consultations. An example is the investigation of the status and control of a patient's hypertension or diabetes.

Emergency Care

Problems addressed in the *emergency care* phase include those involving head and neck pain or infection. They are treated before routine dental problems but after acute problems involving the patient's systemic health. Clinical judgment is exercised to determine the relative importance of systemic problems and dental emergency problems. A review of this topic is found in the text by Little and Falace.[1]

Treatment Plan Presentation

The *treatment plan presentation* (and patient acceptance of the treatment plan) should precede all nonemergency dental care. Presentation and discussion of the proposed treatment are the basis of informed consent and must not be overlooked. In addition to the primary or optimal treatment plan, the dentist should be prepared to present alternative plans that may be indicated based on extenuating circumstances, such as patient finances or the therapeutic response of teeth crucial to the success of the plan.

Disease Control

The *disease control* phase consists of treatment designed to arrest active disease. Examples include endodontic treatment to control infection; periodontal treatment to control inflammation; and restorative care, linked with behavior modification, to control caries. Treatment in this phase is aimed at the control of active disease, so that the disease processes would not progress even if no treatment beyond disease control were provided.

Reevaluation

The *reevaluation* phase consists of a formal reassessment, during which the dentist decides if all factors, including such criteria as the patient's treatment goals, oral hygiene, behavior modification, and response to periodontal therapy, warrant continuing with the original treatment plan. This is an important phase of treatment because it provides a predetermined point at which both patient and clinician may elect to alter or even discontinue treatment.

Definitive Care

The *definitive care* phase is the final phase of treatment preceding maintenance care. Many of the procedures accomplished within the disease-control phase, such as removal of carious tooth structure and placement of direct restorations, achieve both disease control and definitive restoration; however, a number of procedures that go beyond the treatment of active disease are possible. These include procedures designed to enhance function and esthetics, such as orthodontics, surgery, prosthodontics, and cosmetic restorative procedures. Treatment sequencing for most of these modalities is beyond the scope of this text; a detailed and comprehensive review is provided by Stefanac and Nesbit.[2]

Maintenance Care

Maintenance care is an ongoing phase designed to maintain the results of the previous treatment and prevent recurrence of disease. The maintenance phase generally focuses on the maintenance of periodontal health; the prevention, detection, and treatment of caries; and the prevention of dental attrition, erosion, and abrasion.

Dental History and Chief Complaint

The key to successful treatment planning lies in identifying the problems that are present and formulating a treatment plan that addresses each problem, so that each phase of treatment is designed to lead to the final, optimal treatment goal. The dentist who follows this approach begins by listening carefully to the patient and asking relevant questions. A thorough dental history serves as a guide for the clinical examination.

The dental history is divided into three components: chief complaint, dental treatment, and symptoms related to the stomatognathic system. The chief complaint is addressed first and is recorded in the dental record in the patient's own words. By discussing the patient's chief concern at the outset, the dentist accomplishes two important goals. First, the patient feels that his or her problems have been recognized, and the doctor-patient relationship begins positively; second, by writing out the chief complaint, the dentist ensures that it will not be omitted from the problem list. It is not uncommon to encounter a patient who has a multitude of significant dental problems but only a minor chief complaint. If the dentist focuses too quickly on the other problems and omits a discussion of the chief complaint, the patient may question the dentist's ability and desire to resolve the patient's chief concern.

A brief history of past dental treatment can provide useful information. The number and frequency of past dental visits reflect the patient's dental awareness and the priority he or she places on oral health. The dentist should elicit information about the past treatment of specific problems, as well as the patient's tolerance for dental treatment. All of this information can be of use in developing the treatment plan.

Questions about previous episodes of fractured or lost restorations, trauma, infection, sensitivity, and pain can elicit information that will alert the dentist to possible problems and guide him or her during the clinical and radiographic examination. Patients may not volunteer this information; hence, specific questions regarding thermal sensitivity, discomfort during chewing, gingival bleeding, and pain are warranted. When there is a history of symptoms indicative of pulpal damage or incomplete tooth fracture, specific diagnostic tests should be performed during the clinical examination.

Clinical Examination

For the purpose of restorative treatment planning, the intraoral assessment involves an examination of the periodontium, dentition, and occlusion. Specific diagnostic tests may be performed as indicated, and a radiographic examination is completed. The dentist should be sure to complete one portion of the evaluation before beginning another aspect of the examination. The findings from each area are placed under the appropriate heading in the problem list. Some problems may be noted in the evaluation of more than one system. For example, gingival bleeding and periodontal inflammation resulting from the impingement of a restoration on the periodontal attachment would be noted in both the periodontal examination and the evaluation of the existing restorations. At this stage, such duplication of effort is acceptable in the interest of completeness.

The following sections describe the elements of the intraoral examination used to establish the restorative dentistry problem list (see box).

Evaluation of the Dentition

Caries Risk and Plaque
An assessment of caries risk (see chapter 4) should be accomplished, and the presence of plaque should be documented with a standardized plaque index. The O'Leary index, for example, is a simple, effective measure of plaque accumulation.[3] The use of a standardized index permits an objective assessment of plaque accumulation. Depending upon initial

---

Elements of the Clinical Examination

I. Evaluation of the dentition
  - Assessment of caries risk and plaque
  - Caries lesion detection and assessment of disease activity
  - Assessment of the pulp
  - Evaluation of existing restorations
  - Evaluation of the occlusion and occlusal contours
  - Evaluation of axial tooth surfaces
  - Assessment of tooth integrity and fractures
  - Evaluation of esthetics

II. Evaluation of the periodontium
  - Assessment of disease activity
  - Evaluation of the structure and contour of bony support
  - Mucogingival evaluation
  - Assessment of tooth mobility

III. Evaluation of radiographs

IV. Evaluation of diagnostic casts (may include a diagnostic mounting in centric relation and use of a facebow)

---

findings, a dietary analysis and/or unstimulated salivary flow rate determination may be indicated. The determination of baseline caries risk and plaque levels at the time of initial examination provides a basis for communication with the patient and other clinicians and permits assessments of changes over time. This is important information in establishing a prognosis for restorative care and provides criteria for deciding whether treatment should progress beyond the disease-control phase into the definitive rehabilitation stage.

The levels and location of plaque should be established at the outset of the examination. At the conclusion of the examination appointment, the patient may be given a toothbrush and floss and asked to clean the teeth as well as possible. Reassessment immediately after the cleaning will establish the patient's hygiene ability and reveal the nature of hygiene instructions needed. A patient who sincerely tries to remove plaque but is unsuccessful in certain areas requires instruction in technique, whereas the patient who demonstrates effective hygiene while in the office but consistently presents with high plaque levels has a problem with motivation. This information is important in designing the treatment plan: a plan requiring a great deal of patient participation and compliance would not be appropriate for a patient with inadequate motivation, while a motivated patient who is teachable may well be suited to such a plan.

One of the most reliable indicators of future caries activity is the presence of an existing or recently treated caries lesion.[4] Three additional factors that heighten the risk of caries are: (1) a large number of cariogenic bacteria, (2) frequent ingestion of cariogenic sugars, and (3) a restricted flow of saliva.[5] Patients demonstrating active caries should receive an evaluation that entails more than simply a determination of levels and location of plaque.[6] Both a diet survey and a salivary flow assessment are useful in determining the patient's susceptibility to caries and the caries-related prognosis for restorative treatment.

Diet has been shown to be one of the most significant factors in caries risk. A review of more than 100 studies by van Palenstein Helderman et al[7] demonstrated that the frequency and duration of refined carbohydrate exposure is more predictive of caries occurrence than *Streptococcus mutans* counts. Using a diet survey, the patient itemizes all food and drink intake for a specified period (generally 1 week). From this diary, the dentist can identify the contribution of specific dietary habits to the patient's caries risk and can direct the patient's attention to these areas. The identification and management of episodic sugar and carbohydrate intake (snacking), as well as overall carbohydrate consumption, should be the focus of dietary intervention.[8,9]

Xerostomia, or dry mouth, is associated with increases in the number of cariogenic bacteria and increased caries activity.[10] Saliva provides lubrication; promotes oral clearance of fermentable carbohydrates, sugars, and acids; and possesses antimicrobial components and buffering agents.[10,11] Saliva is critical to tooth remineralization because it is a source of calcium, phosphates, and proline-rich proteins active in recrystalization of the tooth surface.[11] The patient's health status, medications, aging, and iatrogenic changes can alter salivary flow and composition and, thereby, caries risk status. Consideration should be given to assessing salivary flow rates in all caries-active patients. There is not complete agreement as to the minimum salivary flow rate necessary to maintain oral health. Some authorities suggest that less than 0.1 to 0.2 mL/min unstimulated flow is the criterion for hypofunction.[12,13] However, others correlate clinical symptoms of hypofunction, such as dysphasia, dysphagia, xerostomia, and a higher incidence of caries lesions and/or candidiasis with an unstimulated flow rate of less than 0.2 mL/min.[14,15]

Because the character of the microflora determines the cariogenicity of the plaque, periodic assessment of the number of cariogenic bacteria present in the plaque can indicate alterations in the caries susceptibility of patients at high risk of developing caries.[16] Although higher levels of *S mutans* (greater than 10^6 CFU/mL of saliva) are not consistently indicative of caries activity, estimates of the number of bacteria are more useful for predicting the absence, rather than the presence, of an active infection.[17] By monitoring the levels at baseline and over time, the dentist can assess the effectiveness of caries management measures.

Once plaque assessments have been completed, an examination of other areas can be accomplished. The visual examination of the dentition should be conducted in a dry field, with adequate lighting, using a mirror and explorer. Ideally, the dentist will employ some form of magnification to aid in the examination. A number of products providing 2 to 4 times magnification are commercially available. Some magnifying lenses attach to eyeglasses and can be removed, while others are built directly into the lenses of specially constructed eyeglasses (see Fig 6-68). The use of magnification, with adequate lighting significantly enhances the ability of the clinician to detect subtle signs of disease. If the presence of plaque and calculus partially obscures the dentition, debridement is required to accomplish a thorough examination.

Detection of Caries Lesions

The terms *carious lesion* and *caries lesion* are both acceptable to describe the effect of the caries process on a tooth, and both terms will be used interchangeably throughout this textbook.

Caries lesions may be classified by location into two broad categories: smooth-surface lesions (including those involving proximal surfaces, root surfaces, and lesions on other smooth surfaces) and pit and fissure caries lesions. Detection of caries lesions requires both clinical (visual and tactile) and radiographic examinations.

Pit and fissure caries lesions. Pit and fissure caries lesions are generally found in areas of incomplete enamel coalescence. These areas are most commonly found on the occlusal surfaces of posterior teeth, the lingual surfaces of maxillary anterior teeth and maxillary molars, and the buccal pits of molars. Because pit and fissure lesions may begin in small enamel defects that lie in close approximation to the dentinoenamel junction, they may be difficult to detect. A pit and fissure lesion must be fairly extensive to be detected radiographically; these lesions generally appear as crescent-shaped radiolucencies immediately subjacent to the enamel[18] (Figs 2-1a to 2-1c).

Historically, tactile examination with firm application of a sharp explorer into the fissure was the clinical technique most commonly used by dentists in the United States to locate pit and fissure lesions.[19] A sticky sensation on removal of the explorer has been the classic sign of pit and fissure caries. Clinical studies, however, have shown this method to be

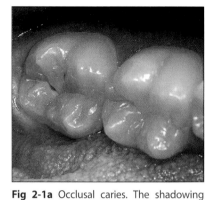

Fig 2-1a Occlusal caries. The shadowing around the stained pits in the second molar indicates the presence of carious dentin at the base of the fissure.

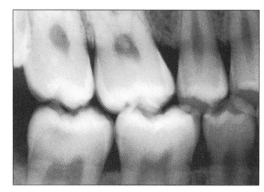

Fig 2-1b The caries lesion shown in Fig 2-1a extends well into dentin.

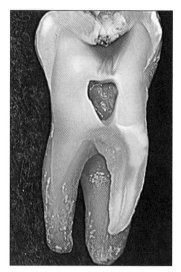

Fig 2-1c The typical pattern of an occlusal caries lesion in cross section.

unreliable, producing many false-positive and false-negative diagnoses.[20] In addition, an explorer can cause cavitation in a demineralized pit or fissure, precluding the possibility of re-mineralization.[20–23]

Visual observation, with magnification, of a clean, dry tooth has been found to be a reliable, nondestructive method of detecting pit and fissure caries lesions,[20–23] which appear as gray or gray-yellow opaque areas that show through the enamel (see Fig 2-1a). However, stain within a fissure is not indicative of carious dentin at the base of the fissure.

Fiber-optic transillumination may be helpful in visualizing pit and fissure and other types of caries lesions. A variety of new technologies are being evaluated for detection of caries lesions. A comprehensive discussion of these new technologies can be found in chapter 4.

When the presence of pit and fissure lesions is uncertain and the patient will be available for recall evaluations, a sealant may be placed over the suspect area. Clinical investigation by Mertz-Fairhurst et al[24] indicates that sealed caries lesions do not progress. However, placement of sealants in fissures over known carious dentin cannot be recommended at present, as the risk of sealant loss makes this an injudicious practice. Mertz-Fairhurst et al[24] found the placement of a conservative amalgam or resin composite restoration, followed by the placement of a resin fissure sealant over the margins of the restoration and remaining fissures, to be a predictable and relatively conservative treatment for such lesions.

Smooth-surface caries lesions. Of the three types of smooth-surface caries lesions, proximal lesions are the most difficult to detect clinically. Generally inaccessible to both visual and tactile examination, proximal caries lesions in posterior teeth are usually detected radiographically. Proximal lesions in anterior teeth may be detected radiographically or with visual examination using transillumination (Fig 2-2). Root caries lesions located on facial or lingual surfaces of the roots present few diagnostic problems. When root-surface lesions occur proximally, however, they are not readily visible on clinical examination and are generally detected through the radiographic examination (Fig 2-3). Smooth-surface caries lesions occurring on enamel in nonproximal areas are not difficult to detect clinically. These lesions, which are most commonly found in patients with high levels of plaque and a cariogenic diet or deficient salivary flow, occur on the facial and lingual enamel surfaces and are readily accessible during visual and tactile examination.

Dental Pulp

Evaluation of pulpal vitality in every tooth is not warranted; however, each tooth that will undergo extensive restoration, as well as all teeth that are critical to the plan of treatment and teeth with pulps of questionable vitality, should be tested.

The application of cold is a valuable method of vitality testing. Canned refrigerants present minimal risk to teeth and restorations. A cotton pellet saturated with an aerosol

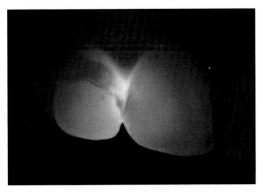

Fig 2-2 Proximal caries lesion is detected in an anterior tooth with the use of transillumination.

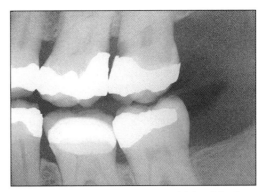

Fig 2-3 Root caries lesion that would be difficult to detect in a routine clinical examination is revealed in a radiograph.

refrigerant spray, such as tetrafluoroethane, is placed on the tooth to determine its vitality. A similar test can be performed by placing a "pencil of ice" (made by freezing water inside a sterilized anesthetic cartridge) against a tooth.

An additional vitality test involves the use of an electric pulp tester. While it can provide information regarding pulp vitality, this test has limitations; it cannot be used in a wet field or on teeth with metallic proximal surface restorations unless measures are taken to insulate adjacent teeth. Furthermore, the numeric scale of the instrument does not reflect the health of the pulp or its prognosis. The electric pulp tester is merely a means of determining whether the tissue within the pulp senses electrical current. A high score may be due to the presence of a partially necrotic pulp or extensive reparative dentin, or it may be the result of poor contact between the tooth and the pulp tester.

When the results of pulp tests are not congruent with the clinical impression, additional tests are indicated. When neither thermal nor electric pulp tests provide a clear picture of pulp vitality, and a restoration is indicated, the preparation can be initiated without the use of anesthetic. This is termed a *test cavity*. If pain or sensitivity is elicited when dentin is cut with a bur, pulpal vitality is confirmed. The restoration may then be completed after administration of local anesthetic.

Pulp vitality should be determined prior to restorative treatment. It is professionally embarrassing to discover that a recently restored tooth was nonvital prior to restoration and subsequently became symptomatic, requiring endodontic treatment and a replacement restoration.

It is advantageous to ascertain the pulpal prognosis of a tooth prior to restorative treatment. When pulpal prognosis is uncertain or guarded, it is often best to perform endodontic therapy before extensive restorative treatment. If the endodontic treatment is completed before restorative care, the

repair or replacement of a recently completed large restoration may be avoided.

Planning for endodontic treatment and presenting it as part of the original treatment plan is generally more acceptable to the patient than presenting this treatment option after treatment has begun. An added benefit is that the endodontic prognosis can be established before the dentist commits to restorative care.

When endodontic therapy is required, the feasibility of completing the endodontic procedures should be determined early in the course of treatment. The more critical the tooth is to the overall success of the treatment, the more important it becomes to complete the necessary endodontic treatment early in the treatment schedule. It is poor planning to rely on a tooth in the treatment plan when that tooth cannot be successfully treated with endodontics.

Endodontic diagnosis can be challenging. A thorough discussion of this subject can be found in the text by Cohen and Burns.[25]

When a posterior tooth has received endodontic treatment, placement of a complete–cuspal-coverage restoration is generally indicated to prevent fracture.[26] When an anterior tooth has received endodontic treatment, the least invasive form of restoration that satisfies the esthetic and functional needs of the patient is indicated.[27] If sufficient enamel and dentin remain for support, a bonded restoration, such as a resin composite or a ceramic veneer, is preferred. If there is insufficient support for such a restoration after removal of carious tooth structure or defective restorations or following endodontic access preparation, a ceramic or metal-ceramic crown is the restoration of choice. A post is indicated only when a crown is needed and there is insufficient tooth structure to provide support for the crown.[27] When a post is needed, preparation of a small post space preserves dentin and provides optimal fracture resistance for the tooth[28] (see chapter 20).

Existing Restorations

In the course of the intraoral examination, the serviceability of existing restorations must be evaluated. The following general criteria are used to evaluate existing restorations: (1) structural integrity, (2) marginal opening, (3) anatomic form, (4) restoration-related periodontal health, (5) occlusal and interproximal contacts, (6) caries lesions, and (7) esthetics.

Structural integrity. The structural integrity of a restoration should be evaluated to determine whether it is intact or whether portions of the restoration are partially or completely fractured or missing. The presence of a fracture line dictates replacement of the restoration. If voids are present, the dentist must exercise clinical judgment in determining whether their size and location will weaken the restoration and predispose it to further deterioration or recurrent carious involvement.

Marginal opening. Few restorations have perfect margins, and the point at which marginal opening dictates replacement of the restoration is difficult to determine. For amalgam restorations, it has been demonstrated that marginal ditching neither implies the presence nor necessarily portends the development of caries lesions[29]; therefore, its existence does not dictate the replacement of amalgam restorations. Because the margins of amalgam restorations become relatively well sealed by the accumulation of corrosion products, a general guideline has been to continue to observe the restoration unless signs of recurrent caries lesions are present. An accumulation of plaque in the marginal gap is also an indication for repair or replacement of an amalgam restoration. It has been suggested that noncarious marginal gaps in amalgam may be repaired with a resin sealant to enhance the longevity of the restoration.[30] The long-term clinical efficacy of this method has yet to be documented, but there is some in vitro evidence of its benefit.[31] A recent long-term, retrospective clinical study[32] indicated that the repair of local defects in amalgam restorations is an effective alternative to restoration replacement.

For restorations that do not seal by corrosion, a marginal gap into which the end of a sharp explorer may penetrate should be considered for repair, or the restoration should be replaced. This is especially true for resin composite restorations, because bacterial growth has been shown to progress more readily adjacent to resin composite than to amalgam or glass-ionomer materials.[33] An increased susceptibility to caries has been reported in resin composite restorations whose marginal gaps exceeded 100 to 150 µm (see Figs 2-6a and 2-6b).[34]

The presence of a marginal gap is less critical for restorations with anticariogenic properties (eg, glass-ionomer cement). Both in vitro[35–39] and in vivo[40–44] studies have shown that tooth structure adjacent to glass-ionomer restorations is less susceptible to caries attack than that adjacent to either resin composite or amalgam restorations. Consequently, restorations with anticariogenic properties generally should be replaced not because of marginal ditching but rather when a frank caries lesion has occurred or when some other defect indicates the need for treatment. In anterior teeth, replacement is indicated when the tooth structure adjacent to the marginal gap becomes carious or when marginal staining is esthetically unacceptable.

Anatomic form. Anatomic form refers to the degree to which the restoration duplicates the original contour of the intact tooth. Common problems include overcontouring, undercontouring, uneven marginal ridges, inadequate facial and lingual embrasures, and lack of occlusal or gingival embrasures. Many restorations exhibit one or more of these problems yet adequately serve the needs of the patient and do not require replacement. The critical factor in determining the need for replacement is not whether the contour is ideal but whether pathosis has resulted, or is likely to result, from the poor contour.

Restoration-related periodontal health. Examination of restorations must include an assessment of the effect that existing restorations have on the health of the adjacent periodontium. Problems commonly encountered in this area are (1) surface roughness of the restoration, (2) interproximal overhangs, and (3) impingement of the restoration margin on the zone of attachment, called the *biologic width* or the *dentogingival junction* (the area, approximately 2 mm in the apicocoronal dimension, occupied by the junctional epithelium and the connective tissue attachment) (see Fig 1-31).

All three of these phenomena can cause inflammation within the periodontium.[45–47] If restorative material extends vertically or horizontally beyond the cavosurface margin in the region of the periodontal attachment or impinges on the biologic width, the health of the periodontal tissue should be assessed (Fig 2-4). If other local etiologic factors have been removed and periodontal inflammation persists in the presence of these conditions, treatment should be initiated. In the case of overhanging restorations, pathosis may be eliminated and the restoration may be made serviceable simply by removing the overhang. If the periodontal inflammation fails to resolve, the restoration should be replaced. In the case of

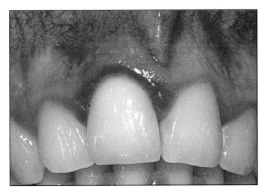

Fig 2-4 The periodontal inflammation is caused by the encroachment of the crown margins into the periodontal attachment area of the right maxillary central incisor.

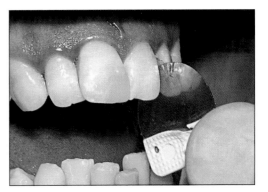

Fig 2-5 An interproximal contact–smoothing device is useful for removing irregularities that impede the passage of floss.

biologic width impingement, space for a healthy periodontal attachment must be gained through surgical crown lengthening or a combination of orthodontically forced eruption and surgical crown lengthening.

Inflammatory changes suggestive of biologic width violations are common on the facial aspects of anterior teeth that have been restored with crowns. On occasion, however, evaluation of the marginal areas reveals inflammation even when an adequate space remains between the crown margin and the periodontal attachment apparatus, leaving the clinician puzzled as to the cause of the problem. If periodontal inflammation persists in the apparent absence of local etiologic factors, including biologic width impingement, the dentist should evaluate the entire cervical circumference of the restoration. Inflammatory changes on the facial aspect of a restoration are sometimes a manifestation of interproximal inflammation. Further evaluation may reveal an interproximal violation of biologic width from which the inflammatory reaction has extended to the more visible facial areas.

Even in the absence of impingement on biologic width, open or rough subgingival margins can harbor sufficient bacterial plaque to generate an inflammatory response. Gingival inflammation around a crown may also be due to an allergic reaction to a material in the crown. Nickel alloy in a cast restoration often causes such reactions.

During the assessment of existing restorations or the planning of future restorations, the location of margins is an important consideration. Supragingival margins result in significantly less gingival inflammation than do subgingival margins.[48] Supragingival margins should be the goal when overriding concerns (eg, esthetics or requirements for resistance and retention) do not contraindicate their use.

Occlusal and interproximal contacts. The dentist should assess all interproximal contacts with thin dental floss. In addition, the patient should be queried regarding any problems encountered in the passing of floss through the contacts during home hygiene procedures. Contacts that do not allow the smooth passage of floss must be altered, or the restoration must be replaced, to permit the use of floss. The use of an interproximal contact–smoothing device is often effective in eliminating roughness that impedes the passage of floss (Fig 2-5).

Contacts that are open or excessively light should be evaluated to determine whether pathosis, food impaction, or annoyance to the patient has resulted. When any of these problems is present, steps should be taken to alleviate them. Generally, the placement or replacement of a restoration is required to establish an adequate proximal contact.

When an open contact is found, an attempt should be made to determine its cause. If occlusal contacts have moved a tooth and a restoration is to be placed to close the proximal contact, the occlusal contacts must be altered to prevent the open contact from recurring after the placement of the new restoration.

The occlusal contacts of all restorations should be evaluated to determine whether they are serving their masticatory function without creating a symptomatic or pathogenic occlusion. In the absence of periodontally pathogenic bacteria, traumatic occlusion has not been found to initiate loss of periodontal attachment.[49–51] However, in a susceptible host and in the presence of periodontal pathogens, occlusal trauma can play a role in the progression of periodontal disease.[52–54] Existing restorations located in teeth exhibiting significant attachment deficits should be examined closely for the presence of hyperocclusion. Restorations in which occlusal contacts are

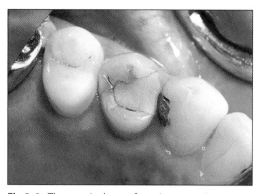

Fig 2-6a The marginal gap of a resin composite restoration is stained. Note the shadow indicating that caries has affected the dentin.

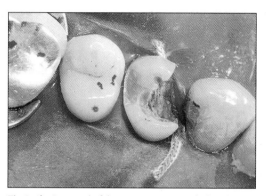

Fig 2-6b Removal of the restoration reveals that there is extensive carious dentin.

creating primary occlusal trauma should be altered or replaced, as necessary, to resolve the problem. Restorations that are in significant infraocclusion may permit the supraeruption of teeth and should be considered for replacement.

Recurrent caries lesions. The evaluation for carious tooth structure around existing restorations focuses on an examination of the margins. The dentist must use a combination of visual, tactile, and radiographic examinations to detect the presence of caries lesions. A radiolucent area surrounding a radiopaque restoration or the presence of soft tooth structure generally indicates a caries lesion and warrants either repair or replacement of the restoration.

Discoloration in the marginal areas is a sign that is more difficult to interpret. It often indicates leakage of some degree. In nonamalgam restorations without anticariogenic properties, discoloration that penetrates the margin often indicates the need for replacement of the restoration (Figs 2-6a and 2-6b). This is not a definite indication, however, and clinical judgment is required. In restorations with anticariogenic properties, leakage and stain may be observed with less concern for carious involvement, leaving esthetics as the primary consideration. This is not to imply that restorative materials with caries-resistant properties are immune to caries, however. Caries lesions have been documented adjacent to glass-ionomer restorations.[41,55] If the tooth structure adjacent to the margin of a restoration appears to be carious (either with undermined enamel or frank cavitation), rather than simply discolored, the restoration should be replaced.

For amalgam restorations, the decision to replace a restoration when there is discoloration in the adjacent tooth structure is less clear because corrosion products may discolor tooth structure, even in the absence of caries lesions, especially

when little dentin is present. When there is no apparent communication between the cavosurface margin and the stained area, and when the discoloration is primarily gray, then metal "show-through" should be suspected and observation is warranted (Fig 2-7). When the discolored area appears yellow or brown and appears to communicate with the cavosurface margin, replacement of the restoration is indicated (Fig 2-8).

Esthetics. The esthetic evaluation of existing restorations is highly subjective. When the functional aspects of a restoration are adequate, it is often best to simply inquire whether the patient is satisfied with the esthetic appearance of the existing restorations. If the patient expresses dissatisfaction with the appearance of a restoration, the dentist must determine whether improvement is feasible. Care should be taken to ascertain the reason that the original restoration had less-than-optimal esthetics. An underlying problem may preclude improvement of the original esthetic problem, and an equally unsatisfactory result may occur in the replacement restoration.

When replacing a restoration for esthetic reasons only, the dentist must carefully explain the risks (eg, endodontic complications) incurred in replacement.

Some of the more common esthetic problems found in existing restorations are *(1)* display of metal, *(2)* discoloration or poor shade match in tooth-colored restorations, *(3)* poor contour in tooth-colored restorations, and *(4)* poor periodontal tissue response in anterior restorations. (See chapter 3 for further discussion of esthetic problems.)

Occlusion, Occlusal Wear, and Erosion

The occlusion can have significant effects on the restorative treatment plan. The following factors should be evaluated in the course of the occlusal examination: *(1)* occlusal interfer-

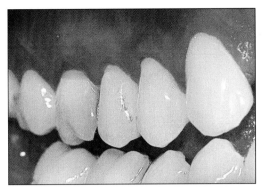

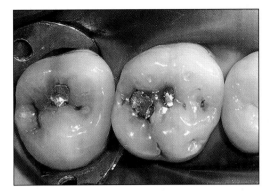

Fig 2-7 The shadow in the mesiofacial aspect of the maxillary first molar is caused by amalgam that shows through the translucent enamel. No caries lesion is present.

Fig 2-8 The shadow located on the mesiolingual cusp adjacent to the larger occlusal amalgam restoration on the maxillary right first molar indicates the presence of carious dentin.

ences between the occlusion of centric relation (CR) and that of maximum intercuspation (MI); *(2)* the number and position of occlusal contacts, as well as the stress placed on the occlusal contacts in MI; *(3)* the amount and pattern of attrition of teeth and restorations resulting from occlusal function and parafunction; and *(4)* the interarch space available for placement of needed restorations.

Occlusal interferences. Most people have some difference between the positions of CR and MI and have no consequent pathosis, indicating that the existence of a discrepancy between these positions is not, in itself, an indication for occlusal equilibration. Findings from the occlusal examination that should be recorded in the restorative dentistry problem list and do warrant treatment with occlusal adjustment are the following: *(1)* signs and symptoms of occlusal pathosis resulting from discrepancies between the occlusion of CR and MI (eg, mobility, excessive wear of teeth in the areas of interference between CR and MI, or periodontal ligament soreness); and *(2)* the need to restore the majority of the posterior occlusion.

This second factor does not imply the restoration of the majority of the posterior teeth but rather the restoration of the majority of the occlusal contacts. For example, insertion of a three-unit fixed partial denture in the mandibular right quadrant and several large restorations in the maxillary left quadrant results in the restoration of the majority of the occlusal contacts for the posterior teeth. There is no reason to fabricate the occlusion of the new restorations to duplicate the interferences that existed preoperatively. In such a case, occlusal equilibration should be completed prior to the restorative treatment. Through adjustment of only a very few occlusal contacts on teeth not involved in restorations

and subsequent fabrication of the new restorations in CR, the occlusions of CR and MI become coincident.

Occlusal contacts. The number and position of occlusal contacts in the MI position, the force of the occlusal load, and the manner in which opposing teeth occlude in excursive function strongly influence the selection of restorative materials, as well as the design of the preparation and restoration. As the number of missing teeth increases, so does the proportion of the occlusal load borne by each tooth. As occlusal stress increases, the dentist is forced to select the strongest of the available restorative materials and to design restorations that will provide the greatest strength in the areas of maximum stress. Likewise, the greater the potential for the patient to function on the restorations in lateral excursions, the greater the need for strength in the restorative material and the greater the imperative to select a material that will function without causing injury to the opposing dentition.

Wear. The clinician must be concerned with the abrasive potential that various restorative materials have on the opposing dentition. Wear (attrition and abrasion) is a progressive phenomenon characterized by the loss of anatomic tooth form. This process may result from physiologic or pathologic causes. Physiologic wear is generally considered a slow, progressive surface degradation of tooth form manifesting as a flattening of cusp tips of posterior teeth and incisal mamelons of anterior teeth.[56,57] When wear becomes excessive, it presents restorative difficulties. Excessive occlusal wear is caused primarily by occlusal parafunction. In these instances, facets on opposing teeth match well, indicating the predominant pattern of parafunctional activity. Because altering occlusal parafunctional habits is extremely difficult, prevention of

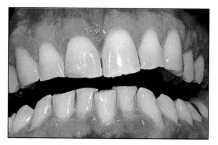

Fig 2-9a The significant occlusal attrition is caused by a habit of parafunctional grinding in a patient younger than 30 years of age.

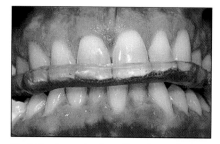

Fig 2-9b An occlusal acrylic resin appliance is used to minimize the abrasive trauma generated by the parafunctional grinding habit.

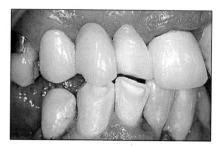

Fig 2-10 Extensive tooth structure has been lost in the mandibular teeth because of wear caused by the opposing porcelain fixed partial denture.

excessive occlusal wear is accomplished with the use of an occlusal resin appliance (Figs 2-9a and 2-9b). The dentist should identify patients who demonstrate signs of excessive occlusal wear (especially patients who exhibit these signs at an early age) and include occlusal appliance therapy in the treatment plan.

The restorative materials used in dentistry today have varying abrasive potential. No single variable is predictive of abrasivity; it is a function of a number of mechanical properties.[58] Hardness is a useful indicator, but the best predictor of wear is the relative clinical performance of the various materials. In clinical determinations of wear behavior, occlusal contact of enamel to amalgam causes only slightly greater wear to the amalgam than enamel-to-enamel contact causes to enamel. The amalgam causes less wear to the opposing dentition than does enamel.[59] The wear rate of resin composite depends on the nature of the resin composite. Microfilled resins exhibit wear behavior similar to that of enamel, while hybrid resins exhibit more wear and generate more wear to opposing enamel than does either amalgam or enamel.[60] Polished cast gold is more wear resistant than enamel or amalgam and generates minimal wear of opposing tooth structure.

Ceramic restorations have demonstrated a consistent ability to severely abrade the enamel of the opposing dentition[56,61] (Fig 2-10). Manufacturers have produced newer generations of dental ceramics called *low fusing ceramic materials*, claiming that they are less abrasive to the opposing natural dentition than the conventional porcelains. Several authors have supported this hypothesis[62–65]; however, just as many have contradicted it.[66–68] Some have even reported that the low fusing porcelains can result in significantly greater enamel wear than conventional porcelain.[67,69]

Minimizing wear of enamel by dental ceramics can best be accomplished by the following[70]:

1. Ensure anterior guidance that discludes posterior teeth in excursive movements.
2. Eliminate occlusal interferences.
3. Use gold alloys in functional bruxing areas.
4. If occlusion is on a ceramic surface, use small-particle veneering porcelains on the occluding surfaces.
5. Polish ceramic surfaces periodically.
6. Adjust occlusion periodically if needed.

Occasionally, the presence of abrasive substances in the mouth is the cause of excessive occlusal wear. When the vocation or lifestyle of a patient frequently places him or her in contact with airborne abrasives, prevention of wear is difficult. Education of the patient and use of an occlusal resin appliance will decrease the occlusal abrasion; however, decreasing the patient's exposure to the causative agent is the only reliable means of reducing the problem.

Erosion. Another form of tooth loss that often mimics wear is caused by chemical erosion. Erosion can result from habits such as sucking lemons or swishing carbonated beverages or from the introduction of gastric acid into the oral cavity, which can occur with repeated regurgitation. Gastroesophageal reflux disease, frequently referred to as GERD, occurs in the presence of an incompetent esophageal sphincter and is a common cause of acid-related erosion of the dentition. While the dentist may be the first to detect the signs of this condition, referral to a physician to manage the disease is in order.

Bulimia is another condition that may be detected by the dentist first. The frequent forced regurgitation associated with this disorder results in acidic dissolution of exposed tooth surfaces and can have devastating effects on the dentition.

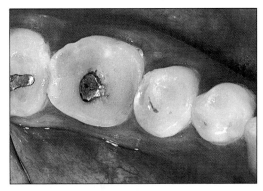

Fig 2-11a In the absence of facets that would indicate occlusal wear, significant loss of tooth structure is evidence of a chemical erosive process. Note both the amalgam restoration situated above the surrounding tooth structure and the smooth, glasslike character of the dentin. Also, note the cratering pattern of the buccal cusp tips of the premolars.

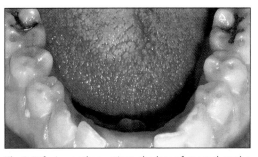

Fig 2-11b In another patient, the loss of enamel on the buccal surfaces of the posterior teeth is suggestive of soft drink swishing.

Chemical erosion can be distinguished from mechanical wear by the location and character of the defects. Erosive lesions have a smooth, glassy appearance. When found on the occlusal surfaces of posterior teeth, these lesions are characterized by concave defects into which abrasive agents are unlikely to penetrate. Severely "cupped out" cusp tips and teeth that have restorations standing above the surrounding tooth structure are clinical findings commonly associated with chemical erosion (Figs 2-11a and 2-11b).

Erosion lesions appearing primarily on the lingual surfaces of maxillary teeth and the occlusal surfaces of posterior teeth in both arches are characteristic of erosion caused by gastric acid. Smooth lesions on the facial surfaces might be of chemical or mechanical origin. In instances of uncertainty, questions related to habits may elucidate the cause of mechanical abrasion, while a thorough history and medical evaluation may reveal the presence of acid-related erosion. When bulimia is the underlying problem, detection is often difficult. The dentist must be tactfully candid in discussing this possible etiology. Regardless of the cause of the loss of tooth structure, the primary cause should be determined and resolved before rehabilitative therapy is undertaken. A thorough review of the loss of tooth structure from wear and erosion has been published by Verrett.[57]

Interarch space. When the dentist determines that significant loss of occlusal tooth structure has occurred and pulpal sensitivity has arisen, or that teeth have been so weakened by abrasion or erosion as to be at risk for fracture, restorative treatment is indicated. The dentist must evaluate the occlusion at MI and determine whether sufficient space exists for the placement of the restoration. If inadequate space is available, the dentist must either gain space for adequate tooth reduction and restoration resistance form by surgical crown lengthening, shorten the opposing tooth, or select a different restorative option that requires less bulk of material for resistance. Recognition of the space inadequacy prior to tooth preparation is essential.

In those cases in which generalized wear or erosion has resulted in the loss of an extensive amount of tooth structure, the dentist is faced with a significant restorative problem. In these instances, sufficient interarch space is often not available to restore the lost tooth structure without increasing the vertical dimension of occlusion, a complex restorative process involving more than a consideration of the mechanics of individual tooth restoration.

Axial Tooth Surfaces

Unlike changes in occlusal contours, the alteration of the axial contours of teeth is not due to tooth-to-tooth abrasion. Although it is generally due to erosion or toothbrush-related abrasion, occlusally generated stresses may contribute to this phenomenon in some instances. The term *abfraction* is applied to those noncarious lesions thought to have a combined cause of abrasion and occlusally induced tooth flexure.[71–74] Preventive treatment for cervical abrasion is directed at altering the habit or other factor(s) causing the problem. Modification of tooth brushing habits and the use of minimally abrasive toothpastes with a neutral pH can reduce the rate of erosion and abrasion. If abfraction is suspected, treatment should include the nighttime wear of an occlusal resin appliance.

Noncarious cervical lesions should be included on the problem list to alert the patient to the problem and to ensure that the dentist addresses the possible causes and considers restorative treatment options. In the absence of symptoms, the extent of the lesion should be assessed and restorative intervention should be a matter of clinical judgment. A prudent approach would be to restore the area when tooth loss has progressed to the point that the normal tooth contour could be replaced with restorative material without leaving the restorative material too thin to withstand functional and abrasive stresses. The reader is referred to a 2003 paper on diagnosis and treatment of noncarious cervical lesions[75] and to chapter 14 for a detailed discussion of etiology and treatment.

Tooth Integrity and Fractures

Tooth fractures are either complete or incomplete. A 2004 study[76] presented the risk indicators and incidence of complete cusp fractures in posterior teeth. The authors concluded that fewer than 10% of complete cusp fractures of posterior teeth occur in teeth without restorations and that the greatest risk indicator is the presence of a fracture line that is detectable through tactile examination. An extension[77] of this study looked at the frequency and location of cusp fractures in posterior teeth. Maxillary posterior teeth were found to fracture at approximately the same frequency as mandibular teeth. In the maxillary arch, premolars and molars fractured at about the same rates, with the first molar and first premolar fracturing slightly more often than the second molar and second premolar. In the mandibular arch, molars suffered fractured cusps much more frequently than premolars, with the first molar fracturing about twice as often as the second molar. Fractured cusps in mandibular premolars accounted for less than 1% of all tooth fractures. In both arches, the nonholding cusps (maxillary facial cusps and mandibular lingual cusps) tended to fracture more often than the holding cusps. This trait was more pronounced in the mandibular arch.[77]

Incomplete tooth fractures are most commonly called *cracked teeth*, but several terms have been used over the years.[78,79] *Cracked-tooth syndrome* is a fairly common result of the incomplete fracture of a vital tooth. Patients suffering from cracked-tooth syndrome present with a series of symptoms that include discomfort during chewing, unexplained sensitivity to cold, and pain on application or release of pressure.[80–85]

Cracked-tooth syndrome may be found in restored or unrestored teeth.[86] In restored teeth, it is often associated with existing small-to-medium-sized restorations.[87,88] One study of 51 patients concluded that teeth treated with Class 1 or 2 restorations have a 29 times greater risk for cracks.[84]

Incomplete fractures have been found to occur equally in both the maxillary and mandibular arches. In the maxillary arch, they have been reported to occur with similar frequencies in molars and premolars. In the mandibular arch, molars are the teeth most commonly found to be cracked.[89] Regardless of the location by arch, the cusps most commonly fractured are the nonholding cusps.[89] Often, patients with multiple cracked teeth have parafunctional habits or malocclusions that have contributed to the problem. Cracked-tooth syndrome is an age-related phenomenon; the greatest occurrence is found among patients between 33 and 50 years of age.[86] A recent etiology for an increase in the incidence of incomplete and complete fractures includes intraoral jewelry, especially in the tongue.[90]

Cracked-tooth syndrome is often difficult to diagnose. The patient is frequently unable to identify the offending tooth, and evaluation tools, such as radiographs, visual examination, percussion, and pulp tests, are typically nondiagnostic. The two most useful tests are transillumination and the "biting test."

Many teeth contain cracks and craze lines, most of which cause no symptoms; however, transillumination of a severely cracked tooth generally presents a distinctive appearance that permits the clinician to distinguish minor cracks from those deep enough to result in symptoms. When a tooth with a severe crack is transilluminated from either the facial or lingual direction, light transmission is interrupted at the point of the crack. This results in the portion of the tooth on the side away from the light appearing quite dark. The transition from bright illumination on one side of the tooth to darkness on the other is sudden rather than gradual, occurring abruptly at the point of the fracture.

The biting test is the most definitive means of localizing the crack responsible for the patient's pain. By having the patient bite a wooden stick, rubber wheel, or one of the commercially available instruments designed for that purpose (eg, Tooth Slooth, Professional Results), the dentist is generally able to reproduce the patient's symptom and identify not only the cracked tooth but also the specific portion of the tooth that is cracked. Crunchy food, placed sequentially on suspect teeth, has also been suggested as a diagnostic aid.[91] Once the offending tooth has been identified, tooth preparation often allows visualization of the crack (Fig 2-12; see also Fig 1-8).

Where direct diagnostic methods prove unsuccessful, indirect methods may be used. Orthodontic bands may be placed on suspected teeth to prevent separation of the crack during function. If the patient's symptoms subside, the diagnosis of cracked-tooth syndrome has been made.

In the treatment of incomplete tooth fracture, the tooth sections are splinted together with a complete-cuspal-coverage restoration.[83,87] Although a full-veneer crown is the treatment of choice, cuspal coverage and protection may also be accomplished with the use of an amalgam restoration[92] or an indirectly fabricated onlay of metal, ceramic, or resin composite. Because of their potential to lose bond integrity over time, bonded intracoronal restorations presently are not considered to be adequate for long-term resolution of the problem.[83,93,94]

While the diagnoses of incomplete tooth fractures has historically been symptom based, the dental operating microscope with its high magnification capability allows the dentist a new level of increased diagnostic sensitivity. An excellent review on the use of the surgical optical microscope in the diagnosis of early enamel and dentin cracks is available.[95]

Esthetic Evaluation

In addition to an esthetic evaluation of existing restorations, an assessment of the esthetics of the entire dentition should be completed. Because dental esthetics is a subjective area, patients should be questioned about any dissatisfaction they may have regarding the esthetics of their dentition. In the absence of complaints by the patient, the dentist's impressions regarding esthetic problems should be tactfully conveyed to determine whether the patient would like the esthetic problems addressed. The dentist, who has studied dental esthetics, is often better able than the patient to determine how dental procedures might enhance the patient's appearance. If an agreement is reached between the patient and dentist as to the existence of specific esthetic problems, the problems should be included on the restorative dentistry problem list.

Commonly encountered esthetic problems that are related to or may be addressed by restorative dentistry include: (1) stained or discolored anterior teeth; (2) unesthetic contours in anterior teeth (eg, unesthetic length, width, incisal edge shape, or axial contours); (3) unesthetic position or spacing of anterior teeth; (4) caries lesions and unesthetic restorations; (5) excessive areas of dark space in the buccal corridors due to a constricted arch form; and (6) unesthetic color and/or contour of tissue adjacent to anterior restorations. This last problem includes excessive gingival display, occasionally referred to as the "gummy smile." (See chapter 3 for a thorough discussion of esthetic considerations in diagnosis and treatment planning.)

The restorative treatment of esthetic problems may range from conservative therapy, such as bleaching, to more invasive measures, such as the placement of resin or ceramic veneers and posterior restorations or complete-coverage crowns. Additionally, adjunctive periodontal, endodontic, or

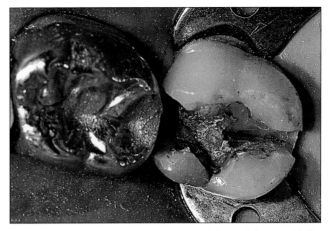

Fig 2-12 The mesiodistal crack in the pulpal floor of the mandibular right second molar caused sharp pain upon chewing. The tooth is to be restored with an onlay to splint the tooth together during function, relieve the patient's symptoms, and prevent propagation of the crack.

orthodontic procedures may be helpful, depending on the nature of the original problem. Esthetic restorations are discussed in subsequent chapters.

Evaluation of the Periodontium

From a restorative dentistry perspective, the periodontium must be evaluated primarily for two reasons: (1) to determine the effect that the periodontal health of the teeth will have on the restorative dentistry treatment plan, and (2) to determine the effect that planned and existing restorations will have on the health of the periodontium.

Evaluation of the periodontium consists of a clinical assessment of attachment levels, bony topography, and tooth mobility; a qualitative assessment of tissue health; and a radiographic evaluation of the supporting bone. The assessment of attachment levels involves periodontal probing of the entire dentition with both a straight probe for determination of vertical probing depths and a curved probe to explore root concavities and furcation areas. Any bleeding induced by gentle probing should be noted. A variety of tests are available to aid in determining the presence and identity of periodontal pathogens; however, the most consistent clinical indicator of inflammation is bleeding on probing.[96] Bleeding on probing does not always indicate the presence of active periodontal disease, but active disease has been consistently found to be absent when there is no bleeding on probing.[96]

The qualitative assessment of periodontal tissue health calls for a subjective assessment of the inflammatory status of the tissue; tissue color, texture, contours, edema, and sulcular

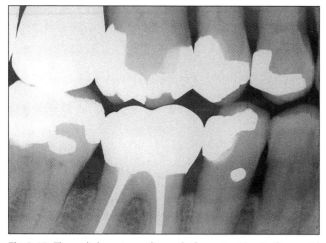

Fig 2-13 The radiolucent area beneath the restoration in the mesial surface of the maxillary first molar is radiographic burnout. No carious tooth structure is present.

exudates are noted. The presence of specific local factors, such as plaque and calculus, and their relationship to tissue inflammation should be noted. Abnormal mucogingival architecture, such as gingival dehiscences and areas of minimal attached gingiva, should be recorded. This is especially true when these anomalies are noted in the proximity of existing or planned restorations.

During examination of the periodontium, the dentist must not only be cognizant of periodontal inflammation adjacent to existing restorations but also estimate the location of margins for future restorations and their potential for impinging on the biologic width. Review of radiographs, especially correctly angulated bite-wing radiographs, during the periodontal examination enables the dentist to assess the relationship of existing and planned restorations to bone levels and to correlate radiographic signs with clinical findings.

When the clinical and radiographic portions of the periodontal examination have been completed, a periodontal prognosis should be established for all teeth; special attention should be given to teeth involved in the restorative dentistry treatment plan. Teeth requiring restorative treatment that have a guarded periodontal prognosis should be noted in the restorative dentistry problem list. Until the periodontal prognosis becomes predictably positive, the restorative treatment of teeth with a guarded prognosis should be as minimal as possible, and treatment planning that relies on these teeth must remain flexible.

Evaluation of Radiographs

The radiographic examination is an essential component of the comprehensive evaluation. Problems detected during the

evaluation of radiographs are listed under the appropriate headings on the problem list (eg, restorative, endodontic, periodontal).

Although radiographs can provide valuable information for use in diagnosis and treatment planning, exposure of patients to ionizing radiation must be minimized; therefore, discretion is required when the dentist orders radiographs. There are no inflexible rules for radiographic evaluation; rather, clinical judgment should be exercised. The goal is to minimize unnecessary exposure and cost but to avoid underutilization, which could result in inadequate diagnosis. The use of patient-specific criteria is the key. Different patients have different requirements both in terms of the radiographic views needed and the frequency with which radiographs should be repeated.

A reasonable guideline to follow is that all dentate patients should initially have a radiographic series completed that reveals the periapical areas of the entire dentition. This will permit detection of central lesions not visible on bite-wing radiographs and will serve as a baseline, allowing the clinician to assess changes over time. Although it is not common to discover pathoses by using panoramic films or complete-mouth radiograph series, it has been reported that approximately 85% of central jaw lesions are apparent in views of the apical areas of the dentition but are not visible on bite-wing radiographs.[97] For patients with periodontal disease, periapical radiographs are indicated. For patients with no significant periodontal pathoses, a panoramic radiograph provides the necessary view. For all patients with approximating teeth, a series of films is indicated to show the proximal areas of posterior teeth. Bite-wing radiographs serve this purpose.

The frequency with which radiographs should be updated is a matter of clinical judgment. The dentist should assess the etiologic factors present and determine whether new disease is likely to have occurred since the last radiographic examination. The dentist must weigh the risk of undetected disease against the cumulative risk of radiation exposure. A suggested guideline is to make new bite-wing radiographs of caries-active adults on an annual basis and of caries-inactive adults every 2 to 3 years.[98] Patients may be considered minimally susceptible to caries if they have had no caries lesions in recent years, demonstrate low plaque levels, have adequate salivary flow, have a noncariogenic diet, and exhibit no clinically discernible caries lesions. Periapical radiographs of the entire dentition should be repeated only as dictated by the specific needs of the treatment to be accomplished. For example, a patient under active treatment or maintenance for periodontal disease may require an updated radiographic series every 2 to 3 years to reevaluate bony contours, while another patient whose disease processes are controlled may require subsequent periapical radiographic updates only every 4 to 5 years.

In evaluating radiographic findings for restorative purposes, the dentist should note open interproximal contacts, marginal openings, overhanging restorations, periapical radiolucencies and radiopacities, and radiolucencies within the body of the tooth. The dentist must interpret "abnormal" radiographic findings with caution. Many phenomena that are detectable radiographically can also be detected clinically and should be verified clinically before treatment is planned. This is especially true when the clinician evaluates radiolucencies that appear to represent carious tooth structure but may in fact represent nonpathologic structures. An example of this is the radiographic phenomenon commonly known as "burnout" (Fig 2-13). Burnout is a radiolucency that is not caused by demineralization but instead occurs when the x-ray beam traverses a portion of the tooth with less thickness than the surrounding areas. It is most commonly found near the cervical area of a tooth and may be caused by concavities in the tooth or the angulation of the beam, but it is also related to the portion of the tooth not covered with enamel or by alveolar bone.

The dentist must be careful not to mistakenly diagnose as demineralized tooth structure a decrease in radiopacity resulting from an abraded area. Likewise, the dentist must be cautious in diagnosing carious tooth structures beneath existing restorations, because certain radiolucent dental materials have a radiographic appearance similar to that of demineralized tooth structure. A comprehensive review of dental radiology has been provided by Goaz and White.[99]

Evaluation of Diagnostic Casts

The dentist can gain valuable information through an evaluation of diagnostic casts. By examining diagnostic casts of the dentition, the dentist can see areas that are visually inaccessible during the clinical examination. Facets and marginal openings that may be difficult to discern intraorally are readily visible on the diagnostic casts. Facets on the casts of the dentition can be aligned to provide a guide to dynamic occlusal relationships. In addition, the dentist may use gypsum casts to complete diagnostic preparations and diagnostic waxups, simulating planned treatment. Where removable partial dentures are indicated, survey and design procedures may be completed on the diagnostic casts before restorative treatment is planned. The requirements of removable partial denture design may thus be considered during the planning of restorative care.

Although not every case requires the evaluation of casts mounted on a semiadjustable articulator, cases involving multiple missing teeth or the restoration of a significant portion of the occlusion should be evaluated with diagnostic casts mounted in CR. If multiple teeth are missing, the articulator maintains the correct interarch relationship, permitting buccal and lingual views of interarch spaces. Using a semiadjustable articulator that provides a reasonable approximation of the patient's intercondylar distance, condylar inclination, lateral guidance, and hinge axis of rotation, the dentist can simulate the patient's mandibular movements. This enables the clinician to assess the occlusal scheme and to plan restorative care accordingly.

Treatment Plan

Having completed a comprehensive examination, the dentist documents problems related to restorative dentistry on the restorative dentistry problem list (Fig 2-14). Each problem on the list is then reevaluated. After consideration, some of the problems may be deleted. For example, a tooth with a defective restoration may also have a significant loss of periodontal attachment and, therefore, a poor periodontal prognosis. In such a case, the defective restoration is initially considered a problem, but, in view of the periodontal condition, the tooth would be planned for extraction rather than restoration. The defective restoration is then omitted from the restorative problem list. Sometimes the treatment planned to address a problem may lead to additional problems. For example, reducing an extruded tooth to the level of the occlusal plane may result in the need for elective endodontic treatment, surgical crown lengthening, and a full-coverage restoration.

Once the final problem list is formulated, the next step is to establish a plan for the treatment of each problem on the list. The treatment planned for each problem should be based on current research evidence to the extent possible.[100] Caries should be treated as a disease using a medical model,[101,102] and interventions to stop demineralization and bring about remineralization should be planned for early caries lesions.[102–104] (See chapter 4 for an in-depth review of current strategies for caries management.) A problem list worksheet (Fig 2-15) is a useful tool to help organize the planning of treatment for each problem. It consists of an unsequenced list of problems and their associated solutions. Later, during the sequencing process, this list of treatments will be integrated into the comprehensive treatment plan.

Planning the restoration of individual teeth is the "nuts and bolts" of restorative dentistry treatment planning. It requires the consideration of four primary factors as well as a number of modifying factors. The primary considerations are: *(1)* the amount and form of the remaining tooth structure; *(2)*

PATIENT: Blank, Felina D.

PROBLEM LIST

Chief complaint: "My tooth hurts every time I chew, and lately iced tea has made it hurt, too."

Medical/systemic: Hypertension. Present blood pressure: 155/95.

Restorative (also see charting):

- Incomplete tooth fracture of mesiolingual cusp, #19
- Caries lesions, #20, #21, #28 (high caries risk)
- Defective restorations, #2, #12
- Facial, noncarious cervical lesion, #12
- Worn incisal edges, #6 to #11
- Fluorosis stain, #8
- Biologic width impingement, #3, distal
- Patient wishes to whiten maxillary anterior teeth

Periodontal:

- AAP Case Type I (see periodontal charting form)
- Generalized marginal gingivitis
- Generalized minimal bone loss with 3- to 4-mm pockets
- Vertical defect, #3, distolingual (5 mm)
- Biologic width problem, #3, distal
- Plaque and calculus: Generalized interproximal plaque in all posterior sextants (Modified O'Leary index: 50% plaque free), subgingival calculus revealed on bite-wing radiographs of #19 and #30; supragingival calculus present on lingual surfaces of mandibular anterior teeth

Endodontic: None

Prosthodontic: Missing, #29

Orthodontic: None

Occlusion: Supraeruption, #4; excessive wear, #6 to #11

Temporomandibular dysfunction: None

Oral surgery: None

Fig 2-14 Example of a problem list.

PATIENT: Blank, Felina D.

PROBLEM LIST WORKSHEET

Problem	Treatment
Chief complaint: cracked #19	• Gold onlay
Hypertension	• Referral to physician for evaluation and treatment
Caries	• Educate patient: snacking, hygiene techniques, home fluoride use • Rx: neutral sodium fluoride (1.1%) gel or dentifrice • If caries continues, complete caries risk assessment (diet survey, *mutans* culture) • #20, #21: Class 5 resin-modified glass-ionomer restorations
Defective restorations	• #2: MOD amalgam • #4: Porcelain-fused-to-metal (PFM) crown (shorten to level occlusal plane) • #12: MO resin composite
Abrasion: #12	• Class 5 resin composite restoration
Wear: #6 to #11	• Protective acrylic resin occlusal splint
Fluorosis: #8	• Microabrasion
Biologic width: #3	• Surgical crown lengthening
Patient desires to lighten maxillary anterior teeth	• Home bleaching #5 to #12
Periodontal inflammation associated with local factors	• Patient education and hygiene instruction; goal: 90% plaque-free index • Prophylaxis; scaling/root planing in mandibular sextants and any areas not responding to initial care • Reevaluate; goal: eliminate bleeding on probing • Surgical crown lengthening #3: osseous recontouring and soft tissue excision
Missing: #29	• Fixed partial denture (FPD) #28 to #30; PFM retainer #28, 3/4 retainer #30
Supraeruption: #4	• Shorten #4 when PFM crown is completed

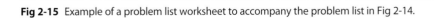

Fig 2-15 Example of a problem list worksheet to accompany the problem list in Fig 2-14.

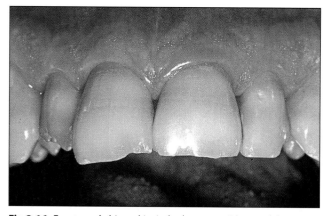

Fig 2-16 Facets and chipped incisal edges are evidence of the severe stresses placed on these anterior teeth by parafunction. Although they demonstrate tetracycline staining and possess a largely intact facial surface, these teeth would be poor candidates for veneer restorations. Complete-coverage restorations are indicated if the patient wishes to mask the tetracycline staining.

the functional needs of each tooth; (3) the esthetic needs of each tooth; and (4) the final objective of the overall treatment plan.

Remaining Tooth Structure

The quantity and location of remaining tooth structure determine the resistance features available for the restoration and thus greatly influence the restorative design. These factors determine not only the resistance to displacement of the restoration, but also the fracture resistance of the remaining tooth structure. The clinician should select the restoration that provides the best retention of the restoration and the optimal protection of the remaining tooth structure, using the least invasive design possible.

For the restoration of posterior teeth, an intracoronal restoration with amalgam or resin composite is generally the most conservative choice, and both materials have proven to be clinically successful. When the width of the intracoronal preparation of a posterior tooth exceeds one third of the intercuspal width, the tooth becomes significantly more susceptible to cuspal fracture and the concern becomes not only restoration failure but also tooth fracture.[105]

Even more significant to the fracture resistance of the tooth than restoration width is the depth of the preparation.[106] In instances of deep and/or wide preparations, the clinician must assess the need for occlusal coverage to protect the fracture-prone portions of the tooth. Often the assessment of remaining tooth structure and integrity can be accomplished only after removing the existing restoration and any defective tooth structure. For occlusal coverage, choices

include cuspal-coverage amalgam, partial veneer restorations (eg, onlays, three-quarter crowns, or seven-eighths crowns), and complete crowns. The clinician should resist the temptation to progress immediately to a complete crown and instead should select the most conservative choice that satisfies the needs of the individual tooth and the overall treatment plan.

The quantity of remaining tooth structure has an equally important effect on the choice of restorations for anterior teeth. For conservative interproximal restorations in anterior teeth, resin composite is almost always indicated because sufficient tooth structure is generally available for effective resin-enamel and resin-dentin bonding. When extensive facial tooth structure has been esthetically compromised but the facial enamel and the majority of the lingual aspect of the tooth remain intact, a ceramic veneer affords a conservative alternative to a complete crown. The veneer satisfies the esthetic requirement but is considerably less invasive than complete coronal coverage. When the facial enamel has been destroyed, significant lingual tooth structure has been lost, occlusal stress is exceptionally heavy, or there is very darkly pigmented dentin, veneers are not a viable option and complete crowns are required (Fig 2-16).

Functional Needs

The choice of restorative materials and the design of restorations must accommodate the functional needs of the individual patient. This precludes the use of a cookbook approach to treatment planning and requires that the clinician assess the circumstances peculiar to each tooth before planning restorative procedures. The functional and parafunctional stresses of the occlusion are significant considerations in this decision process. For example, a patient with average-strength musculature, an anterior-guided disclusion of posterior teeth in excursions, and minimal tendency toward parafunction may require only an intracoronal amalgam or resin composite restoration to restore mesial and distal surfaces of a posterior tooth. In a similar circumstance, a patient with heavy musculature, signs of parafunctional activity, and no anterior-guided disclusion may require a cast-metal restoration that covers the entire occlusal surface to minimize the chances of tooth fracture.

A useful guide in making decisions about material selection and restoration design is the evidence of functional demand provided by the existing dentition. Patients who present with a dentition exhibiting minimal destruction are good candidates for conservative, directly placed restorations. Patients whose teeth exhibit severe wear facets or considerable loss of tooth structure from occlusal attrition are best served by materials high in strength and wear resistance, such as cast-metal restorations.

Restorations placed due to noncarious cervical lesions pose little dilemma in terms of restorative choices. Any of the restorative materials suited to the restoration of Class 5 areas will serve satisfactorily. Glass-ionomer restorative materials have proven to be effective in the restoration of Class 5 areas, providing longevity in excess of 10 years.[107] Resin-modified glass-ionomer restorative materials provide an alternative to conventional glass-ionomer cements and have been shown to demonstrate exceptional retention. One study[108] found a retention rate of 98% after 3 years and a second, independent study[109] found 100% retention after 5 years. Improvements in the performance of resin adhesives have made the retention of resin composites and polyacid-modified resin composite restorations predictable as well. A number of investigators have reported retention rates for resin composite restorations of over 95% after 3 years.[110,111] The glass-ionomer materials offer the anticariogenic advantage of fluoride release, while the materials containing greater amounts of resin composite generally provide better esthetics and wear resistance.

The patient's level of caries activity will influence the selection of restorative materials. Patients whose caries risk assessment indicates a high potential for caries are good candidates for treatment with anticariogenic restorative materials, as well as the use of a caries management protocol.[112] Conventional glass-ionomer cements have been found through clinical study to provide an anticariogenic effect.[40–44] Resin-modified glass-ionomer materials have been found to inhibit simulated caries in vitro[35–39] and have been shown to possess anticariogenic properties in the clinical environment.[41,112] None of the anticariogenic restorative materials presently available is able to withstand the stresses of occlusal function.

Esthetic Needs

Establishing the patient's esthetic priorities is essential in planning restorative care. In most instances, the dentist will have the choice of a tooth-colored or a non–tooth-colored restoration for a given situation. Because non–tooth-colored materials (ie, metals) are generally superior in strength and durability, they are the materials of choice when strength and wear resistance are the overriding considerations. With the patient's input, the clinician must decide which requirement is more important, durability or esthetics.

For intracoronal, directly placed restorations in the anterior area of the mouth, resin composites are the obvious choice. They can be made to match most teeth in color and have been shown to provide an average service life of 43.5 to 72 months.[113,114] In stress-bearing areas in the posterior aspect of the mouth, amalgam is the material of choice for direct intracoronal restorations. Although resin composites have been steadily improving in terms of physical properties and have good wear resistance, clinical research indicates that they have not quite matched the success of amalgam for use in posterior teeth.[115,116] In the posterior area of the mouth, on those occasions when esthetic concerns take priority and when occlusal stresses are minimal to moderate, resin composite is the restorative material of choice.

As with large amalgam restorations, large resin composite restorations do not fare as well in clinical studies as do more conservative restorations.[117,118] Where full or partial occlusal coverage is required, amalgam has been found to yield favorable results, routinely providing service in excess of 10 years[119,120] (Fig 2-17); cast-metal restorations offer even greater longevity and should receive special consideration for patients with parafunctional habits (see chapter 19).[121,122] When occlusal coverage is required in an area of esthetic concern, the clinician may choose between an all-ceramic and a metal-ceramic restoration. All-ceramic restorations generally provide a superior esthetic result, while the metal substructure of metal-ceramic restorations offers tremendous strength. However, recent improvements in the fabrication techniques of high-alumina ceramics have produced high-purity alumina copings that have the potential to replace the metal copings for the metal-ceramic crowns.[123] These copings are made through a slip-cast technique (In-Ceram Alumina [Vident]) or a computer-aided milling process (Procera AllCeram [Nobel Biocare]).[123] These crowns have demonstrated flexural strengths four to six times greater than conventional feldspathic and pressed porcelain systems.[124] The strongest of the ceramic cores is zirconia, which has a strength that approaches seven times that of conventional porcelains.[58] Unfortunately, as the strength of the core ceramic increases, the esthetic value decreases. A moderate-strength ceramic core, IPS Empress 2 (Ivoclar Vivadent), has good esthetics with or without veneering porcelains and is also twice as strong as the traditional porcelains and about one half as strong as the zirconia.[58,124] Giordano[124] reports a success rate of about 97% for Procera from 2-year data in the United States and 5-year data from Europe and a 98% success rate for In-Ceram from 7-year data with anterior and posterior crowns. A recent study[125] found 56 of 58 all-ceramic restorations created with computer-aided design/computer-assisted manufacture (CAD-CAM) were clinically successful at the 3-year recall. Other studies evaluating crown survival and clinical success provide favorable data for these stronger ceramic systems.[125–129] Successful restorations depend on the choice of system that fits the clinical situation, proper preparation of the tooth, the careful laboratory fabrication of the restoration, and careful insertion technique.[130,131] Even though there has been marked

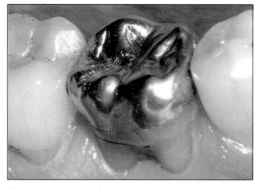

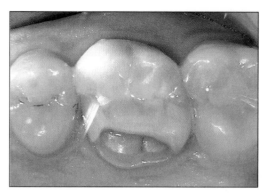

Fig 2-17 Example of a large cuspal-coverage amalgam restoration. This restoration is 6 years old.

Fig 2-18 Example of a catastrophic failure of an all-ceramic crown. The crown is 5 years old. The failure is probably due to inadequate tooth preparation of the palatal cusp and excessive occlusal forces. The thin porcelain is visible at the mesial aspect of the fracture.

improvement in the strength of all-ceramic restorations, they are still subject to fracture (Fig 2-18). At this time, patients exhibiting signs of high occlusal stress are better served with metal-ceramic or gold alloy restorations.

Intracoronal ceramic restorations have proven quite successful, with one clinical study finding a 93% success rate over a 6-year time span for leucite-reinforced pressed ceramic inlays (IPS Empress, Ivoclar Vivadent).[132] A study involving 232 inlays made from either a heat-pressed ceramic (Dicor, Dentsply), a leucite-reinforced ceramic material (IPS Empress), or a conventional feldspathic porcelain found a 98% success rate over an average of 28 months.[133] Although clinical studies have found relatively little difference in survival between the stronger and the weaker ceramics when they are used as intracoronal restorations, the same is not true in occlusal coverage situations. Secondarily polymerized resin composites have been found to provide excellent performance in intracoronal applications but have not yet proven to be of sufficient durability to serve in occlusal coverage restorations where occlusal stress is a significant factor (see chapter 18).[134,135]

All-ceramic materials and fiber-reinforced resin materials have been marketed for use in the fabrication of fixed partial dentures. One recent clinical study reported a 93% success rate from 30 posterior lithia disilicate–based core ceramic fixed partial dentures after 2 years.[136] In a retrospective study of In-Ceram Alumina–core fixed partial dentures, Olsson et al[137] found successful results for anterior fixed partial dentures and promising success rates for alumina-core posterior fixed partial dentures. Another study demonstrated a 90% success rate with In-Ceram Alumina posterior fixed partial dentures.[138] Another promising technology is the computer-aided milling

of single, large zirconia blanks for the cores of three-unit posterior prostheses. Although promising results are beginning to appear, more long-term clinical data is required to support the use of all-ceramic core materials as an alternative to metal or metal-ceramic for posterior fixed partial dentures. With regard to the single missing tooth, osseointegrated dental implants are replacing the traditional fixed partial denture as the treatment of choice in appropriate clinical situations.

Final Treatment Objective

The anticipated ultimate outcome of restorative and prosthodontic rehabilitation is the final factor to consider when the design of a restoration is planned and the restorative material is selected. Teeth that may require one type of restoration to restore health and function may require a different treatment to meet the needs of the final treatment plan. For example, if implant treatment is planned or if no prosthodontic replacement is planned for teeth that are missing, the teeth adjacent to the edentulous area may require only conservative restorative care for the treatment of small caries lesions. In a different treatment plan that calls for replacement of the missing teeth with a removable partial denture, surveyed indirect restorations may be required for the teeth adjacent to the edentulous area. In a third variation of the same case, missing teeth may be replaced with a fixed partial denture and the teeth in question may be needed as fixed partial denture abutments.

When the final treatment objective has been visualized, it is often possible to identify certain teeth as key teeth, the retention and restoration of which are crucial to the success of the treatment plan. These teeth are often potential prosthodontic abutments and/or canine teeth. Because the success of the total treatment plan often hinges on these teeth, it is crucial to ascertain their periodontal and endodontic prognosis and to plan the restorative treatment that provides the best long-term prognosis. This may dictate an aggressive restorative design to achieve the most predictable success for these key teeth.

The following example serves to illustrate this principle. A hypothetical patient has a freestanding second molar that contains a defective mesio-occlusodistal (MOD) amalgam restoration. Although the facial wall location slightly undermines the facial cusp, a replacement amalgam restoration appears likely to function adequately. In the comprehensive treatment plan, the tooth will serve as a distal abutment for a removable partial denture. With mere replacement of the defective amalgam restoration, the tooth is at some risk for cuspal fracture in the future. Fracture of the tooth would necessitate fabrication of a crown beneath the removable partial denture. By planning a crown prior to fabrication of the removable partial denture, a treatment plan somewhat more aggressive than would be dictated by the needs of the individual tooth, the prognosis for the ultimate treatment objective becomes more predictable and the risk of compromising the final result is reduced. This does not mean that every removable partial denture abutment should receive a crown, but it is intended to convey the importance of planning for predictable longevity in key teeth.

Treatment Sequence

When the completed treatment has been envisioned and the design of the restorations required to address each problem on the restorative dentistry problem list has been established, the final step in establishing the restorative dentistry treatment plan is sequencing the treatment. Proper sequencing of all procedures involved is often critical to successfully achieving the treatment goals. The dentist must not only be able to envision the ultimate outcome of treatment but he or she must also understand the order in which the procedures must be performed to achieve that outcome. Considerable thought is required to understand and plan a treatment sequence that avoids unnecessary complication.

Most restorative treatment will fall into the categories of disease control or definitive rehabilitative treatment discussed at the beginning of the chapter. Restorative treatment aimed at controlling active disease generally consists of direct restorative procedures using amalgam, resin composite, or glass-ionomer materials. The sequence of treatment within the disease-control phase is dictated by three considerations:

(1) severity of the disease process (ie, the most symptomatic tooth, the tooth with the deepest lesion, or the most debilitated tooth is restored first); (2) esthetic needs; and (3) effective use of time. At each appointment, treatment is rendered in the area in the most acute need of restorative treatment. When possible, the restorations should be completed quadrant by quadrant to optimize the use of time.

Treatment provided in the definitive rehabilitative phase goes beyond that needed for the stabilization of active disease and includes restorative treatment designed primarily to enhance esthetics (eg, ceramic veneers) and to provide optimum function (eg, replacement of missing teeth using fixed partial dentures) and resistance to oral stresses (eg, cast restorations).

One of the primary benefits of segregating the restorative treatment into these categories is that a formal reevaluation is completed at the end of the disease-control phase, before progressing into the definitive treatment phase. This approach incorporates into the plan the opportunity to modify or curtail restorative treatment after the control of caries and the replacement of defective restorations. There can be many reasons for altering the original treatment plan, including the patient's desires, disease risk, failure to accomplish disease control, finances, or the doctor-patient relationship.

The patient's financial situation or third-party payment guidelines may dictate that treatment be divided into stages and completed over a period of time. Organization of treatment in phases serves the patient's most urgent needs first, directing resources into the management of active disease and allowing less acute problems to be addressed as finances permit.

As previously emphasized, treatment planning for restorative dentistry requires that the dentist recognize the sequence in which restorative care should be provided within the context of the overall plan. It is not enough to be able to envision the final goal of treatment; one must be able to visualize each step that must be accomplished to achieve this goal. The following example illustrates this point.

A patient presented stating that he wished to "close the spaces" between his front teeth (Fig 2-19a). Upon evaluation, this seemingly simple request revealed a complex set of problems. The dentist recognized the problem associated with the patient's chief complaint: diastemata resulting from a tooth-size vs jaw-size discrepancy. The dentist also recognized other esthetic problems associated with the anterior teeth (Fig 2-19b): fluorosis-related discolorations of the teeth and incomplete exposure of the crowns of the anterior teeth due to altered passive eruption of the maxillary lateral incisors.

The dentist considered possible solutions to the diastema problem. The two most common solutions to this type of space-related problem are *(1)* closure of the spaces by the placement of restorations, and *(2)* orthodontic retraction of the maxillary teeth, creating a smaller arch perimeter and reducing or eliminating the spaces between the teeth. An occlusal analysis revealed that the maxillary-mandibular dental relationships would not permit retraction of the maxillary anterior teeth (see Fig 2-19b). Thus, complete space closure would require filling all of the open spaces with tooth-colored restorative materials. A space analysis and a diagnostic waxup revealed that closure of all of the spaces would result in excessive (unesthetic) widening of the maxillary lateral incisors and canines. Complete space closure would be esthetically acceptable only if it were accomplished by adding a small amount of restorative material to all of the maxillary anterior teeth. The two options available were *(1)* partial closure of the diastemata with tooth-colored restorative material, leaving small spaces between the maxillary lateral incisors and canines, or *(2)* orthodontic redistribution of the existing spaces, followed by complete space closure using tooth-colored restorations placed on all six maxillary anterior teeth.

When presented with these possibilities, the patient stated that he would prefer complete space closure and would be willing to undergo orthodontic treatment to accomplish this. The dentist then visualized the optimal treatment goal and realized that the maxillary lateral incisors would need to be moved to a more distal position to equalize the anterior spacing. This was added to the problem list. Visualizing the distal movement of the maxillary lateral incisors, the dentist realized that the positions of the mandibular lateral incisors would interfere with this movement. This presented a new problem, which was added to the problem list. The dentist considered two options: *(1)* orthodontic movement of the mandibular lateral incisors, or *(2)* alteration of the contour of the mandibular lateral incisors to accommodate the repositioning of the maxillary lateral incisors. The orthodontic movement required to reposition the mandibular lateral incisors was deemed unfeasible, and so the second option was selected.

Having determined the feasibility of orthodontic space redistribution for the maxillary anterior teeth, the dentist visualized the final result. Increasing the width of the anterior teeth using tooth-colored restorations (ceramic veneers) would increase the tooth-width to tooth-height ratio, making the maxillary lateral incisors appear unesthetically short and wide. Diagnostic periodontal probing and bone sounding procedures were completed to address this newfound problem. The relative locations of the cementoenamel junctions and the distances from the gingival crest to the osseous crests of the mandibular lateral incisors were determined. It was decided that the ideal solution for the "short tooth" problem of the mandibular lateral incisors was to expose the complete crown

of these teeth through surgical crown lengthening before ceramic veneer placement. This plan was presented and was accepted by the patient.

In stepwise fashion, the entire problem complex was broken down into its individual components. Each component and its proposed solution were assessed. Any new problems that were created by proposed treatment were considered. The final chain of treatment was established and presented to the patient. By recognizing which form of treatment was required to address each component problem, the dentist was able to plan the entire sequence before initiating treatment. All of the proposed procedures were completed, and the treatment of the patient's anterior esthetic problem was realized (Figs 2-19c to 2-19h).

The Dental Record

Accurate and descriptive record keeping is essential to quality dental care. The dental chart should include findings from the history and examination, the problem list, the treatment plan, and a description of the treatment accomplished. This record serves several purposes:

1. Organization and documentation of the examination findings, the problem list, the treatment plan, and the treatment rendered
2. Documentation for third-party payment, if applicable
3. Legal purposes
4. Forensic purposes

Organizing and documenting the examination findings and the problem list enable the dentist to evaluate the patient's dental problems and plan the treatment when the patient is no longer present. Once treatment has begun, documentation of the sequenced treatment plan also permits the dentist to review the anticipated treatment without the need to reconsider the entire treatment planning process. Dental records should include the following information:

1. Charting of examination findings, including existing restorations and dental relationships (eg, diastemata, dentoalveolar extrusion, tilted teeth), existing periodontal and endodontic conditions, occlusal relationships, and caries lesions and defective restorations
2. Medical history and consultations
3. Problem list
4. Treatment plan
5. Description of treatment provided

Fig 2-19a The patient wished to close the diastemata adjacent to the maxillary lateral incisors.

Fig 2-19b A close-up view reveals, in addition to the diastemata and discolored anterior teeth, the unesthetically short clinical crowns of the maxillary lateral incisors. For better space distribution prior to ceramic veneer fabrication, the maxillary lateral incisors need to be repositioned distally and their crowns lengthened. The mandibular canines are obstructing movement of the maxillary lateral incisors into the desired locations.

Fig 2-19c The maxillary lateral incisors have been repositioned orthodontically. Space was created by odontoplasty of the mandibular canines, followed by resin composite restorations. The space redistribution permits diastema closure to be completed by adding restorative material to all six anterior teeth, which avoids the problem of making any single tooth excessively wide.

Fig 2-19d Mucogingival flap elevation reveals the osseous crest to be immediately adjacent to the cementoenamel junctions of the maxillary lateral incisors. This anatomic relationship is responsible for the gingiva covering a portion of the crowns of these teeth.

Fig 2-19e Ostectomy and osteoplasty have created approximately 3 mm of space for the combination of sulcus depth, connective tissue attachment, and epithelial attachment. This space will allow the gingival crest to reside at the level of the cervical margin of the veneers, displaying the entire crown of each tooth.

Fig 2-19f Three months after surgery, healing is complete and the teeth are ready for veneer preparation.

Fig 2-19g One month after veneer placement (maxillary first premolar to first premolar). The spaces have been closed, and the fluorosis-related discoloration has been eliminated.

Fig 2-19h The patient was extremely satisfied with the final results of his multidisciplinary treatment.

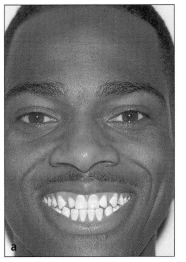

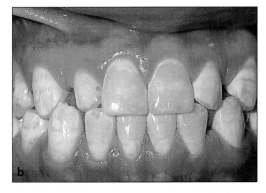

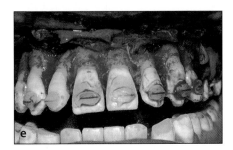

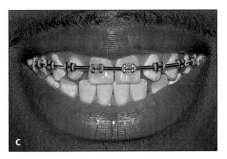

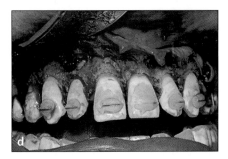

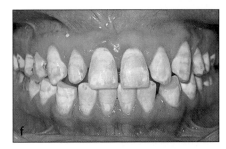

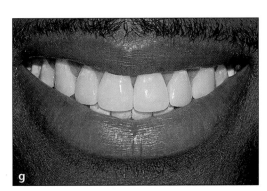

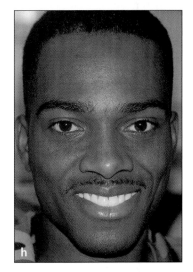

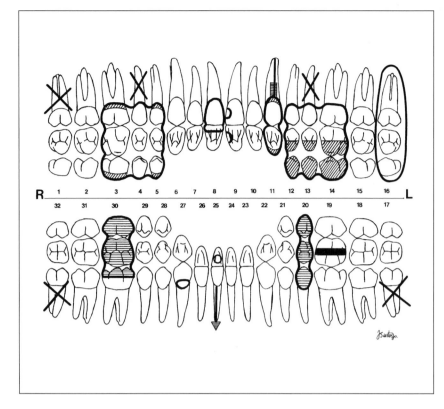

Fig 2-20 Example of a pictorial charting system used to record dental restorations. Any system that distinguishes among the various restorations is acceptable. In this example, tooth 1 is missing; tooth 4 has been replaced with a metal-ceramic fixed partial denture that extends from tooth 3 to tooth 5 with ceramic occlusal coverage; tooth 8 has a facial veneer; tooth 9 has a mesial resin composite restoration; tooth 11 has been endodontically treated and has a post and metal-ceramic crown; tooth 13 has been replaced by a metal-ceramic fixed partial denture that extends from tooth 12 to tooth 14 with metal occlusal coverage; tooth 16 is impacted; tooth 17 is missing; tooth 19 has an MOD amalgam restoration; tooth 20 has been restored with a metal crown; tooth 25 has been endodontically treated, received a retrograde restoration, and has a resin composite restoration in the lingual access opening; tooth 27 has a facial tooth-colored restoration; tooth 30 has a metal three-quarter crown; and tooth 32 is missing.

6. Informed-consent documentation
7. Follow-up assessment

In addition to the usual typed or handwritten entries in a dental record, pictorial charting is an efficient means of recording a great deal of information in a small area (Figs 2-20 and 2-21). Intraoral imaging devices, either conventional cameras or videographic recording devices, provide an extremely effective means of recording findings and documenting treatment and are an ideal complement to a pictorial charting system. These offer the added advantage of simplifying communication with the patient and third-party funding agencies.

The format used to document the care provided should reflect an orderly and logical diagnostic and treatment sequence. A method commonly used in medicine that satisfies this requirement is the SOAP format. *SOAP* is an acronym for the steps involved whenever any treatment is rendered. *S* refers to subjective findings. This includes a summary of the patient's chief complaint, a description of his or her symptoms, and any other relevant information the patient provides. The patient's own words should be used as much as possible. The *O* refers to objective findings. These include examination findings and the results of consultations and diagnostic tests. *A* refers to the assessment, which is the dentist's diagnosis, based on the subjective and objective findings

present. The *P* refers to the plan of treatment (when the treatment is rendered immediately, it refers to the procedures, or the treatment itself). An example of the use of the SOAP format is provided (see box).

S: Patient presents complaining of a "toothache that began yesterday and has hurt all night." (Patient points to tooth 30). Patient states that ice water reduces the pain.

0: Teeth 27 to 30 are within normal limits (WNL) to percussion, palpation, and periodontal exam and are vital and normal to cold testing. Tooth 31 is painful to percussion and pain is alleviated with the application of cold. Radiographs of teeth 27 to 31 are unremarkable, except for a deep mesio-occlusal amalgam restoration on tooth 31.

A: Tooth 31 has irreversible pulpitis.

P: Patient advised of diagnosis. Patient consents to endodontic treatment on tooth 31. Patient reappointed for pulpectomy on tooth 31 at 3:00 PM today.

The SOAP format is an excellent guide in the performance and documentation of care when a challenging diagnostic problem presents itself; however, it is less suited to the routine restorative care provided based on the treat-

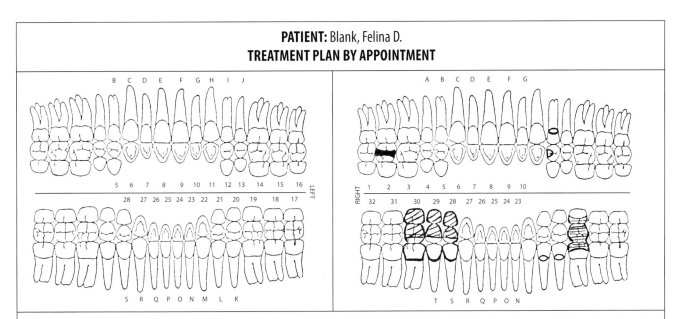

PATIENT: Blank, Felina D.
TREATMENT PLAN BY APPOINTMENT

REMARKS

Appt	Problem	Treatment	Time	Total cost	Patient cost	Insur. code	Comp. date
1	CC: #19 Hypertension	Discuss & defer until after med Tx Refer to Dr Dogood	30 min				
2	Tx plan Caries Periodontics	Present Tx plan Counseling; diet and hygiene instruction Plaque index; prophylaxis; scale/root plane mandibular posterior sextants	Dr: 30 min Hygiene: 60 min				
3	Cracked: #19	Prep gold onlay	45 min				
4	Defective restorations #2, #12	#2: MOD amalgam #12: MO resin composite #12: Class 5 resin composite	60 min				
5	Caries: #20, #21 #19	Resin-modified glass ionomer, Class 5 facial #20, #21 Deliver #19 gold onlay	60 min				
6	Biologic width: #3	Crown-lengthening surgery	45 min				
7	Biologic width: #3	Postop evaluation (1 week)	10 min				
8	Reevaluation	Perio and hygiene reeval; confirm definite phase plan	20 min				
9	Missing: #29 Supraerupted: #4	Prep FPD, #28–#30 Shorten	2 h				
10	Missing: #29	Deliver FPD, #28–#30 Impression for occlusal splint	90 min				
11	Wear: #6–#11	Deliver occlusal splint	30 min				
12	Fluorosis: #8	Microabrasion; maxillary impression for bleaching stent	30 min				
13	Color: maxillary anterior teeth	Deliver bleaching stent & give use instructions	15 min				
14	Color: maxillary anterior teeth	Reevaluate bleaching results; reinforce hygiene	10 min				
15	Maintenance	Prophylaxis; fluoride; reexamination	Dr: 10 min Hygiene: 30 min				

Fig 2-21 Example of a combined written and pictorial treatment planning sheet. The pictorial charts are for use in recording both completed treatment *(left)* and treatment yet to be accomplished *(right)*. Once completed, the treatment charted in pencil on the right may be erased. The remarks section is for making comments, generally in pencil (erased and updated as needed). The area below the remarks section is for the sequenced treatment plan. A treatment planning sheet such as this allows for quick review of the overall treatment plan and provides a profile of the current status of treatment.

ment plan. When a straightforward diagnosis is made in the absence of symptoms and patient complaint, a more concise form of documentation is appropriate (see box).

DX: Caries in tooth 3, vital to cold and asymptomatic.
TX: Tooth 3: MOD amalgam (Tytin), Amalgambond, rubber dam. Local anesthesia: 36 mg lidocaine, with 0.018 mg epinephrine.
Plan: Reappoint for preparation of veneers for teeth 5 to 12.

There are times when the identification of a deceased individual must be accomplished through the use of dental records. A complete record of the dentition and restorations, a radiographic survey, and photographic records are useful for identification purposes.

The dental record is a legal document. The nature and clarity of the entries made should reflect the knowledge that it may be needed in a court of law to document examination findings, informed consent, and treatment completed. The records should be accurate and should contain the elements listed above. They should not contain erasures or text that has been obliterated by any means. If errors are made, a single line should be drawn through the mistake and the change should be initialed and dated. In the retrospective review of a legal investigation, the descriptiveness and clarity of the record is often held to be an indication of the quality of care provided.

Summary

Treatment planning for restorative dentistry can be a complex undertaking. Use of a logical and orderly problem-oriented approach can simplify the process. The following principles have been offered as guidelines:

1. Be aware of pathoses that may be encountered and be able to distinguish the normal from the abnormal and stable from risk-prone situations.
2. Organize abnormal findings into a problem list.
3. Envision an overall restorative goal for the patient. This is the anticipated final state of rehabilitation. Not every patient can be restored to the ideal, but each patient has an optimum state of health that can be obtained, given his or her circumstances.
4. Determine a treatment plan for each problem, so that each treatment contributes to the achievement of the anticipated ultimate treatment goal. This is the linchpin of restorative treatment planning. It requires that the dentist consider a number of factors before selecting the optimum

restorative option. Chief among these considerations are the overall goal of treatment; the functional and esthetic needs of each restorative situation (using the existing dentition and restorations as an indicator of the performance of future restorations); the strengths and weaknesses of the various restorative materials available; and the amount and location of remaining tooth structure.

5. Recognize the sequence of steps needed to achieve a specific restorative objective. The dentist must know, for example, that a tooth fractured at the level of the osseous crest and in need of a crown will require endodontic treatment, a post and core, and crown lengthening surgery before fabrication of the final restoration.
6. Sequence the treatment based on a logical model. Control active disease processes first, beginning treatment with teeth in the most acute need of care. Complete as much care as is feasible in each sextant at the same appointment. Establish a restorative prognosis for key teeth early in the treatment schedule. Consider nondental factors (especially third-party payment guidelines and time-related limits) when planning the treatment schedule.

References

1. Little JW, Falace DA. Dental Management of the Medically Compromised Patient, ed 6. St Louis: Mosby, 2002.
2. Stefanac SJ, Nesbit SP. Treatment Planning in Dentistry. St. Louis: Mosby, 2001.
3. O'Leary TJ, Drake RB, Naylor JE. The plaque control record. J Periodontol 1972;43:38.
4. Disney JA, Graves RC, Stamm JW, Bohannan HM, Abernathy JR, Zack DD. The University of North Carolina Caries Risk Assessment study: Further developments in caries risk prediction. Community Dent Oral Epidemiol 1992;20:64–75.
5. Wyatt C, MacEntee M. Dental caries in chronically disabled elders. Spec Care Dentist 1997;17(6):196–202.
6. Caries diagnosis and risk assessment. A review of preventive strategies and management. J Am Dent Assoc 1995;126(suppl):1S-24S.
7. Van Palenstein Helderman WH, Matee MIN, van der Hoeven JS, Mikx FHM. Cariogenicity depends more on diet than the prevailing mutans streptococcal species. J Dent Res 1996;75:535–545.
8. Mendoza M, Mobley CL, Hattaway K. Caries risk management and the role of dietary assessment [abstract 33]. J Dent Res 1995;74:16.
9. Mobley CC. Nutrition and dental caries. Dent Clin North Am 2003;47:319–336.
10. Stack KM, Papas AS. Xerostomia: Etiology and clinical management. Nutr Clin Care 2001;4:15–21.
11. Kaufman E, Lamster IB. The diagnostic applications of saliva—A review. Crit Rev Oral Biol Med 2002;13:197–212.
12. Ship JA, Fox PC, Baum BJ. How much saliva is enough? Normal function defined. J Am Dent Assoc 1991;122:63–69.
13. Valdez IH, Fox PC. Diagnosis and management of salivary dysfunction. Crit Rev Oral Biol Med 1994;4:271–277.

14. Dodds M, Suddick R. Caries risk assessment for determination of focus and intensity of prevention in a dental school clinic. J Dent Educ 1995;59:945–956.

15. Navazesh M, Christensen C, Brightman V. Clinical criteria for the diagnosis of salivary gland hypofunction. J Dent Res 1992;71:1363–1369.

16. Van Houte JH. Bacterial specificity in the etiology of dental caries. Int Dent J 1980;30:305–326.

17. MacEntee MI, Clark DC, Glick N. Predictors of caries in old age. Gerontology 1993;10:90–97.

18. Wenzel A, Larsen MJ, Fejerskov O. Detection of occlusal caries without cavitation by visual inspection, film radiographs, xeroradiographs and digitized radiographs. Caries Res 1991;25:365–371.

19. Chan DCN. Current methods and criteria for caries diagnosis in North America. J Dent Educ 1993;57:422–427.

20. Bader JD, Brown JP. Dilemmas in caries diagnosis. J Am Dent Assoc 1993;124:48–50.

21. Bergman G, Linden LA. The action of the explorer on incipient caries. Sven Tandlak 1969;62:629–634.

22. Dodds MWJ. Dilemmas in caries diagnosis—Applications to current practice and need for research. J Dent Educ 1993;57:433–438.

23. Ekstrand K, Qvist V, Thylstrup A. Light microscope study of the effect of probing in occlusal surfaces. Caries Res 1987;21:368–374.

24. Mertz-Fairhurst E, Curtis JW, Ergle JW, Rueggeberg FA, Adair SM. Ultraconservative and cariostatic and sealed restorations: Results at year 10. J Am Dent Assoc 1998;129:55–66.

25. Cohen S, Burns RC. Pathways of the Pulp, ed 8. St Louis: Mosby, 2002.

26. Sorenson JA, Martinoff MD. Intracoronal reinforcement and coronal coverage: A study of endodontically treated teeth. J Prosthet Dent 1984;51:780–784.

27. Trope M, Maltz DO, Tronstad L. Resistance to fracture of restored endodontically treated teeth. Endod Dent Traumatol 1985;1:108–111.

28. Trabert KC, Caputo AA, Abou-Rass M. Tooth fracture: A comparison of endodontic and restorative treatments. J Endod 1978;4:341–345.

29. Kidd EAM, O'Hara JW. The caries status of occlusal amalgam restorations with marginal defects. J Dent Res 1990;69:1275–1277.

30. Summitt JB, Osborne JM. Initial preparations for amalgam restorations: Extending the longevity of the tooth-restoration unit. J Am Dent Assoc 1993;123:67–73.

31. Roberts HW, Charlton DG, Murchison DF. Effect of flowable resin on leakage at amalgam margin defects [abstract 3779]. J Dent Res 2000;79(special issue):616.

32. Smales RJ, Hawthorne WS. Long-term survival of repaired amalgams, recemented crowns and gold castings. Oper Dent 2004;29:249–253.

33. Svanberg M, Mjör IA, Orstavik D. Mutans streptococci in plaque from margins of amalgam, composite and glass ionomer restorations. J Dent Res 1990;69:861–864.

34. O'Neal SJ, Miracle RL, Leinfelder KF. Evaluating interfacial gaps for esthetic inlays. J Am Dent Assoc 1993;124:48–54.

35. Gilmour ASM, Edmunds DH, Newcombe RG. Prevalence and depth of artificial caries-like lesions adjacent to cavities prepared in roots and restored with a glass ionomer or a dentin-bonded composite material. J Dent Res 1997;76:1854–1861.

36. Hara AT, Turssi CP, Serra MC, Nogueira MCS. Extent of the cariostatic effect on root dentin provided by fluoride-containing restorative materials. Oper Dent 2002;27:480–487.

37. Nagamine M, Itota T, Torii Y, Irie M, Staninec M, Inoue K. Effect of resin-modified glass ionomer cements on secondary caries. Am J Dent 1997;10:173–178.

38. Souto M, Donley KJ. Caries inhibition of glass ionomers. Am J Dent 1994;7:122–124.

39. Tantbirojn D, Douglas WH, Versluis A. Inhibitive effect of a resin-modified glass ionomer cement on remote enamel artificial caries. Caries Res 1997;31:275–280.

40. Donly KJ, Segura A, Wefel JS, Hogan MM. Evaluating the effects of fluoride-releasing dental materials on adjacent interproximal caries. J Am Dent Assoc 1999;130:817–825.

41. Haveman CW, Summitt JB, Burgess JO, Carlson K. Three restorative materials and topical fluoride gel used in xerostomic patients. A clinical comparison. J Am Dent Assoc 2003;134:177–184.

42. McComb D, Erickson RL, Maxymiw WG, Wood RE. A clinical comparison of glass ionomer, resin-modified glass ionomer and resin composite restorations in the treatment of cervical caries in xerostomic head and neck radiation patients. Oper Dent 2002;27:430–437.

43. Qvist V, Laurberg L, Poulsen A, Teglers PT. Longevity and cariostatic effects of everyday conventional glass-ionomer and amalgam restorations in primary teeth: Three year results. J Dent Res 1997;76:1387–1396.

44. Tyas M. Cariostatic effect of glass ionomer cement: A five year clinical study. Aust Dent J 1991;36:236–239.

45. Maynard JG, Wilson RD. Physiologic dimensions of the periodontium fundamental to successful restorative dentistry. J Periodontol 1979;50:170–174.

46. Than A, Duguid R, McKendrick AJW. Relationship between restorations and the level of periodontal attachment. J Clin Periodontol 1982;9:193–202.

47. Waerhaug J. Effect of rough surfaces upon the gingival tissues. J Dent Res 1956;35:323–327.

48. Löe H. Reaction of marginal periodontal tissue to restorative procedures. Int Dent J 1968;18:759–778.

49. Glickman I. Inflammation and trauma from occlusion, co-destructive factors in chronic periodontal disease. J Periodontol 1963;34:5–10.

50. Waerhaug J, Hansen ER. Periodontal changes incident to prolonged occlusal overload in monkeys. Acta Odontol Scand 1966;24:91–105.

51. Waerhaug J. The angular bone defect and its relationship to trauma from occlusion and downgrowth of subgingival plaque. J Clin Periodontol 1979;6:61–82.

52. Kantor M, Polson A, Zander H. Alveolar bone regeneration after removal of inflammatory and traumatic factors. J Periodontol 1976;47:687–695.

53. Lindhe JA. Influence of trauma from occlusion on the progression of experimental periodontitis in beagle dogs. J Clin Periodontol 1974;1:3–14.

54. Pihlstrom B, Anderson K, Aeppli D, Schaffer E. Association between signs of trauma from occlusion and periodontitis. J Periodontol 1986;57:1–6.

55. Mjor I. Glass-ionomer cement restorations and secondary caries: A preliminary report. Quintessence Int 1996;27:171–174.

56. Oh WS, DeLong R, Anusavice KJ. Factors affecting enamel and ceramic wear: A literature review. J Prosthet Dent 2002;87:451–459.

57. Verrett RG. Analyzing the etiology of an extremely worn dentition. J Prosthodont 2001;10:224–233.

58. Anusavice KJ. Phillips' Science of Dental Materials, ed 11. St Louis: Saunders, 2003.

59. Lambrechts P, Braem M, Vanherle G. Evaluation of clinical performance for posterior composites and dentin adhesives. Oper Dent 1987;2:53–78.

60. Lutz F, Kreci I, Barbakow F. Chewing pressure versus wear of composites and opposing enamel cusps. J Dent Res 1992;71:1525–1529.

61. Monasky DE, Taylor DF. Studies on the wear of porcelain, enamel and gold. J Prosthet Dent 1971;25:299–306.

62. Imai Y, Suzuki S, Fukishima S. Enamel wear of modified porcelains. Am J Dent 2000;13:315–323.

63. Metzler KT, Woody RD, Miller AW 3rd, Miller BH. In vitro investigation of the wear of human enamel by dental porcelain. J Prosthet Dent 1999;81:356–364.

64. Sorensen JA, Sultan E, Condon JR. Three-body in vitro wear of enamel against dental ceramics [abstract 909]. J Dent Res 1999;78(SI):219.

65. Sorensen JA, Berge HX. In vivo measurement of antagonist tooth wear opposing ceramic bridges [abstract 2942]. J Dent Res 1999; 78(SI):473.

66. al-Hiyasat AS, Saunders WP, Smith GM. Three-body wear associated with three ceramics and enamel. J Prosthet Dent 1999;82: 476–481.

67. Clelland NL, Agarwala V, Knobloch LA, Seghi RR. Relative wear of enamel opposing low-fusing dental porcelain. J Prosthodont 2003;12:168–175.

68. Clelland NL, Agarwala V, Knobloch LA, Seghi RR. Wear of enamel opposing low-fusing and conventional ceramic restorative materials. J Prosthodont 2001;10:8–15.

69. Magne P, Oh WS, Pintado MR, DeLong R. Wear of enamel and veneering ceramics after laboratory and chairside finishing procedures. J Prosthet Dent 1999;82:669–679.

70. Anusavice KJ, Esquivel-Upshaw JF. Less abrasive ceramic esthetic materials. In: Duke ES (ed). The Changing Practice of Restorative Dentistry. [Proceedings of the 5th Annual Indiana Conference, 8–10 June 2000, Indianapolis, IN]. Indianapolis: Indiana University School of Dentistry, 2002:216–236.

71. Heymann HO, Sturdevant JR, Bayne S, et al. Examining tooth flexure effects. J Am Dent Assoc 1991;122:41–47.

72. Kuroe T, Hidemi I, Caputo AA, Konuma M. Biomechanics of cervical tooth structure lesions and their restoration. Quintessence Int 2000;31:267–274.

73. Lee WC, Eakle WS. Possible role of tensile stress in the etiology of cervical lesions of teeth. J Prosthet Dent 1984;52:374–380.

74. Whitehead SA, Wilson NHF, Watts DC. Development of noncarious cervical notch lesions in vitro. J Esthet Dent 1999;11:332–337.

75. LittleStar ML, Summitt JB. Non-carious cervical lesions: An evidenced-based approach to their diagnosis. Tex Dent J 2003;120: 972–980.

76. Bader JD, Shugars DA, Martin JA. Risk indicators for posterior tooth fracture. J Am Dent Assoc 2004;135:883–892.

77. Bader JD, Shugars DA, Sturdevant JR. Consequences of posterior cusp fracture. Gen Dent 2004;52:128–131.

78. Ellis SG. Incomplete tooth fracture—Proposal for a new definition. Br Dent J 2001;190:424–428.

79. Rivera EM, Williamson A. Diagnosis and treatment planning: Cracked tooth. Tex Dent J 2003;120:278–283.

80. Cameron CE. Cracked tooth syndrome. J Am Dent Assoc 1964;68: 405–411.

81. Cameron CE. The cracked tooth syndrome: Additional findings. J Am Dent Assoc 1976;93:971–975.

82. Cohen SN, Silvestri AR. Complete and incomplete fractures of posterior teeth. Compend Contin Educ Dent 1984;5:652–663.

83. Lynch CD, McConnell RJ. The cracked tooth syndrome. J Can Dent Assoc 2002;68:470–475.

84. Ratcliff S, Becker IM, Quinn L. Type and incidence of cracks in posterior teeth. J Prosthet Dent 2001;86:168–172.

85. Stanley HR. The cracked tooth syndrome. J Am Acad Gold Foil Oper 1968;11:36–47.

86. Hiatt WH. Incomplete crown-root fracture in pulpal-periodontal disease. J Periodontol 1973;49:369–379.

87. Guthrie RC, Difiore PM. Treating the cracked tooth with a full crown. J Am Dent Assoc 1991;122:71–73.

88. Langouvardos P, Sourai P, Douvitsas G. Coronal fractures in posterior teeth. Oper Dent 1989;14:28–32.

89. Cavel WT, Kelsey WP, Blankenau RJ. An in vivo study of cuspal fracture. J Prosthet Dent 1985;53:38–42.

90. De Moor RJ, De Witt AM, De Bruyne MA. Tongue piercing and associated oral and dental complications. Endod Dent Traumatol 2000;16:232–237.

91. Albers HF. Treating cracked teeth. ADEPT Report 1994;4:17–24.

92. Davis R, Overton JD. Efficacy of bonded and non-bonded amalgam in the treatment of teeth with incomplete fractures. J Am Dent Assoc 2000;131:469–478.

93. Eakle WS. Effect of thermocycling on fracture strength and microleakage in teeth restored with a bonded composite resin. Dent Mater 1986;2:114–117.

94. Hansen EK. In vivo cusp fracture of endodontically treated premolars restored with MOD amalgam or MOD resin fillings. Dent Mater 1988;4:169–173.

95. Clark DJ, Sheets CG, Paquette JM. Definitive diagnosis of early enamel and dentin cracks based on microscopic evaluation. J Esthet Restor Dent 2003;15:391–401.

96. Polson AM, Caton JG. Current status of bleeding in the diagnosis of periodontal disease. J Periodontol 1985;56(suppl):1.

97. Bhaskar SN. Radiographic Interpretation for the Dentist. St Louis: Mosby, 1986.

98. US Department of Health and Human Services. The Selection of Patients for X-ray Examination: Dental Radiographic Examination. US Dept of Health and Human Services Publication (FDA), 1987:87–88.

99. Goaz PW, White SC (eds). Oral Radiology: Principles and Interpretation, ed 4. St Louis: Mosby, 2000.

100. Garcia LT, Summitt JB. The role of research evidence in clinical practice [guest editorial]. Tex Dent J 2003;120:942–943.

101. Anderson MH, Bales DJ, Omnell K-A. Modern management of dental caries: The cutting edge is not the dental bur. J Am Dent Assoc 1993;124:37–44.

102. Holleron BW, Porteous NB, Amaechi BT. Treating caries as a disease and restoring carious teeth via remineralization. Tex Dent J 2003; 120:946–957.

103. Nicholson JW. Evidence-based approach to minimal restorative intervention for early carious lesions. Tex Dent J 2003;120: 960–969.

104. Hudson P. Conservative treatment of the Class I lesion: A new paradigm for dentistry. J Am Dent Assoc 2004;135:760–764.

105. Larson TO, Douglas WH, Geistfeld RE. Effects of prepared cavities on the strength of prepared teeth. Oper Dent 1981;6:2–5.

106. Blaser PK, Lund MR, Cochran MA, Potter RH. Effect of designs of Class 2 preparations on the resistance of teeth to fracture. Oper Dent 1983;8:6–10.

107. Matis BA, Cochran M, Carlson T. Longevity of glass-ionomer restorative materials: Results of a 10-year evaluation. Quintessence Int 1996;27:373–382.

108. Duke ES, Robbins JW, Summitt JB, et al. Clinical evaluation of Vitremer in cervical abrasions and root caries [abstract 2578]. J Dent Res 1998;77:954.

109. Boghosian A, Ricker J, McCoy R. Clinical evaluation of a resin-modified glass ionomer restorative: 5-year results [abstract 1436]. J Dent Res 1999;78:285.

110. Robbins JW, Duke ES, Schwartz RS, Summitt JB. 3-year clinical evaluation of a dentin adhesive system in cervical abrasions [abstract 1436]. J Dent Res 1995;74:164.

111. Trevino DF, Duke ES, Robbins JW, Summit JB. Clinical evaluation of Scotchbond Multi-Purpose adhesive system in cervical abrasions [abstract 3037]. J Dent Res 1996;75:397.

112. Haveman CW. Xerostomia management in the head and neck radiation patient. Tex Dent J 2004;121:482–497.

113. Friedl K-H, Hiller K-A, Schmalz G. Placement and replacement of composite restorations in Germany. Oper Dent 1995;20:34–38.

114. Qvist V, Qvist J, Mjör IA. Placement and longevity of tooth-colored restorations in Denmark. Acta Odontol Scand 1990;48:305–311.

115. Pink FE, Minder NJ, Simmonds S. Decisions of practitioners regarding placement of amalgam and composite restorations in a general practice setting. Oper Dent 1994;19:127–132.

116. Bogacki RE, Hunt RJ, del Aguila M, Smith WR. Survival analysis of posterior restorations using an insurance claims database. Oper Dent 2002;27:488–492.58.

117. Barnes DM, Blank LW, Thompson VP, et al. A five-and eight-year clinical evaluation of a posterior resin composite. Quintessence Int 1991;22:143–154.

118. Statement on posterior resin-based composites. ADA Council on Scientific Affairs; ADA Council on Dental Benefit Programs. J Am Dent Assoc 1998;1627–1628.

119. Robbins JW, Summitt JB. Longevity of complex amalgam restorations. Oper Dent 1988;13:54–57.

120. Smales R. Longevity of cusp-covered amalgams: survival after 15 years. Oper Dent 1991;16:17–20.

121. Bentley C, Drake CW. Longevity of restorations in a dental school clinic. J Dent Educ 1986;50:594–600.

122. Leempoel PJB, Eschen S, DeHaan AFJ, Van't Hof MA. An evaluation of crowns and bridges in a general dental practice. J Oral Rehabil 1985;12:515–518.

123. McLean JW. Evolution of dental ceramics in the twentieth century. J Prosthet 2001;85:61–66.

124. Giordano R. A comparison of all-ceramic restorative systems: Part 2. Gen Dent 2000;48:38–45.

125. Reich SM, Wichmann M, Rinne H, Shortall A. Clinical performance of large, all-ceramic CAD/CAM-generated restorations after three years: A pilot study. J Am Dent Assoc 2004;135:605–612.

126. Boening KW, Wolf BH, Schmidt AE, Kastner K, Walter MH. Clinical fit of Procera AllCeram crowns. J Prosthet Dent 2000;84:419–424.

127. Haselton DR, Diaz-Arnold AM, Hillis SL. Clinical assessment of high-strength all-ceramic crowns. J Prosthet Dent 2000;83:396–401.

128. McLaren EA, White SN. Survival of In-Ceram crowns in a private practice: A prospective clinical trial. J Prosthet Den 2000;83: 216–222.

129. Van Dijken JWV, Hasselroth L, Ormin A, Olofsson A-L. Clinical evaluation of extensive dentin/enamel bonded all-ceramic onlays and onlay-crowns [abstract 2713]. J Dent Res 1999;78:444.

130. Esquivel-Upshaw JF, Anusavice KJ. Ceramic design concepts based on stress distribution analysis. Compend Contin Educ Dent 2000;21:649–654.

131. Goodacre CJ, Campagni WV, Aquilino SA. Tooth preparations for complete crowns: An art form based on scientific principles. J Prosthet Dent 2001;85:363–376.

132. Frankenberger R, Rumi K, Kramer N. Clinical evaluation of leucite reinforced glass ceramic inlays and onlays after six years [abstract 1623]. J Dent Res 1999;78:308.

133. Schmalz G, Federlin M, Hiller K-A, Felden A. Retrospective clinical investigation on ceramic inlays and partial crowns [abstract 455]. J Dent Res 1996;75:74.

134. Christensen G. Filled polymer crowns. Clinical Research Associate's Newsletter 1998;22(10):1–3.

135. Hannig M. Five-year clinical evaluation of a heat- and pressure-cured composite resin inlay system [abstract 1908]. J Dent Res 1996;75:256.

136. Esquivel-Upshaw JF, Anusavice KJ, Young H, Jones J, Gibbs C. Clinical performance of a lithia disiliate–based core ceramic for three-unit posterior FPDs. Int J Prosthodont 2004;17:469–475.

137. Olsson KG, Furst B, Andersson B, Carlsson GE. A long-term retrospective and clinical follow-up study of In-Ceram Alumina FPDs. Int J Prosthodont 2003;16:150–156.

138. Vult von Steyern P, Johnsson O, Nilner K. Five-year evaluation of posterior all-ceramic three-unit (In-Ceram) FPDs. Int J Prosthodont 2001;14:379–384.

Esthetic Considerations in Diagnosis and Treatment Planning

J. William Robbins

Because beauty is primarily a matter of personal taste modified by social norms, visualizing beauty is a subjective experience. Creating a beautiful smile requires the dentist to dip into these subjective waters. This chapter provides a comprehensive and, when possible, evidence-based set of guidelines that will enable dentists to provide esthetic as well as functional dentistry.

Esthetic Parameters

Face Height

The face can be divided vertically into thirds, and the length of the middle third of the face should approximately equal the lower third of the face when measured in repose[1] (Fig 3-1). The midface is measured from glabella, the most prominent point of the forehead between the eyebrows, to subnasale, the point below the base of the nose. The lower face is measured from subnasale to soft tissue menton, which is the lower border of the chin.

Variations from the norm can reflect a continuum from underdevelopment to hypertrophic development of either one or both arches. However, regarding esthetic diagnoses that impact dental treatment, excessive length of the lower third of the face is most common. The long lower face is commonly the result of vertical maxillary excess and, in many cases, is accompanied by excess gingival display in the maxilla during full smile.

Lip Length

The length of the upper lip is measured from subnasale to the inferior border of the upper lip in repose (Fig 3-2a). The average length of the upper lip is 20 to 22 mm in the young adult female and 22 to 24 mm in the young adult male.[2] The upper lip tends to lengthen with age.[3] When a patient presents with excess gingival display (more than 2 mm of gingiva exposed above the maxillary central incisors during full smile), lip length may be part of the etiology (Fig 3-2b).

Lip Mobility

Mobility of the upper lip is measured from repose position to high smile position. The average lip mobility is 6 to 8 mm. In the patient with excess gingival display in full smile, hypermobility of the upper lip may be a contributing factor.

Symmetry

Outline symmetry is essential at the midline[4]; the maxillary central incisors should be mirror images of each other. Additionally, a line drawn between the maxillary central incisors should be perpendicular to the horizon[5] (Fig 3-3). Finally, the maxillary dental midline should be coincident with the facial midline.[6] Asymmetry at the midline creates a visual tension in the observer, resulting in an unacceptable esthetic presentation. As the eye moves peripherally from the

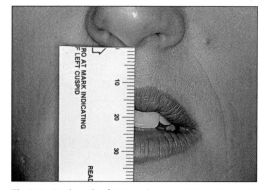

Fig 3-1 The length of the middle third of the face should equal the length of the lower third of the face.

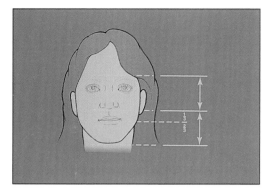

Fig 3-2a Lip length of 18 mm (average, 20 to 22 mm in females) causes gingival display in full smile.

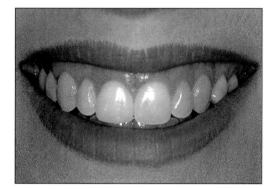

Fig 3-2b Approximately 2 mm of gingival display in full smile.

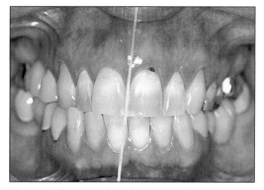

Fig 3-3 Midline canted in relation to the horizon.

midline, deviations from perfect symmetry (eg, notched edges or slight differences in edge lengths) become desirable.[7]

Incisal Plane

The incisal plane should be parallel to the horizon; the interpupillary line is helpful in making this determination.[7] However, if the interpupillary line is not parallel to horizon, it should not be used. The incisal plane is evaluated from cusp tip of the maxillary right canine to cusp tip of the maxillary left canine. Although the incisal plane must be parallel to the horizon, it is generally not flat, but has a curve that parallels the curve of the lower lip in full smile. In addition, it should not be canted up or down from right to left.

It is important not to perpetuate or create a canted incisal plane with restorations. If the interpupillary line is parallel to

the horizon, the corners of the mouth should be pulled outward so that the upper lip parallels the interpupillary line (Fig 3-4). The relationship between the incisal plane and the interpupillary line, via the upper lip, can then be visualized. To transfer this information to an articulator, a facebow may be used, as long as the horizontal member of the facebow is made parallel to the horizon before attaching the bite fork. An incisal plane relationship bite may also be used. A bite registration paste is placed between the maxillary and mandibular incisors. A long cotton-tipped applicator is then embedded in the bite registration paste and set parallel to the horizon (Fig 3-5). This relationship bite can then be used to mount the maxillary cast with an accurate incisal plane orientation to the maxillary member of the articulator (Fig 3-6).

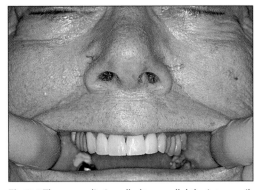

Fig 3-4 The upper lip is pulled to parallel the interpupillary line. The vermilion border of the upper lip is then used to evaluate the cant of the incisal plane and posterior occlusal plane in relation to the horizon.

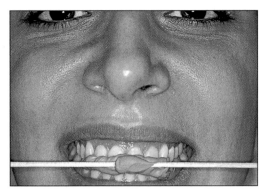

Fig 3-5 Bite registration paste is placed between maxillary and mandibular anterior teeth, and a cotton-tipped applicator is embedded in the paste. The cotton-tipped applicator is then paralleled with the interpupillary line, and the paste is allowed to set.

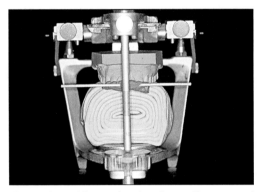

Fig 3-6 The stick bite is placed on the maxillary cast, and the stick is set parallel to the maxillary member of the articulator to orient the cast for mounting.

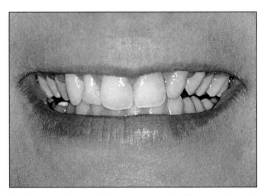

Fig 3-7 A patient with excess space in the buccal corridors.

Posterior Occlusal Plane

The buccal cusp tips of the maxillary posterior teeth should provide a visual progression from the canine cusp tips, with no step up or step down. In addition, the posterior occlusal plane should not be canted up or down from right to left.[5]

It is important not to perpetuate or create a canted posterior occlusal plane. The same techniques used to ensure an accurate mounting of the incisal plane are used for the posterior occlusal plane.

Buccal Corridor

The buccal corridor is the space between the buccal surfaces of the maxillary posterior teeth and the cheek. In full smile, the buccal corridor is almost filled with teeth. However, a minimal negative space frames the maxillary posterior teeth and is desirable.[5]

Excess buccal corridor space (Fig 3-7) is usually due to a developmental problem, such as a constricted maxillary arch. Inadequate space in the buccal corridor is usually due to bulky posterior restorations.

Lower Lip

In full smile, the incisal edges of the maxillary anterior teeth ideally are cradled by the lower lip[8,9] (Figs 3-8a and 3-8b). The smile may also be very pleasing when a space exists between the lower lip and the maxillary incisal edges, as long as the space is uniform from right to left (Fig 3-9). Conversely, none of the incisal edges of the maxillary anterior teeth should be concealed by the lower lip in full smile.

If there is a reverse incisal edge curve in relation to the lower lip, or a significant space between the lower lip and the maxillary incisal edges during full smile, esthetics may be enhanced with increased incisal edge length. Conversely, if

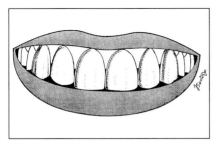

Fig 3-8a Ideal maxillary incisal edge position in relation to the lower lip.

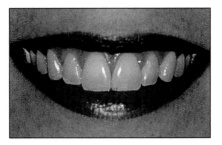

Fig 3-8b Ideal incisal edge position in relation to the lower lip. Ideal relationship between the upper lip and the gingival line.

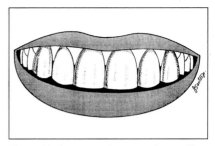

Fig 3-9 Uniform space between the maxillary incisal edges and the lower lip.

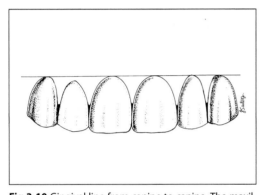

Fig 3-10 Gingival line from canine to canine. The maxillary lateral incisors can fall on this line or be up to 1.5 mm below it.

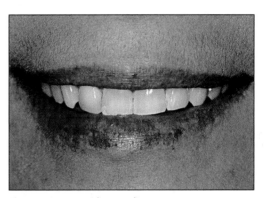

Fig 3-11 Patient with upper lip asymmetry.

incisal edges of maxillary anterior teeth are hidden by the lower lip during full smile, there is likely a problem with the vertical position of the maxilla. The cause may be dentoalveolar extrusion (overeruption of maxillary anterior teeth), vertical maxillary excess, or both.

Upper Lip

In full smile, the upper lip should ideally translate up to the gingival line[8] (see Fig 3-8b). This occurs in approximately 70% of the population. Approximately 10% have a high smile line, and approximately 20% have a low smile line.[9] To evaluate the gingival line, a straight line is drawn from the tooth-gingiva interface of the right maxillary canine to the tooth-gingiva interface of the left maxillary canine. The tooth-gingiva interface of both central incisors should be on this line. The tooth-gingiva interface of the lateral incisors may either fall on the gingival line or be up to 1.5 mm below it (Fig 3-10).[10]

If the upper lip does not translate up to the gingival line during full smile, some of the clinical crowns of the maxillary anterior teeth remain covered. This results in a loss of dynam-

ics in the smile. If, in full smile, the upper lip translates above the gingival line, the result is gingival display above the clinical crowns. Gingival display of 2 mm or more above the gingival line results in compromised esthetics.

Lip Asymmetry

If a patient displays an upper lip asymmetry during full smile (Fig 3-11), it does not generally influence treatment. However, if a patient has an asymmetric upper lip translation, resulting in excess gingival display on one side, esthetic crown lengthening surgery may be accomplished to provide more symmetry in the posterior gingival display. Any time a patient has an upper lip asymmetry, he or she should be advised of the condition before restoration of the maxillary anterior teeth, because the brighter restored teeth will draw attention to the smile and accentuate the asymmetry.

If a patient has a lower lip asymmetry during full smile that results in a unilateral increase in negative space between the maxillary incisal edges and the lower lip, smile symmetry is lost (see Fig 3-31b). When restoring maxillary anterior teeth in this circumstance, consideration is given to subtly length-

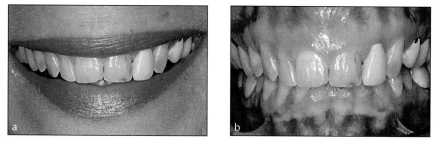

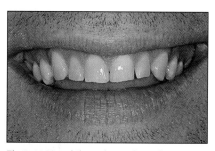

Figs 3-12a and 3-12b Note step up from maxillary left canine to maxillary left first premolar.

Fig 3-13 Note bilateral step down from maxillary canines to maxillary first premolars.

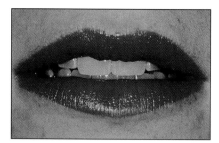

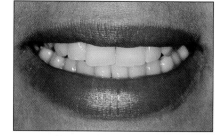

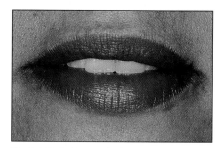

Fig 3-14 Three millimeters of display of maxillary central incisors in repose.

Fig 3-15a Patient in the "E" position.

Fig 3-15b Patient in the "F" position.

ening the incisal edges on the affected side to minimize the unilateral asymmetry. This is first accomplished in a diagnostic waxup from which provisional restorations are fabricated. The patient can then make the decision regarding the incisal edge configuration of the final restorations.

Lip asymmetries, which can play a significant role in the final restorative result, are commonly overlooked.

Incisal Edge Placement of Maxillary Central Incisors

Determining the correct position of the incisal edges of the maxillary central incisors is essential and the first step in the provision of anterior restorative dentistry. The following five guidelines are used to determine the correct incisal edge position.

1. In full smile, the incisal edges of the maxillary anterior teeth should be cradled by the lower lip[8,9] (see Fig 3-8b).
2. In full smile, the buccal cusp tips of the posterior maxillary teeth should provide a visual progression from the canine cusp tip, with no step up or step down[5] (Figs 3-12 and 3-13).

3. In gentle repose (have the patient say "M" or "Emma"), approximately 3 to 4 mm of the incisal edges of the maxillary central incisors should be displayed in the young adult female (Fig 3-14). In the young adult male, approximately 1 to 2 mm of the incisal edges should be displayed. After age 40, the amount of incisal edge display decreases approximately 1 mm per decade.[3]
4. When the patient says "E," a space between the upper and lower lips should be apparent (Fig 3-15a). If less than 50% of the space is occupied by the maxillary central incisors, the teeth can possibly be lengthened esthetically. However, if more than 70% of the space is occupied by the maxillary central incisors, lengthening of the maxillary anterior teeth will probably not be esthetically pleasing (Kois J, oral communication, 1999).
5. When the patient says "F" or "V," the incisal edges of the maxillary central incisors should lightly touch the wet/dry border of the lower lip[11] (Fig 3-15b).

Steps 1 through 4 are used together to develop an approximation of the correct incisal edge position for the diagnostic waxup. At this point, incisal edge position is dictated strictly by esthetics. After tooth preparation, provisional restorations

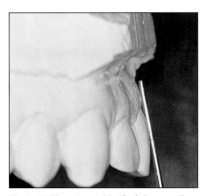

Fig 3-16 The gingival half of the maxillary central incisor is parallel to and continuous in contour with the surface of the gingival tissue overlying the alveolus.

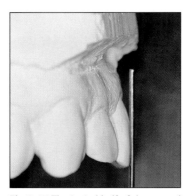

Fig 3-17 The incisal half of the central incisor is contoured to feel comfortable to the patient during lip closure and speech.

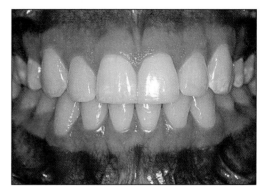

Fig 3-18 The gingival zenith is slightly distal to the midline on the maxillary central and lateral incisors.

that have been fabricated using the diagnostic waxup are placed. The final incisal edge position is then developed dynamically, over time, in the provisional restorations to ensure suitable function and phonetics as well as esthetics. Step 5 is helpful in assessing phonetics with lengthened provisional restorations.

Facial Contour of Maxillary Incisors

Divide the facial surface of the maxillary central incisor into two planes. The gingival half of the tooth should be parallel to and continuous in contour with the surface of the gingival tissue overlying the alveolus[12] (Fig 3-16). The incisal half is tapered back for ease in speaking and swallowing (Fig 3-17).

Facial overcontouring of a partial- or full-coverage restoration in the gingival half can result in chronic gingival inflammation. Facial overcontouring in the incisal half may result in lip pressure, causing linguoversion of the overcontoured teeth or interference with the lip closure path.

Lingual Contour of Maxillary Incisors

Incorrect spacing between maxillary and mandibular anterior teeth may cause a lisp. A lisp can occur with too much or too little space, although it occurs most commonly with too little space.

If a patient develops a lisp after placement of provisional or definitive restorations, the position of the incisal edges of the mandibular incisors in relation to the maxillary central incisors when the patient makes an "S" sound must be determined. If the mandibular incisor approximates the cingulum or lingual concavity of the maxillary incisor, the lisp is most commonly corrected by increasing the lingual concavity of the maxillary incisors. If, however, the mandibular incisor approximates the incisal edge of the maxillary central incisor during the "S" sound, the lisp can most commonly be corrected by changing the length of the maxillary central incisors.

Gingival Zenith

The long axes of the maxillary anterior teeth are distally inclined. Therefore, the gingival contour adjacent to the maxillary incisors is not a symmetric rounded arch form. Rather, the marginal gingiva has a parabolic shape with the high point (gingival zenith) slightly distal to the midline of the tooth[10] (Fig 3-18).

In gingival recontouring surgery, the gingival zenith should not be overemphasized. Although a distalized zenith is more common, many patients prefer a more symmetric gingival architecture.

Interproximal Contact Areas

Maxillary interproximal contact areas become progressively more gingival from central incisor to canine (Fig 3-19). The interproximal contact between the maxillary central incisors is in the incisal third of the teeth. However, the interproximal contact between the central and lateral incisors is at the junction of the incisal and middle thirds; it is slightly more gingival between the lateral incisors and the canines.[7]

If the interproximal contact extends too far incisally, a closed and unnatural-appearing incisal embrasure results. If the interproximal contact does not extend far enough gingivally, an open gingival embrasure, or black triangle, results.

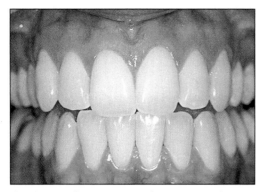

Fig 3-19 Maxillary interproximal contact areas become progressively more gingival from central incisor to canine, and incisal embrasures increase in depth from midline to canine.

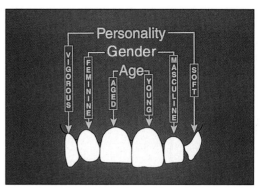

Fig 3-20 The Lombardi matrix describes characteristics associated with different incisal edge configurations.

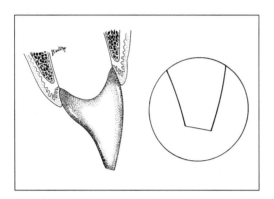

Fig 3-21 Maxillary incisal edge.

Incisal Embrasures

The incisal embrasures increase from maxillary central incisor to canine (see Fig 3-19). While the incisal embrasure between the maxillary central incisors is minimal, the incisal embrasure between the maxillary central and lateral incisors is more pronounced and between the lateral incisors and canines is the most pronounced.

Uniform incisal embrasures, from maxillary canine to canine, are esthetically unnatural.

Maxillary Incisal Edge Configuration and Tooth Morphology

In nature, it is impossible to determine gender based on tooth shape or incisal edge relationships.[9] However, tooth morphology and tooth-to-tooth relationships do convey information, albeit subjective, about the individual. In 1973, based on the writings of Frush and Fisher,[13,14] Lombardi[5] described relationships for fabricating complete dentures. His matrix is equally relevant for the dentulous patient today (Fig 3-20).

Using the Lombardi matrix, it is possible to characterize the teeth in the diagnostic waxup, the provisional restorations, and, ultimately, the definitive restorations.

Maxillary Incisal Edge Shape (Buccolingual)

Natural maxillary incisal edges, in a buccolingual direction, are not rounded but rather are sharp. Due to wear, the incisofacial line angle in adults is relatively sharp and blends into a 1-mm lingual facet before dropping off to the concave lingual surface (Fig 3-21).

Rounded maxillary incisal edges give the restoration an unnatural appearance due to the light reflection off a curved surface.

Halo Effect

The natural incisal edge anatomy of the maxillary incisor commonly imparts a thin, white, opaque "halo effect" at the incisal edge that frames the incisal translucency (Fig 3-22). The halo effect is incorporated into porcelain restorations by

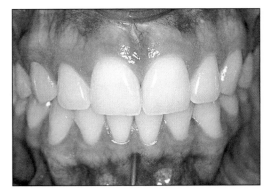

Fig 3-22 "Halo effect" in natural maxillary incisors.

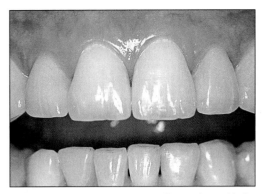

Fig 3-23 Porcelain veneers on maxillary and mandibular teeth. Note the natural appearance of the maxillary incisal edges with halo effect. (Porcelain veneers by Gilbert Young, CDT, GNS Dental Laboratory.)

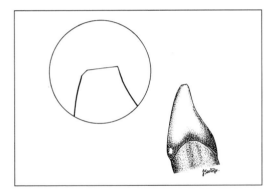

Fig 3-24 The incisal edge of a mandibular incisor. Note the pitch of the incisal table and the bevel of the incisofacial line angle.

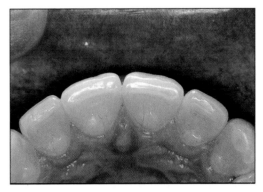

Fig 3-25 Incisal view of natural maxillary incisors. Note the flat facial surfaces, bold mesial line angles, slightly less bold distal line angles, and deep facial embrasures.

building the sharp incisal edge anatomy into the crown or porcelain veneer (Fig 3-23).

Mandibular Incisal Edge Shape

The incisal edge of the mandibular incisor should have a narrow, but defined, flat incisal table. This incisal table should be slightly canted facially. This is referred to as the *pitch* of the incisal table. The facial incisal line angle should be slightly beveled (Becker I, oral communication, 1997) (Figs 3-23 and 3-24).

This incisal edge configuration not only enhances esthetics but also improves function. As the mandible moves forward, the disclusion occurs efficiently on the leading incisofacial line angle of the mandibular incisor, rather than dragging on the broader facial surface.

Outline Symmetry

The distal surfaces of the maxillary central and lateral incisors should be similar in outline form, as should the distoincisal line angles of these teeth[5] (see Fig 3-22).

The outline symmetry of the maxillary central and lateral incisors should be similar. A large outline discrepancy (eg, a peg-shaped lateral incisor) negatively affects the beauty of the smile.

Facial Contour of the Maxillary Incisors

The facial surfaces of the maxillary incisors should not be rounded mesiodistally but rather should be flat, with resulting bold mesial and distal line angles and deep facial embrasures (Fig 3-25). Restorations with rounded facial surfaces look unnatural; facial embrasures are not well defined, resulting in a lack of visual distinction of the maxillary anterior teeth.

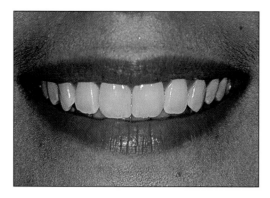

Fig 3-26 A smile that demonstrates the principle of gradation. The maxillary central incisor is visually the widest tooth, followed by the lateral incisor, the canine, and so on distally. The distal half of the canine must not be visible when viewed from the front to maintain the principle of gradation.

Outline Form of Maxillary Canines

The distal half of the maxillary canine should not be visible when viewed from the front[7] (Fig 3-26). As the eye moves laterally from the midline, each tooth should appear proportionately narrower than its mesial neighbor. This is termed the *principle of gradation*.[5] After placement of porcelain restorations on the maxillary teeth, the most common offender of this principle is the canine tooth. It appears too wide in relation to both the lateral incisor and the first premolar because the mesiodistal height of contour is too distal.

Correct placement of the mesiodistal height of contour on the facial surface of canine restorations involves the skills of both the dentist and the laboratory technician. First, the dentist must remove sufficient tooth structure on the distofacial half of the tooth to allow the technician to create the correct facial contours. Second, the technician must visualize the case from the front during final contouring of the restorations to ensure that the principle of gradation is heeded.

Color

In dentistry, color is described in four dimensions. *Hue* is the basic color of the tooth and is usually in the yellow range. *Chroma* is the saturation or intensity of the hue. *Value* is a measure of the brightness of the tooth; a high-value tooth appears bright while a low-value tooth appears darker. Finally, *maverick colors* are concentrated areas of color that are different from the overall background color.

Natural teeth are polychromatic. They generally have higher chroma in the gingival third, transitioning to a lower chroma and higher value in the middle third. The incisal third is characterized by the transition to incisal translucency, which is commonly framed by the halo effect (see Fig 3-22). Maverick colors can appear anywhere, and they individualize the tooth.

The chroma of the maxillary lateral incisor is commonly the same as that of the central incisor; however, the value of the lateral incisor is commonly slightly lower. In the maxillary canine, the chroma is generally higher, especially in the gingival third, and the value is lower. Incisal translucency is usually minimal in the maxillary canine, and seldom does the halo effect occur.

Polychromicity in the individual tooth and between neighboring teeth is essential in porcelain restorations if natural beauty is the goal.

Color Modifiers

It has been stated that hair color, skin color, and lipstick color all significantly affect shade selection when restorations are being placed in the esthetic zone.[11] Of these modifiers, skin color is by far the most important. A given tooth shade will look lighter and higher in value in a patient with darker skin. Conversely, the same tooth shade will appear yellower and lower in value in a patient with very light skin.

When choosing a tooth shade for a patient with variable skin color, for instance, a Caucasian patient with a deep tan, the impact of the skin color must be discussed with the patient prior to treatment. If porcelain restorations are placed while the skin is tanned, the restorations will appear to become more yellow and lower in value as the skin color lightens.

Image

The overall presentation of the smile can be described as the *image*. Miller[8] discusses the differences between the "natural image" and the "media image." With the media image, the teeth are generally more symmetric, monochromatic, and very high in value. The natural image incorporates asymmetries, polychromicity, and lower value with higher chroma. Dentists commonly make esthetic choices for patients based on their own notions of beauty rather than on the patient's desires.[15] When restoring maxillary anterior teeth, it is essen-

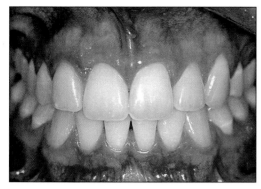

Fig 3-27 Young teeth demonstrate higher value, lower chroma, higher surface texture, and lower luster.

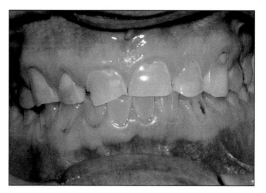

Fig 3-28 Older teeth demonstrate lower value, higher chroma, lower surface texture, and higher luster.

tial that the dentist understand the overall image that the patient desires.

To maximize predictability when placing anterior restorations, the issue of overall smile presentation first must be developed to the patient's satisfaction in the provisional restorations.

Age Characteristics of Teeth

Both tooth color and surface texture relate information about the age of the patient (Figs 3-27 and 3-28).

Chroma and Value

The value, or brightness, of a tooth is higher in young patients and decreases with age. Conversely, the chroma, or color saturation, is lower in young patients and increases with age.[4]

Surface Texture

Surface texture is higher in the young patient and decreases as the patient ages.[4] The surface luster is a function of the amount of surface texture. Therefore, the young tooth with greater surface texture has a lower luster. As the surface texture is worn away with age, the surface luster increases.

It is important to communicate with the laboratory technician about texture and luster. For example, porcelain veneers with low value, low surface texture, and high luster are not appropriate for a 25-year-old patient.

Individual Tooth Length and Proportion

The maxillary central incisor is the centerpiece of the smile. The average length of the maxillary central incisor is 10 to 11 mm (Figs 3-29a to 3-29c).[16] The ratio of height to width in

the maxillary central incisor should be approximately 1.2 to 1.0. In other words, the width of the central incisor should be approximately 75% of its height.[16]

When evaluating a smile, the dentist must start with the position and size of the maxillary central incisor. It is difficult, if not impossible, to develop optimum esthetics with short maxillary anterior teeth.

Tooth-to-Tooth Proportions

The principle of gradation[5] states that as the eye moves laterally from the midline, each tooth should appear proportionately narrower than its mesial neighbor. There has been much discussion about what this mesiodistal proportion should be. The golden proportion (1.618:1.0), which was formulated as one of Euclid's elements, has been proposed.[17] Viewed from the front, the maxillary central incisor would be 1.618 times wider than the lateral incisor, the lateral incisor would be 1.618 times wider than the visual width of the canine, and so on as the eye moves distally. However, developing esthetic proportions is not that simple. In a patient with a very tapered maxillary arch, the maxillary central incisors will appear wide, and the teeth may approximate the golden proportion. However, in a patient with a very square maxillary arch form, the golden proportion would result in unesthetically wide central incisors. To some degree, the width of the central incisor, in relation to the lateral incisor, is also a matter of personal taste. The golden proportion produces very bold central incisors,[5,18] which appeals to some individuals. However, in natural teeth situated in natural arch forms, the golden proportion seldom occurs. The natural proportion of the width of the maxillary central incisor to the lateral incisor, when measured with a caliper, is approximately 1.2 to 1.0.[15] The golden proportion

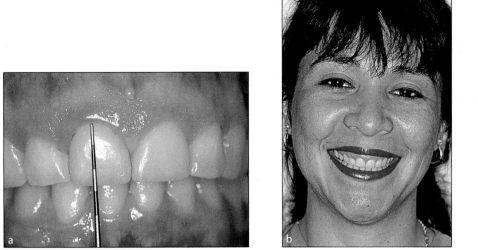

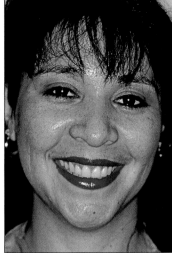

Figs 3-29a and 3-29b Short maxillary central incisor measuring 8 mm due to altered passive eruption.

Fig 3-29c After esthetic crown lengthening to treat altered passive eruption.

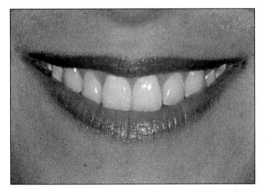

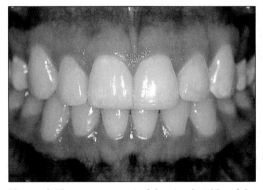

Fig 3-30a Note the beauty and proportionality of this natural smile.

Fig 3-30b The measurement of the visual widths of the maxillary central incisor and maxillary lateral incisor reveals a natural proportion of central incisor to lateral incisor of 1.4 to 1.0.

is not based on actual tooth measurements, but on the tooth proportions when viewed from the front. This proportion is approximately 1.4 to 1.0 in nature (Figs 3-30a and 3-30b).

Because dental esthetics is a matter of taste, the ultimate decision on widths and proportions must be developed in provisional restorations.

Principle of Illumination

Visually, light objects are perceived to approach the viewer and dark objects to recede from the viewer.[5] This principle must be considered when high value porcelain or resin composite restorations are placed only on maxillary anterior teeth, because the result may be an unesthetic visual separation of the anterior and posterior teeth. A visual coupling of the front and back of the mouth may require placement of restorations on one or more maxillary premolars (Figs 3-31a and 3-31b).

Law of the Face

The face of a tooth is that portion of the facial surface bound by transitional line angles when viewed from the front.[4] To make teeth of dissimilar widths appear similar, the apparent faces should be made equal.

To make an anterior tooth appear wider, the transitional facial line angles are moved into the interproximal facial embrasures. Conversely, to make an anterior tooth appear narrower, the transitional line angles are moved closer to the tooth midline (Figs 3-32a to 3-32d).

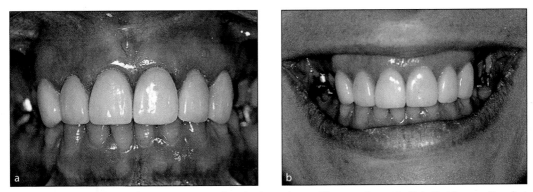

Figs 3-31a and 3-31b Porcelain veneers were placed only on the maxillary anterior teeth. Note that the maxillary first premolars are virtually invisible when viewed from the front. This results in a loss of visual coupling of the front and the back of the mouth. Note also lower lip asymmetry.

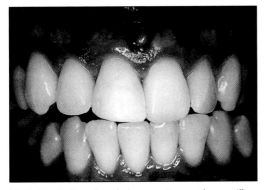

Fig 3-32a A direct bonded restoration on the maxillary right central incisor appears too wide.

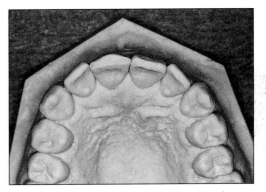

Fig 3-32b The cast of the patient in Fig 3-32a demonstrates that the mesiofacial and distofacial transitional line angles are too far into the facial embrasures, resulting in a visual widening of the tooth.

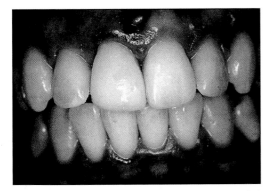

Fig 3-32c After replacement of the direct bonded restoration on the right central incisor. The tooth now appears narrower.

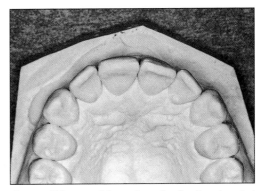

Fig 3-32d The cast of the patient after the direct bonded restoration was replaced. Note the narrower appearance of the tooth because the mesiofacial and distofacial transitional line angles are closer together.

Conclusion

The provision of esthetic and functional restorative dentistry must be based on a set of guidelines founded on the best clinical science available. These guidelines can then be used to determine a patient's overall orofacial presentation and to guide the diagnostic waxup. Based on the diagnostic waxup, the provisional restorations are fabricated and placed. It is at this point that the "eye of the artist" becomes helpful for developing the final shade, shape, contour, and incisal edge configuration of the provisional restorations, which will serve as the blueprint for the final restorations.

References

1. Proffitt WM. Contemporary Orthodontics, ed 2. St Louis: Mosby, 1992:150.
2. Peck S, Peck L, Kataja M. The gingival smile line. Angle Orthod 1992;62:91–100.
3. Vig RG, Brundo GC. The kinetics of anterior tooth display. J Prosthet Dent 1978;39:502–504.
4. Heymann HO. The artistry of conservative esthetic dentistry. J Am Dent Assoc 1987;(special issue):14E–22E.
5. Lombardi RE. The principles of visual perception and their clinical application to denture esthetics. J Prosthet Dent 1973;29:358–382.
6. Brisman AS. Esthetics: A comparison of dentists' and patients' concepts. J Am Dent Assoc 1980;100:345–352.
7. Williams HA, Caughman WF. Principles of esthetic dentistry: Practical guidelines for the practitioner. In: Clark JW (ed). Clinical Dentistry. New York: Harper & Row, 1976:1–20.
8. Miller CJ. The smile line as a guide to anterior esthetics. Dent Clin North Am 1989;33:157–164.
9. Tjan AHJ, Miller GD, The JGP. Some esthetic factors in a smile. J Prosthet Dent 1984;51:24–28.
10. Allen EP. Surgical crown lengthening for function and esthetics. Dent Clin North Am 1993;37:163–179.
11. Pound E. Applying harmony in selecting and arranging teeth. J Am Dent Assoc 1957;55:181–191.
12. Croll BM. Emergence profiles in natural tooth contour. Part 1: Photographic observations. J Prosthet Dent 1989;62:4–10.
13. Frush JP, Fisher RD. Introduction to dentogenic restorations. J Prosthet Dent 1955;5:586–595.
14. Frush JP, Fisher RD. How dentogenic restorations interpret the sex factor. J Prosthet Dent 1956;6:160–172.
15. Goldstein R. Study of need for esthetics in dentistry. J Prosthet Dent 1969;21:589–598.
16. Gillen RJ, Schwartz RS, Hilton TJ, Evans DB. An analysis of selected normative tooth proportions. Int J Prosthodont 1994;7:410–417.
17. Levin EI. Dental esthetics and the golden proportion. J Prosthet Dent 1978;40:244–252.
18. Preston JD. The golden proportion revisited. J Esthet Dent 1993;5:247–251.

Caries Management: Diagnosis and Treatment Strategies

J. Peter van Amerongen
Cor van Loveren
Edwina A. M. Kidd

Traditional caries management has consisted of the detection of caries lesions followed by immediate restoration. In other words, caries was managed primarily by restorative dentistry. However, when the dentist takes the bur in hand, an irreversible process begins. Placing a restoration does not guarantee a sound future for the tooth; on the contrary, it may be the start of a restorative cycle in which the restoration will be replaced several times. The decision to initiate invasive treatment should be preceded by a number of questions: Is a lesion present, and if so, how far does it extend? Is the caries active or not? Is a restoration required, or could the process be arrested by noninvasive treatments? Sometimes the decision to restore may be based on questionable diagnostic criteria.[1]

The introduction of adhesive restorative materials has allowed dentists to make smaller preparations, which has led to preservation of hard dental tissues and, along with declining disease prevalence, has allowed elimination of Black's principle of "extension for prevention." Maximum tooth structure is preserved. However, this approach, sometimes described as a "dynamic treatment concept," does not prevent repeated treatment procedures and the occurrence of iatrogenic damage (Fig 4-1).

The recommended treatment strategy is based on a proper diagnosis of caries, taking into account the dynamics of the caries process. The activity of caries should be determined, and causative factors should be evaluated. Caries risk should be assessed before treatment is considered, and treatment should include

regimens to arrest the caries process by redressing the imbalance between demineralization and remineralization.[2]

The treatment goal in caries management should be to prevent new lesions from forming and to detect lesions sufficiently early in the process so that they can be treated and arrested by nonoperative means.[2] Such management requires skill and is time-consuming and worthy of appropriate compensation. If these attempts fail, high-quality restorative dentistry will be required to restore the integrity of the tooth surface.

Etiology

The factors involved in the caries process, which include the tooth, dental plaque, and diet, were presented in the 1960s in a model of overlapping circles.[3] Since then, the model has been supplemented with the factors of time, fluoride, saliva, and social and demographic factors (Fig 4-2). At first sight, these circles constitute a simple model to explain caries risk, which is represented by the overlap of the three inner circles. When one of the risk factors increases, the respective circle becomes larger, as does the overlap of the circles, indicating increased caries risk. If there is, for instance, hyposalivation, the saliva circle will tighten the three inner circles, enlarging the overlap, again indicating a greater risk. Inversely, the model explains why reduction in any risk factor decreases caries risk.

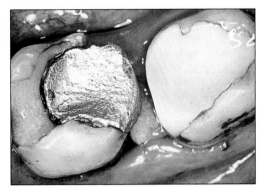

Fig 4-1 Iatrogenic damage caused by repeated treatment procedures.

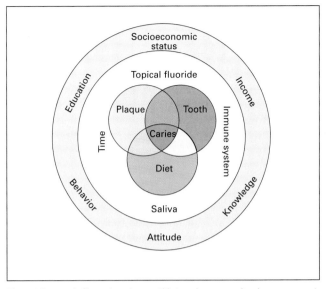

Fig 4-2 Factors influencing the equilibrium between the three prerequisites for the caries process as first described by Keyes and Jordan.[3]

Dental Plaque

The prevalence of mutans streptococci and lactobacilli is associated with dental caries.[4–6] *Streptococcus mutans* is involved in caries lesion formation from its initiation, while lactobacilli flourish in a carious environment and contribute to caries progression. Dental plaque may be more cariogenic locally where mutans streptococci and lactobacilli are concentrated, but in everyday practice it is difficult for the dentist to identify cariogenic plaque to make this knowledge useful in treating individual patients. Plaque can be sampled and mutans streptococci and lactobacilli can be quantified, but the procedure is quite complicated and requires the support of a microbiologic laboratory. It is easier to count mutans streptococci and lactobacilli in saliva, and kits are commercially available for this purpose. However, these counts do not give site-specific information and are poor predictors for high caries activity in general, although low counts or absence of mutans streptococci are good predictors of low caries activity.[7]

High numbers of mutans streptococci and lactobacilli are probably the consequence of a high sugar intake and the resulting periods of low pH levels in dental plaque.[8,9] Inversely, it has been shown that restriction of sugar intake reduces the numbers of mutans streptococci and lactobacilli.[8,10] In one study of individuals complying with a Weight Watchers diet, the numbers of mutans streptococci and lactobacilli were reduced by half.[11] A comparable reduction was found in subjects who reduced their sugar intake frequency from 7.2 to 1.8 times a day.[12] Interestingly, after a period of sugar restric-

tion, the pH response to glucose was reduced in buccal[13] but not in interdental plaque.[12] Apparently, the reductions in numbers of mutans streptococci and lactobacilli are insufficient to reduce the acidogenicity of interdental plaque.[12]

The oral flora colonizes on teeth continuously, but it takes up to several days before the dental plaque contains enough acidogenic bacteria to lower plaque pH to the level that causes demineralization.[14] Theoretically, plaque removal every second day would be sufficient. If the dentition is professionally cleaned, an even lower frequency of home-care cleaning has been demonstrated to prevent caries.[15,16] But we have only to consider the caries prevalence in the prefluoride era to realize that few people are capable of cleaning their teeth to a level adequate to prevent caries.

Teeth

Teeth consist of a calcium phosphate mineral that demineralizes when the environmental pH lowers. As the environmental pH recovers, dissolved calcium and phosphate can reprecipitate on remaining mineral crystals. This process is called *remineralization*. Remineralization is a slower process than demineralization. When remineralization is given enough time, it can eliminate the damage done during demineralization, but in the absence of this the caries process will progress and a lesion will develop. Dentin is more vulnerable than enamel because of structural differences and impurities in the lattice. For many years, much emphasis was given to the preeruptive effect of fluoride improving the quality of the dental hard tissues. However, it is now clear that posteruptive use of fluoride is far more protective against caries.[17–19]

Diet

Dietary carbohydrates are necessary for the bacteria to produce the acids that initiate demineralization. In general, dietary advice for caries prevention is based on three principles: (1) the drop in pH lasts for approximately 30 minutes; (2) the frequency of intake is more important than the quantity; and (3) the stickiness of foods is an important factor in their cariogenicity. It has become obvious, however, from many epidemiologic studies that where fluoride is used daily, sugar consumption and caries prevalence have become independent for many individuals. Even when there was a significant correlation between sugar consumption and caries prevalence, the caries-preventive effect of sugar restriction was small. For instance, in Basel, Switzerland, wartime restriction reduced sugar supply from about 40 to 16 kg per person per year, but the number of caries-free children rose only from approximately 3% to 15%.[20,21] At that time, the improvement seemed impressive, but it was dwarfed by the effect of nationwide use of fluoride. With this evidence, the role of dietary counseling in caries prevention should be reexamined. This does not negate the value of diet analysis and advice for patients presenting with multiple carious lesions, but the importance of the proper use of fluoride should also be emphasized.

Information gathered with the reliable pH-telemetry method has revealed that a pH drop induced by eating may last for hours if there is no stimulation of the salivary flow.[14,22,23] Even the consumption of an apple can depress the pH for 2 hours or longer.[14] Long pH depressions will be most prevalent in areas where saliva has little or no access, and these areas are the most caries-prone. It is unknown how much additional harm is caused by a second sugar intake during such a period of low pH or how beneficial it is to omit a second sugar intake during that period. Foods believed to be "good" for teeth may not be better than foods that are supposedly "bad." A chocolate and caramel bar might be considered bad because it feels sticky. In reality, however, the caramel dissolves and leaves the mouth relatively quickly, whereas potato chips, generally considered less harmful, take a longer time to clear the mouth.[24] During this retention, the carbohydrate fraction may be hydrolyzed to simple sugars, providing a substrate for the acidogenic bacteria.[25]

All the uncertainties about the determinants of the cariogenicity of foods make it impossible to provide strict dietary guidelines. To snack in moderation, limited to 3 or 4 snacks a day, is the only wise recommendation.

Time

Time affects the caries process in several ways. When caries was commonly considered to be a chronic disease, time was introduced to indicate that the substrate (dietary sugars) must be present for a sufficient length of time to cause demineralization.[26] Now we know that caries is not a chronic disease and that its effects can be arrested or completely repaired if enough time is given for remineralization. Finally, it is clear that caries lesions do not develop overnight, but take time; in fact, it may take years for cavitation to occur. This potentially gives the dentist and the patient ample time for preventive treatment strategies.

Fluoride

Experiments have shown that fluoride protects enamel more effectively when it is present in the ambient solution during acid challenges than when it is incorporated into the enamel lattice.[17] The mechanism by which fluoride inhibits demineralization is reprecipitation of dissolved calcium and phosphate, which prevents these constituents from being leached out of the enamel into the plaque and saliva.[19] Part of the reprecipitation takes place at the surface of the tooth. This narrows the pores in the enamel surface that provide diffusion pathways for the acids produced in the dental plaque to penetrate into the enamel. Acid penetration is thus hampered. In addition, during periods where the ambient pH is higher than 5.5, fluoride will facilitate remineralization, promoting lesion arrest and repair. A lack of fluoride constitutes a caries risk.

The retention of fluoride in the mouth is site-specific. In plaque and saliva and in dentin samples fixed in dental splints, most fluoride was found on the labial surfaces of maxillary incisors and buccal surfaces in the mandibular molar region after rinsing with a fluoride solution.[27,28] In addition, it was observed that fluoride from passively dissolving fluoride tablets remained highly concentrated only at the site of tablet dissolution. There was very little or no transport of fluoride between the right and the left sides of the mouth and between the maxillary and mandibular arches.[27] Because of this, localized caries lesions in the mouth may be related to an insufficient spread of fluoride when subjects use fluoride toothpaste. Certainly, when patients use fluoride toothpaste they should be encouraged to spit out any excess rather than to rinse vigorously with water.

Saliva

The important role of saliva is clearly demonstrated by the rampant caries that may occur in subjects with compromised

Table 4-1 Percentages of 6- and 12-year-old caries-free children and mean dmfs and DMFS scores in children who were not caries free in 1989, 1993, and 1996, according to socioeconomic level[29]

	6-year-old children					12-year-old children				
Socioeconomic status	%	d	m	f	dmf ± SD	%	D	M	F	DMF ± SD
Low										
1989	43	4.7	0.6	2.8	8.2 ± 8.5	46	0.2	0.0	3.4	3.6 ± 2.2
1993	39	4.8	0.3	2.7	7.8 ± 9.0	67	0.1	0.0	3.9	4.0 ± 3.1
1996	49	5.0	1.1	3.5	9.6 ± 9.8	50	0.1	0.0	3.1	3.2 ± 2.4
Medium										
1989	60	3.4	0.8	1.3	5.5 ± 6.9	49	0.2	0.1	3.5	3.9 ± 2.7
1993	69	4.0	0.3	1.4	5.8 ± 7.5	61	0.3	0.0	2.5	2.8 ± 1.9
1996	79	3.7	0.9	0.4	4.9 ± 5.3	89	0.0	0.0	3.6	3.6 ± 2.6
High										
1989	77	1.5	0.0	0.6	2.1 ± 1.3	59	0.9	0.2	1.8	2.9 ± 2.0
1993	77	2.5	0.2	1.7	4.4 ± 3.5	63	0.3	0.0	1.7	2.1 ± 1.6
1996	84	1.6	0.9	2.2	4.7 ± 5.1	86	0.3	0.0	2.0	2.3 ± 2.1

dmfs = decayed, missing, or filled surfaces in primary teeth; DMFS = decayed, missing, or filled surfaces in permanent teeth.

Table 4-2 Time line of strongest clinical predictors of caries incidence[7]

	Age (y)						
	0 and 1	2–5	6–9	10–13	14–21	22–45	> 45
Dentition	Primary	Primary	Mixed dentition	Mixed dentition	Early permanent	Mature permanent	Mature permanent and gingival recession
Predictor*	Mutans streptococci	**dmfs, especially primary incisors;** mutans streptococci and lactobacilli	**dmfs, especially primary molars;** first molar occlusal morphology; DMFS	**DMFS, especially first permanent molars;** first molar occlusal morphology; incipient smooth surface lesions	**Incipient smooth surface lesions;** DMFS	Not studied	Coronal and root DMFS; number of teeth; periodontal disease

dmfs = decayed, missing, or filled surfaces in primary teeth; DMFS = decayed, missing, or filled surfaces in permanent teeth.
*The strongest predictors are in bold.

salivary flow. These subjects lack the protective qualities of saliva, of which the flow rate and buffering capacity may be the most important. Both help to neutralize and clear the acids and carbohydrates from dental plaque. Clearance, however, is not uniform throughout the mouth and may be slowest at the labial aspects of the maxillary incisors and buccal aspects of the mandibular molars. Other sites in the dentition may not be easily accessible to saliva as a result of an individual's anatomy, including interproximal spaces and fissures. Dental plaque in a cavitated area of a tooth may also be protected from salivary clearance.

The sites that are difficult for saliva to reach may also be difficult to reach with mechanical cleaning devices, such as a toothbrush or dental floss. Plaque and food may adhere for long periods of time in these areas, making these sites more prone to caries. Furthermore, this caries risk factor may be easily overlooked in children, whose teeth appear to be clean as judged from the sites that are easily cleaned. These children may even brush their teeth twice daily and have only a moderate number of sugar intake episodes per day. The most feasible way to prevent caries lesions at these sites is by thorough oral hygiene measures and use of a fluoride-containing toothpaste so that plaque is removed and fluoride is applied.

Social and Demographic Factors

Many studies have shown that, at least in the western world, dental caries is more prevalent in lower socioeconomic categories, in less affluent areas, and among some ethnic minorities (Table 4-1).[29] Differences related to the socioeconomic status are very clear for the primary dentition and less clear for the permanent dentition, although this pattern may differ in other parts of the world. Studies have shown that for the prediction of caries lesion development, social and demographic factors may be successful in very young children without a long dental history, but for older children, clinical parameters are more predictive.[30,31] In the elderly population, however, root caries lesion development again seems to be more prevalent in people from lower socioeconomic backgrounds.

Caries Prediction

To make the most appropriate treatment decisions, a good estimate of the caries risk is necessary. Indicators of past caries experience are the strongest predictors, and the status of the most recently erupted or exposed surfaces is a strong predictor for the newly emerging surfaces. One very elegant review plots the strongest clinical predictors against age and dentition (Table 4-2).[7] The sensitivity and specificity of the predictors varied from 0.60 to 0.80, indicating that 20% to 40% of the children who developed caries lesions during the study were not identified as being at high risk for caries and that 20% to 40% of the children who were not caries active were, in contrast, predicted to develop caries lesions. In addition, it is important to recognize that none of the studies in the review were designed to predict the progression rate of carious demineralization at a specific site. So, even if it could be predicted that an individual would develop caries lesions, the lesion that is going to progress cannot be confidently identified.

Rate of Caries Lesion Progression

The decline in caries prevalence has been accompanied by a change in lesion behavior. Caries lesions progress more slowly than they did several decades ago, probably due to increased use of fluoride, which delays lesion progression. It is clear that the progression rate is not the same for each site. Little is known about the progression rate of fissure caries lesions. Longitudinal epidemiologic data from the 1950s, when fluoride was not yet widely used, showed that it took approximately 1 year for an enamel fissure lesion to develop into a dentinal lesion.[32] More recent data from the same geographic area, after the introduction of fluoride toothpaste, showed that 50% of the enamel fissure lesions had progressed to involve dentin within 2 years while 75% had become dentinal lesions after 4 years.[33] Data from Switzerland showed that, for permanent first molars, approximately 10%, 20%, and 45%, respectively, of sound fissures, fissures with a yellowish discoloration, and fissures with a dark discoloration progressed to carious dentin or tooth restoration in 4 years.[34] These progression rates were slightly lower than those found by the same investigators 10 years earlier. It is the experience of many clinicians that not all initial fissure

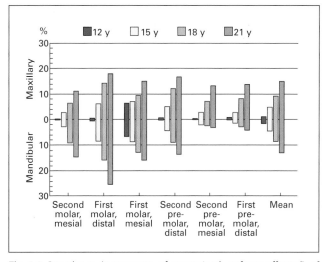

Fig 4-3 Prevalence (percentage of approximal surfaces affected) of dentinal lesions in the respective approximal surfaces in different age groups. (Data from Mejàre et al.[41])

lesions will develop to involve the dentin, but that a number of them may become arrested. In populations in which not all fissure lesions develop into open cavities, the dentist will be confronted with clinically undetected carious dentin at the base of occlusal fissures. This is not a new phenomenon; it was discussed as early as 1931.[35] Today, reported prevalence rates vary greatly.[36,37]

Based on epidemiologic data from the 1950s, the progression rates of proximal caries lesions from initial enamel lesions to involve dentin in the permanent dentition was estimated to be 2 years at age 7 and approximately 4 years at age 12.[32] Data collected after fluoride supplementation became available showed a progression rate of 3 to 4 years for proximal caries lesions to reach the dentin in 12-year-olds.[38] Shwartz et al[39] concluded from data collected in Sweden and the United States that it takes an average of 4 years for caries lesions to progress through the proximal enamel of permanent teeth. The progression rate seemed to be independent of the number of decayed, missing, or filled surfaces (DMFS) of the individuals.

Not all caries lesions progress, however. In one study, more than 50% of initial proximal caries lesions in 13-year-old children had not advanced during a 3-year period.[40] The majority of the lesions that progressed were found in the children who had the highest number of lesions at the start of the study, which probably reflects the difference between caries-active and caries-inactive children. Recently, Mejàre et al[41] published data on the caries lesion prevalence on the proximal surfaces of the posterior teeth at various ages (Fig 4-3). The prevalence was low, with the distal surfaces of the first molars being the most prone to developing caries lesions.

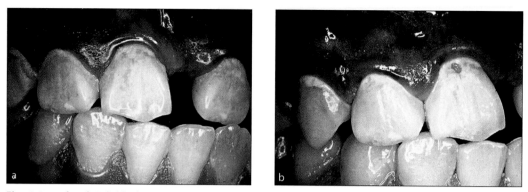

Figs 4-4a and 4-4b Reliable detection of caries lesions can be obstructed by plaque. *(a)* Plaque covers labial surfaces and conceals a cavity in the maxillary right central incisor. *(b)* The same surface, cleaned, reveals the cavitated lesion. (Courtesy of K. R. Ekstrand.)

Caries lesions on free smooth surfaces seem to progress more slowly than on proximal surfaces or in fissures. Many lesions do not progress into the dentin and even show regression to sound enamel.[32,42–44] In one study, dentists were asked at what point they would treat small noncavitated lesions on the buccal surfaces of teeth. Approximately 40% indicated that they would use a preventive rather than an operative strategy.[45] This indicates that many dentists believe that they are well able to judge the severity of buccal lesions and to monitor lesion development.

Altogether, the evidence indicates that the decline in caries prevalence has been accompanied by a decline in caries lesion progression rates. Between the initiation of caries and the involvement of dentin in the caries process, there is ample time for a preventive management strategy. This implies that the early lesion should be detected so that preventive treatment can arrest its progress and bring about remineralization. If this strategy is successful, operative intervention will not be required.

Detection and Diagnosis

When a dentist identifies a caries lesion, it is a change in mineral content that is detected. The dentist must also determine whether the lesion is active or arrested before a logical management plan can be proposed; the dynamics of the caries process must be recognized.[2]

Detection

Teeth must be clean for the clinical detection of caries lesions. Otherwise, reliable detection may be obstructed by the presence of plaque (Figs 4-4a and 4-4b). The teeth are cleaned and an air/water syringe used so that the tooth surface may be dried. This drying has two functions: the first is to remove saliva, which can obscure a lesion; the second is to dry a white spot lesion. Removing water from the porous tissue in this way enables the dentist to gauge how far through the enamel a lesion has progressed. A white spot lesion visible on a wet tooth surface indicates that demineralization is over halfway through the enamel, possibly extending into dentin. A white spot lesion that becomes visible only after thorough air-drying will be less than halfway through enamel.

The dentist also requires bite-wing radiographs to assist in the detection of proximal caries lesions, occlusal caries lesions, and recurrent caries. The radiographs should be obtained using a film holder and beam-aiming device to take the guesswork out of tube alignment and allow comparable views to be taken on subsequent occasions. Because lesions confined to enamel on radiographs should be managed by preventive treatment, monitoring them is important.

Pit and Fissure Lesions

Detection of carious structure in fissures and pits is most often performed by visual inspection. Good lighting and dry, clean teeth are prerequisites. It appears that any sign of visible cavitation in the occlusal surface corresponds to progression of the lesion into the dentin.[46,47] When occlusal surface caries was recorded visually using a caries score ranking system (Table 4-3), a high correlation with the histologic depth of the lesions into enamel and dentin was found (Table 4-4).[48,49]

A clear, ranked caries lesion scoring system is useful for subsequent assessment and monitoring. Careful examination of bite-wing radiographs is also important, although enamel lesions will not be visible. Carious dentin, however, can usually be detected, and such lesions are often large (Fig 4-5). Bite-wing radiographs can be considered to provide a safety-

Table 4-3	Criteria for visual examination of caries lesions[5,6]	
Score	**Criteria**	
0	No or slight change in enamel translucency after prolonged air drying (> 5 s)	
1	Opacity or discoloration hardly visible on the wet surface but distinctly visible after air drying	
2	Opacity or discoloration distinctly visible without air drying	
3	Localized enamel breakdown in opaque or discolored enamel and/or grayish discoloration from the underlying dentin	
4	Cavitation in opaque or discolored enamel, exposing the dentin	

Table 4-4	Criteria for the histologic examination of fissure caries lesions[5,6]	
Score	**Criteria**	
0	No enamel demineralization or a narrow surface zone of opacity (edge phenomenon)	
1	Enamel demineralization limited to the outer half of the enamel layer	
2	Demineralization involving enamel and outer third of the dentin	
3	Demineralization involving the middle third of the dentin	
4	Demineralization involving the pulpal third of the dentin	

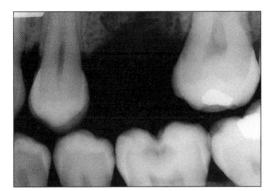

Fig 4-5 The radiograph as "safety net": Occlusal carious dentin is well detected (mandibular left first molar).

Table 4-5	Criteria for the radiographic examination of fissure caries lesions[5,6]	
Score	**Criteria**	
0	No radiolucency visible	
1	Radiolucency visible in the enamel	
2	Radiolucency visible in the dentin but restricted to the outer third of the dentin	
3	Radiolucency extending to the middle third of the dentin	
4	Radiolucency in the pulpal third of the dentin	

net function for occlusal lesions.[48,50,51] For assessment and monitoring, a ranked scoring system can be used (Table 4-5).

Tactile examination of fissures with a dental explorer has been advocated for many decades (even centuries) as an important method to detect caries lesions, but research has shown this to be an unwise practice. The method is inaccurate,[52] and, worse, the explorer can damage a white spot lesion by breaking through the relatively intact surface zone (Fig 4-6).[53] Vigorous use of a sharp explorer can cause a cavity that will subsequently trap dental plaque and encourage lesion progression. Detection of fissure caries lesions should rely on sharp eyes, not sharp explorers.

Lesions Involving Proximal Surfaces

When there is contact between proximal surfaces, the radiograph is the most accurate method for detecting demineralization. In the premolar and molar regions, lesion progression or arrest can be monitored, provided that appropriate film holders and beam-aiming devices have been used to ensure

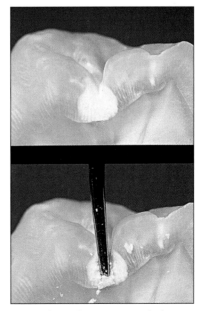

Fig 4-6 The explorer tip can easily damage white spot lesions.

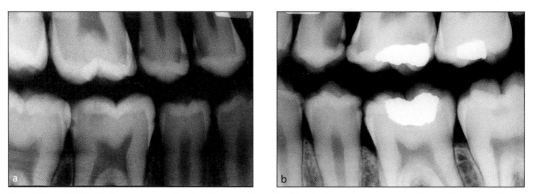

Figs 4-7a and 4-7b Radiographs showing proximal demineralizations in the outer enamel, to the dentinoenamel junction, and in the outer and inner half of dentin. (Occlusal lesions are visible on the mandibular left second molar and right first and second molars, and recurrent caries lesion under the restoration on the maxillary left first molar.)

that subsequent bite-wing radiographs are taken at approximately the same angulation.[54] The radiograph should be examined carefully to determine whether caries lesions are present in the outer enamel, at the dentinoenamel junction, in the outer half of dentin, or in the inner half of dentin (Figs 4-7a and 4-7b).

For detection of proximal lesions in anterior teeth, the fiber-optic transillumination technique is particularly appropriate and convenient.[55] With this technique, a fine light, coned down to a 0.5-mm diameter, is transmitted through a contact area. A lesion appears as a dark shadow. It is difficult, however, to discriminate between demineralization extending just into enamel and that progressing further into dentin, especially in the posterior areas.

Finally, use of an orthodontic separator has been advocated in some cases to allow the dentist to see more clearly and to gently feel for a break in the enamel surface.[56]

Lesions in Smooth, Free Surfaces

Lesions in smooth, free surfaces, whether in the enamel of the crown or the dentin of the root, can be detected easily with visual inspection. The surface to be examined must be cleaned, dried, and well illuminated.

New Detection Devices

There has been much research interest in developing electronic and optical caries diagnostic methods capable of quantifying the size of the carious lesion.[57] Electronic caries monitors are based on the principle that porous caries lesions have lower conductive values than intact tooth structures.[58] Various optical methods, including several laser systems, are also promising.[59–63]

It is an attractive concept to have a machine with a digital readout that will give a valid result and take the subjectivity

out of caries lesion detection. However, the readings must be consistent between different models of the same instrument, the same operator on different occasions, and different operators. Although these instruments cannot make the clinical judgment of lesion activity when used once, a valid and reproducible method could be used longitudinally to measure lesion progression or arrest.

The DIAGNOdent instrument (KaVo) is a laser-based instrument described here because at this moment it is one of the few commercially available modern tools to aid the diagnosis of occlusal caries. It is an adjunct to visual inspection and radiographic examination. The tip emits light and gathers fluorescent photons. The intensity of the gathered light appears to depend on bacterial porphyrins within the lesion and appears to indicate the size and depth of the caries lesion. Results seem more reliable with advanced lesions than with white spot lesions, and the instrument can be confused by staining and calculus, interpreting them as demineralized tooth structure. This serves to emphasize that any machine is an aid to diagnosis; it will not yet dispense with logical human thought.

Diagnosis

What is the difference between lesion detection and diagnosis? In the mouth, caries is a ubiquitous, natural process that does not have to progress.[64] Detecting mineral loss resulting from the caries process is only the first step. If this information is to be useful, it must be determined whether the detected lesion is arrested or active. If the lesion is arrested, no treatment is required except for esthetic or functional reasons; if the lesion is active, treatment, which may include operative dentistry, is needed to arrest lesion progression. Thus, diagnosis adds the dimension of lesion activity to detection.[65]

Table 4-6	Parameters concerning caries activity
Immediate past caries experience	Development of new lesions within a certain period of time
Progression of the lesions	Progression or arrest of previously registered lesions
Appearance of the lesions/cavities	Structure: shiny, matte, smooth, cavitated Consistency: hard, soft Moistness: wet, dry Color: white, yellow, brown, black
Location of the lesions/cavities	Lesions only on sites of predilection or on sites not normally affected by caries
Presence of plaque/gingivitis	Lesion covered or not covered by plaque; gingival inflammation near the lesion or not

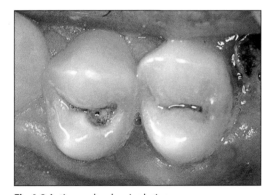

Fig 4-8 Active occlusal caries lesion.

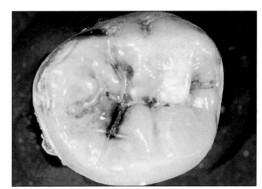

Fig 4-9 Arrested lesions.

Assessing Caries Activity

There are some features of individual lesions that indicate whether a lesion is active or arrested. Some of these features will be obvious the first time a dentist and patient meet. However, most patients see their dentist at regular intervals. Thus, the initial diagnosis can and should be refined at recall, and these visits provide the opportunity to assess the effects of preventive treatment. Has a lesion, previously diagnosed as active, apparently arrested? Table 4-6 lists some of the parameters relevant in the assessment of caries activity.

Following are discussions of the individual sites where caries may affect teeth, as well as definitions of the features of active and arrested lesions.[66] Difficulties in making this distinction are highlighted.

Occlusal lesions. The visual and radiographic features of occlusal caries lesions were presented in Tables 4-3 and 4-5. The following features indicate lesion activity:

- White spot lesions that have a matte or visibly frosted surface or are plaque covered. This can be noticed after drying or application of a disclosing solution.[67]
- Cavitated lesions, including microcavities and cavities exposing dentin (Fig 4-8).
- Lesions visible in dentin on bite-wing radiographs.[68]

The following feature indicates that the lesion may be arrested:

- White or brown spot lesions with a shiny surface (Fig 4-9)[67]

Proximal lesions. Diagnosis of lesion activity is more difficult when the adjacent tooth precludes a direct visual assessment. (The radiographic features are presented in chapter 2 and in preceding paragraphs.) The presence or absence of a cavity is relevant to lesion activity, but this unfortunately cannot be judged from the radiograph. For an active caries lesion to be

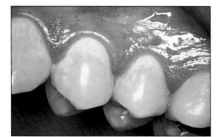

Fig 4-10 Matte, white, active cervical lesions.

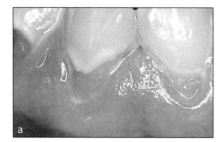

Figs 4-11a and 4-11b Cavitated, active cervical lesions.

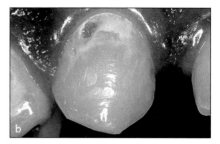

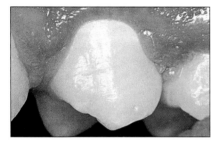

Fig 4-12 Shiny, white, arrested cervical lesion.

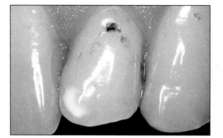

Fig 4-13 Brown, arrested lesion.

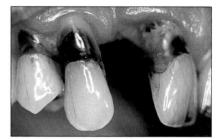

Fig 4-14 Arrested root caries lesions.

arrested, plaque must be removed regularly from the cavity, but on a proximal surface, there is no access for the toothbrush, and even the most fastidious of flossers will only skate over the surface.

The following tend to indicate lesion activity:

- A patient with proximal lesions on the radiograph who is at high risk for caries[69]
- A proximal lesion present radiographically and persistent gingival inflammation despite the patient's attempts to remove plaque with dental floss[70]
- A lesion not present at previous examination

The following features indicate that the lesion may be arrested:

- Successive, reproducible, bite-wing radiographs showing no lesion progression
- A patient who is now judged to be at low risk for caries because, following preventive treatment, he or she presents with no new lesions

Smooth, free surface lesions. These are probably the most straightforward lesions for assessing activity because they are the most visible. Of all lesions, these are the ones most likely to be arrested by preventive treatment alone. Indeed, they act as a barometer that a patient can and should monitor in the quest for dental health.

The following indicate lesion activity:

- White spot lesions close to the gingival margin that have a matte or visibly frosted surface; these are often plaque-covered (Fig 4-10).
- Cavitated, plaque-covered lesions with or without exposed dentin; if dentin is exposed and soft, the dentin is heavily infected and the lesion is active (Figs 4-11a and 4-11b).

The following indicate that the lesion is arrested:

- Shiny white or brown lesions, often well exposed due to recession; the lesions are not plaque-covered (Fig 4-12).
- Cavitated lesions, often dark brown, with hard dentin at their bases; the lesions are not plaque-covered and are often remote from the gingival margin (Fig 4-13).

Root caries. Active lesions are:

- Close to the gingival margin and plaque-covered
- Soft or leathery in consistency

Arrested lesions are:

- Often at some distance from the gingival margin and not covered with plaque (Fig 4-14)
- As hard as the surrounding healthy root surface[71]

Color is unreliable in differentiating active from inactive lesions. While arrested lesions may be dark, so may the soft dentin in some active lesions. The research community has yet to fully explain why demineralized dentin is brown.

Recurrent caries. A caries lesion at the margin of a restoration is called *recurrent caries*, and its diagnosis on various tooth surfaces is the same as that described previously for primary lesions. The bite-wing radiograph is very important in the diagnosis of recurrent caries lesions because they often form cervical to an existing proximal restoration, in the area of plaque stagnation. Lesions that are obviously in dentin as seen radiographically tend to be cavitated and active. However, research has shown that ditching and staining around an amalgam restoration[72] and staining around a tooth-colored restoration[73] are not reliable indicators of an active caries lesion beneath a restoration.

Assessing Caries Risk

Caries risk may be defined as the probability of an individual developing a certain number of caries lesions reaching a given stage of disease progression during a specified period.[74]

It is useful for the dentist to be able to assess caries risk so that preventive treatments, which are time-consuming and therefore expensive, can be targeted appropriately. Thus, the dentist might like to make the following prediction: This patient will develop new cavities within the next 12 months unless something is done to prevent it.

Because caries is a multifactorial disease, it is probably not surprising that it is difficult to predict accurately. Clinical and radiographic examination and dental history are the most important sources of information. Thus, a person with no active lesions, few or no restorations, and no history of needing restorations replaced may safely be designated as currently at low risk. On the other hand, a person with multiple active lesions, a heavily restored mouth, and a history of repeated replacement of restorations may be designated as being at high risk. This means that instead of concentrating on predicting the future, dentists should concentrate on controlling the caries lesions their patients have at present. The linchpin of the preventive approach is proper self-care, and this also helps to prevent future lesions.

In addition to clinical evidence, the following are relevant to caries risk:

- Plaque control
- Use of fluoride
- Dietary habits
- Saliva

- Medical history
- Social history

Unfortunately, none of these factors, either singly or in combination, will predict caries risk accurately.

However, identification of these risk factors as they relate to the individual patient may be of great use to the dentist in explaining the lesions that are present. This is useful because some factors need to be modified in order to reduce risk. A frequently consumed sweet drink is a good example of this. Other factors cannot be modified, and this may affect the preventive management regimen and the prognosis. For instance, a patient with reduced salivary flow due to Sjögren syndrome is, and will remain, at high risk for caries.

Identifying the Risk Factors

Dental Plaque
Dental plaque is *the* risk factor for dental caries.[75] All patients with active lesions should be shown the relationship of disclosed plaque in the mouth to the lesions that are present. This makes advice on tooth cleaning relevant to the patient and specific to the lesion.

Note should be taken of the following experimental evidence[76]:

- Fluoride concentration of toothpaste. Check that the patient is using a toothpaste containing fluoride (1,100 to 1,500 ppmF for children older than 7 years of age and adults).
- Frequency of brushing. Fluoride-containing toothpaste should be used twice a day, including last thing at night.
- Tooth brushing in children. Check that a parent or caregiver is helping a child to brush and supervising the amount of toothpaste on the brush for children younger than 7 years of age. The adult should "finish off" the brushing, paying particular attention to occlusal surfaces of erupting teeth.
- Rinsing behavior. Ask whether large volumes of water are used to wash away excess toothpaste. The message should be, "Spit, don't rinse."
- Ability to remove plaque. When plaque is disclosed, *can* the patient remove it? On a subsequent visit, *has* he or she removed plaque? The answer to the second question defines the patient's motivation rather than his or her ability with a toothbrush.

It should also be remembered that placing a dental appliance, such as an orthodontic appliance[77] or a partial denture,[78] in the mouth can encourage plaque retention and explain the development of caries lesions.

Use of Fluoride

Check the following:

- Does the patient's toothpaste contain fluoride?
- Is a fluoride-containing mouthwash being used?
- Does the patient live in an area in which the water is fluoridated?

The patient with multiple lesions is unlikely to live in an area with fluoridated water and is probably not using a fluoride-containing mouthwash. It is also possible that he or she has selected (perhaps unwittingly) a nonfluoride toothpaste.

Diet

The diet of a patient presenting with multiple lesions, whether white spots or cavities, should be analyzed for frequency of sugar intake. An inappropriate dietary habit, such as a sweet drink frequently consumed, will often be obvious.[79]

Saliva

A dry mouth predisposes to high caries risk,[80] and measuring salivary flow (stimulated and unstimulated) is useful because a low flow rate may explain multiple lesions. The four most common causes of dry mouth are:

1. Medications, such as antidepressants, antipsychotics, tranquilizers, antihypertensives, and diuretics.
2. Sjögren syndrome, which affects the salivary and lacrimal glands, leading to a dry mouth and dry eyes. Rheumatoid arthritis may indicate the presence of this disorder.
3. Eating disorders, which may induce hyposalivation; combined with a poor diet, this can lead to extensive caries.[81]
4. Radiation therapy in the region of the salivary glands for a head and neck malignancy, which often induces xerostomia.

Patients with multiple caries lesions will have high salivary counts of mutans streptococci and lactobacilli. Many research studies have shown that these counts help predict caries risk.[82] This large volume of work appears to show that, in individual patients, low counts are often good predictors of low risk, but that the opposite is not necessarily true. Therefore, the routine use of salivary counts for the prediction of risk status is not recommended.

Medical History

Medically compromised and handicapped people may be at high risk for developing caries, and the onset of such problems may explain a change in a patient's caries status.[83] For these patients, oral hygiene may be difficult, and long-term use of medicines can be a problem if the medicines are sugar-based[84] or cause reduced salivary flow.[43]

The most important caries risk factor in a medical history is the complaint of dry mouth,[43] discussed previously. It is important to realize that the medical history is a factor that can change. A vigilant dentist will detect such changes and assist the patient with the potential dental consequences.

Social History

Many studies[85,86] have shown that social deprivation can predispose to caries. Other diseases, such as coronary heart disease and some cancers, are also prevalent in socially deprived people. The dentist may notice high caries rates in siblings, and the patient or parent may possess little knowledge of dental disease. Concern about dental health may be low and dental visits irregular.

Putting It All Together

The dentist is now in a position to categorize caries risk status. The following is a possible approach[87]:

Caries Inactive/Caries Controlled

These patients present with no new lesions and need only encouragement to continue good oral hygiene with a fluoride-containing toothpaste.

Caries Active, But All Relevant Risk Factors Can Potentially Be Changed

These patients present with lesions. Mechanical plaque control should be improved and consideration given to supplementing fluoride toothpaste with mouthwashes and/or chairside fluoride applications. Where diet investigation shows multiple sugar attacks, advice should be given as to how this might be improved.

Caries Active, But Some Risk Factors Cannot Be Changed

These cases are difficult because the progress that can be made will depend very much on individual circumstances. For instance, if disability is preventing adequate plaque control, is it possible for a caregiver to help? Social deprivation and level of education may mean the preventive treatment required is not considered of sufficient importance by the patient, and it may, indeed, be unaffordable. A dry mouth is often permanent, and preventive treatments, plaque control including professional tooth cleaning, use of fluoride, dietary modification, and stimulation of salivary flow all may play a role.

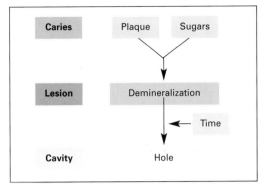

Fig 4-15 Caries presented as a one-way process.

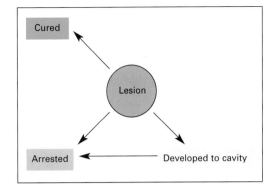

Fig 4-16 A caries lesion presented as dynamic.

Caries Active, But Some Risk Factors Have Not Been Identified

This is the most frustrating group for the dentist. Something has been missed, so the detective work must continue, and the case must be managed as with the preceding group.

Treatment Strategy

Traditionally, radiographic evidence of demineralization in enamel or to the dentinoenamel junction led to the immediate decision to place a restoration. Such management is still an accepted part of some state board examinations. However, contemporary research has shown that this is not the optimal approach. Radiographs may reveal demineralization, but this does not necessarily mean that there is an active lesion. If the lesion is arrested, it requires no treatment. The management of an active lesion should be directed to redressing the imbalance of demineralization and remineralization. This management may arrest the lesion so that a restoration is never required.

Caries is often presented as a one-way process: sugar in the presence of plaque causes demineralization that presents as a dull, white lesion. As the process progresses, a hole or cavity results (Fig 4-15). In fact, caries is a dynamic process in which periods of demineralization and remineralization alternate depending on the oral environment. It may be possible to cure or arrest an early lesion (Fig 4-16).

Caries lesions are detected at a relatively late point of development. This may be due to difficulties in detecting the early lesion or it may be because the patient did not visit the dentist early in the lesion process. Although this may suggest the value of a rigorous, invasive approach, it is preferable to select a treatment option that is as conservative as possible, because of the iatrogenic damage that may occur during preparation. Lussi and Gygax[87] showed that during the preparation of a proximal surface, the neighboring surface was damaged 100% of the time, despite very careful operating procedures.

The treatment should be based on interpretation of the activity of the lesion and on future caries risk. Figure 4-17 demonstrates a decision-making tree for occlusal fissure lesions with different features leading to different treatment options dependent upon lesion activity and risk assessment.

Although lesions that are cavitated are treated traditionally by preparation and restoration, a preventive treatment approach is often successful, especially when the lesion is in a free, smooth surface. When a lesion is present in an occlusal or proximal surface, it will often be difficult to arrest lesion progression because of the difficulty of removing plaque.

Caries is caused by a multifactorial process, and its management should reflect this.[88] The general approach to active caries should be preventive treatment,[15] including plaque control, use of fluoride, and dietary modification. Restoration makes up only one part of a strategy to facilitate plaque control.

Causal (Noninvasive or Preventive) Treatment

When causal (which includes noninvasive or preventive) treatment is considered, it is still relevant to ask what effects preventive treatment has on initial demineralized lesions and on cavities: Can they be cured (healed) or merely arrested?

Initial Lesions

Von der Fehr et al[89] and Koch[90] have shown that normal individuals can be turned into individuals with high caries risk. Within a short period of time, numerous initial caries lesions can develop when oral hygiene is withdrawn and a sugar-rich diet is offered.[89,90] However, when effective oral hygiene and

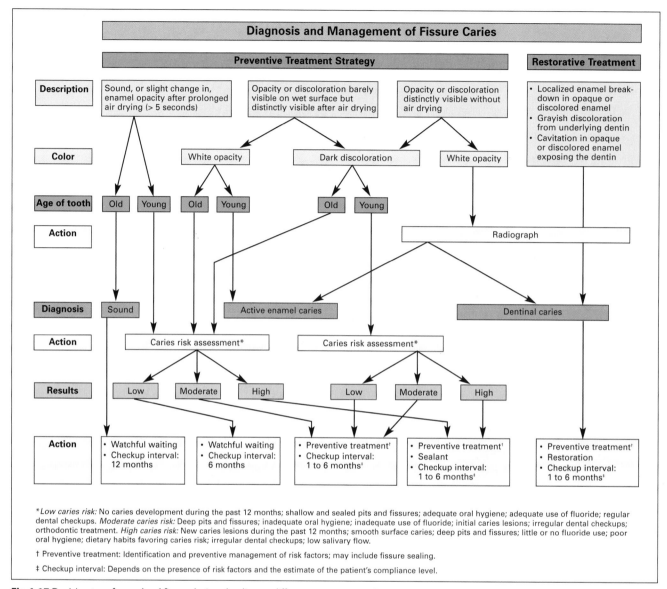

Fig 4-17 Decision tree for occlusal fissure lesions leading to different treatment options.

application of topical fluoride are instituted and a normal, less sugar-rich diet is consumed, reversal of the situation seems possible; after a period of time, the initial lesions are no longer visible. But are they healed or controlled? Thylstrup et al[91] demonstrated that in the very early lesion, only the external microsurface is dissolved by plaque. When the plaque is removed mechanically at this stage, the eroded area will change from the chalky white appearance of the earlier active lesion into a hard and shiny surface. It has been suggested that this phenomenon is caused by wear and polishing and not by recovery of the carious surface.[91]

Further progression of the lesion leads to deeper surface and subsurface dissolution. Intervening in the process with

plaque removal, fluoride application, and a better diet leads again to wear and a polished surface and a slowly remineralizing subsurface lesion.[91] Although these lesions decrease in depth and width with time, they may remain visible as shiny white lesions, commonly seen on facial surfaces. In this case, the lesion cannot be considered completely recovered, but it can be concluded that the caries process has ceased. These arrested lesions may be seen throughout life as whitish or brownish "scar tissue" (Figs 4-18a and 4-18b). Research has shown that these areas are more resistant to a subsequent caries attack than sound enamel.

The average speed of progression of caries lesions on different surfaces has been determined.[92,93] On proximal and

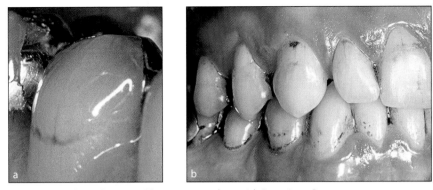

Figs 4-18a and 4-18b Arrested lesions seen as brownish "scar tissue."

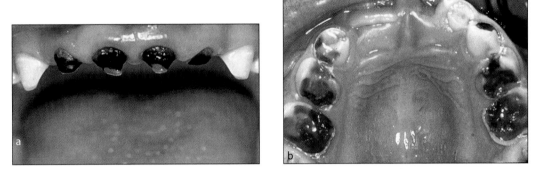

Figs 4-19a and 4-19b Arrested caries lesions in the primary dentition.

free, smooth areas, caries proceeds slowly. It is thus reasonable to postpone restorative intervention. A procedure whereby the patient is examined regularly ("watchful waiting") creates the opportunity for arrest and remineralization. "Watchful waiting" implies that nothing is done, but in fact it is based on the intellectual decision not to restore because of knowledge of the caries process. The dentist is performing active preventive treatment by helping the patient to improve oral hygiene, by applying fluoride, and by encouraging the patient to modify his or her diet. These measures should always be carried out when active noncavitated lesions exist. But what should be done when further progression has led to a cavity?

Cavitated Lesions

Several authors have shown that when an occlusal lesion has cavitated, the dentin is always involved in the process.[46,47] Moreover, these lesions, mostly detectable on radiographs, contain many microorganisms and are therefore considered active.[48–51,59]

It is not difficult to imagine that measures directed to a thorough removal of plaque are ineffective on the occlusal surface because the bristles of the toothbrush cannot get into the undermined cavity. Proximal cavitations are also difficult to reach. Dental floss will skim the surface but will not have access to the cavitated area. However, where there are cavitated areas on free, smooth surfaces, the situation is different. Those areas are easily reached by the toothbrush but may be difficult to clean due to undermining of the enamel. Removal of the overhanging enamel margins must be considered to aid in keeping the whole area free of plaque. Cavities in these surfaces, cleaned twice daily with a fluoride toothpaste, can be arrested and converted into leathery or hard lesions[66,94] (see Figs 4-13 and 4-14). When the activity of highly infected caries lesions is decreased and finally arrested, the carious layers contain few bacteria that can be cultivated.[95–98] Although occlusal or proximal caries lesions cannot be approached by preventive measures alone, in primary molars this method can be successful. Therefore, undermined enamel margins should be eliminated, so that when plaque is removed, fluoride can be applied easily to the carious dentin. Under ideal conditions, carious dentitions can be managed so that caries is arrested and demineralization and remineralization are in equilibrium (Figs 4-19a and 4-19b).

Preventive Management Strategies

The most plausible explanation for the decline of caries prevalence is the steady improvement in oral hygiene, which results in regular (at least partial) removal of dental plaque, combined with a regular daily administration of fluoride, provided via toothpaste.[18,99] A recently published analysis of data derived from a sample of 1,450 preschool children studied in the British National Diet and Nutrition Survey confirmed the significant caries-inhibiting effect of tooth brushing with a fluoride dentifrice twice daily. On a population basis, sugar-containing foods and drinks were not associated with caries experience, unless children brushed once a day or less.[100] Thus, the cornerstone of any preventive strategy for the management of caries is oral self-care: twice-daily, careful cleaning of the teeth with a toothbrush and an effective fluoride toothpaste. Additionally, dental floss should be used, but patients should be instructed carefully and the frequency should be recommended individually. In areas where the water is fluoridated to optimal levels, twice-daily careful cleaning of the teeth with a fluoride toothpaste is a safe and effective preventive treatment and caries management strategy.[101–103]

If caries or caries lesion progression is not prevented, the reasons should be carefully examined (Fig 4-20). A first step in this procedure is to carefully assess the quality of the oral hygiene. If hygiene is adequate, it is appropriate to evaluate whether additional risk factors such as multiple intake episodes of sugar-containing foods and drinks are present. If so, these risks must be reduced as much as possible. In the meantime, the patient can be helped with professionally applied preventive measures such as topical application of concentrated fluoride solutions, gels, or varnishes or chlorhexidine gels or varnishes. Salivary flow can be stimulated by daily use of sugar-free chewing gum. When no additional risks can be identified, the fluoride supply must be intensified, perhaps by adding a third daily fluoride application in the form of additional brushing, mouthwash, or tablet.

If the daily oral hygiene procedures are inadequate, an attempt should be made to determine whether the problem is due to an inability to use a toothbrush or whether the patient simply is noncompliant. The dentist should apply disclosing solution to the teeth and watch as the patient demonstrates the oral hygiene procedures. If he or she is not able to remove the plaque, the patient should be taught alternative methods. Sometimes a patient can be helped by professionally applied preventive measures. If a patient is able to remove plaque but is not motivated to do so, the dentist must try to determine the reasons. The patient may not be convinced of the necessity for thorough plaque removal. This puts the dentist in the realm of behavior modification, a subject not within the scope of this textbook but an important part of dental practice.

Professionally Applied Preventive Measures

Professionally applied topical fluorides in solutions, gels, or varnishes have been shown to be effective in many clinical trials.[104,105] The effectiveness seems not to depend on the method of application, the use of additional fluoride supplements, or baseline caries prevalence. A recent meta-analysis revealed a 22% to 26% overall caries-inhibiting effect for fluoride gel treatments.[105–107] Chlorhexidine has also been successfully applied to prevent caries but is not shown to be more effective than fluoride.[107] Applications of chlorhexidine in either gel or varnish form are more laborious and less palatable than fluoride applications and must be performed every 3 to 4 months. In addition, they have been shown to reduce caries only in those who harbor 10^6 mutans streptococci or more per milliliter of saliva. To select these patients, the number of mutans streptococci should be quantified in saliva.

With the decline in caries prevalence, the professionally applied preventive treatments do not seem appropriate on a population basis. In a population with, for example, a mean caries incidence of 0.25 DMFS per year, a preventive treatment with 22% effect would theoretically save 0.055 DMFS per year per individual. In the total population, 36 treatments would be needed to prevent 1 DMFS per year. With a low caries activity, the cost-effectiveness ratio is unfavorable. Based on cost-effectiveness calculations, an individual can decide whether he or she is willing to pay for professionally applied treatments to prevent tooth decay.

Sealants

Fissures are more susceptible to caries attack than smooth surfaces because fissure anatomy favors plaque maturation and retention.[108] When active fissure caries has been diagnosed or if a high risk has been established and fissures have susceptible morphologic characteristics, sealants may be indicated (see Fig 4-17). After acid etching, a lightly filled resin fissure sealant or a flowable resin composite is used to penetrate the fissures and prevent plaque accumulation. This is especially important during the period of tooth eruption, although the application of sealants in suspect fissures is also advisable in older patients with high caries risk.[109] Advantages of fissure sealants are that no irreversible interventions are necessary, active dentin lesions inadvertently covered by the resin do not progress further, and the possible development of new lesions in other sites of the fissure is prevented. Sealants have been used successfully for many years.[110] Concern has been expressed about placement of sealants over

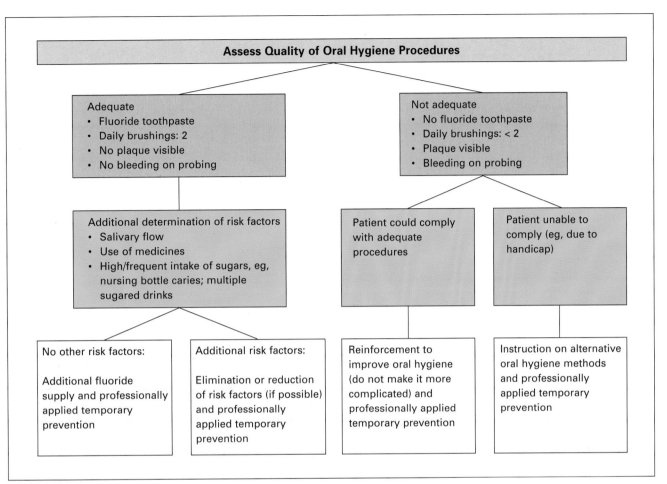

Fig 4-20 Assessment of oral hygiene procedures when caries or caries progression is not prevented.

undetected dentin caries lesions. However, there is ample evidence that caries lesions does not progress as long as the fissure remains sealed.[111–114] Sealed, radiographically evident caries lesions has been shown in one study not to progress over a 10-year period.[115,116] Also, sealed restorations placed directly over frankly cavitated lesions arrested the progress of these lesions. Sealing of restorations, therefore, appears to be very effective in conserving sound tooth structure, protecting the margins of restorations, and preventing recurrent caries.[116]

But do not forget: no sealant without reinforcement of prevention!

Symptomatic (Invasive or Restorative) Treatment

It is necessary to have well-defined criteria for the decision to restore a tooth due to caries. The most important reason for placing a restoration is to aid plaque control. Elderton and Mjör[117] formulated the following indications for restorative treatment:

- The cavitated tooth is sensitive to hot, cold, sweetness, etc.
- Occlusal and proximal lesions extend deep into dentin (and cannot be reached by the toothbrush).
- The pulp is endangered.
- Previous attempts to arrest the lesion have failed, and there is evidence that the lesion is progressing (such evidence usually requires an observation period of months or years).
- The patient's ability to provide effective home care is impaired.
- Drifting is likely to occur through loss of proximal contact.
- The tooth has an unesthetic appearance.

Treatment will be directed in such a way that infected dental tissue is removed and the remaining cavity is adapted so that the restorative material can be optimally placed. The particular preparation methods and restorative procedures are discussed in the following chapters.

Most dentists enjoy the technical, esthetic, and intellectual challenges of restorative dentistry. However, before invasive procedures are initiated, noninvasive options must be explored and preventive measures taken. Restorative dentistry is one part of preventive treatment. Above all, it must be remembered that caries is a dynamic process, and its diagnosis requires the determination of caries activity and risk assessment.

References

1. Elderton RJ. Principles in the management of dental caries. In: Elderton R (ed). The Dentition and Dental Care. Oxford: Heinemann Medical Books, 1990.

2. Lagerlöf F, Oliveby A. Clinical implications: New strategies for caries treatment. In: Stookey GK (ed). Early Detection of Dental Caries. Indianapolis: Indiana University, 1996:297–321.

3. Keyes PH, Jordan HV. Factors influencing the initiation, transmission and inhibition of dental caries. In: Harris RJ (ed). Mechanisms of Hard Tissue Destruction. New York: Academic Press, 1963:261–283.

4. Carlsson J, Grahnen H, Jonsson G. Lactobacilli and streptococci in the mouth of children. Caries Res 1975;9:333–339.

5. Keene H, Shklair I. Relationship of Streptococcus mutans carrier status to the development of caries lesions in initially caries free recruits. J Dent Res 1974;53:1295–1299.

6. Loesche W. Dental Caries: A Treatable Infection. Springfield, IL: Thomas, 1982.

7. Powell LV. Caries prediction: A review of the literature. Community Dent Oral Epidemiol 1998;26:361–371.

8. De Stoppelaar JD, Van Houte J, Backer Dirks O. The effect of carbohydrate restriction on the presence of Streptococcus mutans, Streptococcus sanguis and iodophylic polysaccharide-producing bacteria in human dental plaque. Caries Res 1970;4:114–123.

9. McDermid AS, McKee AS, Ellwood DC, Marsh PD. The effect of lowering the pH on the composition and metabolism of a community of nine oral bacteria grown in a chemostat. J Gen Microbiol 1986;132:1205–1214.

10. Krasse B. The effect of the diet on the implantation of caries inducing streptococci in hamsters. Arch Oral Biol 1967;10:215–226.

11. Andréen I, Köhler B. Effects of Weight Watchers' diet on salivary secretion rate, buffer effect and number of mutans streptococci and lactobacilli. Scand J Dent Res 1992;100:93–97.

12. Wennerholm K, Birkhed D, Emilson CG. Effects of sugar restriction on Streptococcus mutans and Streptococcus sobrinus in saliva and dental plaque. Caries Res 1995;29:54–61.

13. Scheie AA, Arneberg P, Orstavik D, Afseth J. Microbial composition, pH-depressing capacity and acidogenicity of 3-week smooth surface plaque developed on sucrose-regulated diets in man. Caries Res 1984;18:74–86.

14. Imfeld T. Identification of Low Risk Dietary Components. Basel: Karger, 1983.

15. Axelsson P, Lindhe J. Effect of controlled oral hygiene procedures in caries and periodontal diseases in adults. J Clin Periodontol 1978; 5:133–151.

16. Axelsson P, Lindhe J, Nyström B. On the prevention of caries and periodontal disease. Results of a 15 year longitudinal study in adults. J Clin Periodontol 1991;18:182–189.

17. Øgaard B, Rølla G, Ruben J, Dijkman T, Arends J. Microradiographic study of demineralization of shark enamel in a human caries model. Scand J Dent Res 1988;96:209–211.

18. Rølla G, Øgaard B, de Almeida Cruz R. Clinical effect and mechanism of cariostatic action of fluoride-containing toothpastes: A review. Int Dent J 1991;41:171–174.

19. ten Cate JM, Duijsters PPE. The influence of fluoride in solution on tooth enamel demineralization. I. Chemical data. Caries Res 1983; 17:193–196.

20. Gülzow H-J, Maeglin B, Mühlemann R, Ritzel G, Staheli D. Caries morbidity and caries incidence in 7- to 15-year-old Basel schoolchildren in 1977 after 15 years of drinking-water fluoridation [in German]. SSO Schweiz Monatsschr Zahnheilkd 1982;92:255–266.

21. König KG. Changes in the prevalence of dental caries: How much can be attributed to changes in diet? Caries Res 1990;24(suppl 1):16–18.

22. Jensen ME, Schachtele CF. Plaque pH measurements by different methods on the buccal and proximal surfaces of human teeth after a sucrose rinse. J Dent Res 1983;62:1058–1061.

23. Jensen ME, Wefel JS. Human plaque pH responses to meals and the effects of chewing gum. Br Dent J 1989;167:204–208.

24. Kashket S, Van Houte J, Lopez LR, Stocks S. Lack of correlation between food retention on the human dentition and consumer perception of food stickiness. J Dent Res 1991;70:1314–1319.

25. Lingstrom P, Birkhed D. Plaque pH and oral retention after consumption of starchy snack products at normal and low salivary secretion rate. Acta Odontol Scand 1993;51:379–388.

26. Newbrun E. Cariology. Baltimore: Williams & Wilkins, 1978.

27. Dawes C, Weatherell JA. Kinetics of fluoride in the oral fluids. J Dent Res 1990;69(special issue):638–644.

28. Vogel GL, Carey CM, Ekstrand J. Distribution of fluoride in saliva and plaque fluid after a 0.2% NaF rinse: Short term kinetics and distribution. J Dent Res 1992;71:1553–1557.

29. Truin GJ, König KG, Bronkhorst EM, Frankenmolen F, Mulder J, van't Hof MA. Time trends in caries experience of 6- and 12-year-old children of different socioeconomic status in The Hague. Caries Res 1998;32:1–4.

30. Demers M, Brodeur J-M, Mouton C, Simard PL, Trahan L, Veilleux G. A multivariate model to predict caries increment in Montreal children aged 5 years. Community Dent Health 1992;9:273–281.

31. Grindefjord M, Dahlöf G, Nilsson D, Modéer T. Prediction of dental caries development in 1-year-old children. Caries Res 1995;29: 343–348.

32. Backer Dirks O. Posteruptive changes in dental enamel. J Dent Res 1966;45(suppl):503–511.

33. Van Palenstein Helderman WH, Ter Pelkwijk L, Van Dijk JW. Caries in fissures of permanent first molars as a predictor for caries increment. Community Dent Oral Epidemiol 1989;17:282–284.

34. Marthaler TM, Steiner M, Bandi A. Will discolored molar fissures within 4 years become carious more frequently than nondiscolored ones? Observations from 1975 to 1988 [in German]. Schweiz Monatsschr Zahnmed 1990;100:841–846.

35. Hyatt TP. Observable and unobservable pits and fissures. Dent Cosmos 1931;73:586–592.

36. Creanor SL, Russell JI, Strang DM, Stephen KW, Burchell CK. Prevalence of clinically undetected occlusal dentin caries in Scottish adolescents. Br Dent J 1990;169:126–129.

37. Weerheijm KL, Kidd EA, Groen HJ. The effect of fluoridation on the occurrence of hidden caries in clinically sound occlusal surfaces. Caries Res 1997;31:30–34.
38. Bjarnason S, Kingman A. Caries progression in populations with different caries prevalence. Caries Res 1991;25:215.
39. Shwartz M, Gröndhal H-G, Pliskin JS, Boffa J. A longitudinal analysis from bitewing radiographs of the rate of progression of proximal carious lesions through human dental enamel. Arch Oral Biol 1984; 29:529–536.
40. Gröndhal H-G, Hollender L, Malmcrona E, Sundquist B. Dental caries and restorations in teenagers. II. A longitudinal radiographic study of the caries increment of proximal surfaces among urban teenagers in Sweden. Swed Dent J 1977;1:51–57.
41. Mejàre I, Källestål C, Stenlund H, Johansson H. Caries development from 11 to 22 years of age: A prospective radiographic study. Prevalence and distribution. Caries Res 1998;32:10–16.
42. Groeneveld A. Longitudinal study of prevalence of enamel lesions in a fluoridated and non-fluoridated area. Community Dent Oral Epidemiol 1985;13:159–163.
43. Kidd EAM, Joyston-Bechal S. Saliva and caries. In: Kidd EAM, Joyston-Bechal (eds). Essentials of Dental Caries. Oxford: Oxford University Press, 1997:66–78.
44. Saxer UP, Marthaler TM. Caries increase over 10 years in young adults with and without a prevention program during the mandatory school year (II) [in German]. Quintessenz 1982;4:833–840.
45. Nuttal NM, Fyffe HE, Pitts NB. Caries management strategies used by a group of Scottish dentists. Br Dent J 1994;176:373–378.
46. Ekstrand KR, Kuzmina I, Bjørndal L, Thylstrup A. Relationship between external and histologic features of progressive stages of caries in the occlusal fossa. Caries Res 1995;29:243–250.
47. van Amerongen JP, Penning C, Kidd EAM, ten Cate JM. An in vitro assessment of the extent of caries under small occlusal cavities. Caries Res 1992;26:89–93.
48. Ekstrand KR, Ricketts DNJ, Kidd EAM. Reproducibility and accuracy of three methods for assessment of demineralization depth on the occlusal surface: An in vitro examination. Caries Res 1997;31:224–231.
49. Ekstrand KR, Ricketts DNJ, Kidd EAM, Qvist V, Schou S. Detection, diagnosing, monitoring and logical treatment of occlusal caries in relation to lesion activity and severity: An in vivo examination with histological validation. Caries Res 1998;32:247–254.
50. Espelid I, Tveit AB, Fjelltveit A. Variations among dentists in radiographic detection of occlusal caries. Caries Res 1994;28:169–175.
51. van Amerongen JP, van Amerongen-Pieko A, Penning C. Validity of caries diagnosis in molars with discolored fissures by radiography. J Dent Res 1993;72:344.
52. Penning C, van Amerongen JP, Seef RE, ten Cate JM. Validity of probing for fissure caries diagnosis. Caries Res 1992;26:445–449.
53. Ekstrand KR, Qvist V, Thylstrup A. Light microscope study of the effect of probing in occlusal surfaces. Caries Res 1987;21:368–374.
54. Pitts NB, Kidd EAM. Some of the factors to be considered in the prescription and timing of bitewing radiography in the diagnosis and management of dental caries. J Dent 1992;20:74–84.
55. Mitropoulos CM. The use of fibre-optic transillumination in the diagnosis of posterior-proximal caries in clinical trials. Caries Res 1985;19:379–384.
56. Rimmer PA, Pitts NB. Temporary elective tooth separation as a diagnostic aid in general practice. Br Dent J 1990;169:87–92.
57. Verdonschot EH, Angmar-Månsson B. Advanced methods of caries diagnosis and quantification. In: Fejerskov O, Kidd EAM (eds). Dental Caries. Copenhagen: Blackwell Munksgaard, 2003:129–139.
58. Ricketts DNJ, Kidd EAM, Liepins PJ, Wilson RF. Histological validation of electrical resistance measurements in the diagnosis of occlusal caries. Caries Res 1996;30:148–155.
59. Angmar-Månsson B, Al-Khateeb S, Tranaeus S. Monitoring the caries process. Optical methods for clinical diagnosis and quantification of enamel caries. Eur J Oral Sci 1996;104:480–485.
60. Longbottom C, Pitts NB, Reich E, Lussi A. Comparison of visual and electrical methods with a new device for occlusal caries detection. Caries Res 1998;32:297.
61. Lussi A, Imwinkelried S, Longbottom C, Reich E. Performance of a laser fluorescence system for detection of occlusal caries. Caries Res 1998;32:297.
62. Lussi A, Pitts N, Hotz P, Reich E. Reproducibility of a laser fluorescence system for detection of occlusal caries. Caries Res 1998;32:297.
63. Reich E, Al Marrawi F, Pitts N, Lussi A. Clinical validation of a laser caries diagnosis system. Caries Res 1998;32:297.
64. Fejerskov O. Concepts of dental caries and their consequences for understanding the disease. Community Dent Oral Epidemiol 1997; 25:5–12.
65. Featherstone JDB. Clinical implications: New strategies for caries prevention. In: Stookey GK (ed). Early Detection of Dental Caries. Indianapolis: Indiana University, 1996:287–295.
66. Nyvad B, Fejerskov O. Assessing the stage of caries lesion activity on the basis of clinical and microbiological examination. Community Dent Oral Epidemiol 1997;25:69–75.
67. Carvalho JC, Thylstrup A, Ekstrand K. Results after 3 years non-operative occlusal caries treatment of erupting permanent first molars. Community Dent Oral Epidemiol 1992;20:187–192.
68. Ricketts DNJ, Kidd EAM, Beighton D. Operative and microbiological validation of visual, radiographic and electronic diagnosis of occlusal caries in non-cavitated teeth judged to be in need of operative care. Br Dent J 1995;79:214–220.
69. Lunder N, von der Fehr FR. Proximal cavitation related to bitewing image and caries activity in adolescents. Caries Res 1996;30:143–147.
70. Ekstrand KR, Brunn C, Brunn M. Plaque and gingival status as indicators for caries progression on proximal surfaces. Caries Res 1998;32:41–45.
71. Hellyer PH, Beighton D, Heath MR, Lynch E. Root caries in older people attending a general dental practice in East Sussex. Br Dent J 1990;169:201–206.
72. Kidd EAM, Joyston-Bechal S, Beighton D. Marginal ditching and staining as a predictor of secondary caries around amalgam restorations: A clinical and microbiological study. J Dent Res 1995; 74:1206–1211.
73. Kidd EAM, Beighton D. Prediction of secondary caries around tooth-colored restorations: A clinical and microbiological study. J Dent Res 1996;75:1942–1946.
74. Hausen H. Caries prediction. In: Fejerskov O, Kidd EAM (eds). Dental Caries. Copenhagen: Blackwell Munksgaard, 2003:327–341.
75. Fejerskov O, Manji F. Reactor paper: Risk assessment in dental caries. In: Bader JD (ed). Risk Assessment in Dentistry. Chapel Hill, NC: University of North Carolina Dental Ecology, 1990:215–217.
76. Davies RM, Davies GM, Ellwood RB. Prevention. Part 4: Toothbrushing: What advice should be given to patients? Br Dent J 2003;195:135–141.

77. Zachrisson BK, Zachrisson S. Caries incidence and orthodontic treatment with fixed appliances. Scand J Dent Res 1971;79:183–192.

78. Drake CW, Beck JD. The oral status of elderly removable partial denture wearers. J Oral Rehabil 1993;20:53–60.

79. Kidd EAM, Nyvad B. Caries control for the individual patient. In: Fejerskov O, Kidd EAM (eds). Dental Caries. Copenhagen: Blackwell Munksgaard, 2003:303–312.

80. Tenovuo J. Salivary parameters of relevance for assessing caries activity in individuals or populations. Community Dent Oral Epidemiol 1997;25:82–86.

81. Montgomery MT, Ritvo J, Ritvo J, Weiner K. Eating disorders; phenomenology, identification and dental intervention. Gen Dent 1988; 36:485–488.

82. Van Houte J. Microbiological predictors of caries risk. Adv Dent Res 1993;7:87–96.

83. Shou L. Social and behavioural aspects of caries prediction. In: Johnson NW (ed). Dental Caries: Markers of High and Low Risk Groups and Individuals. Cambridge: Cambridge University Press, 1991: 172–197.

84. Hobson P. Sugar-based medicines and dental disease. Community Dent Health 1985;2:57–62.

85. Beal JF. Social factors and preventive dentistry. In: Murray JJ (ed). Prevention of Oral Disease. Oxford: Oxford University Press, 1996:216–233.

86. Hunt RJ. Behavioural and sociodemographic risk factors for caries. In: Bader JD (ed). Risk Assessment in Dentistry. Chapel Hill, NC: University of North Carolina Dental Ecology 1990:29–34.

87. Lussi A, Gygax M. Iatrogenic damage to adjacent teeth during classical proximal box preparation. J Dent 1998;26:435–441.

88. Benn DK. Practical evidence-based management of the initial caries lesion. J Dent Educ 1997;61:853–854.

89. Von der Fehr FR, Löe H, Theilade E. Experimental caries in man. Caries Res 1970;4:131–136.

90. Koch G. Importance of early determination of caries risk. Int Dent J 1988;38:203–210.

91. Thylstrup A, Bruun C, Holman L. In vivo caries models—Mechanisms for caries initiation and arrestment. Adv Dent Res 1993;8:144–157.

92. Pitts NB, Kidd EAM. The prescription and timing of bitewing radiography in the diagnosis and management of dental caries: Contemporary recommendations. Br Dent J 1992;172:225–227.

93. Pitts NB, Kidd EAM. Some of the factors to be considered in the prescription and timing of bitewing radiography in the diagnosis and management of dental caries. J Dent 1992;20:74–84.

94. Nyvad B, Fejerskov O. Active root surface caries converted into inactive caries as a response to oral hygiene. Scand J Dent Res 1986;94:281–284.

95. Nyvad B, Fejerskov O. An ultrastructural study of bacterial invasion and tissue breakdown in human experimental root surface caries. J Dent Res 1990;69:2218–2225.

96. Parikh SR, Massler M, Bahn A. Microorganisms in active and arrested carious lesions of dentin. N Y State Dent J 1963;29:347–355.

97. Sarnat H, Massler M. Microstructure of active and arrested dentinal caries. J Dent Res 1965;44:1389–1401.

98. Schüpbach P, Guggenheim B, Lutz F. Human root caries: Histopathology of arrested lesions. Caries Res 1992;26:153–164.

99. Brathall D, Hänsel-Petersson G, Sundberg H. Reasons for the caries decline: What do the experts believe? Eur J Oral Sci 1996;104: 416–422.

100. Gibson S, Williams S. Dental caries in preschool children: Associations with social class, toothbrushing habit and the consumption of sugars and sugar containing foods. Caries Res 1999;33:101–113.

101. Murray JJ, Breckon JA, Reynolds PJ, Tabari ED, Nunn JH. The effect of residence and social class on dental caries experience in 15–16-year-old children living in three towns (natural fluoride, adjusted fluoride and low fluoride) in the north east of England. In: Murray JJ (ed). The Prevention of Dental Disease, ed 2. Oxford: Oxford Medical, 1989.

102. O'Mullane D, Whelton H. Caries prevalence in the Republic of Ireland. Int Dent J 1994;44:387–391.

103. Pendrys GP, Katz RV, Morse DE. Risk factors for enamel fluorosis in a fluoridated population. Am J Epidemiol 1994;140:461–471.

104. Marthaler T. Clinical cariostatic effects of various fluoride methods and programs. In: Ekstrand J, Fejerskov O, Silverstone LM (eds). Fluoride in Dentistry, ed 1. Copenhagen: Munksgaard, 1988:252–275.

105. Ripa LW. Review of the anticaries effectiveness of professionally applied and self-applied topical fluoride gels. J Public Health Dent 1989;49(special issue):297–309.

106. Clark DC, Hanley JA, Stamm JW, Weinstein PL. An empirically based system to estimate the effectiveness of caries-preventive agents. Caries Res 1985;19:83–95.

107. Van Rijkom HM, Truin GJ, van't Hof MA. A meta-analysis of clinical studies on the caries-inhibiting effect of chlorhexidine treatment. J Dent Res 1996;75:790–795.

108. Ripa LW. Sealants revisited: An update of the effectiveness of pit and fissure sealants. Caries Res 1993;27:77–82.

109. Ripa LW, Leske GS, Varma OA. Longitudinal study of the caries susceptibility of occlusal and proximal surfaces of first permanent molars. J Public Health Dent 1988;48:8–13.

110. Simonsen R. Retention and effectiveness of dental sealant after 15 years. J Am Dent Assoc 1991;122:34–42.

111. Handelman S, Washburn F, Wopperer P. Two-year report of sealant effect on bacteria in dental caries. J Am Dent Assoc 1976;93: 967–970.

112. Handelman S. Effect of sealant placement on occlusal caries progression. Clin Prev Dent 1982;4:11–16.

113. Mertz-Fairhurst E, Schuster G, Fairhurst C. Arresting caries by sealants: Results of a clinical study. J Am Dent Assoc 1986;112: 194–197.

114. Mertz-Fairhurst EJ, Adair SM, Sams DR, et al. Cariostatic and ultraconservative sealed restorations: Nine-year results among children and adults. J Dent Child 1995;62:97–107.

115. Briley JB, Dove SB, Mertz-Fairhurst EJ. Radiographic analysis of previously sealed carious teeth [abstract 2514]. J Dent Res 1994;73: 416.

116. Mertz-Fairhurst EJ, Curtis JW Jr, Ergle JW, Rueggeberg FA, Adair SM. Ultraconservative and cariostatic sealed restorations: Results at year 10. J Am Dent Assoc 1998;129:55–66.

117. Elderton RJ, Mjör IA. Treatment planning. In: Hörsted-Bindslev P, Mjör IA (eds). Modern Concepts in Operative Dentistry. Copenhagen: Munksgaard, 1988.

Pulpal Considerations

Thomas J. Hilton
James B. Summitt

Because caries is a bacterial infection, it has a deleterious effect on the pulp, ranging from mild inflammation to pulpal death. In addition, virtually all restorative procedures cause pulpal irritation. As discussed in chapter 1, the pulp has inherent defense mechanisms to limit damage caused by irritants. There are also a number of dental procedures performed with the goal of preserving pulpal health. Most of these procedures attempt to provide a barrier to external irritants by placing a protective sealer or liner on the cavity walls.

Before placing or cementing a restoration into a cavity preparation, the clinician must decide if a cavity base or a protective cavity sealer or liner should be placed. While seemingly simple, this decision has been complicated by an ever-increasing number of products for sealing and lining. This chapter reviews pulpal considerations relevant to operative dentistry, including the effects of cavity preparation, caries, and restorative materials on the pulp. In addition, it defines the various protective materials, describes the ways they interact with and provide protection for the pulp, reviews the properties of current materials, and discusses the changes that have occurred in this area of operative dentistry in recent years.

Physiologic Considerations

The physiology of the pulp is influenced by several factors that form the basis for the decision to use a sealer, liner, and/or base.

Remaining Dentinal Thickness

No material that can be placed in a tooth provides better protection for the pulp than dentin. Dentin has excellent buffering capability to neutralize the effects of cariogenic acids,[1p42–43] and it insulates the pulp from temperature increases during cavity preparation.[2] The remaining dentinal thickness (RDT), from the depth of the cavity preparation to the pulp, is the single most important factor in protecting the pulp from insult.[1p41,3] In vitro studies have shown that a 0.5-mm thickness of dentin reduces the effect of toxic substances on the pulp by 75% and a 1.0-mm thickness reduces the effect of toxins by 90%.[4] Little pulpal reaction occurs when there is an RDT of 2 mm or more.[1p41] The greatest impact on the pulp occurs when the RDT is no more than 0.25 to 0.3 mm.[3,5] Conservation of remaining tooth structure is more important to pulpal health than is replacement of lost tooth structure with a cavity liner or base.

Causes of Pulpal Inflammation

Like other soft tissues, the pulp reacts to an irritant with an inflammatory response.[6] It was previously believed that pulpal inflammation was the result of toxic effects of dental materials.[7,8] More recent evidence, however, demonstrates that pulpal inflammatory reactions to dental materials are mild and transitory; significant adverse pulpal responses occur more as the result of pulpal invasion by bacteria or their toxins (Fig 5-1a).[3,9–14] Even early enamel caries lesions that extend less than one fourth of the way to the dentinoenamel junction (DEJ) have been shown to induce a slight pulpal reaction, particularly when the caries lesion has advanced rapidly. This is probably due to an increase in the permeability of enamel, allowing the transmission of stimuli along enamel rods.[15,16]

As a lesion progresses deeper into the tooth, pulpal reaction increases.[15] When actual pulpal encroach-

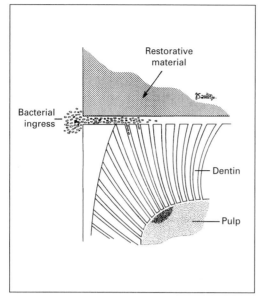

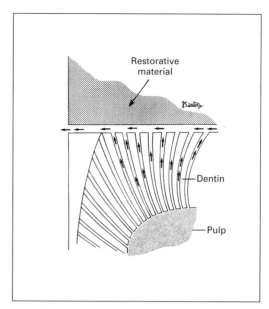

Fig 5-1a Bacteria will penetrate the marginal gap and dentinal tubules from the saliva, which may cause pulpal irritation, pulpal necrosis, or recurrent caries.

Fig 5-1b If a restoration is not well sealed, fluid flows out of the dentinal tubules and into the space between the restorative material and the tooth surface *(arrows)*. A stimulus such as heat or cold causes a change in the flow rate, which is interpreted by mechanoreceptors as pain.

ment by bacteria and/or their toxins has taken place, severe inflammation or pulpal necrosis frequently occurs.[12] The outward flow of fluid through dentinal tubules does not prevent bacteria or their toxins from reaching the pulp and initiating pulpal inflammation.[17] The caries process also induces the formation of reparative dentin and reactive dentin sclerosis, which increases the protective effects of the remaining dentin.[18]

When bacterial contamination is prevented, favorable responses have been found in pulpal tissue adjacent to many restorative materials. Those materials include amalgam, light-activated resin composite, autocured resin composite,[19] zinc phosphate cement, silicate cement,[11] glass-ionomer cement, and acrylic resin.[20] Acid etching of dentin has long been considered detrimental to the pulp, but the pulp can readily tolerate the effects of low pH if bacterial invasion is prevented[10,19,21] and resin components are precluded from traversing the dentinal tubules and entering the pulp.[5,22]

A number of instrumentation techniques elicit pulpal responses as well. The most common are rotary instruments used in high- and low-speed handpieces for tooth preparation. Tooth preparation can be traumatic to the pulp, and a number of factors affect pulpal reaction. The degree of pulpal reaction is dependent on the amount of friction and desiccation.[23,24] One retrospective study indicated that high-speed preparation, with the use of light force (1 to 3 oz), new burs,

air coolant, and intermittent water spray from the air-water syringe, rarely led to a need for postrestoration endodontic therapy.[25] However, the key to controlling both friction and desiccation is water spray at the site of contact between the bur and tooth structure. While some research has shown that this is more important than the amount of water that is used on a rotating bur,[24] another study has demonstrated that increased water spray volume can significantly reduce pulpal temperature rises caused by friction.[2] Frictional heat generated by tooth preparation can result in burn lesions in the pulp and abscess formation.[26] While it is often advantageous to refine aspects of a cavity preparation without water spray in order to aid visibility, this must be done conservatively. The pulp can tolerate dry preparation in a limited area, but the severity of the pulpal reaction increases as the area of dentin subjected to preparation without water spray increases.[24] Another consequence of desiccating dentin in a preparation is that dentinal fluid is lost from the tubules. The lost fluid may be replaced with chemicals that can elicit a harmful pulpal reaction.[24]

The temperature rise is considerably greater when enamel or a combination of enamel and dentin is prepared versus preparation of dentin alone.[27] Additionally, research has shown that pressure applied during rotary instrumentation has a greater effect on temperature rise than does rotational speed,[27] which is probably why preparation using low-speed rotary instrumentation has been shown to be more traumatic to the pulp than high-speed preparation.[26] Diamond burs tend to produce more temperature increase than do carbide burs,[26] and the reaction of the pulp tends to increase as the depth of the cavity preparation increases. Considering the latter two findings, it should not be surprising that an occasional consequence of full-coverage restorations is pulpal necrosis.[28–30] Research has shown that 3% to 22% of teeth with full-coverage crowns require endodontic therapy.[29–31] It is clear that the combination of reducing water coolant and RDT and increasing bur speed and pressure can produce a significant increase in temperature during tooth preparation.[2,26,27,32] Therefore, the keys to minimizing adverse pulpal reaction from rotary instrumentation are the following:

• Adequate air-water coolant spray
• Light pressure
• Sharp rotary cutting instruments
• Preservation of tooth structure

Two relatively new methods for tooth preparation are available—lasers and kinetic cavity preparation, also known as *air abrasion*. Animal studies have shown that air abrasion cavity preparation is no more traumatic to the pulp than rotary instrumentation.[32,33] Likewise, the use of a variety of lasers, including CO_2, Er:YAG, Nd:YAG, and free-electron lasers (FEL), on tooth structure has demonstrated minimal pulpal response, comparable to that of high-speed rotary instrumentation.[34–37] The key to minimizing thermal pulpal insult during tooth preparation with a laser preparation, as with preparation using rotary instrumentation, is the use of water coolant.[38]

One other modality commonly used in conjunction with operative dentistry—electrosurgery to remove gingival tissue for enhanced access during tooth preparation and impression making—may affect the dental pulp. Several animal studies have shown that as long as the contact of the electrosurgical probe is with intact enamel, little or no pulpal reaction ensues. However, if the probe contacts a metallic restoration, adverse and often severe pulpal reaction results.[39–42] This adverse reaction occurs regardless of whether a cavity base is present or not.[42] The pulpal response is more severe with increased contact time (longer than 0.4 seconds)[40] and decreased dentin thickness between the metallic restoration and the pulp.[39,42]

Causes of Pulpal Pain

The causes of pulpal pain and sensitivity, while not fully explained, are becoming better understood. Increased intrapulpal pressure on nerve endings, secondary to an inflammatory response, is one mechanism that may explain pain as a result of bacterial invasion.[1p9] However, this interpretation fails to explain sensitivity that occurs in the absence of inflammation. The explanation for pulpal pain in the absence of inflammation that is most accepted is the *hydrodynamic theory*.[43] In a vital tooth with exposed dentin, there is a constant slow movement of fluid outward through the dentinal tubules (Fig 5-1b). The hydrodynamic theory proposes that when a stimulus causes the slow fluid movement to become more rapid, nerve endings in the pulp are deformed, creating a response that is interpreted as pain. Stimuli such as tooth preparation, air drying, and application of cold have been suggested as causes of this sudden, rapid movement of fluid.[43]

Causes of Thermal Sensitivity

Prevention of postoperative thermal sensitivity has long been a rationale for the placement of cavity bases beneath metallic restorations. Initial in vivo research documenting the alleged problem was sparse and poorly controlled. Although one study showed reduced postoperative sensitivity when thick cement bases were used,[44] another demonstrated that, by 6 months postoperatively, few patients had thermal sensitivity regardless of whether a cavity base had been placed.[45] In one survey, 50% of patients questioned 24 hours after restoration placement reported some discomfort, but 78% of these patients described the discomfort as mild and fleeting.[46] Several more recent studies have demonstrated that a significant majority of patients receiving amalgam restorations do not experience postoperative thermal sensitivity, regardless of lesion depth or the absence or presence of a particular cavity sealer or liner. Of those patients with postoperative thermal discomfort, almost all describe it as minor, and it has almost always disappeared within 30 days.[47–52] Any discussion of the need for protection against postoperative thermal sensitivity must be tempered by the understanding that the prevalence and magnitude of this problem have likely been overestimated.

Theory of Thermal Shock

There are two theories about the cause of thermal sensitivity (usually to cold) following restoration placement and, consequently, two philosophies about how to best address the problem. The first theory states that sensitivity is the result of direct thermal shock to the pulp via temperature changes transferred from the oral cavity through the restorative material,[53,54] especially when remaining dentin is thin. Protection from this insult would then be provided by an adequate thickness of an insulating material with low thermal diffusivity.[54,55] It has been noted that resin composite exhibits such low thermal diffusivity that a thermal insulating base should be unnecessary in conjunction with resin composite restorations.[55,56] Use of an insulating base for thermal protection would, therefore, be limited to metallic restorative materials that exhibit higher rates of temperature transfer.

When a base is used to provide insulation to counter thermal sensitivity in amalgam restorations, the thickness of the material must be minimized in areas subject to occlusal loading. Research has shown that, as the thickness of the base increases, the fracture resistance of the overlying amalgam decreases.[57,58] Because temperature diffusion through amalgam to the floor of the cavity preparation is effectively reduced by 0.50 to 0.75 mm of basing material, if a base is used, its thickness should be restricted to that dimension.[55] Modulus of elasticity is the key property that determines how effectively a base or liner will support an amalgam restoration; a high modulus of elasticity indicates stiffness, while a low modulus of elasticity indicates flexibility. As the modulus of elasticity of a basing material decreases, the resistance to fracture of overlying amalgam decreases.[57–59]

Theory of Pulpal Hydrodynamics

The more widely accepted theory of thermal sensitivity holds that temperature sensitivity is based on pulpal hydrodynamics. Most restorations have a gap between the wall of the preparation and the restorative material that allows the slow outward movement of dentinal fluid (see Fig 5-1b). Cold temperatures cause a sudden contraction of this fluid, resulting in a rapid increase in the flow, which is perceived by the patient as pain.[43] As dentin nears the pulp, tubule density and diameter increase,[1p38] as does permeability,[60] thus increasing both the volume and flow of pulpal fluid susceptible to the hydrodynamic effects of cold temperatures. This may explain why deeper restorations are sometimes associated with more problems of sensitivity.

According to this theory, if the tubules can be occluded, fluid flow is prevented and a cold temperature does not induce pain. The operative factor in reducing sensitivity to thermal change thus becomes effective sealing of dentinal tubules rather than placement of an insulating material of a certain thickness.[43] Scanning electron microscopic observations have revealed significantly higher numbers of open tubule orifices in hypersensitive dentin, lending credence to this theory.[61,62]

* The theory of pulpal hydrodynamics has gained general acceptance in recent years and has changed the direction of restorative procedures away from thermal insulation and toward dentinal sealing. Thus, there is increasing emphasis on the integrity of the interface between restorative material and cavity preparation.

Cavity Sealers, Liners, and Bases

The terms *varnish*, *sealer*, *liner*, and *base*, used to describe a variety of materials, have been a source of confusion in dental literature. In 1995, McCoy[63] provided the following definitions for these terms.

1. Cavity sealers: Materials in this category provide a protective coating to the walls of the prepared cavity and a barrier to leakage at the interface of the restorative material and the walls. The term *sealer* implies total prevention of leakage, but, in fact, the barrier provides various degrees of seal. Sealers usually coat all walls of a cavity preparation. Commonly used sealers fall into two categories:
   a. Varnish: A natural rosin or gum (such as copal), or a synthetic resin, dissolved in an organic solvent such as acetone, chloroform, or ether[64]
   b. Adhesive sealers: The adhesive systems designed to provide sealing as well as bonding at the interface between restoration and cavity preparation walls
2. Cavity liners: Cement or resin coating of minimal thickness (usually less than 0.5 mm) to achieve a physical barrier to bacteria and their products and/or to provide a therapeutic effect, such as an antibacterial or pulpal anodyne effect. Liners are usually applied only to dentin cavity walls that are near the pulp.
3. Cavity bases: Materials to replace missing dentin, used for bulk buildup and/or for blocking out undercuts in preparations for indirect restorations.

Knowledge of the properties and indications for the materials in each category will aid the practitioner faced with an array of choices.

Cavity Sealers

Cavity sealers provide a protective coating for freshly cut tooth structure of the prepared cavity. The tooth-restoration interface has always been considered critical in dentistry, a fact apparent in the profession's emphasis on marginal adaptation of dental restorations. The concern is that any interfacial gap, even one not readily apparent under magnification, will allow microleakage. Kidd[65] defined microleakage as the passage of bacteria, fluids, molecules, or ions along the interface of a dental restoration and the wall of the cavity preparation. This process is theorized to cause marginal discoloration, secondary caries, and pulpal pathosis. A summary of

Table 5-1	Tooth-Restoration Interface: Materials and Clinical Failures						
	Composite			Amalgam	Glass ionomer		
Study	Secondary caries	Marginal gap/fracture	Marginal discoloration	Secondary caries	Secondary caries	Marginal gap/fracture	Marginal discoloration
Friedl et al[66]	40%	18%	—	—	—	—	—
Browning and Dennison[67]	28.6%	14.1%	21.7%	—	—	—	—
Mjör and Qvist[68]	62%	—	—	70%	—	—	—
Mjör and Toffenetti[69]	44%	6%	9%	—	—	—	—
Mjör[70]	33%	—	—	—	50%	5%	3%

some retrospective studies on the causes of clinical failure of existing restorations is provided in Table 5-1.

Clearly, the junction between the restorative material and tooth structure is the source of a considerable number of restoration failures; providing a seamless transition from restoration to tooth structure has long been a goal in dentistry. Cavity sealers, used to fulfill this function, take two forms: varnishes and adhesive sealers.

Varnishes

As previously discussed, varnish is a natural gum (such as copal), a rosin, or a synthetic resin dissolved in an organic solvent, such as acetone, chloroform, or ether, that evaporates, leaving behind a protective film.[64] It is used as a barrier against the passage of bacteria and their by-products into dentinal tubules, and it reduces the penetration of oral fluid at the restoration-tooth interface. This film is very thin, usually 2 to 5 μm, and provides no thermal insulation.[71–73]

Copal varnishes were used for many years to fill the gap at the amalgam-tooth interface until corrosion products formed to reduce it.[71,74,75] Varnishes have also been used as barriers against the passage of irritants from cements and bacteria into dentinal tubules.[71] Two applications have been shown to be more effective than a single coat, but a third application does not significantly improve the coating of the cavity walls.[76] Copal varnish is capable of reducing dentin permeability by 69%[77] and significantly reducing microleakage for 4 to 6 months.[78–80] Although its use has diminished in recent years, varnish has commonly been used under amalgam restorations and before cementation of indirect restorations with zinc phosphate cement. Placement of copal varnish before crown cementation with zinc phosphate does not have a detrimental effect on retention.[81]

Adhesive Sealers

The most recent materials to be used as cavity sealers have a demonstrated multisubstrate bonding ability that allows the restorative material to adhere to tooth structure. Examples include adhesive bonding systems, resin luting cements, and glass-ionomer luting cements. The benefits of using adhesive bonding systems (described in chapter 8) to attach resin composite materials to tooth structure are well documented and accepted. It is well established that acid etching will promote a reliable, durable bond to enamel.[10] Its mechanism of action (ie, the diffusion of polymerizable monomers into porosities and channels established in enamel and dentin as a result of the demineralizing action of acid) is well accepted. Bonding systems also provide a chemical bond between the unfilled resin of the adhesive system and the resin composite. Enamel's more consistent and highly mineralized structure provides a more reliable bond than that achieved to dentin.

Researchers and clinicians have worked to develop cavity sealers that can improve the seal provided by cavity varnishes for amalgam restorations. Some studies have demonstrated that varnishes reduce, but do not eliminate, microleakage around amalgam restorations,[78,82,83] while other studies have shown no benefit or even increased microleakage when a varnish is used.[84–86] Because of postplacement amalgam marginal leakage, the duration of which is prolonged when the slower-corroding high-copper alloys are used, more effective and longer-lasting sealers have been sought. This has led to the frequent use of adhesive resins in conjunction with amalgam restorations.[87] At least one study has shown an adhesive to be inferior to varnish in the seal it provides[88]; others have shown adhesives and varnishes to exhibit similar degrees of microleakage,[89,90] while still others have shown adhesive resin to impart no greater seal than when no sealer at all is used.[84,91] However, numerous studies have shown resin adhesives to provide a significant reduction in leakage.[79,80,92–100]

While not unanimous, there is compelling evidence that adhesive resins used as sealers reduce interfacial microleakage compared to either unsealed or varnish-sealed amalgam restorations when evaluated in the short term (24 hours to 14 days). Superior sealing of dentinal tubules by bonding resins compared to varnish has also been demonstrated.[80,92,97,100] Animal research has demonstrated that dentin primers alone or in conjunction with dentin adhesives can significantly reduce dentin sensitivity[101] and that they have good pulpal compatibility when used in cavity preparations.[102,103] However, modern adhesives continue to exhibit significant leakage when cavity margins are on dentin or cementum.[104–107] Most in vitro research on the use of bonding systems with amalgam restorations is of short duration, and uncertainty exists concerning the durability of the bonded interface between amalgam and tooth structure. Studies have found that both interfacial and dentinal tubule leakage increase significantly over periods of 1 month to 1 year after placement of the resin bonding/sealing resin and amalgam.[81,93,97,98]

Most important, numerous controlled clinical trials have failed to demonstrate a decrease in postoperative sensitivity with the use of adhesive agents under amalgam restorations compared with the use of either traditional sealers and liners or no cavity sealer at all.[47,49–52,108–111] These results are consistently found regardless of cavity depth and remaining dentin thickness.[50,51]

Given these facts, there are some concerns about the use of adhesive resins under amalgam restorations. The insoluble adhesive layer may act as a barrier to prevent amalgam corrosion products from ultimately sealing the tooth-restoration interface. As a result, the dentin bonding resins may potentially put the patient at greater risk in the long term for marginal leakage and recurrent caries. In addition, bonding resins are much more technique sensitive than varnishes,[107,112] and bonding systems are more expensive and time-consuming.[113] Researchers have also noted the tendency of self-curing adhesive sealers used in conjunction with amalgam restorations to spread to adjacent tooth surfaces, potentially giving rise to periodontal problems.[52] Additional potential drawbacks to the use of adhesive sealers with amalgam include pooling of resin, resulting in radiographic artifacts,[114] and incorporation of sealer into the amalgam during condensation,[115] leading to significant loss of amalgam strength.[116,117]

These considerations need to be weighed against clinical research evaluating the performance of bonded amalgam restorations. A number of studies have demonstrated clinical performance of bonded restorations that is comparable to that of nonbonded restorations.[47,52,109,111] One recently reported trial demonstrated equal performance of complex amalgam restorations (including at least one proximal surface and one cusp), using either pin retention or adhesive bonding over 6 years.[111] Those outcomes are encouraging, because bonded amalgam restorations permit minimal tooth preparation rather than necessitating the removal of sound tooth structure to develop traditional resistance and retention form. However, the results of the clinical studies that have been done should be interpreted with some caution, as most have evaluated relatively low numbers of restorations and, with the exception of the 6-year study of large restorations cited above, have been of short duration (3 years or less) and have tested mostly small-to-moderate-sized restorations. With these precautions in mind, it should be noted that evidence is accumulating to support the use of adhesive sealers in conjunction with amalgam restorations.

Cavity Liners

Cavity liners are placed with minimal thickness, usually less than 0.5 mm, and provide some type of therapeutic benefit, such as fluoride release, dentinal seal provided by adhesion to tooth structure, and/or antibacterial action that promotes pulpal health.[63]

Calcium Hydroxide

Calcium hydroxide [$Ca(OH)_2$] has long been used as a liner because of its pulpal compatibility and purported ability to stimulate reparative dentin formation with direct pulpal contact.[1p42–43] However, research has shown that not all formulations of calcium hydroxide have a stimulatory effect on human pulpoblasts.[118] There is a growing belief that reparative dentin formation is assisted, rather than stimulated, and that this is due to the antibacterial action of calcium hydroxide, which reduces or eliminates the inflammatory effects of bacteria and their by-products on the pulp.[12,43,119,120] Recent research has also indicated that calcium hydroxide may release growth factors from dentin that can assist in pulp healing.[120]

Conventional formulations of calcium hydroxide liners have demonstrated poor physical properties.[57,121p218] High solubility of some calcium hydroxide liners may lead to contamination of bonding resins and result in increased marginal leakage.[122] High solubility may also result in softening of the liner and in material loss under poorly sealed restorations.[43,123] Visible light–activated calcium hydroxide products have overcome most of these deficiencies. They exhibit improved physical properties[124] and significantly reduced solubility.[121p218] While modulus of elasticity of the light-activated products has

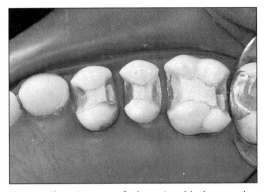

Fig 5-2a The primary use for bases is to block out undercuts in divergent preparations. Glass-ionomer bases are used here to block out undercuts in inlay preparations.

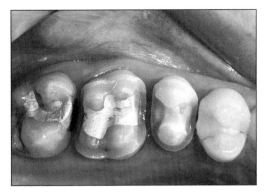

Fig 5-2b Glass-ionomer bases are used in this case to block out undercuts in porcelain onlay preparations.

been shown to increase relative to conventional calcium hydroxide in one study,[125] in another it was lower,[124] with a resulting reduced ability to support an overlying amalgam restoration.[126] These unfavorable physical properties restrict calcium hydroxide use to application over the smallest area that would suffice to aid in the formation of reparative dentin when a known or suspected pulp exposure exists.

Glass Ionomer

Glass ionomer has been used as a cavity liner in an attempt to take advantage of two highly desirable properties: chemical bond to tooth structure and fluoride release.[121p284] Although fluoride release from glass ionomer decreases with time,[127] sustained release has been demonstrated[128] with corresponding uptake into adjacent tooth structure.[129] This is thought to aid in anticariogenic activity.[130] Like zinc phosphate, glass ionomer is quite acidic on initial mixing but tends to neutralize within 24 hours.[116] Pulpal response to both visible light–activated and conventional glass-ionomer formulations has been shown to be favorable,[19,131–133] probably because glass ionomer decreases interfacial bacterial penetration.[132] The exact mechanism by which this is achieved is uncertain, but it may be due to one or more of the following: fluoride release, initial low pH,[134] chemical bond to tooth structure (physically excluding bacteria),[132] or release of a metal cation.[135,136] Both visible light–activated and conventional glass-ionomer liners exhibit good physical properties, with the conventional version exhibiting reduced interfacial gap formation,[137] a higher modulus of elasticity,[138] and subsequently improved support for amalgam restorations.[126] Glass ionomer has been shown to reduce microleakage under amalgam restorations.[84,139] Conventional glass ionomers are relatively soluble in an acidic environment and are susceptible to rapid surface deterioration when subjected to acid etching.[140] Visible light–activated

glass ionomers show improved resistance to acid solubility[124] while maintaining fluoride release and bond to tooth structure.[138] Therefore, the visible light–activated formulations are more desirable for use with resin composite restorations.

Glass-ionomer cements (GICs) have been recommended as liners under resin composite restorations to reduce microleakage. The use of GIC as an intermediate layer between dentin and resin composite, particularly in Class 5 restorations, is often referred to as the *sandwich technique*. Glass ionomer use, most often in conjunction with Class 2 resin composite restorations, is sometimes called the *bonded-base technique*. Both techniques can be "open," in which the GIC at the gingival margin is exposed, or "closed," in which the GIC is completely covered by resin composite. GIC liners, both visible light–cured and autocured, have been studied extensively for their ability to seal the interface between resin composite and the cavity preparation. The preponderance of in vitro evidence indicates that GIC liners perform at least as well as, and in most cases significantly better than, bonding resins used alone to seal the restoration-tooth interface. This is probably due to the delayed set and increased strain capacity provided by the GIC. In addition, the open sandwich or bonded-base restoration appears to be superior to the closed technique in achieving this superior seal.[141–150] The use of the open sandwich technique with posterior resin composite restorations is discussed in greater detail in chapter 10.

Cavity Bases

As previously stated, cavity bases are used as dentin replacement materials, allowing for less bulk of restorative material or blocking out undercuts for indirect restorations[63] (Figs 5-2a and 5-2b). Although cavity bases generally are not used for pulpal protection or health, they are briefly described here.

Zinc Oxide–Eugenol and Zinc Phosphate Cements

Zinc oxide–eugenol and zinc phosphate cements have been used for a number of years for bases under a variety of restorative materials. Although both provide excellent thermal insulation[11,55] and zinc phosphate cement exhibits superior physical properties,[1p200] their use has diminished in recent years with the growing question of their benefit to pulpal health and with the advent of materials that are adhesive to dentin and release fluoride.[151]

Glass Ionomer

As previously discussed, glass-ionomer materials have excellent mechanical properties, with the conventional versions offering excellent modulus of elasticity and restoration support. As a result, glass ionomers can be used as cavity bases as well as cavity liners.

Guidelines for Basing, Lining, and Sealing

Clinicians must always consider the limitations of currently available materials. The best possible base for any restoration is sound tooth structure. The following are guidelines for placement of bases, liners, and sealers:

1. Do not remove sound tooth structure to provide space for a base. Maintaining sound dentin will enhance restoration support and provide maximum dentin thickness for pulpal protection.
2. Use bases as indicated for buildup materials and block-out materials for cemented indirect restorations. If used for direct amalgam restorations or bonded restorations, minimize the extent of the base. Basing a preparation to "ideal" depth and internal form is contraindicated.[152] Bases in cavity preparations for amalgam restorations and bonded resin or ceramic restorations lead to decreased bulk of restorative material and increased potential for restoration fracture.
3. Use the minimum thickness of liner necessary to achieve the desired result. For liners under amalgam restorations, this should not exceed 0.5 mm.[153]
4. Research support is growing for the use of adhesive sealers (dentin bonding agents) under metallic restorations; long-term clinical evidence is still not strong.

Direct and Indirect Pulp Capping

Pulp capping is defined as "endodontic treatment designed to maintain the vitality of the endodontium."[154] Several favorable conditions must be present before considering direct or indirect pulp capping:

1. The tooth must have a vital pulp and no history of spontaneous pain.[154]
2. Pain elicited during pulp testing with a hot or cold stimulus should not linger after stimulus removal.
3. A periapical radiograph should show no evidence of a periradicular lesion of endodontic origin.
4. Bacteria must be excluded from the site by the permanent restoration.

If these conditions can be met, an indirect pulp capping procedure is preferable to a direct pulp capping procedure. An indirect pulp capping procedure allows a protective thickness of dentin to remain adjacent to the pulp. Not only does this provide the advantages previously described for maintaining dentin (as RDT), but because RDT is directly related to odontoblast survival, reparative dentin formation is also enhanced.[3] In addition, avoiding pulpal exposure means that there is less chance for infected debris to be introduced into the pulp to cause an inflammatory reaction.[3,155] Avoiding pulpal exposure also means there is no concern for hemorrhage from the pulp, a factor that has been associated with decreased success rates in direct pulp capping.[156–159]

Because of the uncertainty for success with either indirect or direct pulp capping procedures, pulpal health should be monitored for several months in teeth that are to receive indirect restorations or serve as abutments for fixed or removable partial dentures. If the pulpal status of a tooth is uncertain, the clinician should consider endodontic therapy before initiating restorative treatment.

Direct Pulp Capping

Animal studies have demonstrated that direct pulpal exposures can heal normally, but a bacteria-free environment is required.[160] The adverse consequences of bacterial contamination of the pulp have been well documented.[10–12,19,20] Therefore, the only reasonable chance that a direct pulp cap has to permit formation of a dentin bridge and to maintain pulp vitality is under the most ideal conditions. If a large number of bacteria from a caries lesion or exposure to the oral flora have contaminated the pulp, the likelihood of regaining or maintaining a healthy pulp is slight. In addition, aged pulps have increased fibrosis and a decreased blood supply,[161] and thus a decreased ability to mount an effective response to invading microorganisms.[159]

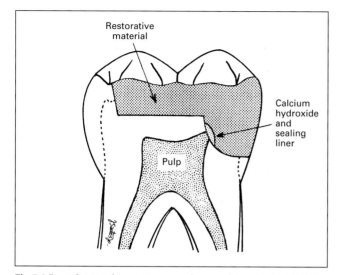

Fig 5-3 For a direct pulp capping procedure, a calcium hydroxide lining material is placed on the exposed pulpal tissue and a small amount of surrounding dentin. A sealing liner and/or a sealing restoration is then placed to seal out bacteria and their by-products.

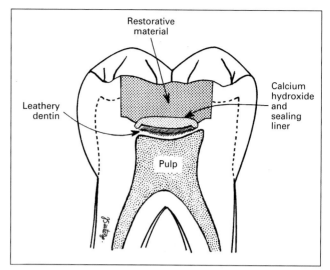

Fig 5-4 In an indirect pulp capping procedure, all carious, demineralized dentin is removed in the periphery of the preparation, but a small amount of demineralized dentin is left immediately over the area of the pulp. A calcium hydroxide lining material is placed to cover the remaining demineralized dentin. A sealing liner and/or a sealing restoration is then placed to seal out bacteria and their by-products.

In one clinical study of direct pulp capping involving 38 patients over 3 years, no relationship was found between success and factors such as patient age, tooth type, or size of exposure.[157] However, in a larger study of both direct and indirect pulp capping involving 592 patients over a 24-year period, age, tooth type, and extent of exposure did have a bearing on success.[162] As previously stated, the degree of bleeding affects the success of direct pulp capping; increased bleeding is associated with increased likelihood of failure.[156–158]

Direct pulp capping should be attempted only when a small mechanical exposure of an otherwise healthy pulp occurs. The tooth must be isolated with a rubber dam, and adequate hemostasis must be achieved. The exposure should be covered with calcium hydroxide because of its documented ability to provide the highest percentage of success[154,157,163,164] (Fig 5-3). It must be possible to restore the tooth with a well-sealed restoration that will prevent subsequent bacterial contamination.

Indirect Pulp Capping

An indirect pulp capping procedure (Fig 5-4) should be considered when there is a radiographically evident, deep caries lesion encroaching on the pulp and the tooth has no history of spontaneous pain and responds normally to vitality tests. Pulp exposure must be avoided; if it occurs, it should be regarded as an iatrogenic event. A direct pulp capping procedure

should be necessary only if the operator inadvertently exposes the pulp in attempting an indirect pulp capping procedure. With a deep caries lesion, the indirect pulp capping procedure is always preferred to a direct pulp capping procedure.

In the procedure (Figs 5-5 and 5-6), after the initial entry into the carious dentin (see Fig 5-5c), a spoon excavator or large round bur, rotating very slowly in a low-speed handpiece, should be used to excavate the caries-softened dentin (see Fig 5-6e). Demineralized dentin not near the pulp should be completely removed, leaving hard, sound dentin. As the excavation of carious dentin nears the pulp, caution must be exercised to avoid pulp exposure. If a bur has been used to excavate softened dentin, a spoon excavator may be used to aid in tactile detection of softened dentin. The wet (soft, amorphous) carious dentin should be removed; as the pulp is approached, the dry, fibrous, demineralized dentin that gives some moderate resistance to gentle scraping with a spoon excavator should be allowed to remain.

Caries-disclosing dyes may be used to assist in excavation of carious dentin (see Figs 5-5e to 5-5g and 5-6b to 5-6f). Studies have demonstrated the benefit of these dyes to aid in identification and removal of demineralized dentin[165] and to greatly reduce remaining viable bacteria.[166] It must be recognized that the dyes stain not only demineralized dentin, but also anything porous, such as debris that may have been left in the cavity preparation. In addition, noncarious deep dentin will absorb the dye[167–169] because of the increased number

Fig 5-5 Indirect pulp capping procedure, mandibular left first molar.

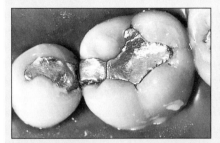

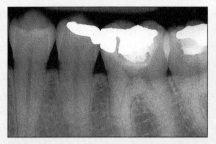

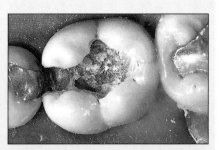

Fig 5-5a Mandibular first molar with deep recurrent carious involvement. Preoperative evaluation indicated vital pulpal tissue and no history of spontaneous pain.

Fig 5-5b Preoperative radiograph shows demineralized dentin around the base, under the amalgam, with carious demineralization advancing toward the pulp chamber.

Fig 5-5c The old restoration and base are removed, revealing soft, carious dentin.

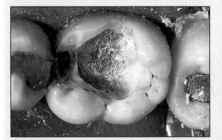

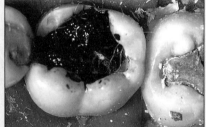

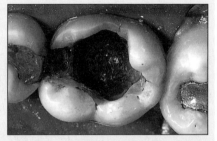

Fig 5-5d The preparation is widened to enable removal of a large amount of carious dentin and some undermined enamel.

Fig 5-5e A cotton pellet, saturated with a blue caries-disclosing dye solution (Cari-D-Tect, Gresco Products), is placed so that the dye coats all areas of the preparation. The cotton pellet is left in place for 10 seconds and removed. The area is then washed with air/water spray.

Fig 5-5f The preparation after being washed. Note the remaining large amount of demineralized dentin, as revealed by the blue dye. The stained dentin is checked for softness, and softened dentin is removed with a large round bur rotating very slowly. The dye is then reapplied and rinsed, and additional softened dentin, as disclosed by the dye, is removed.

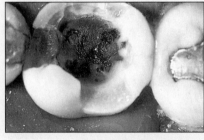

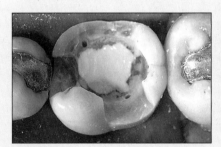

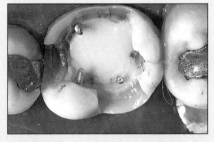

Fig 5-5g Most of the demineralized dentin has been removed. Only a small amount of dye-stained dentin is left; this dentin is believed to immediately overlie the pulp.

Fig 5-5h A calcium hydroxide liner (Dycal, Caulk/Dentsply) is placed over the remaining demineralized dentin.

Fig 5-5i A glass-ionomer liner (Vitrebond, 3M) is placed over the calcium hydroxide liner. The glass-ionomer liner provides some seal and improved strength for amalgam condensation.

Fig 5-5 *(continued)*

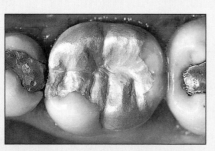

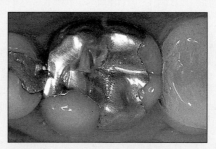

Fig 5-5j The completed amalgam restoration immediately after placement.

Fig 5-5k The restoration after 7 years of service.

Fig 5-6 *Indirect pulp capping procedure, mandibular right second molar.*

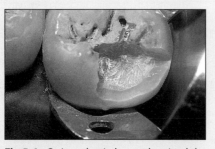

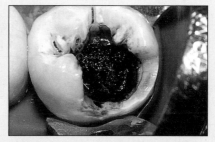

Fig 5-6a Carious dentin has undermined the distolingual cusp of the mandibular second molar. Overlying enamel and some carious dentin have been removed.

Fig 5-6b Caries-disclosing dye is applied.

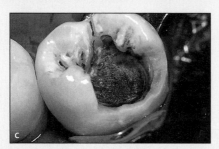

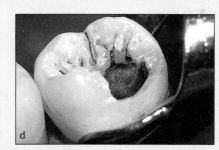

Figs 5-6c and 5-6d Dye-stained carious dentin.

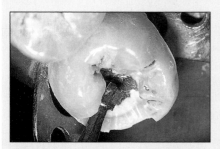

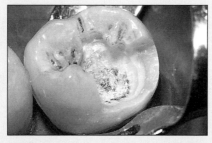

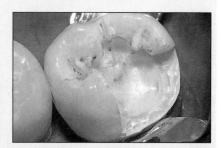

Fig 5-6e A large round bur (No. 8, Midwest), rotating very slowly, is used to remove the soft, dye-stained, carious dentin.

Fig 5-6f After several applications of caries-disclosing dye and removal of caries-softened dentin, only a small amount of dye-stained dentin remains, adjacent to the pulp chamber.

Fig 5-6g Calcium hydroxide and glass-ionomer liners are applied over the remaining demineralized dentin.

Protocol for Indirect Capping Procedures

Diagnosis

The preoperative status of the pulp and periradicular tissues should be evaluated carefully. The tooth is a candidate for indirect pulp capping only if the following conditions exist:

1. There is no history of spontaneous pulpal pain.
2. Pulpal vitality has been confirmed with thermal or electric pulp testing.
3. There is no history of pain that lingers after the tooth has returned to mouth temperature following the application of a hot or cold stimulus.
4. Pain elicited during pulp testing with a hot or cold stimulus does not linger after the tooth returns to mouth temperature.
5. A periapical radiograph shows no evidence of a periradicular lesion of endodontic origin.

Treatment

1. Isolation: After administering anesthetic, isolate the tooth with a rubber dam.
2. Preparation: Prepare the tooth for the final restoration, leaving demineralized dentin only in the area immediately adjacent to the pulp. Use a caries-disclosing dye if necessary to ensure complete carious dentin removal (other than that immediately adjacent to the pulp). After this is accomplished, use a spoon excavator or a large round bur in a low-speed handpiece at very low speed. Use very gentle, featherweight strokes over the area of the demineralized dentin to remove only the wet (soft, amorphous) carious dentin. Leave the dry, fibrous, demineralized dentin that gives some moderate resistance to gentle scraping with a spoon excavator.
3. Lining: Place a calcium hydroxide liner over the remaining demineralized dentin. If additional sealing is indicated, use a glass-ionomer liner.
4. Restoration:
   a. Direct restorations: For direct restorations (bonded amalgam, composite, glass ionomer), place the final restoration. If time does not allow for placement of a final restoration at the first appointment, a glass ionomer or reinforced zinc oxide–eugenol provisional restoration should be placed and the patient reappointed for the final restoration as soon as possible. The indirect pulp capping liner should not be disturbed during the subsequent restoration process.
   b. Indirect restorations: For indirect restorations (cast-metal restorations, ceramic onlays, or crowns), place a definitive buildup (bonded amalgam, composite, glass ionomer) at the appointment in which the indirect pulp capping procedure was performed if time allows. Delay placement of the final restoration for 4 to 8 months. Before proceeding with the definitive restoration, ensure normal pulp vitality.

Precautions

1. Use care in removing carious dentin near the pulp to prevent accidental pulp exposure.
2. If a temporary restoration has previously been placed over an indirect pulp capping liner and the tooth is re-entered for a restorative procedure, do not remove the indirect pulp capping material.
3. Prior to excavation, use tactile exploration to confirm that dye-stained dentin lacks hardness.

and size of the dentinal tubules in deep dentin; if this dye-stained sound dentin is removed, pulp exposure will result. If the operator uses a caries-disclosing dye, he or she must be aware of this characteristic of dye use in deep dentin. There has been concern that, when using a dentin bonding system, the previous use of caries-disclosing dyes can reduce the strength of the bond to dentin and increase microleakage at the interface of the bonded restoration with the wall of the cavity.[170] However, the preponderance of evidence indicates that neither of these should be a concern.[171–173]

In the procedure, carious dentin is removed except for the last portion of firm, leathery carious dentin immediately overlying the pulp; this layer is left because its removal would likely expose the pulp. At this point, a calcium hydroxide liner is placed over the demineralized area of dentin (see Fig 5-5h). Placement of calcium hydroxide over this layer of leathery dentin has been shown to virtually eliminate all remaining bacteria and render the residual carious dentin operationally sterile.[174–176] If any vital bacteria remain, a well-sealed restoration should isolate them from life-sustaining substrate and prevent further acid production, thereby arresting the caries process.[177,178] These facts argue against a two-step procedure in which the tooth is re-entered for the purpose of excavating the remaining acid-affected dentin to confirm reparative dentin formation. This procedure risks creating a pulp exposure and causing further traumatic insult to the pulp.[179] A glass-ionomer liner may be placed over the calcium hydroxide liner to improve strength during amalgam condensation and to enhance the seal (see Figs 5-5i and 5-6g). The definitive restoration should then be placed (see Fig 5-5j). This restoration should be placed to minimize microleakage at the interface of the restoration with the cavity preparation walls.

Calcium Hydroxide vs Dentin Bonding Agents

It has been suggested that dentin bonding agents may be used for direct and indirect pulp capping.[180,181] The rationale is based on the belief that an effective, permanent seal against bacterial invasion is provided and will promote pulpal healing. This theory is supported by a number of studies. Animal research has shown good compatibility of mechanically exposed pulps to visible light–activated resin composites when bacteria are excluded.[119] In addition, adhesive resins and pulpal tissues were shown to be compatible for up to 90 days when the smear layer was removed from cavity walls before the application of a dentin adhesive, confirming the ability of the bonding agents to minimize bacterial invasion for this period of time.[102,103,182] Several animal studies have shown that while calcium hydroxide may result in faster dentin bridge formation, adhesives can be successfully associated with dentin bridge formation and that this can occur without long-term pulpal inflammation.[156,183–186] Many components of dentin bonding agents are directly toxic to pulp cells,[187–189] but their release is rapid and slows dramatically with time, so these materials are not thought to be chronic sources of potentially toxic resin components.[190]

Clinical success of direct pulp capping with adhesive resins following traumatic pulp exposure[180] and exposure during excavation of carious dentin has been described.[181] In a clinical study of 64 cases of direct pulp capping with a dentin bonding agent following exposure during removal of carious dentin, it was reported that 60 of the teeth were vital 1 year later. In this same study, the pulps of six caries-free third molars were intentionally exposed with a bur and capped with a dentin bonding agent; the teeth were extracted up to 1 year later for histologic evaluation. All cases revealed dentin bridge formation and no inflammatory changes in the pulp.[191]

However, a number of in vivo studies counter the claims of success of direct pulp capping with adhesive sealers. In an animal study comparing direct pulp capping with conventional and visible light–activated calcium hydroxide to direct capping with a resin bonding agent, dentin bridges formed in almost all teeth in which the capping material was calcium hydroxide but in only a minority of those in which the capping material was resin adhesive.[192] It is important to note that the results of pulp capping studies using animals do not directly translate to comparative outcomes in humans.[22] The animal studies showing successful direct pulp capping with dentin bonding agents have invariably been accomplished in an environment not contaminated by bacteria.[102,103,156,183–186,193,194] When the exposed pulps of experimental animals were intentionally contaminated to simulate the clinical setting, the majority of direct pulp caps accomplished with adhesive sealers failed (75%), with resulting pulpal death or failure to form dentin bridges; most of the contaminated pulps capped with calcium hydroxide succeeded (77%).[158] Recent animal studies have confirmed the superiority of calcium hydroxide over adhesive resin sealers for capping inflamed pulps.[195,196]

Several human studies have also shown calcium hydroxide to perform better than adhesive resin sealers for direct pulp capping. One study showed mixed results with pulp capping using a dentin bonding agent.[197] Two other studies showed no evidence of dentin bridge formation in the exposures capped with a total-etch adhesive resin, while all of the calcium hydroxide–capped pulps demonstrated repair and dentin bridge formation.[198,199] Similar results have been found with a self-etching adhesive system. Human premolars that received pulp caps with a self-etch adhesive showed persistent inflammation and no dentin bridge formation, while those pulps capped with a calcium hydroxide preparation demonstrated pulp repair and dentin bridge formation.[22] Several other studies with human subjects have shown very high failure rates when adhesive sealers were used for pulp capping, especially when the adhesive sealers were compared with calcium hydroxide preparations.[193,197–199]

Although clinical success has been reported for direct pulp capping with dentin bonding agents,[191] most of these recommendations are empirical and are based on case reports in which clinical signs and symptoms were used to determine pulpal status.[180,181] However, controlled clinical trials have shown that there is no correlation between clinical findings and the actual condition of the pulp as determined by histologic examination. In fact, ailing pulps can be vital and cause no symptoms, even when the potential for recovery is poor.[22,200]

There are additional concerns regarding indirect and/or direct pulp capping procedures using dentin bonding resins. In vitro microleakage tests showing imperfect seals with dentin bonding agents have been criticized as being invalid because many dye tracer molecules are orders of magnitude smaller than the oral bacteria that cause pulpal inflammation.[103] These tests, therefore, may not be reliable indicators of the ability of bacteria to penetrate dentin toward the pulp. In addition, the outward flow of dentinal fluid in vivo partially opposes the diffusion of toxins into dentin,[201] and those toxins that ultimately reach the pulp are diluted and removed by the circulation.[202] However, while pathogenic intraoral bacteria may be larger than the initial interfacial gaps associated with dentin bonding agents, key components of pulpal inflammation are bacterial by-products,[203] the molecules of which are much smaller than the bacteria.

Interconnecting microporosities within the hybrid layer, created by dentin bonding resins in the etchant-demineralized dentin surface, have been shown to be permeable to very small molecules via "nanoleakage."[204,205] This demonstrates the potential for diffusion of even smaller water molecules, which could then lead to the hydrolysis of exposed collagen fibers within the hybrid layer.[206] Likewise, nearly all dye molecules are at least as large as, if not larger than, glucose, which allows for the possibility that bacteria present in the smear layer or in caries-affected dentin could be sustained by the diffusion of this nutrient. Finally, gap formation seen at the tooth-restoration interface in a number of studies indicates the presence of openings considerably larger than bacteria, viruses, and endotoxins.[142,207–212] It would seem reasonable to assume that dye penetration between dentin and the bonding resin would indicate an imperfect seal, ultimately leading to bacterial penetration, especially as the size of the interfacial gap and subsequent leakage is increased by thermal stress.[213]

Numerous studies have found a significant loss of bond strength of adhesive resins to human carious dentin vs sound dentin,[62,214–216] leading to further questioning of the integrity of the bond and subsequent ability to prevent bacterial invasion of a carious substrate. Proponents of the use of dentin bonding agents for direct pulp capping point to the shortcomings of calcium hydroxide in this role, including breakdown when acid etchants are used, dissolution under leaking restorations, interfacial failure during amalgam condensation, and the presence of tunnel defects in reparative dentin that remain open from the pulp to the medicament interface, allowing recurring microleakage of bacteria to the pulp.[217] The ultimate failure of calcium hydroxide is thought to be its inability to provide a seal against microleakage.[182] These are all valid concerns; methods for gaining the maximum benefit from calcium hydroxide in direct pulp capping while compensating for its shortcomings are described at the end of this chapter.

The success of dentin bonding agents for pulp capping depends on the quality and durability of the bond and requires that their placement have no deleterious effects on the pulp.

Quality and Durability of the Bond

Improvements in dentin bonding agents have been dramatic. However, in vitro research has demonstrated that modern dentin bonding resins leak almost immediately when bonded to superficial dentin.[104–107] The anatomy of dentin near the pulp can have an even greater adverse impact on bond formation. As tooth preparation nears the pulp, more area of a cut dentin surface is taken up by tubules and less by intertubular dentin.[218] The collagen of intertubular dentin is required for the formation of a hybrid layer or hybrid zone,

which is thought to be a primary means by which modern bonding resins adhere to dentin.[219] In addition, the bond immediately adjacent to dentinal tubules is often loose, allowing fluid shift and leakage of substrates due to a cuff of collagen-poor peritubular dentin.[220] Bond strengths of dentin bonding agents to surfaces of cut dentin are directly related to the area of sound dentin minus the area of the tubules,[221] since resin tags in the dentinal tubules contribute little to the bond strength.[222] It is, therefore, not surprising that dentin bonding agents show significantly reduced bond strength to deep dentin compared to superficial dentin.[221–225] In addition, as demonstrated by in vitro studies, the bond degrades with time.[97,206,226,227] Bond degradation with time and function has also been demonstrated in a human clinical trial.[228,229] This is significant because animal studies of pulpal compatibility are short term (21 to 90 days)[11,102,103,182]; studies have not provided long-term in vivo evaluation of the effectiveness of bonding systems as barriers to bacterial penetration.

Effect of Dentin Bonding Agent Application on Pulp

Modern dentin bonding systems require conditioning that removes the dentinal smear layer, usually through acid etching.[102,103,107,219] Acid etching of dentin has been demonstrated in multiple animal studies not to cause pulpal damage.[19,21,102,103,230] However, removal of the smear layer before placement of a dentin bonding resin and resin composite restoration significantly increased dentinal fluid flow and pulpal nerve firing in dogs[231] and pulp inflammation in humans.[232] The increased dentinal fluid flow that can result from opening the dentinal tubules may also cause fluid contamination, poor bonding, and fluid-filled gaps, which can allow bacterial penetration into dentinal tubules if the restorative material provides an imperfect seal.[220] These bacteria and their toxins can progress to the pulp despite the outward flow of dentinal tubular fluid.[17] Dentinal tubules opened by acid etching have been shown to allow the passage of adhesive sealer particulates into the human dental pulp, eliciting foreign body responses that inhibit dentin bridge formation.[5,197] Finally, applying acid to exposed pulps tends to increase bleeding, which inhibits good adhesion to dentin adjacent to the exposure.[185,193]

Many components of modern dentin bonding resins, primarily unpolymerized monomers, are toxic to cells[187,189,233,234] and capable of diffusing into the dental pulp.[235] Cellular toxicity decreases with improved degree of cure of the resin, since fewer unpolymerized monomers are available to leach from the adhesive resin.[236] Greater RDT and dentinal fluid flow significantly reduce diffusion to the dental pulp and help to decrease the toxic effects of these components.[237]

Although the concentration at which they reach the pulp is difficult to determine with certainty,[187] research has indicated that reducing RDT to 0.5 mm allows reactions to range from mild biologic responses[238] to mild toxic reactions after 12 hours to significant toxicity after 24 hours.[237] The presence of pulpal inflammation and direct placement of adhesives on pulp tissue, such as would occur with direct pulp capping, will exacerbate these responses.[237,238] The inward diffusion of these components is not prevented by intrapulpal pressure, even at a level of intrapulpal pressure that would simulate that of an inflamed pulp.[239] More important, at certain concentrations, most resin components in dentin bonding agents inhibit pulp T lymphocytes, leading to speculation that immunosuppression of pulpal immunocompetent cells may enhance potential for bacterial injury to pulpal tissues.[188]

Another issue in placing bonding resins directly on pulpal tissue is heat generation from a quartz tungsten halogen (QTH) curing light. An intrapulpal temperature increase of more than 20°F (11.2°C) has been shown to cause irreversible damage in vivo.[240] One study investigated the temperature rise in a bonding resin during polymerization with a QTH curing light.[241] An increase of 18.2°C was found with a 10-second cure, and a 25.2°C increase was detected with a 20-second cure. Because most bonding resins require a 20-second cure, there is potential for the pulp to be exposed to dangerous heat levels. Light-emitting diode (LED) curing lights have been shown to produce less heat than QTH lights; plasma arc curing (PAC) lights and high-intensity QTH (HQTH) lights have been shown to produce significantly more heat.[242]

The Future of Direct Pulp Capping Materials

A number of materials are being investigated for future use as direct pulp capping agents. Hydroxyapatite elicited a better pulpal response than calcium hydroxide in one animal study, because the hydroxyapatite acted as a scaffold for dentin formation.[243] In another animal study, bone morphogenetic protein (BMP) and bone sialoprotein (BSP) were more effective for inducing reparative dentin than was calcium hydroxide.[244]

However, the material that has shown the most promise is mineral trioxide aggregate (MTA), a combination of tricalcium silicate, tricalcium aluminate, tricalcium oxide, and silicate oxide. This material demonstrates a high pH similar to calcium hydroxide, exhibits compressive strength comparable to reinforced zinc oxide–eugenol, and is radiopaque.[245] It also displays some antibacterial activity and has shown significantly decreased microleakage compared to amalgam and two temporary restorative materials (Super-EBA [Harry J. Bosworth] and IRM [Caulk/Dentsply]).[246,247] Good biocompatibility in cell cultures has been demonstrated.[248] Animal studies have

shown good pulp healing following pulp capping with MTA, with MTA demonstrating similar healing mechanisms to those of calcium hydroxide.[155,249,250] The authors of one report noted that calcium hydroxide is released during the setting of MTA and suggested that to be the reason for the success of MTA.[155] Additionally, MTA has been shown to stimulate dentin bridge formation in primate animal studies.[251,252]

To date, virtually all of the in vivo research regarding MTA has been in animals, and, as previously stated, correlation of results of studies of pulp capping between animal and human studies is often lacking. Although one human study comparing pulp capping with MTA vs calcium hydroxide indicated MTA might be superior, it must be kept in mind that that study was done using noncarious teeth and without salivary contamination; no assessment for bacterial contamination was performed, and so few teeth were evaluated that no conclusion could be supported by statistical analysis.[253] Given the lack of human clinical research regarding MTA, the known success rate of calcium hydroxide, and the disadvantage MTA demonstrates with its extended setting time of 2 hours, 45 minutes,[254] it is advisable to wait for further research support before using MTA as a pulp-capping agent.

Antibacterial Efficacy of Restorative Materials

One of the keys to any successful restoration, but particularly for a tooth that has undergone a pulp capping procedure, is the ability to exclude bacteria and their by-products from entry into the pulp.[11,154] Of particular concern are the cariogenic bacteria, which tend to invade the interface between the restoration and the cavity preparation. Ultimately, these bacteria may lead to recurrent caries, and, if they reach the pulp in sufficient quantities, they will cause inflammatory and ultimately pathologic responses.[11] In particular, *Streptococcus mutans* is often used in in vitro studies evaluating the efficacy of restorative materials against bacteria, since this organism is associated with recurrent caries[255] (see chapter 4).

The discussion so far has focused on the materials placed immediately adjacent to the site of near or actual pulp exposure. However, the seal provided by the restorative material will also affect the ultimate success of the procedure. Restorative materials can effectively prevent bacterial contamination by one of two means: providing an impermeable seal with the cavity walls to physically exclude bacteria and the toxins they produce, or possessing antibacterial properties to destroy bacteria entering the restoration-tooth interface. No material yet provides an impermeable seal that can ensure the physical exclusion of bacteria.

Amalgam

Although typically not considered a material possessing anti-bacterial properties, dental amalgam has demonstrated varying levels of antibacterial activity.[256–259] This activity has been attributed to a variety of elements released from amalgam, including copper, mercury, zinc, silver, and chloride compounds. A number of studies have shown that amalgam is effective against cariogenic bacteria, including *S mutans*, *Actinomyces viscosus*, and *Lactobacillus* spp.[256–259]

S mutans thrive and produce lactic acid in an acidic environment.[260] The tooth-amalgam interface has a decreased pH,[261] which results in demineralization of tooth structure.[262] In vivo studies have shown that metallic solutions of copper, silver, and zinc are all capable of reducing acid production in plaque.[263] In one case, ions of these metals reduced acid production more than did fluoride in a comparable concentration.[264] All of these ions are released by amalgam and would, therefore, be present at the tooth-restoration interface.[256–259]

In addition to its antibacterial properties, amalgam is the only restorative material in which the marginal seal improves with time. This is due to the acidic environment and low oxygen concentration that exists in the amalgam–to–cavity wall gap, which promotes corrosion. In conventional amalgam, the gamma-2 phase forms SnO_2, $SnCl_2$, and $Sn(OH)_2Cl$, which slowly fill the interfacial gap. In high-copper alloys, in which there is no gamma 2, the eta phase (Cu_6Sn_5) corrodes to form CuO_2 and $CuCl_2$, but this occurs much more slowly. Corrosion in high-copper alloys may take twice as long as in conventional alloys to produce the same level of seal.[265]

Glass Ionomer

Glass ionomer has the ability to decrease bacterial penetration,[132] possibly through its fluoride release, initial low pH,[134] physical exclusion of bacteria,[132] or release of a metal cation.[135,136] Whatever the mechanism, glass-ionomer restorative and liner/base materials inhibit cariogenic bacteria[138] and demineralization at tooth-restoration interfaces.[266,267] In vivo plaque studies assessing the level of cariogenic bacteria invariably show significantly lower levels of these organisms adjacent to glass ionomer compared to either resin composite or amalgam.[268–270]

Resin Composite

In contrast to amalgam and glass ionomer, resin composite is most dependent on the formation of an impermeable seal to exclude bacterial penetration. This is because, as shown in in vitro bacterial inhibition studies, there is little, if any, inhibitory effect demonstrated by resin composite against cariogenic bacteria,[136] and, therefore, there is little resistance to secondary caries activity.[267] This is true even if a resin composite contains fluoride.[267] In fact, research has indicated that certain monomers released from resin composite actually stimulate cariogenic bacteria growth.[271] In vivo plaque studies have demonstrated that levels of cariogenic bacteria in the plaque present on surfaces of resin composite restorations are significantly higher than on either amalgam or glass ionomer.[269–273] While certain adhesive systems are similar to resin composite in that they demonstrate no bacterial inhibition,[274] some glutaraldehyde-containing bonding systems have shown an inhibitory effect on cariogenic organisms.[274,275] As previously stated, the quality and durability of adhesive bonding to dentin is questionable, and an impermeable seal is not achieved. Because resin composite does not have the ability to inhibit cariogenic bacteria, placement of a resin composite restoration with a dentin margin in a tooth that has been treated with pulp capping may decrease the chances of successful treatment.

Summary

1. Most operative procedures are traumatic to the pulp, and the effects are at least somewhat cumulative. Excessive heat and dehydration should be avoided. Questionable teeth should receive pulp vitality testing before undergoing clinical procedures.
2. Because, in direct pulp capping, no dentin remains between the capping material and the pulp, the problem of exposure of pulpal tissues and surrounding vital dentin to caustic or toxic materials is significant. The effects of thermal and chemical insults are magnified with an exposed vital pulp. Of the materials currently available, calcium hydroxide remains the material of choice for direct pulp capping, and it should be used with very specific clinical procedures and excellent isolation. Indirect pulp capping is preferred to direct pulp capping; with proper diagnosis and good clinical procedure, direct pulp capping should rarely be required.

3. Calcium hydroxide is also the material of choice for indirect pulp capping. If the restoration–to–cavity wall interface is well sealed, calcium hydroxide eliminates or greatly reduces the numbers of vital bacteria in the remaining demineralized dentin. Dentin bonding resins adhere poorly to carious dentin, provide a poor seal, and impart little to no antimicrobial activity.

4. Drawbacks attributed to the use of calcium hydroxide as a pulp capping agent include dissolution with acid etching, degradation under leaking restorations, and interfacial failure during amalgam condensation. While the most significant drawback of calcium hydroxide is its inability to provide a permanent seal against bacterial invasion, the integrity and durability of the bond achieved with dentin adhesives is questionable as well. Although there is potential as a possible future treatment modality, the lack of long-term documentation of clinical success for pulp capping with dentin bonding resins in controlled clinical trials should be weighed against literature that demonstrates 75% to 90% success for up to 12 years when calcium hydroxide is used.[132,154,157,276]

5. When calcium hydroxide is used as a pulp capping material, it should be limited to as small an area as possible, and some method of protecting it should be considered during subsequent restorative procedures. Placement of a glass-ionomer lining material over the calcium hydroxide provides a combination of clinically proven materials associated with clinical success in pulp capping. Calcium hydroxide provides antibacterial properties; glass ionomer provides resistance to acids, condensation pressures, and dissolution, as well as a fluoride source in the event of leakage and adhesion to tooth structure. A well-sealed restoration should then be placed to further reduce the potential for microleakage and enhance the success of the pulp cap.

References

1. Stanley HR. Human Pulp Response to Restorative Dental Procedures. Gainesville, FL: Storter, 1981.
2. Öztürk B, Üsümez A, Öztürk AN, Ozer F. In vitro assessment of temperature change in the pulp chamber during cavity preparation. J Prosthet Dent 2004;91:436–440.
3. Murray PE, About I, Lumley PJ, Franquin JC, Remusat M, Smith AJ. Cavity remaining dentin thickness and pulpal activity. Am J Dent 2002;15:41–46.
4. Meryon SD. The model cavity method incorporating dentine. Int Endod J 1988;21(2):79–84.
5. de Souza Costa, do Nascimento A, Texeira R. Response of human pulps following acid conditioning and application of a bonding agent in deep cavities. Dent Mater 2002;18:543–551.
6. Weine FS. Endodontic Therapy, ed 3. St Louis: Mosby, 1982:118.
7. Stanley HR. Pulpal responses to ionomer cements—Biological characteristics. J Am Dent Assoc 1990;120:25–29.
8. Stanley HR, Going RE, Chauncey HH. Human pulp response to acid pretreatment of dentin and to composite restoration. J Am Dent Assoc 1975;91:817–825.
9. Bergenholtz G, Lindhe J. Effect of soluble plaque factors on inflammatory reactions in the dental pulp. Scand J Dent Res 1975; 83(3):153–158.
10. Brannstrom M, Nordenvall KJ. Bacterial penetration, pulpal reaction and the inner surface of Concise enamel bond. Composite fillings in etched and unetched cavities. J Dent Res 1978;57:3–10.
11. Cox CF, Keall CL, Keall HJ, Ostro E, Bergenholtz G. Biocompatibility of surface-sealed dental materials against exposed pulps. J Prosthet Dent 1987;57:1–8.
12. Watts A, Paterson RC. Bacterial contamination as a factor influencing the toxicity of materials to the exposed dental pulp. Oral Surg Oral Med Oral Pathol 1987;64:466–474.
13. Bergenholtz G, Spångberg L. Controversies in endodontics. Crit Rev Oral Biol Med 2004;15:99–114.
14. Ritter AV, Swift EJ. Current restorative concepts of pulp protection. Endod Top 2003;5:41–48.
15. Bjorndal L, Darvann T, Thylstrup A. A quantitative light microscopic study of the odontoblast and subodontoblastic reactions to active and arrested enamel caries without cavitation. Caries Res 1998;32:59–69.
16. Brannstrom M, Lind PO. Pulpal response to early dental caries. J Dent Res 1965;44:1045–1050.
17. Vojinovic O, Nyborg H, Brannstrom M. Acid treatment of cavities under resin fillings: Bacterial growth in dentinal tubules and pulpal reactions. J Dent Res 1973;52:1189–1193.
18. Stanley HR, Pereira JC, Spiegel E, Broom C, Schultz M. The detection and prevalence of reactive and physiologic sclerotic dentin, reparative dentin and dead tracts beneath various types of dental lesions according to tooth surface and age. J Oral Pathol 1983; 12:257–289.
19. Nordenvall KJ, Brannstrom M, Torstensson B. Pulp reactions and microorganisms under ASPA and Concise composite fillings. ASDC J Dent Child 1979;46:449–453.
20. Brannstrom M, Vojinovic O. Response of the dental pulp to invasion of bacteria around three filling materials. ASDC J Dent Child 1976; 43:83–89.
21. Kurosaki N, Kubota M, Yamamoto Y, Fusayama T. The effect of etching on the dentin of the clinical cavity floor. Quintessence Int 1990;21:87–92.
22. de Souza Costa CA, Lopes do Nascimento AB, Teixeira HM, Fontana UF. Response of human pulps capped with a self-etching adhesive system. Dent Mater 2001;17:230–240.
23. Hamilton AI, Kramer IR. Cavity preparation with and without waterspray. Effects on the human dental pulp and additional effects of further dehydration of the dentine. Br Dent J 1967;123:281–285.
24. Langeland K, Langeland LK. Cutting procedures with minimized trauma. J Am Dent Assoc 1968;76:991–1005.
25. Lockard MW. A retrospective study of pulpal response in vital adult teeth prepared for complete coverage restorations at ultrahigh speed using only air coolant. J Prosthet Dent 2002;88:473–478.
26. Stanley HR Jr, Swerdlow H. Reaction of the human pulp to cavity preparation: Results produced by eight different operative grinding techniques. J Am Dent Assoc 1959;58(5):49–59.

27. Peyton FA, Henry EE. The effect of high speed burs, diamond instruments and air abrasive in cutting tooth tissue. J Am Dent Assoc 1954;49:426–435.

28. Karlsson S. A clinical evaluation of fixed bridges, 10 years following insertion. J Oral Rehabil 1986;13:423–432.

29. Valderhaug J, Jokstad A, Ambjornsen E, Norheim PW. Assessment of the periapical and clinical status of crowned teeth after 25 years. J Dent 1997;25:97–105.

30. Saunders WP, Saunders EM. Prevalence of periradicular periodontitis associated with crowned teeth in an adult Scottish subpopulation. Br Dent J 1998;185:137–140.

31. Felton D, Madison S, Kanoy E, Kantor M, Maryniuk G. Long term effects of crown preparation on pulp vitality [abstract 1139]. J Dent Res 1989;68(special issue):1009.

32. Laurell KA, Carpenter W, Daugherty D, Beck M. Histopathologic effects of kinetic cavity preparation for the removal of enamel and dentin. An in vivo animal study. Oral Surg Oral Med Oral Pathol 1995;80:214–225.

33. James VE, Schour I. Early dentinal and pulpal changes following cavity preparations and filling materials in dogs. Oral Surg Oral Med Oral Pathol 1955;8:1305–1314.

34. Dostalova T, Jelinkova H, Krejsa O, et al. Dentin and pulp response to Erbium:YAG laser ablation: A preliminary evaluation of human teeth. J Clin Laser Med Surg 1997;15(3):117–121.

35. Powell GL, Morton TH, Larsen AE. Pulpal response to irradiation of enamel with continuous wave CO_2 laser. J Endod 1989;15:581–583.

36. Sonntag KD, Klitzman B, Burkes EJ, Hoke J, Moshonov J. Pulpal response to cavity preparation with the Er:YAG and Mark III free electron lasers. Oral Surg Oral Med Oral Pathol 1996;81:695–702.

37. Srimaneepong V, Palamara JE, Wilson PR. Pulpal space pressure and temperature changes from Nd:YAG laser irradiation of dentin. J Dent 2002;30:291–296.

38. Attrill DC, Davies RM, King TA, Dickinson MR, Blinkhorn AS. Thermal effects of the Er:YAG laser on a simulated dental pulp: A quantitative evaluation of the effects of a water spray. J Dent 2004; 32:35–40.

39. D'Souza R. Pulpal and periapical immune response to electrosurgical contact of cervical metallic restorations in monkeys. Quintessence Int 1986;17:803–808.

40. Krejci RF, Reinhardt RA, Wentz FM, Hardt AB, Shaw DH. Effects of electrosurgery on dog pulps under cervical metallic restorations. Oral Surg Oral Med Oral Pathol 1982;54:575–582.

41. Robertson PB, Luscher B, Spangberg LS, Levy BM. Pulpal and periodontal effects of electrosurgery involving cervical metallic restorations. Oral Surg Oral Med Oral Pathol 1978;46:702–710.

42. Spangberg LS, Hellden L, Robertson PB, Levy BM. Pulpal effects of electrosurgery involving based and unbased cervical amalgam restorations. Oral Surg Oral Med Oral Pathol 1982;54:678–685.

43. Brannstrom M. Communication between the oral cavity and the dental pulp associated with restorative treatment. Oper Dent 1984; 9:57–68.

44. Miller BC, Charbeneau GT. Sensitivity of teeth with and without cement bases under amalgam restorations: A clinical study. Oper Dent 1984;9:130–135.

45. Piperno S, Barouch E, Hirsch SM, Kaim JM. Thermal discomfort of teeth related to presence or absence of cement bases under amalgam restorations. Oper Dent 1982;7(3):92–96.

46. Silvestri AR Jr, Cohen SH, Wetz JH. Character and frequency of discomfort immediately following restorative procedures. J Am Dent Assoc 1977;95:85–89.

47. Belcher MA, Stewart GP. Two-year clinical evaluation of an amalgam adhesive. J Am Dent Assoc 1997;128:309–314.

48. Browning WD, Johnson WW, Gregory PN. Postoperative pain following bonded amalgam restorations. Oper Dent 1997;22:66–71.

49. Gordan VV, Mjor IA, Hucke RD, Smith GE. Effect of different liner treatments on postoperative sensitivity of amalgam restorations. Quintessence Int 1999;30:55–59.

50. Gordan VV, Mjor IA, Moorhead JE. Amalgam restorations: Postoperative sensitivity as a function of liner treatment and cavity depth. Oper Dent 1999;24:377–383.

51. Kennington LB, Davis R, Murchison DF, Langenderfer WR. Short-term clinical evaluation of post-operative sensitivity with bonded amalgams. Am J Dent 1998;11:177–180.

52. Mahler DB, Engle JH, Simms LE, Terkla LG. One-year clinical evaluation of bonded amalgam restorations. J Am Dent Assoc 1996; 127:345–349.

53. Going RE. Cavity liners and dentin treatment. J Am Dent Assoc 1964;69:415–422.

54. Peters DD, Augsburger RA. In vitro cold transference of bases and restorations. J Am Dent Assoc 1981;102:642–646.

55. Harper RH, Schnell RJ, Swartz ML, Phillips RW. In vivo measurements of thermal diffusion through restorations of various materials. J Prosthet Dent 1980;43:180–185.

56. Drummond JL, Robledo J, Garcia L, Toepke TR. Thermal conductivity of cement base materials. Dent Mater 1993;9:68–71.

57. Farah JW, Clark AE, Mohsein M, Thomas PA. Effect of cement base thicknesses on MOD amalgam restorations. J Dent Res 1983;62: 109–111.

58. Hormati AA, Fuller JL. The fracture strength of amalgam overlying base materials. J Prosthet Dent 1980;43:52–57.

59. Pierpont W, Gray S, Hermesch C, Hilton T. Effect of various bases on the fracture resistance of amalgam [abstract 981]. J Dent Res 1993;72:226.

60. Pashley DH. Clinical considerations of microleakage. J Endod 1990; 16:70–77.

61. Duke ES, Lindemuth JS. Variability of clinical dentin substrates. Am J Dent 1991;4:241–246.

62. Yoshiyama M, Masada J, Uchida A, Ishida H. Scanning electron microscopic characterization of sensitive vs. insensitive human radicular dentin. J Dent Res 1989;68:1498–1502.

63. McCoy RB. Bases, liners and varnishes update. Oper Dent 1995; 20:216.

64. Anusavice KJ. Phillips' Science of Dental Materials, ed 10. Philadelphia, Saunders, 1996:545.

65. Kidd EA. Microleakage: A review. J Dent 1976;4:199–206.

66. Friedl K-H, Hiller K-A, Schmalz G. Placement and replacement of composite restorations in Germany. Oper Dent 1995;20:34–38.

67. Browning WD, Dennison JB. A survey of failure modes in composite resin restoration. Oper Dent 1996;21:160–166.

68. Mjör IA, Qvist V. Marginal failures of amalgam and composite restorations. J Dent 1997;25(1):25–30.

69. Mjör IA, Toffenetti F. Placement and replacement of resin-based composite restorations in Italy. Oper Dent 1992;17:82–85.

70. Mjör IA. Glass-ionomer cement restorations and secondary caries: A preliminary report. Quintessence Int 1996;27:171–174.

71. Craig RG. Restorative Dental Materials, ed 9. St. Louis: Mosby-Year Book, 1993:203–207.

72. Phillips RW. Skinner's Science of Dental Materials, ed 9. Philadelphia: Saunders, 1991.

73. Summitt JB. On bases, liners, and varnishes [letter]. Oper Dent 1994;19:35.

74. Andrews JT, Hembree JH. Marginal leakage of amalgam alloys with high content of copper: A laboratory study. Oper Dent 1980;5:7.

75. Lin JHC, Marshall GW, Marshall SJ. Microstructures of Cu-rich amalgams after corrosion. J Dent Res 1983;62:112–115.

76. Pashley DH, O'Meara JA, Williams EC, Kepler EE. Dentin permeability: Effects of cavity varnishes and bases. J Prosthet Dent 1985;53:511–516.

77. Pashley DH, Livingston MJ, Outhwaite WC. Rate of permeation of isotopes through human dentin, in vitro. J Dent Res 1977;56:83–88.

78. Fitchie JG, Reeves GW, Scarbrough AR, Hembree JH. Microleakage of a new cavity varnish with a high-copper spherical amalgam alloy. Oper Dent 1990;15:136–140.

79. McComb D, Ben-Amar A, Brown J. Sealing efficacy of therapeutic varnishes used with silver amalgam restorations. Oper Dent 1990;15:122–128.

80. Moore DS, Johnson WW, Kaplan I. A comparison of amalgam microleakage with a 4-META liner and Copal varnish. Int J Prosthodont 1995;8:461–466.

81. Felton DA, Kanoy BE, White JT. Effect of cavity varnish on retention of cemented cast crowns. J Prosthet Dent 1987;57:411–416.

82. Pashley DH, Depew DD. Effects of the smear layer, copalite, and oxalate on microleakage. Oper Dent 1986;11:95–102.

83. Sneed WD, Hembree JH Jr, Welsh EL. Effectiveness of three cavity varnishes in reducing leakage of a high-copper amalgam. Oper Dent 1984;9:32–34.

84. Marchiori S, Baratieri LN, de Andrada MA, Monteiro S Jr, Ritter AV. The use of liners under amalgam restorations: An in vitro study on marginal leakage. Quintessence Int 1998;29:637–642.

85. Mazer RB, Rehfeld R, Leinfelder KF. Effect of cavity varnishes on microleakage of amalgam restorations. Am J Dent 1988;1:205–208.

86. Wright W, Mazer RB, Teixeira LC, Leinfelder KR. Clinical microleakage evaluation of a cavity varnish. Am J Dent 1992;5:263–265.

87. Christensen G. Product use survey—1995. Clin Res Assoc Newsletter 1995;19(10):1–4.

88. Mahler DB, Engle JH, Adey JD. Bond strength and microleakage of amalgam adhesives [abstract 42]. J Dent Res 1992;71(special issue):111.

89. Dutton FB, Summitt JB, Garcia-Godoy F. Effect of a resin lining and rebonding on the marginal leakage of amalgam restorations. J Dent 1993;21:52–56.

90. Stefanoni JI, Abate PF, Polack MA, Macchi RL. In vitro marginal leakage in amalgam restorations [abstract 37]. J Dent Res 1996;75:1063.

91. Oliveira HP, Araujo MAJ, Figueiredo MOG. Adhesive amalgam: A microleakage study [abstract 69]. J Dent Res 1996;75:1086.

92. Ben-Amar A, Liberman R, Rothkoff Z, Cardash HS. Long term sealing properties of Amalgambond under amalgam restorations. Am J Dent 1994;7:141–143.

93. Cao DS, Hollis RA, Christensen RP, et al. Shear strength and microleakage of 23 adhesives for amalgam bonding [abstract 1760]. J Dent Res 1995;74(special issue):231.

94. Chang JC, Chan JT, Chheda HN, Iglesias A. Microleakage of a 4-methacryloxyethyl trimellitate anhydride bonding agent with amalgams. J Prosthet Dent 1996;75:495–498.

95. Hollis RA, Hein DK, Rasmussen TE, et al. Shear strength and microleakage of 14 amalgam bonding adhesives [abstract 2958]. J Dent Res 1996;75(special issue):387.

96. Meiers JC, Turner EW. Microleakage of dentin/amalgam alloy bonding agents: Results after 1 year. Oper Dent 1998;23:30–35.

97. Saiku JM, St Germain HA Jr, Meiers JC. Microleakage of a dental amalgam alloy bonding agent. Oper Dent 1993;18:172–178.

98. Tangsgoolwatana J, Chochran MA, Moore BK, Li Y. Microleakage evaluation of bonded amalgam restorations: Confocal microscopy versus radioisotope. Quintessence Int 1997;28:467–477.

99. Tjan AHL, Tan DE, Sun JC, Tjan AH. Marginal leakage of amalgam restorations pretreated with various liners. Am J Dent 1997;10:284–286.

100. Turner EW, St Germain HA, Meiers JC. Microleakage of dentin-amalgam bonding agents. Am J Dent 1995;8:191–196.

101. Watanabe T, Sano M, Itoh K, Wakumoto S. The effects of primers on the sensitivity of dentin. Dent Mater 1991;7:148–150.

102. Suzuki S, Cox CF, White KC. Pulpal response after complete crown preparation, dentinal sealing, and provisional restoration. Quintessence Int 1994;25:477–485.

103. White KC, Cox CF, Kanca J 3rd, Dixon DL, Farmer JB, Snuggs HM. Pulpal response to adhesive resin systems applied to acid-etched vital dentin: Damp versus dry primer application. Quintessence Int 1994;25:259–268.

104. Hilton TJ, Schwartz RS, Ferracane JL. Microleakage of four Class II resin composite insertion techniques at intraoral temperature. Quintessence Int 1997;28:135–144.

105. Pameijer CH, Wendt SL Jr. Microleakage of "surface-sealing" materials. Am J Dent 1995;8:43–46.

106. Strydom C, Retief DH, Russell CM, Denys FR. Laboratory evaluation of the Gluma 3-step bonding system. Am J Dent 1995;8:93–98.

107. Tay FR, Gwinnett AJ, Pang KM, Wei SHY. Variability in microleakage observed in a total-etch wet-bonding technique under different handling conditions. J Dent Res 1995;74:1168–1178.

108. Browning WD, Johnson WW, Gregory PN. Clinical performance of bonded amalgam restorations at eighteen months [abstract 427]. J Dent Res 1997;76(special issue):67.

109. Mahler DB, Engle JH. Clinical evaluation of bonding amalgam in traditional Class I and Class II restorations. J Am Dent Assoc 2000;131:43–49.

110. Mazer RB, Leinfelder KF, Barnette JH. Post-operative sensitivity and margin adaptation of amalgam and composite restorations treated with ProBond adhesive [abstract 748]. J Dent Res 1995;74(special issue):105.

111. Summitt JB, Burgess JO, Berry TG, Robbins JW, Osborne JW, Haveman CW. Six-year clinical evaluation of bonded and pin-retained complex amalgam restorations. Oper Dent 2004;29:261–268.

112. Hilton TJ, Schwartz RS. The effect of air thinning on dentin adhesive bond strength. Oper Dent 1995;20:133–137.

113. Christensen GJ. Should you and can you afford to bond amalgams? J Am Dent Assoc 1994;125:1381–1382.

114. Tyler DW, Thurmeier J. Amalgam bonding: Visualization and clinical implications of adhesive displacement during amalgam condensation. Oper Dent 2001;26:81–86.

115. Boston DW. Adhesive liner incorporation in dental amalgam restorations. Quintessence Int 1997;28:49–55.

116. Charlton DG, Moore BK, Swartz ML. Direct surface pH determinations of setting cements. Oper Dent 1991;16:231–238.

117. Millstein PL, Naguib GH. Effects of two resin adhesives on mechanical properties of set amalgam. J Prosthet Dent 1995;74:106–109.

118. Hanks CT, Bergenholtz G, Kim JS. Protein synthesis in vitro, in the presence of Ca(OH)$_2$-containing pulp-capping medicaments. J Oral Pathol 1983;12:356–365.

119. Cox CF. Biocompatibility of dental materials in the absence of bacterial infection. Oper Dent 1987;12:146–152.

120. Murray PE, Windsor LJ, Smyth TW, Hafez AA, Cox CF. Analysis of pulpal reactions to restorative procedures, materials, pulp capping, and future therapies. Crit Rev Oral Biol Med 2002;13:509–520.

121. Craig RG. Restorative Dental Materials, ed 8. St. Louis: Mosby, 1989.

122. Krejci I, Lutz F. Mixed Class V restorations: The potential of a dentine bonding agent. J Dent 1990;18:263–270.

123. Pereira JC, Manfio AP, Franco EB, Lopes ES. Clinical evaluation of Dycal under amalgam restorations. Am J Dent 1990;3:67–70.

124. Tam LE, Pulver E, McComb D, Smith DC. Physical properties of calcium hydroxide and glass-ionomer base and lining materials. Dent Mater 1989;5:145–149.

125. Lewis BA, Burgess JO, Gray SE. Mechanical properties of dental base materials. Am J Dent 1992;5:69–72.

126. Pierpont WF, Gray SE, Hermesch CB, Hilton TJ. The effect of various bases on the fracture resistance of amalgam. Oper Dent 1994;19:211–216.

127. Olsen BT, Garcia-Godoy F, Marshall TD, Barnwell GM. Fluoride release from glass ionomer–lined amalgam restorations. Am J Dent 1989;2:89–91.

128. Mitra SB. In vitro fluoride release from a light-cured glass-ionomer liner/base. J Dent Res 1991;70:75–78.

129. Geiger SB, Weiner S. Fluoridated carbonatoapatite in the intermediate layer between glass ionomer and dentin. Dent Mater 1993;9:33–36.

130. Garcia-Godoy F, Jensen ME. Artificial recurrent caries in glass ionomer–lined amalgam restorations. Am J Dent 1990;3:89–93.

131. Gaintantzopoulou MD, Willis GP, Kafrawy AH. Pulp reactions to light-cured glass ionomer cements. Am J Dent 1994;7:39–42.

132. Heys RJ, Fitzgerald M. Microleakage of three cement bases. J Dent Res 1991;70:55–58.

133. Hosoda H, Inokoshi S, Shimada Y, Harnirattisai C, Otsuki M. Pulpal response to a new light-cured composite placed in etched glass-ionomer lined cavities. Oper Dent 1991;16:122–129.

134. DeSchepper EJ, Thrasher MR, Thurmond BA. Antibacterial effects of light-cured liners. Am J Dent 1989;2(3):74–76.

135. Meryon SD, Jakeman KJ. Zinc release from dental restorative materials in vitro. J Biomed Mater Res 1986;20:285–291.

136. Scherer W, Lippman N, Kaim J. Antimicrobial properties of glass-ionomer cements and other restorative materials. Oper Dent 1989;14:77–81.

137. Irie M, Suzuki K. Marginal gap formation of light-activated base/liner materials: Effect of setting shrinkage and bond strength. Dent Mater 1999;15:403–407.

138. Burgess JO, Barghi N, Chan DCN, Hummert T. A comparative study of three glass ionomer base materials. Am J Dent 1993;6:137–141.

139. Arcoria CJ, Fisher MA, Wagner MJ. Microleakage in alloy-glass ionomer lined amalgam restorations after thermocycling. J Oral Rehabil 1991;18:9–14.

140. Smith GE. Surface deterioration of glass-ionomer cement during acid etching: An SEM evaluation. Oper Dent 1988;13:3–7.

141. Aboushala A, Kugel G, Hurley E. Class II composite resin restorations using glass-ionomer liners: Microleakage studies. J Clin Pediatr Dent 1996;21(1):67–71.

142. Ciucchi B, Bouillaguet S, Delaloye M, Holz J. Volume of the internal gap formed under composite restorations in vitro. J Dent 1997;25:305–312.

143. Friedl K-H, Schmalz G, Hiller K-A, Mortazavi F. Marginal adaptation of composite restorations versus hybrid ionomer/composite sandwich restorations. Oper Dent 1997;22:21–29.

144. Kemp-Scholte CM, Davidson CL. Complete marginal seal of Class V resin composite restorations effected by increased flexibility. J Dent Res 1990;69:1240–1243.

145. Miller MB, Castellanos ER, Vargas MA, Denehy GE. Effect of restorative materials on microleakage of Class II composites. J Esthet Dent 1996;8(3):107–113.

146. Prati C, Nucci C, Davidson CL, Montanari G. Early marginal leakage and shear bond strength of adhesive restorative systems. Dent Mater 1990;6:195–200.

147. Sidhu SK, Henderson LJ. In vitro marginal leakage of cervical composite restorations lined with a light-cured glass ionomer. Oper Dent 1992;17:7–12.

148. Trushkowsky RD, Gwinnett AJ. Microleakage of Class V composite, resin sandwich, and resin-modified glass ionomers. Am J Dent 1996;9:96–99.

149. Wells DL, Davis RD, Osborne PB. Effect of dentin treatment on the cervical marginal integrity of Class II composite restorations [abstract 199]. J Dent Res 1998;77(special issue):130.

150. Yap AUJ, Mok BYY, Pearson G. An in vitro microleakage study of the "bonded-base" restorative technique. J Oral Rehabil 1997;24:230–236.

151. Manders CA, Garcia-Godoy F, Barnwell GM. Effect of a copal varnish, ZOE or glass ionomer cement base on microleakage of amalgam restorations. Am J Dent 1990;3:63–66.

152. Robbins JW. The placement of bases beneath amalgam restorations: Review of literature and recommendations for use. J Am Dent Assoc 1986;113:910–912.

153. Eames WB, Scrabeck JG. Bases, liners and varnishes: Interviews with contemporary authorities. Gen Dent 1980;33:201–207.

154. Baume LJ, Holz J. Long term clinical assessment of direct pulp capping. Int Dent J 1981;31(4):251–260.

155. Horsted-Bindslev P, Lovschall H. Treatment outcome of vital pulp treatment. Endod Top 2002;2:24–34.

156. Cox CF, Hafez AA, Akimoto N, Otsuki M, Suzuki S, Tarim B. Biocompatibility of primer, adhesive and resin composite systems on non-exposed and exposed pulps of non-human primate teeth. Am J Dent 1998;11(special issue):S55–S63.

157. Matsuo T, Nakanishi T, Shimizu H, Ebisu S. A clinical study of direct pulp capping applied to carious-exposed pulps. J Endod 1996;22:551–556.

158. Pameijer CH, Stanley HR. The disastrous effects of the "total etch" technique in vital pulp capping in primates. Am J Dent 1998;11(special issue):S45–S54.

159. Swift EJ, Trope M, Ritter A. Vital pulp therapy for the mature tooth—Can it work? Endod Top 2003;5:49–56.

160. Paterson RC. Bacterial contamination and the exposed pulp. Br Dent J 1976;140(7):231–236.

161. Bernick S, Nedelman C. Effect of aging on the human pulp. J Endod 1975;1(3):88–94.

162. Reuver J. 592 pulp cappings in a dental office—A clinical study (1966–1990) [in German]. Dtsch Zahnärztl Zeitschr 1992;47:29–32.

163. Fitzgerald M, Heys RJ. A clinical and histological evaluation of conservative pulpal therapy in human teeth. Oper Dent 1991;16:101–112.

164. Weine FS. A preview of the canal-filling materials of the 21st century. Compend Contin Educ Dent 1992;13:688–698.

165. Starr CB, Langenderfer WR. Use of a caries-disclosing agent to improve dental residents' ability to detect caries. Oper Dent 1993;18:110–114.

166. Boston DW, Graver HT. Histological study of an acid red caries-disclosing dye. Oper Dent 1989;14:186–192.

167. Ansari G, Beeley JA, Reid JS, Foye RH. Caries detector dyes—An in vitro assessment of some new compounds. J Oral Rehabil 1999;26:453–458.

168. Kidd EAM, Joyston-Bechal S, Beighton D. The use of a caries detector dye during cavity preparation: A microbiological assessment. Br Dent J 1993;174:245–248.

169. Yip HK, Stevenson AG, Beeley JA. The specificity of caries detector dyes in cavity preparation. Br Dent J 1994;176:417–421.

170. Demarco FF, Matos AB, Matson E, Powers JM. Dyes for caries detection influence sound dentin bond strength. Oper Dent 1998;23:294–298.

171. Kazemi RB, Meiers JC, Peppers K. Effect of caries disclosing agents on bond strengths of total-etch and self-etching primer dentin bonding systems to resin composite. Oper Dent 2002;27:238–242.

172. Piva E, Meinhardt L, Demarco FF, Powers JM. Dyes for caries detection: Influence on composite and compomer microleakage. Clin Oral Investig 2002;6:244–248.

173. el-Housseiny AA, Jamjoum H. The effect of caries detector dyes and a cavity cleansing agent on composite resin bonding to enamel and dentin. J Clin Pediatr Dent 2000;25:57–63.

174. Dumsha T, Hovland EJ. Evaluation of long-term calcium hydroxide treatment in avulsed teeth—An in vivo study. Int Endod J 1995;28:7–11.

175. Fairbourn DR, Charbeneau GT, Loesche WJ. Effect of improved Dycal and IRM on bacteria in deep carious lesions. J Am Dent Assoc 1980;100:547–552.

176. Leung RL, Loesche WJ, Charbeneau GT. Effect of Dycal on bacteria in deep carious lesions. J Am Dent Assoc 1980;100:193–197.

177. Mertz-Fairhurst EJ, Curtis JW Jr, Ergle JW, Rueggeberg FA, Adair SM. Ultraconservative and cariostatic sealed restorations: Results at year 10. J Am Dent Assoc 1998;129:55–66.

178. Mertz-Fairhurst EJ, Schuster GS, Williams JE, Fairhurst CW. Clinical progress of sealed and unsealed caries. Part I: Depth changes and bacterial counts. J Prosthet Dent 1979;42:521–526.

179. Dumsha T, Hovland E. Considerations and treatment of direct and indirect pulp-capping. Dent Clin North Am 1985;29:251–259.

180. Kanca J 3rd. Replacement of a fractured incisor fragment over pulpal exposure: A case report. Quintessence Int 1993;24:81–84.

181. Prager M. Pulp capping with the total-etch technique. Dent Econ 1994;84(1):78–79.

182. Cox CF, Suzuki S. Re-evaluating pulp protection: Calcium hydroxide liners vs. cohesive hybridization [review]. J Am Dent Assoc 1994;125:823–831.

183. Gerbo L, Cox CF, Suzuki S, Suzuki SH. Histologic pulp response of a dentin bonding system [abstract 937]. J Dent Res 1993;72(special issue):220.

184. Kitasako Y, Inokoshi S, Fujitani M, Otsuki M, Tagami J. Short-term reaction of exposed monkey pulp beneath adhesive resins. Oper Dent 1998;23:308–317.

185. Kitasako Y, Inokoshi S, Tagami J. Effects of direct resin pulp capping techniques on short-term response of mechanically exposed pulps. J Dent 1999;27:257–263.

186. Olmez A, Oztas N, Basak F, Sabuncuoglu B. A histopathologic study of direct pulp-capping with adhesive resins. Oral Surg Oral Med Oral Pathol Oral Radiol Endod 1998;86(1):98–103.

187. Hanks CT, Strawn SE, Wataha JC, Craig RG. Cytotoxic effects of resin components on cultured mammalian fibroblasts. J Dent Res 1991;70:1450–1455.

188. Jontell M, Hanks CT, Bratel J, Bergenholtz G. Effects of unpolymerized resin components on the function of accessory cells derived from the rat incisor pulp. J Dent Res 1995;74:1162–1167.

189. Rathbun MA, Craig RG, Hanks CT, Filisko FE. Cytotoxicity of a BIS-GMA dental composite before and after leaching in organic solvents. J Biomed Mater Res 1991;25:443–457.

190. Ferracane JL, Condon JR. Rate of elution of leachable components from composite. Dent Mater 1990;6:282–287.

191. Kashiwada T, Takagi M. New restoration and direct pulp capping systems using adhesive composite resin. Bull Tokyo Med Dent Univ 1991;38(4):45–52.

192. Pitt Ford TR, Roberts GJ. Immediate and delayed direct pulp capping with the use of a new visible light-cured calcium hydroxide preparation. Oral Surg Oral Med Oral Pathol 1991;71:338–342.

193. Stanley HR, Pameijer CH. Dentistry's friend: Calcium hydroxide. Oper Dent 1997;22:1–3.

194. Tarim B, Hafez AA, Suzuki SH, Suzuki S, Cox CF. Biocompatibility of compomer restorative systems on nonexposed dental pulps of primate teeth. Oper Dent 1997;22:149–158.

195. Murray PE, Hafez AA, Smith AJ, Cox CF. Identification of hierarchical factors to guide clinical decision making for successful long-term pulp capping. Quintessence Int 2003;34:61–70.

196. Trope M, McDougal R, Levin L, May KN, Swift EJ. Capping the inflamed pulp under different clinical conditions. J Esthet Restor Dent 2002;14:349–357.

197. Tay FR, Gwinnett AJ, Wei SH. Ultrastructure of the resin-dentin interface following reversible and irreversible rewetting. Am J Dent 1997;10:77–82.

198. Hebling J, Aparecida Giro EM, de Souza Costa CA. Biocompatibility of an adhesive system applied to exposed human dental pulp. J Endod 1999;25:676–682.

199. Pereira JC, Segala AD, Costa CA. Human pulp response to direct capping with an adhesive system—Histologic study [abstract 1329]. J Dent Res 1997;76(special issue):180.

200. Horsted-Bindslev P, Vilkinis V, Sidlauskas A. Direct capping of human pulps with a dentin bonding system or with calcium hydroxide cement. Oral Surg Oral Med Oral Pathol Oral Radiol Endod 2003;95:591–600.

201. Vongsavan N, Matthews B. The permeability of cat dentine in vivo and in vitro. Arch Oral Biol 1991;36:641–646.

202. Pashley DH. The influence of dentin permeability and pulpal blood flow on pulpal solute concentrations. J Endod 1979;5:355–361.

203. Bergenholtz G, Cox CF, Loesche WJ, Syed SA. Bacterial leakage around dental restorations: Its effect on the dental pulp. J Oral Pathol 1982;11:439–450.

204. Sano H, Takatsu T, Ciucchi B, Horner JA, Matthews WG, Pashley DH. Nanoleakage: Leakage within the hybrid layer. Oper Dent 1995;20:18–25.

205. Sano H, Yoshiyama M, Ebisu S, et al. Comparative SEM and TEM observations of nanoleakage within the hybrid layer. Oper Dent 1995;30:160–167.

206. Watanabe I, Nakabayashi N. Bonding durability of photocured Penyl-P in TEGDMA to smear layer–retained bovine dentin. Quintessence Int 1993;24:335–342.

207. Coli P, Brannstrom M. The marginal adaptation of four different bonding agents in Class II composite resin restorations applied in bulk or in two increments. Quintessence Int 1993;24:583–591.

208. Finger WJ, Fritz U. Laboratory evaluation of one-component enamel/dentin bonding agents. Am J Dent 1996;9:206–210.

209. Prati C, Nucci C. Marginal gap, microleakage and shear bond strength of adhesive restorative systems [abstract 1036]. J Dent Res 1989;68(special issue):996.

210. Sorensen JA, Munksgaard EC. Relative gap formation adjacent to ceramic inlays with combinations of resin cements and dentin bonding agents. J Prosthet Dent 1996;76:472–476.

211. Symons AL, Wing G, Hewitt GH. Adaptation of eight modern dental amalgams to walls of Class I cavity preparations. J Oral Rehabil 1987;14:55–64.

212. Tjan AH, Bergh BH, Lidner C. Effect of various incremental techniques on the marginal adaptation of Class II composite resin restorations. J Prosthet Dent 1992;67:62–66.

213. Bullard RH, Leinfelder KF, Russell CM. Effect of coefficient of thermal expansion on microleakage. J Am Dent Assoc 1988;116:871–874.

214. Frankenberger R, Sindel J, Kramer N, Petschelt A. Dentin bond strength and marginal adaptation: Direct composite resins vs ceramic inlays. Oper Dent 1999;24:147–155.

215. Nakajima M, Sano H, Burrow MF, et al. Tensile bond strength and SEM evaluation of caries-affected dentin using dentin adhesives. J Dent Res 1995;74:1679–1688.

216. Nakajima M, Sano H, Zheng L, Tagami J, Pashley DH. Effect of moist vs. dry bonding to normal vs. caries-affected dentin with Scotchbond Multi-Purpose Plus. J Dent Res 1999;78:1298–1303.

217. Cox CF, Subay RK, Ostro E, Suzuki S, Suzuki SH. Tunnel defects in dentin bridges: Their formation following direct pulp capping. Oper Dent 1996;21:4–11.

218. Garberoglio R, Brannstrom M. Scanning electron microscopic investigation of human dentinal tubules. Arch Oral Biol 1976;21:355–362.

219. Nakabayashi N, Ashizawa M, Nakamura M. Identification of a resin-dentin hybrid layer in vital human dentin created in vivo: Durable bonding to vital dentin. Quintessence Int 1992;23:135–141.

220. Pashley DH. Clinical correlations of dentin structure and function. J Prosthet Dent 1991;66:777–781.

221. Suzuki T, Finger WJ. Dentin adhesives: Site of dentin vs bonding of composite resins. Dent Mater 1988;4:379–383.

222. Tao L, Pashley DH. Shear bond strengths to dentin: Effects of surface treatments, depth and position. Dent Mater 1988;4:371–378.

223. Mitchem JC, Gronas DG. Effect of time after extraction and depth of dentin on resin dentin adhesives. J Am Dent Assoc 1986;113:285–287.

224. Panighi MM, Allart D, Jacquot BM, Camps J, G'Sell C. Influence of human tooth cryopreservation on dentin bond strength. Dent Mater 1997;13:56–61.

225. Tagami J, Tao L, Pashley DH, Hosoda H, Sano H. Effects of high-speed cutting on dentin permeability and bonding. Dent Mater 1991;7:234–239.

226. De Munck J, Van Meerbeek B, Yoshida Y, et al. Four-year water degradation of total-etch adhesives bonded to dentin. J Dent Res 2003;82:136–140.

227. Armstrong SR, Vargas MA, Fang Q, Laffoon JE. Microtensile bond strength of a total-etch 3-step, total-etch 2-step, self-etch 2-step, and a self-etch 1-step dentin bonding system through 15-month water storage. J Adhes Dent 2003;5:47–56.

228. Hashimoto M, Ohno H, Kaga M, Endo K, Sano H, Oguchi H. In vivo degradation of resin-dentin bonds in humans over 1 to 3 years. J Dent Res 2000;79:1385–1391.

229. Hashimoto M, Ohno H, Kaga M, Endo K, Sano H, Oguchi H. Resin-tooth adhesive interfaces after long-term function. Am J Dent 2001;14:211–215.

230. Brannstrom M, Vojinovic O, Nordenvall KJ. Bacteria and pulpal reactions under silicate cement restorations. J Prosthet Dent 1979;41:290–295.

231. Hirata K, Nakashima M, Sekine I, Mukouyama Y, Kimura K. Dentinal fluid movement associated with loading of restorations. J Dent Res 1991;70:975–978.

232. Murray PE, Smyth TW, About I, Remusat R, Franquin JC, Smith AJ. The effect of etching on bacterial microleakage of an adhesive composite restoration. J Dent 2002;30:29–36.

233. Lefebvre CA, Schuster GS, Rueggeberg FA, Tamareselvy K, Knoernschild KL. Responses of oral epithelial cells to dental resin components. J Biomater Sci Polym Ed 1996;7:965–976.

234. Ratanasathien S, Wataha JC, Hanks CT, Dennison JB. Cytotoxic interactive effects of dentin bonding components on mouse fibroblasts. J Dent Res 1995;74:1602–1606.

235. Gerzina TM, Hume WR. Diffusion of monomers from bonding resin–resin composite combinations through dentine in vitro. J Dent 1996;24:125–128.

236. Caughman WF, Caughman GB, Shiflett RA, Rueggeberg F, Schuster GS. Correlation of cytotoxicity, filler loading and curing time of dental composites. Biomaterials 1991;12:737–740.

237. Bouillaguet S, Wataha JC, Hanks CT, Ciucchi B, Holz J. In vitro cytotoxicity and dentin permeability of HEMA. J Endod 1996;22:244–248.

238. Hanks CT, Wataha JC, Parsell RR, Strawn SE, Fat JC. Permeability of biological and synthetic molecules through dentine. J Oral Rehabil 1994;21:475–487.

239. Gerzina TM, Hume WR. Effect of hydrostatic pressure on the diffusion of monomers through dentin in vitro. J Dent Res 1995;74:369–373.

240. Zach L, Cohen G. Pulp response to externally applied heat. Oral Surg Oral Med Oral Pathol 1965;19:515–530.

241. Puckett A, Thompson N, Phillips S, Reeves G. Heat generation during curing of a dentin adhesive and composite [abstract 1380]. J Dent Res 1965;74(special issue):184.

242. Ozturk B, Ozturk AN, Üsümez A, Üsümez S, Ozer F. Temperature rise during adhesive and resin composite polymerization with various light curing sources. Oper Dent 2004;29:325–332.

243. Hayashi Y, Imai M, Yanagiguchi K, Viloria IL, Ikeda T. Hydroxyapatite applied as direct pulp capping medicine substitutes for osteodentin. J Endod 1999;25:225–229.

244. Goldberg M, Six N, Decup F, et al. Application of bioactive molecules in pulp-capping situations. Adv Dent Res 2001;15:91–95.

245. Torabinejad M, Hong CU, Pitt Ford TR, Kettering JD. Cytotoxicity of four root end filling materials. J Endod 1995;21:489–492.

246. Torabinejad M, Rastegar AF, Kettering JD, Pitt Ford TR. Bacterial leakage of mineral trioxide aggregate as a root-end filling material. J Endod 1995;21:109–112.

247. Torabinejad M, Watson TF, Pitt Ford TR. Sealing ability of a mineral trioxide aggregate when used as a root end filling material. J Endod 1993;19:591–595.

248. Saidon J, He J, Zhu Q, Safavi K, Spångberg LS. Cell and tissue reactions to mineral trioxide aggregate and Portland cement. Oral Surg Oral Med Oral Pathol Oral Radiol Endod 2003;95:483–489.

249. Tziafas D, Pantelidou O, Alvanou A, Belibasakis G, Papadimitriou S. The dentinogenic effect of mineral trioxide aggregate (MTA) in short-term capping experiments. Int Endod J 2002;35:245–254.

250. Dominguez MS, Witherspoon DE, Gutmann JL, Opperman LA. Histological and scanning electron microscopy assessment of various vital pulp-therapy materials. J Endod 2003;29:324–333.

251. Ford TR, Torabinejad M, Abedi HR, Bakland LK, Kariyawasam SP. Using mineral trioxide aggregate as a pulp-capping material. J Am Dent Assoc 1996;127:1491–1494.

252. Torabinejad M, Chivian N. Clinical applications of mineral trioxide aggregate. J Endod 1999;25:197–205.

253. Aeinehchi M, Eslami B, Ghanbariha M, Saffar AS. Mineral trioxide aggregate (MTA) and calcium hydroxide as pulp-capping agents in human teeth: A preliminary report. Int Endod J 2002;36:225–231.

254. Torabinejad M, Hong CU, McDonald F, Pitt Ford TR. Physical and chemical properties of a new root-end filling material. J Endod 1995;21:349–353.

255. Wallman-Bjorklund C, Svanberg M, Emilson CG. *Streptococcus mutans* in plaque from conventional and from non-gamma-2 amalgam restorations. Scand J Dent Res 1987;95:266–269.

256. Morrier JJ, Suchett-Kaye G, Nguyen D, Rocca JP, Blanc-Benon J, Barsotti O. Antimicrobial activity of amalgams, alloys and their elements and phases. Dent Mater 1998;14:150–157.

257. Nunez LJ, Schmalz G, Hembree J. Influence of amalgam, alloy, and mercury on the in vitro growth of *Streptococcus mutans*: I. Biological test system. J Dent Res 1976;55:257–261.

258. Orstavik D. Antibacterial properties of and element release from some dental amalgams. Acta Odontol Scand 1985;43:231.

259. Updegraff DM, Chang RW, Joos RW. Antibacterial activity of dental restorative materials. J Dent Res 1971;50:382–387.

260. Harper DS, Loesche WJ. Growth and acid tolerance of human dental plaque bacteria. Arch Oral Biol 1984;29:843–848.

261. Marek M, Hochman RF. Mechanism of crevice corrosion of dental amalgam [abstract 166]. J Dent Res 1975;54(special issue):242.

262. McTigue D, Brice C, Nanda CR, Sarkar NK. The in vivo corrosion of Dispersalloy. J Oral Rehabil 1984;11:351–359.

263. Afseth J, Oppermann RV, Rolla G. The in vivo effect of glucose solutions containing Cu++ and Zn++ on the acidogenicity of dental plaque. Acta Odontol Scand 1980;38:229–233.

264. Oppermann RV, Johansen JR. Effect of fluoride and non-fluoride salts of copper, silver and tin on the acidogenicity of dental plaque in vivo. Scand J Dent Res 1980;88:476–480.

265. Ben-Amar A, Cardash HS, Judes H. The sealing of the tooth/amalgam interface by corrosion products. J Oral Rehabil 1995;22:101–104.

266. Donly KJ, Gomez C. In vitro demineralization-remineralization of enamel caries at restoration margins utilizing fluoride-releasing composite resin. Quintessence Int 1994;25:355–358.

267. Gilmour AS, Edmunds DH, Newcombe RG. Prevalence and depth of artificial caries-like lesions adjacent to cavities prepared in roots and restored with a glass ionomer or a dentin-bonded composite material. J Dent Res 1997;76:1854–1861.

268. Svanberg M, Krasse B, Ornerfeldt HO. Mutans streptococci in interproximal plaque from amalgam and glass ionomer restorations. Caries Res 1990;24:133–136.

269. Svanberg M, Mjor IA, Orstavik D. Mutans streptococci in plaque from margins of amalgam, composite, and glass-ionomer restorations. J Dent Res 1990;69:861–864.

270. Zalkind M, Keisar O, Ever-Hadani P, Sela M. Accumulation of *Streptococcus mutans* on light-cured composites and amalgam: An in vitro study. J Esthet Dent 1998;10(4):187–190.

271. Hansel C, Leyhausen G, Mai UE, Geurtsen W. Effects of various resin composite (co)monomers and extracts on two caries-associated micro-organisms in vitro. J Dent Res 1998;77:60–67.

272. Skjorland KK. Plaque accumulation on different dental filling materials. Scand J Dent Res 1973;81:538–542.

273. Skjorland KK, Sonju T. Effect of sucrose rinses on bacterial colonization on amalgam and composite. Acta Odontol Scand 1982;40:193–196.

274. Carvalhaes Fraga R, Freitas Siqueira JJ, de Uzeda M. In vitro evaluation of antibacterial effects of photo-cured glass ionomer liners and dentin bonding agents during setting. J Prosthet Dent 1996;76:483–486.

275. Meiers JC, Miller GA. Antibacterial activity of dentin bonding systems, resin-modified glass ionomers, and polyacid-modified composite resins. Oper Dent 1996;21:257–264.

276. Haskell EW, Stanley HR, Chellemi J, Stringfellow H. Direct pulp capping treatment: A long-term follow-up. J Am Dent Assoc 1978;97:607–612.

Nomenclature and Instrumentation

James B. Summitt

Basic to any science is a language understood by the members of the community of the discipline. This chapter is devoted to a review of the language of operative dentistry and to the basic instrumentation of that discipline. *Operative dentistry* today may be defined as that part of restorative dentistry involving assessment, prevention, and treatment of diseases and defects of the hard tissues of individual teeth to maintain or restore functional, physiologic, and esthetic integrity and health.

Nomenclature and Classification of Caries Lesions and Cavity Preparations

Systems for Naming and Numbering Teeth

Each tooth may be identified by its location in the mouth and by its individual name. Examples include the *maxillary right central incisor* and the *mandibular left second premolar*. Areas of the mouth are referred to by arch (*maxillary* or *upper* and *mandibular* or *lower*) and by the side of the patient's midline (left and right) (Fig 6-1). Each arch is divided in half at the midline, forming four *quadrants* (maxillary right and left quadrants and mandibular right and left quadrants). In addition, each tooth is identified as *primary* or *permanent*. Finally, the individual name of the tooth, eg, *molar* or *central incisor*, completes the

identification. Examples of complete tooth names are *mandibular left permanent first molar* and *maxillary right primary canine*.

Because their names are cumbersome, teeth are frequently referred to by number. The tooth-numbering systems primarily used today are the Universal system and the Fédération Dentaire Internationale (FDI) system (Fig 6-2). In the Universal system, the numbering begins with the maxillary (upper) right third molar (tooth 1), proceeds around the arch to the maxillary left third molar (tooth 16), then to the mandibular (lower) left third molar (tooth 17) and around the mandibular arch to the mandibular right third molar (tooth 32).

In the FDI system, the first digit of the tooth number represents a quadrant (1, maxillary right; 2, maxillary left; 3, mandibular left; and 4, mandibular right). The second digit represents the tooth (1, a central incisor, regardless of the arch or quadrant; 2, lateral incisor; 3, canine; and so on to 8, third molar). The maxillary left first premolar would be identified as tooth 24; the mandibular right second molar would be identified as tooth 47.

Incisors and canines are referred to as *anterior teeth*, regardless of the arch; premolars and molars are *posterior teeth*.

In addition to quadrants, the mouth may also be divided into *sextants*, or sixths. There are three sextants in each arch, with divisions between the canines and first premolars—the maxillary right, anterior, and left sextants and the mandibular right, anterior, and left sextants.

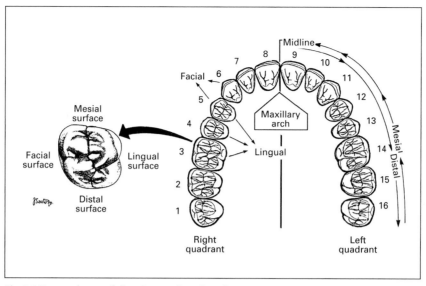

Fig 6-1 Nomenclature of directions and tooth surfaces.

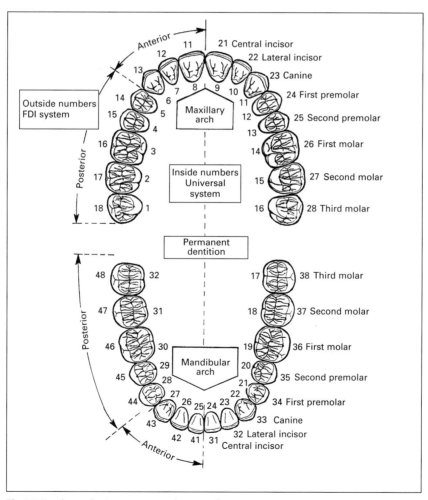

Fig 6-2 Tooth-numbering systems and nomenclature.

Fig 6-3 Directions, features, and tooth surfaces of anterior teeth.

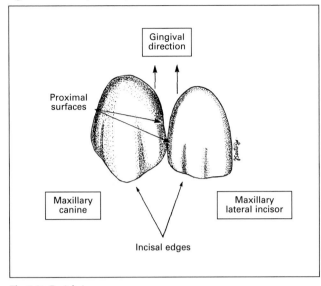

Fig 6-3a Facial view.

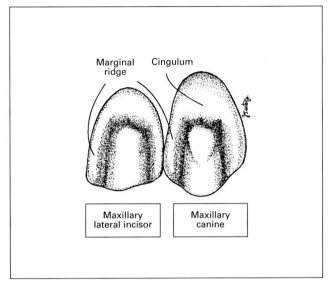

Fig 6-3b Lingual view.

Fig 6-4 Directions, features, and tooth surfaces of posterior teeth.

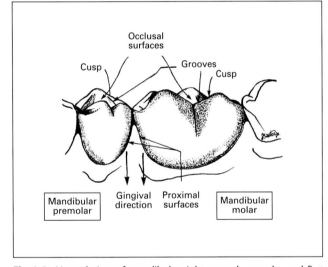

Fig 6-4a Lingual view of mandibular right second premolar and first molar.

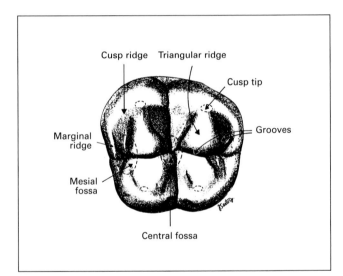

Fig 6-4b Occlusal view of mandibular right molar.

Nomenclature of Tooth Surfaces and Cavity Preparations

The surfaces of the teeth are identified by their locations. Any surface or movement toward the midline of the arch is referred to as *mesial* (see Fig 6-1). A surface or movement away from the midline is *distal*. Surfaces and movements toward the tongue are termed *lingual*; those that are in the direction of the cheek or lips are termed *facial*. For the ante-rior teeth, facial may be referred to as *labial* (toward the lips); for posterior teeth, facial may be referred to as *buccal* (toward the cheek).[1]

On any tooth, gingival refers to an area or movement toward the gingiva (Figs 6-3 and 6-4). A distinction is made, however, between the chewing surfaces of posterior teeth, which are called *occlusal* (see Figs 6-4a and 6-4b) and the biting edges of anterior teeth, which are called *incisal* (see Figs 6-3a and 6-3b). A proximal surface is one that faces an adja-

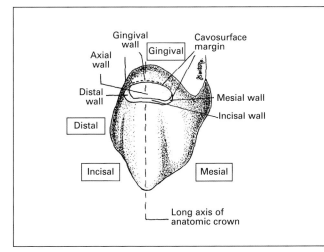

Fig 6-5 Class 5 cavity preparation in an anterior tooth (maxillary canine, facial view). In a posterior tooth, there would be an occlusal wall instead of an incisal wall.

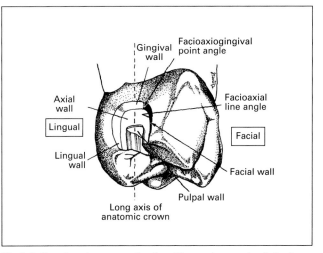

Fig 6-6 Class 2 cavity preparation (maxillary molar, proximal view).

cent tooth; it may be further identified as mesial or distal.[1] The contact between two adjacent teeth is referred to as the *interproximal contact.*

The anatomic contour of anterior teeth is less complicated than that of posterior teeth, in which the occlusal surfaces are characterized by grooves, cusp tips and ridges, marginal ridges, and fossae. *Marginal ridges* (both mesial and distal) border the lingual surfaces of anterior teeth (see Fig 6-3b) and the occlusal surfaces of posterior teeth (see Fig 6-4b). A *groove* is a linear channel between enamel elevations, such as cusps and/or ridges. A *fissure* is a developmental linear cleft usually found at the base of a groove; it is commonly the result of the lack of fusion of the enamel of adjoining dental cusps or lobes. A *pit* is a small depression in enamel, usually located in a groove and often at the junction of two or more fissures. A *fossa* is a hollow, rounded, or depressed area in the enamel surface of a tooth. For example, a mesial fossa lies just distal to a mesial marginal ridge (see Fig 6-4b).[1]

With the advent of bonding restorative materials to teeth, walls of cavity preparations are less distinct than they are in preparations for restorations that are retained by mechanical undercuts in the preparation walls or by nonadhesive cements. The walls of cavity preparations, however, are generally referred to by the same terms as the surface features of the teeth, for example, the gingival and distal walls (Figs 6-5 to 6-9). Exceptions are the *pulpal wall* (or floor), which is only in the occlusal portion of a preparation and is the wall adjacent or nearest to the pulp chamber of the tooth (see Figs 6-6 and 6-7), and the *axial wall,* which, in all other areas of a

preparation, is the wall adjacent or nearest to the pulp chamber or pulp canal(s) and is approximately parallel to the long axis of the tooth (see Figs 6-5, 6-6, and 6-9).[1]

The junction of two walls in a cavity preparation is called a *line angle.*[1] Again, in preparations for bonded restorations, line angles may not be well defined, but the names for line angles may be used to refer to general areas of the preparation. For example, the meeting of the facial and axial walls forms the facioaxial (or axiofacial) line angle (see Fig 6-6). Similarly, the junction of three walls is referred to as a *point angle.* For example, the junction of the facial, axial, and gingival walls creates the facioaxiogingival (or axiofaciogingival or gingivofacioaxial) point angle. Again, the junction of two walls is often rounded, so it does not actually form a line, but it is still referred to as a line angle; likewise, a point angle is usually not a sharp point.

The *margins* (or *cavosurface angles*[1]) of a preparation, which are formed by the junction of a cavity wall and an external tooth surface, are identified by the names of the adjacent walls (eg, incisal margin, mesial margin, or gingival margin).

The *anatomic crown* of a tooth is the portion that extends from the cementoenamel junction, or cervical line, to the occlusal surface or incisal edge; it is covered by enamel (Figs 6-10 and 6-11). The *clinical crown* is the portion that is visible in the oral cavity.[1] Depending on the tooth, the clinical crown may include only part of the anatomic crown (see Fig 6-10) or it may include all of the anatomic crown and part of the root (see Fig 6-11).

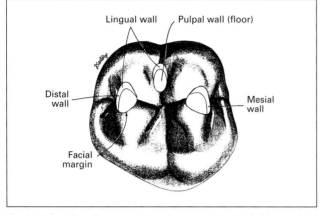

Fig 6-7 Class 1 cavity preparations in a posterior tooth. The occlusal surface of this mandibular right molar is viewed slightly from the facial aspect (occlusofacial), so the facial wall is hidden from view.

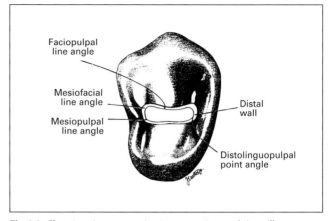

Fig 6-8 Class 1 cavity preparation in a posterior tooth (maxillary premolar, occlusal view). In a direct restoration (such as for amalgam), the facial and lingual walls would be parallel or convergent for retention of the amalgam. The walls of a preparation for bonded resin composite could diverge as shown here or by considerably more, because the restoration would be bonded to the enamel and dentin.

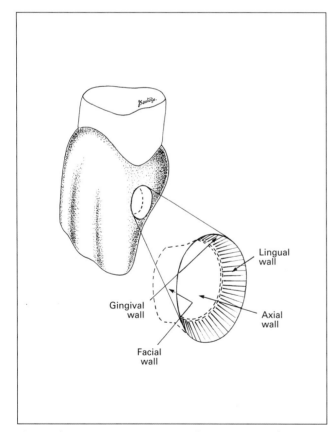

Fig 6-9 Class 3 cavity preparation (maxillary incisor, mesiofacial view). The preparation is for a bonded, tooth-colored restoration.

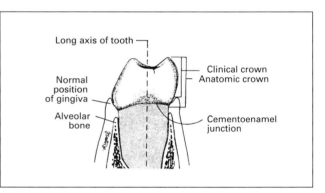

Fig 6-10 Anatomic and clinical crowns of a mandibular molar with the periodontal attachment at the normal, healthy level.

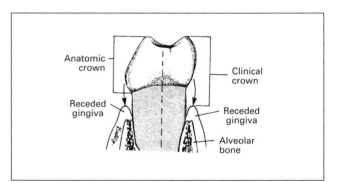

Fig 6-11 Anatomic and clinical crowns of a mandibular molar with the periodontal attachment at a more apical level (periodontal recession). With loss of gingival height comes an increase in the length of the clinical crown, but the anatomic crown, which is defined by the cementoenamel junction (or cervical line), stays constant. The occlusogingival dimension of the anatomic crown can be reduced by loss of occlusal tooth structure from wear or erosion.

Fig 6-12 Classification of cavity preparations.

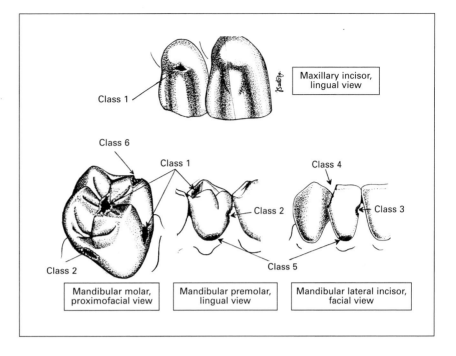

Class 1

Maxillary incisor, lingual view

Class 6

Class 1

Class 4

Class 2

Class 3

Class 5

Class 2

Mandibular molar, proximofacial view

Mandibular premolar, lingual view

Mandibular lateral incisor, facial view

Classification of Caries Lesions and Tooth Preparations

Near the beginning of the 20th century, G. V. Black,[2] who is known as the father of operative dentistry, classified caries lesions into groups according to their locations in permanent teeth. The same classification is used to refer to cavity preparations, because the location of carious tooth structure is a major factor in the design of the cavity preparation and the selection of instruments (Fig 6-12).

Class 1 (I) lesions occur in pits and fissures on the facial, lingual, and occlusal surfaces of molars and premolars and, less often, the lingual surfaces of maxillary anterior teeth (most frequently lateral incisors, less frequently central incisors, rarely canines) (see Figs 6-7 and 6-8).

Class 2 (II) lesions occur in the proximal surfaces of the posterior teeth (molars and premolars). If a proximal surface of a posterior tooth is involved in a restoration, it is a Class 2 restoration (see Fig 6-6).

Class 3 (III) lesions occur in the proximal surfaces of anterior teeth (central and lateral incisors and canines). Class 3 cavities do not involve an incisal angle (see Fig 6-9).

Class 4 (IV) lesions occur in the proximal surfaces of anterior teeth when the incisal angle requires restoration. The angle may have to be removed because of its fragility or for proper placement of the restoration, or it may have been fractured by trauma (Fig 6-13).

Class 5 (V) lesions occur in smooth facial and lingual surfaces in the gingival third of teeth. Class 5 lesions begin close to the gingiva and may involve a cementum or dentin surface as well as enamel (see Fig 6-5).

Class 6 (VI) lesions are in pit or wear defects on the incisal edges of anterior teeth or the cusp tips of posterior teeth (Fig 6-14).

In addition to being named for their classifications, cavity preparations and restorations are named for the tooth surfaces involved. For example, a restoration involving the mesial and occlusal surfaces of a posterior tooth is called a *mesio-occlusal Class 2 restoration*; simply saying *mesio-occlusal restoration* identifies it as a Class 2 restoration because the proximal surface of a posterior tooth is involved. A preparation or restoration involving the mesial, occlusal, distal, and facial surfaces of a posterior tooth is called a *mesio-occlusodistofacial preparation* or *restoration*.

For brevity's sake, the names of the surfaces are often abbreviated (distal, *D*; lingual, *L*; facial, *F*; mesial, *M*; incisal, *I*; occlusal, *O*). A mesio-occlusal restoration in a posterior tooth would be abbreviated *MO*, and a distolingual restoration in an anterior tooth is abbreviated *DL*.

Black's Steps in Cavity Preparation

Treatment modalities for dental caries other than surgical removal of lesions are discussed in chapter 4. When it has been determined that nonsurgical means of treating caries lesions will not suffice, however, restorative therapy is indicated. This involves the surgical removal of carious tooth structure and restoration of the tooth to its original anatomic form

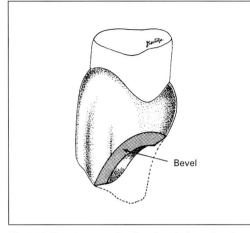

Fig 6-13 Class 4 preparation for a bonded, tooth-colored restoration. Maxillary incisor, facial view.

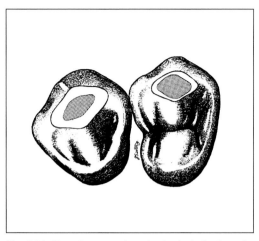

Fig 6-14 Class 6 preparations in the incisal edge of a maxillary canine and the cusp tip of a premolar (incisal/occlusal view). The dotted area of the preparation represents dentin; the clear area of the preparation represents enamel. The preparations have no mechanical, or undercut, retention; they are for bonded, tooth-colored restorations.

with a suitable restorative material. The design of the cavity preparation is determined first by the location of the caries lesion(s) in the tooth. The shape or outline of the cavity preparation, as it meets the external surface of the tooth, is referred to as *outline form*. Other factors influencing the design include the need to obtain access for the instruments as the operator is preparing the cavity or placing the restoration (*convenience form*) and the need to provide retention for the restorative material (*retention form*). Also required is resistance to stresses on the restoration and the tooth from forces of biting and chewing (*resistance form*). Because cavity preparation is a surgical procedure in which a mistake can mean injury to living tissue, it is essential that the operator be knowledgeable and highly skilled.

Sequential steps for cavity preparation were established by Black.[2] Black's steps represent a systematic, scientific procedure for efficiency in cavity preparation. Although the technology of bonding restorative materials to enamel and dentin was not available to Black, his steps of cavity preparation are generally as appropriate today as they were when he formulated them:

1. *Establish outline form*. Outline form is based primarily on the location and extent of the caries lesion, tooth fracture, or erosion. In carious teeth, the outline form is established after penetration into carious dentin and removal of the enamel overlying the carious dentin. The extent of carious dentin should be a primary determinant of the outline

form of the preparation; the final outline is not established until the carious dentin and, usually, its overlying enamel have been removed.

2. *Obtain resistance form*. Resistance for the remaining tooth structure and for the restoration must be designed in the preparation, so that the restoration will be resistant to displacement and both the tooth and the restoration will be resistant to fracture during function.

3. *Obtain retention form*. Retention may be obtained through mechanical shaping of the preparation to retain the restoration and/or via bonding procedures that attach the restorative material to tooth structure.

4. *Obtain convenience form*. Convenience form allows adequate observation, accessibility, and ease of operation during preparation and restoration of the tooth. Convenience form that involves the removal of sound, strong tooth structure should be limited to that which is necessary.

5. *Remove remaining carious dentin*. Removal of remaining carious dentin applies primarily to that in the deepest part (pulpally) of the preparation. Other carious tooth structure was removed when the outline form was established.

6. *Finish enamel walls and cavosurface margins*. For indirect restorations (those requiring the making of an impression and fabrication of a stone duplicate of the preparation or the creation of a digital image), finishing involves making the walls relatively smooth. For direct and indirect restorations not utilizing bonding, finishing involves removing any unsupported, weak, or fragile enamel and making the

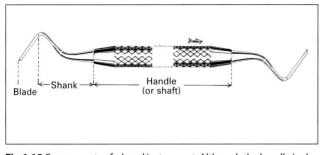

Fig 6-15 Components of a hand instrument. Although the handle is also called a shaft, that designation is little used.

Fig 6-16 Blade bevels. Most hand cutting instruments not only have a bevel on the end of the blade but also have bevels on the sides. Although most of the work of a hand cutting instrument is accomplished with the end of the blade, the sides may also be used to plane or scrape walls and margins. (In the drawing on the right, the blade is lying face down.)

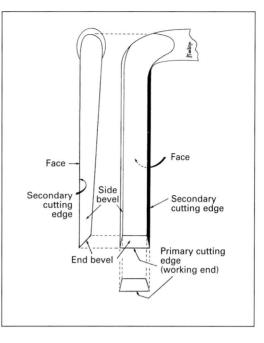

cavosurface margin smooth and continuous to facilitate finishing of restoration margins. For bonded resin composite restorations, enamel that is not supported by dentin and is not going to be exposed to significant occlusal loading is frequently allowed to remain in place and is reinforced by bonding to its internal surface.

7. *Clean the preparation*. Black referred to this step as "performing the toilet of the cavity." It includes washing or scrubbing away any debris in the preparation and drying the preparation. Afterward, the cavity is inspected for any remaining debris, fragile enamel, and demineralized tooth structure and altered if necessary; then the restoration is placed.

Instrumentation

Hand Instruments

Black[2] organized not only the classification of cavity preparations and their parts, but also the naming and numbering of hand instruments. *Cutting instruments*, which he also called *excavators*, were to be used in shaping the tooth preparation. All other hand instruments are grouped into the noncutting category.

Metals

For many years, carbon steel was the primary material used in hand instruments for operative dentistry because carbon steels were harder and maintained sharpness better than stainless steels. Stainless steels are now the preferred materials for hand instruments, because all instruments must be sterilized with steam or dry heat between patients and because the properties of stainless steels have improved. There are literally hundreds of formulas for stainless steels,[3] all incorporating a significant amount of chromium, some carbon, and iron. Chromium imparts corrosion resistance and brightness to the metal; carbon imparts hardness.

Cutting Instruments

Before rotating instruments were available, dentists could cut well-shaped cavity preparations using sharp hand instruments alone. The process was slow. The advent of the dental handpiece in 1871,[4] first attached to a foot-operated engine, allowed increased speed of tooth preparation. Most tooth preparation today is accomplished with rotary instruments, but hand cutting instruments are still important for finishing many tooth preparations. Few preparations involving a proximal surface can be completed properly without the use of hand cutting instruments. It is crucial that hand instruments used for cutting tooth structure or carving restorative materials be sharp.

Design. Hand cutting instruments are composed of three parts: *handle* (or *shaft*), *shank*, and *blade*[2] (Fig 6-15). The *primary cutting edge* of a cutting instrument is at the end of the blade (called the *working end*), but the sides of the blade are usually beveled and also may be used for cutting tooth structure (Fig 6-16). The shank joins the blade to the handle of the

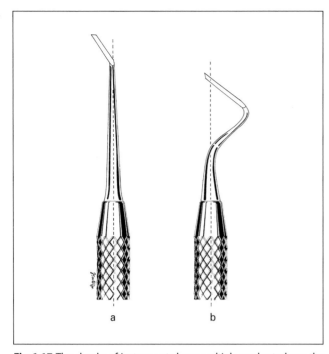

Fig 6-17 The shanks of instruments have multiple angles to keep the working end of the instrument within 2.0 to 3.0 mm of the long axis of the handle. (a) The working end of this instrument is not close to the long axis of the handle, and the instrument is, therefore, not balanced. (b) The shank of this instrument has two angles in it so that the working end is brought near (within 2.0 mm) to the long axis of the handle; this provides balance to facilitate control of the instrument during the application of force. The instrument is said to be contra-angled.

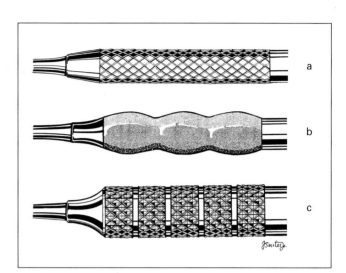

Fig 6-18 Instrument handle configurations. Instrument handles are available from most manufacturers in a variety of designs and diameters. (a) Standard stainless steel handle has a diameter of approximately 6.4 mm. (b) Padded handles are available; the diameter of the illustrated padded handle is approximately 8 mm. (c) Handles with larger diameters are said to be more ergonomic; the diameter of the one illustrated is approximately 9.5 mm.

instrument and is angled to keep the working end of the blade within 2.0 to 3.0 mm of the axis of the handle (Fig 6-17). This angulation is intended to provide balance, so that when force is exerted on the instrument it is not as likely to rotate, which would decrease the effectiveness of the blade and could possibly cause damage to the tooth or soft tissue. Figure 6-17a illustrates an instrument that has a single angle at the junction of the blade and the shank. Because the working end of the blade is not aligned with the handle, the instrument is said to be out of balance. Such an instrument may still be useful in tooth preparation. Its blade will usually be relatively short, and it will usually be used with minimal force. Figure 6-17b shows a shank that has two angles to bring the cutting edge into near alignment with the long axis of the handle to provide balance.

A variety of handle configurations is available (Fig 6-18). Padded handles (Fig 6-18b) are said to increase operator comfort and grip during use. Most metal handles today are round and have knurled areas for improved grip. The standard metal handle has a diameter of approximately one-fourth inch (6.4 mm). Although little research support can be

found, handles with larger diameters, such as the three-eighths-inch (9.5-mm) diameter handle illustrated in Fig 6-18c, are said to be more ergonomic and less likely to contribute to the development of carpal tunnel syndrome. A handle with an intermediate diameter (five-sixteenths inch or 7.9 mm) is also available. The larger diameters are encouraged primarily for dental hygienists, who spend a large part of their day using hand instruments. A drawback to the use of larger handles in operative dentistry is the space they consume in an instrument tray.

Nomenclature. The terminology organized by Black[2] in the early part of the last century is still used today with minor modifications. Most names Black assigned to cutting instruments were based on the appearance of the instrument, such as *hatchet, hoe, spoon,* and *chisel.* For an instrument that did not have the appearance of a commonly used item, Black based the name on the intended use, for example, *gingival margin trimmer.* Black called all cutting instruments used for tooth preparation *excavators,* and he referred to instruments as *hatchet excavators, spoon excavators,* etc. The term *exca-*

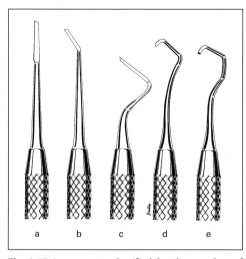

Fig 6-19 Instruments classified by the number of angles in the shank: (a) straight; (b) monangle; (c) binangle; (d) triple-angle; (e) quadrangle.

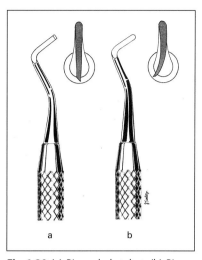

Fig 6-20 (a) Binangle hatchet. (b) Binangle spoon. A double-ended hatchet or spoon would have a left-cutting end and a right-cutting end (see Fig 6-21).

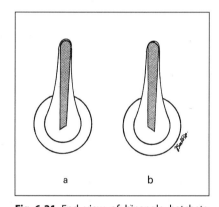

Fig 6-21 End view of binangle hatchets, paired: (a) right-cutting; (b) left-cutting. A double-ended binangle hatchet has left-cutting and right-cutting ends.

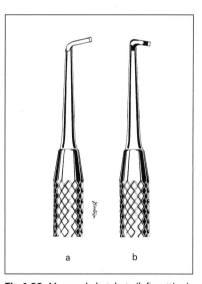

Fig 6-22 Monangle hatchets (left-cutting).

vator is still applicable, but in the day-to-day language of operative dentistry, it is little used. In catalogs of instruments, however, cutting instruments are often indexed as excavators.

Black combined the name of each instrument with a designation of the number of angles in the shank of the instrument. Shanks may be *straight*, *monangle* (one angle), *binangle* (two angles), *triple-angle* (three angles), or *quadrangle* (four angles) (Fig 6-19). The term *contra-angled* refers to a shank in which two or more angles are necessary to bring the working end into near alignment (within 2.0 to 3.0 mm) with the axis of the handle (see Fig 6-17b).

Hatchet. In a *hatchet* (also called an *enamel hatchet*), the blade and cutting edge are on a plane with the long axis of the handle; the shank has one or more angles (Figs 6-19e, 6-20a, 6-21, and 6-22). The face (see Fig 6-16) of the blade of the hatchet will be directed either to the left or the right in relation to the handle, and the instrument is usually supplied in a double-ended form. Therefore, there are left-cutting and right-cutting ends of the double-ended hatchet.

Chisel. A *chisel* has a blade that is either aligned with the handle (Figs 6-19a, 6-23, and 6-24d), slightly angled (Figs

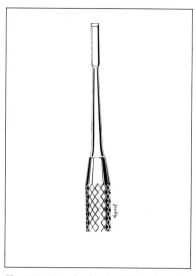

Fig 6-23 Straight chisel with bevels on the sides of the blade, to give secondary cutting edges, as well as on the end (primary cutting edge).

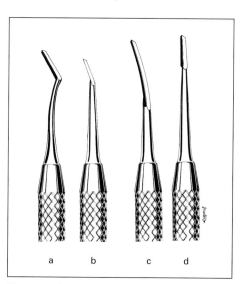

a   b   c   d

Fig 6-24 Chisels: (a) binangle; (b) monangle; (c) Wedelstaedt; (d) straight. The blades for a, c, and d are slightly rotated to visualize the face, as well as the side bevel.

6-19b, 6-24a, and 6-24b), or curved (Fig 6-24c) from the long axis of the handle, with the working end at a right angle to the handle.

Hoe. A *hoe* has a cutting edge that is at a right angle to the handle, like that of a chisel. However, its blade has a greater angle from the long axis of the handle than does that of the chisel; its shank also has one or more angles (Figs 6-15, 6-19c, and 6-25). A general guideline for distinguishing between a hoe and a chisel will be given later in the chapter.

Spoon. The blade of a *spoon* is curved, and the cutting edge at the end of the blade is in the form of a semicircle (Figs 6-20b and 6-26b); this gives the instrument an outer convexity and an inner concavity that make it look somewhat like a spoon. Like the hatchet, the spoon has a cutting edge at the end of its blade that is parallel to the handle of the instrument; therefore, there are left-cutting and right-cutting spoons. The shank of some spoons holds a small circular, or disk-shaped, blade at its end, and the cutting edge extends around the disk except for its junction with the shank; these are called *discoid spoons* (Figs 6-26a and 6-26c).

Gingival margin trimmer. A *gingival margin trimmer* is similar to an enamel hatchet, except that the blade is curved and the bevel for the cutting edge at the end of the blade is always on the outside of the curve; the face of the instrument is on the inside of the curve (Figs 6-27 and 6-28). Gingival margin trimmers, like hatchets and spoons, come in pairs (left

cutting and right cutting) (see Fig 6-27), but there are also mesial gingival margin trimmers and distal gingival margin trimmers (see Fig 6-28). Thus, a set of gingival margin trimmers is composed of four instruments: left-cutting and right-cutting mesial gingival margin trimmers and left-cutting and right-cutting distal gingival margin trimmers. Because these are usually double-ended instruments, one instrument is a mesial gingival margin trimmer (with left- and right-cutting ends), and the other is a distal gingival margin trimmer (with left- and right-cutting ends). Figure 6-28a illustrates a mesial left-cutting gingival margin trimmer. Figure 6-28b illustrates a distal left-cutting gingival margin trimmer. Contrasted with these is a right-cutting hatchet (see Fig 6-28c). Gingival margin trimmers have many uses in addition to trimming gingival margins (Fig 6-29).

Off-angle hatchet. Black's instrument names apply to instruments that have cutting edges that are either parallel or at a right angle to the handle. Instruments have been developed that have blades rotated 45 degrees from the plane of the long axis of the handle; these are called *off-angle hatchets*.

Usage. Hand cutting instruments are, for the most part, made in pairs, and, as with the gingival margin trimmers, most instruments used today are double-ended and will have one of the pair on each end (see Figs 6-15, 6-21, and 6-27). A cutting instrument may be used with horizontal strokes, in which the long axis of the blade is directed at between 45 and 90 degrees to the surface being planed or scraped (see Fig

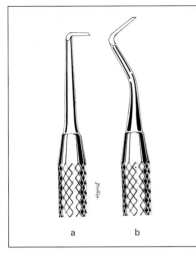

Fig 6-25 Hoes: (a) monangle; (b) binangle. The blade of a hoe has an angle from the long axis of the handle of greater than 12.5 centigrades; in contrast, the blade of a chisel will have an angle from the long axis of the handle of 12.5 centigrades or less (see Figs 6-33 and 6-34).

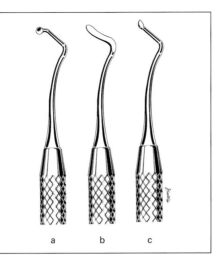

Fig 6-26 Spoons: (a) triple-angle discoid spoon; (b) binangle spoon (or regular spoon or banana spoon); (c) binangle discoid spoon. Spoons are used in tooth preparation for removing (or "spooning out") carious dentin.

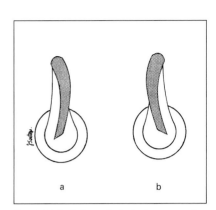

Fig 6-27 End view of gingival margin trimmers, paired: (a) right-cutting, (b) left-cutting. A double-ended gingival margin trimmer has both left-cutting and right-cutting ends, but there must be two double-ended gingival margin trimmers to complete a set, one double-ended mesial gingival margin trimmer and one double-ended distal gingival margin trimmer.

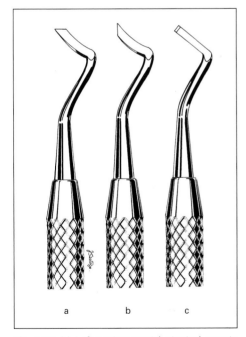

Fig 6-28 (a) Left-cutting mesial gingival margin trimmer. (b) Left-cutting distal gingival margin trimmer. (c) Right-cutting binangle hatchet.

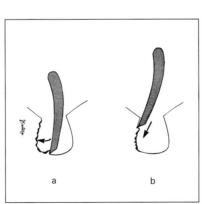

Fig 6-29 (a) Gingival margin trimmer being used in a proximal box of a Class 2 preparation with a horizontal (left or right) stroke to scrape (plane) a gingival wall and margin. (b) Gingival margin trimmer being used with a vertical, or chopping, stroke to plane a facial or lingual wall and margin. A hatchet could be used in a similar way.

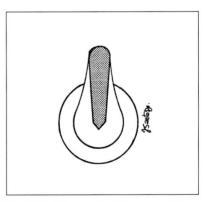

Fig 6-30 Bi-beveled cutting edge. These instruments are useful in placing retention points in some direct gold (gold foil) preparations but have little use in any of the preparations described in this book.

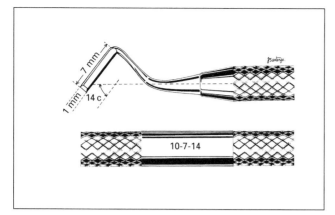

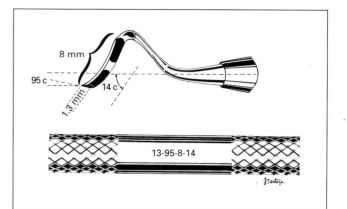

Fig 6-31 Black's three-number formula for instruments that have a primary cutting edge (working end) that is at a right angle (90 degrees) to the long axis of the blade: The first number is the width of the blade in tenths of a millimeter; the second number is the length of the blade in millimeters; and the third number is the blade angle, the angle the blade makes with the long axis of the handle, in centigrades. The complete name of the instrument illustrated would be binangle hatchet, 10-7-14. The formula would be the same if the blade were rotated 90 degrees on the shank to form a hoe, but the name would be different. Assuming the instrument illustrated is double-ended, the right-cutting end is shown.

Fig 6-32 Black's four-number formula for instruments that have a primary cutting edge (working end) that is not at a right angle to the long axis of the blade: The first number is the width of the blade in tenths of a millimeter; the second number is the cutting edge angle, the angle the primary cutting edge makes with the long axis of the handle, in centigrades; the third number is the length of the blade in millimeters; and the fourth number is the blade angle, the angle the blade makes with the long axis of the handle, in centigrades. Illustrated is the right-cutting end of a distal gingival margin trimmer, 13-95-8-14.

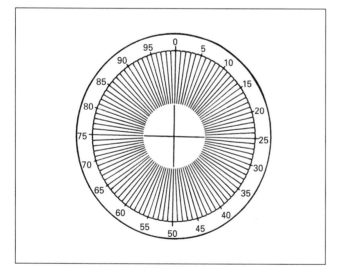

Fig 6-33 Centigrade scale. The circle is divided into 100 units.

6-29a), or with vertical or chopping strokes, in which the blade is nearly parallel to the wall or margin being planed (see Fig 6-29b). For horizontal (scraping) or vertical (chopping) strokes, the acute angle of the cutting edge is intended for use. The acute angle is the junction of the face of the blade with the bevel; in other words, the bevel is on the back of the blade, not the face of the blade. A double-ended hatchet,

gingival margin trimmer, or spoon will have one end that is designated as right cutting and one that is designated as left cutting. In a double-ended hoe, in addition to allowing vertical or chopping strokes, one end is intended for pulling strokes (beveled end or end with distal bevel) and the other is intended for pushing strokes (contrabeveled end or end with mesial bevel).

The cutting edges of most hand cutting instruments used today are single beveled, as are all of those described here (see Fig 6-16). Double-beveled, or bi-beveled, cutting edges are also available but have limited application in contemporary operative dentistry (Fig 6-30). These instruments usually have narrow blades and are used for tasks such as adding mechanical retention points in areas of preparations that cannot be reached by a bur.

Numeric formulas. The configuration of the shanks combined with the appearance of the blade or the use of the instrument produces names such as *straight chisel, monangle chisel, binangle hoe,* and *triple-angle hatchet.* These are descriptive terms, but they are imprecise because they do not indicate sizes or angles. For more complete identification of hand cutting instruments, Black[2] developed a system of assigning numeric formulas to instruments (Figs 6-31 and 6-32). The formulas make use of the metric system. For designating

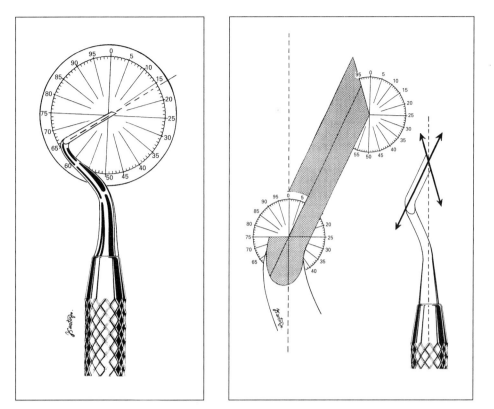

Fig 6-34 (*left*) Centigrade scale inset to show angulation indicator of 16.0 centigrades for the blade angle of this hoe (three-number formula). The vertical axis (0.0 centigrades) is the axis of the instrument's handle. If the blade of the instrument were 1.4 mm wide and 10.0 mm long, the formula for the instrument would be 14-10-16.

Fig 6-35 (*right*) Centigrade scales inset to show angulation indicators of 7.0 centigrades for the blade angle and 95.0 centigrades for the cutting edge angle of this gingival margin trimmer (four-number formula). The vertical axis (0.0 centigrades) is the axis of the instrument's handle. If the blade were 1.5 mm wide and 10.0 mm long, the formula for the instrument would be 15-95-10-7.

the degree of angulation, centigrades are used. Centigrades are based on a circle divided into 100 units (Fig 6-33), as opposed to the 360-degree circle ordinarily used to designate angles. In a centigrade circle, a right angle has 25.0 centigrades.

Three-number formula. For instruments in which the primary cutting edge (at the end of the blade) is at a right angle to the long axis of the blade, Black developed a formula that has three numbers (see Fig 6-31). The first number is the width of the blade in tenths of a millimeter; the second is the length of the blade in millimeters, and the third is the angle (in centigrades) made by the long axis of the blade and the long axis of the handle (Fig 6-34).

Four-number formula. For instruments in which the cutting edge at the end of the blade is not at a right angle to the long axis of the blade, such as gingival margin trimmers, Black designed a four-number formula (see Fig 6-32). The first number is the width of the blade in tenths of a millimeter; the second number is the angle (in centigrades) that the primary cutting edge (working end) makes with the axis of the handle (Fig 6-35); the third number is the length of the blade in millimeters; and the fourth number is the angle (in centigrades) that the long axis of the blade makes with the handle. In mar-

gin trimmers, a cutting edge angle of greater than 90 centigrades is intended for distal gingival margins (see Fig 6-32); an angle of 85 centigrades or less is intended for mesial gingival margins.

Chisel vs hoe. Although Black defined a chisel as having a blade that is aligned with the handle or slightly curved from it, terminology has evolved so that a chisel may also have a blade that is angled from the handle up to 12.5 centigrades.[5] A chisel with a blade angled more than 3 or 4 centigrades from the axis of the handle must be binangle for the instrument to be balanced.

If the blade is angled more than 12.5 centigrades, the instrument is defined as a hoe. In a curved or angled chisel or a hoe, a blade with its primary cutting edge (and its face) on the side of the blade toward the handle is said to be *beveled*, or to have a *distal bevel* (see Figs 6-24a to 6-24c); a blade with its primary cutting edge (and its face) on the side of the blade away from the handle is said to be *contrabeveled*, or to have a *mesial bevel* (see Fig 6-19c).

Recommended instrument kit. Black recommended a long set of 96 cutting instruments, a university set of 44 cutting instruments, or a short set of 25 cutting instruments. Because

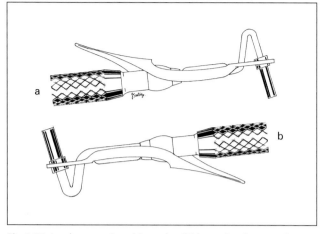

Fig 6-36 Amalgam carriers: (a) regular; (b) large. Amalgam carriers are usually supplied as double-ended instruments. They are available in several different diameters; for example, mini is 1.5 mm; regular (medium) is 2.0 mm; large is 2.5 mm; and jumbo is 3.0 to 3.5 mm. These are the approximate inside diameters of the cylinders of amalgam carriers and may vary slightly from manufacturer to manufacturer.

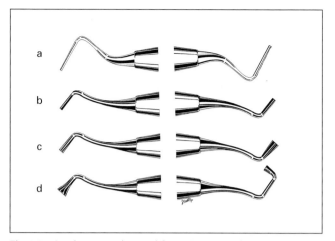

Fig 6-37 Condensers with round faces: (a) SA1, with 0.5- and 0.6-mm diameter faces; (b) SA2, with 0.7- and 1.0-mm faces; (c) SA3, with 1.5- and 2.0-mm faces; (d) SA4, with a 2.5-mm face on the binangle end and a 1.5-mm face on the triple-angle or back-action end.

bonding technology and high-speed handpieces were not available, the dental materials of the time were more limited, and a primary restorative material was direct gold; the longevity of restorations depended on the retention and resistance form developed with hand cutting instruments.

With access to advanced materials and technology, current use of hand cutting instruments is greatly diminished. The kit recommended in this chapter has only 12 hand cutting instruments (six double-ended instruments). Because it is now recognized that there is no need to plane walls and floors of cavity preparations to smoothness with hand instruments for a restoration to perform well, hand cutting instruments play only a small, albeit important, part in cavity preparation. If burs alone were used for shaping proximal preparations, excessive sound tooth structure would have to be removed from the tooth being restored or the bur would damage the adjacent tooth. Hand cutting instruments enable the dentist to shape and refine small proximal boxes without damaging adjacent teeth.

Hatchets, hoes, chisels, and gingival margin trimmers have straight cutting edges and are designed to plane enamel and dentinal walls and margins in shaping cavity preparations, especially in areas of the preparation that cannot be reached with a bur. Spoons, on the other hand, have rounded cutting edges; their intended use is the removal of carious dentin. Although slowly rotating round burs are most useful in removing carious dentin, a spoon gives more tactile sensation and is preferred by many operators.

Noncutting Instruments

Non–tooth-cutting hand instruments are similar in appearance to cutting instruments, except that the blade used for tooth preparation is replaced with a part that has a totally different use. In noncutting instruments such as burnishers and condensers, the blade is replaced by a *nib* or *point*.[2] The flat end of the nib of a condenser is called the *face*. Amalgam carvers have carving blades instead of tooth-cutting blades.

Condensers, carvers, and burnishers are used to place dental amalgam and, to a certain extent, resin composite restorative materials. Plastic filling instruments are used to place resin composite and glass-ionomer materials, provisional restorative materials, and sometimes cavity-basing materials into tooth preparations. Spatulas may be necessary for mixing cavity-lining and cavity-basing materials; provisional restorative materials; and cements for luting inlays, onlays, and crowns.

Amalgam carriers. For silver amalgam restorations, amalgam is placed into the preparation with an *amalgam carrier*, an instrument with a hollow cylinder that is filled with amalgam (Fig 6-36). A plunger operated with a finger lever pushes the amalgam out of the carrier into the preparation.

Condensers. *Condensers* are used to compress amalgam or to push resin composite or glass-ionomer materials into all areas of the preparation. The working ends, or nibs, of condensers may be any shape, but usually they are round with flat ends (faces). Figure 6-37 shows four round condensers of

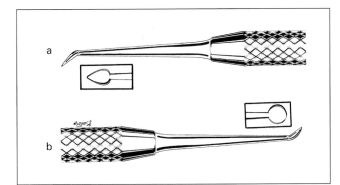

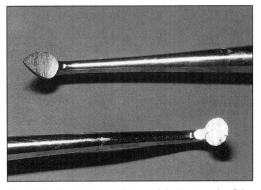

Fig 6-38a Cleoid-discoid carver: (a) cleoid end; (b) discoid end. This type of carver is a double-ended instrument. *Cleoid* means claw shaped. Both shapes are useful in carving occlusal surfaces of amalgam restorations. The point of the cleoid carver is used to carve the bases of grooves in the occlusal amalgam, and the tip is usually very slightly rounded so the grooves that it carves won't be sharp.

Fig 6-38b Cleoid *(top)* and discoid *(bottom)* ends of the cleoid-discoid carver.

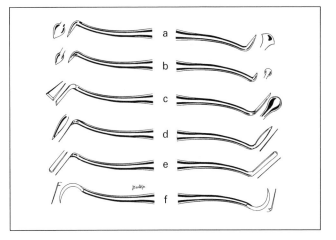

Fig 6-39 Amalgam carvers: (a) large cleoid-discoid (Tanner No. 5 [5T]) carver; (b) small cleoid-discoid (UWD5) carver; (c) Walls No. 3 carver; (d) Hollenback No. ½ carver; (e) interproximal carver (IPC); (f) No. 14L sickle-shaped carver.

different sizes and configurations. Other commonly used condenser nibs are triangular, rectangular, or diamond shaped. Amalgam is condensed by pushing the condenser directly into the preparation and confining the amalgam between the condenser face and the preparation floor through vertical pressure (vertical condensation). The amalgam is condensed against the vertical walls of the preparation (lateral condensation) by angling the nib and using the end for condensation, or by lateral, or side-to-side, movements of the condenser, using the sides of the nib to condense the amalgam.

The condensation pressure applied to the amalgam with a condenser depends on the size of the face and the amount of force used by the operator. For small condensers, such as the SA1 condenser (see Fig 6-37a), little force is needed. The nibs of the SA1 condenser are 0.5 and 0.6 mm in diameter. For larger condensers, such as the SA3 (see Fig 6-37c), with nib diameters of 1.5 and 2.0 mm, a significant amount of force (6 to 8 lbs) gives optimum condensation.

When condensers are used in placing resin composite or glass-ionomer materials, the resin material is not actually con-

densed, but is pushed or patted into all areas of the preparation with the largest condenser face that will fit into the area.

Carvers. *Carvers* are used to shape amalgam and resin composite and other tooth-colored materials after they have been placed in tooth preparations. Figures 6-38a and 6-38b show the shapes of the blades of a cleoid-discoid carver. Figure 6-39 illustrates six commonly used carvers. In general, when a convex amalgam contour is being carved, a concave-shaped carver facilitates the shaping or carving. Likewise, a convex carver facilitates carving of a concave shape. A convex carver may be used to carve a convex surface; the surface is carved tangentially, with multiple strokes. Whether a carver is used to carve amalgam or resin composite, it is important that the blade be sharp.

The cleoid-discoid (or discoid-cleoid) carvers shown in Figs 6-39a and 6-39b are used primarily for occlusal carving in amalgam restorations. The Walls No. 3 carver (see Fig 6-39c) is useful for carving occlusal surfaces; the end that is shaped like a hoe is also useful for shaping cusps and for carving facial and lingual surfaces of large amalgam restorations. The Hol-

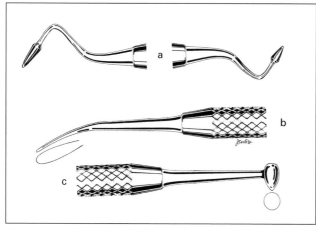

Fig 6-40 Burnishers: (a) PKT3 (rounded cone-shaped) burnisher, designed by Peter K. Thomas as a waxing instrument but useful in placing direct restorations as well; its rounded end and cone shape allow it to serve most functions that a small ball-shaped burnisher would serve, plus others; (b) beavertail (No. 2) burnisher; (c) football or ovoid (No. 30) burnisher. The ovoid burnisher, available in various sizes (eg, 28, 29, and 31), can be used for final condensation of amalgam and the initial shaping of the occlusal anatomy in amalgam. The beavertail and ovoid burnishers are useful for burnishing margins of cast-gold restorations.

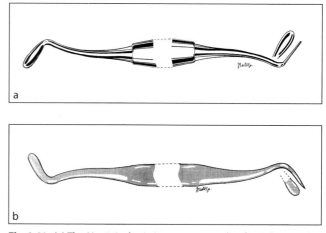

Fig 6-41 (a) The No. 1-2 plastic instrument, made of stainless steel, is useful for placing a rubber dam, placing and shaping resin composite and other tooth-colored restorative materials, and packing gingival retraction cord into the sulcus around a crown or abutment preparation before an impression is made. Some cord-packing instruments are similar to the No. 1-2 plastic instrument but may have serrated ends to provide better control of the cord. (b) A plastic instrument made of hard plastic, rather than metal, is preferred by some operators for placing resin composites.

lenback No. ½ carver (see Fig 6-39d) is useful for occlusal, proximal, and axial (facial and lingual) surfaces; several larger Hollenback carvers, with the same general shape, are also available. The interproximal carver (IPC) (see Fig 6-39e) has very thin blades and is extremely valuable for carving proximal amalgam surfaces near the interproximal contact area. Other uses for this instrument include placing and shaping resin composite and glass ionomer and pushing retraction cord into a gingival sulcus. The No. 14L carver (see Fig 6-39f) can be used to carve proximal surfaces, or it may be used for carving convex facial and lingual surfaces of very large amalgam restorations. The No. 14L carver has a very strong, hollow-ground triangular blade, so it can be used to remove amalgam overhangs from completely set amalgam.

Although most of the shaping of resin composite restorations should be completed before the material is polymerized and most operators prefer to use rotary instruments for postpolymerization shaping, several amalgam carvers are also useful for carving resin composite. The discoid carvers are especially useful for lingual concavities of anterior teeth; cleoid and discoid carvers and the hoe-shaped end of the Walls No. 3 carver are useful for occlusal surfaces of posterior resin composite restorations. Another carver very useful for resin composite restorations is a disposable scalpel blade (No. 12 or No. 12b blade) mounted in a scalpel handle.

Burnishers. *Burnishers* are used for several functions. The word *burnish* is defined as "to make shiny or lustrous, especially by rubbing; to polish"; and "to rub (a material) with a tool for compacting or smoothing or for turning an edge."[6] Burnishing is probably used in all of those ways in dentistry. Two frequently used double-ended burnishers are illustrated in Fig 6-40.

One use of burnishers is to shape metal matrix bands so that they impart more desirable contours to restorations. Large burnishers are used with considerable force to pinch off freshly condensed amalgam at the margins, or, in other words, to impart some condensation and to begin shaping the occlusal surfaces of amalgam restorations. After the amalgam has been carved, a burnisher may be used with a gentle rubbing motion to smooth the surface. The PKT3 (P. K. Thomas No. 3) burnisher (see Fig 6-40a) and some other burnishers are also useful for sculpting occlusal anatomy in posterior resin composite restorations prior to polymerization of the resin.

Burnishers are used to "bend" cast gold near the margin to narrow the gap between the gold and the tooth. This closing of a marginal gap is best accomplished with a narrow burnisher, such as the side of a beavertail burnisher, used with heavy force in strokes parallel to the margin but about 1.0 or 1.5 mm away from it. If burnishing is accomplished directly

Fig 6-42 Spatulas: (a) No. 24, a flexible spatula, is used for luting cements such as zinc phosphate and glass ionomer; (b) No. 24A is thicker, for more rigidity; (c) No. 313 is used for cavity liners, such as the calcium hydroxide liners.

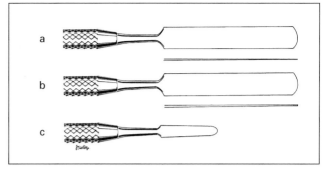

on a thin gold margin, the gold can be bent severely and may break.

Plastic instruments. Plastic instruments (or plastic filling instruments) are so named because they were originally designed to use with plastic restorative materials, such as the silicates and acrylic resins used in the middle of the 20th century. They are currently used to carry and shape tooth-colored restorative materials such as resin composites and glass-ionomer restorative materials. Many specially designed instruments are available, in a myriad of shapes and sizes, for contouring resin composite and resin-modified glass ionomer prior to curing. A plastic instrument with a large, slightly curved paddle-shaped blade (Barghi No. 1, American Eagle; or Performa No. 1, Bisco) is very useful for placing and contouring large, anterior resin composite restorations or veneers.

A commonly used plastic instrument is the No. 1-2 (Fig 6-41a). The double-ended instrument has a nib or blade on each end, one at a 90-degree angle to the other. Other double-ended plastic instruments have a blade-type nib on one end and a condenser nib on the other. The bladed plastic instruments have many uses in operative dentistry in addition to carrying and contouring restorative materials. The IPC (see Fig 6-39e), for instance, is preferred by some operators for packing knitted cord and placing and shaping resin composite.

These instruments are now available in both hard plastic and metal, and metal instruments are available with several different coatings on blades or nibs to prevent resin materials from sticking to them. The original rationale for using an instrument made of plastic (Fig 6-41b) was to eliminate abrasion of metal by the quartz in resin composites, which caused grayness in the tooth-colored material. Because of changes in the inorganic fillers used in many of today's resin composites, the problem of metal abrasion and graying is unusual and material-specific, so even a stainless steel instrument functions well to carry and shape resin composite.

Cement spatulas. A variety of materials in operative dentistry require mixing, some on a glass slab, others on a paper pad. Several spatulas are available, and they vary in size and thickness (Fig 6-42). The larger cement spatulas were originally designed for mixing luting cements and the smaller spatulas for cavity liners, but with the advent of resin luting cements, the smaller spatulas are frequently used for mixing small amounts of those materials. The thinner spatulas are flexible; the thicker ones are rigid. Selection of a rigid or flexible cement spatula is dependent on the desired viscosity of the cement and personal preference.

Sharpening of Hand Instruments

To assess sharpness, the user of the instrument should look at the cutting edge in bright light; the presence of a "glint" indicates that the edge is dull or rounded (Figs 6-43a and 6-43b). Alternatively, the dentist can pull the instrument across hard plastic, such as the handle of a plastic mouth mirror or an evacuator tip. A dull blade will slide across the plastic; a sharp blade will cut into the surface, stopping movement. A specially made, sterilizable, sharpness-testing stick is also available (Figs 6-44a and 6-44b) (Dalron Test Stick, American Eagle or Miltex).

Sharpening is performed in different ways for different hand instruments. When chisels, hatchets, hoes, and margin trimmers are sharpened, the cutting-edge bevel is placed flat against a flat stone, which is on a stable surface, and the instrument is pushed or pulled so that the acute cutting angle is moved forward, with fairly heavy force on the forward stroke, and with little or no force on the back stroke (Figs 6-45 and 6-46). Usually, unless the instrument has been badly neglected, only two or three forward strokes are required. Because the bevels of these instruments should usually make a 45-degree angle with the face of the blade, the blade should make a 45-degree angle with the surface of the sharpening stone (Figs 6-46 and 6-47).

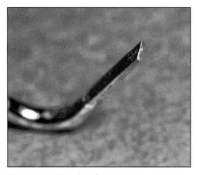

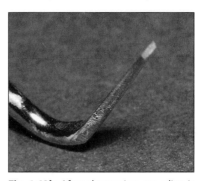

Fig 6-43a The glint from the cutting edge of this hoe indicates that the blade is quite dull.

Fig 6-43b After sharpening, no glint is noticeable.

Fig 6-44 The sharpness-testing stick is a hard plastic stick used for testing the sharpness of instruments. For testing sharpness, the blade should be applied to the stick at an angle that is similar to that applied during use and pulled or pushed in a direction that is similar to the direction of its intended use.

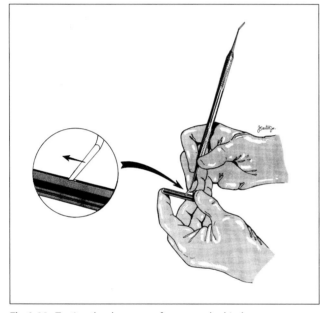

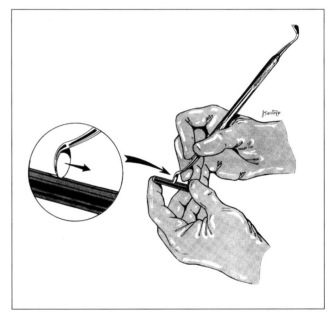

Fig 6-44a Testing the sharpness of a monangle chisel.

Fig 6-44b Testing the sharpness of the discoid end of Walls No. 3 carver.

When spoons, discoid carvers, and cleoid carvers are sharpened, the instrument is rotated as the blade is advanced on the flat stone (Fig 6-48). The bevel is at 45 degrees, or slightly more or less, to the face, and the instrument is advanced on the stone with the bevel against the surface of the stone and the cutting edge of the instrument perpendicular to the path of advancement. When a blade with a rounded edge is being sharpened, the handle cannot simply be twirled to achieve the desired rotation, but must actually be swung in an arc to keep the cutting edge of the blade perpendicular to the direction of the stroke, and the bevel parallel with and against the surface of the stone.

The discoid carver and spoon may be sharpened with a continuous rotation of the blade; the shank moves clockwise from the 9 o'clock position to the 3 o'clock position in one motion. For the cleoid carver, however, the rotation begins with the shank in the 9 o'clock position and continues clockwise only until the bevel just next to the point is ground (see Fig 6-48); to sharpen the other side of the cleoid, the rotation begins with the shank at the 3 o'clock position and continues counterclockwise to the point. If sharpening both sides of a cleoid carver creates a sharp point at its tip, the junction of the bevels at the point should be slightly rounded.

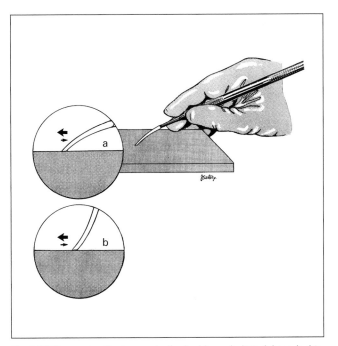

Fig 6-45 Sharpening the two ends of a double-ended Wedelstaedt chisel: (a) sharpening the contrabevel end (inside or mesial bevel); (b) sharpening the bevel end (outside or distal bevel). The end bevel (for the primary cutting edge or working end) of each blade is placed flat on the stone; the blade will make a 45-degree angle with the stone. In the primary sharpening stroke, the cutting edge is moved forward. Unless the instrument is very dull, only two or three fairly heavy forward strokes will be necessary to sharpen the cutting edge.

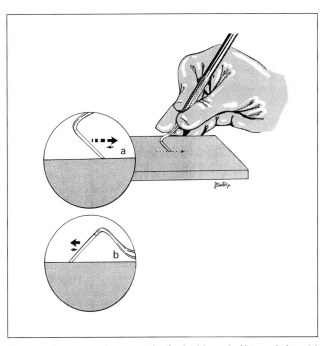

Fig 6-46 Sharpening the two ends of a double-ended binangle hoe: (a) sharpening the bevel end (outside or distal bevel); (b) sharpening the contrabevel end (inside or mesial bevel). The primary bevel is always flat against the stone; the face of the blade is up.

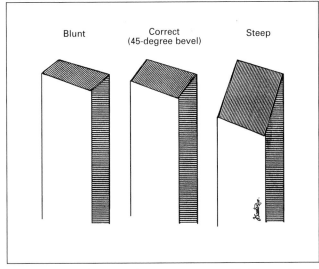

Fig 6-47 Bevels of sharpened cutting instruments. Working end bevels of chisels, hatchets, and hoes, as well as the bevels of amalgam carvers, should be at approximately 45 degrees to the face of the blade. The cutting edge at the left is too blunt, the center blade has a correctly angled cutting edge, and the cutting edge at the right is too acute and will dull rapidly.

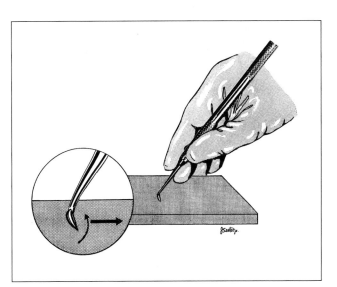

Fig 6-48 Sharpening a cleoid carver. The handle is swung in an arc to rotate the blade as the bevel is pulled forward on the stone. This movement is used to keep the cutting edge perpendicular to the direction of the stroke.

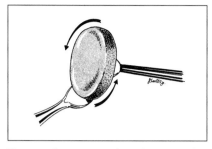

Fig 6-49 Sharpening a discoid spoon with a rotating sharpening stone. A discoid spoon may also be sharpened on a flat stone; the blade is rotated as it is pulled with the cutting edge forward. If the face is ground with a rotating stone, the blade will be thinned and could be more likely to break during use.

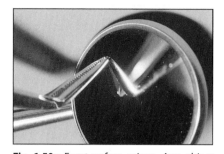

Fig 6-50a Front-surface mirror. Any object touching the mirror, such as the tips of the cotton forceps, will appear to be touching itself.

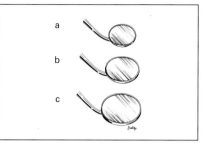

Fig 6-50b Mouth mirrors: (a) No. 2 ($^5/_8$-inch diameter); (b) No. 4 ($^7/_8$-inch diameter); (c) No. 5 ($^{15}/_{16}$-inch diameter).

The blade of a discoid spoon may be sharpened by grinding the face of the blade with a rotating stone (Fig 6-49). This method of sharpening also thins the blade, and care must be taken to avoid rendering the blade so thin that it could easily break.

Sharpening machines are available. A slowly rotating sharpening wheel is employed by one type of machine; an oscillating flat stone, or hone, is used by another. These machines are useful for sharpening instruments between patients and before sterilization.

When instruments are sharpened during an operative procedure, they should be sharpened with a sterile stone. When a stone is sterilized, it should not have oil in or on it, because the oil may thicken during the sterilization process and form a shellac-like coating that will prevent the abrasion needed for sharpening. A good substitute for oil is water. Stones lubricated with water should be washed well or cleaned in an ultrasonic cleaner after use to remove the metal filings prior to sterilization. A flat, white Arkansas stone or fine synthetic sharpening stone should be made a part of the operative dentistry instrument kit so that it is available during each procedure.

Mirrors, Explorers, Periodontal Probes, and Forceps

Mirrors, explorers, periodontal probes, and forceps are basic instruments that will be needed during each appointment for diagnosis or treatment.

Mirrors. For every procedure performed in the mouth, the dentist must have clear and distinct vision of the field. Wherever possible, the field should be viewed with direct vision. When needed, the mouth mirror allows the operator to visualize areas of the mouth that he or she would not otherwise be able to see. It also allows the operator to maintain a body position that will reduce health problems associated with poor posture.

Almost as important as its allowing indirect visualization of obscure areas of the mouth is the mirror's function as a reflector of light into the area being examined or treated. A mirror that is positioned properly allows the operator to visualize the field of operation in the mirror and, at the same time, reflects the operating light into that area. To accomplish this, the light should be positioned behind and directed just to the side of the operator's head and into the mirror.

The mouth mirror can also serve as a retractor of soft tissue (tongue, cheeks, or lips) to aid access and visualization.

For clarity of vision, the reflective surface of the mirror should be on the external surface of the glass. This type of mirror is called a front-surface mirror (Fig 6-50a). Mouth mirrors are usually round and come in a variety of sizes (Fig 6-50b). The most widely used sizes for adults are the No. 4 and No. 5. For constricted areas in posterior regions of the mouth, when a rubber dam is in place, a smaller mirror, such as a No. 2, is helpful.

Explorers. Explorers are pointed instruments used to feel tooth surfaces for irregularities and to determine the hardness of exposed dentin. The explorer that is used most often is the shepherd's hook, or No. 23, explorer (Fig 6-51a). Another useful shape is a cowhorn explorer, which provides improved access for exploring proximal surfaces (Fig 6-51b). The No. 17 explorer is also useful in proximal areas (Fig 6-51c).

Periodontal probes. Periodontal probes are designed to detect and measure the depth of periodontal pockets. In

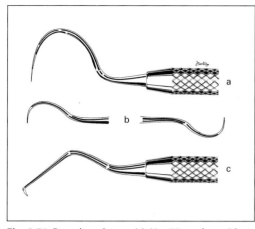

Fig 6-51 Dental explorers: (a) No. 23 explorer (shepherd's hook); (b) 3CH explorer (cowhorn or pigtail); (c) No. 17 explorer.

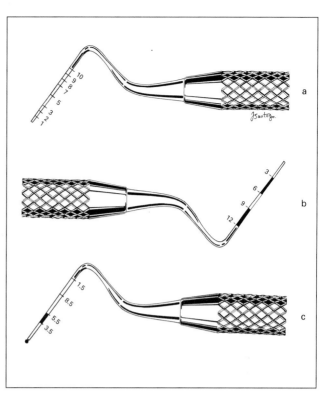

Fig 6-52 Periodontal probes: (a) QOW probe (Michigan O probe with Williams markings); (b) PCP12 probe (Marquis markings); (c) PSR (periodontal screening and recording) probe.

operative dentistry, they are also used to determine dimensions of instruments and of various features of preparations or restorations. There are many periodontal probe designs; the differences are in the diameters, the position of the millimeter markings, the configuration of the markings (eg, whether they are notched or painted), and the design of the tip. Three commonly used probes are illustrated in Fig 6-52.

Forceps. Forceps of various kinds are useful in operative dentistry. Cotton forceps are used for picking up small items, such as cotton pellets (small cotton balls), and carrying them to the mouth (Fig 6-53). Other forceps useful in operative dentistry include hemostatic forceps (hemostats) (Fig 6-54) and articulating paper forceps (Fig 6-55). A hemostat locks tightly, so it is often helpful in placing or removing items used to confine amalgam for condensation. Articulating paper forceps are designed to carry an inked tape to the mouth to mark the contacts of teeth in opposing arches during closure.

Instrument Grasps

The operator should master two basic instrument grasps, the pen grasp, which provides more flexibility of movement, and the palm or palm-thumb grasp, which provides limited movement but controlled power. Usually only one-handed grasps are used, but occasionally two-handed instrumentation is needed to make refinement of a preparation more precise (Fig 6-56).

Pen grasp. This is the most frequently used instrument grasp in operative dentistry. The pen grasp is actually different from the way one would grasp a pen (Fig 6-57); the handle of the instrument is engaged by the end, not the side, of the middle finger; this provides more finger power. The pen grasp is initiated by placement of the instrument handle between the thumb and index finger; the middle finger engages the handle near the shank or the shank itself (Figs 6-57 and 6-58). The ring finger is braced against the teeth to stabilize instrument movement (see Figs 6-58a and 6-58b).

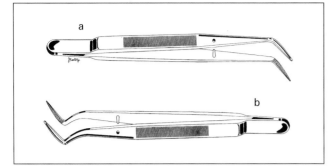

Fig 6-53 Cotton forceps: (a) College (No. 17); (b) Meriam (No. 18).

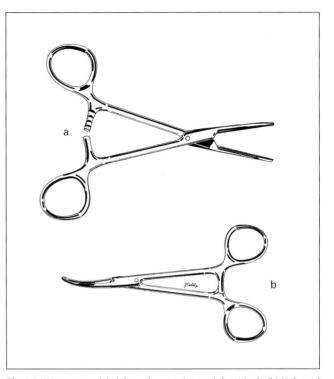

Fig 6-54 Hemostats: (a) Halstead mosquito straight, 6-inch; (b) Halstead mosquito curved, 5-inch.

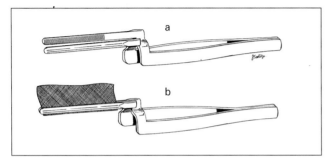

Fig 6-55 Articulating paper forceps: (a) Forceps handles provide a spring that keeps the jaws closed together; they are opened (as shown) by squeezing the handle. (b) The entire length of the piece of articulating paper or tape is supported by the jaws of the forceps.

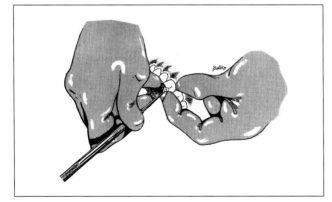

Fig 6-56 Two-handed instrumentation. The use of both hands can make refinement of a preparation more precise. The right hand is thrusting and rotating the instrument while the index finger of the left hand guides and assists the motion of the working end to refine a proximal margin of a Class 2 preparation. A similar dual-handed action is useful for condensing amalgam; it allows increased condensation force to be controlled.

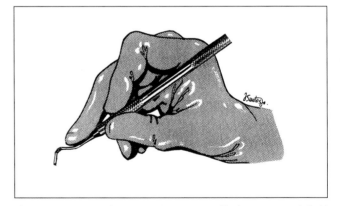

Fig 6-57 Pen grasp. The pen grasp is not actually the way a pen is held for writing. The instrument is held between the index finger and thumb, and the middle finger is placed atop the handle or shank, nearer the working end of the instrument, to provide more force, or thrust, directed toward the working end of the instrument.

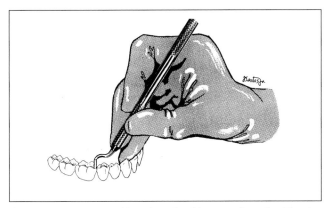

Fig 6-58a Pen grasp used in a chopping (downward) motion. The ring finger is resting on the incisal edges of the anterior teeth. During the use of any instrument in the mouth (with the exception of the mirror), a firm rest must be achieved on teeth or attached gingival tissue.

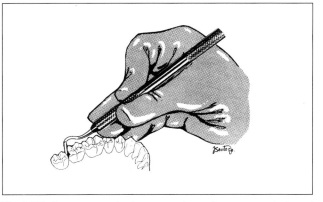

Fig 6-58b Pen grasp as the instrument is used more posteriorly and with a side-to-side or scraping motion. The small finger and ring finger are resting on the facial and occlusal surfaces, respectively.

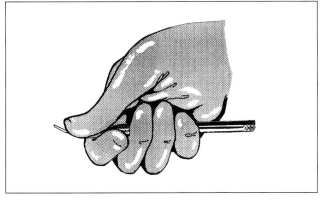

Fig 6-59 Palm-thumb grasp. The instrument is grasped much nearer to its end than in the pen grasp, so that the thumb can be braced against the teeth to provide control during movement of the instrument.

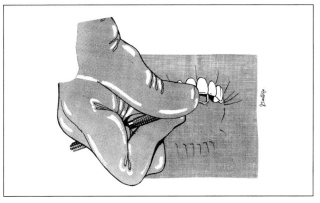

Fig 6-60 The palm-thumb grasp is used frequently when a hand cutting instrument, such as a gingival margin trimmer, is used in Class 3 preparations that have lingual access. The thumb is resting on the incisal edges of the teeth. The palm-thumb grasp is also used frequently with the Wedelstaedt chisel, usually for facial access in posterior and anterior operations, and occasionally for lingual access.

Palm or palm-thumb grasp. In this grasp, the thumb serves as a brace (Fig 6-59). Side-to-side, rotating, or thrusting movements of the instrument by the wrist and fingers are controlled by the thumb, which is firmly in contact with the teeth (Fig 6-60).

Instrument Motions

The following are some of the many motions used with hand instruments:

- *Chopping* (in the direction of the working end of the instrument, or parallel to the long axis of the blade)
- *Pulling* (toward the operator's hand)
- *Pushing* (away from the hand)

- *Rotating*
- *Scraping* (with the blade directed at an angle between 45 and 90 degrees to the surface being scraped and moved side to side or back and forth on the surface)
- *Thrusting* (forcibly pushing against a surface)

Rotating Instruments

Handpieces

In dentistry, two basic types of handpiece are used, the straight handpiece (Fig 6-61) and the contra-angle handpiece (Fig 6-62). In the straight handpiece, the long axis of the bur is the same as the long axis of the handpiece. The straight

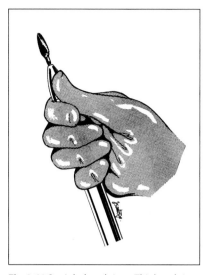

Fig 6-61 Straight handpiece. This handpiece is used occasionally in the mouth, but it is more frequently used extraorally, for tasks such as making adjustments to removable prostheses or adjusting and repolishing a cast-gold or ceramic restoration prior to insertion. The bur installed in this handpiece is a tree-shaped denture bur.

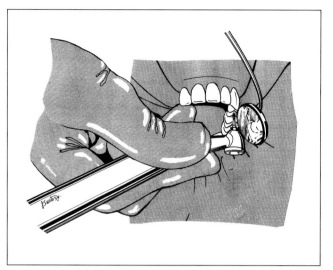

Fig 6-62 Contra-angle handpiece. This is a high-speed contra-angle handpiece, which is used with small-diameter burs for rapid cutting of tooth structure or restorations. A low-speed contra-angle is also useful for removal of carious dentin, with a slowly rotating round bur, and for shaping and polishing with abrasive disks and impregnated rubber polishers. Some operators also prefer the low-speed contra-angle for refining tooth preparations.

handpiece is used more frequently for laboratory work but is occasionally useful clinically.

The primary handpiece used in the mouth is the contra-angle handpiece. As with hand instruments, *contra-angle* indicates that the head of the handpiece is angled first away from, and then back toward, the long axis of the handle. Also as with hand instruments, this contra-angle design is intended to bring the working point (the head of the bur) to within a few millimeters of the long axis of the handle of the handpiece to provide balance.

There are two types of contra-angle handpieces, which are classified by their speed potential. Low-speed contra-angle handpieces have a typical free-running speed range of 500 to 15,000 rpm; some are able to slow to 200 rpm, and others are able to achieve speeds of 35,000 rpm. High-speed handpieces have a free-running speed range greater than 160,000 rpm, and some handpieces attain free-running speeds up to 500,000 rpm.[7] In the United States, most dentists are accustomed to air-turbine high-speed handpieces. The speed of these handpieces during tooth preparation is 180,000 rpm and lower, depending on the application pressure and the power of the handpiece. For air-turbine handpieces, speeds during tooth preparation are significantly less than their free-running speeds.

Electric handpieces (powered by an electric motor instead of an air-turbine) have been used for some time in Europe, and their use is rapidly growing in the United States. Most electric handpieces achieve free-running speeds of 200,000 rpm, an ideal speed for cutting enamel. Electric handpieces are very efficient in preparing teeth.

High-speed techniques are generally preferred for cutting enamel and dentin. Penetration through enamel and extension of the cavity outline are more efficient at high speed. Small-diameter burs should be used in the high-speed handpiece. High speed generates considerable heat, even with small-diameter burs, and should be used with air and water coolant sprays[8] and high-efficiency evacuation. For refining preparations, a high-speed handpiece may be slowed considerably and used with only air coolant and a gentle brushing or painting motion in which each application of the bur to the tooth is brief. This technique allows visualization and prevents overheating.[9]

Low-speed contra-angle handpieces, with round burs rotating very slowly, are used for removal of carious dentin. Low-speed contra-angle handpieces are also used for various finishing and polishing procedures that use abrasive disks, points, or cups.

Fig 6-63 Typical dimensions (and ANSI/ADA standard dimension tolerances), in millimeters, of the three common bur designs: (a) straight handpiece bur; (b) latch-type bur for latch-type contra-angle handpiece; (c) friction-grip bur for friction-grip contra-angle handpiece.[10,11]

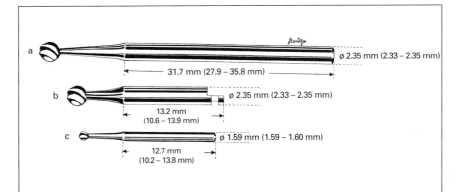

Fig 6-64 Parts of a rotary cutting instrument (bur).

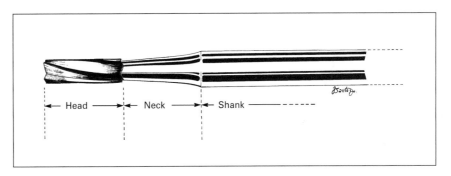

There are two types of contra-angles based on their bur-locking, or chucking, mechanisms for the low-speed handpiece: a friction-grip chuck and a latch-type chuck. The shanks of the burs that fit into each of these types of contra-angle chuck are shown in Fig 6-63. The high-speed handpiece will receive only the friction-grip bur.

Burs

Hand-rotated dental instruments are known to have been used since the early 1700s. The foot engine came into use in dentistry in 1871 and the electric engine in 1872.[4] The most significant advance, which has made present-day high-speed cutting possible, is the tungsten carbide bur, which became available in 1947.[10]

Burs have three major parts, the head, the neck, and the shank (Fig 6-64). For the different types of handpieces or handpiece heads, there are burs with different designs and dimensions (see Fig 6-63).

The head of a bur is the portion that cuts. The cutting action is produced by blades on the head, and the blades are produced by cuts made into the head. The angle of the cutting edge of a blade (edge angle) is usually not acute; the angle is in the range of 90 degrees to provide strength to the blade and longevity of cutting efficiency of the bur. A cross section of a typical six-bladed bur is shown in Fig 6-65; the names of the faces and angles of the blades are also shown. The bur in Fig 6-65 has a negative rake angle, as do most burs used in dentistry.[10] The negative rake angle increases the life expectancy of the bur and provides for the most effective performance in low- and high-speed ranges.

A positive rake angle would produce a more acute edge angle. Positive rake angles may be used to cut softer, weaker substances, such as soft carious dentin. If a blade with a positive rake angle were used to cut a hard material, such as sound enamel or dentin, it would dig in, leaving an irregularly cut surface, and the cutting edges of the blades would chip and dull rapidly.

The basic shapes of tooth-preparation burs used in operative dentistry are shown in Fig 6-66. Many other shapes are available; most are modifications of these five. Numbering systems have been introduced to describe the shapes of dental burs. The original system, introduced by SS White Dental Manufacturing, had nine shapes based on the burs available at that time.[10] That system has been modified and expanded as new burs have been developed. The American National Standards Institute/American Dental Association (ANSI/ADA) specification[11] provides standard characteristics for dental burs; this specification lists both the US numbers and the

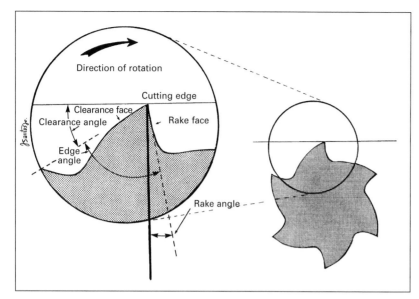

Fig 6-65 Typical bur head, viewed from the end of the bur nearest the handpiece.[5,10]

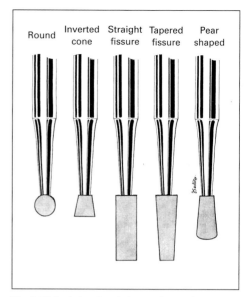

Fig 6-66 Basic bur head shapes for tooth preparation. Most burs used for tooth preparation are modifications of these burs. The primary modifications are lengthening of the bur heads and rounding ends or corners to allow preparations to be cut without sharp line angles.

International Standards Organization (ISO) numbers for dental burs.

Prior to the advent of high-speed handpieces, it was found that additional cuts across the blades of a dental bur increased cutting efficiency; these cuts were called *crosscuts*. Today, with high-speed handpieces, crosscut burs are not normally of any benefit.

Table 6-1 shows diagrams, US bur sizes, and the head diameters of many available regular carbide tooth-preparation burs. ISO sizes for each type of bur can be calculated from the diameter: A bur with a diameter of 0.8 mm will have an ISO size of 008; a diameter of 1.0 mm will have an ISO size of 010. The ISO sizes are combined with the shape of the bur, so an ISO inverted cone 006 is an inverted cone bur with a 0.6-mm major diameter; from Table 6-1, it can be determined that an ISO inverted cone 006 corresponds with a US No. 33½ bur.

It is useful to know the diameters and lengths of the burs used in tooth preparation so that they can be used as gauges of depth and distance. Bur-head lengths may vary from manufacturer to manufacturer, so it is best to measure the individual burs being used and to use their dimensions as references for measuring preparation dimensions.

Another type of bur that is very useful in operative dentistry is the trimming and finishing bur. These burs come in a variety of shapes and sizes; the heads of some trimming and finishing burs are shown in Table 6-2. Trimming and finishing burs are excellent for making very smooth cuts in tooth preparations, for adjusting occlusion in enamel or of a restoration, and for contouring and finishing restorations. Trimming and finishing burs have more blades than tooth-preparation burs, and the more blades, the smoother the cut surface that can be attained. The number of blades necessary for a desired surface smoothness varies with the diameter of the bur; typical trimming and finishing burs have 8 to 12, 16 to 20, and 30 blades.

Many designs of trimming and finishing burs are available for shaping and contouring esthetic restorations. One extremely useful type of trimming and finishing bur that is available with 8, 16, or 30 blades is a straight-sided taper with a safe (noncutting) end (called esthetic trimming, or ET, burs from Brasseler). This bur is designed so that the end will rest on the tooth surface without cutting tooth structure and allow contouring of the adjacent restoration; it is available in several different lengths and diameters, as well as with the different numbers of blades.

Table 6-1	**Shapes and diameters of regular carbide burs used for tooth preparation (US designations*)**

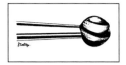

Round

Bur size	1/16	1/8	1/4	1/2	1	2	3	4	5
Diameter (mm)	.30	.40	.50	.60	.80	1.0	1.2	1.4	1.6

Bur size	6	7	8	9	11
Diameter (mm)	1.8	2.1	2.3	2.5	3.1

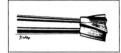

Inverted cone

Bur size	33½	34	35	36	37	39	40
Diameter (mm)	.60	.80	1.0	1.2	1.4	1.8	2.1

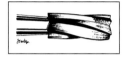

Straight fissure†

Bur size	55½	56	57	58	59	60
Diameter (mm)	.60	.80	1.0	1.2	1.4	1.6

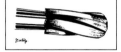

Straight fissure, rounded end (straight dome)†

Bur size	1156	1157	1158
Diameter (mm)	.80	1.0	1.2

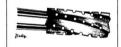

Straight fissure, crosscut†

Bur size	556	557	558	559	560
Diameter (mm)	.80	1.0	1.2	1.4	1.6

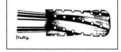

Straight fissure, rounded end, crosscut (straight dome crosscut)

Bur size	1556	1557	1558
Diameter (mm)	.80	1.0	1.2

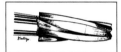

Tapered fissure†

Bur size	168	169	170	171
Diameter (mm)	.80	.90	1.0	1.2

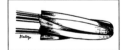

Tapered fissure, rounded end (tapered dome)†

Bur size	1169	1170	1171
Diameter (mm)	.90	1.0	1.2

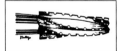

Tapered fissure, crosscut†

Bur size	699	700	701	702	703
Diameter (mm)	.90	1.0	1.2	1.6	2.1

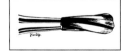

Pear†

Bur size	329	330	331	332
Diameter (mm)	.60	.80	1.0	1.2

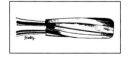

Long inverted cone, rounded corners (amalgam preparation)

Bur size	245	246
Diameter (mm)	.80	1.2

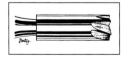

End-cutting

Bur size	956	957
Diameter (mm)	.80	1.0

*Adapted from American National Standards Institute/American Dental Association Specification 23 and catalogs of Midwest Dental Products and Brasseler.
†Some sizes available with a long head (L).

Table 6-2	Shapes and diameters of some of the available 12-bladed carbide finishing burs used for smooth cuts in tooth preparation and for finishing restorations (US designations)*						

Egg

Bur size	7404	7406	7408				
Diameter (mm)	1.4	1.8	2.3				

Bullet

Bur size	7801	7802	7803				
Diameter (mm)	.90	1.0	1.2				

Needle

Bur size	7901	7902	7903				
Diameter (mm)	.90	1.0	1.2				

Round

Bur size	7002	7003	7004	7006	7008	7009	7010
Diameter (mm)	1.0	1.2	1.4	1.8	2.3	2.7	3.1

Flame

Bur size	7102	7104	7106	7108			
Diameter (mm)	1.2	1.4	1.8	2.3			

Cone

Bur size	7202	7204	7205	7206			
Diameter (mm)	1.0	1.4	1.6	1.8			

Long pear (inverted taper)

Bur size	7302	7303	7304				
Diameter (mm)	1.0	1.2	1.4				

Straight fissure

Bur size	7572	7583					
Diameter (mm)	1.0	1.2					

Taper

Bur size	7702	7713					
Diameter (mm)	1.0	1.2					

*Adapted from catalogs of Midwest Dental Products and Brasseler.

Diamonds. Used increasingly in operative dentistry, diamond burs are especially useful for preparations for bonded restorations. Several manufacturers produce diamonds that mimic the shapes of many of the carbide burs. Diamond burs cut tooth structure well and are acceptable substitutes for carbide burs, but many of the smaller sizes are not available as diamond burs. Diamond burs with fine-grit diamond surfaces are also useful for contouring and polishing esthetic restorations.

Air-Abrasion Technology

In the 1940s, an instrument called the Airdent (SS White) was introduced as a means of cavity preparation.[12] Because all restorations placed at that time depended on cavity preparation shape for retention, and as the Airdent did not prepare undercuts in preparations, the technology soon lost favor. When it was reintroduced in the 1980s, it received a greater

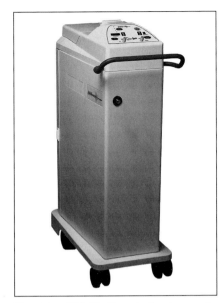

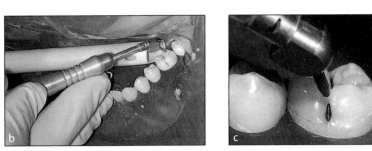

Fig 6-67a KCP FlexiJet air-abrasion cavity preparation unit from American Medical Technologies.

Figs 6-67b and 6-67c Air-abrasion handpiece in use for a small Class 1 cavity preparation for resin composite.

degree of acceptance because bonded restorations had become routine.[13] Etched enamel and dentin, rather than the shape of the cavity preparation, give retention to many restorations. A large number of air-abrasion units are being marketed for opening fissures, for some cavity preparations, and to facilitate repair of existing restorations with bonding technology (Figs 6-67a to 6-67c).

Magnifiers

The quality, and therefore the serviceability and longevity, of dental restorations is dependent on the ability of the operator to see what he or she is doing. One of the primary advantages of the rubber dam in operative dentistry is improvement of the visualization of the operating field. Most current contra-angle handpieces have fiber-optic systems by which lights are placed in the contra-angle heads to improve visualization of the operating field.

Magnification devices are extremely helpful in restorative procedures, and some form of magnification is recommended for every dentist providing restorative dentistry services.[14] Available magnification devices run the gamut of effectiveness and expense. Among the finest magnifiers are the telescopes (Figs 6-68a to 6-68c), which are the most expensive. Less expensive loupes are available from several manufacturers (Figs 6-69a to 6-69c).

In choosing a magnification device, the operator is wise to select one that gives a focal distance in the range of 10 to 14 inches. The 2.0- to 4.0-diopter range is recommended. In addition, magnifiers are available that are mounted into the lenses of eyeglasses (see Fig 6-68a) or that flip down either from the glasses frames (see Fig 6-68b) or a headband (see Figs 6-68c and 6-69a to 6-69c).

Suggested Operative Dentistry Instrument Kit

A compact assembly of hand instruments that will satisfy most operators' needs during any amalgam, resin composite, glass-ionomer, ceramic, or cast-gold restorative procedure is presented here. This kit is especially useful for dental schools and large group practices. Dental students, residents, and practitioners have used the kit, and, although another instrument may have to be added for a specific situation from time to time, the kit will more than suffice for most procedures. The kit was designed with the sequence of most operative procedures in mind.

In slots (in this order, from left to right, with the open well to the rear):

- Mirror (No. 5 with handle)
- Explorer–periodontal probe (XP23/QOW)
- Cotton forceps (college, with serrations)
- Plastic instrument, No. 1-2
- Spoon, discoid, $11\frac{1}{2}$-7-14
- Hatchet, 10-7-14
- Hoe, 12-10-16
- Gingival margin trimmer, 10-80-7-14
- Gingival margin trimmer, 10-95-7-14
- Wedelstaedt chisel, 10-15-3
- Applicator/spatula (American Eagle or Miltex)
- Condenser, SA1 (American Eagle or Miltex)
- Condenser, SA2 (American Eagle or Miltex)
- Condenser, SA3 (American Eagle or Miltex)
- Burnisher, beavertail-ovoid, 2/30
- Burnisher, PKT3
- Barghi No. 1 (paddle-shaped for composite) (American Eagle)
- Carver, cleoid-discoid, UWD5
- Carver, Walls No. 3
- Carver, Hollenback No. $\frac{1}{2}$
- Carver, interproximal (IPC)
- Carver, No. 14L
- Articulating paper forceps
- Carrier, amalgam, medium/large

In well of tray:

- Scalpel handle, No. 3, flat
- Sharpening stone, flat, Arkansas or ceramic
- Tofflemire retainer, straight
- Tofflemire retainer, contra-angle
- Amalgam well, stainless steel, small (American Eagle or Miltex)

Therefore, instrument sequence in the kit proceeds from the mirror and explorer for examination, to the plastic instrument used to facilitate dam placement as well as for placement of materials, to tooth preparation instruments, to restoration placement instruments. The kit uses a 26-slot tray with a small well (open, boxlike section) from American Eagle. American Eagle has this tray and others available with customizable color-coded tabs to facilitate replacement of similarly color-coded instruments into the correct positions in the tray.

Clipped to lid of tray:

- Hemostat, mosquito, 5-inch curved
- Scissors, Quimby

Sterilized separately and available for each operative procedure:

- Anesthetic syringe
- Rubber dam kit (forceps; punch; frame; 1 each of clamps W2A, 27, and 212SA; and 2 W8ASA clamps [Hu-Friedy])
- Brasseler bur block (No. A600) with burs arranged in the following order (Fig 6-70):
  - Friction-grip burs, No. $\frac{1}{8}$, $\frac{1}{4}$, 1, 2, $33\frac{1}{2}$, 56, 169L, 170, 329, 330, 7404, OS1F, 7803, 7901, ET9F
  - Latch burs, No. 2, 4, 6, 8
  - Mandrel for pop-on disks

Sterilized separately and available for occasional use:

- Condenser, SA4
- Hemostat, mosquito, 5-inch straight
- Mirror, No. 2 (on handle)
- Proximal contact disks (Thierman Products or Centrex) (see chapter 7)
- Rubber dam clamps, 00, W1A, W8A
- Scaler, McCalls, SM13s-14s
- Spatula, No. 24 (or 324)

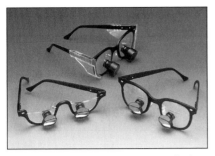

Fig 6-68a Binocular telescopes (in-the-lens type) manufactured by SurgiTel Systems, General Scientific Corp.

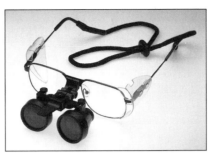

Fig 6-68b Binocular telescopes (frame-mounted flip-down type) manufactured by Sheer Vision.

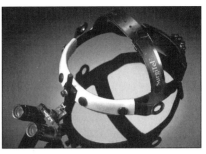

Fig 6-68c Binocular telescopes (head-band flip-down type) manufactured by SurgiTel Systems, General Scientific Corp.

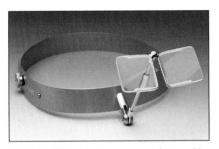

Fig 6-69a Binocular loupes manufactured by Almore International.

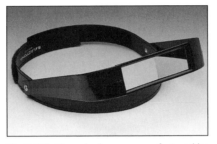

Fig 6-69b Binocular loupes manufactured by Universal Dental.

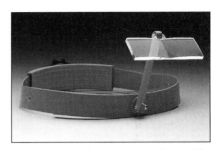

Fig 6-69c Binocular loupes manufactured by Edroy Products.

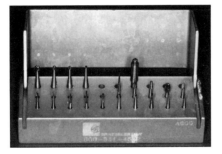

Fig 6-70 Bur block (No. A600, Brasseler), containing the burs listed in the instrument kit recommended in this chapter.

References

1. Glossary of Operative Dentistry Terms, ed 1. Washington, DC: Academy of Operative Dentistry, 1983.
2. Black GV. A Work on Operative Dentistry. Chicago: Medico-Dental Publishing, 1908.
3. Metals Handbook, ed 10, vol 1. Materials Park, OH: American Society of Metals International, 1990:841–842, 908–909.
4. Ring ME. Dentistry, an Illustrated History. New York: Abrams, 1985:251.
5. Charbeneau GT. Principles and Practice of Operative Dentistry, ed 3. Philadelphia: Lea & Febiger, 1988.
6. Webster's Ninth New Collegiate Dictionary. Springfield, MA: Merriam-Webster, 1988.
7. Young JM. Dental air-powered handpieces: Selection, use, and sterilization. Compend Contin Educ Dent 1993;14:358–366.
8. Lauer H, Kraft E, Rothlauf W, Zwingers T. Effects of the temperature of cooling water during high-speed and ultrahigh-speed tooth preparation. J Prosthet Dent 1990;63:407–414.
9. Bouschor CR, Matthews JL. A four-year clinical study of teeth restored after preparation with an air turbine handpiece with an air coolant. J Prosthet Dent 1966;16:306–309.
10. Sturdevant CM, Roberson TM, Heymann HO, Sturdevant JR. The Art and Science of Operative Dentistry, ed 3. St Louis: Mosby, 1995.
11. American National Standards Institute/American Dental Association Specification No. 23 (Revised) for Dental Excavating Burs. Chicago: American Dental Association, 1982.
12. Black RB. Technique for nonmechanical preparation of cavities and prophylaxis. J Am Dent Assoc 1945;32:955–965.
13. Goldstein RE, Parkins FM. Air-abrasive technology: Its new role in restorative dentistry. J Am Dent Assoc 1994;125:551–557.
14. Christensen GJ. Magnification. Clin Res Assoc Newsletter 1990; 14(10):1.

Field Isolation

James B. Summitt

There are many ways to isolate an area of the mouth or a tooth so that restorative services can be performed without interference from soft tissues, the tongue, saliva, or other fluids. Various tongue- and cheek-retracting devices and suction methods may be used; some of these are discussed later in this chapter. By far the most complete method of obtaining field isolation is the rubber dam, the primary subject of this chapter.

Rubber Dam

Sanford C. Barnum is credited with introducing the rubber dam to the dental profession in 1864.[1] For many years, the rubber dam has been recognized as an effective method of obtaining field isolation, improving visualization, protecting the patient, and improving the quality of operative dentistry services. It has been demonstrated that most patients prefer the use of the rubber dam for restorative procedures.[2–4] The dam has been acknowledged as an important barrier for prevention of microbial transmission from patients to members of the dental care team. In addition, it is medicolegally prudent to use a dam for procedures in which small objects, such as dental burs or endodontic files, could be aspirated by the patient.

Experts in restorative dentistry[5,6] have emphatically stated that the use of the rubber dam not only boosts the quality of restorations but also increases quantity of restorative services because patients are unable to talk or expectorate when the dam is in place. They have further stated that the operating field can only be maintained free of saliva and other contaminants with the dam in place, and the field is more accessible, airborne debris is reduced, and the patient feels more comfortable.

Complete isolation is important for the operative field, but not specifically the use of the rubber dam. One study[7] evaluated longevity and performance of facial cervical resin composite restorations: two thirds were performed with rubber dam isolation, and one third with thorough isolation using saliva ejector, cotton rolls, and gingival retraction cord. In 3 years, there was no significant difference in performance of the restorations between the two groups, and more than 95% of the restorations were completely retained; of those placed using non–rubber dam isolation methods, all were retained at 3 years.

There is evidence supporting rubber dam use during resin bonding procedures involving enamel. Barghi et al[8] used cotton roll isolation or rubber dam isolation in bonding resin composite buttons to facial enamel surfaces of teeth that were to be extracted. They found shear bond strengths to be significantly greater when rubber dam isolation was used. The same group, using similar techniques, showed that rubber dam isolation significantly reduced microleakage of resin composite buttons bonded to etched enamel[9] and that salivary contamination may affect the bond strength provided by some dentin bonding systems.[10]

Table 7-1	Available rubber dam thicknesses (gauges)*	
Gauge	**Thickness (range)***	
Thin	0.006 (0.005–0.007) inch	
Medium	0.008 (0.007–0.009) inch	
Heavy	0.010 (0.009–0.015) inch	
Extra heavy	0.012 (0.0115–0.0135) inch	
Special heavy	0.014 (0.0135–0.0155) inch	

*Thickness ranges listed by Hygenic.

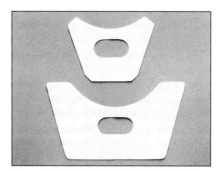

Fig 7-1 Rubber dam napkins (Hygenic) for longer procedures. Napkins provide padding between the rubber dam and the face and lips, making the dam more comfortable for the patient. The small napkin is for use with rubber dam frames. The larger napkin is for use with strap- or harness-type rubber dam holders.

Most dentists are taught the use of the rubber dam in dental school, and many suffer tremendous frustrations during rubber dam applications. For the dam to be used and to actually save chair time, the practitioner must be able to apply it quickly and easily. This chapter is designed to describe methods that facilitate use of the rubber dam.

Instruments and Materials

Rubber Dam Material

Rubber dam materials are currently available in an array of colors, ranging from green to lavender to gray to ivory. It is important in operative dentistry to use a dam color that contrasts with the color of teeth; the ivory-colored dam is therefore not recommended for operative dentistry procedures. The original gray dam is still available, but the bright colors have gained popularity. Some operators use the gray dam because they believe that it is better for matching shades in tooth-colored restorations. Because shades of restorative materials are selected prior to rubber dam placement and tooth color changes with the enamel desiccation that accompanies rubber dam use, the restorative shade is probably not affected by the use of a brightly colored rubber dam.

Rubber dam material is available in rolls, either 5 or 6 inches wide, from which squares may be cut. It is also available in sheets that are 5 inches square, usually used for children, and 6 inches square.

Rubber dam material is available in several thicknesses, or gauges (Table 7-1). The heavy and extra heavy gauges are recommended for isolation in operative dentistry. If the rubber of the heavier gauges is passed through the interproximal tooth contacts in a single thickness and not bunched in the contacts, the heavy dams are no more difficult to apply than are the thinner materials, and heavier dams are less likely to tear. The heavier materials provide a better seal to teeth and retract tissues more effectively than the thinner materials.

Rubber dam material has a shelf life of more than a year, but aging is accelerated by heat. Extra boxes of dam material can be stored in a refrigerator to extend the shelf life. Dam material that has exceeded its shelf life becomes brittle and tears easily; unfortunately, this is usually noticed during dam application. A simple test for the resistance of rubber dam material to tearing is to attempt to tear a sheet grasped with thumbs and index fingers; a strong dam will be very difficult to tear. Brittle dam material should be discarded. If the material was recently purchased, it should be returned to the supplier for replacement.

Napkin

The rubber dam napkin is a piece of strong, absorbent cloth or paper placed between the rubber dam and the patient's face. The napkin provides greater comfort for the patient, especially during unusually long procedures. Napkins are available in two shapes (Fig 7-1). The smaller napkin is usually used with rubber dam frames; the larger provides padding for the side of the face when retracting straps are used.

Punch

At least two types of rubber dam punches are available (Figs 7-2a and 7-2b). The Ainsworth-type punch, which is made by several manufacturers, is excellent if it is well made. The Ivory punch (Heraeus Kulzer) is also excellent and has a self-centering coned piston, or punch point, that helps to prevent partially punched holes (Fig 7-3). Punches should have hard-

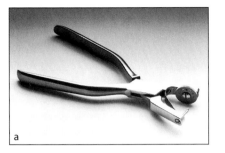

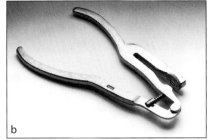

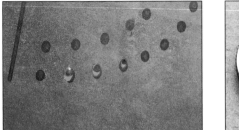

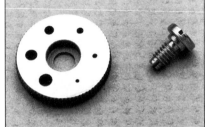

Fig 7-2a Ainsworth-design (Hygenic) rubber dam punch.

Fig 7-2b Ivory-design rubber dam punch.

Fig 7-3 *(left)* Partially punched holes. Stretched rubber dam shows the flaps of dam material left when holes are incompletely punched. The flaps will prevent proper seal. If the flaps are torn off, ragged edges can lead to tearing of the dam during application.

Fig 7-4 *(right)* The cutting table, or anvil, of a rubber dam punch should have a range of hole sizes. Pictured is the cutting table from an Ivory punch.

ened steel cutting tables (or anvils) with a range of hole sizes so that the dam will seal against teeth of various cervical dimensions (Fig 7-4).

Occasionally, the rim of a hole may be damaged because the rotating cutting table was not snapped completely into position before an attempt was made to punch a dam. Holes must be cleanly cut; incompletely punched holes (see Fig 7-3) will allow tearing of the dam during application or will affect the ability of the dam to seal.

A damaged hole rim in the cutting table will cause incomplete cutting. A damaged wheel should usually be replaced; the manufacturer of the punch can replace a damaged wheel.

Hole-Positioning Guides

Although many operators punch the holes without a positioning aid, most find it helpful to have some form of guide to determine where the holes should be punched. There are several ways to mark a rubber dam so that holes can be located optimally.

Teeth as a guide. The teeth themselves, or a stone cast of the teeth, can be used in marking the dam. To use this method, the dam is held in the desired position in the mouth, or on the stone cast, over the teeth to be included in the isolation. The cusp tips of posterior teeth and incisal edges of anterior teeth can be visualized through the dam, and the centers of the teeth are marked on the dam with a pen. An advantage of this method is precise positioning of the marks even when teeth

are malaligned. Its disadvantages include the time-consuming nature of the procedure and the inability to punch a dam before the patient is seated.

Template. Templates are available to guide the marking of the dam (Fig 7-5). These templates are approximately the same size and shape as the unstretched rubber dam itself. Holes in each template correspond to tooth positions. The template is laid over the dam, and a pen is used to mark through selected holes onto the dam. With the template, the dam can be marked and punched before the patient is seated.

Rubber dam stamp. Rubber stamps provide a very convenient and efficient way of marking the dam for punching (Fig 7-6). There are commercially available stamps, or stamps can be made by any rubber stamp manufacturer from a pattern such as the one shown in Fig 7-7 or any custom design. Dams should be prestamped by an assistant so that the marks for the maxillary central incisors are positioned approximately 0.9 inch from the top of the dam. Exceptions to normal tooth position are easily accommodated.

Rubber Dam Holders

Strap holders. Strap holders such as the Woodbury holder or retractor (Fig 7-8), available from Suter Dental, provide the most cheek and lip retraction, access, and stability, but may cause the most discomfort to the patient. A rubber dam nap-

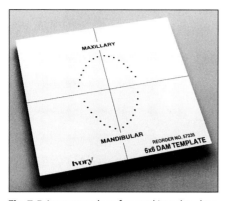

Fig 7-5 Ivory template for marking the dam. Marks corresponding to the teeth to be isolated are made on a 6.0-inch rubber dam through the holes with a felt-tipped or ballpoint pen.

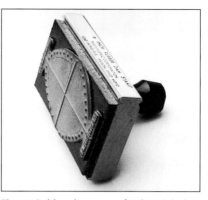

Fig 7-6 Rubber dam stamp for the adult dentition.

kin is a necessity for patient comfort when a strap holder is used. The Woodbury retractor grasps the dam material with spring-loaded clips. When posterior teeth are isolated with a Woodbury-type holder, a tuck or fold in the dam may be needed (Fig 7-9).

Frame holders. Frame holders are exemplified by the Young frame (Young Dental) and the Nygaard-Ostby frame (Figs 7-10a to 7-10d). A U-shaped Young frame is made by several manufacturers in both metal and plastic. The Young-type frames are available in both adult and child sizes. A plastic frame is advantageous when radiographs will be a part of the procedure because it is radiolucent. The plastic frames do not, however, stand up to heat sterilization as well as metal frames, and they have a shorter life span. Metal frames are less bulky and last for years.[11] They are available with balls on the ends to protect the patient in the event that the frame is inadvertently pushed toward the eyes.

The Young frame is usually positioned on the outside surface of the dam so that it is not in contact with the patient's face. The Nygaard-Ostby frame is normally positioned on the tissue surface or inside surface of the dam and touches the patient's face (or the rubber dam napkin). All frames have points or pegs over which the dam material is stretched to provide a clear operating field and to hold the frame in position. Some Young-type frames come with a hook on each side for attachment of a strap. The strap is run around the back of the head and can be tightened to pull the frame posteriorly to better retract lips and cheeks. If the operator doesn't find the strap useful, the hooks may be cut off, leaving an additional point on each side of the frame for attachment of the dam.

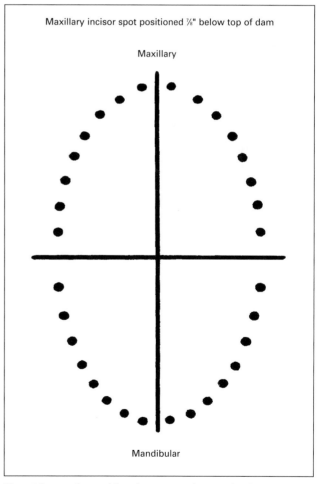

Fig 7-7 Pattern for a rubber dam stamp. This may be duplicated and taken to a rubber stamp manufacturer.

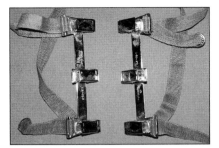

Fig 7-8 Strap- or harness-type rubber dam holders provide excellent lip and cheek retraction. Pictured is a Woodbury retractor.

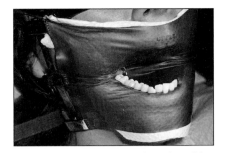

Fig 7-9 A fold or tuck is made in the rubber dam to provide an uncluttered operating field.

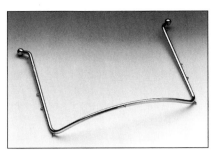

Fig 7-10a Metal Young frame with eye protectors.

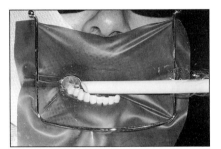

Fig 7-10b Young frame inserted into the external surface of the dam.

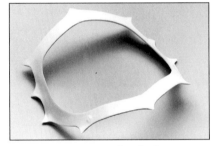

Fig 7-10c Plastic Nygaard-Ostby frame.

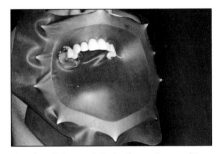

Fig 7-10d Nygaard-Ostby frame inserted into the internal surface of the dam.

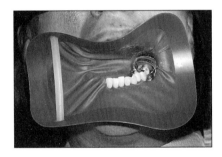

Fig 7-11 In the HandiDam, the frame is an integral part of the dam.

Preattached frames. One commercially available rubber dam (HandiDam, Aseptico) comes with a built-in frame and a rod for insertion to keep the dam open (Fig 7-11).

Clamp Forceps

Ivory-type clamp forceps (Fig 7-12a) are available from several manufacturers and with differently angled beaks. Ivory forceps (Heraeus Kulzer) have stabilizers that prevent the clamp from rotating on the beaks (Fig 7-12b). This is usually advantageous, but it limits the use of these forceps to teeth that are within a range of normal angulation.

Stokes-type clamp forceps (Fig 7-12c), which have notches near the tips of their beaks in which to locate the holes of a rubber dam clamp (Fig 7-12d), allow a range of rotation for the clamp so that it may be positioned on teeth that are mesially or distally angled.

Either of these types of clamp forceps will serve the practitioner well, and selection should be based on personal preference. The Ivory-type forceps are probably the most popular because of cost.

Fig 7-12a Ivory forceps.

Fig 7-12b Stabilizers near the tips of the Ivory-type forceps limit rotation of the clamp when it is held by the forceps.

Fig 7-12c Stokes-type forceps.

Fig 7-12d The tip design of the Stokes forceps provides more freedom for rotation of the clamp while it is held by the forceps.

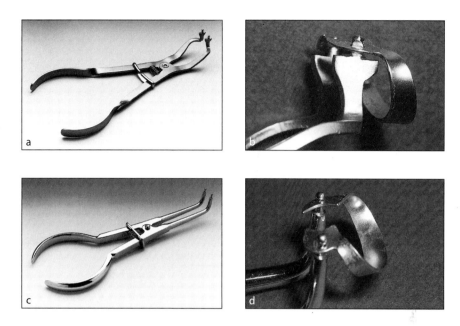

Clamps

Rubber dam clamps are the usual means of retaining the rubber dam. The three basic types of clamps and their parts are shown in Fig 7-13. When a posterior segment is isolated, the clamp is usually placed on the distalmost exposed tooth (Fig 7-14). The clamp may also be placed on an unexposed tooth (one for which a hole has not been punched) (Fig 7-15).

There are clamps with jaw sizes to fit every tooth. Some clamps simply have a number designation; others have a W in front of the number. The W indicates that the clamp is wingless (see Fig 7-13b); those clamps that do not bear a W have wings (see Fig 7-13a) so that the dam may be attached to the wings before the clamp is placed on the tooth (Fig 7-16).

Although in recent years manufacturers have reduced the number of clamps they produce, a variety of clamp designs remain available. For the practice of operative dentistry, the number of clamps should be limited to a few that will satisfy most needs; these may be kept in the instrument kit and sterilized along with the other operative dentistry instruments. Clamps that will serve in most situations and are recommended for inclusion in operative dentistry instrument kits are listed in Table 7-2 and shown in Fig 7-17.

Supplemental clamps, to be available on the rare occasions when the usual clamps will not suffice, should be packaged and sterilized separately. Recommended supplemental clamps are listed in Table 7-3 and shown in Fig 7-18.

No. W8A clamp. Although Ivory modified the design of the No. W8A clamp several years ago so that the jaw points do not extend so severely in a gingival direction, some No. W8A clamps still have points that extend farther gingivally than is desirable. The jaws of a No. W8A clamp, for most applications, should be approximately horizontal (Fig 7-19) prior to expansion of the clamp for placement on a tooth. As the jaws are spread, the angle of the jaws will change to a gingival orientation; this is usually desirable, but before the clamp is expanded, the jaws should have little or no gingival angulation.

For No. W8A clamps in which the jaws have a significant gingival angulation, a modification procedure is recommended (Figs 7-19a to 7-19c) unless deep subgingival placement of the points is needed. This modification may be made with a stone used in a low-speed handpiece or a finishing bur used in a high-speed handpiece. After the modification is made, the points, which have been sharpened by the modification procedure, must be blunted to prevent damage to tooth surfaces.

The No. W8ASA clamp (Fig 7-20) is available from Hu-Friedy. This design incorporates most of the advantages of the modification of the No. W8A described above and in Fig 7-19.

Butterfly clamps. Most of the clamps listed in Tables 7-2 and 7-3 may act as rubber dam retainers (placed on the distal tooth or teeth to hold the dam on the quadrant or arch) or as

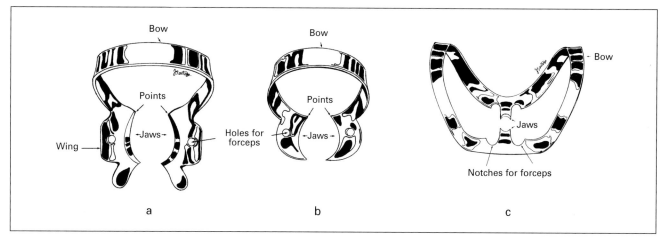

Fig 7-13 (a) Winged rubber dam clamp; (b) wingless rubber dam clamp; (c) butterfly rubber dam clamp.

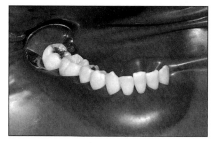

Fig 7-14 Isolated mandibular right quadrant. The clamp is positioned on the distalmost exposed tooth.

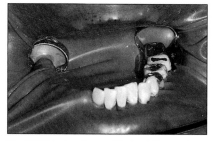

Fig 7-15 Isolated mandibular left quadrant with a second clamp placed on an unexposed molar on the right side of the mouth to give additional access to the lingual surfaces of the teeth in the left quadrant. The dam has been loosely stretched over the unexposed tooth to prevent the clamp from initiating a tear. The mirror and other instruments will now be unimpeded when the defective lingual margin of the crown on the first molar is treated.

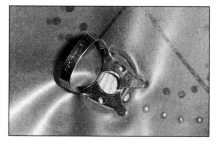

Fig 7-16 Winged clamp attached to the rubber dam. The edges of the hole are stretched over the wings of the clamp.

Table 7-2	Clamps recommended for inclusion in operative dentistry instrument kits		
Wingless clamps	Winged clamps	Tooth fit	Comment
W8A, W8ASA,* or B1	8A	Molar	
	27*	Molar	Bow extended distally in 27
W2A*	2A	Premolar	
212SA*		Premolar, canine, and incisor	For Class 5 isolation

*Clamps recommended to be available for routine use.
All clamps except B1 and W8ASA are from Ivory catalog (Heraeus Kulzer).
B1 is from Hygenic, and W8ASA is from Hu-Friedy.

Table 7-3	Supplemental clamps recommended for availability on request		
Wingless clamps	Winged clamps*	Tooth fit	Comment
W0	00†	Small incisor	
W1A†	1A	Premolar	Gingivally angled jaws
W14A†	14A†	Molar	For partially erupted molar

*Same clamps as in first column but with wings.
†Clamps recommended to be available to supplement clamps listed in Table 7-2.
All clamps are from Ivory catalog (Heraeus Kulzer).

Fig 7-17 *(left)* Clamps recommended for routine use: *(top row, left to right)* No. W8A, B1, 27; *(bottom row)* No. W2A and No. 212SA retractor.

Fig 7-18 *(right)* Recommended supplemental clamps: *(left to right)* No. 00 (for mandibular incisors and other small teeth), No. W14A (for partially erupted molars), and No. W1A (for premolars with subgingival margins).

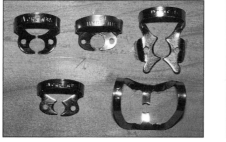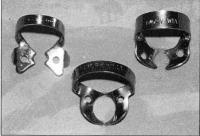

Fig 7-19 Modification recommended for No. W8A clamps, to thin the jaws and reduce the extension of the jaw points toward gingival tissue.

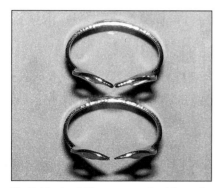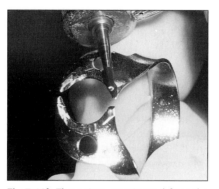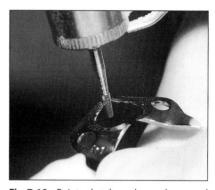

Fig 7-19a *(top)* Clamp as received from the manufacturer; *(bottom)* clamp that has been modified.

Fig 7-19b The points are trimmed from the tissue side so that gingival extension is reduced and jaws are thinned. The bur being used in the high-speed handpiece is a No. 7803 bullet-shaped finishing bur.

Fig 7-19c Points that have been sharpened during modification must be dulled. If the points are left sharp, they can damage the surface of the tooth.

Fig 7-20 No. W8ASA clamp (Hu-Friedy). This clamp features most of the benefits of the modified W8A clamp shown in Fig 7-19.

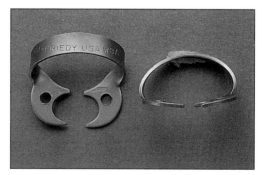

rubber dam and gingival tissue retractors (to retract the dam and tissues away from a preparation margin in the cervical area of a tooth). One clamp, however, the butterfly clamp, No. 212SA (Fig 7-21a), is designed to serve as a retractor only. Because of its double bow and the closeness of the points of each jaw, this clamp must be stabilized on the tooth (Fig 7-21b), or it may rock mesiodistally during the procedure and damage the root. For retraction for a facial Class 5 restoration, dental impression compound (such as red or green compound, Kerr/Sybron) should be used under the

bows of the clamp on the occlusal (or incisal) and lingual aspects of the teeth to provide stabilization.

The double bow of the No. 212SA clamp precludes placement of two clamps on adjacent teeth. When two Class 5 restorations are to be placed on adjacent teeth, two No. 212SA clamps may be modified (Fig 7-21c); one of the bows of each clamp is cut off so that the remaining bow of one clamp extends to the right and the bow of the other extends to the left. If these clamps are stabilized with modeling compound, adjacent Class 5 restorations may be accomplished

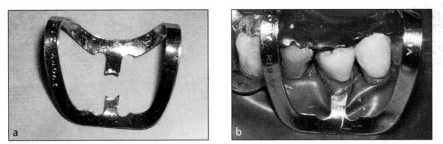

Figs 7-21a and 7-21b No. 212SA clamp (or retractor) for retracting the gingival tissue and rubber dam.

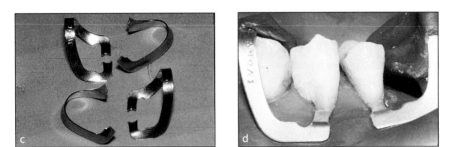

Figs 7-21c and 7-21d Two No. 212SA retractors may be modified to give two clamps for tissue and dam retraction for side-by-side restorations. The No. 212SA and the modified No. 212SA retractors must be stabilized with modeling compound, or the jaws will damage tooth surfaces.

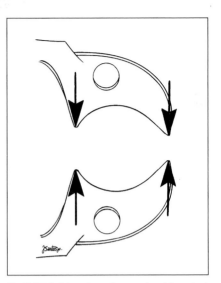

Fig 7-22 Rubber dam clamps should contact the tooth at the mesial and distal extent of the jaws. This four-point contact provides stability, or resistance to rotation or dislodgment, for the clamp.

simultaneously (Fig 7-21d). A No. 212SA clamp or a modified No. 212SA clamp may be used on one root of a molar that has a long clinical crown as well as on single-rooted teeth.

Tooth contact. An important consideration when a clamp is selected is that only its jaw points contact the tooth; this gives four-point contact (Fig 7-22). No clamp jaw can ever be contoured to fit a tooth precisely, nor is there any reason for a clamp to fit precisely because the dam, not the clamp, creates the seal. Molar clamps should have accentuated arches between the jaw points to ensure that the points are in contact with the tooth, even in teeth with very convex cervical areas. The distance between the points of a jaw, along with the strength of the bow of the clamp, determines the stability of the clamp. If there is contact between the tooth and any other part of the clamp's jaw, the contact points are brought closer together, thus reducing the stability of the clamp and allowing it to rotate on the tooth and, occasionally, to be dislodged from the tooth. Four-point contact is, therefore, very desirable.

The strength or temper of the bow of the clamp should also be maintained. Clamps should be expanded with the clamp forceps no more than is necessary for the clamp to be passed over the facial and lingual heights of contour of the tooth. If a clamp has been overexpanded, it will grasp the tooth with less strength and is more likely to be dislodged. Occasionally, the jaws of clamps that have been overexpanded may be squeezed together so that enough of the strength returns, but it is usually best to discard a clamp that has been overexpanded.

Floss ligatures. Many clinicians and dental schools recommend that dental floss be attached to every clamp used in the mouth to allow retrieval if the clamp is dislodged or breaks. Certainly, it is wise to attach floss to the clamp that is positioned in the mouth prior to application of the dam. After dam placement is completed, however, the floss causes leakage if it extends under the dam or is in the way if left to dangle in the operating field. A solution is to attach the floss to the clamp during application of the dam (see Fig 7-35a) and to cut and detach the floss from the clamp after the dam is in place. If the clamp dislodges or breaks after the dam is in place, it will either be catapulted from the mouth by the tension of the dam or be trapped by the dam so that it cannot be swallowed or aspirated.

When a winged clamp is attached to the dam during placement of the clamp onto a tooth, the attachment of a floss ligature to the clamp is redundant. Floss also need not be attached to a second clamp placed for retraction after the dam is in place.

Fig 7-23 *Alternative methods for dam retention.*

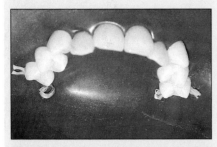

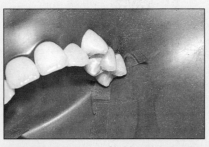

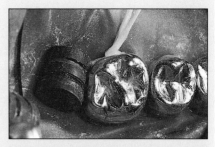

Fig 7-23a Dental tape placed doubly through the contact distal to the distalmost exposed tooth.

Fig 7-23b Short strip of rubber dam used to retain the dam.

Fig 7-23c Anesthetic cartridge plunger tied around the distal tooth with floss.

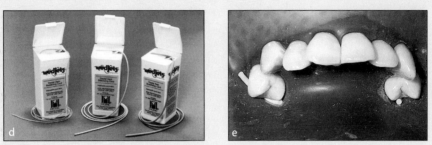

Figs 7-23d and 7-23e Elastic cord used as a rubber dam retainer.

Other Retainers

Other methods are sometimes used for rubber dam retention:

1. Dental floss or tape is placed doubly through a contact and then cut to a short length so that it does not impede access (Fig 7-23a).
2. A short strip of rubber dam material is cut from the edge of the rubber dam, stretched and carried through the contact, and then allowed to relax to retain the dam (Fig 7-23b).
3. Floss is tied to a sterilized rubber plunger from an anesthetic cartridge or similar item and then tied around the most distal isolated tooth (Fig 7-23c).
4. Elastic cord, eg, Wedjets (Hygenic), is placed interproximally to retain the dam (Figs 7-23d and 7-23e).

Modeling Compound

Modeling compound may be used as an adjunct to the application of any clamp as a retainer or retractor. It is especially useful and necessary for anchoring and stabilizing the No. 212SA retainer (see Figs 7-21b and 7-21d).

For stabilizing a clamp, use of modeling compound, either red or green (Kerr/Sybron), is recommended. The clamp is positioned appropriately on the tooth and held in position with a finger until stabilization is completed. There are several effective methods for applying compound to stabilize a clamp. One of these techniques allows the practitioner to have prewarmed modeling compound immediately available and avoids the use of a flame. With this technique, modeling compound is placed into a plastic syringe, such as a large Monoject or impression syringe, which is then placed in a water bath at the appropriate temperature for the type of modeling compound used. The diameter of the aperture of the tip should be made larger to allow the softened compound to be ejected easily from the syringe. When the clamp is positioned, the practitioner removes the syringe with the prewarmed modeling compound from the water bath and flows it into the desired area to stabilize the clamp.

Another technique involves the use of the compound in the stick form. A stick is held over a low alcohol flame and rotated and moved back and forth so that the length to be softened is heated evenly (Fig 7-24a). After the surface is softened, the stick is withdrawn from the flame to allow the heat to diffuse to the center of the stick. When the length is warmed to the center, there will no longer be a core of unsoftened compound to support the shape, and the softened length will sag or droop (Fig 7-24b). If the stick has been overheated, so that it elongates in addition to drooping, it should be tempered in a container of water. Before the compound is taken to the mouth, the surface should be briefly reheated to enhance adhesion of the compound to the retracting clamp and teeth.

Fig 7-24 *Use of modeling compound to stabilize a No. 212SA retractor.*

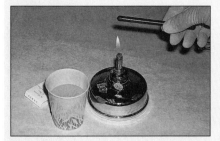

Fig 7-24a The compound stick is warmed in an alcohol flame.

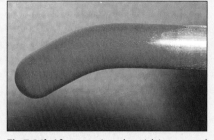

Fig 7-24b After warming, the stick is removed from the flame and held until the heat has diffused to the center of the stick so that the warmed end of the stick begins to droop.

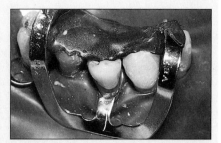

Fig 7-24c Use of compound to stabilize a No. 212SA retractor is completed.

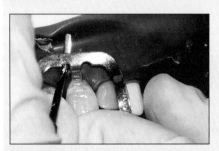

Fig 7-24d Removal of the clamp with forceps may be hampered by the compound on the lingual aspect. If so, a facial notch of the clamp may be engaged with an instrument such as a plastic instrument.

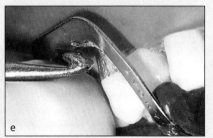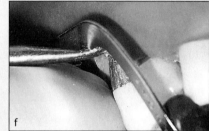

Figs 7-24e and 7-24f A No. 0 crochet hook (with handle made of laboratory acrylic) or a No. 34 surgical elevator modified to mimic a No. 0 crochet hook may be used to engage a notch of the clamp. Such a modified surgical elevator is manufactured by Hu-Friedy.

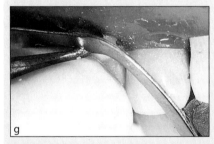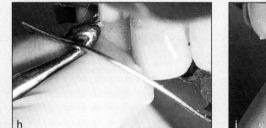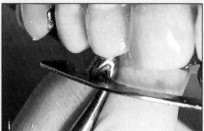

Figs 7-24g to 7-24i The facial jaw of the clamp is then pulled facially away from the tooth surface and rotated occlusally or incisally to quickly remove the clamp and the stabilizing compound.

The compound should be applied to the retainer and teeth in a location as far away from the area to be restored as possible. The stick is then twisted and pulled away, leaving softened compound in place. The compound should be shaped and molded with damp, gloved fingers into embrasures and made to contact a large area of the clamp and the lingual surfaces of the teeth. It should then be cooled with the air syringe for 20 seconds or more. Stabilization of the retracting clamp is then completed (Fig 7-24c); the finger holding the clamp may now be released, and the clamp is tested for stability.

Compound should be kept away from the planned area of operation so that it will not inhibit access; in that regard, for a facial restoration, compound should be confined to the occlusal (or incisal) and lingual surfaces. Full advantage should be taken of the lingual surfaces for maximum dependability of attachment of the compound to the teeth. When the lingual surfaces are covered by the compound, the lingual notches for the clamp forceps will be covered. To remove the clamp with forceps, the operator would have to chip away the compound to expose a lingual notch. In a simpler method, an instrument is used to pull the facial jaw of the clamp away from the facial surface and then occlusally (incisally) (Figs 7-24d to 7-24i).

Fig 7-25 *Inverting instruments. Note the tip of the air syringe in each instance; a high-volume stream of air is used to dry the tooth and dam surfaces to facilitate inversion.*

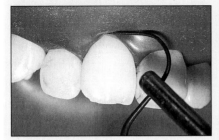

Fig 7-25a No. 23 explorer.

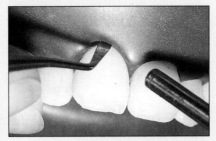

Fig 7-25b No. 1-2 plastic instrument.

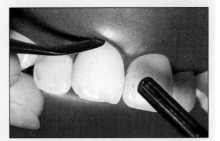

Fig 7-25c Beavertail burnisher.

Fig 7-26 Wooden wedges are used to protect the dam from being cut during a procedure that involves the use of burs or cutting instruments near the dam.

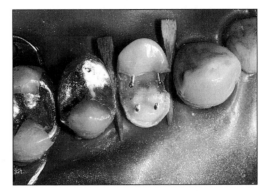

Inverting Instrument

Almost any instrument may be used for inverting the dam. Commonly used instruments include explorers such as the No. 23 (Fig 7-25a), plastic filling instruments such as the No. 1-2 (Fig 7-25b), or a beavertail burnisher (Fig 7-25c). Dental tape or floss used interproximally is also useful for dam inversion.

Wedge

The wooden wedge, which is used to stabilize a matrix and hold it against the gingival margin of a cavity preparation involving a proximal tooth surface, is also useful for protecting the dam (Fig 7-26) when rotary cutting instruments are used in proximal areas. Placement of water-soluble rubber dam lubricant on the wedge enhances the ease of wedge placement.

Scissors

Scissors are often useful in preparing the dam for insertion and are a necessity for cutting the dam for removal. Blunt-ended scissors are preferred by many operators, but other scissors, such as sharp crown and collar scissors and Quimby scissors (see Fig 7-40b), will also serve well. Scissors used for cutting rubber dams must be sharp, or they will frustrate the operator.

Dental Tape and Floss

Waxed tape or floss, not unwaxed floss, is recommended for flossing the dam through interproximal contacts. Waxed tape, or ribbon floss (see Fig 7-35f), will carry more of a septum through a contact in a single pass than will the narrower floss, but the tape must be maintained flat and not bunched up, or it will be difficult to pass through the contact.

Proximal Contact Disk

A proximal contact disk (Thierman Products or Centrix) is used to plane rough enamel, amalgam, or resin composite contacts so that the floss will pass through without shredding and so that the dam can be flossed through without tearing (Figs 7-27a to 7-27c). The plane metal disk, without abrasive, is recommended. This instrument should not be used in a contact that involves a gold casting because it can cut into the gold and produce additional obstruction to passage of the floss through the contact.

The disk is placed into the occlusal embrasure and rocked facially and lingually as it is pushed firmly, but with control, gingivally. If it cannot be worked through the contact, the teeth should be separated slightly with a plastic instrument placed snugly into the gingival embrasure and torqued slight-

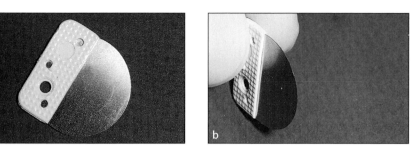

Figs 7-27a and 7-27b Proximal contact disk or plane with handle (Thierman Products).

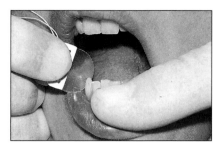

Fig 7-27c The proximal contact disk is used to plane rough contact.

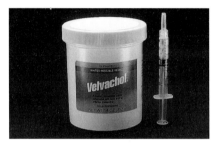

Fig 7-28 A water-soluble rubber dam lubricant, such as Velvachol, can be loaded into a syringe, such as a 3.0-mL disposable syringe. The lubricant can be dispensed from the syringe onto the tissue surface (underside) of the rubber dam or onto a glove for coating of the dam adjacent to the holes.

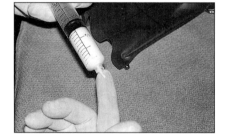

Fig 7-29a Water-soluble lubricant can be carried to the dam with a finger.

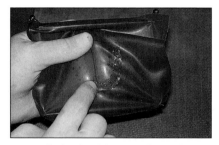

Fig 7-29b The dam lubricant is layered on the tissue surface of the dam in the area of the holes.

ly while the disk is being pushed into the contact from the occlusal embrasure. Several passes of the disk through the contact will usually plane it smooth.

Lubricant

Rubber dam lubricant makes a significant difference in the ease with which the dam is applied. A water-soluble lubricant is preferred. A product that has proven especially suitable for lubricating the rubber dam is Velvachol water-miscible vehicle (Healthpoint) (Fig 7-28). Velvachol is a pharmaceutical product manufactured as a water-soluble ointment base, but it is an excellent dam lubricant. Petroleum-based lubricants, such as Vaseline (Chesebrough-Pond's), should be avoided as rubber dam lubricants because they are difficult to remove from the dam after application and therefore can impede bonding procedures and make inversion of the dam more difficult.

Water-soluble lubricant is applied in a thin coat in the area of the holes on the tissue surface of the dam before it is taken to the mouth (Figs 7-29a and 7-29b). The lubricant makes passage of the dam through the interproximal contacts much easier, and the dam will often pass through the contacts in a

single layer without the use of floss. If additional lubrication is desired, lubricant may be applied to the teeth prior to placement of the dam.

A lubricant for the lips will make the patient more comfortable during the procedure. A petroleum-based lubricant, such as Vaseline, cocoa butter, silicate lubricant, or lip balm, functions well as a lip lubricant.

Application and Removal

Preparation of the Mouth

Teeth should be cleaned, if necessary, and contacts should be checked with floss. The rapid passage of dental floss through each contact that will be involved in the isolation is very important and, if accomplished as a part of the routine, will save chair time. Any rough contact should be smoothed with the proximal contact disk (see Fig 7-27), not only to facilitate dam placement but also to enable the patient to clean each interproximal area during routine flossing.

If a restorative procedure that involves an occlusal surface is planned, centric occlusion (maximum intercuspation) con-

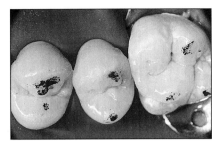

Fig 7-30 The centric occlusion markings were protected by a light-cured resin or varnish during dam placement; had the markings not been protected, the placement procedure would likely have erased them.

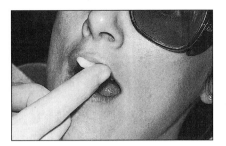

Fig 7-31 Lips are lubricated with petroleum-based lubricant prior to placement of the rubber dam.

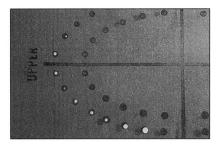

Fig 7-32 Varying hole sizes are used to seal the dam around various sizes of teeth.

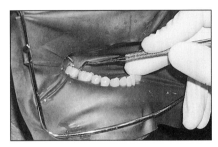

Fig 7-33 The incisal edges of the anterior teeth are used as a finger rest.

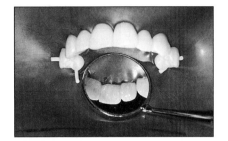

Fig 7-34 In isolation for an anterior restoration, the anterior teeth and first premolars are exposed to provide anchorage of the dam and to leave adequate working room on the lingual aspect of the anterior teeth.

tacts may be marked with articulating paper or tape prior to application of the dam. Centric occlusion markings may be coated with a clear light-cured resin or varnish to protect them from being rubbed off. An applicator or brush containing the liquid resin should be touched to the enamel adjacent to the markings and the material allowed to flow across the markings prior to curing (Fig 7-30).

If lips are to be lubricated, this should be accomplished prior to application of the dam (Fig 7-31).

Preparation of the Dam

Use of a prestamped dark (gray or green), heavy (or extra heavy) gauge dam material is recommended. Various hole sizes should be used to ensure a seal around the variety of tooth sizes (Fig 7-32). For example, an Ivory punch has six hole sizes, numbered 1 (smallest) through 6 (largest) (see Fig 7-4). Hole sizes recommended are 5 for clamped molars; 4 for other molars; 3 for premolars, canines, and maxillary central incisors; and 2 for maxillary lateral incisors and mandibular incisors.

Slight variation from the recommended hole sizes may be needed, depending on the size of individual teeth, operator preference, and gauge of the dam, but a range of hole sizes should be used to prevent leakage between the dam and the teeth.

For operative procedures involving posterior teeth, the tooth or teeth to be restored should be exposed, as well as at least one tooth posterior to the most distal tooth to be restored, if possible. In addition, all teeth around to the central or lateral incisor on the opposite side of the same arch should be exposed. This extension of the area of isolation to the opposite side will hold the dam flat in the arch to give room for fingers and instruments in the area of the teeth to be restored. It will also expose teeth in the anterior area for finger rests during the operation (Fig 7-33).

For anterior restorations, exposure of the first premolar through the first premolar on the opposite side is recommended (Fig 7-34). This will provide room for the mirror and for hand instruments on the lingual aspect of the anterior teeth.

When a prestamped dam or a template is used, holes should be punched away from the spots to accommodate atypical alignment of teeth. In addition, when the dam is being prepared to provide isolation for Class 5 restorations, the hole for the tooth to receive a facial Class 5 restoration should be punched approximately 1.0 mm facial to the spot to allow retraction with the No. 212SA clamp. No holes should be punched for missing teeth.

After the dam is punched, the tissue side of the dam should be lubricated with a water-soluble lubricant. A small dollop of lubricant is applied to the tissue surface and smeared over the surface of the dam in the area of the holes (see Fig 7-29). The rubber dam frame can then be attached to the top and bottom of the dam, leaving a relaxed area or "pouch" of dam material between the top and bottom (see Fig 7-35b). Attaching the dam to the frame in this way holds the edges of the dam away from the holes for better visualization during application.

Placement of the Dam

If a local anesthetic agent has been administered to provide pulpal anesthesia for the tooth or teeth being restored, at least a portion of the gingival tissue will have also been anesthetized. If an inferior alveolar block has been given, the lingual nerve will almost always have been anesthetized as well, so the gingival tissue lingual to the mandibular posterior teeth will also have been anesthetized. If infiltration anesthesia has been administered to maxillary teeth, the facial gingival tissue will have been anesthetized. For application of a rubber dam clamp, the portions of the gingival tissue that have not been anesthetized along with the delivery of pulpal anesthesia will not normally need to be anesthetized. When the clamp is applied, as long as the points of the clamp's jaw are firmly on the tooth and have not penetrated gingival tissue, the patient may feel some discomfort for a few seconds where the jaws are pressing against tissue. This pressure discomfort will usually disappear within 1 minute due to "pressure anesthesia," and injection anesthesia for the gingival tissue is usually unnecessary. If additional gingival anesthesia is necessary, topical anesthetic solutions or gels may suffice.

When the clamp is applied to the tooth with the clamp forceps, the clamp should be expanded only enough to allow it to pass over the crown of the tooth. Overexpansion of the clamp will permanently distort it so that it will be weak, unstable, and more likely to dislodge from the tooth.

There are several methods of dam placement:

Dam over clamp. A wingless clamp is placed on the tooth. It is recommended that a finger be maintained over the inserted clamp to prevent its dislodgment until its stability on the tooth has been confirmed. The operator checks stability by engaging the bow of the clamp with an instrument and firmly attempting to pull it occlusally (Fig 7-35a). If the clamp rotates on the tooth, it is not stable and should be repositioned or replaced.

The top and bottom attachment points of the Young frame are engaged at the top and bottom of the dam to give a slackness or pouching of the dam (Fig 7-35b). The tissue side of the dam is lubricated in the area of the holes. Then, with a finger on each side of the distal hole in the dam, the dentist (or assistant) stretches the dam so that the hole is enlarged and appears to be an open slit; the hole is then carried over the bow and jaws of the clamp (Fig 7-35c). The hole at the opposite end of the row (usually for the lateral or central incisor on the opposite side) is then passed over the appropriate tooth, and the septa are worked through the interproximal contacts.

A gloved fingernail used to slightly separate the anterior teeth is very helpful, and floss is rarely needed to carry the dam through anterior interproximal contacts (Fig 7-35d). To use the "fingernail technique," the edge of the septum is positioned at the incisal extent of the contact and pulled gingivally with fingers on the facial and lingual aspects. This method also can frequently facilitate septum passage through interproximal contacts of posterior teeth.

Good lubrication of the dam is necessary for easy and quick application. The dam should be passed through each contact in a single layer. This may be accomplished by stretching a septum over one of the teeth adjacent to the contact and sliding the edge of the rubber to the contact so that a leading edge of dam is touching the contact (Fig 7-35e).

In posterior areas, the leading edge should be touching the occlusal portion of the contact in the occlusal embrasure. Waxed tape (ribbon floss) or waxed floss may then be used to move the dam progressively through the contact (Figs 7-35e to 7-35g). Tape will carry more of the rubber through the contact in a single pass than will floss. If tape is used, like the rubber, it should be taken through the contact in a single layer, not twisted or bunched up.

If the dam goes through with one pass of the floss, the floss should be removed from the contact without pulling the rubber back out. To accomplish this, the tail of the floss that is on the lingual side of the teeth is doubled back across the occlusal embrasure of the contact so that both ends are on the facial aspect; then the tape is pulled facially through the contact. If only a portion of the septum goes through the contact with the first pass of the floss or tape, the floss should be doubled back and passed through the contact again; it is then pulled facially out of the gingival embrasure (Fig 7-35h). The tape should be passed through repeatedly until the entire septum has been carried through the contact.

Winged clamp in dam. Prior to lubrication of the dam, the clamp is placed into the distal hole so that the hole is stretched over the wings of the clamp from its tissue side (Figs

Fig 7-35 Dam over clamp method of dam application.

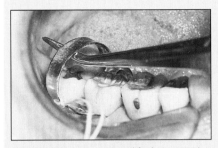

Fig 7-35a The clamp (modified No. W8A) is tested for stability. To do so, the operator attempts to pull the bow occlusally.

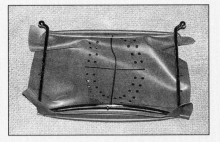

Fig 7-35b The dam is fitted loosely on the frame.

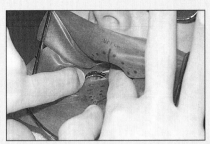

Fig 7-35c The distal hole of the dam is carried over the bow of the clamp.

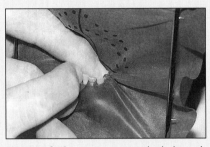

Fig 7-35d The septa are worked through anterior contacts as a gloved fingernail is used to slightly separate teeth.

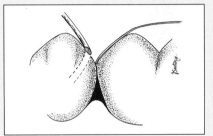

Fig 7-35e The leading edge of the dam is touching the occlusal aspect of the interproximal contact; floss is on the adjacent tooth.

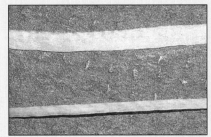

Fig 7-35f Waxed dental tape, or ribbon floss *(top)*, if it is not folded or bunched, will carry more of the dam septum through the contact in a single pass than will waxed floss *(bottom)*, but either type will serve the purpose.

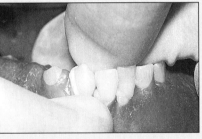

Fig 7-35g The dam septum is lying on the mesial aspect of the mandibular first premolar, with its leading edge at the mesial contact; the floss is lying on the distal aspect of the canine, ready to move to the contact, meeting the dam there. The floss will then carry at least a portion of the septum through the contact.

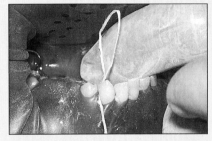

Fig 7-35h The floss has been doubled back to the facial aspect and passed through the contact again, carrying another portion of the septum through the contact. The floss is then removed from the contact; one or both of the tails of the floss are pulled facially away from the teeth.

Fig 7-36 *Winged clamp in dam method of dam application.*

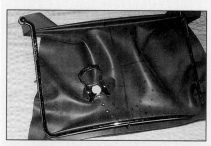

Fig 7-36a A winged clamp (No. 27) is inserted into the distal hole of the dam.

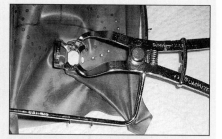

Fig 7-36b The clamp-dam-frame assembly is carried to the mouth as a unit.

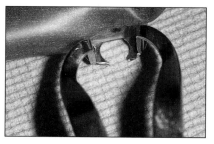

Fig 7-37a Wingless clamp in dam method of dam application. Shown is the clamp in the dam.

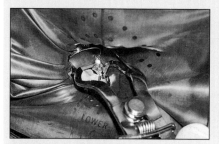

Fig 7-36c The clamp is placed on the mandibular second molar.

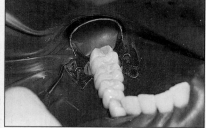

Fig 7-36d The dam has been applied to the quadrant, and a No. 1-2 plastic instrument is used to pull the edges of rubber off the wings of the clamp.

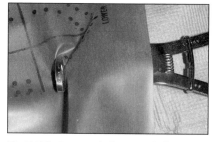

Fig 7-37b Dam and clamp with forceps in place.

7-16 and 7-36a). The dam is then lubricated, and the frame is attached. The forceps are inserted into the holes of the clamp, and the clamp, dam, and frame are carried as a unit into place (Figs 7-36b and 7-36c). After the stability of the clamp is confirmed, the dam material on the wings of the clamp is pulled off the wings with finger tension or with a bladed instrument such as a plastic instrument (Fig 7-36d). The remainder of the dam is placed as previously described.

Wingless clamp in dam. The distal hole of the lubricated dam is passed over the bow of a wingless clamp, such as the modified No. W8A, so that the hole comes to rest at the junction of the bow and the jaw arms (Fig 7-37a). The frame is not attached to the dam at this point. The dam is gathered up and elevated to expose the jaw arms of the clamp, and the forceps are then inserted into the forceps holes (Figs 7-37a and 7-37b). The gathered dam is carried to the mouth with one hand and the forceps with the other. After the clamp is applied to the distal tooth and the dam has been pulled over the jaws of the clamp, the frame is attached and the other teeth are isolated as previously described.

Clamp after dam. The dam is applied to the teeth and then the clamp is placed. This technique, occasionally necessary, is the most difficult.

Completion of Application

Application of the napkin. For longer procedures, the use of a rubber dam napkin is recommended. The napkin may be positioned before or after the dam is in place on the teeth. For placement of the napkin after the dam has been applied, the frame is removed, the napkin is placed so that its edges remain on the skin and not in the mouth, and the frame is replaced.

Adjustment of the dam in the frame. The frame and dam are adjusted so that there is a minimum of folds and wrinkles and so that the dam does not obstruct the nostrils.

Washing of the dam. The dam and isolated teeth are washed with an air/water spray to remove the lubricant. After they are washed, the dam and teeth should be dried with air from the air syringe.

Fig 7-38a Without inversion of the dam, positive pressure under the dam, created by tongue movement, swallowing, etc, will cause leakage of saliva into the operating field.

Fig 7-38b With inversion of the dam, positive pressure under the dam only causes the dam to seal more tightly against the tooth, preventing leakage.

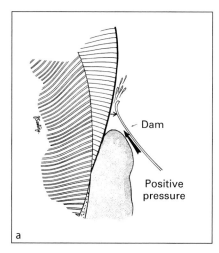 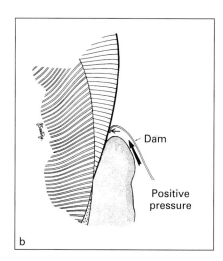

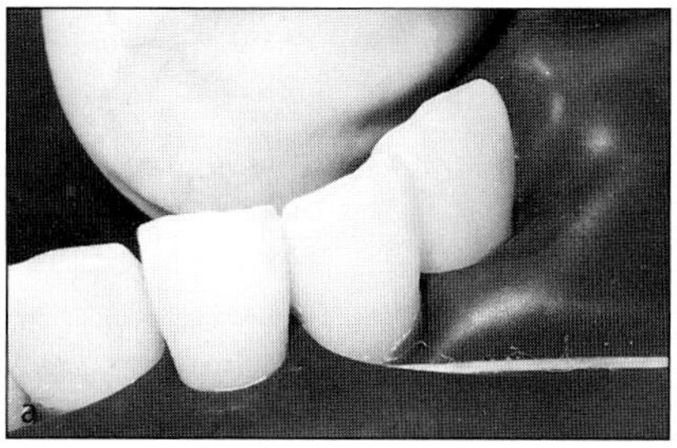

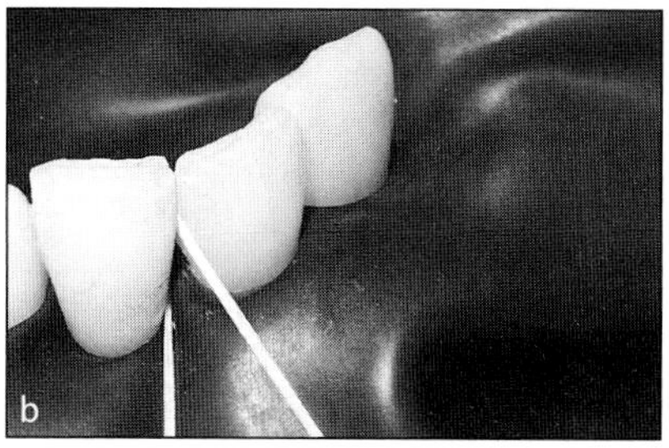

Fig 7-39a Floss is used to invert the dam in an interproximal area.

Fig 7-39b Floss is "rolled out" to the facial aspect to prevent reversal of the inversion it accomplished.

Inversion of the dam. The dam should be inverted around the necks of the teeth, at least in the area of the tooth or teeth to be restored. The edge of the dam that is against the tooth acts as a valve. If the edge is directed occlusally (Fig 7-38a), when a positive pressure is created by the tongue and cheeks under the dam, the valve opens, and saliva and other liquids under the dam are pushed between the tooth and dam to flood the operating field; then when a negative pressure is created under the dam, the valve closes and the saliva is trapped in the field. When the dam is inverted, a positive pressure under the dam simply serves to push the valve more tightly against the tooth (Fig 7-38b) so that no flooding of the field occurs.

Almost any instrument may be used to tuck the edge of the dam gingivally (see Figs 7-25a to 7-25c). A steady, high-volume stream of air should be directed at the tip of the instrument used to invert the dam, and the instrument should be moved along the margin of the dam so that the inversion is progressive.

Floss may be used to invert the dam in interproximal areas (Fig 7-39a). When it is used to carry the edge of the dam gingivally, the floss should not then be pulled occlusally for removal because it will frequently pull the edge of the dam with it, eliminating the inversion. Instead, the floss can be doubled over on itself on the lingual aspect and passed again through the contact. Then one end is pulled in a facial direction so that the floss rolls from the sulcus, leaving the dam inverted (Fig 7-39b). In this floss-facilitated inversion, a steady stream of air is as helpful as it is when inversion is accomplished with an instrument. The dam inverts more easily when the surfaces of the tooth and adjacent dam are dry.

Protection of the Dam

Torn dams provide poor isolation, so expenditure of a little effort to prevent tearing is worthwhile. An example of protection would be the use of a wedge interproximally when rotary instruments are used in the proximity of the dam. Another example is the use of a second clamp to retract the dam below a margin that is near, or below, the level of the gingival crest (see Fig 7-46).

Removal of the Dam

The interproximal septa are stretched and clipped with scissors (Figs 7-40a and 7-40b). The scissors are held so that the tips are not in contact with any tissue (Fig 7-40b). When all septa are cut, the clamp is removed with the forceps and the dam is snapped from the teeth.

After the dam is free from the mouth, the teeth should be examined to ensure that no rubber remains around them or in the contacts. The frame should be removed from the dam, and the dam should be laid flat on a surface and examined to ensure that no pieces are missing (Figs 7-41a and 7-41b). If a

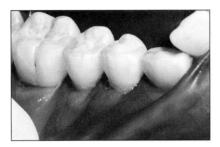

Fig 7-40a To remove the dam, the interproximal septa are stretched for cutting.

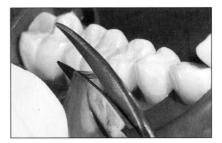

Fig 7-40b One blade of the scissors is used to pull the dam well away from any tissue before the septum is cut.

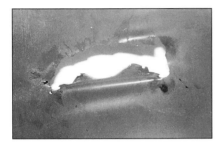

Fig 7-41a While the dam is on the frame, it is difficult to determine if any portion is missing.

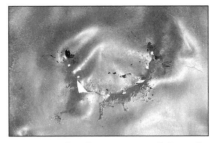

Fig 7-41b The dam is removed from the frame and laid on a flat surface. Note that a portion of dam is missing.

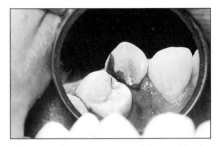

Fig 7-41c The missing piece is located in the mouth and removed.

piece is missing and unaccounted for, the mouth should be reexamined in the area of the missing piece of dam; any remnant should be removed (Fig 7-41c). A small piece of dam left subgingivally can cause inflammation, gingival abscess, or even significant loss of periodontal support.

Special Considerations

Bite Block

Patients often have difficulty keeping their mouths open or are uncomfortable with wide opening. A rubber bite block can relieve their discomfort, allow them to relax musculature, and permit them to keep the mouth open without effort. Bite blocks are available in a variety of sizes (Figs 7-42a and 7-42b). A piece of floss or tape may be attached to the bite block to allow retrieval if necessary (Fig 7-42c). Figures 7-43a and 7-43b show placement of the bite block after the dam is in place.

Isolation for a Fixed Partial Denture

Whenever possible, it is best to achieve isolation without incorporating a fixed partial denture into the isolated operating field. When a fixed partial denture must be included, there are several techniques that can be used; they are all somewhat time-consuming but often valuable. Two methods are described.

Cyanoacrylate method (Fig 7-44). Holes for the teeth are punched in the dam. The holes for the abutment teeth are connected with a cut that is in an arc to give a "tongue" of dam material between the holes. The tongue of material is folded back, and a piece of dam material is attached with cyanoacrylate glue over the opening left when the tongue was folded back. This piece is glued into place so that there is a slit connecting the abutment holes and a tongue of material that is free to swing down over the attached piece of dam material.

The dam is inserted over all teeth for which holes have been punched, and the tongue of material is pulled under the pontic(s) and glued into place on the added piece of dam. Tension on the tongue while the glue is setting (10 to 15 seconds) will ensure that the dam is tight around the abutments after tension is released.

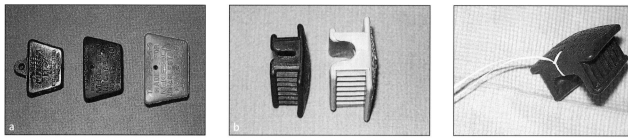

Figs 7-42a and 7-42b Rubber bite blocks are available in various sizes.

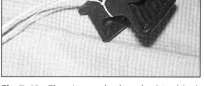

Fig 7-42c Floss is attached to the bite block for emergency retrieval if necessary.

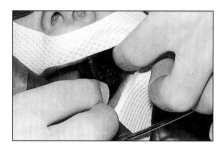

Fig 7-43a A bite block is inserted on the patient's left side after a rubber dam is applied to isolate the right quadrant.

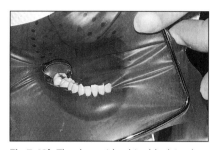

Fig 7-43b The dam with a bite block in place aids access to the field and increases patient comfort.

Ligation of septa around the retainer-pontic connectors (Fig 7-45). This procedure is for three-unit fixed partial dentures or splinted teeth. Holes are punched for each abutment, and, for three-unit fixed partial dentures, another hole is punched for the pontic. A piece of floss or suture material is used to tie through the holes so that the septum between adjacent holes is stretched around the retainer-pontic connector. If floss is used, a "floss-feeder," made for carrying floss under bridge pontics for oral hygiene measures, may be used to guide the floss under the pontic and pull it through. If suture material is used, the suture needle may be blunted and used for that purpose.

Use of Multiple Clamps

In addition to the clamp on the distal tooth, which retains the posterior portion of the dam, a second (or third) clamp is often needed. When the No. 212SA or other butterfly clamp (retractor) is used to retract tissue and dam for a Class 5 or other restoration, it is almost invariably used in addition to the posterior clamp. If a cavity that is at least partly subgingival is to be prepared, a clamp on that tooth will prevent the dam from riding up over the margin (Fig 7-46).

Placement of Clamp Over Dam

When it is desirable to clamp a tooth that was not considered when the dam was punched, the clamp may be applied over the dam (see Fig 7-15). The clamp jaws should be dull, so as not to cut through the dam, and the dam should be stretched loosely over the tooth being clamped, as stretching it tightly will cause the clamp jaw to perforate the rubber, initiating a rip in the dam.

Gingival Relaxation Incisions

When using a No. 212SA retractor for isolation for a Class 5 restoration, the jaw of the retractor should be positioned at least 0.5 mm (preferably 1.0 mm) gingival to the gingival margin of the planned restoration. This can usually be accomplished without laceration of tissue, because the free gingiva is elastic enough to be retracted. If, however, the free gingival margin is fibrous and difficult to displace gingivally, forced retraction could lacerate the tissue. In such a case, it is preferable to make one or two small incisions[12,13] to allow the tissue to be displaced without tearing.

For this technique (sometimes referred to as a miniflap procedure) to be successful, the periodontium must be healthy.

Fig 7-44 *Rubber dam isolation around a fixed partial denture (cyanoacrylate method).*

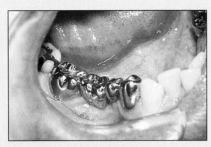

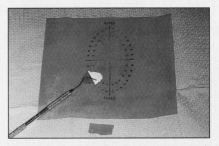

Fig 7-44a A four-unit fixed partial denture extends from the mandibular first premolar to the second molar.

Fig 7-44b The holes for the abutment teeth are connected with an arched cut. Note small piece of dam material at bottom that will be used as shown in Figs 7-44c and 7-44d.

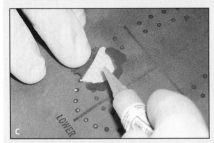

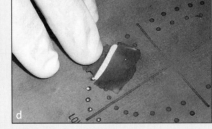

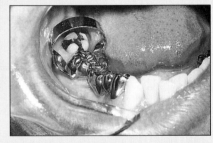

Figs 7-44c and 7-44d A small piece of dam is glued in place.

Fig 7-44e A No. W8A clamp is positioned on the second molar.

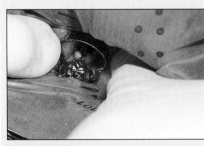

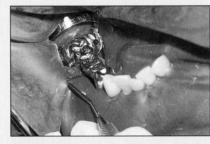

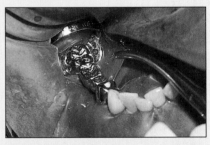

Fig 7-44f The dam is carried to place.

Fig 7-44g The tongue of dam material is tucked under the pontics with a periodontal probe.

Fig 7-44h The tongue of material is grasped and pulled lingually with a hemostat.

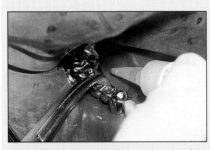

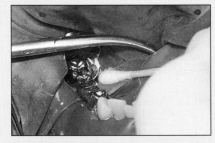

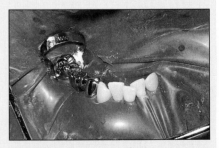

Fig 7-44i Glue is applied for attachment of the rubber dam tongue.

Fig 7-44j The tongue is held in place with a hemostat and a cotton-tipped applicator while the glue sets.

Fig 7-44k Isolation is complete.

Fig 7-45 Isolation around a three-unit fixed partial denture or splinted teeth (ligation method).

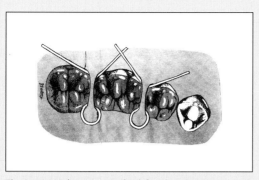

Fig 7-45a Holes are punched for the abutment teeth and pontic, and the dam is positioned. The septa on the mesial aspect of the mesial abutment and the distal aspect of the distal abutment are flossed to place, and then the holes are stretched over the abutments and the pontic.

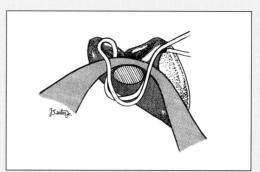

Fig 7-45b A ligature is threaded through an abutment hole on the facial aspect, under the retainer-pontic connector, through the same hole again on the lingual aspect, around the septum, through the pontic hole on the lingual aspect, back under the connector to the facial aspect, and back through the pontic hole.

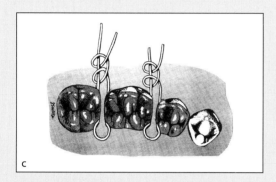

c

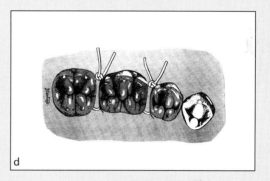

d

Figs 7-45c to 7-45e The ends of the ligatures are tied together to pull the rubber septum tightly around the connector.

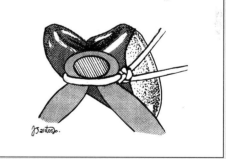

e

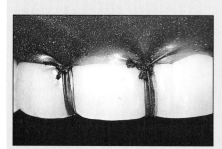

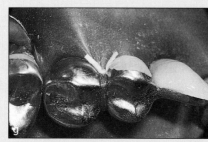
g

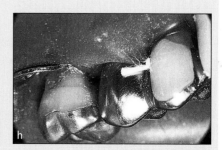
h

Figs 7-45f Sutures have been used for field isolation involving an anterior three-unit fixed partial denture.

Figs 7-45g and 7-45h Floss has been used for isolation involving a cantilevered canine pontic attached to splinted premolars.

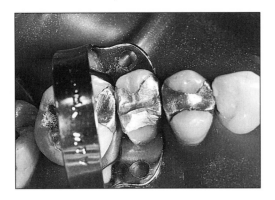

Fig 7-46 A second clamp is in place to retract the dam and give access to the gingival extent of a cusp fracture. A No. W1A clamp was used instead of a No. W2A clamp because of the need for a jaw to be apical to the fracture margin.

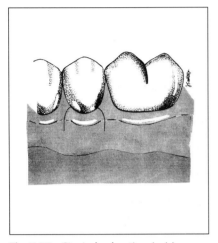

Fig 7-47a Gingival relaxation incisions are made within the keratinized gingival tissue. Either one or both can be made, depending on the amount of release needed for relaxation of the tissue.

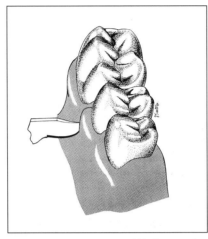

Fig 7-47b The No. 15 scalpel blade is used to make the incision.

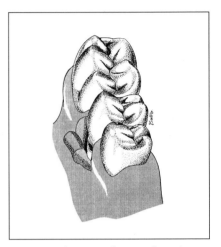

Fig 7-47c The tissue flap is reflected away from the root prior to application of the dam and No. 212SA retractor. The incisions are directed slightly into the papilla and then vertically.

The incisions should be confined to the keratinized tissue and kept as short as possible (just long enough to allow adequate exposure for isolation). Incisions can often be limited to the free gingiva, and, although reattachment to previously unexposed cementum can be expected, unnecessary severing of attachment should be avoided. Full-thickness vertical incisions should be initiated at the mesial and/or distal aspects of the facial surface and should be directed perpendicular to the root and surface of bone, first slightly toward the interproximal papilla, then apically (Figs 7-47a to 7-47c).

The blade of a plastic instrument or a beavertail burnisher may be used to push the tissue and rubber dam back while the facial jaw of the No. 212SA clamp is being situated on the root of the tooth. Again, the jaw should be dull, not sharp, so that it will not damage the root surface. A finger should be used to hold the clamp in place while it is stabilized with compound (see Figs 7-24a to 7-24c). After the restorative procedure is completed, the No. 212SA clamp is removed (see Figs 7-24d to 7-24i), then the dam is removed. Any blood in the area is washed away. The reflected gingival tissue is returned to its original location and held there with a dampened gauze sponge and finger pressure for about 2 minutes to allow initiation of a fibrin clot. As long as the incisions were confined to keratinized tissue, no sutures or periodontal dressing are needed, and healing should proceed uneventfully.

Evacuation of Fluid from Dam

If the dentist must work without an assistant, a very effective method for evacuation of fluid from the rubber dam involves the use of a suction tube anchored within the operating field. One evacuation method that uses a readily available item and is quick and easy involves the modification of a saliva ejector, as described by Lambert.[14] The molded plastic tip is cut off with a pair of crown scissors; then an additional 0.4 inch of

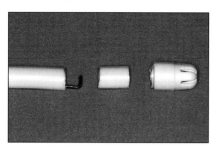
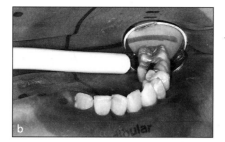
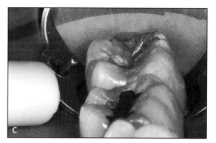

Fig 7-48a For unassisted fluid evacuation from the dam,[14] a saliva ejector is modified. First, the tip is cut off; then another 0.4 inch, except for the wire, is cut off, and the protruding wire is bent at a right angle (in direction of tube) to form an "L"-shaped hook.

Fig 7-48b and 7-48c For fluid evacuation, the wire hook is carried under the jaw of the clamp and allowed to go into the forceps hole of the rubber dam clamp.

Fig 7-49 Sealing of the root concavity. The dam is retracted by the clamp to allow isolation for a large Class 5 restoration; the retraction is apical to the beginning of the root concavity of the furcation. The gap between the dam and the concave root surface is sealed with Cavit, a provisional restorative material that hardens when it comes into contact with moisture.

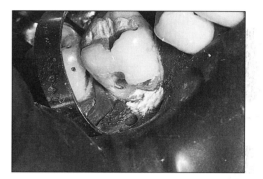

the plastic tube is cut off without cutting the wire within the plastic. The 0.4-inch length of plastic tubing is then pulled off the wire, leaving the wire extending from the end of the tube (Fig 7-48a); using forceps such as hemostats, the wire is bent in its center at a 90-degree angle in the direction of the tube to form an "L" shape. The wire is then carried under the jaw of the clamp and placed into the hole in the jaw of the clamp, usually on the lingual side of the clamped tooth. The taut rubber under the clamp jaw will hold the wire in place in the hole and push the tube against the dam (Figs 7-48b to 7-48c). This method will supply continuous fluid evacuation during the operative procedure.

Sealing a Root Concavity

The rubber dam seals well on convex tooth surfaces. If the dam is retracted so that its edge goes across a root concavity, however, saliva will leak into the operating field. A solution is to seal the gap between the edge of the dam and the concave root surface. This may be accomplished with a provisional restorative material, such as Cavit (ESPE Premier), which hardens with moisture (Fig 7-49).

Repair of a Torn Rubber Dam

A small tear in a dam may often be patched. A piece of dam material is cut to cover the tear and extend 1.0 cm or so beyond the tear on all sides. The piece is attached over the tear with cyanoacrylate glue.

Placement of a Second Dam Over the First

If a dam is torn beyond repair during a procedure, the dentist might choose to remove the dam and replace it. Alternatively, another dam may be placed over the top of the first. Brownbill[15] recommended that this technique be used when there is leakage around teeth through incorrectly sized holes and when strong chemicals are to be used.

Latex Allergies

There is an increasing awareness of latex sensitivity.[16–19] One survey[19] reported 3.7% of patients to have a latex allergy; the investigators recommended careful questioning of patients regarding a history of sensitivity to latex-based products, so that the use of latex products, such as gloves and the rubber dam, may be avoided with these patients.

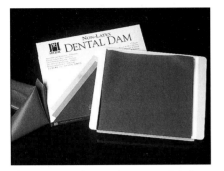

Fig 7-50 Nonlatex dam material from Hygenic. Nonlatex dams should be used for patients with a latex allergy.

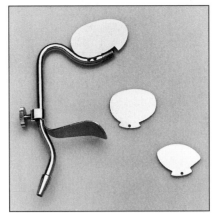

Fig 7-51a The Svedopter tongue-retracting evacuation device is supplied with three sizes of vertical blades.

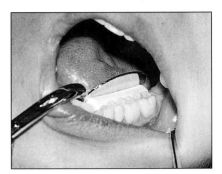

Fig 7-51b The Svedopter is used to hold the tongue away from the operating field.

For latex-sensitive patients, use of a latex dam should be avoided, as should other latex products. Nonlatex dam material is available and should be on hand for latex-allergic patients. Current nonlatex dams (Fig 7-50) have elastic properties very similar to latex. Some dentists have elected to use nonlatex dams exclusively for all their patients.

Summary of Recommendations

Following are some of the procedures that facilitate rubber dam use:

1. Use a heavy-gauge, prestamped dam.
2. Floss through contacts prior to dam placement, planing any contact that shreds or tears the floss.
3. Use a good water-soluble lubricant, such as Velvachol.
4. Use a clamp designed for four-point contact on the tooth, and avoid overexpansion of the clamp so that the clamp will maintain its strength and will be stable as a retainer.
5. Isolate enough teeth to hold the dam on the lingual aspect of the teeth away from the operating field and to provide exposed teeth for finger rests.
6. With waxed floss, floss the dam through interproximal contacts in a single layer and avoid doubling or bunching the dam in the contact.
7. Master the use of modeling compound to stabilize rubber dam retainers when necessary.

Other Methods of Isolation

Svedopter

The Svedopter (Miltex) is probably the most commonly used tongue retraction device (Figs 7-51a and 7-51b). It is designed so that the vacuum evacuator tube passes anterior to the chin and mandibular anterior teeth, over the incisal edges of the mandibular anterior teeth, and down to the floor of the mouth, to either the left or the right of the tongue. A mirror-like vertical blade is attached to the evacuator tube so that it holds the tongue away from the field of operation. Several sizes of vertical blades are supplied by the manufacturer. An adjustable horizontal chin blade is attached to the evacuation tube so that it will clamp under the chin to hold the apparatus in place.

Absorbent cotton rolls are placed adjacent to the Svedopter in the floor of the mouth and in the maxillary buccal vestibule adjacent to the opening of the parotid gland (Stensen's) duct. The Svedopter is especially useful for preparation and cementation of fixed prostheses. It is less effective than the rubber dam for procedures in which total isolation from the fluids and vapors of the oral cavity is desired.

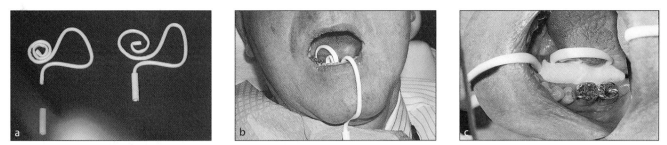

Figs 7-52a to 7-52c The Hygoformic saliva ejector should be routinely rebent to pass under the chin, over the incisal edges of the mandibular incisors, and then down to the floor of the mouth. The apparatus should usually be uncoiled slightly to extend further posteriorly. *(a, left)* Hygoformic saliva ejector as received; *(a, right)* Hygoformic saliva ejector that has been reshaped. *(b, c)* Isolation achieved with the Hygoformic saliva ejector.

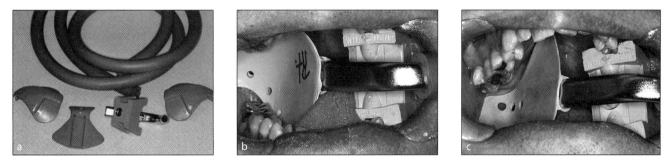

Figs 7-53a to 7-53c The Vac-Ejector provides a bite block, tongue retraction, and suction: *(a)* parts of the Vac-Ejector; *(b)* assembled and in use for isolation in the mandibular right posterior area; if the distal wrap-around needs to be closer to the most distal tooth, the tongue-retracting assembly may be slid more anteriorly on the metal attachment; *(c)* assembled and in use for isolating maxillary right posterior area.

Hygoformic Saliva Ejector

The Hygoformic (Pulpdent) saliva ejector is used in the same way as the Svedopter, but it does not have a reflective blade (Figs 7-52a to 7-52c). It is, however, usually more comfortable and less traumatic to lingual tissues than is the Svedopter. For use, the saliva ejector must be re-formed (rebent) so that the evacuator tube passes under the chin, up over the incisal edges of the mandibular incisors, and then down to the floor of the mouth. The tongue-retracting coil should be loosened, or partially uncoiled, so that it extends posteriorly enough to hold the tongue away from the operating field. The Hygoformic saliva ejector is also used with absorbent cotton for maximum effectiveness.

Vac-Ejector

The Vac-Ejector Moisture Control System (Coltène/Whaledent) is made to facilitate isolation when restoring posterior teeth (Fig 7-53a). The Vac-Ejector incorporates a bite block, tongue retractor for mandibular areas, and high-speed suction attachment. It comes with three flexible deflectors, one for each side when operating in mandibular areas (Fig 7-53b) and one universal deflector for operating on either side in the maxillary arch (Fig 7-53c). The bite block is adjustable, by rotation, for large or small arches; in all photos, it is adjusted for large arches. Although this product appears complex to assemble correctly, operators soon become skilled at rapid assembly.

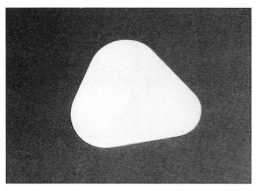

Fig 7-54a A parotid shield is triangular and made of absorbent paper.

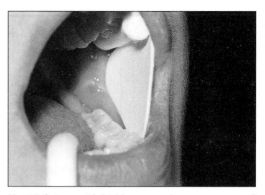

Fig 7-54b A parotid shield may supplement a cotton roll in the buccal vestibule or may be used alone.

Absorbent Paper and Cotton Products

Absorbent materials are important in dentistry. Vacuum apparatuses remove fluids from the operating field by suctioning them; cotton and paper products help control fluids by absorbing them. Several types of absorbent cotton rolls are available in various diameters and lengths. These are placed into areas of the mouth, where salivary gland ducts exit, to absorb saliva and prevent salivary contamination of the operating field.

Isolation using absorbent materials with suctioning devices is less effective than using the rubber dam with suction, but in many procedures, the more complete isolation provided by the dam is unnecessary. In these situations, absorbent products are useful.

Small gauze sponges may be folded or rolled to substitute for cotton rolls. In addition, absorbent paper triangles, or parotid shields, such as Dri-Aid (Lorvic), are useful on the facial aspect of posterior teeth to absorb saliva secreted by the parotid gland (Figs 7-54a and 7-54b).

References

1. Christen AG. Sanford C. Barnum, discoverer of the rubber dam. Bull Hist Dent 1977;25:3–9.
2. Gergely EJ. Rubber dam acceptance. Br Dent J 1989;167:249–252.
3. Reuter JE. The isolation of teeth and the protection of the patient during endodontic treatment. Int Endod J 1983;16:173–181.
4. Stewardson DA, McHugh ES. Patients' attitudes to rubber dam. Int Endod J 2002;35:812–819.
5. Christensen GJ. Using rubber dams to boost quality, quantity of restorative services. J Am Dent Assoc 1994;125:81–82.
6. Small BW. Rubber dam—The easy way. Gen Dent 1999;47:30–33.
7. Trevino D, Duke E, Robbins J, Summitt J. Clinical evaluation of Scotchbond Multipurpose adhesive system in cervical abrasions [abstract 3037]. J Dent Res 1996;75:397.
8. Barghi N, Knight GT, Berry TG. Comparing two methods of moisture control in bonding to enamel: A clinical study. Oper Dent 1991; 16:130–135.
9. Knight GT, Barghi N, Berry T. Microleakage of enamel bonding as affected by moisture control methods [abstract]. J Dent Res 1991; 70:561.
10. Knight GT, Barghi N. Effect of saliva contamination on dentin bonding agents in vivo [abstract 434]. J Dent Res 1992;71:160.
11. Reid JS, Callis PD, Patterson CJW. Rubber Dam in Clinical Practice. Chicago: Quintessence, 1990.
12. Drucker H, Wolcott RB. Gingival tissue management with Class V restorations. J Am Acad Gold Foil Oper 1970;13(1):34–38.
13. Xhonga FA. Gingival retraction techniques and their healing effect on the gingiva. J Prosthet Dent 1971;26:640–648.
14. Lambert RL. Moisture evacuation with the rubber dam in place. J Prosthet Dent 1985;53:749–750.
15. Brownbill JW. Double rubber dam. Quintessence Int 1987;18: 699–700.
16. Fay MF, Beck WC, Checchi L, Winkler D. Gloves: New selection criteria. Quintessence Int 1995;26:27–29.
17. Kosti E, Lambrianidis T. Endodontic treatment in cases of allergic reaction to rubber dam. J Endod 2002;28:787–789.
18. March PJ. An allergic reaction to latex rubber gloves. J Am Dent Assoc 1988;117:590–591.
19. Rankin KV, Jones DL, Rees TD. Latex reactions in an adult dental population. Am J Dent 1993;6:274–276.

Bonding to Enamel and Dentin

Bart Van Meerbeek   *Yasuhiro Yoshida*
Kirsten Van Landuyt   *Jorge Perdigão*
Jan De Munck   *Paul Lambrechts*
Satoshi Inoue   *Marleen Peumans*

After observing the industrial use of phosphoric acid to improve the adhesion of paints and resin coatings to metal surfaces, Buonocore[1] in 1955 applied acid to teeth to "render the tooth surface more receptive to adhesion." Buonocore's pioneering work led to major changes in the practice of dentistry. Today, we are in the age of adhesive dentistry. Traditional mechanical methods of retaining restorative materials have been replaced to a large extent by tooth-conserving adhesive methods. The concepts of large preparations and extension for prevention proposed by Black[2] in 1917 have gradually been replaced by concepts of smaller preparations and more conservative techniques.

Advantages of Adhesive Techniques

Bonded restorations have a number of advantages over traditional, nonadhesive methods. Traditionally, retention and stabilization of restorations often required the removal of sound tooth structure. This is not necessary, in many cases, when adhesive techniques are used. Adhesion also reduces microleakage at the restoration-tooth interface. Prevention of microleakage, or the ingress of oral fluids and bacteria along the cavity wall, reduces clinical problems such as postoperative sensitivity, marginal staining, and recurrent caries, all of which may jeopardize the clinical longevity of restorative efforts.[3,4]

Adhesive restorations better transmit and distribute functional stresses across the bonding interface to the tooth and have the potential to reinforce weakened tooth structure.[5-7] In contrast, a traditional metal intracoronal restoration may act as a wedge between the buccal and lingual cusps and increase the risk of cuspal fracture. Adhesive techniques allow deteriorating restorations to be repaired and debonded restorations to be replaced with little or no additional loss of tooth structure.

Adhesive techniques have expanded the range of possibilities for esthetic restorative dentistry.[8,9] Today's patient pays more attention to esthetics than ever before, and teeth are a key consideration in personal appearance. Tooth-colored restorative materials are used to esthetically restore and/or recontour teeth with little or no tooth preparation. Advances in dental adhesive technology have enabled the dentist to improve facial esthetics in a relatively simple and economical way.

Expanding Indications for Adhesive Dentistry

Adhesive techniques with resin composites were initially used for the replacement of carious and fractured tooth structure or for the filling of erosion or abrasion defects in cervical areas. Modern adhesive techniques also enable restorative material to be added to the tooth for the correction of unesthetic shapes, positions, dimensions, or shades. Resin composite can be used to close diastemata, add length, or mask discoloration.[10-12] Because of the alleged mercury toxicity associated with silver amalgam,[13,14] substantial research is focused on the development of alternatives to amalgam.[15] Posterior resin composites

Table 8-1	Bond energy and bond distance (equilibrium length)[19]	
Bond type	**Bond energy (kJmol⁻¹)**	**Equilibrium length (Å)**
Primary		
Ionic	600–1,200	2–4
Covalent	60–800	0.7–3
Secondary		
Hydrogen	≈50	3
Dipole interactions*	≈20	4
London dispersion*	≈40	<10

*Dipole interactions and dispersion forces are often collectively referred to as *van der Waals forces*.

can be directly or indirectly bonded into Class 1 and Class 2 preparations.

Adhesive techniques are also used to bond anterior and posterior ceramic restorations, such as veneers, inlays, and onlays, with adhesive luting composites. Adhesives can be used to bond silver amalgam restorations; to retain metal frameworks; to adhesively cement crowns and fixed partial dentures; to bond orthodontic brackets; for periodontal or orthodontic splints; to treat dentinal hypersensitivity; and to repair fractured porcelain, amalgam, and resin composite restorations. Pit and fissure sealants utilize adhesion as part of a preventive treatment program. Adhesive materials are often used with core buildup foundations for crowns.

Today, dentists in general practice are still exploring the possibilities of adhesive dentistry. Due to the relatively low costs and improved adhesive techniques, they are pushing the limits of resin composite restorations. Although still very controversial, complete-crown restorations (both direct and indirect) and resin composite fixed partial dentures are allowing adhesive techniques to progressively venture into the domain of prosthetic dentistry.[16] More research, however, is needed to evaluate longevity.

Principles of Adhesion

The word *adhesion* is derived from the Latin word *adhaerere*, which is a compound of *ad*, or *to*, and *haerere*, or *to stick*.[17] Cicero used the expression *haerere in equo*, *to stick to a horse*, to refer to keeping a firm seat.

In adhesive terminology, *adhesion* or *bonding* is the attachment of one substance to another. The surface or substrate that is adhered to is termed the *adherend*. The *adhesive* or *adherent*, or in dental terminology the *bonding agent* or *adhesive system*, may then be defined as the material that,

when applied to surfaces of substances, can join them together, resist separation, and transmit loads across the bond.[17,18] The *adhesive strength* or *bond strength* is the measure of the load-bearing capability of the adhesive. The time period during which the bond remains effective is referred to as its *durability*.[19]

Adhesion refers to the forces or energies between atoms or molecules at an interface that hold two phases together.[17] In debonding tests, adhesion is often subjected to tensile or shear forces, and the mode of failure is quantified. If the bond fails at the interface between the two substrates, the mode of failure is referred to as *adhesive*; if failure occurs in one of the substrates, but not at the interface, it is *cohesive*. The mode of failure is often mixed.

Four theories have been advanced to account for the observed phenomena of adhesion[19]:

1. *Mechanical* theories state that the solidified adhesive interlocks micromechanically with the roughness and irregularities of the surface of the adherend.
2. *Adsorption* theories encompass all kinds of chemical bonds between the adhesive and the adherend, including primary (ionic and covalent) and secondary (hydrogen, dipole interaction, and London dispersion) valence forces (Table 8-1). London dispersion forces are almost universally present because they arise from and depend solely on the presence of nuclei and electrons. The other bond types require appropriate chemical groups to interact.
3. *Diffusion* theories propose that adhesion is the result of bonding between mobile molecules. Polymers from each side of an interface can cross over and react with molecules on the other side. Eventually, the interface will disappear and the two parts will become one.
4. *Electrostatic* theories state that an electrical double layer forms at the interface between a metal and a polymer, making a certain, yet obscure, contribution to the bond strength.

An important requirement for the occurrence of any of these interfacial phenomena is that the two materials being joined must be in sufficiently close and intimate relation. Besides an intimate contact, sufficient wetting of the adhesive will occur only if its surface tension is less than the surface energy of the adherend.[20–22] Wetting of a surface by a liquid is characterized by the contact angle of a droplet placed on the surface.[23] If the liquid spreads completely on the solid surface, this indicates complete wetting, or a contact angle of 0 degrees (Fig 8-1).

According to this theory of wetting and surface energies, adhesion to enamel is much easier to achieve than is adhesion

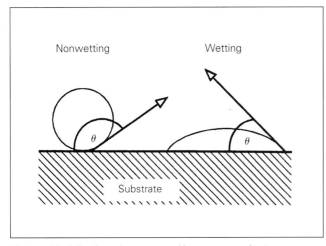

Fig 8-1 Principle of wetting measured by contact angle, θ.

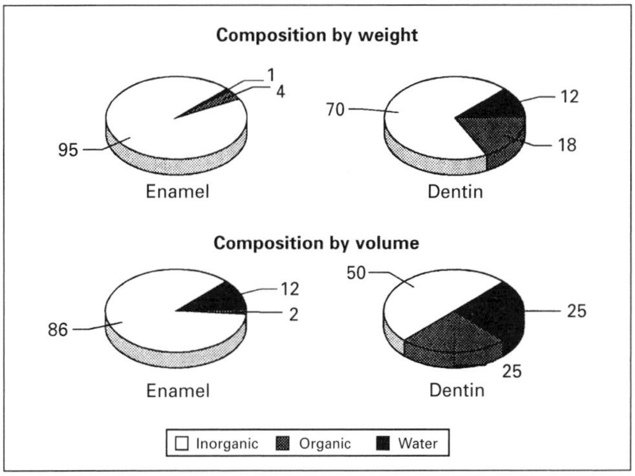

Fig 8-2 Composition of enamel and dentin by weight and volume.

to dentin. Enamel contains primarily hydroxyapatite, which has a high surface energy, whereas dentin is composed of two distinct substrates, hydroxyapatite and collagen, and has a low surface energy. In the oral environment, the tooth surface is contaminated by an organic saliva pellicle with a low critical surface tension (28 dynes/cm),[24] which impairs adequate wetting by the adhesive.[25] Likewise, instrumentation of the tooth substrate during cavity preparation produces a smear layer with a low surface energy. Therefore, the natural tooth surface should be thoroughly cleaned and pretreated before bonding procedures to increase its surface energy and, hence, to render it more receptive to bonding.

Several, if not all, of the mechanisms of adhesion described contribute to some extent to dental bond strength. Glass-ionomer cement is the only restorative material that has been reported to possess an intrinsic self-adhesive capacity to bond to tooth tissue without any pretreatment.[26,27] Other restorative materials with adhesive potential, such as resin composites, require the application of an intermediate resin to unite the tooth substrate with the restorative material. In the case of adhesion to enamel, a resin bonding agent is bonded primarily by micromechanical interlocking with the surface irregularities of the etched substrate. A micromechanical type of bonding is also largely involved in bonding to dentin.[28–32] Although there is some controversy about the contribution of primary chemical bonds to the resin-tooth attachment, secondary, weak London–van der Waals forces may play a contributing role because of the intimate contact between the resin and tooth substrate.[33–37] Recently, the potential of functional monomers in adhesives to chemically interact with residual hydroxyapatite within submicron hybrid layers has regained attention as part of a so-called mild self-etch approach (discussed later in the chapter).[38]

Factors Affecting Adhesion to Tooth Tissue

The strength and durability of adhesive bonds depend on several factors. These include the physicochemical properties of the adherend and the adhesive; the structural properties of the adherend, which is heterogeneous; the formation of surface contaminants during cavity preparation; the development of external stresses that counteract the process of bonding and their compensation mechanisms; and the mechanism of transmission and distribution of applied loads through the bonded joint. Furthermore, the oral environment, which is subject to moisture, physical stresses, changes in temperature and pH, dietary components, and chewing habits, considerably influences adhesive interactions between materials and tooth tissues.[39]

Compositional and Structural Aspects of Enamel and Dentin

Because the composition and structure of enamel and dentin are substantially different, adhesion strategies for the two tooth tissues are also different. The inorganic content of mature enamel is 95% to 98% by weight (wt%) and 86% by volume (vol%); the primary component is hydroxyapatite. The remainder consists of water (4 wt% and 12 vol%) and organic material (1 to 2 wt% and 2 vol%)[40] (Fig 8-2). The major inorganic fraction exists in the form of submicron crystallites, preferentially oriented in three dimensions, in which the spread and contiguous relationship of the crystallites contribute to the microscopic unit, called the *rod* or *prism*.[39,41] The natural surface of enamel is smooth, and the ends of the

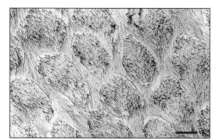

Fig 8-3 Field-emission scanning electron photomicrograph of an acid-etched (Non-Rinse Conditioner, Dentsply) enamel surface disclosing the typical keyhole-shaped enamel prisms or rods. Bar = 2.5 μm.

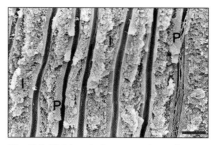

Fig 8-4 Field-emission scanning electron photomicrograph of longitudinally fractured dentinal tubules. I = intertubular dentin; P = peritubular dentin; bar = 5 μm.

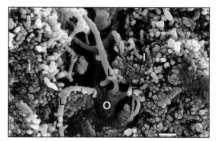

Fig 8-5 Scanning electron photomicrograph demonstrating an odontoblastic process (O) in a dentinal tubule with several lateral branches (L). I = intertubular dentin; bar = 1 μm.

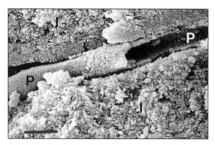

Fig 8-6 Field-emission scanning electron photomicrograph of a fractured dentinal substrate illustrating a tube of highly mineralized peritubular dentin. I = intertubular dentin; P = peritubular dentin; bar = 2 μm.

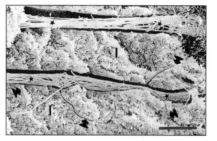

Fig 8-7 Field-emission scanning electron photomicrograph of a fractured dentinal substrate illustrating cross-banded collagen (stars) inside the lumen of two dentinal tubules. Note the microtubules branching off the main tubule (black arrows). I = intertubular dentin; bar = 5 μm.

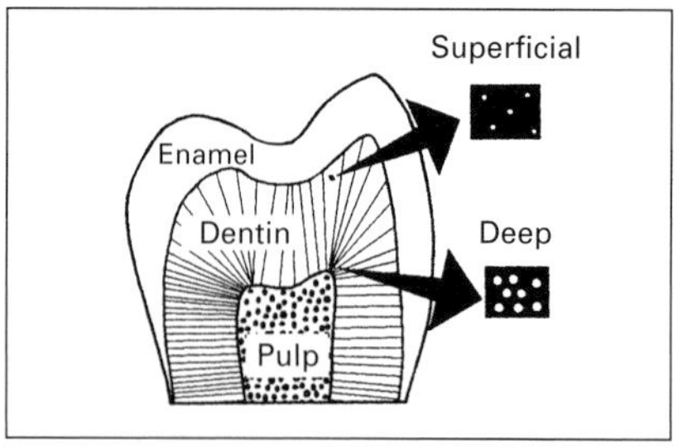

Fig 8-8 Dimension and concentration of dentinal tubules near the dentinoenamel junction (superficial dentin) and near the pulp (deep dentin). (Adapted from Heymann and Bayne.[49] Copyright © 1993 American Dental Association. Reprinted by permission of ADA Publishing, a Division of ADA Business Enterprises, Inc.)

rods are exposed in what has been described as a keyhole pattern (Fig 8-3).[42] Operatively prepared surfaces expose rods in tangential, oblique, and longitudinal planes. Enamel is almost homogeneous in structure and composition, irrespective of its depth and location, except for some aprismatic (prismless) enamel at the outer surface,[39] in which the crystallites run parallel to each other and perpendicular to the surface.

Unlike enamel, dentin contains a higher percentage of water (12 wt%) and organic material (18 wt%), mainly type I collagen,[43] and only about 70 wt% hydroxyapatite (see Fig 8-2).[44] Structurally more important to adhesion are the volumes occupied by the dentinal components. There is, combined, as much organic material (25 vol%) and water (25 vol%) as there is inorganic material (50 vol%).[44] In addition, these constituents are unevenly distributed in intertubular and peritubular dentin (Fig 8-4), so the dentinal tissue is heterogeneous.

Numerous dentinal tubules radiate from the pulp throughout the entire thickness of dentin, making dentin a highly permeable tissue.[45,46] These dentinal tubules contain the odontoblastic processes (Fig 8-5) and form a direct connection to the vital pulp. In contrast to enamel, dentin is a vital and dynamic tissue[47,48] that is able to develop specific defense mechanisms against external injuries. The diameter of the tubules decreases from 2.5 μm at the pulp side to 0.8 μm at the dentinoenamel junction (DEJ). Likewise, the number of tubules decreases from about 45,000/mm² near the pulp to about 20,000/mm² near the DEJ.[45] With an average of 30,000 tubules/mm² in the middle part of cut human dentin, a considerable volume of dentin consists of their lumina. Each tubule is surrounded by a collar of hypermineralized peritubular dentin (Fig 8-6). Intertubular dentin is less mineralized and contains more organic collagen fibrils. Besides an odontoblastic process in the deepest one third of the total tubule length, the tubules are filled with tissue fluid, or so-called dentinal fluid, an organic membrane structure called lamina limitans, and intratubular collagen fibrils of yet unknown origin and function (Fig 8-7).

Because of the fan-shaped radiation of dentinal tubules (Fig 8-8), 96% of a superficial dentin surface is composed of

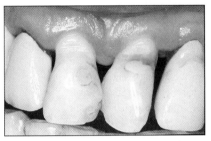

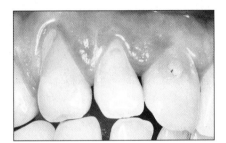

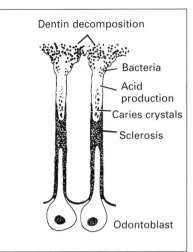

Fig 8-9 Cervical lesions exhibiting sclerotic dentin in combined abrasive (toothbrush) and stress-induced (tooth flexure) lesions.

Fig 8-10 Cervical lesions exhibiting sclerotic dentin in chemically induced erosive lesions.

Fig 8-11 Obstruction of the dentinal tubules by "Whitlockite" or caries crystals. (Adapted from Fusayama,[55] by permission of *Operative Dentistry*, and Ogawa et al.[56])

intertubular dentin; only 1% is occupied by fluid in the dentinal tubules, and 3% by peritubular dentin.[45,49,50] Near the pulp, peritubular dentin represents 66% and intertubular dentin only 12% of the area of a cut surface, while 22% of the surface area is occupied by water. Similar data demonstrate that 3% of the area of a cut surface consists of dentinal tubules in superficial dentin and 25% in deep dentin. A mean diameter of dentinal tubules ranging from 0.63 to 2.37 μm, depending on depth, has been determined by image analysis of transmission electron microscopic (TEM) and scanning electron microscopic (SEM) micrographs.[51] Hence, dentin is an intrinsically wet tissue. Dentinal fluid in the tubules is under a slight, but constant, outward pressure from the pulp. The intrapulpal fluid pressure is estimated to be 25 to 30 mmHg[52] or 34 to 40 cm water.[53]

Changes in Dentinal Structure

Dentin is a dynamic substrate subject to continuous physiologic and pathologic changes in composition and microstructure.[47,54] Dentin that has been violated by caries or has undergone abrasion (Fig 8-9) or erosion (Fig 8-10) may be quite different from unaffected sound dentin. Dentin undergoes *physiologic dentinal sclerosis* as part of the aging process and *reactive sclerosis* in response to slowly progressive or mild irritations, such as mechanical abrasion or chemical erosion.[54] *Tertiary*, or *reparative*, dentin is produced in the pulp chamber at the lesion site in response to insults such as caries, den-

tal procedures, or attrition.[54] Hypermineralization, obstruction of tubules by Whitlockite crystalline deposits (Fig 8-11), and apposition of reparative dentin adjacent to the pulp are well-documented responses to caries.[55,56] Less is known about the compositional and morphologic modifications of dentin that accompany the development of noncarious cervical lesions.[57–59]

Dentinal sclerosis, or the formation of transparent, glasslike dentin, which occurs in the cervical areas of teeth, has several common characteristics. Sclerosis is reported to result from the obstruction of dentinal tubules by apposition of peritubular dentin and precipitation of rhombohedral mineral crystals. The refractive index of the obstructed tubules is similar to that of intertubular dentin, resulting in a glasslike appearance.[58,60–62]

Sclerotic dentin usually contains few, if any, patent tubules and therefore has low permeability[62,63] and tends to be insensitive to external stimuli.[58,59,61,62] The odontoblastic processes associated with sclerotic dentin often exhibit partial atrophy and mineralization.[48,54,64] Heavily sclerotic dentin has areas of complete hypermineralization[60,65] without tubule exposure, even when etched with an acid (Fig 8-12). Some areas show abundant mineral sclerotic casts, which extend from the tubule orifices above the dentin surface and represent mineralized odontoblastic processes (Fig 8-13).

All of these morphologic and structural transformations of dentin, induced by physiologic and pathologic processes, result in a dentinal substrate that is less receptive to adhesive treatments than is normal dentin.[57,58,60,66–68]

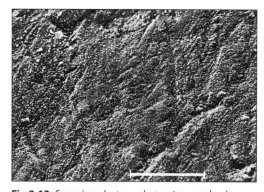

Fig 8-12 Scanning electron photomicrographs demonstrating heavily sclerotic dentin without exposed tubules, despite treatment with 10% citric acid. Bar = 20 μm. (From Van Meerbeek et al.[59] Reprinted with permission from Elsevier Science.)

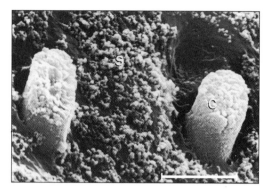

Fig 8-13 Two mineral sclerotic casts (C) extend from the tubules above the acid-etched dentin surface, which is covered by silica particles (S) remaining from the etchant gel. Bar = 2 μm.

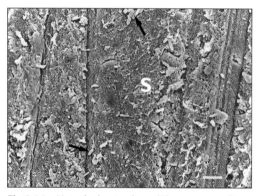

Fig 8-14a Note the bur tracks and the presence of bacteria *(arrows)*. S = smear debris; bar = 3 μm.

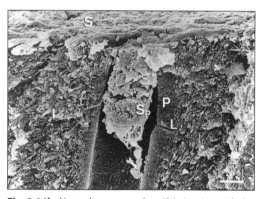

Fig 8-14b Note the smear plug (S_p). I = intertubular dentin; L = lateral tubule branch; P = peritubular dentin; S = smear debris; bar = 1 μm.

The Smear Layer

When the tooth surface is altered by rotary and manual instrumentation during cavity preparation, cutting debris is smeared over the enamel and dentin surfaces, forming what is termed the *smear layer*[69,70] (Figs 8-14a and 8-14b). The smear layer has been defined as "any debris, calcific in nature, produced by reduction or instrumentation of dentin, enamel or cementum,"[71] or as a "contaminant"[72] that precludes interaction with the underlying pure tooth tissue. This iatrogenically produced layer of debris has a great influence on any adhesive bond formed between the cut tooth and the restorative material.[70,73–75]

A variety of instrumentation techniques can be applied to remove carious tooth structure and to make the tooth surface receptive for bonding. Cavity preparation with a diamond or tungsten carbide bur is the most common method. However, bur preparation of cavities often leads to unnecessary removal of sound tooth structure. Moreover, placement of bevels on proximal cavosurface angles is difficult, and adjacent teeth are often damaged by the bur.[76] These drawbacks of rotary instrumentation, along with the current trend toward "minimally invasive" tooth preparation[77–79] have led to the investigation and introduction of new methods as well as the expanded use of previously neglected techniques, such as sono-abrasion, and new techniques, such as air abrasion and laser ablation (Figs 8-15 and 8-16).[75,80]

General Characteristics of the Smear Layer

Most of the time, the tooth surface is covered with a smear layer prior to bonding procedures. As stated previously, the smear layer is an adherent layer of debris and can be found

Fig 8-15 Field-emission scanning electron photomicrographs of dentin surfaces prepared with *(a)* a diamond bur, *(b)* sono-abrasion, *(c)* air abrasion, and *(d)* Er:YAG laser ablation. Cavity preparation alters the outermost layer of tooth structure.

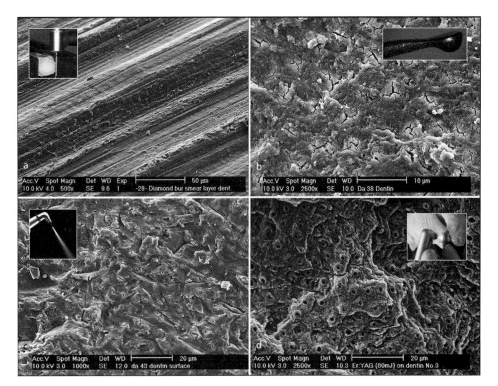

Fig 8-16 Adhesive dentistry requires adhesion-receptive tooth surfaces. On the whole, burs remain the standard preparation tools *(a* and *b)*. However, alternatives, such as sono-abrasion *(c)*, air abrasion *(d* [before abrasion] and *e* [after abrasion]), and laser preparation *(f* to *i)*, have recently gained attention. Every cavity preparation technique has its own advantages and disadvantages.

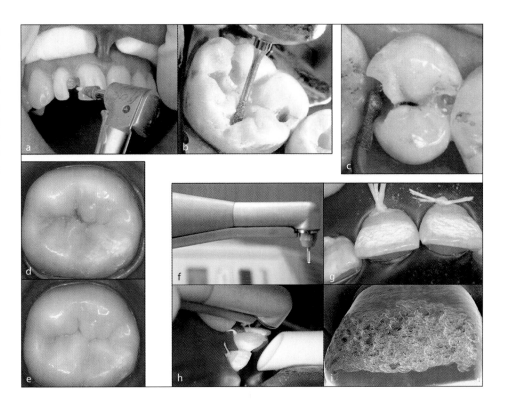

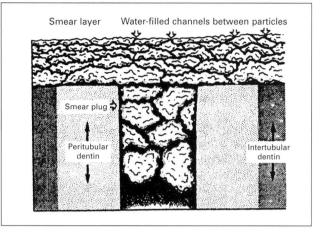

Fig 8-17 Porous smear layer with water-filled channels between the smear particles. (From Pashley et al.[88] Used by permission of *Operative Dentistry*.)

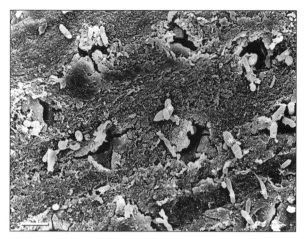

Fig 8-18 Field-emission scanning electron photomicrograph of a dentin surface ground with 600-grit SiC paper under running water. A smear layer covers the entire dentin surface. The dentinal tubules are partially or completely occluded by smear plugs. Note the presence of bacil-like bacteria *(asterisks)*. Bar = 2 μm. (Image from Perdigão.[92])

on tooth surfaces after they have been cut with rotary or hand instruments.[46] Endodontic preparation of a root canal, either by rotary or hand instruments,[81] or extensive root planing in periodontal therapy also produce a smear layer.[82] To obtain satisfactory bonding, the tooth surface should be treated to obtain a clean bonding substrate.

The burnishing action of the cutting instrument generates frictional heat and shear forces, so that the smear layer becomes attached to the underlying surface in a manner that prevents it from being rinsed off or scrubbed away.[46,83,84] In an in vivo study,[85] ethylenediaminetetraacetic acid (EDTA) was found to be the most effective conditioner for removing the smear layer and opening the orifices of the dentinal tubules. In order of increasing effectiveness in removing a smear layer, acidic conditioners include citric, polyacrylic, lactic, and phosphoric acids. Cavity cleansers, such as Tubulicid (Dental Therapeutics) and hydrogen peroxide, were found to have only a slight effect.

The morphologic features, composition, and thickness of the smear layer are determined to a large extent by the type of instrument used, the method of irrigation employed, and the site of tooth substrate at which it is formed.[46,69,86] The smear layer is revealed by SEM to be a 0.5- to 2-μm-thick layer of debris with a mainly granular substructure that entirely covers the dentin (see Fig 8-14b).[69,70,84] The surface of the smear layer generally appears very irregular. Sonication creates a structure partially composed of aggregates of globular subunits approximately 0.05 to 0.1 μm in diameter.[84] The orifices of the dentinal tubules are obstructed by debris tags, called *smear plugs*, that may extend into the tubule to a

depth of 1 to 10 μm (see Fig 8-14b).[84,87] These smear plugs are contiguous with the smear layer. Although smear debris occludes the dentinal tubules with the formation of smear plugs, the smear layer is porous and penetrated by submicron channels, through which small amounts of dentinal fluid are allowed to pass[88] (Figs 8-14b and 8-17). The smear layer is reported to reduce dentinal permeability by about 86%.[89]

The thickness and the morphology of the smear layer likely vary with the method of instrumentation used and with the location within dentin in relation to the pulp. Using light microscopy, Tani and Finger[90] have examined smear layers generated by diamond burs with different grain sizes and by silicon carbide (SiC) papers with varying grit numbers (for research purposes, a smear layer is often created by grinding the tooth surface with SiC paper). They concluded that the smear layer's thickness increases with increasing roughness of the diamond bur or SiC paper.[90]

Due to its small and varying dimensions and its irregular and weak structure, studying the smear layer is rather complicated. Its composition is variable and reflects the composition of the underlying dentin.[50,84] This was confirmed by Ruse and Smith,[91] who used x-ray photoelectron microscopy to examine instrumented dentin. While cutting dentin, the heat and the shear forces produced by the rotary movement of the bur cause dentin debris to compact and aggregate. The smear layer is believed to consist primarily of shattered and crushed hydroxyapatite and fragmented and denatured collagen. In clinical conditions, a smear layer may also be contaminated by bacteria and saliva (Figs 8-14a and 8-18).[46,93,94]

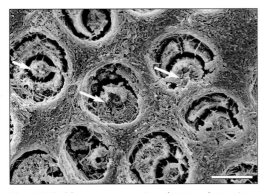

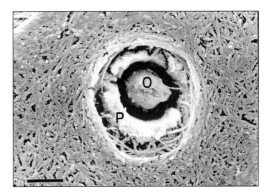

Fig 8-19 Field-emission scanning electron photomicrograph of a dentin surface conditioned with 20% polyalkenoic acid (Cavity Conditioner, GC). This weak acid removed the smear layer but has not opened the tubules completely (*white arrows*). Bar = 2 μm.

Fig 8-20 Field-emission scanning electron photomicrograph illustrating the effect of a 10-second application of 20% polyalkenoic acid (Cavity Conditioner, GC) to dentin. Note that although intertubular collagen was exposed, the fibrils were not completely denuded of hydroxyapatite. O = odontoblast process; P = peritubular dentin; bar = 1 μm.

The smear layer can be a detriment to effective bonding. It has an inherently weak attachment to the underlying dentin[70] and is brittle in nature.[95] In early smear-layer research, non-acidic adhesives, applied without prior etching, did not penetrate profoundly enough to establish a bond with intact dentin. Such bonds were prone to cohesive failure of the smear layer.[87,96]

Two strategies are used to overcome the low attachment strengths of the smear layer: (1) removal of the smear layer prior to bonding (the so-called etch-and-rinse approach), and (2) use of bonding agents that can penetrate the smear layer and incorporate it into the bonding layer (the so-called self-etch approach).[97] Both techniques have been successful.[98]

Removal of the smear layer greatly increases the permeability of the dentinal tubules. Pashley[99] suggested a mainly outward fluid flow under pulpal pressure of 20 to 70 cm/H_2O. When dentin is covered with an iatrogenically produced smear layer and the dentinal tubules are occluded with smear plugs, fluid permeability is substantially reduced.[87] After removal of the smear layer with an acid, dentinal permeability through the dentinal tubules increases by more than 90%.[47,100,101] Because water contamination of bonding was known to lower the bond strength,[102] it was feared that removal of the smear layer and subsequent wetting of the dentin surface would adversely affect bond strength between dentin and resin composites because the dentinal fluid would dilute bonding primers and other bonding resins.[103] However, several contemporary systems have demonstrated the ability to cope with the augmented fluid permeability of dentin, and a high and durable bond strength can be achieved.[104]

The main mechanism of tooth sensitivity is based on hydrodynamic fluid movement. Treatment of tooth surfaces to remove the smear layer can induce tooth sensitivity in vivo.[95,105] It has been suggested that adhesive techniques that require smear-layer removal are associated with more postoperative sensitivity than systems that leave the smear layer in place.[95,106,107] Open dentinal tubules may also permit access to the pulp by bacteria, their by-products, and toxic chemicals such as acids. Although it has been shown that the bonding procedure may cause transient pulpal inflammation, especially in deep cavities, a continuous bacterial irritation due to microgaps and microleakage is more likely to cause pulp damage and postoperative pain.[108]

Advantages and disadvantages of removing the smear layer were discussed by Pashley.[95] The first adhesives achieving clinically acceptable results were based on smear layer removal (etch-and-rinse adhesives), but recently, new smear-layer–incorporating adhesives (self-etch adhesives) have regained popularity.[98]

Complete or partial removal of the smear layer can be achieved by applying acidic or chelating solutions, called *conditioners*. In research conditions, sonication has also been used.[84] The more acidic and aggressive the conditioner, the more completely the smear layer and smear plugs are removed.[85,109] Strong acids not only remove the smear layer, but they also demineralize intact dentin, remove smear plugs to a depth of 1 to 5 μm, and widen the dentinal tubule orifices (see Figs 8-50 to 8-52). Contemporary etch-and-rinse adhesives usually use a 30% to 40% phosphoric acid gel for the conditioning step. Alternatively, maleic, nitric, citric, and tannic acids may be used in varying concentrations. A polyalkenoic acid conditioner used in glass-ionomer restorative techniques also provides clean dentin surfaces, although without substantial dentin demineralization[93] and without rendering dentinal tubules patent (Figs 8-19 and Fig 8-20).[110] In endodontics, chelating agents are widely used to remove

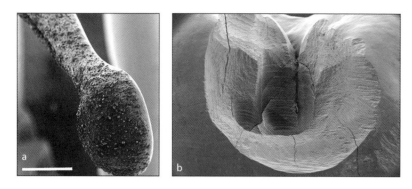

Fig 8-21 Field-emission scanning electron photomicrograph of the diamond-coated tip of the SonicSys system (*a*). The tip is coated with diamonds on only one side to prevent damage to adjacent teeth, and the constricted shape enables easy access in small occlusal and approximal cavities, such as the small Class 2 cavity preparation shown (*b*), which was prepared entirely by sono-abrasion. Bar = 1 mm.

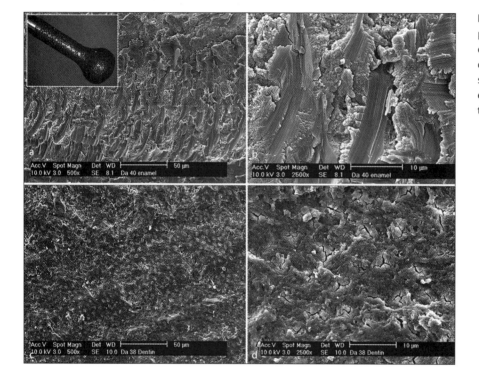

Fig 8-22 Field-emission scanning electron photomicrographs of enamel (*a* and *b*) and dentin (*c* and *d*) surfaces prepared with diamond sono-abrasion. Note the coarse scratches in the enamel. The dentin is covered with a relatively thin smear layer, and the tubules are occluded by smear plugs.

smear debris produced during the canal preparation, whereas sodium hypochlorite is applied to remove organic remnants and bacteria in root canals. Most commonly, a neutral solution of EDTA is used for removing the smear layer in the root canal.[111,112]

Alternative Technologies for Cavity Preparation

Sono-abrasion. Recently, sono-abrasion (SonicSys, KaVo; PiezzonMaster 400TM, EMS) has been introduced as an alternative method of preparing minimally invasive cavities (Fig 8-21). This technique is based on the removal of tooth structure using an air-driven handpiece equipped with a diamond-coated working tip that removes tooth material by ultrasonic kinetic energy. Different sizes and shapes of diamond tips have been designed that enable easy access to occlusal and proximal tooth lesions. As these tips are coated only on one side, damage and trauma to the proximal surface of the adjacent tooth is prevented.[113,114]

Sono-abrasion produces a smear layer because of the semirotary movement of the tip, the very high frequency of oscillations of the tip, and the heat produced (Fig 8-22). Limited research has shown that sono-abraded tooth surfaces are very similar to bur-cut dentin.[75] Van Meerbeek et al[75] reported that sono-abrasion resulted in enamel and dentin surfaces that are as receptive to bonding as bur-cut surfaces. However, they also found that a three-step etch-and-rinse adhesive (OptiBond FL, Kerr), with omission of the acid-conditioning phase, obtains higher bond strengths when bonded to sono-abraded dentin than to bur-cut dentin. This was explained by the relatively high acidity of the primer (pH = 1.78), which

Fig 8-23 *(a)* PrepStart air-abrasion device (Danville Engineering). *(b)* Airflow Prep K1 air-abrasion device (EMS). *(c)* Tips of the PrepStart system with different-size spouts. The narrower the opening, the more precisely tooth structure can be removed. *(d)* Fe-SEM image of aluminum oxide particles (Danville Engineering) at 200× magnification. Note the irregular shape and different sizes of the particles. *(e)* Container of aluminum oxide particles (Danville Engineering). *(f and g)* Air abrasion can be used to open the occlusal fissures, thereby facilitating assessment of caries lesions (shown before and after). These minimally invasive cavities are sealed afterward.

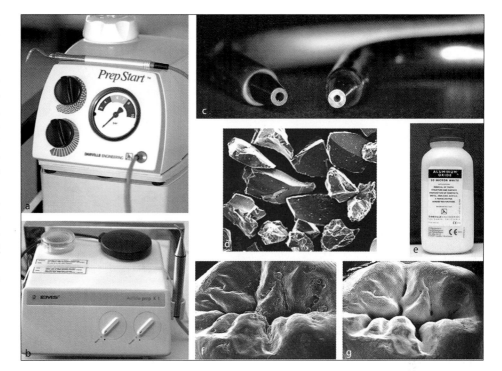

acts as a self-etch adhesive, and by the fact that sono-abrasion produces rather thin smear layers. Pioch and others[115] investigated the interface of an etch-and-rinse adhesive with confocal laser scanning microscopy and did not see any difference between bur-prepared or sono-abraded dentin of primary teeth. They[115] reported comparable microleakage in Class 2 cavities prepared by bur or SonicSys. Their study was confirmed by the findings of Setien et al.[116]

Overall, sono-abrasion may be regarded as a good complement to rotary instruments for cavity preparation. The main advantage is less risk of damage to adjacent teeth.

Air Abrasion. Air abrasion is a relatively old technique that only recently has regained attention in operative dentistry, although it is widely used by prosthodontists and dental technicians to increase surface roughness and enhance adhesion (Fig 8-23). This technique utilizes kinetic energy generated by a high-velocity stream of aluminum oxide particles to prepare hard tooth tissues, while having little effect on gingival tissues. In addition, this technique increases patient comfort by reducing heat, vibration, and noise.[75,117] The main disadvantage of this technique is the large amount of aluminum oxide dust generated and the difficulty in controlling dust particles.

When applied on dentin, air abrasion creates a very irregular surface and a discrete smear layer with smear plugs (Fig 8-24).[75] Intertubular dentin seems to be impact-folded and compressed over the dentinal tubules.[118] Some manufactur-

ers have claimed that an air-abraded tooth surface is more receptive to bonding than an acid-etched surface because a microretentive surface is created by air abrasion. However, several studies have refuted this.[75,116,119,120]

Laser Ablation. Laser technology has gained popularity in recent years, and many applications in dentistry and medicine have been proposed, including removal of carious tooth structure and cavity preparation (Fig 8-25). Like air abrasion, this technique eliminates the noise and vibration of bur cutting, rendering it more tolerable for some patients. In particular, the Er:YAG laser with an ultrashort square pulse technology (wavelength of 2.94 μm) and the Nd:Yag laser may be used as alternative methods of cavity preparation.[121,122]

Laser technology can remove tooth structure effectively and precisely. Lasers work by means of a thermomechanical ablation process that involves microexplosions within the tooth structure.[75] Water cooling is required to prevent cracking and melting of enamel and dentin and to prevent thermal damage to the pulp.[123]

Laser preparation of tooth structure does not produce a smear layer (Fig 8-26).[75,124] SEM characterization of dentin prepared by Er:YAG laser reveals a typical scaly, coarse, and irregular surface due to the microexplosions and volatilization of tooth structure.[75,125–127] As with air abrasion, laser manufacturers often claim that laser pretreatment of tooth structure enhances bonding receptivity of this substrate and that

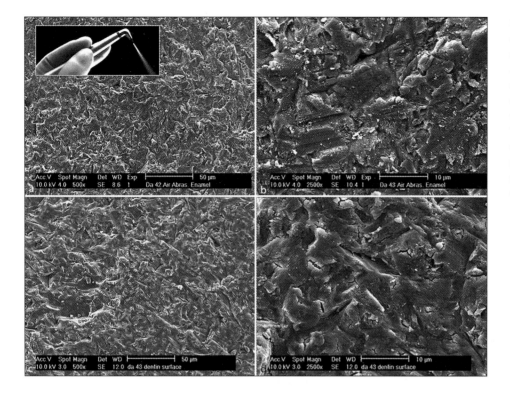

Fig 8-24 Field-emission scanning electron photomicrographs of enamel and dentin prepared by air abrasion. As a result of the kinetic energy of the aluminum oxide particles projected against the tooth surface, tooth material is chipped away. The resultant enamel (*a* and *b*) and dentin (*c* and *d*) surfaces are very irregular and covered with a discrete smear layer. The dentinal tubules are occluded by smear plugs.

"laser etching" can replace an additional conditioning phase (with phosphoric acid).

Many authors have reported possible advantages of laser cavity preparation. The lased surface is rough but not demineralized, and it exhibits patent dentinal tubules that may enhance micromechanical retention.[128,129] According to some authors, laser-prepared dentin produces similar or better results than bur-cut dentin in tests of bond strength and microleakage.[128,130–132] In spite of these favorable findings, however, a number of authors have questioned the usefulness of lasers for removal of tooth structure. Kataumi et al[124] were the first to observe substructural cracks in dentin after the use of an Er:YAG laser. Other authors also mention laser damage of enamel and dentin that results in more fractures within the dentin (Fig 8-27).[75,133–135] Controlled microtensile bond strength tests (µTBS) showed significantly poorer bonding to lased enamel and dentin.[126,134,136]

This structural weakening is not confined to the uppermost layer of dentin. Laser irradiation also modifies and weakens dentin to a depth of 3 to 5 µm, which jeopardizes adhesion of resin composite materials. In addition, TEM investigation of irradiated dentin by Ceballos et al[126] showed a dense but fissured layer devoid of collagen fibrils. Remnants of melted, fused, and denatured collagen fibrils were found only in the basal part of this layer, and they were poorly attached to the underlying intact dentin. Since interfibrillar spaces were lacking in this zone, it is thought that resin infiltration must be impeded, thereby hindering good adhesion.

Mechanical removal of this laser-modified superficial layer or removal by acid etching partially restores bond strengths. Microleakage studies indicate less leakage when lased dentin is acid etched prior to bonding.[137,138]

In conclusion, the currently available lasers do not (yet) offer any advantage over conventional rotary instruments for cavity preparation and may affect the bonding substrate adversely.

Internal and External Dentinal Wetness

The dentinal permeability and, consequently, the internal dentinal wetness depend on several factors, including the diameter and length of the tubules, the viscosity of dentinal fluid and the molecular size of substances dissolved in it, the pressure gradient, the surface area available for diffusion, the patency of the tubules, and the rate of removal of substances by pulpal circulation[139,140] (Fig 8-28). Occlusal dentin is more permeable over the pulp horns than at the center of the occlusal surface; proximal dentin is more permeable than

Figs 8-25a and 8-25b A wide range of different laser devices is commercially available. The main advantages of this rather expensive dental equipment are the precise removal of tooth tissue and the agreeable perception by the patient. However, laser preparation does not yet entail any clinical advantage over other preparation techniques.

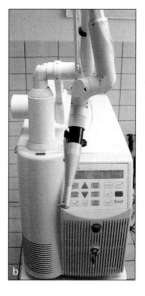

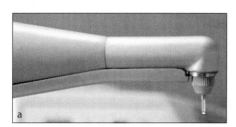

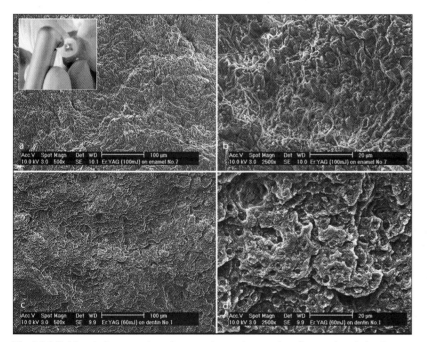

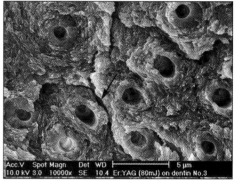

Fig 8-26 Field-emission scanning electron photomicrographs of enamel and dentin prepared by Er:YAG laser. Laser preparation does not yield a smear layer. Note the irregular enamel (*a* and *b*) and dentin (*c* and *d*) surfaces that result from an ablation process of tooth material. Laser preparation gives rise to a microretentive, nondemineralized dentin surface with patent tubules. However, adhesion of composites to laser-treated tooth tissue is jeopardized by structural weakening of the top layer due to microcracks.

Fig 8-27 SEM photomicrograph of laser-conditioned dentin. Note the microcrack *(arrow)* caused by laser irradiation.

occlusal dentin; and coronal dentin is more permeable than root dentin.[141,142] High dentinal permeability allows bacteria and their toxins to easily penetrate the dentinal tubules to the pulp if the tubules are not hermetically sealed.[143]

The variability in dentinal permeability makes dentin a more difficult substrate for bonding than enamel.[47,144] Removal of the smear layer creates a wet bonding surface on which dentinal fluid exudes from the dentinal tubules.[100] This

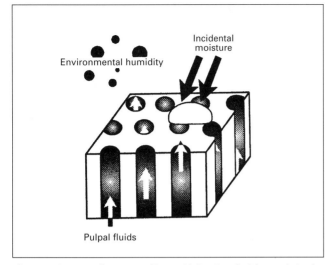

aqueous environment affects adhesion, because water competes effectively, by hydrolysis, for all adhesion sites on the hard tissue.[21,144] Jacobsen and Söderholm[102] showed that water interferes with the polymerization of adhesives, resulting in suboptimal conversion rates. Early dentin bonding agents failed primarily because their hydrophobic resins were not capable of sufficiently wetting the hydrophilic substrate.[145] In addition, bond strengths of several adhesive systems were shown to decrease as the depth of the preparation increased, because dentinal wetness was greater.[88,146–150] No significant difference in bond strengths is observed between deep and superficial dentin when the smear layer is left intact.[96] Bond strengths of more recent adhesive systems that remove the smear layer (etch-and-rinse approach) appear to be less affected by differences in dentinal depth,[66,151,152] probably because their increased hydrophilicity provides better bonding to the wet dentin surface.

Whereas earlier dentin adhesives were too hydrophobic to be successful, recent adhesives tend to be overly hydrophilic, also impairing adhesion. Recently, the so-called all-in-one adhesives have been reported to behave as semipermeable membranes and to absorb moisture from "the outside" as well as from the tooth itself (dentinal tubular fluids).[153–155] As will be described later, this phenomenon is due to the highly hydrophilic nature of one-step self-etch adhesives.[156] Application of an additional hydrophobic resin layer (as part of a two-step self-etch approach) has been shown to improve the dentin seal.

In addition to the adverse effect of internal dentinal wetness, external dentinal wetness, or environmental humidity, has also been demonstrated to negatively affect bond strengths to dentin[157,158] (see Fig 8-28). This is discussed in more detail later in this chapter.

Wetting of the Adhesive

An ideal interface between dental restorative material and tooth tissue would be one that simulates the natural attachment of enamel to dentin at the DEJ.[50] Intimate molecular contact between the two parts is a prerequisite for the development of strong adhesive joints.[18] This means that the adhesive system must sufficiently wet the solid surface, have a viscosity that is low enough to penetrate the microporosities, and be able to displace air and moisture during the bonding process.[159] In one study, the wetting characteristics of six adhesives were compared and judged to be sufficient with contact angles of less than 15 degrees[160] (see Fig 8-1). Primers in current systems usually contain hydrophilic monomers, such as 2-hydroxyethyl methacrylate (HEMA) (see box for list of abbreviations), as surface-active agents to enhance the wettability of the hydrophobic adhesive resins.[161] In addition, solvents in modern primers, such as ethanol or acetone, ensure adequate removal of air and liquid by rapid evaporation.

From polymer chemistry, it is known that polarity and solubility characterize molecular interactions that determine many physical properties, including wetting behavior.[162–164] If an adhesive monomer has a polarity and a solubility similar to those of a polymer substrate, the monomer may act as a solvent for the polymer and infiltrate it. If both parameters are sufficiently different, the monomer and polymer are immiscible.[173]

In dental adhesive technology, the collagen phase of dentin is a polymer, and both the primer and adhesive resin contain monomers that penetrate the exposed collagen layer to form a micromechanical bond. If a given conditioner conveys a specific polarity and solubility to the dentin surface, the primer must match these to achieve penetration. The same is true for the adhesive resin applied to the primed dentin surface.[162,164]

Polymerization Contraction of Restorative Resins

The linking of monomers into polymer chains during polymerization inevitably leads to volume shrinkage.[165–167] Although high filler loading of the restorative resin matrix reduces polymerization contraction, current resin composites shrink 2.9 to 7.1 vol% during free polymerization (values vary depending on test methodology used).[166,168] Contraction stresses within resin of up to 7 MPa have been reported.[169,170]

In clinical situations, the curing contraction is restrained by the developing bond of the restorative material to the cavity

Abbreviations for Chemicals Used in Dental Adhesive Technology*

AA	Acetic acid	MMEM	Mono-methacryloyloxyethylmaleate
4-AET	4-Acryloxyethyltrimellitic acid	MMEP	Mono-2-methacryloxy ethyl phthalate
4-AETA	4-Acryloxyethyl trimeric acid	MPDM	Methacryl propane diol monophosphate
bis-GMA	Bisphenol glycidyl methacrylate	NMENMF	N-Methacryloyloxyethyl-N-methyl formamide
BPDM	Biphenyl dimethacrylate	5-NMSA	N-Methacryloyl-5-aminosalicylic acid
DMA	Dimethacrylate	NPG	N-Phenylglycine
DMAEMA	Dimethylaminoethyl methacrylate	NPG-GMA	N-Phenylglycine glycidyl methacrylate
GPDM	Glycerophosphoric acid dimethacrylate	NTG-GMA	N-Tolylglycine glycidyl methacrylate
HAMA	Hydroxyalkyl methacrylate	PEG-DMA	Polyethylene glycol dimethacrylate
HDMA	Hexanediol dimethacrylate	PENTA	Dipentaerythritol penta acrylate monophosphate
HEMA	2-Hydroxyethyl methacrylate	Phenyl-P	2-Methacryloxy ethyl phenyl hydrogen phosphate
HPMA	Hydroxypropyl methacrylate	PMDM	Pyromellitic acid diethylmethacrylate
MA	Methacrylate	PMGDM	Pyromellitic acid glycerol dimethacrylate
MAC-10	11-Methacryloxy-1 1-undecadicarboxylic acid	PMO-MA	Polymethacryloligomaleic acid
10-MDP	10-Methacryloyloxy decyl dihydrogenphosphate	TBB	Tri-n-butyl borane
4-MET	4-Methacryloxyethyl trimellitic acid	TEG-DMA	Triethylene glycol dimethacrylate
4-META	4-Methacryloxyethyl trimellitate anhydride	TEG-GMA	Triethylene glycol-glycidyl methacrylate
MMA	Methyl methacrylate	UDMA	Urethane dimethacrylate
MDPB	Methacryloyloxydodecylpyridinium bromide		

*Adapted from Van Meerbeek et al[32] and Perdigão.[93]

walls.[171] This restriction induces polymerization contraction stress, which may pull the setting resin composite material away from the cavity walls.[172–174] If the weakest link is the bonding interface with the tooth, the resin-enamel bond may survive the shrinkage, but the weaker resin-dentin interface may not.[172] No current dental resin composite material is free of shrinkage during polymerization,[175] although research is underway to develop low- or nonshrinking materials.[73,175–177] A double ring-opening polymerization process, based on high-strength expandable resin composites used in industry, is being evaluated.[175–178] In addition, a silorane-based composite that polymerizes by a cationic ring-opening process has produced shrinkage values lower than 1 vol% for the first time[179]; however, further testing is needed before it can be released for routine dental use.[180]

Compensation for Polymerization Contraction

Flow

Throughout the entire polymerization process, plastic deformation, or flow, of the resin composite occurs and may partially compensate for the induced shrinkage stress.[172] This irreversible plastic deformation takes place during the early stages of the setting process, when the contraction stress exceeds the elastic limit of the restorative resin. As the setting proceeds, contraction and flow gradually decrease because stiffness increases. Fast-setting light-curing resin composites exhibit less flow-related stress relief, while self-curing or autocuring resin composites give the developing adhesive bond to dentin more time to survive. Only a fraction of the final stiffness is reached by most self-curing resin composites 10 minutes after mixing.[182] Consequently, the combination of a slow curing rate and rapid formation of an adhesive bond is considered favorable for the preservation of marginal integrity.[171]

The apparently superior marginal adaptation of autocuring resin composites can also be explained by the presence of air bubbles, which contribute to the amount of free surface and eventually increase the flow capacity of the resin composite.[183,184]

Restriction of flow is affected by the configuration of the restoration, known as the C-factor. The C-factor is the ratio of bonded (flow-inactive) to unbonded or free (flow-active) surfaces. An increase in the number of bonded surfaces results in a higher C-factor and greater contraction stress on the adhesive bond.[185] Only the free surface of a resin restoration, which is not restricted by bonding to the cavity walls, can act as a reservoir for plastic deformation in the initial stage of polymerization.[172] The higher the ratio of bonded to free resin surfaces, the less flow may compensate for contraction stress (Fig 8-29). For example, to improve marginal integrity of resin composite in a Class 5 restoration, a flatter and more wedge-shaped cavity design would be preferred to the typical butt-joint, five-walled preparation.[186–188] Carrying this a step further, the use of a cavity basin material, such as a glass-ionomer cement, within the cavity preparation (providing a so-called sandwich restoration) decreases the volume of the resin composite portion of the restoration, thus generating more free restorative surface relative to the smaller amount of resin.[173]

Other methods have been used to compensate for polymerization contraction. Bowen[189] has reported that the placement of glass or ceramic blocks into soft resin composite before light curing, displacing as much of the resin composite as possible, results in reduced microleakage. The improvement exhibited by megafilled resin composite restorations was attributed to a decrease in the overall curing contraction of the limited amount of resin composite and a decrease in the coefficient of thermal expansion of the restoration containing the inserts.[190,191]

Prepolymerized resin composite inserts may also be used to help offset polymerization contraction. One example is the addition of prepolymerized resin pieces in the manufacture of microfilled resin composites. At the other extreme are resin composite inlays, which are cemented in the cavity with a luting resin. The use of inlays avoids the direct adverse effect of polymerization contraction on the developing resin-tooth bond. However, the flow-active free surface of the luting resin composite is relatively small at the narrow inlay-tooth marginal gap, yielding a high C-factor. Consequently, the luting resin composite is not likely to provide enough compensation for the shrinkage stress induced by its polymerization.[185] Nevertheless, the incorporation of pores by mixing of the two components and the slow autocuring rate of the dual-cured luting resin may still allow sufficient stress relaxation by flow.[183]

Another strategy for slow curing, to allow more flow to compensate for shrinkage stress, is the so-called soft-start or ramped light-curing technique.[192–194] Curing lights designed for this technique produce low-intensity light (400 mW/cm² or less) during a period of about 10 seconds, after which the light intensity is immediately or exponentially increased to about 800 mW/cm² or more.

The introduction of laser and xenon arc high-powered light-curing technology, a contrasting approach, has elicited much controversy. The theory behind this high-intensity light-curing technology is that curing times can be reduced to 1 to 3 seconds without a decrease of physicomechanical material properties. Advocates of this new light-curing technique recommend placement of small resin composite increments to ensure sufficient polymerization. Evolution of curing technology is expected to continue. The recent development of long-lasting, high-intensity light-emitting diodes (LEDs) has become a useful adjunct to existing curing methods.[195] LED curing units will probably become the standard in the near future because of their many advantages over other light-curing technologies, such as cordless operation, consistent light output, and reduced noise levels.

Hygroscopic Expansion

The effect of polymerization shrinkage is somewhat tempered by fluid absorption, which causes resin composite to swell and may offset some residual elastic stresses. Again, the configuration of the cavity determines the effectiveness of this compensation mechanism.[167,196] Overcompensation may even transform contraction stress into expansion stress. Microfilled resin composites have been shown to absorb nearly two and a half times more water than macrofilled materials because of the greater volume of resin in the microfills.[197]

Very recent research has revealed that the polymerization setting stress within the adhesive is relieved in part due to water absorbed from the dentin (Hashimoto et al, unpublished data, 2005). However, hygroscopic expansion occurs during the days and weeks immediately following placement of the resin composite restoration, after the dentin bonding may already have failed. When this has occurred, hygroscopic expansion may force a Class 5 resin composite restoration to expand beyond the margin of the preparation.[196]

Elasticity

If the resin-tooth bond remains intact, the final stiffness or rigidity of a resin composite may play a compensating role in coping with remaining polymerization contraction stress. Stiffness is quantified by Young's modulus of elasticity, which represents the resistance of a material to elastic deformation.[165] The lower the Young's modulus of a restorative resin, the greater its flexibility and the more capacity it has to reduce remaining contraction stress. Resin composites with a high filler content have a higher Young's modulus of elasticity, which will reduce volumetric contraction (because of the higher filler content relative to the lower resin content), but have higher remaining contraction stress, which may affect the resin-dentin interface.

Viscous adhesive resins produce a rather thick resin bonding layer between the stiff dentinal cavity wall and the shrinking restorative resin composite. Stretching of this intermediate layer (with a low Young's modulus) may provide sufficient elasticity to relieve polymerization contraction stresses of the

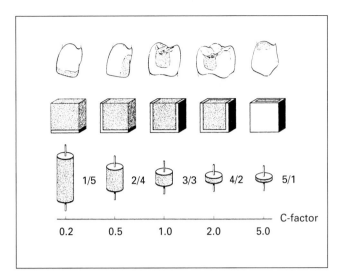

Fig 8-29 Diverse cavity configurations with different C-factors, or ratios of bonded to unbonded (free) surface, and their corresponding clinical cases. (From Feilzer et al.[184] Reprinted with permission.)

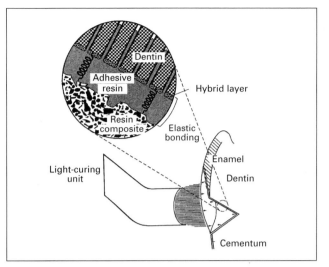

Fig 8-30 Elastic bonding area concept. Use of a relatively thick elastic adhesive may compensate for polymerization shrinkage that occurs in resin composite. Shown is an incrementally filled Class 5 resin composite restoration.

restorative resin composite.[198–200] Based on this theory, an "elastic bonding concept" has been advanced (Fig 8-30). It has been determined that a bonding layer thickness of 125 μm reduces shrinkage stresses below dentin bond strengths, preserving the bond.[201] A flexible intermediate resin layer may also better transmit and distribute stresses induced by thermal changes, water absorption, and occlusal forces across the interface.[200] In addition, a thick adhesive resin layer permits limited inhibition of polymerization by oxygen without impairing the resin-dentin bond.[202]

Support for the elastic bonding concept has been provided by in vitro and in vivo research. When Gluma (Bayer) resin was prepolymerized in a relatively thick layer in an in vitro study,[203,204] less microleakage occurred than when it was left uncured prior to application of the resin composite. Lack of such a built-in polymerization contraction relaxation mechanism might have largely accounted for the high clinical failure rates recorded for Gluma, two experimental total-etch systems, and Gluma 2000.[205]

Clinical trials have reported excellent 7-year results (94% retention rate of Class 5 resin composite restorations) for a three-step etch-and-rinse adhesive that incorporates a particle-filled adhesive resin (OptiBond FL, Kerr), probably the best clinical results ever reported.[206] Likewise, a two-step self-etch adhesive that provides a silica-filled adhesive resin has demonstrated a 100% retention rate at 3 years.[207]

Cervical Sealing

Sealing of cervical marginal gaps with an unfilled low-viscosity resin, applied and cured after the restorative resin has been

cured, is another technique that has been described to overcome the negative effects of polymerization shrinkage and obtain sealed cervical restorations.[189,208] Use of a restorative resin with high elasticity and low curing contraction in combination with such a low-viscosity resin layer may provide sufficient strain relief to compensate for the curing contraction of the unfilled resin layer.[208] However, this technique is laborious and prone to failure in the event of contamination with blood or saliva.

Initial Polymerization

Initiation of polymerization at the resin-tooth interface, directing the shrinking resin material toward the cavity wall rather than away from it, is advantageous.[174] Contraction has always been claimed to occur toward the light source in light-curing resin composites, whereas initial setting has been said to occur in the center of the bulk of material in self-curing resin composites.[173] For both light-curing and self-curing systems, tensile stresses operate across the resin composite–dentin interface, pulling the material away from the cavity walls. Countering the theory that contraction occurs toward the curing light in light-curing systems, a recent study[209] using finite-element analysis showed that the direction of polymerization shrinkage was not significantly affected by the orientation of the incoming curing light. Instead, the cavity shape and the bond quality determined the direction of the polymerization vectors. That study concluded that the contraction patterns between autocuring and photocuring composites were similar.

For many years, Fusayama[210] argued that the initial setting of autocuring resins starts at the dentinal wall because body heat accelerates the chemical reaction. In other words, the shrinking restoration is pulled toward, rather than away from, the cavity base.[172] Evaluation of premolar restorations in vivo showed that the use of chemically cured resin composite did not result in reduced gap formation relative to gaps produced when light-cured composites were used. This study could not confirm the supposed stress-relieving effect of self-curing resin composites.[211]

For light-initiated resin composite polymerization, there is general agreement that the unbonded resin material at the free surface of the restoration sets first when it is exposed to the light source; thus, its flow relaxation capacity is considerably diminished. Incremental layering techniques have been used to minimize the negative effects of light polymerization to increase the actual resin-free area relative to the resin-bonded area.[212–214] This disciplined application technique promotes sufficient polymerization of the deepest material, in contrast to that achieved with the limited light penetration that occurs with bulk placement. The incremental technique has also been hypothesized to result in less stress caused by polymerization contraction, because the flow relaxation capacity is higher and can be used to direct polymerization shrinkage of each increment toward the cavity walls. But the theory that an incremental placement technique reduces stress effects of resin-composite shrinkage is debated.[215] Completeness of cure, adequate adaptation to the cavity walls, and adequate bond formation may still be reasons to use a composite layering technique.[215] Furthermore, improved marginal adaptation of the critical gingivoproximal border of Class 2 resin composite restorations has been described with the use of a three-sited light-curing technique with laterally light-reflecting wedges.[173,216] Once again, however, the benefit of this directed curing technique is no longer generally accepted.[215]

Some adhesive systems are also designed so that chemical polymerization is initiated at the surface of dentin.[217,218] For example, the simplified Gluma 2000 System attempts to impregnate the dentin surface with an amine part of the catalytic system in the form of glycine, which is claimed to establish a chemical bond to collagen.[219] Because camphoroquinone is incorporated as the other part of the catalytic system, and selected methacrylic monomers, such as HEMA and bisphenol glycidyl methacrylate (bis-GMA), are included in the adhesive resin, the polymerization is expected to be initiated at the adhesive interface. This simplified pretreatment technique has proved to be highly effective in reducing the marginal gap in cavities in both enamel and dentin.[219] How-

ever, several in vivo and in vitro reports on the use of amino acids have yielded contradictory results.[205,220,221]

A water-triggered polymerization has been described for the 4-methacryloxyethyl trimellitate anhydride/methyl methacrylate–tri-n-butyl borane (4-META/MMA-TBB) systems, such as Super-Bond D-Liner (Sun Medical) or AmalgamBond (Parkell).[222] Although water and oxygen, which are omnipresent in dentin, are normally expected to affect the polymerization process of bonding resins, they may apparently also act as co-initiators of the polymerization reaction.[223] Effective water-triggered polymerization in deep, tubule-rich dentin has been suggested to direct resin shrinkage toward the dentin surface itself. Imai et al[174] hypothesized that the application of ferric chloride with these adhesive systems to acid etch dentin might promote and initiate resin polymerization at the interface. More research is needed to explore these mechanisms to initiate polymerization at the interface.

Thermal Expansion Coefficient and Thermal Conductivity

Because the coefficient of thermal expansion of resin is about four times that of tooth structure, any bonded resin restoration is likely to suffer from marginal gap formation.[197,224] The microfilled resin composites have a higher coefficient of thermal expansion than do hybrid-type resin composites.[165] However, Harper et al[225] suggested that the dimensional change that occurs in the clinical restoration as a result of temperature fluctuations may not be as great in magnitude as its relatively high coefficient of thermal expansion would suggest. The temperature transfer through resin composite restorations is slower, and the rate of temperature change is lower than in amalgam restorations.[225] Nevertheless, marginal adaptation and microleakage studies have shown that prolonged thermocycling induces percolation under resin composite restorations.[224,226]

Transmission of Stress Across the Restoration-Tooth Interface

The adhesive bond between a restorative material and tooth structure has a biomechanical role in the distribution of functional stress throughout the whole tooth.[144] A true bond will transmit stress applied to the restoration to the remaining tooth structure, and bonded restorations may strengthen weakened teeth.[5,227] Displacement and bending of the cusps may compensate for the contraction stress in Class 2 resin composite restorations,[228] but polymerization contraction may also induce cuspal fracture.[144,168,229] In general, high masticatory stresses are known to reduce the longevity of adhesively bonded restorations.[143,230]

For wedge-shaped cervical lesions, transmission of occlusal loads may affect retention of Class 5 cervical restorations. Noncarious cervical lesions have a multifactorial etiology,[229,231–233] possibly including incisal or occlusal loads that induce compressive and tensile stresses at the DEJ in the cervical region. Adhesively placed cervical restorations are subject to the same stresses,[200,234,235] which may progressively debond the resin restoration and eventually dislodge it. When resin composites with relatively low Young's moduli of elasticity, such as microfilled resin composites, are used, elastic deformation may partially compensate for the induced stress (Fig 8-31). The forces created by compression of the restoration are localized mainly in the bulk of the resin composite as compressive stress and, to a lesser degree, as shear stress at the adhesive interface. When more rigid, denser resin composites are placed, the shear stress at the interface might exceed the compression stress, affecting the bond of resin to dentin. Naturally, this hypothesis can be valid only when the adhesive bond is sufficiently strong. In a clinical study involving Class 5 restorations placed with diverse dentin adhesive systems, the retention rate was found to improve as the Young's moduli of the resin composites declined.[205]

A similar concept of "tooth flexure" has been reported by Heymann et al.[235] It has been suggested that microfilled resin composites compress rather than dislodge during tooth flexure.[236] A high correlation between the modulus of elasticity and marginal leakage was found by Kemp-Scholte and Davidson.[199] They reported that the higher the modulus of elasticity of the resin composite used, the greater the number of cervical gaps.[171] Therefore, microfilled resin composites have commonly been preferred for restorations in wedge-shaped cervical lesions.[208] However, in recent clinical trials, performance of microfilled resin composites was comparable to that of hybrid resin composite materials in Class 5 noncarious cervical lesions at 7 years.[206,237] These findings cast some doubt on the advantages of flexible resin composites in cervical lesions, although benefits may yet appear after a longer term.

Biocompatibility

To the physicochemical aspects of dentin and resin composite restorative materials must be added the biologic concern of biocompatibility. Both dentist and patient are at risk for adverse effects of adhesive materials.

The dissemination of residual monomer molecules to the pulp chamber via the dentinal tubules has been reported to involve a significant degree of cytotoxicity, even in low con-

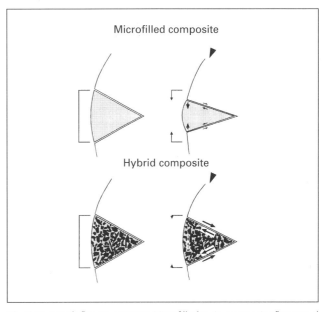

Fig 8-31 Tooth flexure concept. Microfilled resin composite flexes and absorbs some of the force, but the more rigid hybrid resin composite is more likely to be dislodged.

centrations.[238] However, in vivo biocompatibility studies have demonstrated that resin composites, whether fully or partially cured, cause little pulpal irritation if the cavities are sealed to prevent ingress of bacteria from the oral environment.[53,239–241] Fusayama[242] has argued that the fundamental factor involved in pulpal irritation is separation of the resin from dentin. When debonding occurs, thermal and mechanical stresses on the restoration exert a pumping action on the fluid in the gap, pressing irritants or bacterial toxins into the tubules.[242,243]

Some general health concerns have been expressed related to the use of resin composite systems. One concern is that leakage of bisphenol-A from bis-GMA–based resin composites and sealants may have estrogenic effects.[244–249] Söderholm and Mariotti[249] concluded that, considering the dosages and routes of administration and the modest response of estrogenic-sensitive target organs, the short-term risk of estrogenic effects from treatment using bisphenol A–based resins is insignificant and therefore should not be of concern to the general public. Long-term effects need to be investigated further. A "three-finger" syndrome, or contact allergy at the fingertips of clinicians or dental assistants, has been described, although there is currently little experimental data available.[248,250,251] "Noncontact" handling of diverse monomer-based materials, especially primers and adhesive resins, is therefore strongly advised.

Although the biologic evaluation of dentin adhesive systems has received a considerable amount of attention, the results and conclusions of these biocompatibility tests vary widely and do not cover all systems. Therefore, conclusions about the influence of chemical irritants on postoperative sensitivity must be considered premature.[143]

The use of acids on vital dentin has traditionally been avoided because of the fear of pulpal irritation, confusion over the protective function of the smear layer, and the lack of efficacy of the bonding agents.[252–256] Stanley et al[257] reported that acid etching of dentin caused pulpal reactions when the remaining dentin was less than 1 mm thick, but other histopathologic studies[241] have shown that acid etching dentin has no adverse effects. Fusayama[243] has stated that, in the case of carious dentin, diffusion of penetrating acid is largely limited to 10 μm because of the blocking action of odontoblast processes in the tubules of vital teeth and intertubular crystals.

As an in-depth report on the biocompatibility of adhesive materials is beyond the scope of this chapter, reference is made to a recently published book by Schmalz and Arenholt-Bindslev.[258]

An adhesive with alleged therapeutic effects (Clearfil ProtectBond, Kuraray) has been introduced onto the market. This adhesive contains the antimicrobial monomer methacryloyl-oxydodecylpyridinium bromide (MDPB), which is claimed to protect the restored tooth against recurrent caries.[259–261] While the monomer has proven to be strongly antimicrobial, it loses much of its antimicrobial activity after polymerization.[262] Indisputable clinical evidence of the benefit of this antimicrobial effect has not yet been provided.

Adhesion to Enamel and Dentin

Concepts in restorative dentistry are continually changing, and adhesive technology has become increasingly important for two reasons. First, adhesive techniques combined with the use of tooth-colored restorative materials allow clinicians to restore teeth not only anatomically and functionally, but also esthetically, something demanded by many patients. Secondly, today's operative dentistry should primarily involve procedures that are minimally invasive,[77] in a concept referred to as *minimum intervention*.[78] Minimally invasive procedures preserve as much sound tooth structure as possible. In addition, the more recent approach that promotes maintenance and repair[263–266] rather than replacement of the entire restoration has further encouraged the use of adhesive techniques.

The trend toward adhesive dentistry started in the mid-1960s with the advent of the first commercial restorative resin composites, followed in the early 1970s by the introduction of the acid-etch technique in clinical practice. Since then,

there has been continuous progress in developing more refined and diversified restorative resin composites, along with steady improvement in bonding agents. Effective adhesion to enamel was achieved with relative ease and has repeatedly proven to be a durable and reliable clinical procedure. Although adhesion to dentin is not yet as reliable as adhesion to enamel, today's adhesives produce superior results in laboratories[267,268] and improved clinical effectiveness,[205–207,269] and the performance of dentin bonding has approached that of enamel bonding. Early one-step dentin bonding agents became multistep systems with more complicated, time-consuming, and technique-sensitive application procedures. Today, so-called universal, all-purpose, or multipurpose adhesive systems are available that purportedly bond to enamel, dentin, amalgam, metal, and porcelain. In the early 1990s, the selective enamel-etching technique was replaced by a total-etch concept. Since then, universal enamel-dentin conditioners are simultaneously applied to enamel and dentin. Now that adhesives have reached an acceptable bonding effectiveness, most recent efforts have been to simplify the multistep bonding process and to reduce its sensitivity to errors in clinical handling. Although retention is no longer a clinical problem, the difficulty in maintaining sealed margins remains the major factor that shortens clinical longevity.[270,271]

The fundamental principle of adhesion to tooth substrate is based upon an exchange process by which inorganic tooth material is exchanged for synthetic resin.[272] This process involves two phases (Fig 8-32). One phase consists of removal of calcium phosphates, by which microporosities are exposed in both enamel and dentin surfaces. The other, so-called hybridization phase involves infiltration and subsequent in situ polymerization of resin within the created surface microporosities. This results in micromechanical interlocking that is primarily based upon mechanisms of diffusion. While micromechanical interlocking is believed to be a prerequisite to achieve good bonding within clinical circumstances, the potential benefit of additional chemical interaction between functional monomers and tooth substrate components has recently gained new attention.

Bonding to tooth structure can also be achieved directly with glass-ionomer cements. Glass-ionomer–based materials have an auto-adhesive capacity due to their specific chemical formula and structural nature. Parallel with the progress made in resin-based adhesives, glass-ionomer technology has undergone many improvements and modifications to the original chemistry developed in the early 1970s by Wilson and Kent.[273] A recent trend in adhesive material development has been to combine glass-ionomer and resin composite technology in new adhesive systems and restorative materials with mixed characteristics.

Fig 8-32 Schematic representation of the basic mechanism of adhesion to tooth substrate.

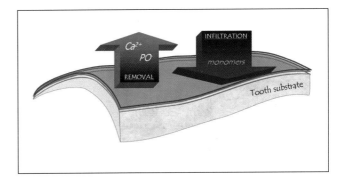

Fig 8-33 Classification of contemporary adhesives according to adhesion strategy and clinical application steps.

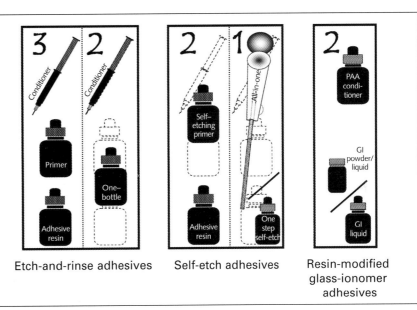

Classifying dental adhesives into different categories is not easy. Several classifications have been suggested in scientific literature in the past. However, no consensus concerning terminology has been reached. Two classifications will be discussed in this chapter. Adhesives used to be categorized according to the order in which they were introduced into the market. This chronological classification is not logical, however, and lacks scientific background. Van Meerbeek et al[75,98,272] have suggested a scientifically based classification with three main groups of adhesives: etch-and-rinse adhesives, self-etch adhesives, and glass-ionomer adhesives (Fig 8-33). This classification is simple and has proved to be reliable and consistent. As it is based on the applied adhesion strategy, this classification provides a dentist or a researcher with background information on the adhesion mechanism and on some characteristics of an adhesive system. Therefore, this scientific classification will be discussed first, followed by the chronological classification for reasons of completeness and historical background.

Adhesion Strategies: Scientific Classification of Modern Adhesives

As previously mentioned, a process by which inorganic tooth material is exchanged for resin is the basis of adhesion to tooth substrate.[96,272] Using contemporary adhesives, the substance exchange between biomaterial and tooth structure is carried out in one, two, or three clinical application steps. Adhesives can further be classified based upon the underlying adhesion strategy, ie, etch-and-rinse, self-etch, and (resin-modified) glass-ionomer adhesives (see Fig 8-33).[272] The degree of substance exchange substantially differs among these adhesives. In general, the degree of exchange induced by etch-and-rinse adhesives exceeds that of self-etch adhesives, although among the latter, systems now exist that intensively interact with tooth structure, even when applied in only a single step.

Table 8-2 Contemporary adhesives categorized according to adhesion strategy and clinical application steps and chronological classification

Brand name	Manufacturer	Brand name	Manufacturer
Etch-and-rinse adhesives		**Two-step self-etch adhesives (sixth generation) (continued)**	
Three-step etch-and-rinse adhesives (fourth generation)		Scotchbond 2 (selective enamel etching)	3M ESPE
All-Bond 2	Bisco	Solobond Plus	Voco
Clearfil Liner Bond	Kuraray	Syntac (Classic) (selective enamel etching)	Ivoclar Vivadent
Denthesive	Heraeus Kulzer		
EBS	ESPE (now 3M ESPE)	Tokuso Mac Bond II	MAC
Gluma CPS	Bayer Leverkusen (now Heraeus Kulzer)	Tyrean	Bisco
		Unifil Bond	GC
OptiBond DC	Kerr		
OptiBond FL	Kerr	*One-step self-etch adhesives (sixth and seventh generation; division is ambiguous and depends on time of market launch)*	
Permagen	Ultradent		
Permaquik	Ultradent	Admira Bond	Voco
Scotchbond MultiPurpose	3M (now 3M ESPE)	Adper Prompt L-Pop	3M ESPE
		AQ Bond	Sun Medical
		Clearfil S³ Bond	Kuraray
Two-step etch-and-rinse adhesives (fifth generation)		Etch&Prime 3.0	Degussa AG
C36 Prime&Bond NT	Dentsply-Detrey	Sustel/F2000 primer-adhesive	3M ESPE
Excite	Ivoclar Vivadent		
Gluma 2000	Bayer	Futurabond	Voco
One Coat Bond	Coltène Whaledent	G-Bond	GC
One-Step	Bisco	Hytac OSB	ESPE (now 3M ESPE)
OptiBond Solo Plus	Kerr	iBond	Heraeus Kulzer
Prime&Bond 2.0	Dentsply-Detrey	One-Up Bond F	Tokuyama
Prime&Bond 2.1	Dentsply-Detrey	One-Up Bond F Plus	Tokuyama
Prime&Bond NT	Dentsply-Detrey	Prime&Bond 2.1 (without etching)	Dentsply-Detrey
Scotchbond 1XT	3M ESPE		
Single Bond (Scotchbond 1)	3M ESPE	Prime&Bond NT (without etching)	Dentsply-Detrey
Solobond M	Voco	Prompt-L-Pop	3M ESPE
Stae	Southern Dental Industries	Prompt-L-Pop (LP2)	3M ESPE
Syntac Single-Component	Ivoclar Vivadent	PSA	Dentsply-Detrey
		Reactmer Bond	Shofu
Syntac Sprint	Ivoclar Vivadent	Xeno III	Dentsply-Detrey
		Xeno IV	Dentsply-Detrey
Self-etch adhesives			
Two-step self-etch adhesives (sixth generation)		**Glass ionomers**	
AdheSE	Ivoclar Vivadent	Fuji 2 LC (GC Dentin Conditioner)	GC
ART Bond	Coltène Whaledent		
Clearfil Liner Bond 2	Kuraray	Fuji Bond LC (GC Cavity Conditioner)	GC
Clearfil Liner Bond 2V	Kuraray		
Clearfil Protect Bond	Kuraray	Fuji Bond LL	GC
Clearfil SE	Kuraray	HIFI Master Palette (HI Tooth Cleanser)	Shofu
Denthesive 2	Heraeus Kulzer		
NRC Prime&Bond NT	Dentsply-Detrey	Imperva Fluorobond	Shofu
One Coat SE Bond	Coltène Whaledent	Ketac-fil (Ketac Conditioner)	ESPE (now 3M ESPE)
OptiBond Solo Plus Self-Etch	Kerr		
		Photac-fil (Ketac Conditioner)	ESPE (now 3M ESPE)
Perme Bond F	Degussa AG		
Prisma Universal Bond 3	Dentsply-Detrey	Reactmer Bond	Shofu
		Vitremer (Vitremer Primer)	3M ESPE
Pro Bond	Dentsply-Detrey		

Smear Layer–Modifying Adhesives

Dentin adhesives that modify the smear layer are based on the concept that the smear layer provides a natural barrier to the pulp, protecting it against bacterial invasion and limiting the outflow of pulpal fluid that might impair bonding efficiency. Efficient wetting and in situ polymerization of monomers infiltrated into the smear layer are expected to reinforce the bonding of the smear layer to the underlying dentin surface, forming a micromechanical and perhaps chemical bond to underlying dentin. Clinically, these systems require selective etching of enamel in a separate step. Most typical in this group are the primers that are applied before the application of polyacid-modified resin composites, or compomers.

The interaction of these adhesives with dentin is very superficial, with only a limited penetration of resin into the dentin surface (Fig 8-34). This shallow interaction of the adhesive system with dentin, without any collagen fibril exposure, confirms the weak acidity of these smear layer–modifying primers. The dentinal tubules commonly remain plugged by smear debris.

Etch-and-Rinse Approach

This adhesion strategy in its most conventional form involves three steps: application of the conditioner or acid etchant, followed by the primer or adhesion-promoting agent, and then the actual bonding agent or adhesive resin (see Fig 8-33). The simplified two-step version combines the second and third step but still follows a separate etch-and-rinse phase.

This etch-and-rinse technique is still the most effective approach to achieve efficient and stable bonding to enamel and only requires two steps. Selective dissolution of hydroxyapatite crystals through etching (commonly with a 30% to 40% phosphoric acid gel) is followed by in situ polymerization of resin that is readily absorbed by capillary attraction within the created etch pits, enveloping individually exposed hydroxyapatite crystals (Fig 8-35). Two types of resin tags interlock within the etch pits. *Macrotags* fill up the space surrounding the enamel prisms, while numerous *microtags* result from resin infiltration/polymerization within the tiny etch pits at the cores of the etched enamel prisms (Fig 8-36). The latter are thought to be the major contributors to retention to enamel.

In dentin, this phosphoric acid treatment exposes a microporous network of collagen with elimination of most or all of the hydroxyapatite (Figs 8-37 and 8-38). High-resolution TEM as well as chemical surface analysis by energy-dispersive x-ray spectroscopy (EDXS) and x-ray photoelectron spectroscopy (XPS) have confirmed that nearly all calcium phosphates are removed (Fig 8-39).[275] As a result, the bonding mechanism of etch-and-rinse adhesives to dentin is primarily diffusion-

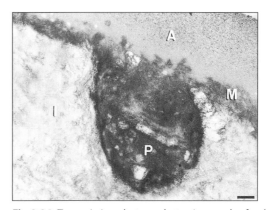

Fig 8-34 Transmission electron photomicrograph of a demineralized specimen showing the resin-dentin interface presented with ProBond. Note the formation of a superficially modified smear layer (M) and smear plug (P). A = adhesive resin; I = intertubular dentin; bar = 200 nm.

based and depends upon hybridization or infiltration of resin within the exposed collagen fibril scaffold (Figs 8-40 to 8-42). True chemical bonding is unlikely because the functional groups of monomers have only weak affinity to the hydroxyapatite-depleted collagen. The limited monomer-collagen interaction might be the principal reason for the so-called nanoleakage phenomenon.[277,278]

The most critical step in the etch-and-rinse approach is application of the primer. When an acetone-based adhesive is used, the highly technique-sensitive wet-bonding technique is mandatory.[279] Gentle postconditioning air-drying of acid-etched dentin (and enamel) followed by a dry-bonding technique may be used with a water- or ethanol-based adhesive.[275,276]

With the two-step etch-and-rinse adhesives (Figs 8-33 and 8-43 to 8-46 and Table 8-2), the primer and adhesive resin are combined into one solution. In conventional three-step systems, the primer ensures efficient wetting of the exposed collagen fibrils, displaces residual surface moisture, transforms a hydrophilic tissue state into a hydrophobic one, and carries monomers into the interfibrillar channels. The adhesive resin fills the pores between the collagen fibrils, forms resin tags that seal the opened dentinal tubules, initiates and advances the polymerization reaction, stabilizes the hybrid layer and resin tags, and provides sufficient methacrylate double bonds for copolymerization with the restorative resin. In simplified one-bottle systems, the functions of the primer and the adhesive resin are combined.

The advantages and shortcomings of three-step and two-step etch-and-rinse adhesives have been summarized elsewhere in separate boxes.

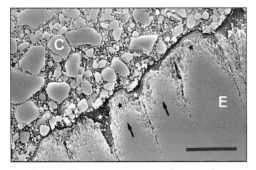

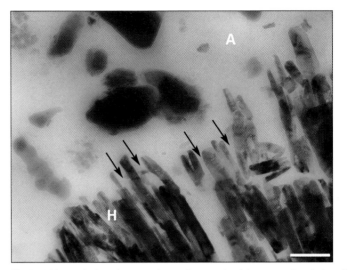

Fig 8-35 Field-emission scanning electron photomicrograph showing a resin-enamel interface subjected to an argon-ion–bombardment procedure when a three-step total-etch adhesive (Scotchbond MultiPurpose Plus, 3M, ESPE) was bonded to 35% phosphoric acid–etched enamel (E). Macrotags *(white stars)* are formed circularly between the longitudinally sectioned enamel prism *(black arrows)* peripheries. Microtags *(black stars)* are formed at the cores of the enamel prisms. C = luting composite; bar = 5 μm. (From Peumans et al.[274] Reprinted with permission from Elsevier Science.)

Fig 8-36 Transmission electron photomicrograph of the enamel-resin interface illustrating the occurrence of micromechanical interlocking of the resin within the etch pits created through conventional phosphoric-acid etching. Macrotags represent the infiltration and in situ polymerization of resin between adjacent enamel prisms. Microtags *(black arrows)* represent resin enveloping individual hydroxyapatite crystals in the enamel-prism cores. A = adhesive resin; H = hydroxyapatite; bar = 200 nm.

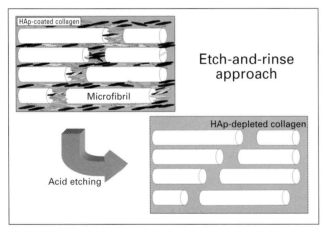

Fig 8-37 Schematic drawing presenting the effect of an etch-and-rinse approach on the hydroxyapatite-collagen arrangement. HAp = hydroxyapatite. (From Van Meerbeek et al.[98] Reprinted with permission.)

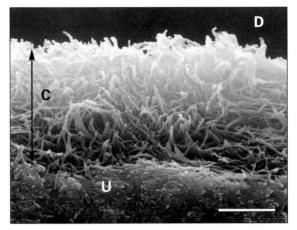

Fig 8-38 Field-emission scanning electron photomicrograph of demineralized dentin. Treatment with 35% phosphoric acid for 15 seconds demineralizes dentin over a depth of 3 to 5 μm, thereby exposing a scaffold of collagen fibrils that is nearly totally depleted of hydroxyapatite. As a consequence, a retentive network with interfibrillar spaces of approximately 20 nm is created. C = Hydroxyapatite-depleted collagen; D = phosphoric acid–etched dentin; U = unaffected dentin; bar = 2 μm. (Image courtesy of Dr Marcos Vargas. From Van Meerbeek et al.[98] Reprinted with permission.)

Fig 8-39 *(a)* TEM photomicrograph of an unstained, nondemineralized 200-nm section through the resin-dentin interface produced by OptiBond Dual-Cure (Kerr). The hybrid layer (H) clearly does not contain any hydroxyapatite, which would have appeared electron dense (dark gray to black) as within the unaffected dentin (D) underneath. EDXS surface mapping confirmed that calcium was below detection limit *(b)*, while only a scarce amount of phosphorous could be detected *(c)*. The latter may also originate from the phosphate-based monomer GPDM, which is a basic constituent of the OptiBond Dual-Cure primer. (From Van Meerbeek et al.[98] Reprinted with permission.)

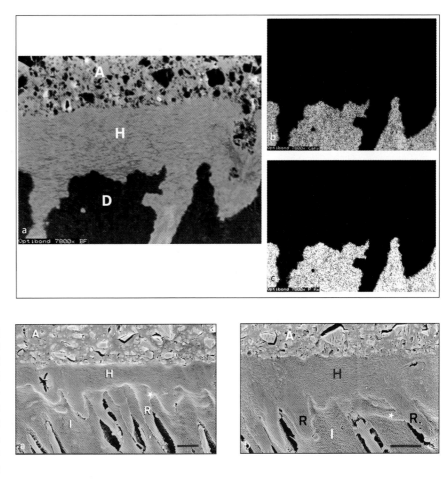

Figs 8-40a and 8-40b Field-emission scanning electron photomicrographs demonstrating the resin-dentin interface produced by Optibond Dual Cure (Kerr) when a 37.5% phosphoric acid was used. Dentin was removed during laboratory processing. A hybrid layer (H) of 4 to 5 µm was formed along with resin tags (R; often particle-filled) into the opened dentinal tubules. A = adhesive resin (particle-filled); I = intertubular dentin (unaffected); white star = micro–resin tag in lateral tubule branch; bar = 5 µm.

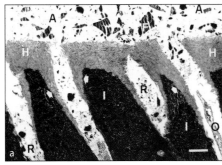

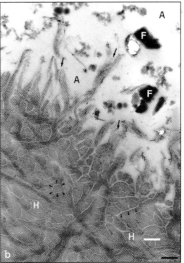

Figs 8-41a and 8-41b Transmission electron photomicrographs of nondemineralized sections demonstrating the resin-dentin interface produced by Optibond Dual Cure (Kerr). The hybrid layer (H) of 3 to 5 µm is loosely organized with longitudinally and cross-sectioned collagen fibrils separated by resin-filled interfibrillar spaces of about 10 to 20 nm *(black arrowheads, b)*. At the transition of the hybrid layer toward the adhesive resin (A), a typical "shag-carpet" appearance can be observed with collagen fibrils directed toward the adhesive resin and often unraveled into their microfibrils *(black arrows, b)*. The hybrid layer extends into the tubule orifice walls, establishing so-called tubule wall hybridization *(thick white arrows, a)*. F = glass filler surrounded by silane coupling agent; I = intertubular dentin (unaffected); O = remnants of odontoblastic process or lamina limitans embedded in the resin tag; R = resin tags (often particle-filled); bar = 2 µm *(a)* and 200 nm *(b)*. (From Van Meerbeek et al.[276] Reprinted with permission.)

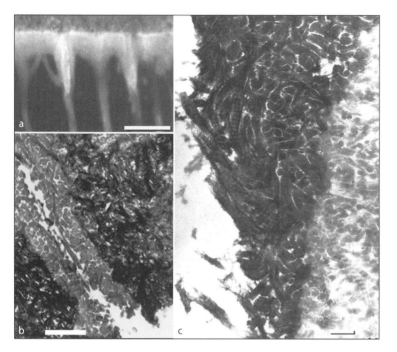

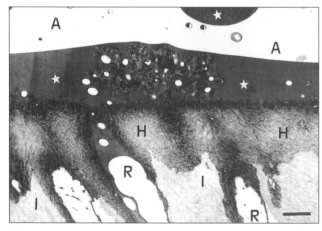

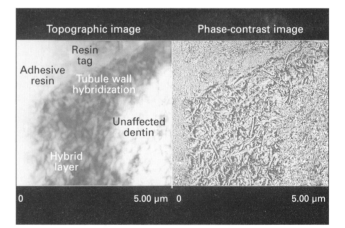

Fig 8-42 *(a)* Laser-scanning confocal photomicrograph illustrating the resin-dentin interface of OptiBond (Kerr). The adhesive resin component of OptiBond has been labeled with rhodamine B. Note the formation of resin microtags in the lateral tubular branches. Bar = 5 μm. *(b)* Detail of transmission electron photomicrograph of a nondemineralized dentin section, showing a resin microtag. A narrow core of resin is surrounded by a hybridized wall (lateral tubule hybridization). Bar = 500 nm. *(c)* Transmission electron photomicrograph of a demineralized and stained dentin section, showing a close-up of the thin hybrid layer produced in the wall of dentinal tubules (tubule-wall hybridization). Note the typical cross banding of the collagen fibrils and their fraying ends ("shag-carpet" appearance). Bar = 300 nm.

Fig 8-43 Transmission electron photomicrograph of a demineralized section demonstrating the resin-dentin interface produced by the "one-bottle" adhesive Single Bond (3M), known as Scotchbond 1 in Europe. Typical is the deposition of an electron-dense phase *(white stars)* on top of the hybrid layer (H) and along the tubule orifice walls, often blocking them. This deposition represents a phase separation of the polyalkenoic acid copolymer (from the other monomers) that reacted with calcium to form a calcium-polycarboxylate salt. Because this phase is rich in carboxylic groups, heavy metals from positive staining (lead citrate and uranyl acetate) are easily picked up, resulting in the heavily stained phase. Fragments of the phase are observed as black globules scattered in the adhesive resin (A). The hybrid layer shows an electron density that gradually becomes less intense toward the lab-demineralized intertubular dentin (I). R = resin tags; bar = 2 μm.

Fig 8-44 Atomic force microscopy tapping-mode images illustrating the resin-dentin interface produced by the one-bottle adhesive Excite (Vivadent). The phase-contrast image results from the interaction of the cantilever tip with the surface; it accentuates the loose collagen fibril arrangement within the hybrid layer with individual collagen fibrils separated by resin-filled interfibrillar spaces. The tubule wall hybridization is obvious.

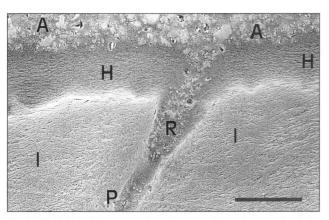

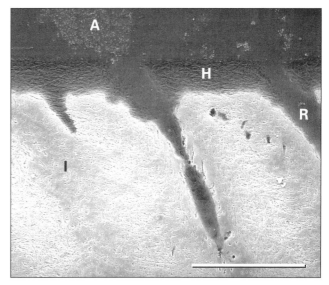

Fig 8-45 Field-emission scanning electron photomicrograph of the resin-dentin interface presented with the one-bottle adhesive Optibond Solo. A = adhesive resin; H = hybrid layer; I = intertubular dentin; P = peritubular dentin; R = resin tag (particle-filled); bar = 5 µm.

Fig 8-46 Field-emission scanning photomicrograph showing a diamond-sectioned interface produced by a two-step etch-and-rinse adhesive (Excite, Ivoclar Vivadent). Morphologically, no significant differences can be found between two- and three-step etch-and-rinse adhesives. A = adhesive resin; H = hybrid layer; I = intertubular dentin; R = resin tag; bar = 10 µm.

Acid Etchants. Generally, an etch-and-rinse procedure involves the use of phosphoric acid with a concentration between 30% and 40%[280] and an etching time of not less than 15 seconds. Washing times of 5 to 10 seconds are recommended to achieve the most receptive enamel surface for bonding.[39,218,281,282] The main objectives of acid conditioning are removing the smear layer (and smear plugs) and rendering enamel and dentin surfaces more receptive for bonding.

Historically, controversy existed about the concentration of phosphoric acid that would provide optimal etching efficacy, because some acids have been reported to form precipitates on the surface that might interfere with resin bonding.[4,283,284] One study showed that 50% phosphoric acid applied for 60 seconds on enamel produces a precipitate of monocalcium phosphate monohydrate that can be rinsed off. A precipitate of dicalcium phosphate dihydrate produced by etching with a less than 27% phosphoric acid was found not to be easily removed.[285] Calcium dissolution and etching depth increase as the concentration of phosphoric acid increases until the concentration reaches 40%; at higher concentrations, a reverse effect is obtained. Although most commercial etchants have concentrations between 30% and 40%, lower concentrations may be used without compromising enamel bond strengths.[286–289]

The etching time has also been reduced from the traditional 60-second application with 30% to 40% phosphoric acid to etching times as brief as 15 seconds. Several laboratory and clinical studies have demonstrated equivalent bonding effectiveness with etching times from 15 to 60 seconds.[40,290,291]

Adequate rinsing is an essential step. Rinsing times of 1 to 3 seconds on flat surfaces have been shown to provide for adequate bond and seal.[281,282] For preparations with more complex form, a rinse time of 5 to 10 seconds is recommended. The use of ethanol to remove residual water from the etched pattern has been reported to enhance the ability of resin monomers to penetrate the etched enamel surface irregularities.[39,292] Modern primers frequently contain drying agents, such as ethanol or acetone, with a similar effect.

In addition to phosphoric acid, other inorganic and organic acids (Fig 8-47) have been advocated for acid etching enamel and dentin and were supplied with specific commercial adhesives.

Conditioning Enamel. Bonding to enamel was established before dentin bonding, and the first bonding systems were intended for enamel only. This enamel bonding technique, known as the *acid-etching technique*, was invented by Buonocore[1] in 1955. He demonstrated a 100-fold increase in retention of small buttons of polymethylmethacrylate to incisors in vivo when enamel was etched with 85% phosphoric acid for 2 minutes. Enamel bonding agents were commonly based on bis-GMA, developed by Bowen[293] in 1962, or urethane dimethacrylate (UDMA) (Fig 8-48). Both monomers are viscous and hydrophobic and are often diluted with other

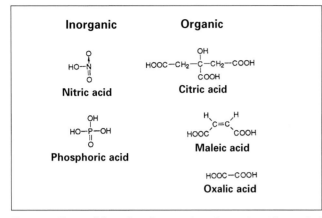

Fig 8-47 Chemical formulas of inorganic and organic acids supplied with etch-and-rinse adhesive systems.

monomers of higher hydrophilicity and lower viscosity, such as triethylene glycol dimethacrylate (TEG-DMA) and HEMA (see Fig 8-48).

Adhesion to enamel is achieved through acid etching of this highly mineralized substrate, which substantially enlarges its surface area for bonding. Further research into the underlying mechanism of the bond suggested that taglike resin extensions were formed and micromechanically interlocked with the enamel microporosities created by etching.[283,286,287]

Enamel etching transforms the smooth enamel surface into an irregular surface with a high surface-free energy (about 72 dynes/cm), more than twice that of unetched enamel.[24] An unfilled or filled liquid acrylic (hydrophobic) resin with low viscosity wets the high-energy surface and is drawn into the microporosities by capillary attraction. After light curing, the bond between enamel and the restorative material is established by polymerization of monomers inside the microporosities and by copolymerization of remaining carbon-carbon double bonds with the matrix phase of the resin composite, producing strong chemical bonds.[214] In addition, the potential for chemical interaction between specific monomers and the etched enamel surface cannot be excluded.[38,217]

Acid etching removes about 10 µm of the enamel surface and creates a microporous layer from 5 to 50 µm deep. Three enamel-etching patterns have been described.[296,297] These include type I, in which there is predominant dissolution of the prism cores; type II, in which there is predominant dissolution of the prism peripheries; and type III, in which no prism structures are evident (Figs 8-49a to 8-49c). Two types of resin tags have been described.[274,298] Macrotags are formed circularly between enamel prism peripheries; microtags are formed at the cores of enamel prisms, where the monomer cures within a multitude of individual crypts formed where

hydroxyapatite crystals have been dissolved (see Figs 8-35 and 8-36). Microtags probably contribute most to the bond strength because of their greater quantity and large surface area.

The effect of acid etching on enamel depends on several parameters[299,300] (see Fig 8-47):

- Type of acid used
- Acid concentration
- Etching time
- Form of the etchant (gel, semigel, or aqueous solution)
- Rinse time
- Method of activation of etching (rubbing, agitation, and/or repeated application of fresh acid)
- Whether enamel is instrumented before etching
- Chemical composition and condition of enamel
- Whether enamel is in primary or permanent teeth
- Whether enamel is prism-structured or prismless
- Whether enamel is fluoridated, demineralized, or stained

An acid gel is generally preferred over a liquid because its application is easier to control.[218]

In vitro shear bond strengths of resin composite to phosphoric acid–etched enamel typically average 20 MPa.[29,287,301] This bond strength is thought to be sufficient to resist the shrinkage stress that accompanies the polymerization of resin composites.[182] Consequently, if the preparation is completely bordered by enamel, acid etching significantly reduces microleakage at the cavosurface interface.[302,303] This enamel etching technique has proven to be a durable and reliable clinical procedure for routine applications in modern restorative dentistry. It is noteworthy that using a modern bond strength technique, ie, µTBS, the microtensile bond strength of an etch-and-rinse adhesive to dentin is commonly higher than that to enamel.[304] This should be attributed to the specific µTBS test set-up and the more brittle nature of enamel, causing adhesive-enamel microspecimens to fail in tension at lower loads than their adhesive-dentin counterparts.

Complete removal of the etchant and dissolved calcium phosphates and preservation of the clean etched field without moisture and saliva contamination are crucial to the longevity of the resin-enamel bond.[300] For this reason, isolation with a rubber dam is preferred over isolation with cotton rolls.[305]

Conditioning Dentin. Conditioning of dentin can be defined as any chemical alteration of the dentin surface by acids (or by a calcium chelator such as EDTA) with the objective of removing the smear layer and simultaneously demineralizing the dentin surface. The use of the term *conditioner* found its

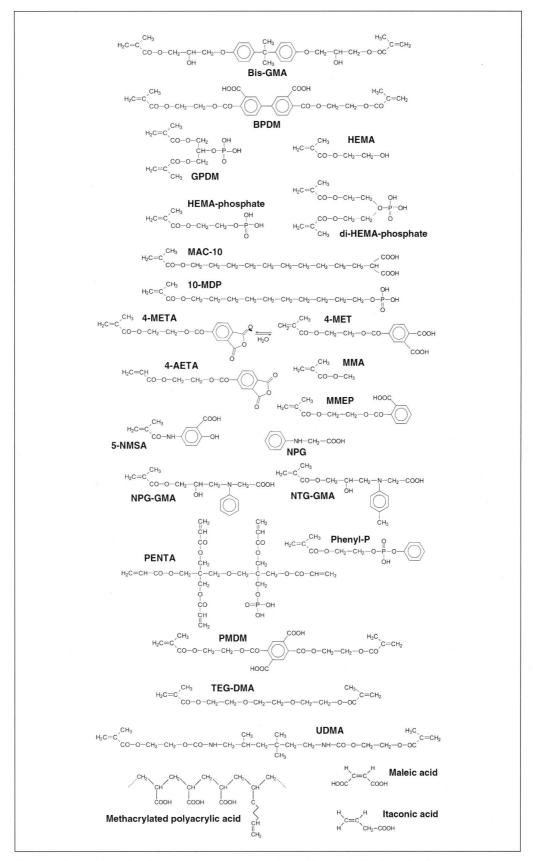

Fig 8-48 Chemical formulas of various monomers commonly used in dental adhesive technology.

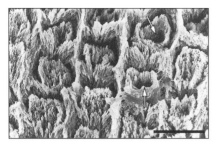

Fig 8-49a Type I enamel-etching pattern *(arrows)*. Etching of prism cores is predominant. Bar = 6 μm.

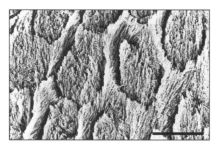

Fig 8-49b Type II enamel-etching pattern. Etching of prism peripheries is predominant. Bar = 6 μm.

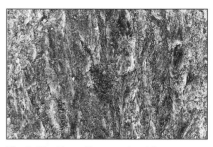

Fig 8-49c Type III enamel-etching pattern. No prism structures are evident. Bar = 6 μm.

origin in the early 1990s, when the application of acid etchants to dentin, particularly in the United States and Europe, was taboo because of its allegedly harmful effects on the underlying pulp. Conditioners are most commonly used as the initial step in the clinical application of etch-and-rinse (previously referred to as *total-etch*) systems and are therefore applied simultaneously to enamel and dentin following the so-called total-etch technique. Various acids, such as citric, maleic, nitric, and phosphoric acids, are supplied in varying concentrations with adhesive systems (see Fig 8-47). After clinical application, these conditioners are generally rinsed off to remove any acid remnants and dissolved calcium phosphates. The only exception was the nitric acid included in ABC Enhanced (Chameleon); the excess etchant was blown off without rinsing. However, this procedure was found to be unfavorable in regard to subsequent resin infiltration.[92,175]

In addition to removing the smear layer, this superficial demineralization process exposes a microporous scaffold of collagen fibrils (Figs 8-50 to 8-53), thus increasing the microporosity of intertubular dentin.[175] Because this collagen matrix is normally supported by the inorganic dentinal fraction, demineralization causes it to collapse[306,307] (Fig 8-54). On intertubular dentin, the exposed collagen fibrils are randomly oriented and are often covered by an amorphous phase with relatively few microporosities and of variable thickness (Fig 8-55). The formation of a relatively impermeable amorphous gel on top of the exposed collagen scaffold has been ascribed to the combined effect of denaturation and collapse of residual smear layer collagen.[31,175,307] Etchants thickened with silica leave residual silica particles deposited on the surface, but the silica does not appear to plug the intertubular microporosities[93] (see Fig 8-51). Sometimes fibrous structures, probably remnants of odontoblastic processes, are pulled out of the tubules and smeared over the surface (Fig 8-56).

The depth of demineralization of the dentin surface depends on several factors, such as the kind of acid and its application time, the acid concentration and pH, and the other components of the etchant such as surfactants, thickeners (silica vs polymer), and modifiers (Table 8-3). Parameters such as osmolality and viscosity may also be involved in the aggressiveness of demineralization.[91,93] The depth of demineralization also appears to be dependent on the distance between tubules: the closer the tubules, the deeper the demineralization. Because acid etching unplugs the dentinal tubules, acid is able to penetrate the tubule to a certain depth (see Figs 8-52 and 8-53). Even when applied to sclerotic dentin, the relatively aggressive phosphoric-acid etching procedure results in the formation of a loosely organized hybrid layer (Fig 8-57). With increasing aggressiveness of the conditioning agent, a circumferential groove may be formed at the tubule orifice, separating a cuff of mineralized peritubular dentin from the surrounding intertubular dentin (Fig 8-58). Alternatively, the mineralized peritubular dentin may be completely dissolved to form a funnel shape (Fig 8-59). In this case, the underlying collagen network, made up primarily of circular collagen fibrils, is exposed (Figs 8-60 and 8-61). The characteristic collagen banding is most visible in the tubule wall.

This demineralization process also changes the surface-free energy of dentin.[21] The high protein content exposed after conditioning with acidic agents is responsible for the low surface-free energy of etched dentin (44.8 dynes/cm), which differentiates it from etched enamel.[144] Wetting of such a low-energy surface is difficult, and adhesion is hard to achieve if the dentin surface energy is not increased by the use of surface-active promoting agents, or primers.[308]

Primers. Primers serve as the actual adhesion-promoting agents and contain hydrophilic monomers dissolved in solvents, such as acetone, ethanol, and/or water. Because of the volatile characteristics of acetone and ethanol, these solvents can displace water from the dentin surface and the moist collagen network, promoting the infiltration of monomers through the nanospaces of the exposed collagen network[309]

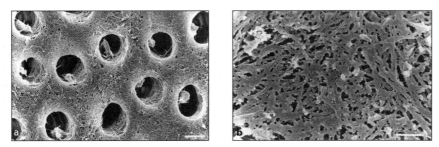

Figs 8-50a and 8-50b Field-emission scanning electron photomicrographs showing the effect of 10% phosphoric acid products All-Etch (Bisco) (a) and Ultra-Etch (Ultradent) (b) on dentin (top view). Note the exposed collagen fibril network almost completely denuded from hydroxyapatite. The pores represent the interfibrillar spaces that were occupied by hydroxyapatite and are now available for resin interdiffusion. The dentinal tubules were unplugged, and peritubular dentin was completely dissolved at the tubule orifices with exposure of circularly oriented collagen. Some remnants of odontoblastic processes remained inside the tubule orifices. Bar = 3 μm (a) and 500 nm (b).

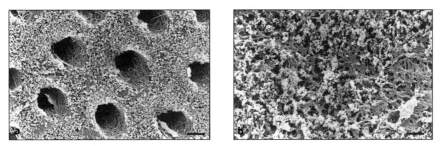

Figs 8-51a and 8-51b Field-emission scanning electron photomicrographs showing the effect of 36% phosphoric acid (DeTrey Etch) on dentin (top view). Note the deposition of silica particles that remained from the acid etchant (thickener) despite it having been thoroughly rinsed off. Nevertheless, higher magnification (b) disclosed that the interfibrillar spaces remained penetrable for resin. Bar = 2 μm (a) and 0.5 μm (b).

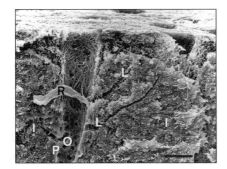

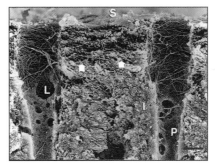

Fig 8-52 Field-emission scanning electron photomicrograph showing the effect of 37% phosphoric acid on dentin (lateral view). Intertubular dentin (I) was etched to a depth of about 2 to 3 μm. The acid penetrated the opened dentinal tubules, exposing primarily circularly oriented collagen fibrils at the dentinal tubule walls. L = lateral tubule branch; O = lateral tubule branch orifice; P = peritubular dentin; R = remnant of odontoblastic process; bar = 3 μm.

Fig 8-53 Field-emission scanning electron photomicrograph demonstrating the effect of 37.5% phosphoric acid (Kerr) on dentin (lateral view). Dentin was demineralized up to a depth of 4 to 5 μm (arrows). The tubule orifice was funneled, with peritubular dentin (P) completely dissolved to a depth of about 6 to 7 μm. I = intertubular dentin; L = orifices of lateral tubule branches; S = silica remaining from the acid etchant; bar = 2 μm.

(see Figs 8-50 to 8-53 and 8-60). Effective primers contain monomers with hydrophilic properties that have an affinity for the exposed collagen fibril arrangement and hydrophobic properties for copolymerization with the adhesive resin.[21] The objective of this priming step is to transform the hydrophilic dentin surface into a hydrophobic and spongy state that allows the adhesive resin to wet and penetrate the exposed collagen network efficiently.[20,163,310,311]

After conditioning, the demineralized collagen network is susceptible to collapse when water is removed by drying. Collapse and subsequent shrinkage of collagen can lead to suboptimal resin infiltration. Depending on the primer, two

213

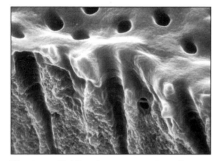

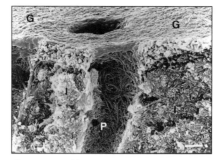

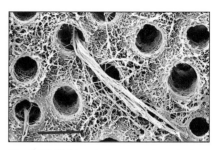

Fig 8-54 Field-emission scanning electron photomicrograph giving a lateral view of phosphoric acid–etched dentin. The exposed collagen network is susceptible to shrinkage and has collapsed due to air drying. Note that no interfibrillar spaces are left and that subsequent resin infiltration will be hindered.

Fig 8-55 Field-emission scanning electron photomicrograph demonstrating the effect of 10% phosphoric acid (All-Etch, Bisco; 15 sec) on dentin (lateral view). Note the formation of a residual smear gel (G) with few microporosities on top of the exposed collagen fibril scaffold. I = intertubular dentin; P = peritubular dentin; bar = 1 μm.

Fig 8-56 Field-emission scanning electron photomicrograph demonstrating the effect of Non-Rinse Conditioner (Dentsply) on dentin (top view). Because of smear layer preparation, a bundle of intratubular collagen was pulled from the dentinal tubule and smeared over the exposed intertubular collagen fibril network. Bar = 5 μm.

Table 8-3	**Etchants ranked by demineralization potency**			
Etchant	**Composition**	**Etch time (sec)**	**pH**	**DID (μm)**
				< 2.0
Clearfil CA Agent (Kuraray)	10% citric acid, 20% calcium chloride	15	–0.10	0.5
Gluma 2000 Solution 1 (Bayer)	1.6% oxalic acid, 2.6% aluminum nitrate, 2.7% glycine	15	1.38	0.7
Mirage ABC Conditioner (Den-Mat)	2.5% nitric acid	15	0.42	0.7
Clearfil CA Agent (Kuraray)	10% citric acid, 20% calcium chloride	40	–0.10	0.9
Amalgambond Universal Dentin Activator (Parkell)	10% citric acid, 3% ferric chloride	10	0.59	1.3
Ultra-etch (Ultradent)	10% phosphoric acid	15	1.31	1.7
Ultra-etch	35% phosphoric acid	15	0.02	1.9
				2.0–3.0
Scotchbond Multi-Purpose Etchant	10% maleic acid	15	0.87	2.1
Mirage ABC Conditioner	2.5% nitric acid	60	0.42	2.2
Mirage ABC Conditioner	10% phosphoric acid	15	*	2.2
Ultra-etch	10% phosphoric acid	30	1.31	2.2
All-etch (Bisco)	10% phosphoric acid	15	0.48	3.0
All-etch without surfactantia (Bisco)	10% phosphoric acid	15	0.78	3.0
All-etch	10% phosphoric acid with surfactans	15	*	3.0
Scotchbond Etching Gel	35% phosphoric acid	15	–0.28	3.0
				> 3.0
Aqueous phosphoric acid solution	10% phosphoric acid	15	0.48	3.2
ESPE Etching Gel	32% phosphoric acid	15	*	3.9
Uni-Etch (Bisco)	32% phosphoric acid with surfactans	15	*	4.0
DeTrey Etch	36% phosphoric acid	15	–0.26	4.3
Mirage ABC Conditioner	10% phosphoric acid	30	*	4.5
Etch-Rite (Pulpdent)	38% phosphoric acid	15	–0.29	4.6
Uni-Etch	32% phosphoric acid	15	–0.17	4.8
Aqueous phosphoric acid solution	37% phosphoric acid	15	–0.43	5.0
Kerr Gel Etchant	37.5% phosphoric acid	15	*	5.6

pH = acidity; DID = depth of intertubular demineralization. From Perdigão.[93]

*pH values not available.

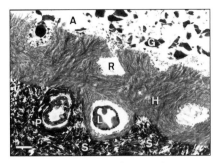

Fig 8-57 Transmission electron photomicrograph of a nondemineralized section demonstrating the resin-dentin interface produced by Optibond Dual Cure applied to sclerotic dentin (S). The hybrid layer (H) reveals a loosely organized collagen network with collagen fibrils separated by resin-filled interfibrillar spaces. Resin tags (R) are embedded in the hybrid layer as they run parallel with the interface. A = adhesive resin; G = glass filler of the particle-filled adhesive resin; L = mineralized remnants of the lamina limitans; P = peritubular dentin; bar = 1 μm.

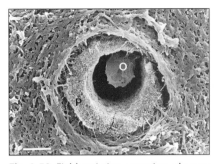

Fig 8-58 Field-emission scanning electron photomicrograph demonstrating the effect of 10% citric acid and 3% ferric chloride (Amalgambond Universal Dentin Activator, Parkell). The etchant was not potent enough to dissolve peritubular dentin (P). O = odontoblast process; bar = 1 μm.

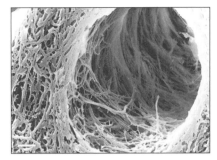

Fig 8-59 Field-emission scanning electron photomicrograph demonstrating the effect of 32% phosphoric acid (Uni-Etch, Bisco) on dentin (top view). The etchant was so aggressive that peritubular dentin was completely dissolved, exposing a circularly oriented network of collagen at the tubule orifice wall. Bar = 500 nm.

techniques (wet and dry bonding) have been proposed to overcome this problem.[272,312] This is discussed in the section on wet vs dry bonding.

HEMA, described as essential to the promotion of adhesion because of its excellent wetting characteristics,[310] is found in the primers of many modern adhesive systems. In addition to HEMA, primers contain other monomers, such as N-tolylglycine glycidyl methacrylate (NTG-GMA), pyromellitic acid diethylmethacrylate (PMDM), biphenyl dimethacrylate (BPDM), and dipentaerythritol penta acrylate monophosphate (PENTA) (see Fig 8-48). Some primers, such as those in All-Bond 2 (Bisco), OptiBond (Kerr), and Clearfil Liner Bond system (Kuraray), also include a chemical or photopolymerization initiator, so that these monomers can be polymerized in situ. More viscous primers, as provided by the so-called one-bottle adhesives, were developed to combine the priming and bonding function, simplifying the bonding technique (see Table 8-2 and Fig 8-33).

Primers have also been used to treat and prevent dentinal hypersensitivity,[313] which is believed to be caused by pressure gradients of dentinal fluid within patent tubules that communicate with the oral environment.[62,314] Primers may induce denaturation and precipitation of proteins from the dentinal fluid and, consequently, decrease dentinal permeability and outward flow of pulpal fluid, reducing the clinical symptoms of hypersensitivity.[313]

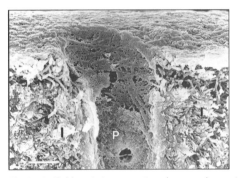

Fig 8-60 Field-emission scanning electron photomicrograph showing a dentin surface etched with 10% phosphoric acid followed by the application of Permagen (Ultradent) primer. The primer did not plug the tubules; the individual collagen fibrils were coated by resin. I = intertubular dentin; P = peritubular dentin; bar = 1 μm.

Adhesive Resin. The adhesive resin, also called the *bonding agent*, is equivalent to former enamel bonding agents and consists primarily of hydrophobic monomers, such as bis-GMA and UDMA, and TEG-DMA as a viscosity regulator, and more hydrophilic monomers, such as HEMA as a wetting agent (see Fig 8-48). The major role of the adhesive resin is to stabilize the hybrid layer and to form resin extensions into the dentinal tubules, called *resin tags* (Figs 8-40 and 8-61).

Adhesive resins can be light curing and/or autocuring. Autocuring adhesive resins have the theoretical advantage of

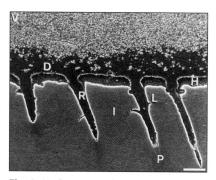

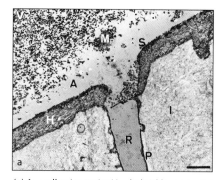

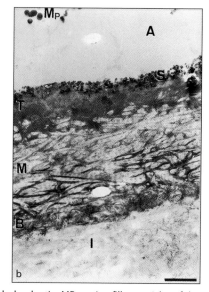

Fig 8-61 Scanning electron photomicrograph demonstrating the resin-dentin interface presented with Clearfil Liner Bond System after an argon-ion–beam etching technique.[32] D = dual-cured adhesive resin; H = hybrid layer; I = intertubular dentin; L = lateral tubule branch; P = peritubular dentin; R = resin tag; V = low-viscosity resin; bar = 5 μm. (From Van Meerbeek et al.[307] Reprinted with permission.)

Figs 8-62a and 8-62b *Transmission electron photomicrographs of a demineralized specimen showing the resin-dentin interface produced by Clearfil Liner Bond System. (From Van Meerbeek et al.[307] Reprinted with permission.)*

(a) A = adhesive resin; H = hybrid layer; I = intertubular dentin; MP = microfiller particles of the low-viscosity resin; P = peritubular dentin; R = resin tag; S = silica particles remaining from the acid etchant; V = low-viscosity resin; bar = 2 μm. *(b)* A = adhesive resin; B = base of the hybrid layer, containing resin-enveloped hydroxyapatite crystals; I = intertubular dentin; M = midzone of the hybrid layer, containing cross-banded collagen fibrils separated by tunnel-like interfibrillar spaces; MP = microfiller particles of the low-viscosity resin; S = silica particles remaining from the acid etchant; T = top of hybrid layer, representing a denatured collagen smear gel; bar = 500 nm.

initial polymerization at the interface due to the higher temperature produced by body heat[210] but the disadvantage of slow polymerization. For light-curing bonding agents, it is recommended that the adhesive resin be polymerized before the application of the restorative resin. In this way, the adhesive resin is not displaced, and adequate light intensity is available to sufficiently cure and stabilize the resin-tooth bond to resist the stresses produced by polymerization shrinkage of the resin composite.[21,203,315] Because oxygen inhibits resin polymerization,[202] an oxygen-inhibited layer of about 15 μm will always be formed on top of the adhesive resin, even after light curing. This oxygen-inhibited layer offers sufficient double MMA bonds (see Fig 8-48) for copolymerization of the adhesive resin with the restorative resin.

Hybridization. Hybridization, or the formation of a hybrid layer, is the process of resin interlocking in the demineralized dentin surface, thereby providing micromechanical retention. This term is commonly used for dentin bonding after acid etching, but it may also be expanded to the micromechanical interaction with enamel, as well as to the interaction layers produced by a self-etch adhesive to enamel and dentin (discussed later in this chapter).

Hybridization in dentin by an etch-and-rinse adhesive occurs following an initial demineralization of the dentin surface

with an acidic conditioner, exposing a collagen fibril network with interfibrillar microporosities that subsequently becomes interdiffused with low-viscosity monomers (Figs 8-62 and 8-63). This zone, in which resin of the adhesive system micromechanically interlocks with dentinal collagen, is termed the *hybrid layer* or *hybrid zone*.

Within the hybrid layer, three different layers or zones initially have been described.[307] With the Clearfil Liner Bond system, the top of the hybrid layer consists of an amorphous electron-dense phase, which has been ascribed to denatured collagen (see Figs 8-62 and 8-63).[307] A more loosely arranged collagen fibril arrangement is seen at the top of the hybrid layer with OptiBond and Super-Bond D-Liner; in this layer, individual collagen fibrils are directed toward the adhesive resin and the interfibrillar spaces are filled with resin (Figs 8-41 and 8-64). With Scotchbond Multi-Purpose and Single Bond (Scotchbond 1 in Europe) (3M ESPE), the hybrid layer was observed to be covered by an amorphous phase that has been attributed to a chemical reaction of a polyalkenoic acid copolymer of the primer with residual calcium (see Fig 8-43). The middle part of the hybrid layer contains cross-sectioned and longitudinally sectioned collagen fibrils separated by electronlucent spaces (see Fig 8-41b). These interfibrillar channels, which have typical dimensions of 10 to 20 nm, represent the areas in which hydroxyapatite crystals have been replaced by

Fig 8-63 Resin-impregnation phase. (From Van Meerbeek et al.[307] Reprinted with permission.)

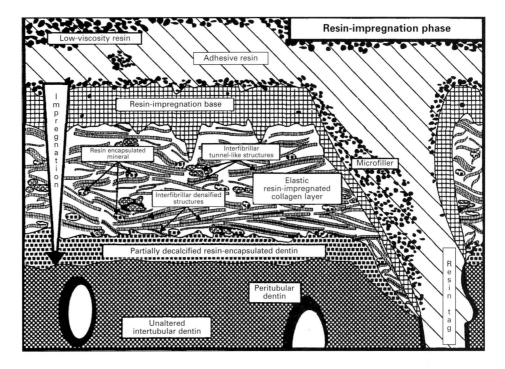

resin as a result of the hybridization process. Residual mineral crystals are sometimes scattered between the collagen fibrils (see Fig 8-62). The base of the hybrid layer is characterized by a gradual transition to the underlying unaltered dentin, with a partially demineralized zone of dentin containing hydroxyapatite crystals enveloped by resin (see Fig 8-62b) or by a more abrupt transition (see Figs 8-41 and 8-64).

This micromechanical bonding mechanism was first described by Nakabayashi et al[30] in 1982 as the formation of a resin-reinforced zone. It took researchers almost 10 years to accept this theory and to further explore this bonding mechanism.[31,93,175,307,316]

A number of questions remain as to which parameters are of primary importance to adhesive efficacy. First, little is known about the impact of collagen denaturation on the durability of the bond. In this respect, Nakabayashi[317] warned that denaturation of collagen by aggressive acid conditioning may cause bond failure in the long term. Evidence of such collagen denaturation was recorded by Shimokobe et al,[318] preliminarily, and by Okamoto et al,[319] when 37% and 40% phosphoric acid, respectively, were applied to demineralized dentinal collagen. Eick et al[175] related the presence of remaining cross banding of collagen fibrils inside the hybrid layer to intact undenatured collagen. However, an absence of collagen banding may also indicate that the fibril structure is in a destabilized state but not necessarily denatured to gelatin.[311,312] Another study using atomic-force microscopy (AFM) revealed the disappearance of the 67-nm banding of collagen after etching and air-drying.[321] Although it was explained as

evidence of denaturation of collagen, the fact that the effect was reversible with the reappearance of collagen banding after storage in water for 1 day most likely indicates that the disappearance of collagen cross banding may be due to contraction of the collagen fibrils. Recent research has provided new insights into the process of collagen disintegration and its immediate effect on bond degradation.[322,323] This will be discussed later in this chapter.

Another parameter in question is the formation of a relatively impermeable amorphous gel on top of the exposed collagen scaffold[31,93,175,307] that might prevent resin from fully penetrating the demineralized dentin. Although not consistently observed, this gel was ascribed to the combined effect of denaturation and collapse of residual smear layer collagen.[307] A brief application of a weak sodium hypochlorite solution has been suggested to remove the gel; this has preliminarily been found to have a favorable effect on dentin bond strength.[324] Others have used sodium hypochlorite to completely dissolve and remove the collagen layer to expose the underlying pure mineralized dentin, to which adhesives could then be bonded directly.[325,326] Because this procedure adds another step to an already technique-sensitive and time-consuming process, this approach was never adopted in routine clinical practice.

Concerns have been raised that aggressive etching of dentin may cause demineralization to a depth that might be inaccessible to complete resin impregnation. If this occurred, a collagenous band at the base of the hybrid layer, not impregnated by resin, would dramatically weaken the resin-

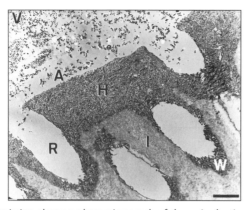

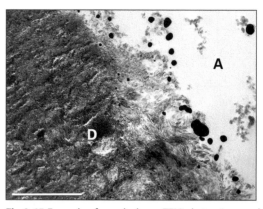

Fig 8-64 Transmission electron photomicrograph of the resin-dentin interface presented with Super-Bond D-Liner after demineralization. A = adhesive resin; H = hybrid layer; I = intertubular dentin; R = resin tag; V = low-viscosity resin; W = hybridized tubule wall; bar = 2 μm.

Fig 8-65 Example of nanoleakage. TEM photomicrograph of a nondemineralized dentin section stained with silver nitrate. Due to its low molecular weight, silver nitrate is capable of penetrating into very small spaces. Such silver tracers are therefore used to search for submicron gaps within the hybrid layer. A = adhesive resin; D = dentin; bar = 2 μm.

dentin bond and, consequently, its durability.[309,319] Incomplete resin penetration has been described as causing a microporous dentinal zone at the base of the hybrid layer[277,328] that is thought to be a pathway for nanoleakage of fluids (Fig 8-65), causing hydrolysis of collagen and a reduction in the longevity of the bond. Microporosities in the hybrid layer have been demonstrated by TEM for some of the first-generation adhesives,[175] and imperfect resin penetration has been reported for some modern adhesive systems.[36,93,175,329] Other modern adhesive systems have been reported to have better sealed interfaces.[275,276,300,331] Another parameter of primary importance to the strength and durability of the resin-dentin bond is the degree of polymerization conversion of resin that has infiltrated the superficially demineralized zone of dentin. Resin monomers might be able to penetrate the demineralized dentin, but if inadequate in situ polymerization occurs, the longevity of the resin-dentin bond may be compromised. The degree of polymerization inside the hybrid layer will depend on the mode of polymerization (light-activated, chemically activated, or both), the site of initial polymerization (interfacial or originating in the adhesive resin), the degree of in situ available double-carbon bonds, and the potential presence of polymerization-inhibiting substances. Besides less degradation-resistant bonding, inadequate in situ polymerization within the hybrid layer may also act as a reservoir for monomer release and thus have cytotoxic potential.[332,333] Finally, water or residual solvent may interfere with optimal hybridization. Water is already present in the hybrid layer. It is also introduced when a wet-bonding technique is used or a water-containing adhesive is applied. In addition, residual amounts of solvents such as ethanol or acetone, if not completely evaporated, may affect resin polymerization inside the

hybrid layer or at least occupy space that optimally should be filled with resin.[309] Water absorbed from the tooth substrate or from the moist oral environment also has a detrimental effect on the bond durability.[323] This will be discussed further in the section on dealing with bond durability and degradation.

All of these concerns in relation to hybridization require consideration and further research, because they will eventually determine the quality of the hybrid layer and consequently the hydrolytic stability of the resin-dentin bond in the oral environment.[66,323]

Resin tag formation. In dentin, the smear layer and smear plugs are removed by acid conditioning and the low-viscosity adhesive resin flows into the dentinal tubules. The polymerized resin extensions are also called *resin tags*.

The formation of resin tags in enamel is considered critical to bond strength, but the contribution to the bond of resin tags in dentin has been a matter of speculation.[50,143,145] Bond strength values drop in deeper dentin where the number and size of dentinal tubules is greater and intertubular dentin occupies less of the total bonding area. This indicates that the presence of intertubular dentin is more important to the bond than the development of resin tags.[96,147,150]

Dentinal resin tags have been observed with cores of resin surrounded by hybridized tubule walls (Figs 8-41, 8-42, 8-64, and 8-66). This phenomenon has been termed *tubule wall hybridization*. It provides a firm attachment of the resin tag to the tubule walls and aids in sealing the tubules and protecting the pulp.

Resin also infiltrates lateral tubule branches and hybridizes their walls (Figs 8-42 and 8-67). A similar attachment of resin tags to the tubule walls through hybridization has been de-

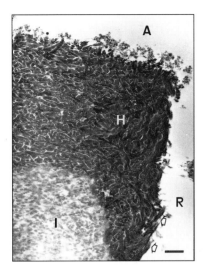

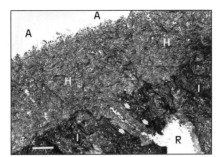

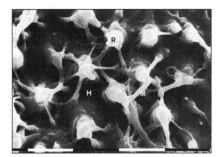

Fig 8-66 Transmission electron photomicrograph of a demineralized section demonstrating the resin-dentin interface produced by Optibond Dual Cure (Kerr). The loosely organized hybrid layer (H) typically contains collagen fibrils separated by resin-filled interfibrillar spaces and extends triangularly into the tubule wall area *(open arrows)*. This tubule wall hybridization firmly attaches the resin tag (R) to the tubule orifice wall and most importantly contributes to a hermetic seal of the tubule. A = adhesive resin; I = lab-demineralized intertubular dentin; bar = 500 nm.

Fig 8-67 Transmission electron photomicrograph of a nondemineralized section demonstrating the resin-dentin interface produced by Optibond Dual Cure. Note the formation of a micro–resin tag *(arrows)* into a lateral tubule branch. A core of resin is surrounded by a hybridized wall (lateral tubule hybridization). A = adhesive resin; H = hybrid layer; I = intertubular dentin; R = resin tag; bar = 1 µm. (From Van Meerbeek et al.[334] Reprinted with permission from Elsevier Science.)

Fig 8-68 Scanning electron photomicrograph of a specimen in which dentin was removed during processing, illustrating the tubule anastomosis concept, as observed with Scotchbond Multi-Purpose. H = hybrid layer, observed from below; M = micro–resin tag in lateral tubule branch; R = resin tag. (From Chappell et al.[335] Reprinted with permission.)

scribed to occur in vivo.[331] The formation of submicron resin tags in lateral tubule branches has also been elegantly illustrated with the tubule anastomosis concept introduced by Chappell et al[335] (Fig 8-68). Such resin tags, which appear to adapt intimately to the inner tubule walls, probably contribute to dentin bonding.[36] In this respect, 15% of the bond strength to dentin obtained with one specific adhesive was ascribed to resin tag formation.[72]

Three-step versus two-step etch-and-rinse. The first effort at simplification of conventional three-step adhesives was to combine the primer and adhesive resin, resulting in two-step etch-and-rinse adhesives (see Fig 8-33). Perdigão et al[336] concluded that the adhesive effectiveness of one-bottle adhesives was unpredictable and highly dependent on the adhesive tested. Labella et al[337] reported that the adaptation of dentin margins in Class 5 restorations was significantly inferior for the one-bottle adhesive OptiBond Solo (Kerr) compared to its three-step precursor OptiBond FL. No differences in marginal adaptation were observed, however, for Single Bond as compared to Scotchbond Multi-Purpose. At the enamel margins, the adaptation did not differ for all four adhesives tested. Blunck and Roulet[338] concluded from their quantitative margin analysis study that some one-bottle adhesives achieved marginal adaptation comparable to that of multibottle adhesives. However, the results obtained with the one-bottle adhesives appeared less consistent than those recorded for multistep adhesives. In general, one-bottle adhesives appear to perform as well as three-step adhesives when bonding to enamel, whereas bonding to dentin still appears to require treatment with a separate application of primer and adhesive. In both in vitro and clinical studies, three-step etch-and-rinse adhesives have demonstrated superior performance compared to two-step etch-and-rinse adhesives.[339–341] The latter are also associated with greater technique sensitivity than their three-step counterparts.[342] Moreover, after aging procedures in durability studies, the bonding integrity of three-step etch-and-rinse adhesives is better maintained.

Therefore, three-step etch-and-rinse adhesives are often considered as the standard. Because two-step etch-and-rinse adhesives do not save time or improve performance, their use is less recommended.

Etch-and-Rinse Adhesives

Three-step etch-and-rinse adhesives

Advantages
- Separate application of conditioner, primer, and adhesive resin
- Low technique sensitivity
- Proven effectiveness of adhesion to enamel and dentin in vitro and in vivo
- Most effective and consistent results
- Best long-term results
- Possibility for particle-filled adhesive ("shock absorber")

Disadvantages
- Risk of overetching dentin (highly concentrated phosphoric-acid etchants), resulting in incomplete resin infiltration
- Time-consuming three-step application procedure
- Postconditioning rinsing required (risk of surface contamination)
- Sensitive to overwet or overdry dentin surface conditions (collagen collapse)
- Weak resin-collagen interaction (which may lead to nanoleakage and early bond degradation)
- Elaborate application procedure

Two-step etch-and-rinse ("one-bottle") adhesives

Advantages
- Basic features of three-step systems
- Simpler application procedure
- Possibility for single-dose packaging
- Consistent and stable composition
- Controlled solvent evaporation (when provided in single-dose packaging)
- Hygienic application (to prevent cross contamination)
- Possibility for particle-filled adhesive ("shock absorber")

Disadvantages
- Application procedure not substantially faster (multiple layers)
- More technique sensitive (multiple layers)
- Risk of a bonding layer that is too thin (no glossy film, no stress-relieving "shock absorber," insufficiently polymerizable due to oxygen inhibition)
- Effects of etch-and-rinse technique
- Risk of overetching
- Postconditioning rinse phase required
- Sensitive to dentin wetness
- Weak resin-collagen interaction
- Collagen collapse
- Lower bonding effectiveness than for three-step etch-and-rinse adhesives in long-term studies

Self-Etch Approach

The self-etch approach is the most promising from a standpoint of user-friendliness and technique sensitivity. Self-etch adhesives do not require a separate etch-and-rinse step. The self-etch concept is not new; it was introduced with an earlier generation of Scotchbond 2–like systems (3M ESPE), such as ART Bond (Coltène), Ecusit Primer-Mono (DMG), and Syntac (Ivoclar Vivadent). However, these systems were advocated for dentin bonding only and therefore required selective enamel etching in a separate step. The current self-etch adhesives can be applied simultaneously on enamel and dentin. This involves a total-etch technique, but the use of the terms *etch-and-rinse* and *self-etch* is preferred to make a clear distinction between the two approaches.

Simplification of the clinical application procedure is obtained by reduction of application steps and by omission of a postconditioning rinsing phase. The clinical application time is reduced; in addition, omission of the etch-and-rinse step reduces the risk of errors during application and manipulation, referred to as *technique sensitivity*. Little is known, however, about the long-term effect of incorporating dissolved hydroxy-

apatite crystals and residual smear layer remnants within the bonding resin or the effects of residual primer/adhesive solvent within the interfacial structure. Residual solvent weakens the bond integrity, provides channels for nanoleakage, and may affect polymerization of the infiltrated monomers. Due to the acidic functional monomers, the resultant interfacial structure becomes more hydrophilic and thus more prone to hydrolytic degradation.[156,157]

A self-etch approach involves two- or one-step application procedures (see Fig 8-33). The self-etch effect is derived from monomers to which one or more carboxylic or phosphate acid groups are added.[275] Depending on the etching aggressiveness, they can be subdivided into strong, intermediary strong, and mild self-etch adhesives (Fig 8-69).

Strong self-etch adhesives usually have a pH of 1 or less (Table 8-4). This high acidity results in rather deep demineralization effects. In enamel, the resulting acid-etch pattern resembles that of a phosphoric-acid treatment using an etch-and-rinse approach.[345,346] In dentin, collagen is exposed and nearly all hydroxyapatite is dissolved (Figs 8-70 to 8-73). Consequently, the underlying bonding mechanism of strong

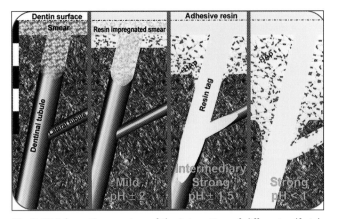

Fig 8-69 Schematic overview of the interaction of different self-etch adhesives with dentin (bar at left represents approximately 5 μm). *(Left)* Unaffected dentin is covered by a smear layer. *(Right)* Interaction of three classes of self-etch adhesives with dentin and the smear layer. Because mild self-etch adhesives do not completely remove the smear layer, a relatively thin submicron hybrid layer is formed without resin tags. The intermediary strong self-etch adhesives remove the smear layer along with a shallow demineralization of dentin. Short resin tags (±10 μm) are formed, and a limited lateral wall hybridization takes place. In the bottom third of the hybrid layer, not all hydroxyapatite crystals have been dissolved. The micromorphologic aspect of strong self-etch adhesives is very similar to that of etch-and-rinse adhesives and is characterized by a 3- to 5-μm-thick hybrid layer, dentinal tubule funneling, extensive resin tags, and tubule wall and lateral tubule wall hybridization. (From De Munck et al.[322] Reprinted with permission.)

Table 8-4	Acidity (pH) of diverse adhesive solutions	
Adhesive	**Classification**	**pH primer***
Adper Prompt L-Pop (3M ESPE)	One-step self-etch	0.4
Prompt L-Pop 2 (3M ESPE)	One-step self-etch	0.8
Xeno III (Dentsply)	One-step self-etch	1.4
i-Bond (Heraeus Kulzer)	One-step self-etch	1.6
Non-Rinse Conditioner (Dentsply)	Two-step self-etch	1.0
AdheSE primer (Ivoclar Vivadent)	Two-step self-etch	1.4
OptiBond Solo Plus SE primer (Kerr)	Two-step self-etch	1.5
Clearfil SE Bond primer (Kuraray)	Two-step self-etch	1.9
Clearfil Protect Bond primer (Kuraray)	Two-step self-etch	2.0
Unifil Bond primer (GC)	Two-step self-etch	2.2
Panavia ED mixed primer (Kuraray)	Two-step self-etch	2.6
OptiBond Solo Plus primer/adhesive (Kerr)	Two-step etch-and-rinse	2.1
Prime&Bond NT primer/adhesive (Dentsply)	Two-step etch-and-rinse	2.2
Scotchbond 1 primer/adhesive (3M ESPE)	Two-step etch-and-rinse	4.7
OptiBond FL primer (Kerr)	Three-step etch-and-rinse	1.8

*Measured in-house using a digital pH meter (Inolab pH Level 2, WTW).

self-etch adhesives is primarily diffusion-based, similar to that of the etch-and-rinse approach. Hybrid layers reach a thickness of 3 to 4 μm and have the typical interfacial characteristics of a loosely organized collagen fibril network with individual fibrils separated by interfibrillar spaces ("shag-carpet" appearance) (Figs 8-71 and 8-72) at the top of the hybrid layer, tubule wall hybridization, and lateral tubule hybridization. Despite the fact that strong self-etching primers are not rinsed off, their interfacial ultramorphologic features closely resemble those of etch-and-rinse systems that use phosphoric acid.

However, the low-pH self-etch adhesives have often been shown to have rather low bond strength values, especially to dentin, and quite a high number of so-called pretesting failures when tested using a microtensile bond strength method.[322,339,340] Besides the high initial acidity that appears to dramatically weaken the bonding performance, another concern is the effect of residual solvent (water) that remains within the adhesive interface and cannot be removed completely. Further study is required to investigate the long-term stability of this strong self-etch approach.

In general, mild self-etch systems have a pH of around 2 (see Table 8-4) and demineralize dentin no deeper than 1 μm (Figs 8-74 to 8-79). This superficial demineralization is incomplete, leaving residual hydroxyapatite still attached to collagen. Nevertheless, sufficient surface porosity is created to obtain micromechanical interlocking through hybridization. The thickness of the hybrid layer is much less than that of the strong self-etch or etch-and-rinse approach, but this has not proven to be important with regard to actual effectiveness of the bond.[322,339,340] The preservation of hydroxyapatite within the submicron hybrid layer may serve as a receptor for additional chemical bonding.[38,345] Carboxylic acid–based monomers, such as 4-methacryloxyethyl trimellitic acid (4-MET), and phosphate-based monomers, such as 2-methacryloxyethyl phenyl hydrogen phosphate (phenyl-P) and 10-methacryloxydecyl dihydrogen phosphate (10-MDP), have chemical bonding potential to the calcium in the residual hydroxyapatite.[38] The weak self-etching effect offers potential advantages: *(1)* dissolution of the smear layer resulting from cavity preparation, *(2)* micromechanical interlocking within etch pits in enamel, and *(3)* shallow micromechanical inter-

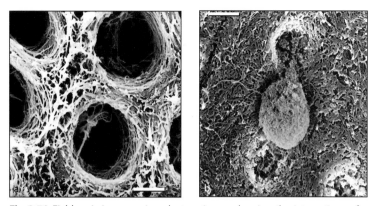

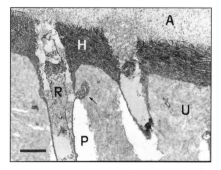

Fig 8-70 Field-emission scanning electron image showing the interactions of a strong (a) and a mild (b) self-etch primer. The strong self-etch primer (Non-Rinse Conditioner) of Prime&Bond NT (Dentsply/Detrey) has removed the smear layer and smear plugs, while exposing the collagen network and widening of the tubule orifices. Conversely, the interaction of the mild self-etch primer of Clearfil Liner Bond 2 (Kuraray) is clearly less intense (b), as very little collagen is exposed and most of the tubules remain occluded with smear plugs. Bar = 2 μm.

Fig 8-71 Transmission electron photomicrograph of a stained, demineralized section showing the interface between dentin and the strong self-etching adhesive Non-Rinse Conditioner/Prime&Bond NT. The acid-resistant 3-μm hybrid layer (H) shows a typical loose organization with collagen fibrils separated by resin-filled interfibrillar spaces. The nanofiller of the adhesive resin (A) did not infiltrate inside the collagen fibril network. Note the lateral tubule hybridization (arrow) with a micro–resin tag surrounded by acid-resistant hybridized lateral tubule walls. U = unaffected lab-demineralized intertubular dentin; P = peritubular dentin that was completely dissolved by the formic-acid lab demineralization process and replaced by epoxy embedding resin; R = resin tag encapsulating remnants of the odontoblastic process or lamina limitans; bar = 1 μm.

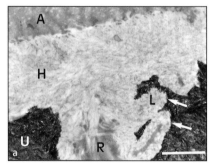

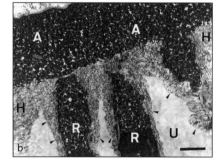

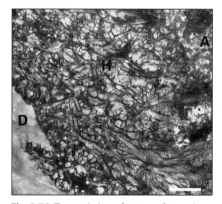

Figs 8-72a and 8-72b Transmission electron photomicrographs illustrating the interface between dentin and the strong self-etching adhesive Prompt L-Pop 1: (a) unstained, nondemineralized section and (b) stained demineralized section. The adhesive resin (A) appears gray in (a) and stains strongly black in (b) due to the phosphate-based composition. As a consequence, the labeled resin can be tracked to the deepest parts of the hybrid layer (H). The hybrid layer is loosely organized with cross- and longitudinally sectioned collagen fibrils separated by resin-filled (black) interfibrillar spaces. Note the extensive tubule wall hybridization (black arrowheads in [b]) and lateral tubule hybridization (white arrows in [a]), revealing that despite the self-etching approach, the adhesive interacted aggressively with dentin, resulting in an interfacial ultrastructure that resembles that typically produced by etch-and-rinse adhesives. A "shag-carpet" appearance can be observed at the transition of the hybrid layer to the adhesive resin. The adhesive resin shows some phase separation between the hydrophobic (methacrylate) and hydrophilic (phosphate) components. L = lateral tubule branch; R = resin tag; U = unaffected intertubular dentin; bar = 2 μm (a) and (b).

Fig 8-73 Transmission electron photomicrograph of a stained demineralized section through the resin-dentin interface produced by a strong one-step self-etch adhesive, Adper Prompt (3M ESPE). Dentin has been relatively deeply demineralized, and no hydroxyapatite crystals remain in the hybrid layer. The demineralization front has stopped abruptly. This image greatly resembles the morphologic aspect of an etch-and-rinse adhesive. A = adhesive resin; H = hybrid layer (±4 μm); D = lab-demineralized dentin; bar = 1 μm.

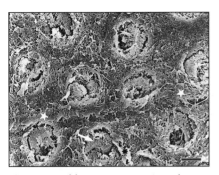

Fig 8-74 Field-emission scanning electron photomicrograph of dentin exposed to Clearfil Liner Bond 2 self-etching primer (Kuraray). Although collagen was partially exposed, residual smear layer remnants were still detected on the surface *(white stars)*, and the dentinal tubules were not completely unplugged *(arrow)*. Bar = 2 μm.

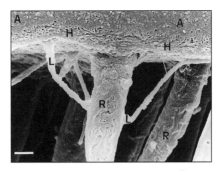

Fig 8-75 Field-emission scanning electron photomicrograph of the resin-dentin interface produced by Clearfil Liner Bond 2 when dentin was completely removed during lab processing. Note that although the tubules were not completely unplugged during the self-etching process, resin tags (R) were formed that incorporated the dissolved smear plugs, together with lateral micro–resin tags (L). The submicron hybrid layer (H) can hardly be detected. A = adhesive resin; bar = 1 μm.

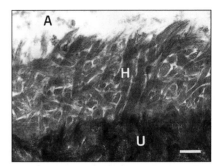

Fig 8-76 Transmission electron photomicrograph of a stained, nondemineralized TEM section illustrating the resin-dentin interface produced by the pioneer of self-etching adhesives, Clearfil Liner Bond 2. An average 0.7-μm-thick hybrid layer (H) consists of cross- and longitudinally sectioned collagen fibrils separated by resin-filled interfibrillar spaces of 10 to 20 nm. A typical "shag-carpet" appearance is formed by collagen fibrils that are directed toward the silica-filled adhesive resin (A) with ends often unraveled into their microfibrils. The transition of the hybrid layer to the unaffected dentin (U) is distinct. Bar = 200 nm.

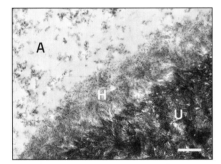

Fig 8-77 Transmission electron photomicrograph of an unstained, nondemineralized section illustrating the interface between dentin and the "moderate" self-etching adhesive Clearfil Liner Bond 2V. A hybrid layer (H) with an average depth of 600 nm was formed with only partial demineralization and exposure of collagen fibrils (not visible because this section was not stained). Hydroxyapatite crystals are clearly scattered within the hybrid layer. A = adhesive resin (particle-filled); U = unaffected intertubular dentin; bar = 500 nm.

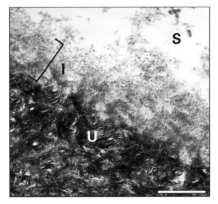

Fig 8-78 Transmission electron photomicrograph of a nondemineralized dentin section, demonstrating the interface with Clearfil SE (Kuraray), a mild two-step self-etch adhesive. A rather shallow hybrid layer of 1 μm has been formed that is only partially demineralized (I), leaving hydroxyapatite crystals available within the hybrid layer. S = silica-filled adhesive; U = unaffected dentin; bar = 1 μm.

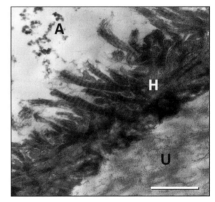

Fig 8-79 Transmission electron photomicrograph of a demineralized and stained section through the resin-dentin interface produced by Clearfil SE (Kuraray). Note the formation of a 1-μm-thick hybrid layer (H) and the typical "shag-carpet" appearance of individual collagen fibrils. These are easily recognizable because of their cross-banded appearance. A = adhesive resin; U = unaffected dentin; bar = 1 μm.

locking through hybridization in dentin. The exposed hydroxyapatite enamel surface and the hydroxyapatite crystals that remained around collagen may be particularly advantageous. They enable more intimate chemical interaction with the functional monomers on a molecular level and may help to prevent or retard marginal leakage phenomena. The challenge is to develop functional monomers that interact with hydroxyapatite in such a way that the resulting calcium-carboxylate or calcium-phosphate bonds are stable long-term within a hydrophilic environment. Retaining the hydroxyapatite may

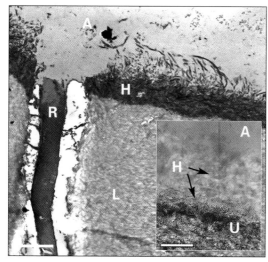

Fig 8-80 Transmission electron photomicrograph of a demineralized and stained section, demonstrating the resin-dentin interface produced by an intermediary strong self-etch adhesive, AdheSE (Ivoclar Vivadent). A relatively thick (2-μm) hybrid layer (H) and resin tags (R) are formed. The insert shows an unstained, nondemineralized TEM section, in which the dentin within the hybrid layer was not completely demineralized. A gradual transition between unaffected dentin (U) and completely demineralized dentin is visible in a small area in the bottom third of the hybrid layer, which still contains residual hydroxyapatite crystals. A = adhesive resin; L = lab-demineralized dentin; bar = 5 μm and 1 μm (insert).

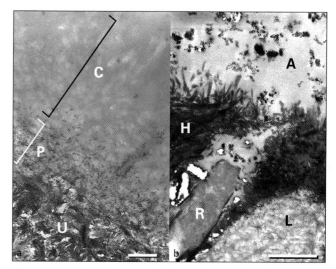

Fig 8-81 TEM photomicrographs of an unstained, nondemineralized section (a) and a stained, demineralized section (b) through the resin-dentin interface produced by the intermediary strong self-etch adhesive, OptiBond Solo Plus Self-Etch (Kerr). The hybrid layer (H) clearly has two zones, one without hydroxyapatite at the top of the hybrid layer and the other containing residual hydroxyapatite at the base of the hybrid layer. Staining disclosed a 2.5-μm-wide homogenous hybrid layer with a typical "shag-carpet" appearance at the transition to the adhesive. A = adhesive resin; C = complete hydroxyapatite depletion; P = partial hydroxyapatite depletion; U = unaffected dentin; L = lab-demineralized dentin; R = resin tags; bar = 1 μm (a) and 2 μm (b). (From Van Meerbeek et al.[98] Reprinted with permission.)

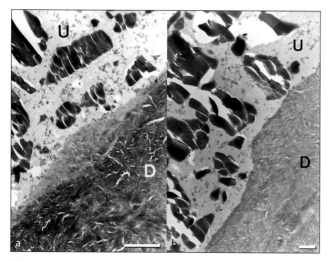

Fig 8-82 Unstained, nondemineralized TEM sections representing the cement-dentin interface when the self-adhesive luting material Unicem (3M ESPE) (U) was applied to bur-cut dentin (a) or to smear layer–free fractured dentin (b). When applied to bur-cut dentin, the gray intermediary zone probably represents the partial infiltration of Unicem components within smear deposited by the diamond on the dentin surface. When Unicem was applied to fractured dentin, it clearly appears to have interacted only very superficially. D = dentin; bar = 2 μm (a) and 1 μm (b). (From Van Meerbeek et al.[98] Reprinted with permission.)

also better protect collagen against hydrolysis and early degradation of the bond.[327,346,347] The weakest property of mild self-etch adhesives remains their bonding potential to enamel. Therefore, the development of monomers with stronger chemical bonding potential to hydroxyapatite is needed.[38]

Some new two-step adhesives, such as AdheSE (Ivoclar Vivadent) and OptiBond Solo Plus Self-Etch (Kerr), cannot be classified as mild or strong. The pH of their self-etching primers is about 1.5 (see Table 8-4), and based upon their interaction with dentin, we refer to them as *intermediary strong* (see Fig 8-69). These adhesives typically produce a dentinal hybrid layer with a completely demineralized top layer and a partially demineralized base (Fig 8-80). Following an etch-and-rinse approach or a strong self-etch approach, the transition of the exposed collagen fibril network to the underlying unaffected dentin is quite abrupt (see Figs 8-38, 8-41a, and 8-46). Following an intermediary strong self-etch approach, the deepest region of the hybrid layer still contains hydroxyapatite, and the transition of the hybrid layer to the underlying unaffected dentin is more gradual (Fig 8-81). These adhesives are more acidic than the mild self-etch adhesives, and better micromechanical interlocking is achieved in

Fig 8-83 Images of an experimental HEMA-free one-step self-etch adhesive. (*a* and *b*) Transmission electron photomicrographs show many droplets entrapped within the adhesive layer. As soon as the solvent starts to evaporate, a phase separation takes place between water and other adhesive ingredients, giving rise to water-filled droplets. These droplets slowly float toward the surface, and may coalesce to form bigger droplets. Upon light curing, they are trapped in the adhesive layer (A). O = oxygen inhibition layer; H = hybrid layer; U = unaffected dentin; bar = 10 µm (*a*) and 1 µm (*b*). (*c*) Light-microscopic image of a drop of uncured adhesive dispensed onto a glass plate. Note the multitude of droplets and the transparent droplet-free halo around the drop. (*d*) Scanning electron photomicrograph of enamel after microtensile bond strength (µTBS) testing, revealing many droplets within the adhesive layer (A). C = composite remnants; bar = 20 µm.

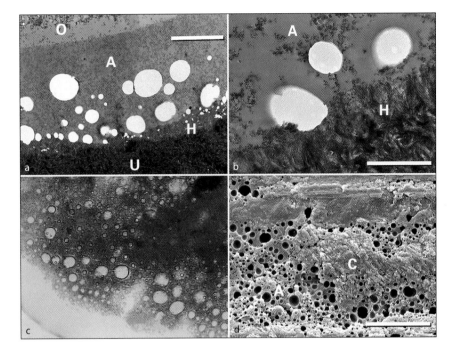

enamel as well as dentin. The residual hydroxyapatite at the hybrid layer base may still allow chemical intermolecular interaction, as was shown before for the mild self-etch adhesives. Based on their level of acidity (see Table 8-4), the one-step self-etch adhesives i-Bond (Heraeus Kulzer) and Xeno III (Dentsply) must also be categorized as intermediary strong self-etch adhesives. Their interfacial interaction is similar to that produced by the intermediary strong two-step self-etch adhesives discussed earlier.

A possible first step toward self-adhesive resin-based restorative materials is Unicem (3M ESPE). This luting material is designed to be applied without any pretreatment. TEM examination of the resultant interface showed only a superficial interaction with dentin (Fig 8-82). When applied to bur-cut dentin, a layer about 0.5 to 1 µm deep appeared less mineralized and most likely represented infiltration of Unicem components and a partially dissolved bur smear layer. This layer did not appear when Unicem was applied to fractured dentin that was free of cutting smear. In this case, the interaction of Unicem with dentin was hard to detect. The actual bonding mechanism of this self-adhesive cement has not been fully investigated.

One-step self-etch adhesives (1-SEAs) are user-friendly, but they have a number of shortcomings. They produce relatively low bond strengths compared to multistep self-etch and etch-and-rinse adhesives.[339,340,348,349] Due to their high hydrophilicity, cured 1-SEAs act as permeable membranes, per-

mitting water movement across the adhesive layer.[106,153–155] Reticular patterns of nanoleakage, so-called water trees, can be found within the adhesive layer of 1-SEAs and are sites of incomplete water removal, suboptimally polymerized resins, and dentinal fluid absorbed from the dentin substrate.[154] The relevance of these water trees remains unclear, but they may function as water ducts, contributing to accelerated degradation of tooth-resin bonds.[156,323,350–352] More recently, complex processes of phase separation have been shown to occur in one-component, HEMA-free self-etch adhesives[353] (Figs 8-83 and 8-84). The explanation for this phenomenon is probably found in the complex mixture of hydrophobic and hydrophilic components, dissolved in an organic solvent (usually ethanol or acetone). Gradual evaporation of solvent sets off the phase separation reaction, in which water probably separates from the other adhesive ingredients. Incorporation of droplets may contribute to bond degradation, and persistence of water in the adhesive layer may also adversely affect bond strength.

Glass-Ionomer Approach

Glass ionomers remain the only materials that are self-adhesive to tooth tissue, in principle without any surface pretreatment. Pretreatment with a weak polyalkenoic-acid conditioner significantly improves their bonding efficiency, however.[107] Hence, this glass-ionomer approach can be achieved following a one- or two-step application procedure (see Fig 8-33). The additional conditioning step is most important when a

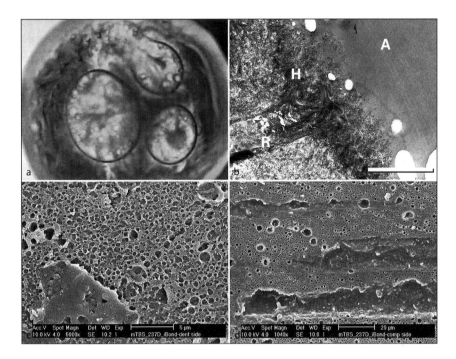

Fig 8-84 iBond, an unfilled, HEMA-free one-step self-etch adhesive. *(a)* Light-microscopic image of a drop of uncured adhesive, dispensed onto a glass plate, revealing a rather vigorous phase-separation reaction taking place. Note how bigger droplets in the top of the image coalesce. *(b)* TEM photomicrograph of a nondemineralized dentin section. Note the droplets trapped in the adhesive layer adjacent to the hybrid layer. A = adhesive resin; H = hybrid layer; R = resin tag; bar = 2 μm. *(c and d)* Field-emission scanning electron images of a dentin specimen after μTBS testing. Note that failure has occurred at the bottom of the adhesive layer, as the main part of the adhesive layer with the droplets is still attached to the resin-composite side of the μTBS specimen.

Self-Etch Adhesives

Two-step self-etch adhesives

Advantages

- No etching, postconditioning rinsing, or drying (which may be difficult to standardize)
- Time-saving application procedure
- Simultaneous demineralization and resin infiltration
- Less sensitivity to diverse dentin-wetness conditions
- Possibility for single-dose packaging
- Consistent and stable composition
- Controlled solvent evaporation (when provided in single-dose packaging)
- Hygienic application (unidose, to prevent cross contamination)
- Possibility for particle-filled adhesive ("shock absorber")
- Effective dentin desensitizer
- Separate adhesive resin (as compared to one-step adhesives)
- Better mechanical strength
- No complex mixtures of hydrophobic and hydrophilic components
- Good performance in vitro and in vivo, approaching bonding effectiveness of etch-and-rinse adhesives, in particular "mild" two-step self-etch adhesives

- Reported reduced postoperative sensitivity
- Excellent 3-year clinical performance for mild two-step self-etch adhesives

Disadvantages

- More elaborate application procedure than one-step solutions
- Incompatibility with autocuring composites (in particular low-pH self-etch adhesives)
- More long-term clinical research required
- Most self-etch systems contain water
- Water influences polymerization adversely
- Reduced shelf life (hydrolysis of monomers)
- Conflicting results in literature concerning bonding effectiveness to enamel, in particular for mild self-etch adhesives
- Bonding effectiveness very dependent on composition of adhesive solution
- High hydrophilicity (due to acidic monomers)
- Promotes water sorption
- Impaired durability

Self-Etch Adhesives *(continued)*

One-Step Self-Etch Adhesives

Advantages
- Most time-efficient application procedure
- No etching, postconditioning rinsing, or drying (which may be difficult to standardize)
- Simultaneous demineralization and resin infiltration
- Less sensitivity to diverse dentin-wetness conditions
- Possibility for single-dose packaging
- Consistent and stable composition
- Hygienic application (unidose, to prevent cross contamination)
- Possibility for particle-filled adhesive ("shock absorber")
- Possibility that phase separation in combination with strong air-blow may help to remove majority of water in adhesive

Disadvantages
- Complex mixes of hydrophobic and hydrophilic components, together with water and high concentrations of solvents

- Prone to phase separation and entrapment of droplets in adhesive layer (when not containing sufficient HEMA)
- More technique-sensitive
- No long-term clinical evaluation
- Less sealing capacity; acts as a semipermeable membrane
- Most self-etch systems contain water
- Water influences polymerization adversely
- Reduced shelf life (hydrolysis of monomers)
- High hydrophilicity (due to acidic monomers)
- Promotes water sorption
- Impaired durabilty
- Incompatibility with autocuring composites
- Insufficient long-term clinical research
- Conflicting results in literature concerning bonding effectiveness to enamel for mild self-etch adhesives
- Bonding effectiveness very dependent on composition of adhesive solution

Mild vs Strong Self-Etch Adhesives

Mild Self-Etch Adhesives (pH ≈ 2)

Advantages
- Hydroxyapatite crystals available within the hybrid layer (chemical interaction potential)
- Relatively good in vitro and in vivo bonding effectiveness

Disadvantages
- Insufficient bonding effectiveness to enamel (although improving)

Strong Self-Etch Adhesives (pH ≈ 1)

Advantages
- Good enamel bonding

Disadvantages
- No hydroxyapatite left throughout hybrid layer
- Reduced shelf life
- More hydrophilic
- Generally lower dentin bond strengths
- Incompatibility with autocuring composites

coarse cutting diamond is used and a thicker, more compact smear layer is produced. In general, a polyalkenoic-acid conditioner is applied for 10 to 20 seconds and then rinsed off, and the tooth is air-dried without dehydrating the surface (Figs 8-19 and 8-85). The polyalkenoic-acid pretreatment is much milder than a traditional phosphoric-acid treatment, and the exposed collagen fibrils are not completely denuded of hydroxyapatite (see Figs 8-20 and 8-85). The increase in bonding efficiency must be attributed to: *(1)* a cleaning effect, by which loose cutting debris is removed; *(2)* a partial demineralization effect, by which the surface area is increased and microporosities are created; and *(3)* chemical interaction of the polyalkenoic acid with residual hydroxyapatite. A network of hydroxyapatite-coated collagen fibrils interspersed with

pores is typically exposed up to 1 μm in depth. TEM and XPS examination have demonstrated that polyalkenoic-acid conditioners cannot be completely rinsed off.[354,355] Up to a 0.5-μm-thick layer, often referred to as the *gel phase,* remains attached to the tooth surface after the conditioner has been rinsed off (Fig 8-86).

The auto-adhesion of glass ionomers to tooth tissue is twofold in nature. First, micromechanical interlocking is achieved by shallow hybridization of the microporous, hydroxyapatite-coated collagen fibril network (see Figs 8-20, 8-85, and 8-86).[354–357] In this respect, glass ionomers can be considered as adhering to tooth tissue through a kind of mild self-etch approach. The basic difference with the resin-based self-etch approach is that glass ionomers are self-etching

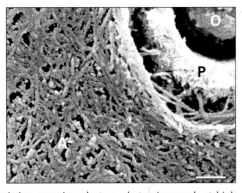

Fig 8-85 Field-emission scanning electron photomicrograph at high magnification of dentin surface conditioned with 20% polyalkenoic acid (A). Along with the removal of the smear layer, polyalkenoic acid superficially demineralizes intertubular dentin, thus exposing a microretentive collagen network. Note that although intertubular collagen was exposed, the fibrils have not been completely denuded of hydroxyapatite crystals. O = odontoblast; P = peritubular dentin; bar = 500 nm.

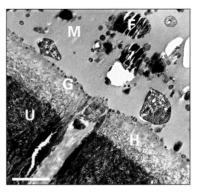

Fig 8-86 Transmission electron photomicrograph of an unstained, non-demineralized dentin section, showing the interaction of dentin with Fuji Bond LC (GC). A partially demineralized hybrid layer (H) of approximately 1 μm is formed. The remaining hydroxyapatite crystals within the hybrid layer function as receptors for chemical bonding with the carboxyl groups of the polyalkenoic acid. On top of the hybrid layer, an amorphous, gray gel phase (G) represents the reaction product formed through interaction of the polyalkenoic acid with calcium that was extracted from the dentin surface. M = resin-modified glass-ionomer matrix; F = resin-modified glass-ionomer filler; bar = 2 μm.

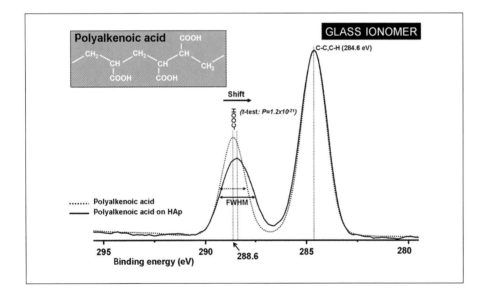

Fig 8-87 XPS narrow-scan spectra of the carbon atom (C 1s) region of the acrylic/maleic polyalkenoic acid copolymer and of the polyalkenoic acid applied on hydroxyapatite.[358] Interaction of the polyalkenoic acid with hydroxyapatite resulted in a significant shift of the peak representing the carboxyl groups (-COO⁻) to a lower binding energy, suggesting the formation of an ionic bond to hydroxyapatite. (From Van Meerbeek et al.[101] Reprinted with permission.)

through the use of a relatively high-molecular-weight (8,000 to 15,000) polycarboxyl-based polymer. Resin-based self-etch adhesives make use of acidic low-molecular-weight monomers.

As the second component of the self-adhesion mechanism, true primary chemical bonding occurs. Ionic bonds form between the carboxyl groups of the polyalkenoic acid and calcium of hydroxyapatite that remained around the exposed surface collagen (Figs 8-87 to 8-89). This was proven for polyalkenoic acids applied to hydroxyapatite,[358] but also to enamel as well as dentin.[359] The application of a polyalkenoic acid to synthetic hydroxyapatite (and dentin/enamel) produced a significant shift of the carboxyl (-COOH) peak to a lower binding energy, indicating that the carboxyl functional group

Fig 8-88 Deconvolution of the shifted carboxyl peak in Fig 8-88 disclosed a peak at 288.6 eV that represents unreacted carboxyl groups and a peak at 288.2 eV that results from carboxyl groups that bonded to calcium of hydroxyapatite.[358] (From Van Meerbeek et al.[101] Reprinted with permission.)

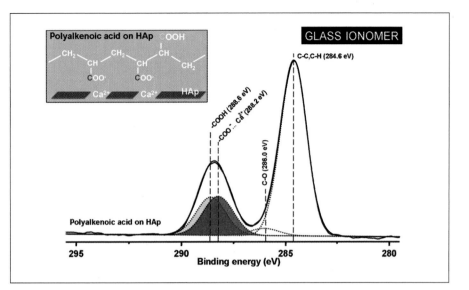

Fig 8-89a Schematic explaining that the shift of the peak representing the carboxyl group (-COO⁻) to a lower binding energy suggests the formation of an ionic bond to calcium of hydroxyapatite. (From Van Meerbeek et al.[98] Used with permission.)

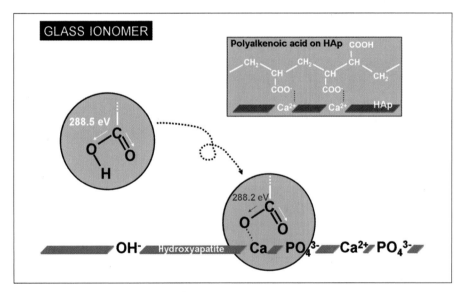

Fig 8-89b Schematic overview demonstrating the typical glass-ionomer reaction between the polyalkenoic acid and hydroxyapatite crystals in enamel and dentin. The multiple carboxylic groups of polyalkenoic acid will ionically bond to calcium, while an ion exchange process goes on. Research has confirmed that this bond is stable and that any decalcification process is rather limited.

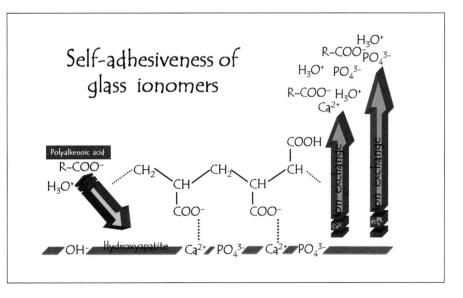

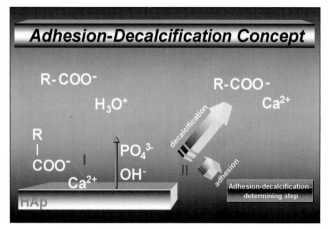

Fig 8-90 Schematic drawing presenting the adhesion-demineralization model that explains why molecules that contain functional carboxyl groups either adhere to or decalcify hydroxyapatite (HAp) tissues.[361] After adhesion to hydroxyapatite, molecules will remain attached to the hydroxyapatite surface depending on the solubility of the calcium salt in their own solution. The second phase is the adhesion-decalcification–determining step. (From Van Meerbeek et al.[98] Reprinted with permission.)

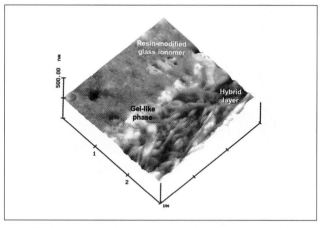

Fig 8-91 Atomic force photomicrograph demonstrating the interface formed at dentin by a glass-ionomer adhesive (Fuji Bond LC). The shallow hybrid layer of about 0.5 µm results from the short (10-second) application of a 20% polyalkenoic acid, by which collagen fibrils are exposed but not completely denuded of hydroxyapatite. The hydroxyapatite crystals remaining around the collagen fibrils serve as receptors for chemical bonding with the carboxyl groups of the polyalkenoic acid. On top of the hybrid layer, a 0.5-µm zone is demarcated from the glass-ionomer matrix. This phase represents the morphologic manifestation of a gelation reaction of the polyalkenoic acid with calcium that was extracted from the underlying dentin surface.

interacted with the hydroxyapatite surface (see Fig 8-87). This interaction was relatively strong, as this peak shift was recorded after ultrasonically rinsing off the polyalkenoic acid solution. This shifted peak at the XPS spectrum in Fig 8-87 represents the binding energy of the carbon atom (C 1s) of the carboxyl group, which is 288.6 eV for the unreacted polyalkenoic acid itself. This binding energy results from the two oxygen atoms that pull on the carbon atom. As explained in Fig 8-89b, when one of the oxygen atoms of the carboxyl functional group of the polyalkenoic acid reacts chemically with calcium of hydroxyapatite, it consumes energy to form an ionic bond with calcium of hydroxyapatite. Consequently, it will then pull less intensely to the carbon atom of the carboxyl group, reducing its binding energy to 288.2 eV. However, the carboxyl peak in Fig 8-87 did not shift entirely to 288.2 eV, indicating that not all carboxyl groups interacted with hydroxyapatite. In fact, deconvolution disclosed that the shifted peak consists of two subpeaks (see Fig 8-88), representing carboxyl groups that interacted with hydroxyapatite (subpeak at 288.2 eV) and those that did not (subpeak at 288.6 eV). It was also demonstrated that the actual molecular formula of the polyalkenoic acid significantly influences the chemical bonding potential.[358,359] XPS clearly showed that a polyalkenoic acid based upon 10:1 acrylic/maleic acid units

Glass-Ionomer Adhesives

Advantages
- Fast and simple application procedure (new liquid-liquid formulation)
- Viscous particle-filled adhesive ("shock absorber")
- Cariostatic/bacteriostatic potential by release of fluoride
- Twofold bonding mechanism
  - Ionic bonding to hydroxyapatite
  - Micromechanical bonding through hybridization
- Highest retention rates in clinical studies

Disadvantages
- Adequate adhesion to enamel requires smear layer removal
- Contains relatively coarse particles that may lead to white lines around restoration margins

has about two thirds of its carboxyl groups bonded to hydroxyapatite vs only half of the carboxyl groups of pure polyacrylic acid.[358,359] Based upon these XPS data,[358,360,361] a so-called adhesion-decalcification model has been proposed that explains why certain acids adhere to tooth structure rather than decalcify it (Fig 8-90). This largely depends on the solubility of the calcium salt that is formed at the hydroxyapatite surface. The more soluble the calcium salts of the acids (or of the adhesive monomer/polymer), the less it will adhere to the mineral substrate. The calcium salts of polyalkenoic acids are only slightly soluble, so they have an adequate chemical-bonding potential to hydroxyapatite-based tissues.

Typical of some glass ionomers is the morphologic manifestation of a gel phase at the interface, as was shown correlatively by TEM (see Fig 8-86) and AFM.[354,362] Correlating TEM and XPS data determined that this gel phase represents the formation of a calcium polycarboxylate salt resulting from either the polyalkenoic acid conditioner or the glass-ionomer material itself.[355] This phase is stable and strong between the shallow 0.5- to 1-μm hybrid layer and the glass-ionomer matrix. In microtensile bond strength testing, the interface typically fractured well above the gel phase within the matrix of the glass-ionomer material.[354] AFM surface analysis confirmed that this gel phase is stronger than the actual glass-ionomer matrix (Fig 8-91).[355] The actual function and contribution of this phase to the bond integrity requires further study.

Development of Adhesives: Chronological Classification

The chronological method of classifying adhesives, also called the "generational" classification system, is described below. This classification is described because it is still frequently referred to in the scientific and commercial literature, although it is inferior to the system already described. The original bonding agents evolved from simple to multistep systems, whereas recent developments have focused on simplification.[334] Only adhesives from the fourth to the seventh generation are currently on the market.

First-Generation Adhesives

Imitating his enamel acid-etching technique, Buonocore et al[363] in 1956 reported that glycerophosphoric acid dimethacrylate (GPDM) (see Fig 8-48) could bond to hydrochloric acid–etched dentin surfaces. However, the bond strengths to dentin attained with this primitive adhesive technique were only 2 to 3 MPa, compared to 15 to 20 MPa to acid-etched enamel, and the bond was unstable in water.[186] Predating Buonocore's experiments, investigators in the early 1950s

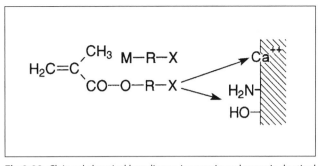

Fig 8-92 Claimed chemical bonding to inorganic and organic dentinal components. (From Asmussen and Munksgaard.[219] Reprinted with permission.)

used the same monomer, GPDM, with the introduction of Severiton Cavity Seal (Amalgamated Dental), an acrylic resin material that could be catalytically polymerized by the action of sulfinic acid.[364,365]

After the failures of this early dentin acid-etching technique, numerous dentin adhesives with complex chemical formulas were designed and developed with the objective of promoting chemical adhesion. Dentin bonding agents were no longer unfilled resins intended purely to enhance wetting of the dentin surface prior to the application of a stiff resin composite. They became bifunctional organic monomers with specific reactive groups that were claimed to react chemically with the inorganic calcium-hydroxyapatite and/or organic collagen component of dentin (Fig 8-92).[366] The traditional concept of molecules with chemical adhesive potential is based on a bifunctional molecule with a methacrylate group, M, linked to a reactive group, X, by an intermediary group, R, or spacer[163,186] (see Fig 8-92). While X is designed for reaction with and/or bonding to dentin, M allows the molecule to polymerize and copolymerize with resin composites. The spacer, R, must be of suitable length and polarity to keep the reactive groups separated.

The development of N-phenylglycine glycidyl methacrylate (NPG-GMA) (see Fig 8-48) was the basis of the first commercially available dentin bonding agent, Cervident (SS White).[367] This first-generation dentin bonding agent theoretically bonded to enamel and dentin by chelation with calcium on the tooth surface and had improved water resistance.[368,369]

Second-Generation Adhesives

Clearfil Bond System F (Kuraray), introduced in 1978, was the first of a large second generation of dentin adhesives that included Bondlite (Kerr/Sybron), J&J VLC Dentin Bonding Agent (Johnson & Johnson Dental), Dentin Adhesit (Ivoclar Vivadent), and Scotchbond (3M). These products were based on phosphorous esters of methacrylate derivatives. Their

Table 8-5	Chemical design of dentin adhesives with potential chemical bonding*
Potential Ca²⁺–bonding dentin adhesives	
M-R$_1$-POYZ	Phosphate group
M-R$_2$-NZ-R$_3$-COOH	Amino acid
M-R$_3$-OH	Amino alcohol
M-R$_4$-COOH	Dicarboxylic acid
^{1}COOH	
Potential collagen-bonding dentin adhesives	
M-R$_1$-NCO	Isocyanate group
M-R$_2$-COCl	Acid chloride
M-R$_3$-CHO	Aldehyde group
M-R$_4$-CO	Carboxylic acid anhydride
^{1}COOH	

*M = methacrylate; R$_{1-4}$ = variable spacers; Y, Z = variable substituents. From Asmussen and Hansen.[163] Reprinted with permission.

adhesive mechanism involved enhanced surface wetting as well as ionic interaction between negatively charged phosphate groups and positively charged calcium.[156,370] Although diverse chemical interactions were postulated with either the inorganic or the organic part of dentin (see Fig 8-92 and Table 8-5) and are theoretically possible, primary chemical adhesion is not thought to play a major role in the bonding process.[20,33,34,36,170,371–374] The second-generation systems had modest bond strengths, seldom exceeding 5 to 6 MPa.[163] In those instances in which higher bond strengths were measured,[28,30] other bonding mechanisms that were unknown at that time were probably involved. Clinical trials of these dentin bonding agents commonly met with poor results.[235,375–378] It was speculated that clinical failure was due to inadequate hydrolytic stability in the oral environment[379,380] and primary bonding to the smear layer rather than to the underlying dentin.[381] The presence of an intermediate smear layer prevents intimate resin-dentin contact, which is a prerequisite for a chemical reaction.[18]

Third-Generation Adhesives

The basis for the third generation of dentin adhesives was established when the Japanese philosophy of etching dentin to remove the smear layer gained acceptance.[382] This dentin acid-etching technique was discouraged in America and Europe until the end of the 1980s because of concerns that acid etchants would induce pulpal inflammation.[257,383–385] The postulated bonding mechanism of the dentin etching technique was that etched dentin would provide micromechanical retention for the restorative resin composite by allowing penetration of the resin bonding agent into the opened dentinal tubules. However, the counterpressure of dentinal

fluid and its abundant presence on the bonding site hindered the micromechanical attachment of the early hydrophobic resins.[50,145] Based on this total-etch concept, Clearfil New Bond (Kuraray) was introduced in 1984. It contained HEMA and 10-MDP (see Fig 8-48), which had long hydrophobic and short hydrophilic active components.

Removal of the smear layer by the use of acids or chelating agents reduces the availability of calcium ions for interaction with chelating surface-active comonomers, such as NPG-GMA (see Fig 8-48). In 1982, Bowen et al[28] tried to supplement the calcium ions by applying an acidic solution of 6.8% ferric oxalate to dentin as an acidic conditioner or cleanser. An insoluble precipitate of calcium oxalates and ferric phosphates was formed on the surface; the precipitate was also expected to seal the dentinal tubules and protect the pulp. The subsequent application of an acetone solution of PMDM mixed with NPG-GMA or its alternative, NTG-GMA (see Fig 8-48), improved bonding to levels of clinical significance.[369] Ferric oxalate sometimes caused black interfacial staining, however, and it was later replaced by aluminum oxalate.[386] But the microretention created by etching dentin probably contributes more to bonding than does the oxalate precipitation,[143] and the precipitate may, in fact, interfere with the interaction of adhesive and dentin.[31]

Extensive research in Japan has demonstrated a favorable effect of 4-META (see Fig 8-49) on bonding to dentin.[30,222,330] 4-META contains both hydrophobic and hydrophilic chemical groups. In 1982, Nakabayashi et al[30] used this system to describe the micromechanical bonding mechanism that is used by current adhesive systems. With this system, dentin is etched with an aqueous solution of 10% citric acid and 3% ferric chloride, followed by the application of an aqueous solution of 35% HEMA and a self-curing adhesive resin containing 4-META, MMA, and tri-n-butyl borane (TBB), the last as a polymerization initiator (see Fig 8-48). Based on this technology, adhesive systems such as C&B Metabond (Sun Medical), Super-Bond D-Liner, and Amalgambond Plus (Parkell) are commercially available and have been reported to yield consistent results in in vitro studies,[387,388] regardless of dentinal depth[152] (see Table 8-2).

Removal of the smear layer with chelating agents such as EDTA was introduced with Gluma. However, irrespective of the use of EDTA, the effectiveness of this system, as mentioned earlier, may have been impaired by the manufacturer's instructions to place the restorative resin composite over an uncured adhesive resin.[203,205,315] Denthesive (Heraeus Kulzer) also used EDTA to pretreat dentin prior to bonding.

Another approach to smear layer treatment was the use of Scotchprep (3M), an aqueous solution of 2.5% maleic acid and 55% HEMA, followed by the application of an unfilled bis-GMA/HEMA adhesive resin (see Figs 8-47 and 8-48 and Table 8-2). The simultaneous etching and impregnation of the dentin surface with this acidic hydrophilic monomer solution enabled more consistent and durable results.[205] In this way, Scotchbond 2 (3M) was in fact the precursor of current self-etch adhesives, although the self-etching primer Scotchprep at that time was advocated for use solely on dentin. Supported by excellent clinical results in diverse clinical trials,[389–391] Scotchbond 2 was the first product to receive provisional acceptance from the American Dental Association, which was followed by full acceptance.[392] Other systems, such as Coltène ART Bond, Superlux Universalbond 2 (DMG), and Syntac (Ivoclar Vivadent) are based on this smear layer–dissolving approach (see Table 8-2).

Other historically popular adhesives belonging to this generation were Prisma Universal Bond (Dentsply) and Tenure (Den-Mat).

Fourth-Generation Adhesives

Significant advances in adhesive dentistry were made with the development of the multistep dentin adhesive systems in the early to mid-1990s. Essential to the enhanced adhesive capacity and responsible for the improved clinical effectiveness of fourth-generation adhesive systems, and still in wide use today, is the pretreatment of dentin with conditioners and/or primers that make the heterogeneous and hydrophilic dentinal substrate more receptive to bonding. In the early 1990s, manufacturers preferentially used the term *conditioner* instead of *etchant*, as these conditioners were to be applied to both enamel and dentin following the total-etch approach. At the time, etching dentin was still a matter of concern among general practitioners in Europe and North America. For the same reason, etchants contained phosphoric acid in a concentration well below 40% or alternative acids (as previously mentioned) with less etching aggressiveness. Today, the fourth-generation adhesives generally come with 30% to 40% phosphoric acid gels and are referred to as *three-step etch-and-rinse adhesives* (see Table 8-2).

A final step in this relatively complex multistep bonding technique involves the application of an unfilled or semifilled low-viscosity adhesive resin that copolymerizes with the primed dentin surface layer and simultaneously offers bonding receptors for copolymerization with the restorative resin composite. With the multistep application procedure for the fourth-generation adhesives, the term *bonding agent* was replaced by the term *adhesive system*.

Representative adhesives in this group include All-Bond 2, OptiBond FL, Permaquik (Ultradent), and Scotchbond Multi-Purpose (see Table 8-2).

Fifth-Generation Adhesives

Because of the complexity and number of steps or compounds involved with the fourth-generation systems, researchers and manufacturers have worked to develop simpler adhesive systems. The objective has been to achieve similar or improved bonding and sealing compared to that provided by the fourth-generation materials, but with fewer "bottles" and/or in less time (see Table 8-2). They utilize a separate etch-and-rinse (total-etch) phase followed by the application of a combined primer-adhesive resin solution. Although most of the fifth-generation systems have fallen somewhat short of their objective, the bond strengths achieved by some systems have been comparable to those of fourth-generation systems. Clinical testing and improvement of these systems continue.

This generation of adhesives is often misleadingly referred to in the literature as one-bottle adhesives. Representative commercial products of this generation include Excite (Ivoclar Vivadent), One-Step (several versions, Bisco), OptiBond Solo (several versions, Kerr), Prime&Bond (several versions, Dentsply), and Single Bond or Scotchbond 1 (several versions) (see Table 8-2).

Sixth-Generation Adhesives

Further demand for simplification has urged manufacturers to develop adhesives with even fewer clinical steps. The sixth generation consists of self-etch adhesives. Sixth-generation adhesives are characterized by the omission of a separate conditioning phase and are composed of two different solutions. Two types of adhesives belong to the sixth generation: those with a self-etching primer and a separate adhesive resin and those that combine the conditioner, primer, and adhesive resin but require mixing. Hence, this generation of adhesives contains two-step self-etch adhesives and one-step, two-component self-etch adhesives, respectively (see Table 8-2).

Similar to the second-generation adhesives, sixth-generation adhesives use the smear layer on enamel and dentin as bonding substrate, and the second generation can therefore be regarded as a precursor to the self-etch adhesives. The main difference between second-generation and sixth-generation adhesives is the acidity of the primer. Whereas the liability of second-generation (smear layer–modifying) adhesives was that they could not etch beyond the smear layer, sixth-generation (smear layer–dissolving) adhesives contain specially developed acidic monomers, such as 4-MET and 10-MDP,[343,393] that render self-etch adhesives much more hydrophilic compared to previous hydrophobic adhesive systems.[156,350] Moreover, in order to ensure etching capability of these monomers, water must be present to act as an ionizing medium.

Bond strengths attained by sixth-generation adhesives vary a great deal and depend on the actual composition of the adhesives. Even though the bond strengths of some two-step self-etch adhesives approach those of fourth- and fifth-generation adhesives, they generally tend toward lower bond strengths and durability.[339,340]

Representative sixth-generation two-step self-etch adhesives include AdheSE, Clearfil SE Bond and Clearfil Protect Bond, OptiBond Solo Plus Self-Etch, and Tyrian SPE One-Step Plus (Bisco) (see Table 8-2). Representative sixth-generation one-step, two-component self-etch adhesives are Adper Prompt L-Pop (3M ESPE), One-Up Bond F (Tokuyama), and Xeno III (see Table 8-2).

Seventh-Generation Adhesives

The latest generation of adhesives consists of single-component, one-step self-etch adhesives. Although fifth-generation adhesives are sometimes misleadingly referred to as one-bottle systems, only seventh-generation adhesives truly belong in that category. Seventh-generation adhesives combine conditioning, priming, and application of adhesive resin, but unlike sixth-generation adhesives they do not require mixing (see Table 8-2). As a consequence, adhesives belonging to this generation are intricate mixes of hydrophilic and hydrophobic components.[353]

So far, a number of shortcomings of the seventh-generation adhesives have been documented. Due to the complex nature of the mixed solutions, they are prone to phase separation and formation of droplets within their adhesive layers.[353] These adhesive layers also can act as semipermeable membranes, permitting bidirectional water currents.[155] In addition, the seventh-generation adhesives have attained consistently lower bond strengths than the fourth- and fifth-generation adhesives.[155,394]

Representative seventh-generation adhesives include Clearfil S[3] Bond (Kuraray), G-Bond (GC), i-Bond, and Xeno IV (Dentsply) (see Table 8-2).

Critical Steps in Adhesion

Isolation

Before any bonding procedure is begun, adequate isolation and moisture control of the substrate to be bonded to must be achieved. Bonding to acid-etched enamel theoretically requires an air-dried surface to allow the photopolymerizable hydrophobic bonding resin to be drawn by capillary attraction into the etched surface.

With dentin bonding, a distinction should be made between internal and external dentinal wetness. Internal dentinal wetness is caused by pulpal fluids that flow from the pulp through the dentinal tubules to exude onto the dentin cavity surface. This internal dentinal wetness and its effects on adhesion to dentin have been thoroughly documented in the literature dealing with the aspects of dentinal permeability by Pashley and colleagues.[31,97] In this respect, first-generation adhesive systems were too hydrophobic to sufficiently wet the etched dentin.[145] As knowledge of the heterogeneous and hydrophilic nature of dentin has become more complete, newer adhesive formulations have been developed for enhanced hydrophilicity and improved wettability.

The external dentinal wetness is related to ambient or environmental humidity (see Fig 8-28), which has been demonstrated to negatively affect bond strengths to dentin.[157,158,395,396] The degree of environmental humidity is high and comparable to that of the oral cavity when no rubber dam is used, whereas with rubber dam use, the environmental humidity is similar to that of the ambient air in the operatory. Bond strengths obtained with most adhesive systems decrease as the level of humidity in air rises, but some systems appear to be more sensitive than others. In this respect, incorporation of polyalkenoic acid copolymers in the Scotchbond products, Scotchbond MultiPurpose and its two-step successor Single Bond (Scotchbond 1 in Europe) (see Fig 8-43), have been reported to have lower moisture sensitivity and better bonding stability over time.[157,275,397] The moisture-stabilizing effect of the polyalkenoic acid copolymer was explained by Eliades[397] following a concept introduced by Peters et al,[398] in which a reversible breaking and reforming of calcium–polyalkenoic acid complexes in the presence of water were suggested to develop a stress-relaxation capacity without rupture of adhesion at any time. Further study of this potentially beneficial effect is needed. Other adhesives that contain methacrylated polyalkenoic acid copolymers are ART Bond and Syntac Single-Component and Syntac Sprint (Ivoclar Vivadent).

Self-etch adhesives are also believed to be less sensitive to humidity, thereby decreasing the need for the use of rubber dam isolation. Besnault and Attal[399,400] showed that Clearfil SE Bond (Kuraray) was less influenced by relative humidity than Scotchbond MultiPurpose. In a study with similar methods, Werner and Tani[401] found that the bond strengths of four self-etch adhesives were not influenced by air humidity.

An accidental form of external dentinal wetness is contamination of the substrate with external fluids, impeding effective contact between the adhesive and the bonding substrate. Salivary contamination is detrimental because saliva contains proteins that may block adequate infiltration of resin into the microretentive porosities created on acid-etched enamel and dentin. Several studies have shown inadequate bonding after blood contamination.[402–404] Because maxillary teeth are more easily isolated, dentin adhesion appears more effective in maxillary teeth than in mandibular teeth.[405] Consistent use of a rubber dam remains the most effective method of moisture control.

Dentin and Pulp Protection

Once the teeth in need of adhesive restoration have been adequately isolated, a decision must be made about the need for any kind of dentin protection.[406] The use of "nonadhesive" liners and bases beneath adhesive restorations is not recommended. Adhesive materials such as glass-ionomer cements can be used (sandwich technique), but in most cases the simple application of an appropriate adhesive is effective.[407] As previously mentioned, studies using microscopic examination have demonstrated that etch-and-rinse adhesives can seal tubules through tubule wall hybridization (see Figs 8-41a, 8-45, 8-57, 8-66, and 8-72b). Murray et al reported no bacterial microleakage in about 80% of Class 5 restorations in an in vivo study that tested several adhesive systems with resin composite or resin-modified glass-ionomer restorations.[407,408]

In a deep cavity preparation with a remaining dentinal thickness of less than 0.5 mm, in very permeable dentin such as that found in young teeth or when the pulp has been exposed, calcium hydroxide remains the material of choice due to its proven pulp-healing properties.[408–414] Its major disadvantage is that it rapidly dissolves if the cavity is not adequately sealed.[407] Therefore, when calcium hydroxide is used, it should be covered by a less-soluble material. A resin-modified glass-ionomer cement is preferred because it allows chemical copolymerization with the adhesive resin and is resistant to acid etching. Because of its high solubility, a calcium hydroxide liner should not be acid etched. It should be used sparingly and limited to the deepest areas of the cavity, over areas of near–pulp exposure, to preserve as much dentinal tissue as possible for bonding. (See chapter 5 for an in-depth discussion of pulpal protection.)

Recent research has focused on the use of adhesive systems as pulp-capping materials, since effective bacterial sealing is considered the primary factor for pulp healing (see chapter 5).[414,415] Although some studies mention healing and repair of the pulp,[416,417] direct application of adhesives onto vital pulp tissues cannot yet be recommended for routine therapy.[395,396,404,405] In spite of the fact that self-etch adhesives are less acidic than phosphoric acid and do not require an additional rinse phase,[395,407] the apparent intrinsic cytotoxicity of their resinous components makes them less appropriate as pulp-capping materials.[395,396,408]

Universal Enamel-Dentin Conditioning

Phosphoric acid alternatives. After the tooth has been adequately isolated and cleaned, a proper etching or conditioning agent must be selected. As mentioned, in most modern adhesive systems, the selective enamel etching technique used by older-generation bonding agents is replaced in smear layer–removing systems by a total-etch concept, in which the conditioner or acid etchant is applied simultaneously to enamel and dentin. As a result, two different microretentive surfaces are exposed in which the adhesive resin will become micromechanically interlocked. Although most research dealing with adhesive techniques has focused on producing good and stable bonds to dentin, the importance of enamel bonding cannot be neglected with the development of new adhesive systems.

Traditionally, enamel was selectively etched with phosphoric acid in a concentration between 30% and 40%. With the introduction of the total-etch technique, less concentrated phosphoric acids or weaker acids such as citric, maleic, nitric, and oxalic acid in varying concentrations have been supplied with adhesive systems (see Fig 8-47). The objective of such universal enamel-dentin conditioning agents is to find the best compromise between etching enamel sufficiently to create a microretentive etch pattern and etching dentin mildly enough to avoid exposure of collagen to a depth that is inaccessible for complete infiltration by resin.[32] However, a few years after the introduction of alternative total etchants into clinical practice, a steadily growing number of clinical trials,[205,263] as well as laboratory studies,[422,423] demonstrated a less consistent and inferior enamel bond with the use of these less aggressive alternative etchants. Two different etchants specifically adapted for enamel and dentin could be used, but this is clinically impractical. Using only a weak acid is acceptable if the enamel surface is mechanically roughened before etching or if the acid gel is rubbed vigorously on the enamel surface. Today, most adhesive systems again use conventional phosphoric acid etchants in concentrations above 30% to etch both enamel and dentin in one application. It is recommended that these etchants be applied first to enamel, so that enamel is etched for at least 15 seconds. Only sclerotic dentin surfaces can be etched longer without the risk of etching too deeply. In fact, this hypermineralized tissue should be etched longer to make it more receptive to bonding.[59]

In all smear layer–removing systems, the conditioner and its by-products should be thoroughly rinsed away before application of the primer and the adhesive resin. For example, failure to rinse off the nitric acid conditioner, as recommended by the manufacturer of ABC Enhanced (Chameleon), resulted in an incomplete resin penetration of the demineral-

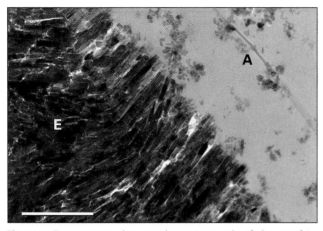

Fig 8-93 Transmission electron photomicrograph of the interface between a two-step self-etch adhesive (Clearfil SE, Kuraray) and enamel. Note the superficial interaction of the adhesive (A) with the enamel (E). Bar = 500 nm.

ized dentin surface layer and minimal hybrid layer formation.[93,334,424] Properly rinsed, the conditioner was sufficient to achieve adequate hybridization.

Self-etch approach on enamel. Self-etching primers have been recommended by manufacturers for use on both enamel and dentin (Fig 8-93 and Table 8-2). Self-etching primers containing acidic monomers (see Fig 8-48) like 4-MET, 10-MDP, and phenyl-P[425] are air dispersed and not rinsed off, simplifying the application procedure. However, controversy exists about their etching efficiency and the resultant enamel bond strength and stability. Results vary with different products. Perdigão et al[426] concluded that although the phenyl-P self-etching primer did not etch enamel as deeply as conventional etchants, Clearfil Liner Bond 2 (Kuraray) demonstrated good bond strengths to enamel. In the measurement of the microtensile bond strength to enamel,[343] two self-etching adhesives, the relatively strong NRC/Prime&Bond NT (Dentsply) and the moderate Clearfil SE Bond, provided bond strengths comparable to those of the conventional three-step total-etch adhesive Optibond FL. Similar results were reported in another study by Kanemura et al,[427] which revealed that two other self-etching adhesives, Clearfil Liner Bond 2 and MacBond 2 (Tokuyama), produced µTBSs to ground enamel that were comparable to those measured for two one-bottle adhesives, One-Step and Single Bond, that involved a separate phosphoric-acid treatment. However, when the self-etching adhesives were directly bonded to unground, intact enamel, the resultant µTBS values were significantly lower.

Long-term clinical trials are needed to confirm this promising enamel bonding effectiveness recorded in vitro. Until then, it remains clinically advisable to use this simplified application technique only on ground enamel. Additionally, the self-etching primer should be actively applied for at least 30 seconds by rubbing the dentin surface with repeated applications of fresh material. Alternatively, a separate conventional etchant can be applied before application of the self-etching primer. However, this should be done solely on enamel, as it was shown that phosphoric-acid etching of dentin followed by the application of a self-etch adhesive negatively affects the bonding effectiveness to dentin.[428]

Very promising clinical data with 100% 3-year retention rates have been reported for the mild two-step self-etch adhesive Clearfil SE Bond.[207,429]

Compomers. Modification of the monomer backbone of conventional resin composites by adding acidic carboxylic groups has led to a new group of adhesive restorative materials. On the basis of their composition, they should be regarded as polyacid-modified resin composites,[430] but products such as Dyract and Dyract AP (Dentsply), Hytac (3M ESPE), Luxat (DMG), and F2000 (3M ESPE) are commercially advertised as *compomers*. This term does not encompass the true characteristics of these materials; it suggests that they originate from combined resin composite and glass-ionomer technology, when in fact they behave more like resin composites. The popularity of the compomers among clinicians must be attributed to their superb clinical handling and simple application method, with only a self-etching primer required to pretreat the enamel and dentin surface. The primers, which like most one-bottle primer/adhesive combinations usually contain acidic monomers dissolved in acetone, are mildly acidic. They interact superficially, to a depth of about 200 nm, with dentin (comparable to the effect seen in Fig 8-34) and are not aggressive enough to expose a highly retentive etch pattern on enamel surfaces. Moreover, two clinical trials reported the occurrence of minimal to severe enamel margin chipping after only 6 months of clinical service, which, if left untreated, could rapidly lead to marginal discoloration and even the development of caries lesions.[431,432] These early enamel margin defects are due to ineffective etching of enamel. The clinical results were confirmed in vitro, where the primer provided with Dyract produced relatively low bond strengths to enamel.[433,434] The clinical effectiveness of these polyacid-modified resin composites is improved by supplementary acid etching of the enamel before primer application, and this is recommended by some manufacturers.

Wet vs Dry Bonding

Surface moisture is an important factor in optimal bonding. On enamel, a dry condition is theoretically preferred. On

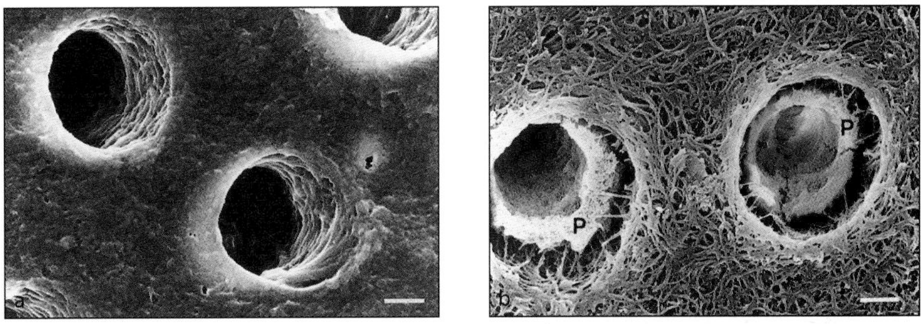

Fig 8-94 Field-emission scanning electron photomicrographs of dentin that was air dried (a) or kept moist (b) after conditioning (top view). P = peritubular dentin; bar = 1 µm.

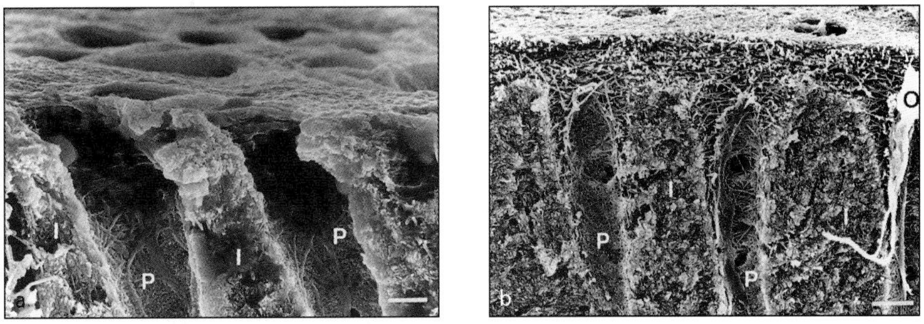

Fig 8-95 Field-emission scanning electron photomicrographs of dentin that was air dried (a) or kept moist (b) after conditioning (lateral view). I = intertubular dentin; O = remnants of odontoblast process or lamina limitans; P = peritubular dentin; bar = 1 µm.

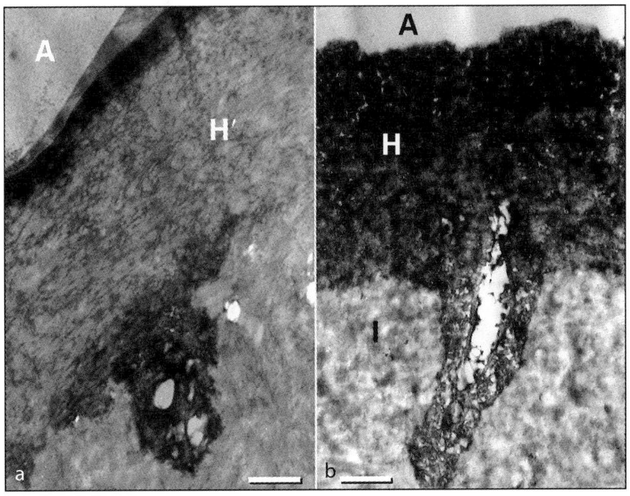

Fig 8-96 Demineralized and stained TEM images of Prime&Bond, an acetone-based adhesive applied to air-dried (a) or blot-dried (b) dentin. Whereas the hybrid layer (H) stains very homogeneously in wet bonding, indicating adequate resin infiltration, only the top of the hybrid layer is stained when the dentin has been air dried before application of the adhesive. This must be explained by suboptimal resin infiltration of the hybrid layer when air dried. As a non–water-containing adhesive is not capable of re-expanding the collagen network, neither primer nor bonding resin is able to penetrate the collapsed network. A = adhesive resin; I = intertubular dentin; H′ = hybridoid zone; bar = 1 µm.

dentin, a certain amount of moisture is needed to avoid collapse of the exposed collagen scaffold, which impedes effective penetration of adhesive monomers (Figs 8-94 to 8-96). Consequently, in the treatment of enamel and dentin, it is difficult to achieve the optimal environment for both substrates. One way to achieve this goal is to keep the substrate field dry and use adhesive systems with water-based primers to rehydrate, and thus re-expand, the collapsed collagen network, enabling the resin monomer to interdiffuse efficiently.[276] The alternative is to keep the acid-etched dentin surface moist and to rely on the water-chasing capacity of acetone-based primers. This clinical technique, commonly referred to as "wet bonding," was introduced by Kanca[435–437] and Gwinnett[438] in the early 1990s.

It is fundamentally important to effective hybridization that the collagen fibril web, deprived of its mineral support following acid treatment, keeps its spongelike quality, allowing interdiffusion of resin monomers in the subsequent priming and bonding steps. Dehydration of the acid-conditioned dentin surface through air-drying is thought to induce surface tension stress, causing the exposed collagen network to collapse, shrink, and form a compact coagulate that is impenetrable to resin.[31,97,329] If some water remains inside the interfibrillar spaces, the loose quality of the collagen matrix

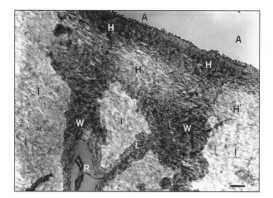

Fig 8-97 Transmission electron photomicrograph of the resin-dentin interface produced by Clearfil Liner Bond System when applied to 35% phosphoric acid–etched dentin. Due to insufficient resin infiltration, a typical hybridoid zone (H′) was formed underneath the top area of the hybrid layer (H), which stained more electron dense, indicating adequate resin infiltration. Compare to Fig 8-62, which shows the resin-dentin interface when Clearfil Liner Bond System was applied, per manufacturer's instructions, following a 20% citric acid solution and resulted in complete resin infiltration. A = adhesive resin; I = lab-demineralized intertubular dentin; L = micro–resin tag in hybridized lateral tubule branch; R = resin tag; W = hybridized tubule wall; bar = 1 μm.

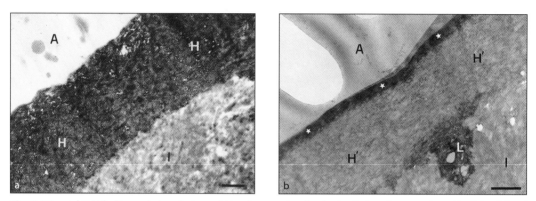

Figs 8-98a and 8-98b Transmission electron photomicrographs of resin-dentin interfaces produced by Prime&Bond applied to moist or blot-dried dentin *(a)* or air-dried dentin *(b)*. Whereas a homogeneously stained hybrid layer (H) is formed with a wet-bonding technique *(a)*, air drying dentin prior to application of the primer/adhesive resin combination resulted in the formation of a collapsed, non–resin-infiltrated collagen or hybridoid zone (H′) *(b)*. In the latter case, resin penetrated only the top part of the exposed collagen fibrils *(white stars)* and at the bottom through a lateral tubule branch (L). A = adhesive resin; I = lab-demineralized intertubular dentin; bar = 1 μm.

is maintained and the interfibrillar spaces are left open.[93,211,436,439,440] An appropriate amount of moisture on the dentin surface has also been reported to promote the polymerization reaction of specific monomers.[223] The wet-bonding technique has repeatedly been reported to increase in vitro bond strengths.[435,436,438,440]

Clinically, a shiny, hydrated surface is seen with moist dentin. Pooled moisture should be removed by blotting or wiped off with a slightly damp cotton pellet. Excess water dilutes the primer and renders it less effective.[291] In some of the currently available adhesive systems, hydrophilic primer monomers are therefore dissolved in volatile solvents, such as acetone and ethanol. These solvents may aid in displacement of the remaining water as well as carrying the polymerizable monomers into the opened dentinal tubules and through the nanospaces of the collagen web.[273] The primer solvents are then evaporated by gentle air-drying, leaving the active primer monomers behind. These monomers have hydrophilic ends with an affinity for the exposed collagen fibrils and hydrophobic ends that form receptors for copolymerization with the adhesive resin. When the water inside the collagen network is not completely displaced, the polymerization of resin inside the hybrid layer may be affected or, at least, the remaining water will compete for space with resin inside the demineralized dentin.[102] The risk that all of the moisture on an overwet dentin surface may not be completely replaced by hydrophilic primer monomers has been well documented for adhesive systems that provide water-free acetone-based primers.[279] In such overwet conditions, excessive water that was incompletely removed during priming appeared to cause phase separation of the hydrophobic and hydrophilic monomer components, resulting in blister and globule formation at the resin-dentin interface. Such interface deficiencies weaken the resin-dentin bond and result in incompletely sealed tubules.[279] On the other hand, even gentle drying of the dentin surface, for times as short as 3 seconds prior to the application of a water-free, acetone-based primer, has been shown to result in incomplete intertubular resin infiltration. Ineffective resin penetration due to collagen collapse has been observed ultramorphologically as the formation of a so-called hybridoid zone (Figs 8-96a, 8-97, and 8-98).[279,331] These hybridoid zones inside the hybrid layer do not appear electron dense on demineralized TEM sections. Consequently, this wet-bonding technique appears to be technique-sensitive, especially in terms of the precise amount of moisture that should be kept on the dentin surface after conditioning.[279,442] In other words, acid-etched dentin should not be kept too wet but also should not be dried too long. A short air blast or blotting of the excess water with a dry sponge or small piece of tissue paper have been recommended as most effective in wet-bonding procedures.

The wet-bonding technique has two other disadvantages of clinical importance. First, acetone quickly evaporates from the primer bottle so that after the primer solution is dispensed in a dappen dish, the primer bottle should immediately be closed and the primer solution immediately applied to the etched surface. Despite careful handling, the composition of the primer solution may change after several uses due to rapid evaporation of solvent. This will increase the ratio of monomers to the acetone content and will eventually affect the penetrability of monomers into the exposed collagen network. To reduce the problem of rapid primer solvent volatilization, special delivery systems have been developed. Examples are the "bubble mixer" syringe system of Permagen (Ultradent); a syringe system with a disposable application brush for Permaquik and PQ1 (Ultradent); or a delivery system with predose, single-use capsules introduced with Optibond Solo, Optibond Solo Plus, Excite, and, recently, G-Bond and i-Bond (see Table 8-2). Another disadvantage of keeping the cavity walls wet after conditioning is that one cannot observe the white, frosted appearance of the enamel that indicates it has been properly etched.

Adhesive systems that provide water-dissolved primers have been demonstrated to bond equally effectively to dry or wet dentin. In one study,[276] the hybridization effectiveness of two three-step smear layer–removing adhesive systems, OptiBond Dual Cure (Kerr) and Scotchbond MultiPurpose, were examined by TEM. No substantial difference in the ultrastructure of the hybrid layer nor signs of incomplete resin penetration or collagen collapse were detected when these water-based adhesives were applied following a wet- or dry-bonding technique. Even excessive postconditioning air-drying of the dentin surface for 15 seconds did not result in the formation of a hybridoid zone.[276,443] When both adhesives were bonded to wet dentin, no morphologic evidence of the overwetting phenomenon was observed.[276,443] This indi-

cates that the two water-based primers were capable of displacing the water that remained as part of the wet-bonding technique as well as the additional amount of water that was introduced with the primers themselves. A self-rewetting effect of the primer, which evidently provides sufficient water to re-expand the air-dried and collapsed collagen scaffold, has been advanced as a reasonable explanation as to why these systems perform equally well in wet and dry conditions. Air-drying of demineralized dentin reduces its volume by 65%, but the original dimensions can be regained after rewetting.[444]

Alternatively, conditioned dentin may be air dried and remoistened with water or an antibacterial solution such as chlorhexidine.[435,438] A study by Perdigão et al[445] has shown that an aqueous HEMA (35%) solution (Aquaprep, Bisco) is effective for rewetting etched dentin. The postconditioning application of the rewetting agent significantly improved the bonding of some simplified adhesives.

Primer Application

Primers should be applied with care to ensure that resin effectively infiltrates the network of interfibrillar collagen channels. A primer application time of at least 15 seconds, as recommended by most manufacturers, should be used to allow monomers to interdiffuse to the complete depth of surface demineralization. When a dry-bonding technique is followed with water-based primers, this 15-second primer application time should allow the collapsed collagen scaffold to re-expand. With a wet-bonding technique, the primer should be applied for at least 15 seconds to displace all remaining surface moisture through concurrent evaporation of the primer solvent carrier. Moreover, water-free, acetone-based primers provided with three- and two-step (one-bottle) etch-and-rinse adhesive systems should be applied generously in multiple layers. After brief, gentle air-drying, the primed surface should appear glossy. The primer should be actively rubbed into the dentin surface with disposable brushes or sponge applicators. This may improve and accelerate the monomer interdiffusion process. The typical "shag-carpet" appearance of collagen fibrils, which are directed up toward the adhesive resin and appear to be frayed into their microfibrils (Figs 8-41b, 8-57, 8-76, 8-79, and 8-99), has been attributed to this active rubbing application method.[276,334,443] A similar pattern of deeply tufted collagen fibrils has been observed to result from citric-acid burnishing of a root surface as part of a tissue regenerative periodontal treatment.[446] The physical rubbing action, combined with the chemical action of citric acid, was found to enhance the removal of chemically dissolved inorganic dentin material and surface debris, exposing a deeply tufted collagen fibril surface topography. Likewise, the combined mechanical/chemical action of rubbing the

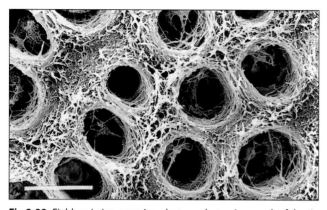

Fig 8-99 Field-emission scanning electron photomicrograph of dentin that was treated with Non-Rinse Conditioner. By actively rubbing the dentin surface, a typical "shag-carpet" appeared with well-opened pores available for interdiffusion. Bar = 5 µm.

dentin surface with a slightly acidic primer probably dissolves additional inorganic dentin material while fluffing and separating the entangled dentin collagen at the surface.

Acid-etched enamel does not need a separate primer application to achieve effective bonding when an unfilled or lightly filled hydrophobic enamel bonding agent is applied on air-dried enamel. On the other hand, primers can be applied on acid-etched enamel without harming the enamel bonding process. In the wet-bonding technique, primers should always be applied on acid-etched enamel to displace any residual surface moisture through concurrent evaporation of the primer's solvent carrier. The primer application should be completed by short and gentle air-drying to volatilize any remaining solvent excess before application of the adhesive resin.

It is noteworthy that some of the current one-step adhesives require a rather strong air-drying technique in order to remove water that has separated from the other adhesive ingredients following a phase separation effect.[353]

Adhesive Resin Application

In the final step of the bonding process, the adhesive layer is placed. Spreading of the adhesive resin over the surface to be bonded should be done by brush thinning rather than by air thinning. The adhesive should be placed and then evenly spread with a brush tip that can be blotted repeatedly with a paper tissue. In this way, the adhesive resin layer will reach an optimal thickness of about 100 µm.[201] When placed in a sufficiently thick layer, the adhesive resin may act as a stress-relaxation buffer (see Fig 8-30) and absorb some of the tensile stresses imposed by polymerization contraction of the resin composite placed over the adhesive resin.[198,200,447,448] Thinning the adhesive resin layer with an air syringe may reduce its thickness too much, decreasing its elastic buffer

potential. In support of this elastic bonding concept, dentin adhesive systems that provide a low-viscosity resin have been reported to produce higher bond strengths and less microleakage.[267,449,450] Microleakage was also found to be reduced when a filled low-viscosity resin was used as an intermediate liner.[268] This elastic bonding concept can be regarded as an efficient means not only to counteract the polymerization contraction stress of the resin composite, but also to aid in absorbing masticatory forces, tooth flexure effects, and thermal cycling shocks, all of which may jeopardize the integrity of the resin-tooth bond.

This innovative concept for relaxation of polymerization shrinkage by elastic compensation was adopted by several modern adhesive systems. Clearfil Liner Bond systems 1 and 2 provide a low-viscosity resin, filled with silanated microfiller and prepolymerized filler at 42 wt%. Optibond DC, Optibond FL, Optibond Solo, and Optibond Solo Plus provide a light-polymerizable adhesive resin that contains radiopaque, fluoride-releasing glass filler particles at 48 wt% (Figs 8-40, 8-41, 8-45, 8-57, and 8-100).[200] A filled adhesive resin is also supplied with other modern adhesives (see Table 8-2). In addition to alleviating stress, these semifilled adhesive resins undergo less polymerization contraction. They have superior physical properties, with a compressive strength approximating that of microfilled resin composites and a Young's modulus of elasticity closer to that of resin composites. They form particle-reinforced resin tags as anchors in the dentinal tubules (see Figs 8-40, 8-41, 8-45, and 8-57). Some may release fluoride to the surrounding demineralized dentin and may provide improved esthetics by preventing the formation of a prism effect or a translucent line around the restoration's margins.[93]

Apart from adhesives that provide low-viscosity particle-filled resins (see Table 8-2), thick adhesive layers are also placed with polyalkenoic acid–based adhesive systems, such as Scotchbond MultiPurpose and Single Bond, and with the more recently developed glass-ionomer–based adhesive system Fuji Bond LC (GC). Excellent clinical results have been reported for Clearfil Liner Bond, Scotchbond MultiPurpose, and Optibond Dual Cure in clinical trials.[269,447,448,451]

Other materials also have stress-relaxing properties. In theory, chemical- and dual-cured adhesive systems that allow small porosities to be mixed in the resin layer and that polymerize more slowly than light-cured materials may also contribute to this stress-relaxation mechanism.[183,211] Adhesive lining cements used under resin composite restorations also act as stress absorbers. The use of an intermediate glass-ionomer liner will reduce the total stiffness and increase the stress-absorption capacity of the restoration. In this respect, resin-modified glass-ionomer cements are preferred over conventional glass-ionomer cements because they can chemical-

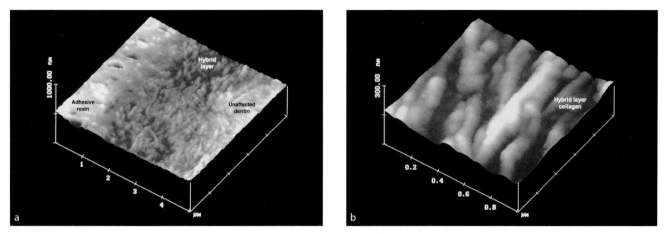

Figs 8-100a and 8-100b Atomic force microscopy tapping-mode images illustrating the resin-dentin interface produced by Optibond Dual Cure.

ly copolymerize with the restorative resin composite placed over the intermediate cement layer. This so-called sandwich technique has been demonstrated to significantly reduce the loss rate of restorations placed with an earlier-generation adhesive, Scotchbond 2, when a resin-modified glass-ionomer liner, Vitrebond (3M ESPE), was used as an intermediate liner.[452]

For light-cured bonding agents, the adhesive resin should always be cured before the application of the restorative resin composite. In this way, the adhesive resin is not displaced when the restorative resin composite is applied, and adequate light intensity is provided to sufficiently cure the adhesive resin layer.[21] Curing the adhesive resin prior to inserting resin composite will stabilize the resin-tooth bond and consequently activate the elastic stress-relaxation mechanism.

Because of oxygen inhibition, the top 15 µm of the adhesive resin will not polymerize[202] but will provide sufficient double methacrylate bonds for copolymerization with the restorative resin. Again, brush thinning rather than air thinning may prevent the film thickness from being reduced to an extent that the air-inhibited layer permeates the whole resin layer, reducing the stress-relaxation capacity and bond effectiveness.[21,453]

Restorative Procedure

As long as resin composites shrink during polymerization, additional clinical measures will be needed to compensate for the polymerization shrinkage.[73,175–177] In addition to building in a flexible stress-absorbing bonding interface, the restorative material should be placed in such a manner that the polymerization-contraction stress is clinically reduced as much as possible. An in vivo study by Perdigão et al[211] showed that, in bulk-filled Class 1 cavities, the dentin-adhesive bond was not

able to withstand polymerization shrinkage stress. Consistent detachment of the adhesive resin from the underlying hybrid layer was observed. In that study, porosities incorporated in relatively thick adhesive resin layers were found to result in less frequent resin-dentin interface separation, providing support for the elastic bonding concept. These observations also confirm the influence of the cavity geometry or configuration on the eventual bond integrity, with Class 1 cavities having the most unfavorable geometry, as previously described[185] (see Fig 8-29).

Bond Durability and Degeneration

The oral cavity is a complex chemical environment, continuously challenging adhesive bonding. Whereas contemporary adhesives can provide a good initial bond to enamel and dentin for composite materials, the long-term durability of bonded restorations is still a hot research topic. Several studies have documented a considerable drop in bond strength after aging.[346,454] Clinical failure of a resin composite restoration occurs more often due to inadequate sealing, with subsequent discoloration of the restoration margins, than to loss of retention.[270,455]

Several degradation mechanisms have been proposed.[323,456] Biomaterial-tooth interfaces are subjected to chemical as well as mechanical degradation. Mechanical stresses exerted at adhesive interfaces are caused not only by chewing forces, but also by temperature-induced contraction and expansion stresses due to differences in the thermal expansion coefficient of resin composite material and tooth structure.[457] These mechanical forces result in crack initiation at the adhesive interface.[304,323,334]

Chemical degradation is mainly triggered by water diffusion into the hybrid and adhesive layers. In addition to water,

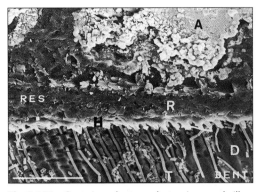

Fig 8-101a Scanning electron photomicrograph illustrating the interface of amalgam (A) and dentin (D). Note the formation of a hybrid layer (H) with resin tags when All-Bond 2 and Dispersalloy are used. R/RES = resin; bar = 30 μm.

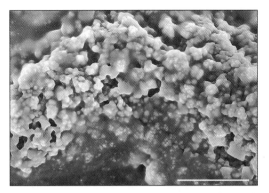

Fig 8-101b Scanning electron photomicrograph revealing the mixture of amalgam particles with resin when All-Bond 2 and Tytin are used. Bar = 7.5 μm.

other components of saliva, such as human and bacterial enzymes, are also thought to contribute to degradation. Resin composite materials are hydrophobic, which prevents water influx, but recent adhesive systems are characterized by increasing hydrophilicity, which favors diffusion processes.[458] Leaching of resin components due to incomplete polymerization also promotes water ingression. Submicron gaps, detected in the hybrid and adhesive layers in TEM sections (see Fig 8-65),[277,278] are thought to function as passages for water and saliva.[351]

In the hybrid layer, both the resin and the collagen fibrils are under attack.[323] Water causes hydrolysis and plasticizing of resin. The same process of hydrolysis jeopardizes collagen polymers that are insufficiently coated with resin, and enzymes enhance this degradation process.[346,352,459] As a result of hydrolysis, smaller breakdown products are formed that leach away, promoting even more water ingression.

Several in vitro and in vivo study protocols have been used to investigate long-term bonding effectiveness.[322,323] Clinical studies are the ultimate test method for bonding effectiveness of adhesives, but in vitro research is more suitable to predict durability in a faster and more economical way and to learn about the degradation processes. De Munck et al[323] concluded in a review article that the most validated in vitro method to assess adhesion durability is storage of microspecimens in water.

After about 3 months, all classes of adhesives exhibited degradation. A comparison of contemporary adhesives revealed that the three-step ethanol- and water-based etch-and-rinse adhesives remain the gold standard in terms of adhesion durability. Any kind of simplification in the clinical application procedure results in a loss of bonding durability. Only two-step self-etch adhesives closely approach this standard.[323]

Amalgam Bonding

Adhesive technology is also used to bond amalgam to tooth structure. Adhesive systems such as All-Bond 2, Amalgambond Plus, Panavia (Kuraray), Scotchbond MultiPurpose Plus (3M ESPE), and Clearfil Liner Bond 2V (Kuraray) have been advocated for bonding amalgam to enamel and dentin. Because amalgam does not allow light transmission, these amalgam bonding systems must have autopolymerizing capability. The nature of the bond between resin and amalgam is not totally understood but appears to involve micromechanical mixing of amalgam with resin during condensation (Fig 8-101).[291] Dhanasomboon and others[460] found that a double application of adhesive to bovine enamel increased the shear-bond strength of bonded amalgam significantly. The first layer was light cured to establish an optimal bond to enamel, and amalgam was mechanically condensed in the second non–light-cured layer, allowing for adequate micromechanical intermingling between the amalgam and the resin.

In vitro bond strengths of amalgam to dentin are generally less than 10 MPa (range, 2 to 20 MPa), which is less than bond strengths of resin composite to dentin.[461–466] A possible problem with the incorporation of resin into amalgam is the potential weakening of the mechanical properties of the amalgam.[467]

The use of amalgam bonding techniques has several potential benefits.[291] Retention gained by bonding lessens the need for removal of tooth structure to gain retention or for retentive devices such as dovetails,[2] grooves, and parapulpal pins.[468,469] Bonded amalgam may increase the fracture resistance of restored teeth,[470] and adhesive resin liners may seal the margins better than traditional cavity varnishes, with decreased risks for postoperative sensitivity and caries recurrence.[464,468,471,472] Most studies agree that the use of adhesives decreases short-term microleakage.[465,466,473–475] It was also suggested that the formation of a hybrid layer by a dentin bonding system prevents permeation of corrosion products of amalgam into the dentinal tubules, avoiding tooth discoloration.[476] Clinical benefit of using amalgam bonding in mechanically retentive cavities has not been proven. No difference in clinical success was found between bonded and nonbonded restorations.[465,477] Although these amalgam bonding techniques have been advocated for repair of existing amalgam restorations with either resin or fresh amalgam,[478,479] several studies have reported poor results in the strengthening of old amalgam restorations.[480–482]

Ceramic Bonding

Adhesion of resin to ceramic materials is important for luting indirect restorations, such as veneers, and inlays and onlays and for repairing fractured porcelain restorations with composite material. Traditional ceramic materials provide a stable and reliable bonding substrate (no inherent wetness) when the bonding substrate is pretreated correctly.[483] New ceramic materials such as aluminum-oxide and zirconium-oxide ceramics have been introduced; these materials require a different approach because they are rather inert.[483,484]

Bonding resin to conventional silica-based ceramics, whether porcelain or glass ceramic, is based on the combined effects of micromechanical interlocking and chemical bonding.[274,485] Porcelain and glass ceramic surfaces are generally etched with hydrofluoric acid and ammonium bifluoride, respectively, to increase the surface area and create microporosities.[486] The adhesive resin flows into the porosities and interlocks, forming strong micromechanical bonds (Figs 8-102 and 8-103).[274] When using these strong acids intraorally, the use of rubber dam is mandatory.[483]

Thorough rinsing followed by ultrasonic cleaning is recommended to remove any remaining acid gel, precipitates, or loose particles, which may weaken the final bond (Fig 8-104). Complete drying of the etched ceramic surface can be obtained by brief immersion in a highly concentrated solution of ethanol.[487] Additional surface roughening can be provided by abrasion with diamond rotary instruments or by air-driven-particle abrasion (sandblasting or air abrasion).[483,484]

Chemical bonding to ceramic surfaces is achieved by silanization with a bifunctional coupling agent. The most commonly used silane in dental applications is γ-methacryloxypropyl-trimethoxysiloane (γ-MPTS).[488] A silane group at one end chemically bonds to the hydrolyzed silicon dioxide at the ceramic surface, and a methacrylate group at the other end

copolymerizes with the adhesive resin[489] (Fig 8-105). In order to be reactive, the silane needs to be hydrolyzed. Silane primers come in single-solution systems (both unhydrolyzed or prehydrolyzed) and in two-component solutions (unhydrolyzed). Single-component systems contain silane in alcohol or acetone and usually require prior acidification of the ceramic surface with hydrofluoric acid to activate the chemical reaction. With two-component silane solutions, the silane is mixed with an aqueous acid solution to hydrolyze the silane so that it can react with the ceramic surface. If not used within several hours, the silane will polymerize to an unreactive polysiloxane.[478] Silane coupling agents usually contain high amounts of solvents, limiting the shelf life of these products.[490]

Silane treatment appears to be critical for optimal adhesion. A good and durable bond will be achieved by combining increasing surface roughness (both by air abrasion and etching) and silanization,[491,492] but several authors have reported sufficient bonding after silanization alone.[493] The bond strengths of resin composites to silica-containing ceramics after etching and silanating are in the range of the resin-enamel bond strengths.[484]

For repairing fractured porcelain, any low-viscosity resin can be applied after appropriate surface treatment. Some manufacturers market special repair kits (eg, Clearfil Repair, Kuraray) containing a silanization primer, hydrofluoric acid, and an adhesive.

Resin composite cements are the material of choice for the adhesive luting of ceramic restorations. They are similar in composition to conventional resin composite restorative materials but are less densely filled and are characterized by higher flow capacity.[484] Considering the limited depth of light curing, the use of a dual-curing cement is recommended.[494] Dual-curing cements provide extended working times and controlled polymerization.[484] Sufficient viscosity of resin composite cements is paramount for good wetting and seating of the restoration, but the filler density determines the shrinkage and mechanical properties.[483,484] Highly filled and therefore viscous cements shrink less during curing, have reduced marginal microleakage, and are more abrasion resistant.[495] Lately, when the ceramic restoration is not too thick (less than 2.5 mm), clinicians tend to lute them using a light-curing micro-hybrid restorative composites that possess better wear resistance.

A different approach is recommended for alumina (eg, In-Ceram Alumina [Vita] and Procera AllCeram [Nobel Biocare]) and zirconium-oxide ceramics (eg, Procera AllZirkon [Nobel Biocare] and LAVA [3M ESPE]). Since chemically reactive silicon dioxide (silica) is not present in alumina or zirconium-oxide ceramics, etching with hydrofluoric acid and silanization do not provide adequate bond strength.[496,497] Surface rough-

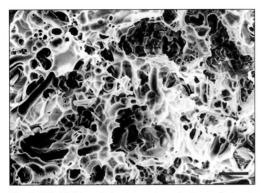

Fig 8-102 Field-emission scanning electron photomicrograph of porcelain etched with 9.6% hydrofluoric acid (Porcelain Etch, Ultradent). Bar = 5 μm.

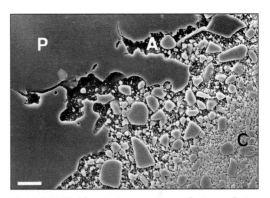

Fig 8-103 Field-emission scanning electron photomicrograph of the porcelain-lute interface. A = adhesive resin (Scotchbond Multi-Purpose Plus); C = luting composite (Opal Luting Composite); P = porcelain (Cosmotech, GC); bar = 5 μm. (From Peumans et al.[274] Reprinted with permission from Elsevier Science.)

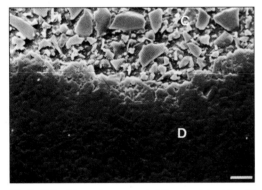

Fig 8-104a Dicor glass ceramic (D) was etched for 60 seconds with 10% ammonium bifluoride, ultrasonically cleaned, and luted with Dicor MGC (C). Postetching ultrasonic cleaning is necessary to remove loose and weakened crystals at the surface to prevent cohesive subsurface failure (see Fig 8-104b).

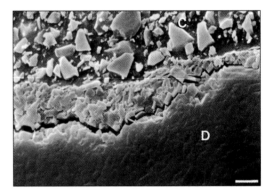

Fig 8-104b Dicor glass ceramic (D) was etched for 60 seconds with 10% ammonium bifluoride and luted with Dicor MGC (C) without ultrasonic cleaning.

Fig 8-105 Silanization of a ceramic surface.

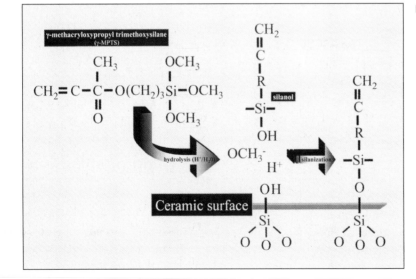

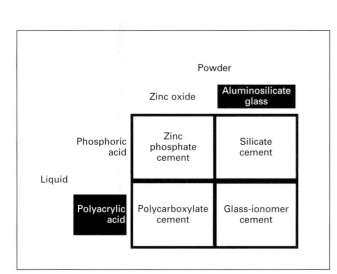

Fig 8-106 Development of glass-ionomer cements from combined technology of silicate and zinc polycarboxylate cements.

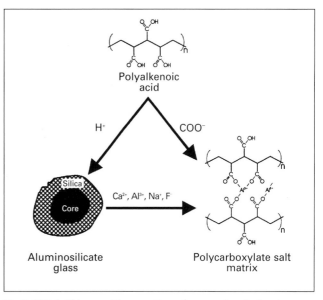

Fig 8-107 Acid-base setting reaction of conventional glass-ionomer cements.

ening can be achieved by air abrasion with aluminum oxide,[496] and tribochemical surface treatment (Rocatec system, 3M ESPE) improves bond strengths to high crystalline ceramics.[498–502] This system uses impact energy to apply a silicate coating to a target surface. Phosphate monomer–based adhesives (Panavia) are effective for bonding to these inert ceramics. It is postulated that 10-MDP has an affinity for aluminum and zirconium oxides.[483]

Glass-Ionomer Cements

Conventional Glass-Ionomer Cements

Glass-ionomer cements were developed in the early 1970s by Wilson and Kent,[273,503] who combined the technology of silicate and zinc carboxylate cements (Fig 8-106). Since that time, glass-ionomer cements have undergone many improvements and modifications of their original chemistry. Conventional glass-ionomer cements contain the ion-leachable fluoroaluminosilicate glass of the silicate cements but avoid their susceptibility to dissolution by substitution of the carboxylic acids from zinc carboxylate cements for phosphoric acid.[504] As stated by McLean et al,[430] a more accurate term for this type of material is *glass-polyalkenoate cement*, because these cements are not true ionomers chemically, but this term has never been as widely used as *glass-ionomer cement*.

The glass is high in aluminum and fluoride, with significant amounts of calcium, sodium, and silica.[505–507] The liquid is typically polyacrylic acid but may contain polymers and copolymers of polyacrylic, itaconic, maleic, or vinyl phosphonic acid.[430,506]

The setting reaction of glass-ionomer cements has been characterized as an acid-base reaction between the glass powder and the polyacid liquid (Fig 8-107). When the powder and liquid are mixed, the fluoroaluminosilicate glass is attacked by hydrogen ions (H^+) from the polyalkenoic acid, liberating Al^{3+}, Ca^{2+}, Na^+, and F^- ions. A layer of silica gel is slowly formed on the surface of unreacted powder, with the progressive loss of metallic ions (Fig 8-108).[508,509] When the free calcium and aluminum ions reach saturation in the silica gel, they diffuse into the liquid and crosslink with two or three ionized carboxyl groups (COO^-) of the polyacid to form a gel. As the crosslinking increases through aluminum ions and the gel is sufficiently hydrated, the crosslinked polyacrylate salt begins to precipitate until the cement is hard (Fig 8-109).

Conventional glass-ionomer cements offer several advantages over other restorative materials. They provide long-term release of fluoride ions, with cariostatic potential, and inherent adhesion to tooth structure.[27,505,509] Because they possess a coefficient of thermal expansion closely approximating that of tooth structure and low setting shrinkage stress, they are reported to provide good marginal sealing, little microleakage at the restoration-tooth interface, and a high

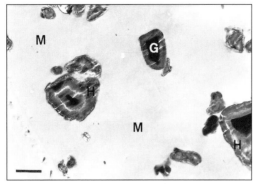

Fig 8-108 Transmission electron photomicrograph showing the ultrastructure of the resin-modified glass-ionomer adhesive Fuji Bond LC. G = core of fluoroaluminosilicate glass filler; H = hydrogel representing the link formed between the matrix and the filler core during the acid-base reaction; M = polycarboxylate salt matrix; bar = 1 μm.

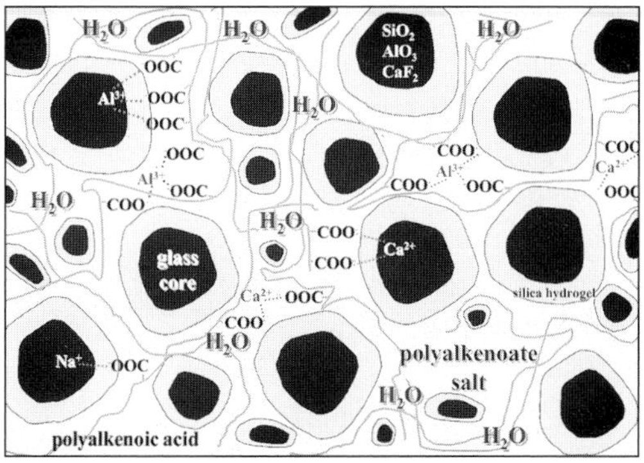

Fig 8-109 The structure of a set glass-ionomer cement.

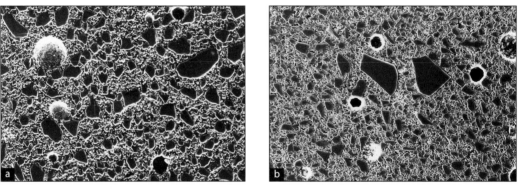

Fig 8-110 Scanning electron photomicrographs of resin-modified glass-ionomer cements after argon-ion–beam etching: *(a)* Photac Bond. *(b)* Vitremer.

retention rate.[504,509] They are biocompatible and have esthetic potential.[504,509]

Despite these important biotherapeutic and clinical advantages, practical difficulties have limited their clinical use.[504,509,510] The material is technically demanding and highly sensitive to changes in its water content. Early moisture contamination disrupts its surface and removes metallic ions, while desiccation causes shrinkage and crazing. Glass-ionomer cements have a short working time but a long setting time, which requires delayed finishing of the restoration. In addition, their physical properties and esthetic potential are inferior to those of resin composites.

Resin-Modified Glass-Ionomer Cements

To overcome the practical limitations of conventional glass-ionomer cements, yet preserve their clinical advantages, con-

ventional glass-ionomer chemistry was combined with methacrylate resin technology; this led to the creation of resin-modified glass-ionomer systems (Fig 8-110).[505,511] They are often incorrectly referred to as light-cured glass-ionomer cements.[27,430,504] The term *dual-cured* is more appropriate, because the original acid-base reaction is supplemented by light-activated polymerization.[505,512]

Generally, these materials still have ion-leachable fluoroaluminosilicate glass in the powder, but they also contain monomers, primarily HEMA, and a photoinitiator, camphorquinone, which are added to the aqueous polyacid liquid.[27,504] In the simplest form of resin-modified glass-ionomer cement, some of the water content of the conventional glass-ionomer cement is replaced by a water-HEMA mixture, while more complex formulations comprise modified polyacids with methacrylate side chains, which can be light polymerized.[505] The first setting reaction is a slow acid-base reaction, typical of conventional glass-ionomer cements (see Fig 8-107). The photoinitiated setting reaction occurs much faster through homopolymerization and copolymerization of methacrylate groups grafted onto the polyacrylic acid chain and methacrylate groups of HEMA (Figs 8-48 and 8-111). With certain materials, such as Fuji II LC (GC) and Vitremer (3M ESPE), a third polymerization initiation is claimed to occur through chemically initiated, free-radical methacrylate curing of the polymer system and HEMA (Table 8-6).[291,504,509]

A diverse group of materials is marketed as resin-modified glass-ionomer cements (see Table 8-6). The products vary from those that closely resemble conventional glass-ionomer cements to those that approximate light-curing resin composites and cure almost exclusively by light-initiated polymerization of free radicals.[291,430,431,509] For the latter, little or no water is present in the system to allow the acid-base reaction typical of glass-ionomer cements.[505] A true resin-modified glass-ionomer cement, then, is defined as a two-part system characterized by an acid-base reaction critical to its cure, diffusion-based adhesion between the tooth surface and the cement, and continuing fluoride release.[430,505]

The underlying mechanism of adhesion of glass-ionomer cements to tooth structure is primarily based on an ion-exchange process, resulting in a shallow demineralization and subsequent infiltration of the tooth surface by the polyalkenoic acid, and in a strong ionic bond between the calcium of the hydroxyapatite and the carboxyl groups of the polyalkenoic molecules (Figs 8-89 and 8-112).[26,27,513,514] It has been postulated that an intermediate adsorption layer of calcium and aluminum phosphates and polyacrylates is formed at the glass-ionomer cement–hydroxyapatite interface.[505,515,516] A reversible breaking and reforming of calcium-carboxyl complexes in the presence of water is suggested to form a dynamic bond.[517] It was only recently that direct evidence of primary chemical bonding of the carboxyl groups of the polyalkenoic acid to calcium of hydroxyapatite could be provided.[358] The interfacial ultrastructure as formed by a resin-modified glass-ionomer adhesive has been documented as well (Figs 8-86 and 8-113).[354]

Clinically, glass-ionomer cement can be used as a luting agent, as a cavity liner or base, as a core buildup material, as a direct restorative material in permanent and primary teeth, as a pit and fissure sealant, as a provisional restorative material, and as a retrograde root-filling material.[291,505,518]

Resin-modified glass ionomers are easier to use than conventional glass-ionomer cements. The supplementary light polymerization allows a longer working time, a rapid hardening on command, and a more rapid early development of strength and resistance against aqueous attack than are found with conventional glass-ionomer cements.[291,431,505]

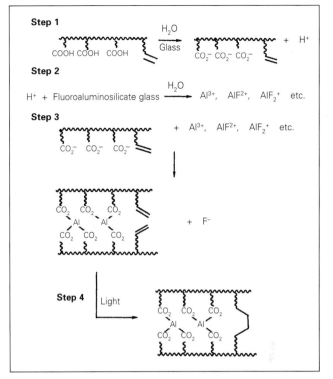

Fig 8-111 Structure of a resin-modified glass-ionomer cement and its probable setting reaction. (From Mitra.[512] Reprinted with permission.)

Mechanical properties such as compressive, tensile, and flexural strengths; fracture toughness; wear resistance; fatigue resistance; bond strengths to enamel, dentin, and other resin-based restorative materials; marginal adaptation; and microleakage are reported to be better than those of conventional glass-ionomer cements.[291,431,505,509,519] They appear to be less sensitive to water, are radiopaque, and offer better esthetic possibilities than do conventional glass-ionomer cements. The fluoride release of resin-modified glass-ionomer cements is reported to be equal to or greater than that of conventional glass-ionomer cements, and the fluoride-releasing property may even be rechargeable.[505,520] Retention rates of more than 90% have been observed for periods up to 5 years in noncarious cervical lesions. A recent review article concluded that glass-ionomer retention rates far exceeded those of other adhesives.[521]

Because of their inferior physical and esthetic properties as compared to resin composites, the primary indications for the resin-modified glass-ionomer materials are restorations for patients at high risk for caries, in areas where esthetics is not a primary concern, in technically difficult areas requiring a capsule application technique, or in the so-called atraumatic restorative treatment (ART) concept.

Table 8-6	Hybrid restorative materials according to their setting mechanism			
		Setting mechanism		
Material	**Manufacturer**	**Acid-base reaction**	**Visible light–initiated polymerization**	**Chemically initiated polymerization**
Resin-modified glass-ionomer cements				
Fuji II LC	GC	✓	✓	✓
Ionosit	DMG	✓	✓	
Photac-Fil Quick	3M ESPE	✓	✓	
Vitremer	3M ESPE	✓	✓	✓
Polyacid-modified resin composites (compomers)				
Compoglass	Ivoclar Vivadent	*	✓	
Dyract	Dentsply	*	✓	
Dyract AP	Dentsply	*	✓	
Elan	Kerr	*	✓	
Hytac Aplitip	3M ESPE	*	✓	
Freedom	STI	*	✓	
F2000	3M ESPE	*	✓	
Geristore	Den-Mat	*	✓	
Glasiosite	Voco	*	✓	
Luxat	DMG	*	✓	

* Claimed but unproven.

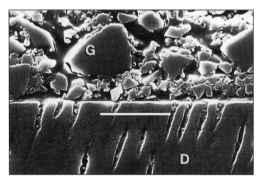

Fig 8-112 Scanning electron photomicrograph of the resin-modified glass-ionomer cement–dentin interface with Fuji II LC. The dentinal tubules appear to be occluded by smear debris. D = dentin; G = resin-modified glass-ionomer cement; bar = 20 μm.

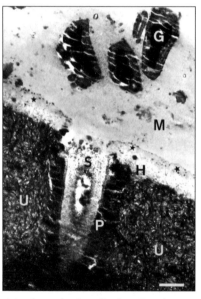

Fig 8-113 Transmission electron photomicrograph of an unstained, nondemineralized section demonstrating the interface formed at dentin by a glass-ionomer adhesive (Fuji Bond LC). The shallow hybrid layer (H) of about 0.5 μm results from the short (10-second) application of 20% polyalkenoic acid, by which collagen fibrils are exposed but not completely denuded from hydroxyapatite (collagen is not visible on this image as the section was not positively stained). The hydroxyapatite crystals remaining around the collagen fibrils served as receptors for chemical bonding with the carboxyl groups of the polyalkenoic acid. On top of the hybrid layer, a 0.5-μm gray zone *(black stars)* typically contains small black globules of yet unknown origin and is clearly demarcated from the glass-ionomer matrix (M). This phase represents the morphologic manifestation of a gelation reaction of the polyalkenoic acid with calcium that was extracted from the underlying dentin surface. G = fluoroaluminosilicate glass filler surrounded by a silica hydrogel; P = peritubular dentin; S = smear occluding the tubule orifice; U = unaffected intertubular dentin; bar = 1 μm.

References

1. Buonocore MG. A simple method of increasing the adhesion of acrylic filling materials to enamel surfaces. J Dent Res 1955;34:849–853.

2. Black GV. A Work on Operative Dentistry in Two Volumes, ed 3. Chicago: Medico-Dental Publishing, 1917.

3. Duke ES. Adhesion and its application with restorative materials. Dent Clin North Am 1993;37:329–340.

4. Phillips RW. Skinner's Science of Dental Materials, ed 8. Philadelphia: Saunders, 1982:25.

5. Eakle WS. Fracture resistance of teeth restored with Class II bonded composite resin. J Dent Res 1986;65:149–153.

6. Hansen EK. In vivo cusp fracture of endodontically treated premolars restored with MOD amalgam or MOD resin fillings. Dent Mater 1988;4:169–173.

7. Morin D, DeLong R, Douglas WH. Cusp reinforcement by the acid-etch technique. J Dent Res 1984;63:1075–1078.

8. Ibsen R, Ouellet D, Strassler H. Clinically successful dentin and enamel bonding. Am J Dent 1991;2:125–131.

9. Strassler HE. Insights and innovations. J Esthet Dent 1991;3:114.

10. Peumans M, Van Meerbeek B, Lambrechts P, Vanherle G. The five-year clinical performance of direct composite additions to correct tooth form and position. I: Esthetic qualities. Clin Oral Investig 1997;1:12–18.

11. Peumans M, Van Meerbeek B, Lambrechts P, Vanherle G. The five-year clinical performance of direct composite additions to correct tooth form and position. II: Marginal qualities. Clin Oral Investig 1997;1:19–26.

12. Peumans M, Van Meerbeek B, Lambrechts P, Vanherle G, Quirynen M. The influence of direct composite additions for the correction of tooth form and/or position on periodontal health. A retrospective study. J Periodont 1998;69:422–427.

13. Leinfelder KF. After amalgam, what? Other materials fall short. J Am Dent Assoc 1994;125:586–589.

14. Mackert JR. Dental amalgam and mercury. J Am Dent Assoc 1991;122:54.

15. Willems G. Multistandard Criteria for the Selection of Potential Posterior Composites [thesis]. Leuven, Belgium: Catholic University of Leuven, 1985.

16. Roeters JJ. Extended indications for directly bonded composite restorations: A clinician's view. J Adhes Dent 2001;3:81–87.

17. Packham DE. Adhesion. In: Packham DE (ed). Handbook of Adhesion, ed 1. Essex, England: Longman, 1992:18.

18. Kinloch AJ. Adhesion and Adhesives. Science and Technology, ed 1. London: Chapman and Hall, 1987.

19. Allen KW. Adsorption theory of adhesion. Theories of adhesion. In: Packham DE (ed). Handbook of Adhesion, ed 1. Essex, England: Longman, 1992:39, 473.

20. Eliades G. Clinical relevance of the formulation and testing of dentine bonding systems. J Dent 1994;22:73–81.

21. Erickson RL. Surface interactions of dentin adhesive materials. Oper Dent 1992;suppl 5:81–94.

22. Ruyter IE. The chemistry of adhesive agents. Oper Dent 1992;suppl 5:32–43.

23. Padday JF. Contact angle measurement. In: Packham DE, ed. Handbook of Adhesion, ed 1. Essex, England: Longman, 1992:88.

24. Jendresen MD, Glantz P-O. Microtopography and clinical adhesiveness of an acid etched tooth surface. An in vivo study. Acta Odontol Scand 1981;39:47–53.

25. Baier RE. Principles of adhesion. Oper Dent 1992;suppl 5:1–9.

26. Akinmade AO, Nicholson JW. Glass-ionomer cements as adhesives. Part I. Fundamental aspects and their clinical relevance. J Mater Sci Mater Med 1993;4:95–101.

27. Mount GJ. Buonocore Memorial Lecture. Glass-ionomer cements: Past, present and future. Oper Dent 1994;19:82–90.

28. Bowen RL, Cobb EN, Rapson JE. Adhesive bonding of various materials to hard tooth tissues: Improvement in bond strength to dentin. J Dent Res 1982;61:1070–1076.

29. Eick JD, Robinson SJ, Chappell RP, Cobb CM, Spencer P. The dentinal surface: Its influence on dentinal adhesion. Part III. Quintessence Int 1993;24:571–582.

30. Nakabayashi N, Kojima K, Masuhara E. The promotion of adhesion by the infiltration of monomers into tooth substrates. J Biomed Mater Res 1982;16:265–273.

31. Pashley DH, Ciucchi B, Sano H, Horner JA. Permeability of dentin to adhesive agents. Quintessence Int 1993;24:618–631.

32. Van Meerbeek B, Inokoshi S, Braem M, Lambrechts P, Vanherle G. Morphological aspects of the resin-dentin interdiffusion zone with different dentin adhesive systems. J Dent Res 1992;71:1530–1540.

33. Eliades G, Palaghias G, Vougiouklakis G. Surface reactions of adhesives on dentin. Dent Mater 1990;6:208–216.

34. Spencer P, Byerley TJ, Eick JD, Witt JD. Chemical characterization of the dentin/adhesive interface by Fourier transform infrared photoacoustic spectroscopy. Dent Mater 1992;8:10–15.

35. Stangel I, Ostro E, Domingue A, et al. Photoacoustic Fourier transform IR spectroscopic study of polymer-dentin interaction. In: Pireaux JJ, Bertrand P, Bredas JL (eds). Polymer-Solid Interfaces. Philadelphia: Institute of Physics Publishing, 1991:157.

36. Tam LE, Pilliar RM. Fracture surface characterization of dentin-bonded interfacial fracture toughness specimens. J Dent Res 1994;73:607–619.

37. Xu J, Butler IS, Gilson DFR, Stangel I. The HEMA interface with dentin and collagen by FT-Raman spectroscopy [abstract 615]. J Dent Res 1995;74:88.

38. Yoshida Y, Nagakane K, Fukuda R, et al. Comparative study on adhesive performance of functional monomers. J Dent Res 2004;83:454–458.

39. Gwinnett AJ. Interactions of dental materials with enamel. Trans Acad Dent Mater 1990;3:30.

40. Nordenvall K-J, Brännström M, Malmgren O. Etching of deciduous teeth and young and old permanent teeth. A comparison between 15 and 60 seconds of etching. Am J Orthod 1980;78:99–108.

41. Lyon D, Darling AI. Orientation of the crystallites in human dental enamel. Br Dent J 1957;102:483.

42. Meckel AH, Grebstein WJ, Neal RJ. Structure of mature human enamel as observed by electron microscopy. Arch Oral Biol 1965;10:775.

43. Linde A. The extracellular matrix of the dental pulp and dentin. J Dent Res 1985;64:523–529.

44. Mjör IA, Fejerskov O, eds. Human Oral Embryology and Histology, ed 1. Copenhagen: Munksgaard, 1986.

45. Garberoglio R, Brännström M. Scanning electron microscopic investigation of human dentinal tubules. Arch Oral Biol 1976;21:355–362.

46. Pashley DH. Smear layer: Physiological considerations. Oper Dent 1984;suppl 3:13–29.

47. Pashley DH. Dentin: A dynamic substrate—a review. Scanning Microsc 1989;3:161–174.

48. Yamada T, Nakamura K, Iwaku M, Fusayama T. The extent of the odontoblast process in normal and carious human dentin. J Dent Res 1983;62:798–802.

49. Heymann HO, Bayne SC. Current concepts in dentin bonding: Focusing on dentinal adhesion factors. J Am Dent Assoc 1993;124:27–36.

50. Pashley DH. Interactions of dental materials with dentin. Trans Acad Dent Mater 1990;3:55.

51. Marchetti C, Piacentini C, Menghini P. Morphometric computerized analysis on the dentinal tubules and the collagen fibers in the dentine of human permanent teeth. Bull Group Int Rech Sci Stomatol Odontol 1992;35:125–129.

52. Van Hassel HJ. Physiology of the human dental pulp. Oral Surg Oral Med Oral Pathol 1971;32:126–134.

53. Otsuki M. Histological study on pulpal response to restorative composite resins and their ingredients [in Japanese]. J Stomatol Soc Jpn 1988;55:203–236.

54. Stanley HR, Pereira JC, Spiegel E, Broom C, Schultz M. The detection and prevalence of reactive and physiologic sclerotic dentin, reparative dentin and dead tracts beneath various types of dental lesions according to tooth surface and age. J Oral Pathol 1983; 12:257–289.

55. Fusayama T. Two layers of carious dentin: Diagnosis and treatment. Oper Dent 1979;4:63–70.

56. Ogawa K, Yamashita Y, Ichijo T, Fusayama T. The ultrastructure and hardness of the transparent layer of human carious dentin. J Dent Res 1983;62:7–10.

57. Duke ES, Lindemuth JS. Polymeric adhesion to dentin: Contrasting substrates. Am J Dent 1990;3:264–270.

58. Duke ES, Lindemuth JS. Variability of clinical dentin substrates. Am J Dent 1991;4:241–246.

59. Van Meerbeek B, Braem M, Lambrechts P, Vanherle G. Morphological characterization of the interface between resin and sclerotic dentine. J Dent 1994;73:141–146.

60. Mjör I. Reaction patterns of dentin. In: Thylstrup A, Leach SA, Qvist V (eds). Dentine and Dentine Reactions in the Oral Cavity. Oxford, England: IRL Press, 1987:27.

61. Yoshiyama M, Masada J, Uchida A. Scanning electron microscope characterization of sensitive vs. insensitive human radicular dentin. J Dent Res 1989;68:1498–1502.

62. Yoshiyama M, Noiri Y, Ozaki K, Uchida A, Ishikawa Y, Ishida H. Transmission electron microscopic characterization of hypersensitive human radicular dentin. J Dent Res 1990;69:1293–1297.

63. Tagami J, Hosoda H, Burrow MF, Nakajima M. Effect of aging and caries on dentin permeability. Proc Finn Dent Soc 1992;88(suppl 1):149–154.

64. Frank RM, Voegel JC. Ultrastructure of the human odontoblast process and its mineralization during dental caries. Caries Res 1980;14:367–380.

65. Ten Cate JM, Jongebloed WL, Simons YM. Adaptation of dentin to the oral environment. In: Thylstrup A, Leach SA, Qvist V (eds). Dentine and Dentine Reactions in the Oral Cavity. Oxford, England: IRL Press; 1987:67.

66. Burrow MF, Takakura H, Nakajima M, et al. The influence of age and depth of dentin on bonding. Dent Mater 1994;10:241–246.

67. Sattabanasuk V, Shimada Y, Tagami J. The bond of resin to different dentin surface characteristics. Oper Dent 2004;29(3):333–341.

68. Tay FR, Pashley DH. Resin bonding to cervical sclerotic dentin: A review. J Dent 2004;32:173–196.

69. Eick JD, Wilko RA, Anderson CH, Sorenson SE. Scanning electron microscopy of cut tooth surfaces and identification of debris by use of the electron microprobe. J Dent Res 1970;49:1359–1368.

70. Pashley DH. Smear layer: An overview of structure and function. Proc Finn Dent Soc 1992;88:215–224.

71. Ishioka S, Caputo AA. Interaction between the dentinal smear layer and composite bond strengths. J Prosthet Dent 1989;61:180–185.

72. Gwinnett AJ. Quantitative contribution of resin infiltration/hybridization to dentin bonding. Am J Dent 1993;6:7–9.

73. Eick JD. Smear layer–materials surface. Proc Finn Dent Soc 1992; 88(suppl 1):225–242.

74. Yazici AR, Ozgunaltay G, Dayangac B. A scanning electron microscopic study of different caries removal techniques on human dentin. Oper Dent 2002;27:360–366.

75. Van Meerbeek B, De Munck J, Mattar D, Van Landuyt K, Lambrechts P. Microtensile bond strengths of an etch&rinse and self-etch adhesive to enamel and dentin as a function of surface treatment. Oper Dent 2003;28:647–660.

76. Lussi A, Gygax M. Iatrogenic damage to adjacent teeth during classical approximal box preparation. J Dent 1998;26:435–441.

77. Degrange M, Roulet JF. Minimally Invasive Restorations with Bonding. Chicago: Quintessence, 1997.

78. Tyas MJ, Anusavice KJ, Frencken JE, Mount GJ. Minimal intervention dentistry—A review. FDI Commission Project 1-97. Int Dent J 2000;50:1–12.

79. Murdoch-Kinch CA, McLean ME. Minimally invasive dentistry. J Am Dent Assoc 2003;134:87–95.

80. Burnett LH Jr, Conceicao EN, Pelinos JE, Eduardo CD. Comparative study of influence on tensile bond strength of a composite to dentin using Er:YAG laser, air abrasion, or air turbine for preparation of cavities. J Clin Laser Med Surg 2001;19:199–202.

81. Sen BH, Wesselink PR, Turkun M. The smear layer: A phenomenon in root canal therapy. Int Endod J 1995;28:141–148.

82. Blomlof JP, Blomlof LB, Lindskog SF. Smear layer formed by different root planing modalities and its removal by an ethylenediaminetetraacetic acid gel preparation. Int J Periodontics Restorative Dent 1997;17:242–249.

83. Berry EA 3rd, von der Lehr WN, Herrin HK. Dentin surface treatments for the removal of the smear layer: An SEM study. J Am Dent Assoc 1987;115:65–67.

84. Pashley DH, Tao L, Boyd L, King GE, Horner JA. Scanning electron microscopy of the substructure of smear layers in human dentine. Arch Oral Biol 1988;33:265–270.

85. Meryon SD, Tobias RS, Jakeman KJ. Smear removal agents: A quantitative study in vivo and in vitro. J Prosthet Dent 1987;57:174–179.

86. Suzuki T, Finger WJ. Dentin adhesives: Site of dentin vs bonding of composite resins. Dent Mater 1988;4:379–383.

87. Prati C. Reaction paper: Mechanisms of dentine bonding. In: Vanherle G, Degrange M, Willems G (eds). Proceedings of the International Symposium on State of the Art on Direct Posterior Filling Materials and Dentine Bonding, ed 2. Leuven, Belgium: Van der Poorten, 1994:171–191.

88. Pashley DH, Horner JA, Brewer PD. Interactions of conditioners on the dentin surface. Oper Dent 1992;suppl 5:137–150.

89. Pashley DH, Livingston MJ, Greenhill JD. Regional resistances to fluid flow in human dentin in vitro. Arch Oral Biol 1978;23:807–810.

90. Tani C, Finger WJ. Effect of smear layer thickness on bond strength mediated by three all-in-one self-etching priming adhesives. J Adhes Dent 2002;4:283–289.

91. Ruse ND, Smith DC. Adhesion to bovine dentin-surface characterization. J Dent Res 1991;70:1002–1008.

92. Perdigão J. An Ultramorphological Study of Human Dentine Exposed to Adhesive Systems [thesis]. Leuven, Belgium: Catholic University of Leuven, 1995.

93. White GJ, Beech DR, Tyas MJ. Dentin smear layer: An asset or a liability for bonding? Dent Mater 1989;5:379–383.

94. Clark-Holke D, Drake D, Walton R, Rivera E, Guthmiller JM. Bacterial penetration through canals of endodontically treated teeth in the presence or absence of the smear layer. J Dent 2003;31:275–281.

95. Pashley DH. Clinical correlations of dentin structure and function. J Prosthet Dent 1991;66:777–781.

96. Tao L, Pashley DH. Shear bond strengths to dentin: Effects of surface treatments, depth and position. Dent Mater 1988;4:371–378.

97. Pashley DH, Carvalho RM. Dentine permeability and dentine adhesion. J Dent 1997;25:355–372.

98. Van Meerbeek B, De Munck J, Yoshida Y, et al. Buonocore memorial lecture. Adhesion to enamel and dentin: Current status and future challenges. Oper Dent 2003;28:215–235.

99. Pashley DH. Dentin bonding: Overview of the substrate with respect to adhesive material. J Esthet Dent 1991;3:46–50.

100. Pashley DH, Michelich V, Kehl T. Dentin permeability: Effects of smear layer removal. J Prosthet Dent 1981;46:531–537.

101. Tagami J, Tao L, Pashley DH, Hosoda H, Sano H. Effects of high-speed cutting on dentin permeability and bonding. Dent Mater 1991;7:234–239.

102. Jacobsen T, Söderholm KJ. Some effects of water on dentin bonding. Dent Mater 1995;11:132–136.

103. Prati C, Pashley DH, Montanari G. Hydrostatic intrapulpal pressure and bond strength of bonding systems. Dent Mater 1991;7:54–58.

104. Shirai K, De Munck J, Yoshida Y, et al. Effect of cavity configuration and aging on the bonding effectiveness of six adhesives to dentin. Dent Mater 2005;21:110–124.

105. Hirata K, Nakashima M, Sekine I, Mukouyama Y, Kimura K. Dentinal fluid movement associated with loading of restorations. J Dent Res 1991;70:975–978.

106. Tay FR, Pashley DH. Aggressiveness of contemporary self-etching systems. I: Depth of penetration beyond dentin smear layers. Dent Mater 2001;17:296–308.

107. Unemori M, Matsuya Y, Akashi A, Goto Y, Akamine A. Composite resin restoration and postoperative sensitivity: Clinical follow-up in an undergraduate program. J Dent 2001;29:7–13.

108. Camps J, Dejou J, Remusat M, About I. Factors influencing pulpal response to cavity restorations. Dent Mater 2000;16:432–440.

109. Calt S, Serper A. Time-dependent effects of EDTA on dentin structures. J Endod 2002;28:17–19.

110. Inoue S, Van Meerbeek B, Abe Y, et al. Effect of remaining dentin thickness and the use of conditioner on micro-tensile bond strength of a glass-ionomer adhesive. Dent Mater 2001;17:445–455.

111. Bogra P, Kaswan S. Etching with EDTA—An in vitro study. J Indian Soc Pedod Prev Dent 2003;21:79–83.

112. Viswanath D, Hegde AM, Munshi AK. The removal of the smear layer using EGTA: A scanning electron microscopic study. J Clin Pediatr Dent 2003;28:69–74.

113. Opdam NJ, Roeters JJ, van Berghem E, Eijsvogels E, Bronkhorst E. Microleakage and damage to adjacent teeth when finishing Class II adhesive preparations using either a sonic device or bur. Am J Dent 2002;15:317–320.

114. Wicht MJ, Haak R, Fritz UB, Noack MJ. Primary preparation of Class II cavities with oscillating systems. Am J Dent 2002;15:21–25.

115. Pioch T, Garcia-Godoy F, Duschner H, Koch MJ, Staehle HJ, Dorfer CE. Effect of cavity preparation instruments (oscillating or rotating) on the composite-dentin interface in primary teeth. Dent Mater 2003;19:259–263.

116. Setien VJ, Cobb DS, Denehy GE, Vargas MA. Cavity preparation devices: Effect on microleakage of Class V resin-based composite restorations. Am J Dent 2001;14:157–162.

117. Malmstrom HS, Chaves Y, Moss ME. Patient preference: Conventional rotary handpieces or air abrasion for cavity preparation. Oper Dent 2003;28:667–671.

118. Mattar Lima D. Airabrasion: Exploring its potential [thesis]. Leuven, Belgium: Catholic University of Leuven, 2002.

119. Jahn KR, Geitel B, Kostka E, Wischnewski R, Roulet JF. Tensile bond strength of composite to air-abraded enamel. J Adhes Dent 1999;1:25–30.

120. Borsatto MC, Catirse AB, Palma Dibb RG, Nascimento TN, Rocha RA, Corona SA. Shear bond strength of enamel surface treated with air-abrasive system. Braz Dent J 2002;13:175–178.

121. Mehl A, Kremers L, Salzmann K, Hickel R. 3D volume-ablation rate and thermal side effects with the Er:YAG and Nd:YAG laser. Dent Mater 1997;13:246–251.

122. Kawaguchi FA, Eduardo CP, Matos AB. Nd:YAG laser influence on microleakage of Class V composite restoration. J Clin Laser Med Surg 2003;21:227–229.

123. Attrill DC, Davies RM, King TA, Dickinson MR, Blinkhorn AS. Thermal effects of the Er:YAG laser on a simulated dental pulp: A quantitative evaluation of the effects of a water spray. J Dent 2004;32:35–40.

124. Kataumi M, Nakajima M, Yamada T, Tagami J. Tensile bond strength and SEM evaluation of Er:YAG laser irradiated dentin using dentin adhesive. Dent Mater J 1998;17:125–138.

125. Ceballos L, Osorio R, Toledano M, Marshall GW. Microleakage of composite restorations after acid or Er:YAG laser cavity treatments. Dent Mater 2001;17:340–346.

126. Ceballos L, Toledano M, Osorio R, Tay FR, Marshall GW. Bonding to Er-YAG-laser-treated dentin. J Dent Res 2002;81:119–122.

127. Ceballos L, Camejo DG, Victoria FM, et al. Microtensile bond strength of total-etch and self-etching adhesives to caries-affected dentine. J Dent 2003;31:469–477.

128. Neev J, Stabholtz A, Liaw LH, et al. Scanning electron microscopy and thermal characteristics of dentin ablated by a short-pulse XeCl excimer laser. Lasers Surg Med 1993;13:353–362.

129. Armengol V, Laboux O, Weiss P, Jean A, Hamel H. Effects of Er:YAG and Nd:YAP laser irradiation on the surface roughness and free surface energy of enamel and dentin: An in vitro study. Oper Dent 2003;28:67–74.

130. Visuri SR, Gilbert JL, Wright DD, Wigdor HA, Walsh JT Jr. Shear strength of composite bonded to Er:YAG laser-prepared dentin. J Dent Res 1996;75:599–605.

131. Kohara EK, Hossain M, Kimura Y, Matsumoto K, Inoue M, Sasa R. Morphological and microleakage studies of the cavities prepared by Er:YAG laser irradiation in primary teeth. J Clin Laser Med Surg 2002;20:141–147.

132. Hossain M, Yamada Y, Nakamura Y, Murakami Y, Tamaki Y, Matsumoto K. A study on surface roughness and microleakage test in cavities prepared by Er:YAG laser irradiation and etched bur cavities. Lasers Med Sci 2003;18:25–31.

133. Martinez-Insua A, Da Silva DL, Rivera FG, Santana-Penin UA. Differences in bonding to acid-etched or Er:YAG-laser-treated enamel and dentin surfaces. J Prosthet Dent 2000;84:280–288.

134. De Munck J, Van Meerbeek B, Yudhira R, Lambrechts P, Vanherle G. Micro-tensile bond strength of two adhesives to Erbium:YAG-lased vs. bur-cut enamel and dentin. Eur J Oral Sci 2002;110:322–329.

135. Giachetti L, Scaminci Russo DS, Scarpelli F, Vitale M. SEM analysis of dentin treated with the Er:YAG laser: A pilot study of the consequences resulting from laser use on adhesion mechanisms. J Clin Laser Med Surg 2004;22:35–41.

136. Kameyama A, Kawada E, Amagai T, Takizawa M, Oda Y, Hirai Y. Effect of HEMA on bonding of Er:YAG laser-irradiated bovine dentine and 4-META/MMA-TBB resin. J Oral Rehabil 2002;29:749–755.

137. Gonzalez Bahillo J, Ruiz Pinon M, Rodriguez Nogueira J, et al. A comparative study of microleakage through enamel and cementum after laser Er:YAG instrumentation in Class V cavity obturations, using scanning electron microscopy. J Clin Laser Med Surg 2002; 20:197–201.

138. De Souza AE, Corona SA, Palma Dibb RG, Borsatto MC, Pecora JD. Influence of Er:YAG laser on tensile bond strength of a self-etching system and a flowable resin in different dentin depths. J Dent 2004; 32:269–275.

139. Pashley DH. The influence of dentin permeability and pulpal blood flow on pulpal solute concentrations. J Endod 1979;5:355–361.

140. Reeder OW, Walton RE, Livingston MJ, Pashley DH. Dentin permeability: Determinants of hydraulic conductance. J Dent Res 1978; 57:187–193.

141. Pashley DH, Andringa HJ, Derkson GD, Derkson ME, Kalathoor SR. Regional variability in the permeability of human dentine. Arch Oral Biol 1987;32:519–523.

142. Pashley DH, Pashley EL. Dentin permeability and restorative dentistry: A status report for the American Journal of Dentistry. Am J Dent 1991;4:5–9.

143. Söderholm K-JM. Correlation of in vivo and in vitro performance of adhesive restorative materials: A report of the ASC MD156 Task Group on Test Methods for the Adhesion of Restorative Materials. Dent Mater 1991;7:74–83.

144. Douglas WH. Clinical status of dentine bonding agents. J Dent 1989;17:209–215.

145. Torney D. The retentive ability of acid-etched dentin. J Prosthet Dent 1978;39:169–172.

146. Mitchem JC, Gronas DG. Effects of time after extraction and depth of dentin on resin dentin adhesives. J Am Dent Assoc 1986;113: 285–287.

147. Pereira PNR, Okuda M, Sano H, Yoshikawa T, Burrow MF, Tagami J. Effect of intrinsic wetness and regional difference on dentin bond strength. Dent Mater 1999;15:46–53.

148. Rueggeberg FA. Substrate for adhesion testing to tooth structure—review of literature. Dent Mater 1991;7:2–10.

149. Stanford JW, Sabri Z, Jose S. A comparison of the effectiveness of dentine bonding agents. Int Dent J 1985;35:139.

150. Tagami J, Tao L, Pashley DH. Correlation among dentin depth, permeability, and bond strength of adhesive resin. Dent Mater 1990;6:45–50.

151. Sano H, Shono T, Sonoda H, et al. Relationship between surface area for adhesion and tensile bond strength—evaluation of a microtensile bond test. Dent Mater 1994;10:236–240.

152. Tao L, Tagami J, Pashley DH. Pulpal pressures and bond strengths of Superbond and Gluma. Am J Dent 1991;4:73–76.

153. Tay FR, King NM, Chan KM, Pashley DH. How can nanoleakage occur in self-etching adhesive systems that demineralize and infiltrate simultaneously? J Adhes Dent 2002;4:255–269.

154. Tay FR, Pashley DH, Yoshiyama M. Two modes of nanoleakage expression in single-step adhesives. J Dent Res 2002;81:472–476.

155. Tay FR, Pashley DH, Suh BI, Carvalho RM, Itthagarun A. Single-step adhesives are permeable membranes. J Dent 2002;30:371–382.

156. Tay FR, Pashley DH. Have dentin adhesives become too hydrophilic? J Can Dent Assoc 2003;69:726–731.

157. Fundingsland JW, Aasen SM, Bodger PD, Cernhous JJ. The effect of high humidity on adhesion to dentine [abstract 1199]. J Dent Res 1992;72:665.

158. Plasmans PJJM, Reukers EAJ, Vollenbrock-Kuipers L, Vollenbrock HR. Air humidity: A detrimental factor in dentine adhesion. J Dent 1993;21:228–233.

159. Terkla LG, Brown AC, Hainisch AP, Mitchem JC. Testing sealing properties of restorative materials against moist dentin. J Dent Res 1987;66:1758–1764.

160. Eliades GC, Caputo AA, Vougiouklakis GJ. Composition, wetting properties and bond strength with dentin of 6 new dentin adhesives. Dent Mater 1985;1:170–176.

161. Hitmi L, Bouter D, Degrange M. Influence of drying and HEMA treatment on dentin wettability. Dent Mater 2002;18:503–511.

162. Asmussen E, Uno S. Solubility parameters, fractional polarities, and bond strengths of some intermediary resins used in dentin bonding. J Dent Res 1993;72:558–565.

163. Asmussen E, Hansen EK. Dentine bonding agents. In: Vanherle G, Degrange M, Willems G (eds). State of the Art on Direct Posterior Filling Materials and Dentine Bonding. Proceedings of the International Symposium Euro Disney, ed 2. Leuven, Belgium: Van der Poorten, 1994:33.

164. Miller RG, Bowles CQ, Chappelow CC, Eick JD. Application of solubility parameter theory to dentin-bonding systems and adhesive strength correlations. J Biomed Mater Res 1998;41:237–243.

165. Braem M. An In-Vitro Investigation into the Physical Durability of Dental Composites [thesis]. Leuven, Belgium: Catholic University of Leuven, 1985.

166. Feilzer AJ, de Gee AJ, Davidson CL. Curing contraction of composites and glass ionomer cements. J Prosthet Dent 1988;59:297–300.

167. Feilzer AJ. Polymerization Shrinkage Stress in Dental Composite Resin Restorations—An In-Vitro Investigation [thesis]. Amsterdam, The Netherlands: University of Amsterdam (ACTA), 1989.

168. Jensen ME, Chan DCN. Polymerization shrinkage and microleakage. In: Vanherle G, Smith DC (eds). Posterior Composite Resin Dental Restorative Materials, ed 1. Utrecht, The Netherlands: Szulc, 1985:243.

169. Bowen RL, Nemoto K, Rapson JE. Adhesive bonding of various materials to hard tooth tissue: Forces developing in composite materials during hardening. J Am Dent Assoc 1983;106:475–477.

170. Hegdahl T, Gjerdet NR. Contraction stresses of composite filling materials. Acta Odontol Scand 1987;35:191–195.

171. Kemp-Scholte CM. The Marginal Integrity of Cervical Composite Resin Restorations [thesis]. Amsterdam, The Netherlands: University of Amsterdam (ACTA), 1989.

172. Davidson CL, de Gee AJ. Relaxation of polymerization contraction stress by flow in dental composites. J Dent Res 1984;63:146–148.

173. Lutz F, Krejci I, Oldenburg TR. Elimination of polymerization stresses at the margins of posterior composite resin restorations: A new restorative technique. Quintessence Int 1986;17:777–784.

174. Imai Y, Kadoma Y, Kojima K, Akimoto T, Ikakura K, Ohta T. Importance of polymerization initiator systems and interfacial initiation of polymerization in adhesive bonding of resin to dentin. J Dent Res 1991;70:1088–1091.

175. Eick JD, Robinson SJ, Byerley TJ, Chappelow CC. Adhesives and nonshrinking dental resins of the future. Quintessence Int 1993;24: 632–640.

176. Ferracane JL. Current trends in dental composites. Crit Rev Oral Biol Med 1995;6:302–318.

177. Stansbury JW. Synthesis and evaluation of new oxaspiro monomers for double ring-opening polymerization. J Dent Res 1992;71: 1408–1412.

178. Stansbury JW, Trujillo-Lemon M, Lu H, Ding X, Lin Y, Ge J. Conversion-dependent shrinkage stress and strain in dental resins and composites. Dent Mater 2005;21:56–67.

179. Eick JD, Byerley TJ, Chappell RP, Chen GR, Bowles CQ, Chappelow CC. Properties of expanding SOC/epoxy copolymers for dental use in dental composites. Dent Mater 1993;9:123–127.

180. Weinmann W, Thalacker C, Guggenberger R. Siloranes in dental composites. Dent Mater 2005;21:68–74.

181. Dauvillier BS, Feilzer AJ. Low-shrinkage dental restorative composite: Modeling viscoelastic behavior during setting. J Biomed Mater Res B Appl Biomater 2005;[Epub ahead of print].

182. Braem M, Lambrechts P, Vanherle G, Davidson CL. Stiffness increase during the setting of dental composite resins. J Dent Res 1987;66:1713–1716.

183. Alster D, Feilzer AJ, De Gee AJ, Mol A, Davidson CL. The dependence of shrinkage stress reduction on porosity concentration in thin resin layers. J Dent Res 1992;71:1619–1622 [erratum 1993;72:87].

184. Feilzer AJ, De Gee AJ, Davidson CL. Increased wall-to-wall curing contraction in thin bonded resin layers. J Dent Res 1989;68:48–50.

185. Feilzer AJ, De Gee AJ, Davidson CL. Setting stress in composite resin in relation to configuration of the restoratives. J Dent Res 1987;66:1636.

186. Asmussen E, Munksgaard EC. Adhesion of restorative resins to dentinal tissues. In: Vanherle G, Smith DC (eds). Posterior Composite Resin Dental Restorative Materials, ed 1. Utrecht, The Netherlands: Peter Szulc, 1985:217.

187. Davidson CL, De Gee AJ, Feilzer A. The competition between the composite-dentin bond strength and the polymerization contraction stress. J Dent Res 1984;63:1396.

188. Hansen EK, Asmussen E. Cavity preparation for restorative resins used with dentin adhesives. Scand J Dent Res 1985;93:474–479 [erratum 1986;94:87].

189. Bowen RL. Bonding agents and adhesives: Reactor response. Adv Dent Res 1988;2:155–157.

190. Bowen RL, Eichmiller FC, Marjenhoff WA. Glass-ceramic inserts anticipated for "megafilled" composite restorations. Research moves into the office. J Am Dent Assoc 1991;122:71, 73, 75.

191. Donly KJ, Wild TW, Bowen RL, Jensen ME. An in vitro investigation of the effects of glass inserts on the effective composite resin polymerization shrinkage. J Dent Res 1989;68:1234–1237.

192. Mehl A, Manhart J, Kremers L. Physical properties and marginal quality of Class-II composite fillings after softstart-polymerization [abstract 2121]. J Dent Res 1997;76:279.

193. Sakaguchi RL, Berge HX. Effect of light intensity on polymerization contraction of posterior composite [abstract 481]. J Dent Res 1997;76:74.

194. Uno S, Asmussen E. Marginal adaptation of a restorative resin polymerised at reduced rate. Scand J Dent Res 1991;99:440–444.

195. Mills RW, Jandt KD, Ashworth SH. Dental composite depth of cure with halogen and blue light emitting diode technology. Br Dent J 1999;186:388–391.

196. Kemp-Scholte CM, Davidson CL. Overhang of Class V composite resin restorations from hygroscopic expansion. Quintessence Int 1989;20:551–553.

197. Asmussen E. Clinical relevance of physical, chemical, and bonding properties of composite resins. Oper Dent 1985;10:61–73.

198. Kemp-Scholte CM, Davidson CL. Complete marginal seal of Class V resin composite restorations effected by increased flexibility. J Dent Res 1990;69:1240–1243.

199. Kemp-Scholte CM, Davidson CL. Marginal integrity related to bond strength and strain capacity of composite resin restorative systems. J Prosthet Dent 1990;64:658–664.

200. Van Meerbeek B, Willems G, Celis JP, et al. Assessment by nano-indentation of the hardness and elasticity of the resin-dentin bonding area. J Dent Res 1993;72:1434–1442.

201. Moon PC, Chang YH. Effect of DBA layer thickness on composite resin shrinkage stress [abstract 1357]. J Dent Res 1992;71:275.

202. Rueggeberg FA, Margeson DH. The effect of oxygen inhibition on an unfilled/filled composite system. J Dent Res 1990;69:1652–1658.

203. Crim GA. Prepolymerization of Gluma 4 sealer: Effect on bonding. Am J Dent 1990;3:25–27.

204. Hansen SE, Swift EJ. Microleakage with Gluma: Effects of unfilled resin polymerization and storage time. Am J Dent 1989;2:266–268.

205. Van Meerbeek B, Peumans M, Verschueren M, et al. Clinical status of ten dentin adhesive systems. J Dent Res 1994;73:1690–1702.

206. Peumans M, De Munck J, Van Landuyt K, Lambrechts P, Van Meerbeek B. Seven-year clinical effectiveness of two 3-step etch-and-rinse adhesives [abstract 147]. IADR-CED/NOF 2005.

207. Peumans M, De Munck J, Van Landuyt K, Lambrechts P, Van Meerbeek B. Three-year clinical effectiveness of a two-step self-etch adhesive in cervical lesions. Eur J Oral Sci 2005. In press.

208. Kemp-Scholte CM, Davidson CL. Marginal sealing of curing contraction gaps in Class V composite resin restorations. J Dent Res 1988;67:841–845.

209. Versluis A, Tantbirojn D, Douglas WH. Do dental composites always shrink toward the light? J Dent Res 1998;77:1435–1445.

210. Fusayama T. Biological problems of the light-cured composite resin. Quintessence Int 1993;24:225–226.

211. Perdigão J, Lambrechts P, Van Meerbeek B, et al. The interaction of adhesive systems with human dentin. Am J Dent 1996;9:167–173.

212. Hansen EK. Effect of cavity depth and application technique on marginal adaptation of resins in dentin cavities. J Dent Res 1986;65:1319–1321.

213. Lutz F, Krejci I, Barbakow F. Quality and durability of marginal adaptation in bonded composite restorations. Dent Mater 1991;7:107–113.

214. Torstenson BC, Odén A. Effects of bonding agent types and incremental techniques on minimizing contraction gaps around resin composites. Dent Mater 1989;5:218–223.

215. Versluis A, Douglas WH, Cross M, Sakaguchi RL. Does an incremental filling technique reduce polymerization shrinkage stresses? J Dent Res 1996;75:871–878.

216. Lutz F, Krejci I, Luescher B, Oldenburg TR. Improved proximal margin adaptation of Class II composite resin restorations by use of light-reflecting wedges. Quintessence Int 1986;17:659–664.

217. Asmussen E, Antonucci JM, Bowen RL. Adhesion to dentin by means of Gluma resin. Scand J Dent Res 1988;96:584–589.

218. Asmussen E, de Araujo PA, Peutzfeldt A. In-vitro bonding of resins to enamel and dentin: An update. Trans Acad Dent Mater 1989;2:36.

219. Asmussen E, Munksgaard EC. Bonding of restorative resins to dentine: Status of dentine adhesives and impact on cavity design and filling techniques. Int Dent J 1988;38:97–104.

220. Jordan RE, Suzuki M, MacLean DF. Early clinical evaluation of Tenure and Scotchbond 2 for conservative restoration of cervical erosion lesions. J Esthet Dent 1989;1:10–13.

221. Perdigão J, Swift EJ. Analysis of dentin bonding systems using the scanning electron microscope. Int Dent J 1994;44:349–359.

222. Nakabayashi N, Nakamura M, Yasuda N. Hybrid layer as a dentin-bonding mechanism. J Esthet Dent 1991;3:133–138.

223. Imai Y, Suzuki A. Effects of water and carboxylic acid monomer on polymerization of HEMA in the presence of N-phenylglycine. Dent Mater 1994;10:275–277.

224. Retief DH. Dentin bonding agents: A deterrent to microleakage? In: Anusavice KJ (ed). Quality Evaluation of Dental Restorations: Criteria for Placement and Replacement. Chicago: Quintessence, 1989:185.

225. Harper RH, Schnell RJ, Swartz ML, Phillips RW. In vivo measurements of thermal diffusion through restorations of various materials. J Prosthet Dent 1980;43:180–185.

226. Porte A, Lutz F, Lund MR, et al. Cavity designs for composite resins. Oper Dent 1984;9:50–56.

227. Gelb MN, Barouch E, Simonsen RJ. Resistance to cusp fracture in Class II prepared and restored premolars. J Prosthet Dent 1986; 55:184–185.

228. McCullock AJ, Smith BGN. In vitro studies of cuspal movement produced by adhesive restorative materials. Br Dent J 1986;161: 405–409.

229. Lambrechts P, Braem M, Vanherle G. Buonocore Memorial Lecture. Evaluation of clinical performance for posterior composite resins and dentin adhesives. Oper Dent 1987;12:53–78.

230. Munksgaard EC, Itoh K, Jorgensen KD. Dentin-polymer bond in resin fillings tested in vitro by thermo- and load-cycling. J Dent Res 1985;64:144–146.

231. Braem M, Lambrechts P, Vanherle G. Stress-induced cervical lesions. J Prosthet Dent 1992;67:718–722.

232. Goel VK, Khera SC, Ralston JL, Chang KH. Stresses at the dentino-enamel junction of human teeth—a finite element investigation. J Prosthet Dent 1991;66:451–459.

233. Lee WC, Eakle WS. Possible role of tensile stress in the etiology of cervical erosive lesions of teeth. J Prosthet Dent 1984;52:374–380.

234. Heymann HO, Sturdevant JR, Brunson WD, Wilder AD, Sluder TB, Bayne S. Twelve-month clinical study of dentinal adhesives in Class V cervical lesions. J Am Dent Assoc 1988;116:179–183.

235. Heymann HO, Sturdevant JR, Bayne S, Wilder AD, Sluder TB, Brunson WD. Examining tooth flexure effects on cervical restorations: A two-year clinical study. J Am Dent Assoc 1991;122:41–47.

236. Bayne SC, Heymann HO, Sturdevant JR, Wilder AD, Sluder TB. Contributing co-variables on clinical trials. Am J Dent 1991;4:247–250.

237. Browning WD, Brackett WW, Gilpatrick RO. Two-year clinical comparison of a microfilled and a hybrid resin-based composite in non-carious Class V lesions. Oper Dent 2000;25:46–50.

238. Anderson DAF, Ferracane JL, Zimmerman E, Kaga M. Cytotoxicity of variably cured light-activated dental composites [abstract 905]. J Dent Res 1988;67:226.

239. Cox CF, Keall CL, Keall HJ, et al. Biocompatibility of surface-sealed dental materials against exposed pulp. J Prosthet Dent 1987;57:1–8.

240. Stanley HR, Bowen RL, Folio J. Compatibility of various materials with oral tissues. II. Pulp responses to composite ingredients. J Dent Res 1979;58:1507–1517.

241. Torstenson BC, Nordenvall KJ, Brännström M. Pulpal reaction and microorganisms under Clearfil Composite Resin in deep cavities with acid etched dentin. Swed Dent J 1982;6:167–176.

242. Fusayama T. Factors and prevention of pulp irritation by adhesive composite resin restorations. Quintessence Int 1987;18:633–641.

243. Fusayama T. A new dental caries treatment system developed in Japan. Proc Jpn Acad 1990;66:121.

244. Mariotti A, Söderholm KJ, Johnson S. The in vivo effects of bisGMA on murine uterine weight, nucleic acids and collagen. Eur J Oral Sci 1998;106:1022–1027.

245. Noda M, Komatsu H, Sano H. HPLC analysis of dental resin composite components. J Biomed Mater Res 1999;47:374–378.

246. Olea N, Pulgar R, Perez P, et al. Estrogenicity of resin-based composites and sealants used in dentistry. Environ Health Perspect 1996;104:298–305.

247. Perez P, Pulgar R, Olea-Serrano F, et al. The estrogenicity of bisphenol A–related diphenylalkanes with various substituents at the central and carbon and the hydroxy groups. Environ Health Perspect 1998;106:167–174.

248. Schuurs AHB, van Amerongen JP. Algemene gezondheidsschade door composietrestauraties. Ned Tijdschr Tandheelk 1996;103: 444–447.

249. Söderholm KJ, Mariotti A. Bis-GMA-based resins in dentistry: Are they safe? J Am Dent Assoc 1999;130:201–209.

250. Katsuno K, Manabe A, Itoh K, et al. A delayed hypersensitivity reaction to dentine primer in the guinea-pig. J Dent 1995;23:295–299.

251. Katsuno K, Manabe A, Kurihara A, et al. The adverse effect of commercial dentine-bonding systems on the skin of guinea pigs. J Oral Rehabil 1998;25:180–184.

252. Ericksen HM. Protection against harmful effects of a restorative procedure using an acid cavity cleanser. J Dent Res 1976;55:281.

253. Fusayama T. The problems preventing progress in adhesive restorative dentistry. Adv Dent Res 1988;2:158–161, discussion 161–163.

254. Michelich V, Schuster GS, Pashley DH. Bacterial penetration of human dentin in vitro. J Dent Res 1980;59:1398–1403.

255. Qvist V, Thylstrup A. Pulpal reactions to resin restorations. In: Anusavice KJ (ed). Quality Evaluation of Dental Restorations: Criteria for Placement and Replacement. Chicago: Quintessence, 1989:291.

256. Stanford JW. Bonding of restorative materials to dentine. Int Dent J 1985;35:133–138.

257. Stanley HR, Going RE, Chauncey HH. Human pulp response to acid pretreatment of dentin and to composite restoration. J Am Dent Assoc 1975;91:817–825.

258. Schmalz G, Arenholt-Bindslev D. Biokompatibilität zahnärztlicher Werkstoffe. Munich: Elsevier, 2005.

259. Imazato S, Kinomoto Y, Tarumi H, Torii M, Russell RR, McCabe JF. Incorporation of antibacterial monomer MDPB into dentin primer. J Dent Res 1997;76:768–772.

260. Imazato S. Antibacterial properties of resin composites and dentin bonding systems. Dent Mater 2003;19:449–457.

261. Kuramoto A, Imazato S, Walls AW, Ebisu S. Inhibition of root caries progression by an antibacterial adhesive. J Dent Res 2005;84: 89–93.

262. Schmalz G, Ergucu Z, Hiller KA. Effect of dentin on the antibacterial activity of dentin bonding agents. J Endod 2004;30:352–358.

263. Bouschlicher MR, Reinhardt JW, Vargas MA. Surface treatment techniques for resin composite repair. Am J Dent 1997;10:279–283.

264. Roeters JJ. A simple method to protect patient and environment when using sandblasting for intraoral repair. J Adhes Dent 2000;2:235–238.

265. Trajtenberg CP, Powers JM. Bond strengths of repaired laboratory composites using three surface treatments and three primers. Am J Dent 2004;17:123–126.

266. Wilson N, Setcos J, Brunton P. Replacement or repair of dental restorations. In: Roulet JF, Fuzzi M (eds). Advances in Operative Dentistry, Vol 2. Challenges of the Future. Chicago: Quintessence, 2001:105–115.

267. Fortin D, Swift EJ, Denehy GE, Reinhardt JW. Bond strength and microleakage of current dentin adhesives. Dent Mater 1994;10: 253–258.

268. Swift EJ Jr, Triolo PT Jr, Barkmeier WW, Bird JL, Bounds SJ. Effect of low-viscosity resins on the performance of dental adhesives. Am J Dent 1996;9:100–104 [erratum 1996;9:following 179].

269. Van Meerbeek B, Peumans M, Gladys S, Braem M, Lambrechts P, Vanherle G. Three-year clinical effectiveness of four total-etch dentinal adhesive systems in cervical lesions. Quintessence Int 1996;27:775–784.

270. Gaengler P, Hoyer I, Montag R, Gaebler P. Micromorphological evaluation of posterior composite restorations—a 10-year report. J Oral Rehabil 2004;31:991–1000.

271. Opdam NJ, Loomans BA, Roeters FJ, Bronkhorst EM. Five-year clinical performance of posterior resin composite restorations placed by dental students. J Dent 2004;32:379–383.

272. Van Meerbeek B, Vargas M, Inoue S, et al. Adhesives and cements to promote preservation dentistry. Oper Dent 2001;suppl 6:119–144.

273. Wilson AD, Kent BE. The glass-ionomer cement, a new translucent cement for dentistry. J Appl Chem Biotechnol 1971;21:313.

274. Peumans M, Van Meerbeek B, Yoshida Y, Lambrechts P, Vanherle G. Porcelain veneers bonded to tooth structure: An ultra-morphological FE-SEM examination of the adhesive interface. Dent Mater 1999;15:105–119.

275. Van Meerbeek B, Conn LJ Jr, Duke ES, Eick JD, Robinson SJ, Guerrero D. Correlative transmission electron microscopy examination of nondemineralized and demineralized resin-dentin interfaces formed by two dentin adhesive systems. J Dent Res 1996;75:879–888.

276. Van Meerbeek B, Yoshida Y, Lambrechts P, et al. A TEM study of two water-based adhesive systems bonded to dry and wet dentin. J Dent Res 1998;77:50–59.

277. Sano H, Shono T, Takatsu T, Hosoda H. Microporous dentin zone beneath resin-impregnated layer. Oper Dent 1994;19:59–64.

278. Sano H, Yoshiyama M, Ebisu S, et al. Comparative SEM and TEM observations of nanoleakage within the hybrid layer. Oper Dent 1995;20:160–167.

279. Tay FR, Gwinnett AJ, Pang KM, Wei SH. Resin permeation into acid-conditioned, moist, and dry dentin: A paradigm using water-free adhesive primers. J Dent Res 1996;75:1034–1044.

280. Silverstone LM. Fissure sealants: Laboratory studies. Caries Res 1974;8:2–26.

281. Summitt JB, Chan DCN, Burgess JO, Dutton FB. Effect of air/water rinse versus water only and of five rinse times on resin-to-etched enamel shear bond strength. Oper Dent 1992;17:142–151.

282. Summitt JB, Chan DCN, Dutton FB, Burgess JO. Effect of rinse time on microleakage between composite and etched enamel. Oper Dent 1993;18:37–40.

283. Gwinnett AJ, Buonocore MG. Adhesion and caries prevention. A preliminary report. Br Dent J 1965;119:77–80.

284. Kellar M, Duke ES. Neutralizing phosphoric acid in the acid etch resin technique. J Oral Rehabil 1988;15:625–630.

285. Chow LC, Brown WE. Phosphoric acid conditioning of teeth for pit and fissure sealants. J Dent Res 1973;52:1158.

286. Barkmeier WW, Erickson RL. Shear bond strength of composite to enamel and dentin using Scotchbond Multi-Purpose. Am J Dent 1994;7:175–179.

287. Gwinnett AJ, Kanca J. Micromorphology of the bonded dentin interface and its relationship to bond strength. Am J Dent 1992;5:73–77.

288. Inoue M, Finger WJ, Mueller M. Effect of filler content of restorative resins on retentive strength to acid-conditioned enamel. Am J Dent 1994;7:161–166.

289. Zidan O, Hill G. Phosphoric acid concentration: Enamel surface loss and bonding strength. J Prosthet Dent 1986;55:388–392.

290. Barkmeier WW, Shaffer SE, Gwinnett AJ. Effects of 15 vs 60 second enamel acid conditioning on adhesion and morphology. Oper Dent 1986;11:111–116.

291. Swift EJ, Perdigão J, Heymann HO. Bonding to enamel and dentin: A brief history and state of the art, 1995. Quintessence Int 1995;26:95–110.

292. Qvist V, Qvist J. Effect of ethanol and NPG-GMA on replica patterns on composite restorations performed in vivo in acid-etched cavities. Scand J Dent Res 1985;93:371–376.

293. Bowen RL [inventor]. Dental filling material comprising vinyl silane, treated fused silica and a binder consisting of the reaction product of bisphenol and glycidyl acrylate. US patent 3066.112, 1962.

294. Buonocore MG, Matsui A, Gwinnett AJ. Penetration of resin dental materials into enamel surfaces with reference to bonding. Arch Oral Biol 1968;13:61–70.

295. Gwinnett AJ, Matsui A. A study of enamel adhesives. The physical relationship between enamel and adhesive. Arch Oral Biol 1967;12:1615–1620.

296. Gwinnett AJ. Histologic changes in human enamel following treatment with acidic adhesive conditioning agents. Arch Oral Biol 1971;16:731–738.

297. Silverstone LM, Saxton CA, Dogon IL, Fejerskov O. Variation in pattern of etching of human dental enamel examined by scanning electron microscopy. Caries Res 1975;9:373–387.

298. Bayne SC, Flemming JE, Faison S. SEM-EDS analysis of macro and micro resin tags of laminates [abstract 1128]. J Dent Res 1982;61:304.

299. Gwinnett AJ. Structure and composition of enamel. Oper Dent 1992;suppl 5:10–17.

300. Tagami J, Hosoda H, Fusayama T. Optimal technique of etching enamel. Oper Dent 1988;13:181–184.

301. Gilpatrick RO, Ross JA, Simonsen RJ. Resin-to-enamel bond strengths with various etching times. Quintessence Int 1991;22:47–49.

302. Crim GA, Shay JS. Effect of etchant time on microleakage. ASDC J Dent Child 1987;54:339–340.

303. Shaffer SE, Barkmeier WW, Kelsey WP. Effects of reduced acid conditioning time on enamel microleakage. Gen Dent 1987;35:278–280.

304. De Munck J, Van Landuyt KL, Coutinho E, et al. Fatigue resistance of dentin/composite interfaces with an additional intermediate elastic layer. Eur J Oral Sci 2005;113:77–82.

305. Barghi N, Knight GT, Berry TG. Comparing two methods of moisture control in bonding to enamel: A clinical study. Oper Dent 1991;16:130–135.

306. Sugizaki J. The effect of the various primers on the dentin adhesion of resin composites—SEM and TEM observations of the resin-impregnated layer and adhesion promoting effect of the primers. Jpn J Conserv Dent 1991;34:228.

307. Van Meerbeek B, Dhem A, Goret-Nicaise M, Braem M, Lambrechts P, Vanherle G. Comparative SEM and TEM examination of the ultrastructure of the resin-dentin interdiffusion zone. J Dent Res 1993;72:495–501.

308. Benediktsson S, Retief DH, Russel CM, Mandras RS. Critical surface tension of wetting of dentin [abstract 777]. J Dent Res 1991;70:362.

309. Jacobsen T, Ma R, Söderholm K-J. Dentin bonding through interpenetrating network formation. Trans Acad Dent Mater 1994;7:45.

310. Nakabayashi N, Takarada K. Effect of HEMA on bonding to dentin. Dent Mater 1992;8:125–130.

311. Nikaido T, Burrow MF, Tagami J, Takatsu T. Effect of pulpal pressure on adhesion of resin composite to dentin: Bovine serum versus saline. Quintessence Int 1995;26:221–226.

312. Jacobsen T, Soderholm KJ, Garcea I, Mondragon E. Calcium leaching from dentin and shear bond strength after etching with phosphoric acid of different concentrations. Eur J Oral Sci 2000;108:247–254.

313. Swift EJ, Hammel SA, Perdigão J, Wefel JS. Prevention of root surface caries using a dental adhesive. J Am Dent Assoc 1994;125:571–576.

314. Brännström M, Linden LA, Astrom A. The hydrodynamics of the dentinal tubule and of pulp fluid. A discussion of its significance in relation to dentinal sensitivity. Caries Res 1967;1:310.

315. Hansen SE, Swift EJ. Microleakage with Gluma: Effects of unfilled resin polymerization and storage time. Am J Dent 1989;2:266–268.

316. Erickson RL. Mechanism and clinical implications of bond formation for two dentin bonding agents. Am J Dent 1989;2:117–123.

317. Nakabayashi N. Bonding of restorative materials to dentine: The present status in Japan. Int Dent J 1985;35:145–154.

318. Shimokobe H, Honda T, Kobayashi Y, et al. Denaturation of dentin collagen by phosphoric acid treatment [abstract 908]. J Dent Res 1988;67:226.

319. Okamoto Y, Heeley JD, Dogon IL, Shintani H. Effects of phosphoric acid and tannic acid on dentine collagen. J Oral Rehabil 1991;18:507–512.

320. Scott PG, Leaver AG. The degradation of human collagen by trypsin. Connect Tissue Res 1974;2:299–307.

321. El Feninat F, Ellis TH, Sacher E, Stangel I. Moisture-dependent renaturation of collagen in phosphoric acid etched human dentin. J Biomed Mater Res 1998;42:549–553.

322. De Munck J, Vargas M, Iracki J, et al. One-day bonding effectiveness of new self-etch adhesives to bur-cut enamel and dentin. Oper Dent 2005;30:39–49.

323. De Munck J, Van Landuyt K, Peumans M, et al. A critical review of the durability of adhesion to tooth tissue: Methods and results. J Dent Res 2005;84:118–132.

324. Ciucchi B, Sano H, Pashley DH. Bonding to sodium hypochlorite treated dentin [abstract 1556]. J Dent Res 1994;73:296.

325. Gwinnett AJ. Altered tissue contribution to interfacial bond strength with acid conditioned dentin. Am J Dent 1994;7:243–246.

326. Wakabayashi Y, Kondou Y, Suzuki K, Yatani H, Yamashita A. Effect of dissolution of collagen on adhesion to dentin. Int J Prosthod 1994;7:302–306.

327. Sano H, Yoshikawa T, Pereira PN, et al. Long-term durability of dentin bonds made with a self-etching primer. J Dent Res 1999;78:906–911.

328. Sano H, Takatsu T, Ciucchi B, Horner JA, Matthews WG, Pashley DH. Nanoleakage: Leakage within the hybrid layer. Oper Dent 1995;20:18–25.

329. Titley K, Chernecky R, Maric B, Smith D. Penetration of a dentin bonding agent into dentin. Am J Dent 1994;7:190–194.

330. Nakabayashi N. Adhesive bonding with 4-META. Oper Dent 1992;suppl 5:125–130.

331. Tay FR, Gwinnett AJ, Pang KM, Wei SHY. Structural evidence of a sealed tissue interface with a total-etch wet-bonding technique in vivo. J Dent Res 1994;73:629–636.

332. Gerzina TM, Hume WR. Effect of dentine on release of TEGDMA from resin composite in vitro. J Oral Rehabil 1994;21:463–468.

333. Gerzina TM, Hume WR. Effect of hydrostatic pressure on the diffusion of monomers through dentin in vitro. J Dent Res 1995;74:369–373.

334. Van Meerbeek B, Perdigão J, Lambrechts P, Vanherle G. The clinical performance of adhesives. J Dent 1998;26:1–20.

335. Chappell RP, Cobb CM, Spencer P, Eick JD. Dentinal tubule anastomosis: A potential factor in adhesive bonding? J Prosthet Dent 1994;72:183–188.

336. Perdigão J, Ramos CJ, Lambrechts P. In vitro interfacial relationship between human dentin and one-bottle dental adhesives. Dent Mater 1997;13:218–227.

337. Labella R, Van Meerbeek B, Yoshida Y, et al. Marginal gap distribution of two-step versus three-step adhesive systems [abstract P35]. Trans Acad Dent Mat 1998;12:237.

338. Blunck U, Roulet J-F. Effect of one-bottle-adhesives on the marginal adaptation of composite resins and compomers in Class V cavities in vitro [abstract 2231]. J Dent Res 1998;77:910.

339. Inoue S, Vargas MA, Abe Y, et al. Microtensile bond strength of eleven contemporary adhesives to dentin. J Adhes Dent 2001;3:237–245.

340. Inoue S, Vargas MA, Abe Y, et al. Microtensile bond strength of eleven contemporary adhesives to enamel. Am J Dent 2003;16:329–334.

341. Van Dijken JWV. Clinical effectiveness of 12 adhesive systems in Class V non-retentive lesions. A 5-year evaluation [abstract 42]. J Dent Res 2001;80:1212.

342. Finger WJ, Balkenhol M. Rewetting strategies for bonding to dry dentin with an acetone-based adhesive. J Adhes Dent 2000;2:51–56.

343. Inoue S, Van Meerbeek B, Vargas M, Yoshida Y, Lambrechts P, Vanherle G. Adhesion mechanism of self-etching adhesives. In: Tagami J, Toledano M, Prati C (eds). Third International Kuraray Symposium of Advanced Dentistry, 3–4 December 1999, Granada, Spain. Como, Italy: Graphice Erredue, 2000:131–148.

344. Pashley DH, Tay FR. Aggressiveness of contemporary self-etching adhesives. Part II: Etching effects on unground enamel. Dent Mater 2001;17:430–444.

345. Van Meerbeek B, Yoshida Y, Inoue S, et al. Bonding mechanism and micro-tensile bond strength of a 4-MET based self-etching adhesive [abstract 249]. J Dent Res 2000;79(special issue).

346. Hashimoto M, Ohno H, Kaga M, Endo K, Sano H, Oguchi H. In vivo degradation of resin-dentin bonds in humans over 1 to 3 years. J Dent Res 2000;79:1385–1391.

347. Hashimoto M, Ohno H, Sano H, et al. Micromorphological changes in resin-dentin bonds after 1 year of water storage. J Biomed Mater Res 2002;63:306–311.

348. Bouillaguet S, Gysi P, Wataha JC, et al. Bond strength of composite to dentin using conventional, one-step, and self-etching adhesive systems. J Dent 2001;29:55–61.

349. Fritz UB, Finger WJ. Bonding efficiency of single-bottle enamel/dentin adhesives. Am J Dent 1999;12:277–282.

350. Tay FR, Pashley DH. Water treeing—a potential mechanism for degradation of dentin adhesives. Am J Dent 2003;16:6–12.

351. Hashimoto M, Ohno H, Sano H, Kaga M, Oguchi H. Degradation patterns of different adhesives and bonding procedures. J Biomed Mater Res 2003;66B:324–330.

352. Hashimoto M, Tay FR, Ohno H, et al. SEM and TEM analysis of water degradation of human dentinal collagen. J Biomed Mater Res 2003;66B:287–298.

353. Van Landuyt K, De Munck J, Snauwaert J, et al. Monomer-solvent phase separation in one-step self-etch adhesives. J Dent Res 2005;84:183–188.

354. Van Meerbeek B, Yoshida Y, Lambrechts P, Vanherle G. Mechanisms of bonding a resin-modified glass-ionomer adhesive to dentin [abstract 2236]. J Dent Res 1998;77(special issue B):911.

355. Van Meerbeek B, Yoshida Y, Inoue S, et al. Interfacial characterization of resin-modified glass-ionomers to dentin [abstract 1701]. J Dent Res 2001;80(special issue):739.

356. Tay FR, Smales RJ, Ngo H, Wei SH, Pashley DH. Effect of different conditioning protocols on adhesion of a GIC to dentin. J Adhes Dent 2001;3:153–167.

357. Yip HK, Tay FR, Ngo HC, Smales RJ, Pashley DH. Bonding of contemporary glass ionomer cements to dentin. Dent Mater 2001;17:456–470.

358. Yoshida Y, Van Meerbeek B, Nakayama Y, et al. Evidence of chemical bonding at biomaterial-hard tissue interfaces. J Dent Res 2000;79:709–714.

359. Fukuda R, Yoshida Y, Nakayama Y, et al. Bonding efficacy of polyalkenoic acids to hydroxyapatite, enamel and dentin. Biomaterials 2003;24:1861–1867.

360. Yoshioka M, Yoshida Y, Inoue S, et al. Adhesion/decalcification mechanisms of acid interactions with human hard tissues. J Biomed Mater Res 2002;59:56–62.

361. Yoshida Y, Van Meerbeek B, Nakayama Y, et al. Adhesion to and decalcification of hydroxyapatite by carboxylic acids. J Dent Res 2001;80:1565–1569.

362. Yoshida Y, Van Meerbeek B, Snauwaert J, et al. A novel approach to AFM characterization of adhesive tooth–biomaterial interfaces. J Biomed Mater Res 1999;47:85–90.

363. Buonocore M, Wileman W, Brudevold F. A report on a resin composition capable of bonding to human dentin surfaces. J Dent Res 1956;35:846–851.

364. McLean JW, Kramer IRH. A clinical and pathological evaluation of a sulphinic acid activated resin for use in restorative dentistry. Br Dent J 1952;93:255.

365. McLean JW. Bonding to enamel and dentin [letter]. Quintessence Int 1995;26:234.

366. Van Meerbeek B, Vanherle G, Lambrechts P, Braem M. Dentin- and enamel-bonding agents. Curr Opin Dent 1992;2:117–127.

367. Bowen RL. Adhesive bonding of various materials to hard tooth tissues. II. Bonding to dentin promoted by a surface-active comonomer. J Dent Res 1965;44:895–902.

368. Alexieva C. Character of the hard tooth tissue-polymer bond. II. Study of the interaction of human tooth enamel and dentin with N-phenylglycine-glycidyl methacrylate adduct. J Dent Res 1979;58:1884–1886.

369. Bowen RL, Marjenhoff WA. Development of an adhesive bonding system. Oper Dent 1992;suppl 5:75–80.

370. Causton BE. Improved bonding of composite restorative to dentine. Br Dent J 1984;156:93–95.

371. Edler TL, Krikorian E, Thompson VP. FTIR surface analysis of dentin and dentin bonding agents [abstract 1534]. J Dent Res 1991;70:458.

372. Spencer P, Wieliczka DM, Meeske J, et al. The resin-dentin interface—morphological and chemical characterization [abstract 44]. J Dent Res 1994;73:107.

373. Van Meerbeek B, Mohrbacher H, Celis JP, et al. Chemical characterization of the resin-dentin interface by micro-Raman spectroscopy. J Dent Res 1993;72:1423–1428.

374. Wolinsky LE, Armstrong RW, Seghi RR. The determination of ionic bonding interactions of N-phenyl glycine and N-(2-hydroxy-3-methacryloxypropyl)-N-phenyl glycine as measured by carbon-13 NMR analysis. J Dent Res 1993;72:72–77.

375. Jendresen MD. Clinical performance of a new composite resin for Class V erosion [abstract 1057]. J Dent Res 1978;57:339.

376. Tyas MJ, Burns GA, Byrne PF, Cunningham PJ, Dobson BC, Widdop FT. Clinical evaluation of Scotchbond: Three-year results. Aust Dent J 1989;34:277–279.

377. Tyas MJ. Three-year clinical evaluation of dentine bonding agents. Aust Dent J 1991;36:298–301.

378. Vanherle G, Lambrechts P, Braem M. An evaluation of different adhesive restorations in cervical lesions. J Prosthet Dent 1991;65:341–347.

379. Eliades GC, Vougiouklakis GJ. 31P-NMR study of P-based dental adhesives and electron probe microanalysis of simulated interfaces with dentin. Dent Mater 1989;5:101–108.

380. Huang GT, Söderholm K-JM. In vitro investigation of shear bond strength of a phosphate based dentinal bonding agent. Scand J Dent Res 1989;97:84–92.

381. Yu XY, Joynt RB, Wieczkowski G, Davis EL. Scanning electron microscopic and energy dispersive x-ray evaluation of two smear layer–mediated dentinal bonding agents. Quintessence Int 1991;22:305–310.

382. Fusayama T, Nakamura M, Kurosaki N, Iwaku M. Non-pressure adhesion of a new adhesive restorative system. J Dent Res 1979;58:1364–1370.

383. Bertolotti RL. Conditioning of the dentin substrate. Oper Dent 1992;suppl 5:131–136.

384. Cox CF. Effects of adhesive resins and various dental cements on the pulp. Oper Dent 1992;suppl 5:165–176.

385. Retief DH, Austin JC, Fatti LP. Pulpal response to phosphoric acid. J Oral Pathol 1974;3:114–122.

386. Bowen RL, Tung MS, Blosser RL, Asmussen E. Dentine and enamel bonding agents. Int Dent J 1987;37:158–161.

387. Perdigão J, Swift EJ, Denehy GE, Wefel JS, Donly KJ. In vitro bond strengths and SEM evaluation of dentin bonding systems to different dentin substrates. J Dent Res 1994;73:44–55.

388. Triolo PT Jr, Swift EJ Jr. Shear bond strengths of ten dentin adhesive systems. Dent Mater 1992;8:370–374.

389. Duke ES, Robbins JW, Snyder DE. Clinical evaluation of a dentinal adhesive system: Three-year results. Quintessence Int 1991;22:889–895.

390. Jordan RE, Suzuki M, Davidson DF. Clinical evaluation of a universal dentin bonding resin: Preserving dentition through new materials. J Am Dent Assoc 1993;124:71–76.

391. Powell LV, Gordon GE, Johnson GH. Clinical comparison of Class V resin composite and glass ionomer restorations. Am J Dent 1992;5:249–252.

392. Council on Dental Materials, Instruments, and Equipment. ADA Clinical Protocol Guidelines for Dentin and Enamel Adhesive Restorative Materials. Chicago: American Dental Association, 1987.

393. Toledano M, Osorio R, de Leonardi G, Rosales-Leal JI, Ceballos L, Cabrerizo-Vilchez MA. Influence of self-etching primer on the resin adhesion to enamel and dentin. Am J Dent 2001;14:205–210.

394. Chan KM, Tay FR, King NM, Imazato S, Pashley DH. Bonding of mild self-etching primers/adhesives to dentin with thick smear layers. Am J Dent 2003;16:340–346.

395. Burrow MF, Taniguchi Y, Nikaido T, et al. Influence of temperature and relative humidity on early bond strengths to dentine. J Dent 1995;23:41–45.

396. Plasmans PJ, Creugers NH, Hermsen RJ, Vrijhoef MM. Intraoral humidity during operative procedures. J Dent 1994;22:89–91.

397. Eliades GC. Reaction paper: Dentine bonding systems. In: Vanherle G, Degrange M, Willems G (eds). Proceedings of the International Symposium on State of the Art on Direct Posterior Filling Materials and Dentine Bonding. Leuven, Belgium: Van der Poorten, 1993:49–74.

398. Peters WJ, Jackson RW, Smith DC. Studies of the stability and toxicity of zinc polyacrylate (polycarboxylate) cements (PAZ). J Biomed Mater Res 1974;8:53–60.

399. Besnault C, Attal JP. Influence of a simulated oral environment on dentin bond strength of two adhesive systems. Am J Dent 2001;14:367–372.

400. Besnault C, Attal JP. Influence of a simulated oral environment on microleakage of two adhesive systems in Class II composite restorations. J Dent 2002;30:1–6.

401. Werner JF, Tani C. Effect of relative humidity on bond strength of self-etching adhesives to dentin. J Adhes Dent 2002;4:277–282.

402. Dietrich T, Kraemer ML, Roulet JF. Blood contamination and dentin bonding-effect of anticoagulant in laboratory studies. Dent Mater 2002;18:159–162.

403. Eiriksson SO, Pereira PN, Swift EJ, Heymann HO, Sigurdsson A. Effects of blood contamination on resin-resin bond strength. Dent Mater 20;2004:184–190.

404. van Schalkwyk JH, Botha FS, van der Vyver PJ, de Wet FA, Botha SJ. Effect of biological contamination on dentine bond strength of adhesive resins. SADJ 2003;58:143–147.

405. Ziemiecki TL, Dennison JB, Charbeneau GT. Clinical evaluation of cervical composite resin restorations placed without retention. Oper Dent 1987;2:27–33.

406. Van Meerbeek B, Perdigão J, Inohoshi S, et al. Pulpareacties enpulpabescherming: Traditionele onderlagen versus dentine hechtlakken. Ned Tijdschr Tandh 1996;103:439–443.

407. Murray PE, Hafez AA, Windsor LJ, Smith AJ, Cox CF. Comparison of pulp responses following restoration of exposed and non-exposed cavities. J Dent 2002;30:213–222.

408. Murray PE, Smith AJ, Windsor LJ, Mjor IA. Remaining dentine thickness and human pulp responses. Int Endod J 2003;36:33–43.

409. de Souza Costa CA, Hebling J, Hanks CT. Current status of pulp capping with dentin adhesive systems: A review. Dent Mater 2000; 16:188–197.

410. de Souza Costa CA, Lopes do Nascimento AB, Teixeira HM, Fontana UF. Response of human pulps capped with a self-etching adhesive system. Dent Mater 2001;17:230–240.

411. Pereira JC, Segala AD, Costa CA. Human pulpal response to direct pulp capping with an adhesive system. Am J Dent 2000;13:139–147.

412. Mestrener SR, Holland R, Dezan E Jr. Influence of age on the behavior of dental pulp of dog teeth after capping with an adhesive system or calcium hydroxide. Dent Traumatol 2003;19:255–261.

413. Hebling J, Giro EM, Costa CA. Human pulp response after an adhesive system application in deep cavities. J Dent 1999;27:557–564.

414. Bergenholtz G. Evidence for bacterial causation of adverse pulpal responses in resin-based dental restorations. Crit Rev Oral Biol Med 2000;11:467–480.

415. Cox CF. Microleakage related to restorative procedures. Proc Finn Dent Soc 1992;88(suppl 1):83–93.

416. Costa CA, Oliveira MF, Giro EM, Hebling J. Biocompatibility of resin-based materials used as pulp-capping agents. Int Endod J 2003;36:831–839.

417. Fujitani M, Shibata S, Van Meerbeek B, Yoshida Y, Shintani H. Direct adhesive pulp capping: Pulpal healing and ultra-morphology of the resin-pulp interface. Am J Dent 2002;15:395–402.

418. Horsted-Bindslev P, Vilkinis V, Sidlauskas A. Direct capping of human pulps with a dentin bonding system or with calcium hydroxide cement. Oral Surg Oral Med Oral Pathol Oral Radiol Endod 2003;96:591–600.

419. do Nascimento AB, Fontana UF, Teixeira HM, Costa CA. Biocompatibility of a resin-modified glass-ionomer cement applied as pulp capping in human teeth. Am J Dent 2000;13:28–34.

420. Kiba H, Hayakawa T, Nakanuma K, Yamazaki M, Yamamoto H. Pulpal reactions to two experimental bonding systems for pulp capping procedures. J Oral Sci 2000;42:69–74.

421. Chen RS, Liu CC, Tseng WY, Jeng JH, Lin CP. Cytotoxicity of three dentin bonding agents on human dental pulp cells. J Dent 2003;31:223–229.

422. Swift EJ, Cloe BC. Shear bond strengths of new enamel etchants. Am J Dent 1993;6:162–164.

423. Triolo PT Jr, Swift EJ Jr, Mudgil A, Levine A. Effect of etching time on enamel bond strengths. Am J Dent 1993;6:302–304.

424. Eick JD, Robinson SJ, Byerley TJ, et al. Scanning transmission electron microscopy/energy-dispersive spectroscopy analysis of the dentin adhesive interface using a labeled 2-hydroxyethylmethacrylate analogue. J Dent Res 1995;74:1246–1252.

425. Watanabe I, Nakabayashi N, Pashley DH. Bonding to ground dentin by a phenyl-P self-etching primer. J Dent Res 1994;73:1212–1220.

426. Perdigão J, Lopes L, Lambrechts P, et al. Effects of self-etching primer on enamel shear bond strengths and SEM morphology. Am J Dent 1997;10:141–146 [erratum 1997;10:183].

427. Kanemura N, Sano H, Tagami J. Tensile bond strength to and SEM evaluation of ground and intact enamel surfaces. J Dent 1999; 27:523–530.

428. Van Landuyt K, Padmini K, De Munck J, Peumans M, Lambrechts P, Van Meerbeek B. Bond strength of a mild self-etch adhesive with and without prior acid-etching. J Dent 2005;[epub ahead of print].

429. Van Meerbeek B, Kanumilli P, De Munck J, Van Landuyt K, Lambrechts P, Peumans M. A randomized controlled study evaluating the effectiveness of a two-step self-etch adhesive with and without selective phosphoric-acid etching of enamel. Dent Mater 2005; 21:375–383.

430. McLean JW, Nicholson JW, Wilson AD. Proposed nomenclature for glass-ionomer dental cements and related materials [guest editorial]. Quintessence Int 1994;25:587–589.

431. Gladys S, Van Meerbeek B, Braem M, Lambrechts P, Vanherle G. Comparative physico-mechanical characterization of new hybrid restorative materials with conventional glass-ionomer and resin composite restorative materials. J Dent Res 1997;76:883–894.

432. Gladys S, Van Meerbeek B, Lambrechts P, Vanherle G. Marginal adaptation and retention of a glass-ionomer, resin-modified glass-ionomers and a polyacid-modified resin composite in cervical Class-V lesions. Dent Mater 1998;14:294–306.

433. Cortes O, Garcia-Godoy F, Boj JR. Bond strength of resin-reinforced glass ionomer cements after enamel etching. Am J Dent 1993;6: 299–301.

434. Fritz U, Finger W, Uno S. Resin-modified glass ionomer cements: Bonding to enamel and dentin. Dent Mater 1996;12:161–166.

435. Kanca J 3rd. Effect of resin primer solvent and surface wetness on resin composite bond strength to dentin. Am J Dent 1992;5:213–215.

436. Kanca J 3rd. Resin bonding to wet substrate. I. Bonding to dentin. Quintessence Int 1992;23:39–41.

437. Kanca J 3rd. Improving bond strength through acid etching of dentin and bonding to wet dentin surfaces. J Am Dent Assoc 1992;123:35–43.

438. Gwinnett AJ. Moist versus dry dentin: Its effect on shear bond strength. Am J Dent 1992;5:127–129.

439. Perdigão J, Swift EJ, Cloe BC. Effects of etchants, surface moisture, and composite resin on dentin bond strengths. Am J Dent 1993;6: 61–64.

440. Perdigão J, Lambrechts P, Van Meerbeek B, Vanherle G, Lopes AB. A field emission SEM comparison of four post-fixation drying techniques for human dentin. J Biomed Mater Res 1995;29:1111–1120.

441. Swift EJ, Triolo PT. Bond strengths of Scotchbond Multi-Purpose to moist dentin and enamel. Am J Dent 1992;5:318–320.

442. Pereira GD, Paulillo LA, De Goes MF, Dias CT. How wet should dentin be? Comparison of methods to remove excess water during moist bonding. J Adhes Dent 2001;3:257–264.

443. Tay FR, Gwinnett AJ, Wei SHY. Micromorphological spectrum from overdrying to overwetting acid-conditioned dentin in water-free acetone-based, single-bottle primer/adhesives. Dent Mater 1996; 12:236–244.

444. Carvalho RM, Pashley EL, Yoshiyama M, et al. Dimensional changes in demineralized dentin [abstract 171]. J Dent Res 1995;74:33.

445. Perdigão J, Van Meerbeek B, Lopes MM, Ambrose WW. The effect of a re-wetting agent on dentin bonding. Dent Mater 1999; 15:282–295.

446. Sterrett JD, Murphy HJ. Citric acid burnishing of dentinal root surfaces. A scanning electron microscopy report. J Clin Periodontol 1989;16:98–104.

447. Bayne SC, Wilder AD, Heymann HO, et al. 1-year clinical evaluation of stress-breaking Class V DBA design. Trans Acad Dent Mater 1994;7:91.

448. Boghosian A. Clinical evaluation of a filled adhesive system in Class 5 restorations. Compend Contin Educ Dent 1996;17:750–752, 754–757.

449. Davidson CL, Abdalla AI. Effect of occlusal load cycling on the marginal integrity of adhesive Class V restorations. Am J Dent 1994;7: 111–114.

450. Fortin D, Perdigão J, Swift EJ Jr. Microleakage of three new dentin adhesives. Am J Dent 1994;7:315.

451. Trevino DF, Duke ES, Robbins JW, Summitt JB. Clinical evaluation of Scotchbond Multi-Purpose Adhesive System [abstract 3037]. J Dent Res 1996;75:397.

452. Powell LV, Johnson GH, Gordon GE. Factors associated with clinical success of cervical abrasion/erosion restorations. Oper Dent 1995; 20:7–13.

453. Tsai YH, Swartz ML, Phillips RW, Moore BK. A comparative study: Bond strength and microleakage of dentin bond systems. Oper Dent 1990;15:53–60.

454. Armstrong SR, Keller JC, Boyer DB. The influence of water storage and C-factor on the dentin-resin composite microtensile bond strength and debond pathway utilizing a filled and unfilled adhesive resin. Dent Mater 2001;17:268–276.

455. Opdam NJ, Roeters FJ, Feilzer AJ, Verdonschot EH. Marginal integrity and postoperative sensitivity in Class 2 resin composite restorations in vivo. J Dent 1998;26:555–562.

456. Santerre JP, Shajii L, Leung BW. Relation of dental composite formulations to their degradation and the release of hydrolyzed polymeric-resin-derived products. Crit Rev Oral Biol Med 2001;12:136–151.

457. Gale MS, Darvell BW. Thermal cycling procedures for laboratory testing of dental restorations. J Dent 1999;27:89–99.

458. Simo-Alfonso E, Gelfi C, Sebastiano R, Citterio A, Righetti PG. Novel acrylamido monomers with higher hydrophilicity and improved hydrolytic stability .1. Synthetic route and product characterization. Electrophoresis 1996;17:723–731.

459. Pashley DH, Tay FR, Yiu C, et al. Collagen degradation by host-derived enzymes during aging. J Dent Res 2004;83:216–221.

460. Dhanasomboon S, Nikaido T, Shimada Y, Tagami J. Bonding amalgam to enamel: Shear bond strength and SEM morphology. J Prosthet Dent 2001;86:297–303.

461. Bagley A, Wakefield CW, Robbins JW. In vitro comparison of filled and unfilled universal bonding agents of amalgam to dentin. Oper Dent 1994;19:97–101.

462. Cooley RL, Tseng EY, Barkmeier WW. Dentinal bond strengths and microleakage of a 4-META adhesive to amalgam and composite resin. Quintessence Int 1991;22:979–983.

463. Hasegawa T, Retief DH, Russell CM, Denys FR. A laboratory study of the Amalgambond Adhesive System. Am J Dent 1992;5:181–186.

464. Pashley EL, Comer RW, Parry EE, Pashley DH. Amalgam buildups: Shear bond strength and dentin sealing properties. Oper Dent 1991;16:82–89.

465. Setcos JC, Staninec M, Wilson NH. A two-year randomized, controlled clinical evaluation of bonded amalgam restorations. J Adhes Dent 1999;1:323–331.

466. Setcos JC, Staninec M, Wilson NH. Bonding of amalgam restorations: Existing knowledge and future prospects. Oper Dent 2000;25:121–129.

467. Charlton DG, Murchison DF, Moore BK. Incorporation of adhesive liners in amalgam: Effect on compressive strength and creep. Am J Dent 1991;4:184–188.

468. Charlton DG, Moore BK, Swartz ML. In vitro evaluation of the use of resin liners to reduce microleakage and improve retention of amalgam restorations. Oper Dent 1992;17:112–119.

469. Ianzano JA, Mastrodomenico J, Gwinnett AJ. Strength of amalgam restorations bonded with Amalgambond. Am J Dent 1993;6:10–12.

470. Eakle WS, Staninec M, Lacy AM. Effect of bonded amalgam on the fracture resistance of teeth. J Prosthet Dent 1992;68:257–260.

471. Edgren BN, Denehy GE. Microleakage of amalgam restorations using Amalgambond and Copalite. Am J Dent 1992;5:296–298.

472. Hadavi F, Hey JH, Ambrose ER, Elbadrawy HE. Effect of different adhesive systems on microleakage at the amalgam/composite resin interface. Oper Dent 1993;18:2–7.

473. Helvatjoglou-Antoniades M, Theodoridou-Pahini S, Papadogiannis Y, Karezis A. Microleakage of bonded amalgam restorations: Effect of thermal cycling. Oper Dent 2000;25:316–323.

474. Neme AL, Evans DB, Maxson BB. Evaluation of dental adhesive systems with amalgam and resin composite restorations: Comparison of microleakage and bond strength results. Oper Dent 2000;25: 512–519.

475. Winkler MM, Moore BK, Rhodes B, Swartz M. Microleakage and retention of bonded amalgam restorations. Am J Dent 2000;13: 245–250.

476. Belli S, Unlu N, Ozer F. Effect of cavity varnish, amalgam liner or dentin bonding agents on the marginal leakage of amalgam restorations. J Oral Rehabil 2001;28:492–496.

477. Mach Z, Regent J, Staninec M, Mrklas L, Setcos JC. The integrity of bonded amalgam restorations: A clinical evaluation after five years. J Am Dent Assoc 2002;133:460–467.

478. Suh BI. All-Bond—fourth generation dentin bonding system. J Esthet Dent 1991;3:139–147.

479. Ozer F, Unlu N, Ozturk B, Sengun A. Amalgam repair: Evaluation of bond strength and microleakage. Oper Dent 2002;27:199–203.

480. Hadavi F, Hey JH, Ambrose ER, Elbadrawy HE. The influence of an adhesive system on shear bond strength of repaired high copper amalgams. Oper Dent 1991;16:175–180.

481. Lacy AM, Rupprecht R, Watanabe L. Use of self-curing composite resins to facilitate amalgam repair. Quintessence Int 1992;23:53–59.

482. Roeder LB, Deschepper EJ, Powers JM. In vitro bond strength of repaired amalgam with adhesive bonding systems. J Esthet Dent 1991;3:126–132.

483. Blatz MB, Sadan A, Kern M. Resin-ceramic bonding: A review of the literature. J Prosthet Dent 2003;89:268–274.

484. Kramer N, Lohbauer U, Frankenberger R. Adhesive luting of indirect restorations. Am J Dent 2000;13(special Issue, Nov):60D–76D.

485. Peumans M, Van Meerbeek B, Lambrechts P, Vanherle G. Factors affecting the efficacy of porcelain veneers: A literature review. J Dent 2000;28:163.

486. El Zohairy AA, de Gee AJ, Mohsen MM, Feilzer AJ. Effect of conditioning time of self-etching primers on dentin bond strength of three adhesive resin cements. Dent Mater 2005;21:83–93.

487. Roulet J-F, Herder S. Bonded Ceramic Inlays. Chicago: Quintessence, 1991.

488. Hooshmand T, van Noort R, Keshvad A. Storage effect of a preactivated silane on the resin to ceramic bond. Dent Mater 2004; 20:635–642.

489. Soderholm KJ, Shang SW. Molecular orientation of silane at the surface of colloidal silica. J Dent Res 1993;72:1050–1054.

490. Chen TM, Brauer GM. Solvent effects on bonding organo-silane to silica surfaces. J Dent Res 1982;61:1439–1443.

491. Thurmond JW, Barkmeier WW, Wilwerding TM. Effect of porcelain surface treatments on bond strengths of composite resin bonded to porcelain. J Prosthet Dent 1994;72:355–359.

492. Kupiec KA, Wuertz KM, Barkmeier WW, Wilwerding TM. Evaluation of porcelain surface treatments and agents for composite-to-porcelain repair. J Prosthet Dent 1996;76:119–124.

493. Hooshmand T, van Noort R, Keshvad A. Bond durability of the resin-bonded and silane treated ceramic surface. Dent Mater 2002;18:179–188.

494. Lambrechts P, Inokoshi S, Van Meerbeek B. Classification and potential of composite luting materials. In: Mormann WH (ed). International Symposium on Computer Restorations. The State of the Art of the CEREC Method. Proceedings. Berlin: Quintessence, 1991:61–90.

495. Hahn P, Attin T, Grofke M, Hellwig E. Influence of resin cement viscosity on microleakage of ceramic inlays. Dent Mater 2001;17: 191–196.

496. Ozcan M, Vallittu PK. Effect of surface conditioning methods on the bond strength of luting cement to ceramics. Dent Mater 2003;19: 725–731.

497. Awliya W, Oden A, Yaman P, Dennison JB, Razzoog ME. Shear bond strength of a resin cement to densely sintered high-purity alumina with various surface conditions. Acta Odontol Scand 1998; 56:9–13.

498. Blixt M, Adamczak E, Linden LA, Oden A, Arvidson K. Bonding to densely sintered alumina surfaces: Effect of sandblasting and silica coating on shear bond strength of luting cements. Int J Prosthodont 2000;13:221–226.

499. Ozcan M, Alkumru HN, Gemalmaz D. The effect of surface treatment on the shear bond strength of luting cement to a glass-infiltrated alumina ceramic. Int J Prosthodont 2001;14:335–339.

500. Valandro LF, Leite FP, Scotti R, Bottino MA, Niesser MP. Effect of ceramic surface treatment on the microtensile bond strength between a resin cement and an alumina-based ceramic. J Adhes Dent 2004;6:327–332.

501. Valandro LF, Della Bona A, Antonio BM, Neisser MP. The effect of ceramic surface treatment on bonding to densely sintered alumina ceramic. J Prosthet Dent 2005;93:253–259.

502. Bottino MA, Valandro LF, Scotti R, Buso L. Effect of surface treatments on the resin bond to zirconium-based ceramic. Int J Prosthodont 2005;18:60–65.

503. Wilson AD, Kent BE. A new translucent cement for dentistry. The glass ionomer cement. Br Dent J 1972;132:133–135.

504. Mitra S. Curing reactions of glass ionomer materials. In: Hunt PR, ed. Glass Ionomers: The Next Generation. Proceedings of the 2nd International Symposium on Glass Ionomers. Philadelphia: International Symposia in Dentistry, 1994:13.

505. Sidhu SK, Watson TF. Resin-modified glass ionomer materials. A status report for the American Journal of Dentistry. Am J Dent 1995;8:59–67.

506. Smith DC. Polyacrylic acid–based cements: Adhesion to enamel and dentin. Oper Dent 1992;suppl 5:177–183.

507. Wilson AD, McLean JW. Glass Ionomer Cement. Chicago: Quintessence, 1988.

508. Ellison S, Warrens C. Solid-State NMR Study of Aluminosilicate Glasses and Derived Dental Cements. Report of the Laboratory of the Government Chemist. London: LGC, 1987.

509. Burgess J, Norling B, Summitt J. Resin ionomer restorative materials: The new generation. J Esthet Dent 1994;6:207–215.

510. Hunt PR, ed. Glass Ionomers: The Next Generation. Proceedings of the 2nd International Symposium on Glass Ionomers. Philadelphia: International Symposia in Dentistry, 1994.

511. Antonucci JM, McKinney JE, Stansbury JW [inventors]. Resin-modified glass-ionomer cement. US patent 160856, 1988.

512. Mitra SB. Adhesion to dentin and physical properties of a light-cured glass-ionomer liner/base. J Dent Res 1991;70:72–74.

513. Lin A, McIntyre NS, Davidson RD. Studies on the adhesion of glass ionomer cements to dentin. J Dent Res 1992;71:1836–1841.

514. Wilson AD, Nicholson JW. Acid-Base Cements. Their Biomedical and Industrial Applications. Cambridge, England: Cambridge University Press, 1993.

515. Mount GJ. An Atlas of Glass-Ionomer Cements. London: Martin Dunitz, 1990.

516. Wilson AD, Prosser HJ, Powis DM. Mechanism of adhesion of polyelectrolyte cement to hydroxyapatite. J Dent Res 1983;62:590–592.

517. Brook IM, Craig GT, Lamb DJ. Initial in-vitro evaluation of glass-ionomer cements for use as alveolar bone substitutes. Clin Mater 1991;7:295–300.

518. McLean JW. Clinical applications of glass-ionomer cements. Oper Dent 1992;suppl 5:184–190.

519. Braem MJA, Gladys S, Lambrechts P, et al. Flexural fatigue limit of several restorative materials [abstract 47]. J Dent Res 1995;74:17.

520. Momoi Y, McCabe JF. Fluoride release from light-activated glass ionomer restorative cements. Dent Mater 1993;9:151–154.

521. Peumans M, Kanumilli P, De Munck J, Van Landuyt K, Lambrechts P, Van Meerbeek B. Clinical effectiveness of contemporary adhesives: A systematic review of current clinical trials. Dent Mater 2005;21:864–881.

Direct Anterior Restorations

David F. Murchison
Joost Roeters
Marcos A. Vargas
Daniel C. N. Chan

Patients demand superior esthetics from anterior restorations. An esthetic restorative material must simulate the natural tooth in color, translucence, and texture,[1] yet also have adequate strength and wear characteristics, good marginal adaptation and sealing, insolubility, and biocompatibility.[2] These materials must also remain color stable and maintain external tooth morphology to provide a lasting esthetic restoration. This chapter addresses the materials and clinical procedures used to place direct esthetic restorations in anterior teeth.

By far the most commonly used restorative materials in the anterior part of the mouth are resin composites (also called *resin-based composites*, *composite resins*, or simply *composites*). Resin composites are currently the direct restorative materials that best fulfill the requirements of excellent esthetics and durability. The longevity of anterior resin composite restorations has been reported to range from 3.3 to 16 years.[3–7] Using actuarial methods to assess the clinical longevity of these restorations, van Noort and Davis[8] calculated the overall probability of survival at 5 years to be 62.9% for Class 3 and 71.8% for Class 5 resin composite restorations. Van Dijken et al[9] reported a higher 5-year success rate for Class 3 resin composite restorations (95%) in a recent prospective clinical trial.

Material Considerations

By definition, a resin composite contains four structural components: polymer matrix, filler particles, a coupling agent, and an initiator. The matrix is the continuous phase to which the other ingredients are added. Most resin composite matrices are based on the bis-GMA (bisphenol-A–glycidyl methacrylate) resin developed by R. L. Bowen of the National Institute of Standards and Technology and patented in 1962. Some resin composites use urethane dimethacrylate (UDMA) instead of bis-GMA, while many now use a combination of the two materials. Recently, some manufacturers have added a portion of TEG-DMA (triethylene glycol dimethacrylate), a low-viscosity resin used as a diluent. Formulation of a material that uses bis-EMA (bisphenol-A–polyethylene glycol diether dimethacrylate) or oxybismethacrylate monomers that will cyclopolymerize can influence handling properties and holds promise to reduce volumetric shrinkage.[10]

Filler particles are usually a type of glass (such as barium or borosilicate glass), zirconium oxide, aluminum oxide, or silicon dioxide added to the matrix to improve its physical properties. The filler improves translucency; reduces the coefficient of thermal expansion; reduces polymerization shrinkage of the composite; and makes the material harder, denser, and more resistant to wear. Generally, the greater the percentage of filler added (by volume or weight), the better the physical properties of the resin composite. However, filler loading has an upper limit, after which the material becomes too viscous for clinical use.

The filler particles are coated with silane, a coupling agent, to promote adhesion to the matrix. Without a coupling agent, the strength of the cohesive mass is reduced, and the filler particles tend to be lost, or "plucked," from the surface as preferential wear occurs in the softer surrounding resin matrix.[11]

The initiator activates the polymerization reaction of resin composite, with camphoroquinone being the most commonly used photoinitiator. Activation may be initiated by chemical reaction of mixed components or through exposure to light of the proper wavelength. Most current resin composite restorative materials require polymerization initiated by exposure to visible light in the range of 460 to 480 nm (blue light).

Physical Characteristics of Resin Composites

Resin composites have steadily improved in recent years; they are now durable, esthetic, and predictable. Used in combination with an adhesive system, resin composite may be reliably and durably bonded to enamel. Although adhesion to dentin is not yet as reliable as adhesion to enamel, advances in the understanding of dentin microstructure, permeability, and the bonded interface have steadily improved the quality and success of adhesive systems in recent years (see chapter 8).

Resin composites have several undesirable characteristics that must be overcome to achieve long-term clinical success. Volumetric shrinkage during polymerization can be as great as 7%[12] and can generate contraction forces of 4.0 to 7.0 MPa,[13–18] leading to cracking and crazing at the enamel margins. Shrinkage stresses that occur in the pre-gel phase of polymerization are effectively relieved by flexure and flow of the material. However, stresses occurring during the post-gel phase are not relieved by material flow, and residual stresses may cause fatigue within the material or at the resin composite–tooth interface over time. These stresses may cause gap formation between the resin composite and the walls of the preparation with the weakest bonds (usually dentin or cementum). Marginal gaps may result in microleakage, sensitivity, staining at the margins of the restoration, and recurrent caries.[19] Recent investigations have determined that nanoleakage at the resin-dentin interface, as well as hydrolytic and enzymatic degradation of collagen bonds, contribute to a weakened adhesive interface over time.[20–22] Incremental curing techniques, enamel bevels, flexible resin liners, and slow-setting resin-modified glass-ionomer liners have all been recommended for use to help offset the effects of polymerization stresses and shrinkage.[23–28] Resin composites have a coefficient of thermal expansion two to six times higher than that of tooth structure.[29p253–254] This means that resin composite expands and contracts at a greater rate than does tooth structure in response to changes in temperature. This mismatch contributes to loss of adhesion and greater microleakage.[19]

The steady improvement in adhesive systems has helped offset some of the inherent problems associated with resin composite. Nonshrinking resin composites and other poten-

tial improvements in resin composites are under development and address different theories of optimizing durability in the challenging oral environment.[26,30–35] Shrinkage stresses are of little concern in direct veneers and Class 4 restorations due to favorable configuration values and minimal stress at the adhesive interface.

Handling Characteristics of Resin Composites

An important factor for the clinician in the selection of a resin composite is the handling of the material. There is a wide variation in the viscosity of resin composites that does not necessarily correlate with the filler content.[36,37] According to their viscosity, resin composites can be classified as either conventional, packable, or flowable. This viscosity has an influence on the adaptation of the material to the cavity wall or previous layer of composite as well as on the presence of porosities and voids. However, when the viscosity is extremely low (thin), as is the case with flowable resin composites, the risk of porosities inside the restoration increases as well.[38]

Materials in the different categories present different degrees of viscosity; this translates to a wide range of consistencies. Additional changes in handling characteristics are observed with variations in temperature and humidity. Ideally, resin composite materials are soft and easily manipulated, do not stick to placement instruments or brushes, and do not slump during placement.

Many instruments, offering a variety of shapes and surface coatings, are available for placing and shaping resin composite materials. The composition of a typical instrument kit contains a bladed instrument, a small, round condenser with round edges, and brushes (Fig 9-1). A gauze pad moistened with alcohol or liquid resin may be used to clean the active part of the instrument during resin composite placement. This will prevent the material from sticking to the instrument. The use of liquid resins as lubricants must be tightly controlled because these materials could potentially dilute the resin composite and bring about a change in physical properties. In addition, alcohol used to clean the instrument should be evaporated to avoid dissolution of the resin.[39]

Optical Characteristics of Resin Composites

Modern resin composite kits sold by dental manufacturers contain multiple shades and various opacities, for the purpose of matching shade and translucency/opacity of both enamel and dentin. Unfortunately, there is great variability among materials and no consensus between manufacturers regarding the degree of translucency/opacity. The combination of

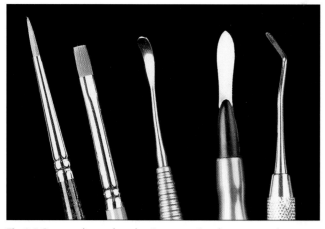

Fig 9-1 Commonly employed resin composite placement and contouring brushes and instruments.

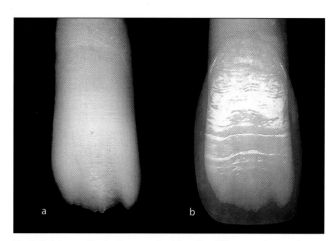

Fig 9-2 Extreme illustration emphasizing the differences in translucency for (a) dentin and (b) enamel (overlay) resin composite compositions. Applying layers with differing chroma and translucency and providing appropriate surface character can greatly enhance the lifelike appearance of anterior restorations.

optical properties of enamel and dentin provide the final appearance of normal tooth structure. These properties are modified by factors such as age, thickness of tissue, and degree and quality of calcification. In a "normal" unworn dentition, dentin provides chroma, opacity, and fluorescence. Enamel modifies the appearance of dentin by providing translucency and opalescence (Fig 9-2a). The terms *dentin* and *opaque*, as they apply to resin composite shades, usually denote highly opaque resins that resemble dentin in opacity/translucency and shade. Overlying the relatively opaque dentin shades, *body* shades represent enamel in opacity/translucency and shade. Manufacturers also provide a group of shades designated as *translucent* or *incisal* with significantly more translucency for the purpose of simulating highly translucent areas (Fig 9-2b)

Microfilled Resin Composites

When microfilled resin composites are manufactured, submicron inorganic filler particles (averaging 0.04 µm) are added to the matrix until the resin composite is very viscous. The resin composite is then polymerized and ground into 5- to 50-µm particles that are incorporated into additional microfilled material to form the restorative material for clinical use (Fig 9-3). In this way, filler content is maximized, polymerization shrinkage is minimized, and the resin composite remains highly polishable.[40]

Microfilled resin composites can be polished to the highest luster and smoothest surface of all the resin composites, and their primary indication is for esthetic areas where this luster is required, such as for Class 5 restorations or direct resin composite veneers. Microfilled resin composites, in general, are not as strong as other classes of the material, however, and are not usually recommended for Class 4 restorations.[29p261,29p275,41–43] Microfills tend to absorb more water than other classes due to their increased resin content, with a resultant decrease in long-term color stability.[44] When a highly polished Class 4 restoration is needed, a hybrid material may be used as a substructure that can be veneered with a microfilled resin composite.[45]

Hybrid Resin Composites

As the name implies, hybrid resin composites contain a blend of submicron (0.04-µm) and small-particle (1- to 4-µm) fillers (see Fig 9-3). The combination of medium and small filler particles allows the highest levels of filler loading among resin composites and a corresponding improvement in physical properties.[46] They can be polished to a fairly high luster, but not to the extent of a microfilled material. Hybrid resin composites are a combination of conventional and microfill technology and are often the materials of choice for Class 3 and 4 restorations. The high filler content also improves the hybrids' resistance to internal discoloration.

In recent years, dental manufacturers have fabricated resin composites in which the average particle size is less than 1 µm. These materials are termed *micro-hybrids* (eg, Esthet-X [Caulk] and Point 4 [Kerr]), or *nano-filled composites*. The goal for the research and development of these materials has been to successfully integrate nanoparticles into filler technology to enhance mechanical properties.[47,48]

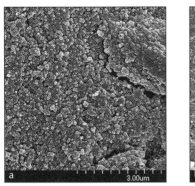
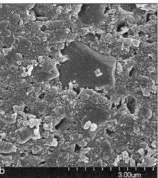

Fig 9-3 Most commonly used classes of resin composite. The microfilled resins (such as Durafill VS [Heraeus Kulzer], *[a]*) contain only submicron particles, while the hybrids (such as Premise [Kerr Dental], *[b]*) contain a combination of submicron particles and particles up to 4 μm in diameter. (Courtesy of Dr Jorge Perdigao.)

Glass-Ionomer Restorative Materials

Glass-ionomer restorative materials are not commonly used when esthetics is a major consideration in anterior restorations. They are often recommended for patients with high caries risk.[49,50] A review of clinical trials that studied the cariostatic effect of fluoride-releasing restorative materials concluded that there is no definite evidence for or against a treatment effect of inhibition of secondary caries by these materials.[51] However, recent studies involving patients at high risk for caries due to xerostomia showed a significant reduction in caries incidence adjacent to resin-modified glass-ionomer restorations, as compared with other restorative materials.[52,53] The traditional chemically cured glass-ionomer materials are not esthetic, but esthetics has been greatly improved in the resin-modified glass-ionomer materials. From a physical property perspective, the resistance against erosive wear of both chemically cured and resin-modified glass-ionomer cements is lower than for resin composites. Recent clinical trials of 5 years' duration have reported high retention rates in Class 5 restorations.[54–56] Though not as color stable nor as durable as resin composites, these materials are suitable for use in visible anterior areas when dentin margins are prevalent or the patient has been identified as being at high risk for developing new caries lesions. Glass-ionomer restorative materials are discussed in more depth in chapter 13.

Class 3 Restorations

Class 3 caries lesions are smooth-surface lesions found on the proximal surfaces of anterior teeth, usually slightly gingival to the proximal contact, but not involving the incisal angle of the tooth. These lesions can usually be detected with an explorer, radiographically, or with transillumination. Clinical changes in translucency may be evident and may be enhanced if light is directed through the proximal area using a focused, intense light source (transillumination). Caries lesions cause a more opaque appearance of tooth structure. Incipient lesions tend to be "V" shaped and confined to enamel; deeper lesions tend to spread within dentin.

Incipient Enamel Caries Lesions

The proximal lesion that is located within enamel and is not cavitated may not necessitate restorative treatment. Although there is no doubt that the lesion is pathologic, research and clinical experience have shown that this lesion is often dormant. Charting it as a lesion that could potentially reactivate and cause a need for restorative treatment is a valid and acceptable procedure.[57,58] Properly addressing caries risk factors for each individual will decrease the chance that future invasive procedures will be necessary. Evidence supports the viability of remineralization of caries lesions in enamel.[59] Chapter 4 contains a more complete discussion of caries and remineralization processes.

Cavitated Enamel Caries Lesions

When the enamel surface is cavitated, it is past the point of remineralization. If the cavitation is very shallow and deeper enamel has been remineralized, a restoration may not be necessary unless the lesion is esthetically displeasing. If the lesion is confined to enamel, enameloplasty or recontouring may be sufficient. If necessary, a conservative cavity preparation may be accomplished with a round tungsten-carbide or diamond bur used in a high-speed handpiece. The finished preparation resembles a saucer and has no retentive undercuts (Fig 9-4). Adhesion to acid-etched enamel provides the necessary retention. Both laboratory and 3-year clinical data have demonstrated the durability of these saucer-shaped restorations.[60,61]

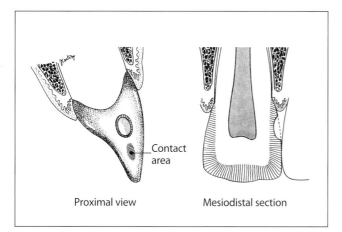

Fig 9-4 Saucer-shaped preparation in enamel. The caries lesion is usually located slightly gingival to the contact area. Every attempt should be made to maintain natural tooth contact between the adjacent teeth during restoration. If no cavitation is present, remineralization is preferable to restoration.

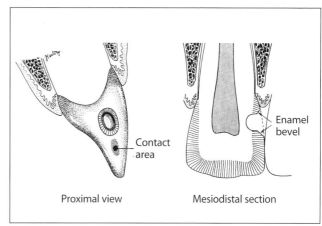

Fig 9-5 This preparation is similar to that in Fig 9-4, except that the axial wall is extended into dentin and the external enamel margins are beveled.

Dentinal Caries Lesions with Peripheral Enamel Margins

The preparation necessitated by dentinal caries lesions is similar to that for enamel lesions except that the axial wall extends into dentin, and the carious dentin—and in many areas, overlying fragile enamel—is removed. Bevels have been advocated by some authors to reduce enamel fracture and provide a gradual shade transition for esthetics.[62,63] However, enamel bonds have been demonstrated clinically to be adequate without bevels.[64,65] An in vitro study using a silver-nitrate tracer revealed no significant differences in marginal microleakage in Class 3 restorations whether or not margins were beveled.[66]

Margins should receive short bevels or chamfers when the gradual blending of enamel and restorative shades would benefit esthetics or when maximum retention is desired (Fig 9-5). In situations in which a Class 3 cavity preparation extends prominently to the facial aspect of a tooth in the esthetic zone, a longer bevel on the facial margins may be employed in order to blend the appearance of the restorative material with that of the tooth structure. Many clinicians advocate an irregular or scalloped pattern for the facial bevel to provide a more inconspicuous margin. If the cervical enamel will be eliminated or compromised by a bevel with a resultant margin in or near dentin, the beveling procedure should be avoided in the cervical area (Fig 9-6). If the margin of the preparation is mostly on enamel, no undercuts, retentive points, or grooves are necessary, as the restoration will be adequately retained by adhesion.[67]

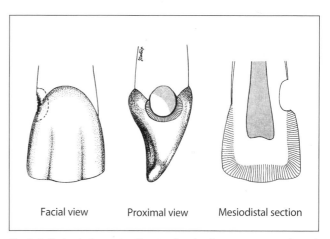

Fig 9-6 Caries lesion extending to the dentin-cementum surface. A bevel is placed only on enamel margins.

Dentinal Caries Lesions with Margins Extending Onto the Root Surface

In areas where there is little or no enamel for bonding, the marginal adaptation of the restoration may be optimized in two distinct ways. For patients with a demonstrated high caries risk, an open sandwich technique using a resin-modified glass-ionomer restorative material may be employed to seal the cervical portion of the restoration. The remaining cavity is then filled with resin composite for improved esthetics.[68] There is debate as to the effectiveness of the open sandwich, with studies showing both advantages and disadvantages to its use.[69–71]

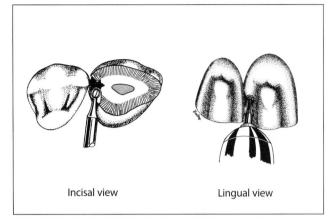

Incisal view   Lingual view

Fig 9-7 Initial penetration should be made through the marginal ridge, near the adjacent tooth but avoiding damage to it. Note the angulation of the long axis of the bur in relation to the location of the lesion.

For patients who do not have significant caries risk, the approach to treating lesions with dentinal margins is simply to employ a fourth- or fifth-generation dentin bonding system and to restore with a resin composite. Because current dentin bonding systems have been demonstrated to be very effective in providing retention, mechanical undercuts at the expense of healthy tooth structure have become unnecessary.[71]

Preparation Approach and Instrumentation

Resin Composite Restorations

Outline form for resin composite restorations is determined solely by the extent of the caries lesion(s) and access for removal of carious tooth structure. There is no need for further extension of the preparation, and the removal of sound tooth structure to gain mechanical undercut retention is contraindicated. The lingual approach is preferred for Class 3 restorations, but it is not always possible, depending on the location of the caries lesion. The number of burs used for cavity preparation should be kept to a minimum. A No. 2 round bur or a No. 329 pear-shaped carbide bur in a high-speed handpiece can be used for initial access to the lesion. Initial penetration should be made through the marginal ridge, near the adjacent tooth but avoiding damage to it (Fig 9-7). The outline form of the preparation is then extended to provide access to the carious dentin. A larger round bur may be used in the low-speed handpiece to excavate demineralized dentin.

The need for enamel bevels has not been clearly demonstrated, but narrow bevels (0.5 to 1.0 mm) may be placed on accessible enamel margins to remove fragile enamel, to make margins smooth, and to enhance esthetics if the margin is in

a visible location. For placing bevels, a flame-shaped finishing bur or fine diamond bur, a gingival margin trimmer, or another hand instrument may be used. Although a very wide bevel should usually be avoided, in situations where maximum esthetics is required, the bevel can be extended to 2 mm or more on the facial surface. The facial bevel may have a scalloped or irregular shape that enhances the visual blend of the restoration with that of the tooth. Adequate depth of this bevel allows proper overlapping of the different opacities of the restorative layers, and the increased length allows a blending transition of the resin material onto the tooth surface.

The appearance of true enamel is more natural and esthetic than that of the most esthetic restorative materials. To preserve facial esthetics, the Class 3 preparation should not be extended onto the facial surface unless necessitated by carious or missing enamel on that surface (Figs 9-8a and 9-8b). Unsupported facial enamel may be left for internal etching and bonding to resin composite[72] (Figs 9-9a to 9-9f). The facial approach for access to carious dentin is indicated only when the caries lesion already involves the facial surface or when the adjacent tooth overlaps the tooth being restored, preventing a lingual approach. The outline should be as conservative as possible, preserving the facial enamel.

Resin-Modified Glass-Ionomer Restorations

Because of their anticaries effect, resin-modified glass-ionomer restorative materials may be used in Class 3 restorations in patients at high risk for caries.[49,73] Preparations for these materials should resemble those for resin composite; no bevels are necessary. The only reason that noncarious tooth structure should be removed is to allow access for excavation of the carious dentin (Figs 9-10a and 9-10b). Because these materials bond to enamel and dentin, the placement of retention grooves or points is not necessary.[74]

Class 4 Restorations

Class 4 restorations are usually necessitated by an injury resulting in a fracture of the incisal angle, a situation plainly visible on clinical examination. In situations in which carious tooth structure is present, radiographs are often helpful to determine the extent of the caries lesion and its proximity to the pulp chamber.

Etiology and Treatment Rationale

A caries-induced Class 4 restoration is usually the result of a large Class 3 caries lesion that has undermined the incisal edge. The need for Class 4 restorations due to traumatic frac-

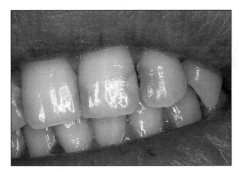

Fig 9-8a Moderate-sized Class 3 caries lesions on the mesial and distal surfaces of the maxillary left central incisor and mesial surface of the lateral incisor.

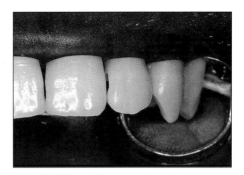

Fig 9-8b After cavity preparation, the labial margins are only slightly visible, and the labial enamel is unsupported by dentin.

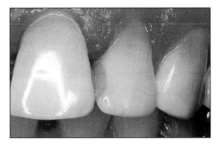

Fig 9-9a A discolored anterior resin composite restoration to be replaced to improve esthetics.

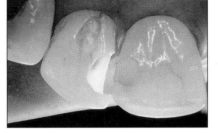

Fig 9-9b Lingual view after existing resin composite was removed, revealing unsupported facial enamel.

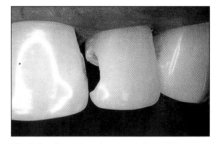

Fig 9-9c Completed preparation with no attempt to remove labial unsupported enamel.

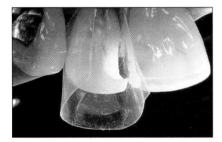

Fig 9-9d Clear matrix and interproximal wedge in place.

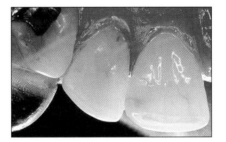

Fig 9-9e Lingual view of the finished and polished resin composite restoration.

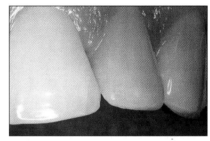

Fig 9-9f Facial view of the Class 3 restoration illustrates the improved esthetic outcome.

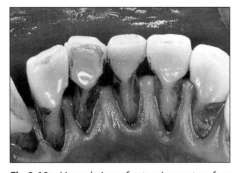

Fig 9-10a Lingual view of extensive root surface exposure and root caries lesions; teeth to be restored with resin-modified glass-ionomer material.

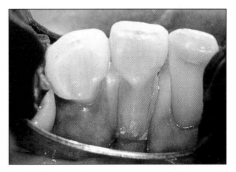

Fig 9-10b Completed excavation of carious tooth structure; the adhesive nature of the restorative material does not demand preparation of mechanical resistance and retention features. (Figs 9-10a and 9-10b courtesy of Dr Robert H. Poindexter.)

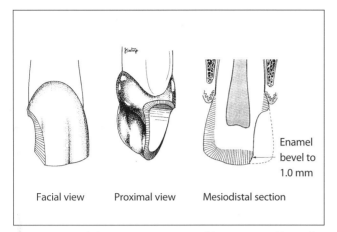

Facial view   Proximal view   Mesiodistal section

Enamel bevel to 1.0 mm

Fig 9-11 Typical Class 4 preparation. Incisal fracture caused by undermining and weakening of incisal enamel associated with a Class 3 lesion may necessitate a Class 4 cavity preparation, which is similar to a Class 3 preparation but includes a portion of the incisal edge.

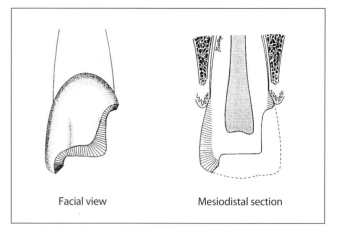

Facial view   Mesiodistal section

Fig 9-12 Class 4 preparation when loss of incisal enamel is extensive.

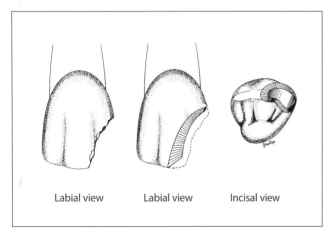

Labial view   Labial view   Incisal view

Fig 9-13a Fractures often require no preparation other than an enamel bevel.

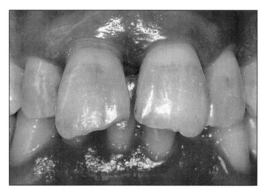

Fig 9-13b Maxillary incisors with fractured mesial angles. The use of a bevel is the only preparation required for these restorations.

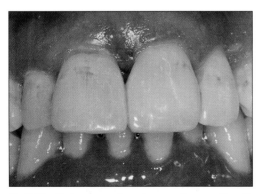

Fig 9-13c Resin composite restores contours and length while closing the midline diastema.

ture occurs most often among children or young adults. The frequency of fractures of permanent incisors in children is reported to range from 5%[32] to 20%.[75] Traumatic fractures are likely to be more horizontal than vertical.

For treating Class 4 caries lesions, the cavity design follows the conventional form of the Class 3 preparation and includes a portion of the incisal edge. Carious tooth structure and weak incisal enamel are removed, and all enamel margins are beveled, with wider bevels placed in the incisal portion of the tooth where the enamel is thicker and the stresses on the restoration are likely to be greater (Fig 9-11). A modified Class 4 preparation with extensive loss of incisal enamel is shown in Fig 9-12.

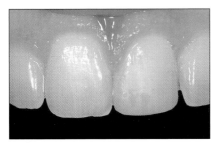

Fig 9-14a Discolored, unesthetic Class 4 restoration that the patient desired to have replaced.

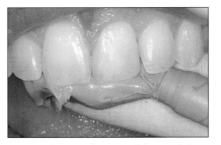

Fig 9-14b Lingual matrix fabricated from impression material to serve as a guide for contours and incisal length.

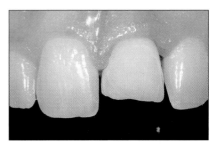

Fig 9-14c The defective restoration is removed, and long, scalloped bevels are placed for retention and esthetic blending of the tooth-restoration interface.

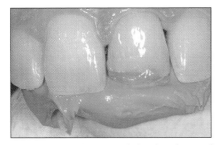

Fig 9-14d Application of the first layer of resin composite to restore lingual incisal contours.

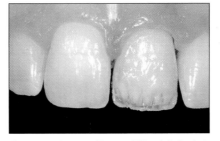

Fig 9-14e A second layer of "dentin" shade is applied to mimic underlying opacity and attempt to mimic the shape of the dental mamelons.

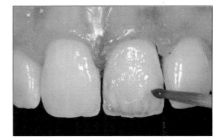

Fig 9-14f Translucent material is applied at the incisal third to imitate incisal translucency.

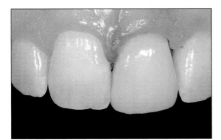

Fig 9-14g An external layer of "enamel" shade of resin composite is feathered onto the facial surface and blended into existing contours for a polychromatic, natural appearance.

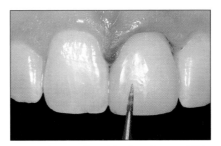

Fig 9-14h A 12-fluted finishing bur establishes final contours and surface characteristics before employing disks and points to provide a final polish.

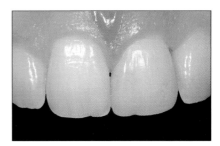

Fig 9-14i The completed restoration with a pleasing color match, surface characterization, and incisal edge morphology yields a highly esthetic outcome.

When a fracture has caused a need for restoration, if there is no carious or pulpal involvement, a bevel is often the only preparation necessary[76] (Figs 9-13a to 9-13c). An enamel bevel of at least 1.0 mm should be placed around the periphery of the cavity where enamel thickness allows. Increasing the width of the bevel beyond 1.0 mm has been shown to provide no additional strength,[77] but a wider bevel may provide a more harmonious esthetic blend between the resin composite and enamel. In cases where esthetics drives the use of a longer bevel, it should present a scalloped or irregular appearance and should blend evenly onto the facial surface (Figs 9-14a to 9-14i). On the lingual surface, where esthetic requirements are less important, the bevel should remain short. If the incisal contact occurs at a marginal area, however, a chamfer may be used to provide greater strength and retention for the restoration. If the original tooth fragment is available after traumatic fracture, the fragment may be reattached to the tooth in some instances by etching and bonding the fractured surfaces.[78–81] Clinical trials have shown these reattachments to be successful, in some cases for more than 7 years.[82,83] Fragment reattachment can often provide a more esthetic result than can a resin composite restoration.

Fig 9-15 *Pins add minimal retention to a Class 3 or Class 4 composite restoration and can create an esthetic problem even if masked with opaque resin.*

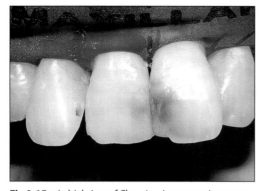

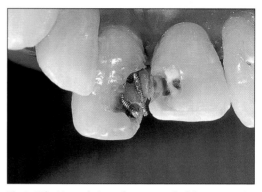

Fig 9-15a Labial view of Class 4 resin composite restoration retained with two pins. Note the wear and color change of the composite material and evidence of corrosion discoloration or recurrent caries.

Fig 9-15b Lingual view after removal of the composite material.

Use of Pins

Retentive pins are not needed in resin composite restorations and should not be used. The adhesive technique provides sufficient retention, and the use of metallic pins in resin composite restorations can greatly reduce the esthetic appearance.[84] A recent study concluded that there was only a small (10%) increase in fracture resistance of large Class 4 resin composite restorations if pins supplemented bonding.[85] Pins in anterior teeth may encroach on the pulp and may discolor the restoration due to corrosion with marginal microleakage. Some clinicians argue that if the adhesive bond is broken, it is better to lose the restoration than to have it held in place by the pins (Fig 9-15).

Techniques for Repair or Correction of Intraoral Restorations

Resin composites are effective for the repair or correction of intraoral restorations for many kinds of materials. By combining chemical bonding techniques as well as macro- and micro-mechanical retention, attachment of the resin composite to the old restoration can be obtained. In many cases, repair or correction requires less preparation and will reduce the risk of damage to the tooth when compared to complete replacement of defective or unesthetic restorations. Macromechanical retention can be created by the preparation of undercuts in the old restoration, which can also improve the resistance form.

Micromechanical retention can be obtained by preparation with a coarse diamond bur or air abrasion. Air abrasion is effective on all resin composites, porcelain, acrylic resins, and met-

als. It may be performed with aluminum oxide particles or with a special aluminum oxide powder that is coated with a layer of silica (CoJet Sand, 3M ESPE).[86] The latter is designed to deposit a layer of silica on the surface of the air-abraded restoration. This may enhance chemical retention and allow silanization. On porcelain and resin composites containing glass, silanization is an effective method to maximize the chemical bond. Some silanes are directly applied to the surface, while others are activated when mixed with specific adhesive primers or resins. On metals, specific metal primers, applied after air abrading, are effective in improving the bond strength.[87]

Direct Resin Composite Veneers

Resin composites may be used for closing diastemata, building up peg-shaped lateral incisors, and/or veneering the labial surfaces of teeth. Direct resin composite veneers offer several advantages over ceramic veneers. Direct veneers generally provide a more conservative approach and can be placed in one visit without laboratory involvement or laboratory fees. Although the chair time required for placement of direct veneers can be considerable, the cost to the patient is generally lower than for ceramic veneers. The lower cost may help to provide an alternate solution for many esthetic problems. Commonly, little or no enamel removal is required (Fig 9-16). Several instruments are useful in placing resin for veneering facial surfaces. Examples include plastic instruments such as the one shown in Fig 9-16b (see also Fig 6-41), a cylindrical or rounded cone-shaped instrument (see Fig 6-40a),

Fig 9-16 *Direct composite veneering technique with the body shade deposited in bulk and distributed by plastic or paddle-shaped instrument. A brush slightly wetted with liquid resin adhesive may also be used for contouring.*

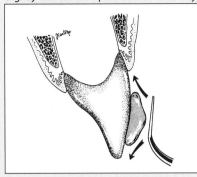

Fig 9-16a Lateral view.

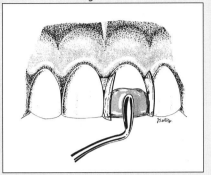

Fig 9-16b Labial view showing the use of clear plastic matrix strips in both interproximal areas.

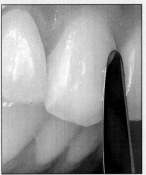

Fig 9-16c A paddle-shaped instrument (Barghi No. 1) is used to apply and contour the resin composite.

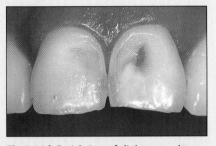

Fig 9-16d Facial view of slight enamel preparation and extent of margins for direct resin composite veneers on maxillary central incisors.

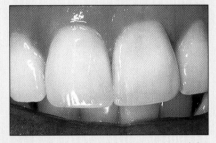

Fig 9-16e Completed direct veneers exhibit excellent esthetics and mask intrinsic stains. (Figs 9-16d and 9-16e courtesy of Dr Nasser Barghi.)

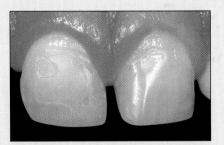

Fig 9-16f External stain, hypocalcification, and discolored restorations on the maxillary central incisors require replacement.

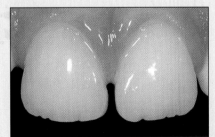

Fig 9-16g Completed direct veneers mask stains and meet esthetic demands in this young patient.

and a thin, slightly curved spatula- or paddle-shaped instrument such as the Barghi No. 1 (Fig 9-16c). Several manufacturers have recently introduced resin composite kits with a greatly expanded range of shades and translucencies, so achieving natural esthetics with resin composite may be easier than in the past. Placement of various shades and opacities in successive layers can result in an intermediate shade. There is

a drawback, however, as resin composite veneers do not maintain their appearance as well over time as do ceramic restorations. The percentage of practitioners providing direct (freehand) resin composite veneers has declined in recent years, with a corresponding increase in the use of porcelain veneer restorations.[88]

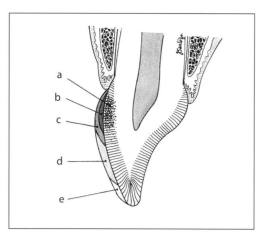

Fig 9-17a Facial veneering and masking of heavy stain/fluorosis using a combination of opaque, cervical, body, and translucent shades. (a) stain/fluorosis; (b) opaque shade; (c) cervical shade; (d) body shade; (e) translucent shade.

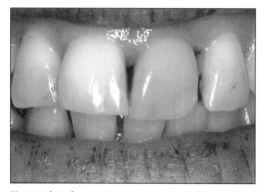

Fig 9-17b Left central incisor is intrinsically discolored and malposed.

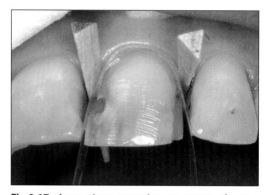

Fig 9-17c Aggressive preparation removes tooth structure to allow layered masking of the darkened tooth stucture.

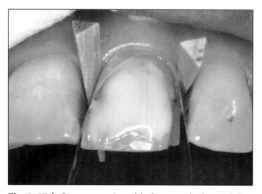

Fig 9-17d Opaque resin added to mask the staining and allow buildup of layers to provide polychromatic layering.

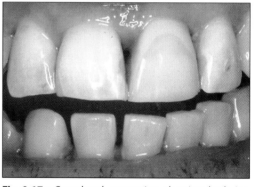

Fig 9-17e Completed restoration showing both improved color and similar incisal edge contours.

To achieve optimal esthetics, direct resin composite veneers should be placed by layering various shades of resin composite or translucent color modifiers to obtain a polychromatic restoration (Fig 9-17a). The tooth surface is etched, and an adhesive is applied. If a tooth shows a dark discoloration, an opaque layer or masking agent may be placed over the adhesive and polymerized (Fig 9-17b to 9-17e). To add a natural look to the cervical or proximal surfaces of teeth, orange or brown tints may be used. These color modifications will influence the surface shade unless the thickness of the resin composite exceeds 2.5 mm.[89] Translucence, the appearance of lobes or mamelons, and/or white or bluish characterization

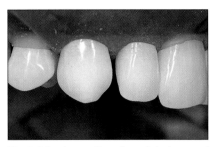

Fig 9-18a A maxillary lateral incisor and canine with an existing diastema to be closed with resin composite.

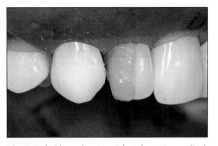

Fig 9-18b Phosphoric acid etchant is applied; no preparation of natural tooth structure is required for adhesion.

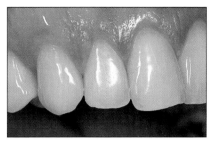

Fig 9-18c Completed diastema closure showing improved esthetics and imperceptible blend of resin composite and natural enamel. Note the translucency of the incisal edge.

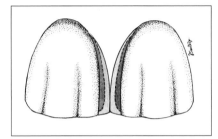

Fig 9-19a Labial view of finished diastema closure showing the use of body and translucent shades to simulate natural tooth color and translucency.

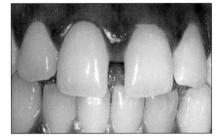

Fig 9-19b Moderate midline diastema. The patient's desire for esthetic improvement may be met with resin composite.

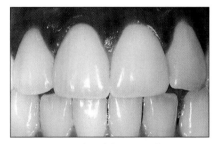

Fig 9-19c Completed diastema closure. Note the physiologic contouring of the cervical aspect of the restorations and the homogenous luster of the composite material and natural tooth surface. (Figs 9-19b and 9-19c courtesy of Dr Robert H. Poindexter.)

of the incisal edge may be added in the incisal third of the composite veneer. An attempt should be made to sculpt the resin composite to desired contours. If the restoration is slightly overcontoured, it may be finished and polished to proper contours. If it is slightly undercontoured in any area, additional resin composite material may be added.

Diastema Closure

The technique for diastema closure is similar to that for placement of direct veneers and Class 4 restorations. In most cases, no tooth structure has to be removed, and the resin composite is retained solely by adhesive bonding (Figs 9-18a to 9-18c). For a small to moderate-sized diastema, resin composite added to the proximal surfaces of the two adjacent teeth will usually suffice (Figs 9-19a to 9-19c). A slight blending of the material onto the facial surface will help achieve a natural transition of shades and improve the esthetic outcome. When closing a diastema, care should be taken to provide the proper tooth contours when placing and finishing the material. This is especially crucial in the gingival embrasure areas. If the diastema exceeds 2.5 mm, it may be necessary to use a combination of direct veneering and orthodontic movement to position the teeth into a more easily managed and esthetically pleasing location. Corrective enameloplasty of the distal-surface contours of the teeth to be restored, followed by building up adjacent teeth, may improve the esthetic outcome.

When diastema closure is performed, occlusal relationships and esthetic proportions, as well as the overall facial esthetics, must be considered. When anterior teeth are widened, it may also be necessary to lengthen them to preserve natural anatomic proportions. If occlusal relationships and facial appearance will allow, the proper tooth length can be established by adding to the incisal edge. It is also possible to improve the length-to-width ratio by surgical crown lengthening in some patients. The desired lengths and widths of teeth should be determined using a diagnostic waxup before treatment is begun (Fig 9-20). A trial application or mock-up, assessing

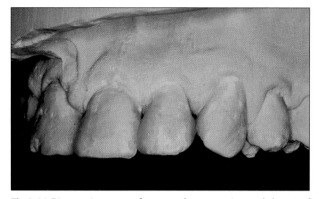

Fig 9-20 Diagnostic waxup of proposed recontouring and closure of diastemata. This treatment-planning procedure may assist in identifying tooth-size discrepancies, areas requiring esthetic recontouring, and gingival height and contour considerations. The cast may also be used for patient education and communication of treatment goals, as well as for fabrication of a lingual matrix and as a chairside guide for direct restorations.

Table 9-1	Dimensional averages (in mm) for maxillary incisors and canines*			
	Males		**Females**	
Tooth	**Length/Width**		**Length/Width**	
Central incisor	10.7	9.4	9.6	9.1
Lateral incisor	9.1	7.5	8.2	7.1
Canine	10.7	8.5	9.2	8.0

*From Gillen et al.[92]

Table 9-2	Length/width and width/width ratios for maxillary incisors and canines*			
	Males			
	Length/ Width	Width/Width Central	Width/Width Lateral	Width/Width Canine
Central incisor	1.15:1	—	1.25:1	1.1:1
Lateral incisor	1.2:1		—	
Canine	1.25:1	—	1.15:1	—
	Females			
	Length/ Width	Width/Width Central	Width/Width Lateral	Width/Width Canine
Central incisor	1.05:1	—	1.3:1	1.15:1
Lateral incisor	1.15:1		—	
Canine	1.15:1	—	1.15:1	—

The length-to-width ratios are for the teeth in the first column.

The width-to-width ratios are between different teeth. Only the larger-to-smaller ratios are listed. For example, the central incisor–to–lateral incisor width ratio is listed, but not the lateral incisor–to–central incisor ratio.

*From Gillen et al.[92]

the esthetic alteration of the shape and color of the proposed veneer, may be accomplished with resin composite applied to unetched teeth.[90,91]

Maintenance of the proper length and width relationships in anterior teeth is very important to achieving an esthetic result for resin composite veneers, porcelain veneers, and diastema closures (see chapter 3). A study evaluating the length and width of anterior teeth revealed that, on average, central incisors and canines are approximately equal in length and are 20% longer than lateral incisors.[92] The proper dimensions, length-to-width ratios, and width-to-width ratios are shown in Tables 9-1 and 9-2.

A periodontal probe or caliper may be used as a measuring device to evenly divide the space to be closed. Diastema closures frequently require augmenting two to six teeth with resin composite to achieve optimal esthetic relationships (Figs 9-21a to 9-21d).

Most diastema closures that require the addition of 1.5 mm or less of material to the proximal enamel can be successfully restored using a relatively translucent enamel shade. Wider diastemata can be difficult because of the disparity in the optical properties of the resin composite material and the tooth structure. To avoid a translucent "shine-through" effect, a relatively opaque dentin shade of resin is added to the proximal surface in a thickness that would approximate the missing dentin. The facial and incisal contours can then be established with an enamel shade of microfilled resin composite to reproduce the surface gloss and translucence of natural tooth structure.

A number of diastema closures may be carefully accomplished without the use of a matrix or a wedge, thus providing better control of proximal contours in the gingival embrasure areas. When restoring adjacent teeth, the proximal contours are best built up one at a time. A sculptable resin composite should be placed on the facial surface of the first tooth and contoured to the shape desired. Care should be taken to achieve the desired proximal contour and tooth width. It is very helpful to measure the width of the restored tooth with calipers and compare it to the adjacent tooth and the remaining space to ensure that the proper symmetry is achieved. Following polymerization, the proximal surface of the first restoration should be finished and polished to the exact contour desired. The contours of the facial surface and incisal edge should be very close to the final desired shape but may be polished at the same time as the adjacent restoration. Fig 9-22 shows a diastema closure without the use of a matrix.

A tight, properly contoured contact can be achieved using a "pull-through" matrix technique. When placing the adjacent restoration, care should be taken to confine both the

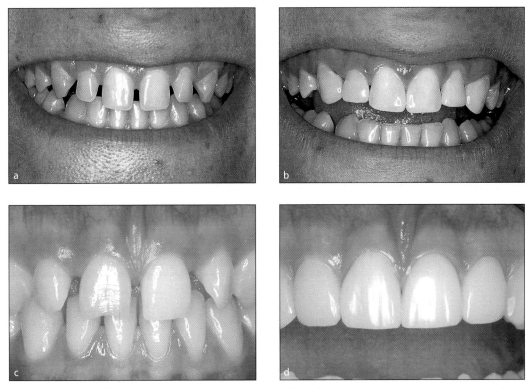

Figs 9-21a to 9-21d Diastema closures frequently require bonding of resin composite to two to six teeth to achieve proper esthetic relationships. Multiple veneers were needed for these two patients.

etchant and the bonding resin to prevent inadvertent splinting. After the adhesive resin is polymerized, a mylar strip is placed in the contact area and the resin composite applied to the facial surface of the second tooth. After the material is blended to contour and shaped against the strip, the strip is slowly pulled to the lingual, drawing the material with it. When the material is midway through the contact, the strip should be removed with a tug, leaving the material in the contact area. Wiping the strip with alcohol-dampened gauze prior to placement may help to release the material from the strip. Using a brush or placement instrument, the facial resin increment can be pushed gently into contact with the already completed restoration on the adjacent tooth and the embrasures then shaped and refined and the composite polymerized. Although the polymerized resin will stick to the adjacent tooth, it can easily be separated by lightly torquing the teeth. Following separation, a mylar strip is reinserted and contoured against the lingual contour of the tooth. A small amount of resin is placed against the strip to fill any deficiencies on the lingual surface, and the lingual portion of the strip is drawn tightly against the cingulum with a thumb or a finger. The strip is then pulled out to the facial, drawing the material into the lingual deficiencies. After polymerization, the teeth are again separated and finishing procedures are initiated.

Shade or Color Selection

Selection of the shade or color of resin composite restorative material is an important and sometimes demanding step in completing an anterior restoration.

Factors Influencing Shade Selection

Proper Lighting

One of the first requirements for a good color match is proper lighting. Commonly used fluorescent tubes emit light with a green tint that can distort color perception. Color-corrected fluorescent tubes that approximate natural daylight are avail-

Figs 9-22a to 9-22s Diastema closure using resin composite. (Courtesy of Dr J. William Robbins.)

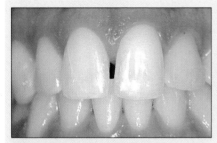

Fig 9-22a The diastema between maxillary central incisors measures slightly more than 1 mm.

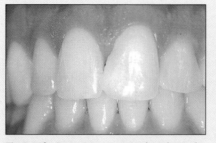

Fig 9-22b Resin composite is placed into the diastema and polymerized to verify shade selection prior to the dehydration of the teeth that accompanies the procedure.

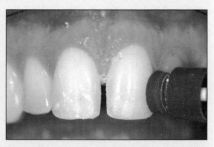

Fig 9-22c Tooth surfaces are cleaned with a slurry of fine pumice.

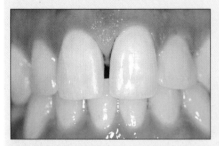

Fig 9-22d Retraction cord has been placed to displace the tissue of the interproximal gingival papilla.

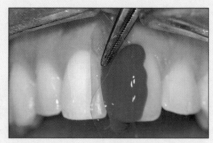

Fig 9-22e Etchant is applied to only one central incisor; the etched area is larger than that needed for attachment of resin composite. A strip of clear, plastic matrix protects the other central incisor from being etched. After 30 seconds of etching, the surface is rinsed and thoroughly dried.

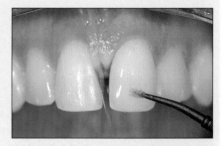

Fig 9-22f Adhesive resin is placed over the etched enamel and light polymerized.

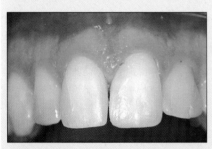

Fig 9-22g Resin composite is placed so that it has slightly greater contour than the desired final restoration.

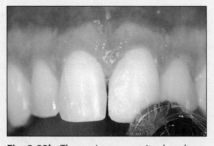

Fig 9-22h The resin composite has been light polymerized.

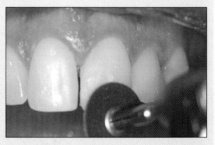

Fig 9-22i The resin composite is contoured with a coarse-grit disk.

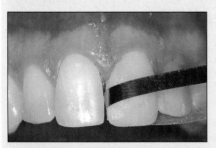

Fig 9-22j The interproximal area is finished so that the resin composite will close one-half of the diastema.

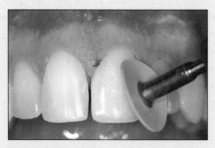

Fig 9-22k Final polishing of the restoration is performed.

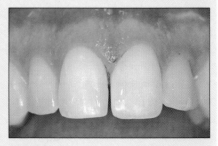

Fig 9-22l The restoration of the left central incisor is complete.

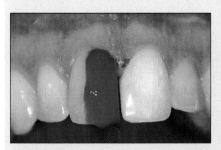

Fig 9-22m The mesial portion of the right central incisor is etched; a plastic matrix strip protects the adjacent tooth from the etchant.

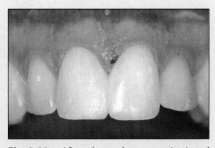

Fig 9-22n After the etchant was is rinsed away, the surface dried, and the resin adhesive applied and polymerized, resin composite was is placed in contact with the adjacent restoration and polymerized.

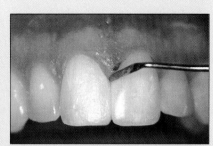

Fig 9-22o The restorations are lightly separated by pushing a thin instrument against the contact from the gingival embrasure.

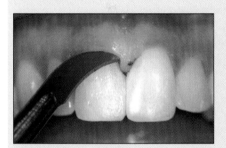

Fig 9-22p The gingival margins of the restoration are shaped with a No. 12 scalpel blade.

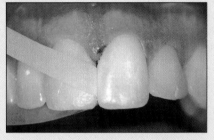

Fig 9-22q The proximal surface, gingival to the interproximal contact, is finished and polished using progressively finer-grit finishing strips.

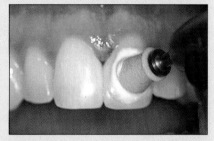

Fig 9-22r Surfaces of the restorations are polished with an aluminum oxide polishing paste.

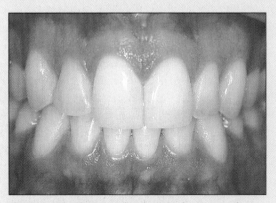

Fig 9-22s The diastema closure procedure is complete.

Clinical Steps for a Direct Resin Composite Veneer

1. Select resin shades prior to dehydration of the tooth.
2. Place a rubber dam and No. 212 (retractor) clamp if desired. If a rubber dam is not used, place gingival retraction cord to control sulcular fluid and retract the gingival tissue.
3. In most cases, the composite material is bonded directly to the tooth surface. If it is necessary to remove tooth structure to establish proper tooth alignment or to create space to mask dark tooth structure, a blunt-ended diamond is recommended. Remove the smallest amount of tooth structure necessary to achieve the desired objective.
4. Etch the tooth surface with an appropriate etchant, such as 37% phosphoric acid. Protect adjacent teeth from the etchant with clear plastic strips.
5. Rinse the tooth thoroughly and dry the etched tooth surface with a stream of air.
6. Place a clear plastic strip or other matrix and wedge interproximally; apply adhesive resin and light cure for the appropriate time (material-specific instructions).
7. Apply opaque resin, if indicated, and light cure.
8. Add the selected resin composite, adapt and contour the material, and light cure for the appropriate length of time.
9. Add additional resin composite as necessary to achieve the proper shape, color, and translucency. Light cure each increment for the appropriate length of time.
10. Contour the gingival margins and remove flash with a No. 12 or 12b scalpel blade.
11. Contour and finish the composite material with a carbide or diamond finishing bur.
12. Repeat the above process on adjacent teeth if indicated.
13. Remove the rubber dam, if used.
14. Check the occlusion and adjust as necessary with finishing burs.
15. Finish and polish with disks, polishing points, etc.
16. Apply low-viscosity rebonding resin (surface sealer) to the restoration surface and margins.

Color-Corrected Lighting[93]

Overhead lights (fluorescent tubes)
Color Rendering Index (CRI): 90 or higher
Spectral energy distribution (SED): natural daylight
Color temperature: 5,500°K
Illumination intensity: approximately 150 to 200 foot-candles at 30 inches above floor

Dental operating light
Illumination intensity: 1,000 to 2,000 foot-candles
Color temperature: optimum 5,000°K, should be adjustable from 4,500°K to 5,500°K to assist in color matching

able and are recommended for dental treatment rooms. The objective is to obtain shadow-free, color-balanced illumination without distracting glare or false colors (see box).[93,94]

If such lighting is not available, color selection can be made near a window. However, even daylight varies considerably from day to day and throughout the day. When shade selection is critical, it is wise to use multiple light sources to choose the best shade and to avoid problems with metamerism, a complication observed when the perceived color of objects (in this case, teeth and resin composite restorations) is different in different light sources.

Color Acuity and Eye Fatigue

When selecting color or shade, the operator should avoid staring at the tooth and shade guide for long periods of time. Staring at these objects during shade selection will cause the colors to blend, resulting in a loss of color acuity. The shade guide should be placed adjacent to the tooth to be restored and then viewed briefly to determine which shade or shades match the color of the tooth; then the eyes should be moved away. Arranging the shade guide based on the value of the shades can also facilitate the shade selection. Ideally, the eyes should be "rested" by viewing the horizon through a window or by looking at an object that is a muted blue, violet, or gray color.

The dental assistant and patient can also assist in shade selection. By viewing the shade guide and tooth from several positions and accepting input from the assistant and patient, the dentist can achieve an acceptable color match.

Achieving Optimal Color Match

The color or shade selection should be accomplished before the restorative procedure is initiated. Therefore, selection is made while the tooth is moist, prior to rubber dam placement or cavity preparation. Desiccation of the tooth causes significant lightening of the tooth color, and the presence of a rubber dam can distort color perception. A prophylaxis cup containing a slurry of pumice may be used to clean the tooth surface and eliminate any stains that may interfere with shade selection.

With proper attention to detail, resin composites allow a very predictable shade match. Most manufacturers provide or recommend a shade guide for their products to offer an approximation of the colors available. The shade guides are only helpful for a general determination of the shade. Most shade guides are made of acrylic resins that have different optical properties than resin composites. As many composites are delivered in Vita shades, porcelain shade guides may also be used. The match between the Vita shade guides and the corresponding shades of resin composites, compomers, and glass ionomers has been shown to be relatively poor.[95] A major drawback of all the shade guides is the fact that the shade of the underlying tooth is not taken into account. There will always be an effect on the shade of the restoration caused by the underlying tooth structure unless the restoration is more than 2.5 mm thick.[89] In order to overcome problems associated with shade guide discrepancies, custom shade-tab disks (approximately 7 mm in diameter and 1 mm in thickness) may be fabricated for each shade of the resin composite material. This disk is then held adjacent to the facial surface within the middle third of the tooth, as well as just lingual to the incisal edge. The selected shade then becomes the overall or basic shade of the restoration.

It is important to realize when using layers of differing opacities that the thickness of each layer will affect the final shade. The ultimate shade selection in very difficult situations is best achieved by producing a mock-up using each of the different layers to accurately match not just a single shade, but also the adjacent tooth structure. The shade can be confirmed with a small amount of resin composite applied as a test shade, placed directly on or adjacent to the tooth and cured. This procedure should only be performed on unetched surfaces to facilitate removal after shade verification. For Class 4 restorations in which no tooth structure will remain lingual or facial to the planned restoration, the test shade should be placed in the approximate thickness of the tooth structure to be replaced to ensure adequate opacity or color density.

Tinting and Opaquing

Many manufacturers of resin composites provide accessory shades that contain a number of intense colors and opaque resins, premixed in syringes, ampules, or bottles. These materials are normally not necessary in conservative Class 3 restorations but can play an important role in large Class 4 restorations, diastema closures, and direct veneers. Opaque shades, or more opaque hybrid resin materials, can be used to block the show-through of darkness from the mouth that

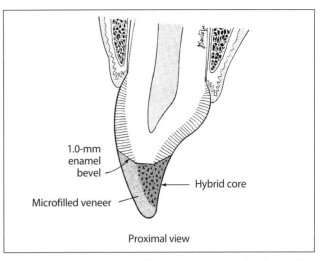

Fig 9-23 Opaque resin or a hybrid core may be used to block the shine-through effect.

may cause a Class 4 restoration to appear too dark or low in value, or too translucent (Fig 9-23). Opaque resins may also be needed to mask discolored tooth structure.

Masking agents should be applied in thin layers to allow sufficient space for the overlying composite to restore translucency. Use of the proper accessory shades can create the appearance of dentin overlaid with enamel. Accessory shades can also be used to recreate the yellow color seen in cervical areas or the translucency that appears in incisal areas. An ochre-shaded resin composite can be used to enhance chroma in the cervical areas, gray or blue may increase the "translucent-incisal" effect, and white can be employed to reproduce a halo. Tints may be used to imitate white or brown spots that appear on adjacent teeth, although with the current ability to bleach teeth, the spots can usually be bleached out or their appearance neutralized with bleaching (see chapter 15).

Matrices

For Class 3 Restorations

With Class 3 restorations, the most commonly used matrix is the clear plastic strip (Figs 9-24a and 9-24b). The clear plastic matrix, when properly wedged, will reduce flash (excess material) at the gingival margin. It is placed between the teeth and adjacent to the cavity preparation. The resin composite may be shaped with a plastic instrument, or the matrix strip may be pulled snugly around the tooth and held in place manually to provide shape to the restoration and intimately adapt the resin composite. An excellent contouring or sculpt-

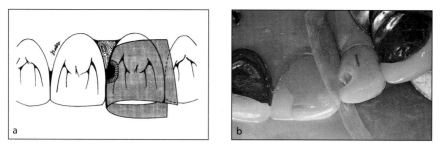

Figs 9-24a and 9-24b Lingual view of matrix and wedge placement for a typical Class 3 resin composite restoration.

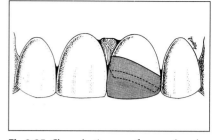

Fig 9-25 Clear plastic crown form and wedge in place for a Class 4 restoration.

ing instrument for resin composite is the interproximal carver described in chapter 6.

For Class 4 Restorations

The majority of Class 4 restorations must be built up incrementally to avoid resin thicknesses of greater than 2.0 mm that would prevent an adequate degree of polymerization of the resin composite. This method usually requires placement of several increments. A clear plastic matrix strip and wedge may be used to achieve proximal contact and contours.

For forming lingual and proximal aspects, one option is to use a portion of a thin, clear plastic crown form positioned to provide support until the lingual and proximal resin has been polymerized (Fig 9-25). The crown form should be trimmed to fit approximately 1.0 mm past the prepared margins. If the crown form is thicker than a clear plastic matrix strip, the contact areas should be thinned with an abrasive disk to allow contact of the restoration with the adjacent tooth. For Class 4 restorations with existing or mock-up resins in place, the clinician may prefer to use polyvinyl-siloxane impression material or putty to provide a lingual matrix that assists in shaping lingual and proximal contours (see Figs 9-14b to 9-14d). For creation of extensive restorations in which lingual contours and/or incisal length need to be changed, these may be developed in wax on a diagnostic cast of the teeth before the lingual matrix is made. The matrix should extend to the facioincisal line angle to guide the shaping of the incisal edge and facilitate the creation of an incisal "halo."

Wedging

Wooden wedges are inserted between the teeth and against the matrix to seal the gingival margin, separate the teeth, protect interproximal gingiva, ensure proximal contact, and push the rubber dam and proximal tissue gingivally to open the gingival embrasure. Prewedging, or placement of the wedge prior to tooth preparation, may be helpful in some situations. This is generally not needed with Class 3 restorations but may be helpful in Class 4 restorations. Prewedging allows greater separation of the teeth and more space to build a contact. Resin composite cannot be condensed against the adjacent tooth, as amalgam can, and depends on the space created by the wedge for achieving contact with the adjacent tooth. If the wedge will cause deformation of the matrix or poor cervical contours, it should not be used, or its use may be delayed until after an increment of resin composite has been placed and sculpted in the cervical portion of the preparation and polymerized.

Placement and Curing of Resin Composite Restorations

Light-cured resin composites are packaged in bulk form in syringes or in unit-dose ampules. The main advantage of purchasing material in bulk is that each unit costs less. However, for direct placement into the preparation, bulk material requires more handling because it must be dispensed and then loaded into a syringe for delivery. Unit-dose ampules allow insertion of the material directly into the preparation, minimizing trapped air bubbles.[96] The ampules also make infection control procedures easier because they are discarded after use and require no disinfection.

Incremental Placement and Curing

Incremental placement and curing of the resin composite may be necessary for large light-cured restorations.[97] Most resin composite should be placed in thicknesses not greater than 2.0 mm. In restorations greater than 2.0 mm in thickness,

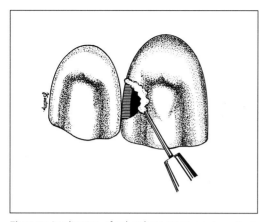

Fig 9-26 Application of gel etchant using a syringe tip. A matrix strip should be placed first to protect the adjacent tooth from the acid.

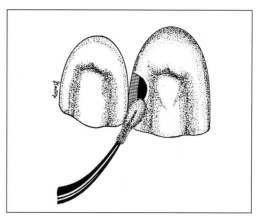

Fig 9-27 The primer and adhesive are placed with disposable brushes or applicators, and the adhesive is light cured in accordance with the manufacturer's protocol.

incremental placement will produce a higher degree of polymerization of the material. Incremental placement has been shown in some studies to offset some of the effects of polymerization stresses,[24,78] but other studies show no difference in bulk placement vs incremental-filling techniques.[45,98]

Incremental placement without loss of restoration strength is possible because of the free radicals available in freshly polymerized resin composite. A thin air- (or oxygen-) inhibited layer remains on the surface of newly polymerized resin. Polymerization of resin composite is initiated and progresses because of free radicals that are formed in the resin monomers. These free radicals are highly reactive to oxygen, and when they come into contact with air at the surface of the resin composite, an unpolymerized, air-inhibited layer is formed.[99] A thin air-inhibited layer contains free radicals and is therefore reactive to new resin composite material applied to it. This provides for formation of a cohesive bond to additional increments. Even in the absence of an air-inhibited layer, if the restoration is freshly placed, free radicals remain that can induce a high degree of chemical attachment for the added increment.[100]

Placement Technique

Class 3 Restorations

The entire cavity preparation, including enamel margins and dentin, is usually etched with phosphoric acid with a concentration of 30% to 40%.[101] Phosphoric acid is most easily dispensed in a gel form with a small syringe (Fig 9-26). Dentin bonding agents provide adhesion with both the enamel and dentin for retention as well as for sealing the cavity-wall inter-

face with the restorative material (see chapter 8 for a complete discussion of dentin adhesives). The dentin adhesive system may be applied and polymerized either before or after the matrix and wedge have been placed (Fig 9-27).

The resin composite–dispensing tip should be inserted into the preparation and the resin composite slowly injected until there is a slight overfill. Small Class 3 preparations can be filled in a single step without incremental placement. For larger Class 3 restorations, placement of multiple increments is recommended to optimize the degree of conversion of the resin composite in deep areas, to minimize the effects of polymerization shrinkage (Figs 9-28a and 9-28b), and to create polychromatic restorations.

After placement, the resin composite is shaped with a plastic instrument or interproximal carver or by pulling the matrix strip tightly around the tooth. The material is light cured with a tungsten-quartz-halogen (TQH) curing light for approximately 40 seconds. When the material has been light cured, the wedge and matrix strip are removed, and the restoration is inspected for voids. If external voids are present, they may be filled with additional resin composite material, which is then light cured.

Large Class 3 restorations often do not blend with the color and translucency of the surrounding tooth structure, and a show-through of the darkness of the mouth can be seen. In order to predictably achieve an imperceptible restoration, the *layering* or *stratified technique* should be employed. The dentin shade selected is typically one or two shades darker than the enamel shade overlying it. The enamel replacement increment should be placed facially over the dentin increment to replace the anatomic enamel, covering the bevel, and possibly feathered over the natural tooth surface.

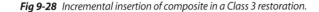

Fig 9-28 Incremental insertion of composite in a Class 3 restoration.

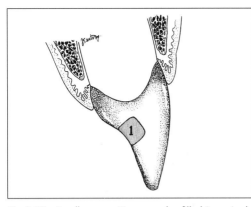

Fig 9-28a Small preparations may be filled in a single increment.

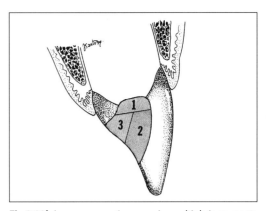

Fig 9-28b Large preparations require multiple increments to minimize the effects of polymerization shrinkage and ensure adequate polymerization.

This facial "enamel" increment should be placed in one application and built to establish the final contour of the restoration. A third enamel-shade increment is then placed over the lingual portion to complete the layering effect.

Class 4 Restorations

An ideal Class 4 restoration is often complicated because of the difficulty in duplicating the natural anatomic contours. When treating a fracture of an incisal edge, a missing Class 4 restoration, or an existing Class 4 restoration that needs replacement, a custom matrix can be fabricated. In one technique, impression material may be formed to provide a lingual matrix. It should cover the lingual and incisal aspects of the tooth to be restored plus the lingual surfaces of one or two adjacent teeth. The matrix should extend facially only far enough to reach the middle of the incisal edge. If tooth structure or a portion of a restoration is missing, then a quick mock-up can be made. Expired resin composite or a seldom-used resin composite shade may be employed for this purpose. The tooth is dried, and composite is applied to form the desired tooth contours and light cured. Care should be taken in shaping the lingual aspect. After polymerization, the occlusion in maximum intercuspation position of the mandible and in excursive mandibular movements should be checked. The lingual contour can be finalized with a round or football-shaped carbide finishing bur. A lingual matrix of impression material that preserves and reproduces the correct lingual contours, anterior guidance, and incisal length in the final restoration can then be made.

Etching procedures are performed and the adhesive system applied. In most cases, resin composite is built up incre-

mentally, layering as necessary to achieve desired coloring, and polymerized. Each increment should be exposed to the curing light for the appropriate material- and curing light–specific time. Inappropriately short curing times or the use of a poorly functioning curing light will result in resin composite restorations with inferior physical properties and an increased chance that unreacted monomer will leach out of the restoration with time. The incremental placement technique allows the clinician to shape the restoration to the desired form and contours. The preparation may be very slightly overfilled to allow subtractive contouring and finishing.

An overlay technique may be used for Class 4 restorations to obtain both strength and a very smooth surface.[102] The bulk of the restoration is built with a hybrid resin composite to provide strength. The final layer is a veneer of microfilled resin composite to provide a smooth, glossy surface. The final layer should be contoured and shaped before polymerization until it closely resembles the desired shape. It is then light polymerized. After any voids are eliminated, the restoration is contoured, finished, and polished.

In order to achieve imperceptible polychromatic restorations, a layering technique employing both enamel and dentin shades is recommended. Selection of dentin and enamel shades is based on the principle of the basic shade and careful observation of the surrounding dentition. Dentin lobes, areas of high translucency, and halos may be incorporated into the restoration. After proper etching and adhesive procedures are complete, the first layer is built up. A thin (0.2- to 0.3-mm) layer of "enamel" shade is placed over the lingual matrix and is limited to the size of the missing tooth portion. The matrix is carried to place in the mouth, taking care to

Clinical Steps for a Class 3 or 4 Resin Composite Restoration

1. Select a shade before dehydration of the tooth.
2. Place a rubber dam.
3. Prewedge if difficulty in achieving proximal contact is anticipated.
4. Initiate the cavity preparation by accessing the caries lesion through the marginal ridge with a No. 329 or 330 bur in a high-speed handpiece. Remove the proximal plate of enamel. Be careful to avoid damaging the adjacent tooth.
5. Remove the carious dentin with a round bur in a low-speed handpiece running at very low speed.
6. Remove unsupported enamel if appropriate, and place bevels with a finishing bur and/or gingival margin trimmer.
7. Etch the enamel. Be careful not to etch the adjacent tooth; protect it with a matrix strip.
8. Place the primer and adhesive, following the manufacturer's instructions.
9. Light cure as indicated.
10. If the preparation is large, place resin composite into the deep areas.
11. Light cure for the appropriate time (material- and curing light–specific).
12. Place a clear plastic strip or other matrix and wedge.
13. Add composite and contour the matrix strip to contain the material in the proper shape.
14. Light cure.
15. Remove the wedge and matrix strip, and inspect the restoration for voids; add resin composite if necessary.
16. Remove gingival flash with a No. 12 or 12b scalpel blade.
17. Remove flash from the other margins, and contour the restoration with a finishing bur, finishing diamond, or abrasive disk.
18. Remove the rubber dam.
19. Check the occlusion and adjust as necessary.
20. Finish and polish with disks, rubber points, etc.
21. Apply etchant to surface and margins; rinse, then apply and cure rebonding resin.

cover the lingual bevel. The increment is light cured for the recommended time and the custom matrix removed. The second increment, using the proper "dentin" shade should be placed to fill the angle produced by the surface of the first increment and wall of tooth structure. The third increment reproduces the dentinal lobes. An interproximal carver instrument or an ovoid-shaped burnisher is useful for forming these lobes, and a brush is useful to smooth the surface. This facial increment should extend over the facial bevel. A view from the incisal edge with an intraoral mirror should be used to evaluate the facial contour of the increment. If a highly translucent area is to be reproduced within the incisal third, an increment of incisal/translucent resin composite is then placed between the lobes and feathered to the incisal edge. A final "enamel" increment is then placed to complete the facial contour of the restoration. After removing the matrix strips, an interproximal carver instrument is used to remove excess and provide final proximal contours prior to curing the increment.

Visible Light–Curing Units

Any light-curing unit with the prescribed wavelength may be used with any resin composite. However, the various commercially available units do not have the same curing capacity. Some units have been shown to cure greater thicknesses of material than others.[93] A light's effectiveness depends on several factors: (1) wavelength of the emitted light (it should be 450 to 500 nm),[103] (2) intensity of the light source, (3) light exposure time, (4) distance from light tip to composite surface, and (5) shade of resin composite. Studies of light-curing units have found that some do not have the correct wavelength, which reduces the effectiveness of the unit.[104]

As a TQH curing unit ages, the bulb and its reflector degrade, reducing light output and curing effectiveness. Friedman[105] examined 67 curing lights in use by dentists around the United States and found bulb blackening in 21 lamps, frosted glass envelopes in 33 lamps, and reflector degradation in 3 lamps.

Because light-curing units can rapidly lose their effectiveness, every office should have a light analyzer (curing radiometer) to evaluate curing lights at least weekly. The bulb and reflector of TQH lights should be examined regularly for signs of degradation, and the light tip should be checked for clarity. The tip of any curing light should also be cleaned of any resin composite or bonding resin that may have touched and adhered to the tip in the course of restoration placement. Bulbs in TQH lights should be replaced when any deterioration is noted.

High-intensity curing lights such as improved conventional TQH lights, blue-light-emitting-diode lights, lasers, and plasma arc lights have been evaluated for curing resin composite materials. (*Laser* is an acronym for "light amplification by stimulated emission of radiation.") Both lasers and plasma arc curing (PAC) light units are able to cure much faster and to a greater degree than the regular halogen light–curing units.[106] However, at present, lasers are expensive to own and maintain, and many practitioners consider them impractical to purchase for light curing alone. The potential advantages and disadvantages of PAC lights are still being investigated.

For a more in-depth discussion of curing lights, see chapter 10.

Finishing and Polishing

Finishing includes the shaping, contouring, and smoothing of the restoration, while polishing imparts a shine or luster to the surface. Sharp amalgam carvers and scalpel blades, such as the No. 12 or 12b, or specific resin carving instruments made of carbide, anodized aluminum, or nickel titanium, are useful for shaping polymerized resins (Fig 9-29). There are many products available for finishing and polishing, including diamond and carbide burs, various types of flexible disks, abrasive-impregnated rubber points and cups, metal and plastic finishing strips, and polishing pastes. The smoothest possible surface is obtained when the resin composite polymerizes against a clear plastic strip without subsequent finishing or polishing.[107,108] However, such a surface has a high resin content and may yield a surface that is less resistant to wear.

The finishing and polishing process can affect many aspects of the final restoration, including surface staining, plaque accumulation, and wear characteristics of the resin composite.[109] Either traumatic finishing technique or overheating can damage the surface of resin composite materials[110,111] and result in accelerated wear.[110,112] A less-than-optimal finishing technique may be one reason that wear of resin composite is often reported to be greatest in the first 6 to 12 months after placement. A low-viscosity surface sealer or rebonding resin, applied after finishing the resin composite, may help stop crack propagation, improve wear resistance, add color stability, and enhance marginal integrity over time.[113]

Instruments

Diamond vs Carbide Burs
The 12-fluted carbide burs have traditionally been used to perform gross finishing of resin composite (Fig 9-30). These finishing burs may be used to develop the proper anatomy for the restoration. The transition from resin to enamel should be slowly smoothed until it is undetectable. These burs can be used dry to better visualize the margins and anatomy being devel-

oped but should be used with light pressure to avoid overheating and possibly damaging the resin composite surface.

Fine finishing diamonds are also available for finishing resin composite restorations and have been found to impart less surface damage to microfilled resin composites than carbide finishing burs.[109,114] They are used in a series of progressively finer abrasive particle sizes.

Disks
One brand of flexible disks (Sof-Lex, 3M) has practically become the standard in finishing and polishing. The disks in one Sof-Lex series have a soft, flexible backing and a series of grits that can provide a smooth, even finish. Another Sof-Lex series, and similar disks made by other manufacturers, have thin plastic or polymeric backings that allow access of the abrasive side into embrasures and interproximal areas. When all four grits are used in sequence, these flexible finishing disks are reported to provide the best surface of any finishing system.[40,115] Sequential use of disks with progressively finer grits produces a smooth, durable finish (Fig 9-31).

Dry finishing with disks used in sequence is reported to be superior or equal to wet finishing for smoothness, hardness, and color stability.[116] However, dry finishing tends to clog disks with abrasive particles and makes the disks work less efficiently.

Impregnated Rubber Points and Cups
A wide variety of rubber finishing and polishing points and cups impregnated with abrasive materials are available. Like disks, rubber cups and points are used sequentially from coarse to fine grit. The coarse grits may be effective for gross reduction and finishing, while the fine grits create a smooth, shiny surface (Figs 9-32a and 9-32b). The primary advantage of rubber points and cups over disks is for providing access to grooves, desirable surface irregularities, and the concave lingual surfaces of anterior teeth.

Finishing Strips
Finishing strips are used to contour and polish the proximal surfaces and margins gingival to the interproximal contact (Fig 9-33). They are available with metal or plastic backings. Most metal-backed strips are used for gross reduction, but care must be taken not to overreduce the restoration; these metal-backed strips will also remove enamel, cementum, and dentin. Plastic strips come in various widths and grits and can be used for both finishing and polishing. Like the flexible disks, finishing strips come in a series of grits, which should be used in series from coarsest to finest.

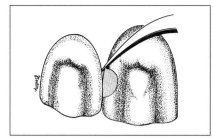

Fig 9-29 Gingival flash is removed with a No. 12 or 12b scalpel blade.

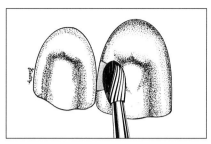

Fig 9-30 A finishing bur or fine diamond is used for gross finishing.

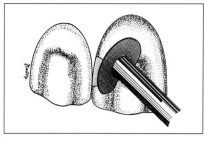

Fig 9-31 Polishing of the final restoration may be accomplished with flexible abrasive disks or abrasive-impregnated rubber points, cups, and/or disks.

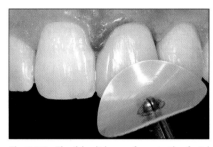

Fig 9-32a Flexible disks conform to the facial contours of the tooth.

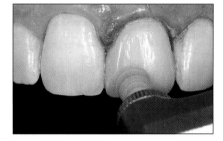

Fig 9-32b Abrasive-impregnated rubber points and/or cups may also be employed for polishing lingual contours and interproximal surfaces that are inaccessible to disks.

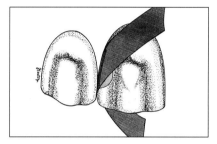

Fig 9-33 Polishing strips are used to contour and polish the proximal surface and margin.

Procedures

A No. 12 or 12b scalpel blade is effective for removing interproximal flash, carving the proximal margins, and otherwise shaping the polymerized resin. Gross reduction and shaping are then performed with diamonds, carbide burs, and/or coarse abrasive disks and strips. Finishing should be done carefully to avoid damaging the surface or margins of the resin composite restoration. Finishing strips can be used on the proximal surfaces and margins so that floss passes over the proximal resin surface smoothly and snaps smoothly through the contact without shredding. After the resin composite is polished with fine abrasive-impregnated disks, strips, or rubber cups or points, a high shine can be added with aluminum-oxide or diamond polishing pastes.

Many operators have observed the development of a "white line" at the margins of resin composite restorations during finishing. The exact cause of this phenomenon is not known, but several investigators and clinicians have put forward possible explanations. One explanation[91,117–119] implicates traumatic finishing leading to microfractures in the resin composite or tooth structure at the interface. Other proposed causes include improperly rotating abrasive disks,[120,121] inadequate polymerization of the resin composite material,[119] and polymerization shrinkage causing microfracture of unsupported or fragile enamel at the margins.[122] When the white line presents an esthetic problem and more conservative procedures such as rebonding do not resolve it, the white area must be removed with a bur and additional composite must be bonded and finished.

Rebonding

Rebonding (also called *surface sealing* or *glazing*) is performed after the restoration is finished and polished. The enamel margins are re-etched, and a coat of unfilled or lightly filled low-viscosity resin is placed over the restoration surface and polymerized. Rebonding has been reported to improve marginal integrity,[123] aid color stability, improve early wear resistance, and help reduce staining of the restoration.[113,124–126] A number of low-viscosity resins, called *surface sealers*, are now available for use in the rebonding procedure.

References

1. Buda M. Form and color reproduction for composite resin reconstruction of anterior teeth. Int J Periodontics Restorative Dent 1994; 14:34–47.

2. Lambrechts P, Willems G, Vanherle G, Braem M. Aesthetic limits of light-cured composite in anterior teeth. Int Dent J 1990;40:149–158.

3. Jokstad A, Mjör IA, Qvist V. The age of restorations in situ. Acta Odontol Scand 1994;52:234–242.

4. Mjör IA. Placement and replacement of restorations. Oper Dent 1981;6:49–54.

5. Mjör IA, Toffenetti F. Placement and replacement of resin-based restorations in Italy. Oper Dent 1992;17:82–85.

6. Smales RJ. Effects of enamel bonding, type of restoration, patient age and operator on the longevity of an anterior composite resin. Am J Dent 1991;4:130–133.

7. Burke FJT, Cheung SW, Mjör IA, Wilson NH. Restoration longevity and analysis of reasons for placement and replacement of restorations provided by vocational dental practitioners and their trainees in the United Kingdom. Quintessence Int 1999;30:234–242.

8. van Noort R, Davis LG. A prospective study of the survival of chemically activated anterior resin composite restorations in general practice: 5-year results. J Dent 1993;21:209–215.

9. van Dijken JW, Olofsson AL, Holm C. 5-year evaluation of Class III composite resin restorations in cavities pre-treated with an oxalic- or a phosphoric acid conditioner. J Oral Rehab 1999;26:364–371.

10. Stansbury JW. Synthesis and evaluation of novel multifunctional oligomers for dentistry. J Dent Res 1992;71:434–437.

11. Leinfelder KF, Suzuki S. In vitro wear device for determining posterior composite wear. J Am Dent Assoc 1999;130:1347–1353.

12. Feilzer AJ, De Gee AJ, Davidson CL. Curing contraction of composites and glass-ionomer cements. J Prosthet Dent 1988;59:297–300.

13. Crim G, Chapman K. Effect of placement techniques on microleakage of a dentin-bonded composite resin. Quintessence Int 1986; 17:21–24.

14. Davidson CL, De Gee AJ. Relaxation of polymerization contraction stresses by flow in dental composites. J Dent Res 1984;63:16–48.

15. Eick JD, Welch F. Polymerization shrinkage of posterior composite resins and its possible influence on postoperative sensitivity. Quintessence Int 1986;17:103–111.

16. Gordon M, Plasschaert A, Saiku J, Pelzner RB. Microleakage of posterior composite resin materials and an experimental urethane restorative material, tested in vitro above and below the cementoenamel junction. Quintessence Int 1986;17:11–15.

17. Lutz F, Krejci I, Oldenburg TR. Elimination of polymerization stresses at the margins of posterior composite resin restorations: A new restorative technique. Quintessence Int 1986;17:777–784.

18. Peutzfeld A. Resin composites in dentistry: The monomer systems. Eur J Oral Sci 1997;105:97–116.

19. Lutz F, Krejci I, Barbakow F. Quality and durability of marginal adaptation in bonded composite restorations. Dent Mater 1991;7: 107–113.

20. Hashimoto M, Tay FR, Ohno H, et al. SEM and TEM analysis of water degradation of human dentinal collagen. J Biomed Mat Res B Appl Biomater 2003;66:287–298.

21. Pashley DH, Tay FR, Yiu C, et al. Collagen degradation by host-derived enzymes during aging. J Dent Res 2004;83:216–221.

22. Tay FR, Hashimoto M, Pashley DH, et al. Aging affects two modes of nanoleakage expression in bonded dentin. J Dent Res 2003; 82:537–541.

23. Alster D, Feilzer AJ, De Gee AJ, Mol A, Davidson CL. The dependence of shrinkage stress reduction on porosity concentration in thin resin layers. J Dent Res 1992;71:1619–1622.

24. Crim GA. Microleakage of three resin placement techniques. Am J Dent 1991;4:69–72.

25. Davidson CL, Feilzer AJ. Polymerization shrinkage and polymerization shrinkage stress in polymer-based restoratives. J Dent 1997; 25:435–440.

26. Eick JD, Robinson SJ, Byerley TJ, Chappelow CC. Adhesives and nonshrinking dental resins of the future. Quintessence Int 1993;24: 632–640.

27. Krejci I, Sparr D, Lutz F. A three sited light curing technique for conventional Class II composite resin restorations. Quintessence Int 1987;18:125–131.

28. Opdam NJM, Roeters JJM, Kuijs R, Burgersdijk RC. Necessity of bevels for box only Class II composite restorations. J Prosthet Dent 1998;80:274–279.

29. Craig RG. Restorative Dental Materials, ed 10. St. Louis: Mosby, 1997.

30. Cipalla AJ. Laser Curing of Photoactivated Restorative Materials. Salt Lake City: ILT Systems, 1994.

31. Feilzer AJ, De Gee AJ, Davidson CL. Influence of light intensity on polymerization shrinkage and integrity of restoration-cavity interface. Eur J Oral Sci 1995;103:322–326.

32. Mehl A, Hickel R, Kunzelmann KH. Physical properties and gap formation of light-cured composite with and without "soft-start" polymerization. J Dent 1997;25:321–330.

33. Sakaguchi RL, Berge H-X. Reduced light energy density decreases post-gel contraction while maintaining degree of conversion in composites. J Dent 1998;26:695–700.

34. Watts DC, Al Hindi A. Intrinsic "soft-start" polymerisation shrinkage-kinetics in an acrylate-based resin composite. Dent Mater 1999; 15:39–45.

35. Stansbury JW, Dickens B, Liu DW. Preparation and characterization of cyclopolymerizable resin formulations. J Dent Res 1995;74: 1110–1115.

36. Opdam NJ, Roeters JJ, Peters TC, Burgersdijk RC, Kuijs RH. Consistency of resin composites for posterior use. Dent Mater 1996; 12:350–354.

37. Tyas MJ, Jones DW, Rizkalla AS. The evaluation of resin composite consistency. Dent Mater 1998;14:424–428.

38. Leevailoj C, Cochran MA, Matis BA, Moore BK, Platt JA. Microleakage of posterior packable resin composites with and without flowable liners. Oper Dent 2001;26:302–307.

39. Tjan AHL, Glancy JF. Effects of four lubricants used during incremental insertion of two types of visible light–activated composites. J Prosthet Dent 1988;60:189–194.

40. Chen RCS, Chan DCN, Chan KC. A quantitative study of finishing and polishing techniques for a composite. J Prosthet Dent 1988; 59:292–298.

41. Goldman M. Fracture properties of composite and glass ionomer dental restorative materials. J Biomed Mater Res 1985;19:771–783.

42. Lambrechts PP, Ameye C, Vanherle G. Conventional and microfilled composite resins. Part II: Chip fractures. J Prosthet Dent 1982;48: 527–538.

43. Tyas MJ. Correlation between fracture properties and clinical performance of composite resins in Class IV cavities. Aust Dent J 1990; 35:46–49.

44. Tyas MJ. Color stability of composite resins: A clinical comparison. Aust Dent J 1992;37;88–90.

45. Winkler MM, Katona TR, Paydar NH. Finite element stress analysis of three filling techniques for Class V light-cured restorations. J Dent Res 1996;75:1477–1483.

46. Shortall AC, Uctasli S, Marquis PM. Fracture resistance of anterior, posterior and universal light activated composite restoratives. Oper Dent 2001;26:87–96

47. Chan DCN, Chung KH, Titus HW, et al. Radiopacity of Ta_2O_5 nanoparticle filled resins [abstract 443]. J Dent Res 1998;77:687.

48. Wellinghoff ST, Dixon H, Nicollela D, et al. Optically translucent composites containing tantalum oxide nanoparticles [abstract 58]. J Dent Res 1998;77:639.

49. Haveman CW, Summitt JB, Burgess JO, Carlson K. Three restorative materials and topical fluoride gel used in xerostomic patients: A clinical comparison. J Am Dent Assoc 2003;134:177–184.

50. Burgess JO, Gallo JR. Treating root surface caries. Dent Clin North Am 2002;46:385–404.

51. Randall RC, Wilson NHF. Glass-ionomer restoratives: A systematic review of a secondary caries treatment effect. J Dent Res 1999; 78:628–637.

52. McComb D, Erickson RL, Maxymiw WG, Wood RE. A clinical comparison of glass ionomer, resin-modified glass ionomer and resin composite restorations in the treatment of cervical caries in xerostomic head and neck radiation patients. Oper Dent 2002;27: 475–479.

53. Haveman CW, Burgess JO, Summitt JB. Clinical comparison of restorative materials for caries in xerostomic patients [abstract 1441]. J Dent Res 1999;78:286.

54. Boghosian AA, Ricker J, McCoy R. Clinical evaluation of a resin-modified glass-ionomer restorative: 5-year results [abstract 1436]. J Dent Res 1999;78(special issue):285.

55. Brackett WW, Gilpatrick RO, Browning WD, Gregory PN. Two-year clinical performance of a resin-modified glass-ionomer restorative material. Oper Dent 1999;24:9–13.

56. Robbins JW, Duke ES, Schwartz RS, Trevino D. Clinical evaluation of a glass ionomer restorative in cervical abrasions [abstract 171]. J Dent Res 1996;75(special issue):39.

57. Eames WB. When not to restore. J Am Dent Assoc 1988;117: 429–432.

58. McDonald SP, Sheiham A. A clinical comparison of non-traumatic methods of treating dental caries. Int Dent J 1994;44:465–470.

59. Silverstone LM. Fluorides and Remineralization: Clinical Uses of Fluorides. Philadelphia: Lea & Febiger, 1985:153–175.

60. Kidd EAM, Roberts GT. The saucer preparation. Part 2. Laboratory evaluation. Br Dent J 1982;153:138–140.

61. Roberts GT. The saucer preparation. Part 1: Clinical evaluation over 3 years. Br Dent J 1982;153:96–98.

62. Fusayama T. Ideal cavity preparation for adhesive composites. Asian J Aesthet Dent 1993;1:55–62.

63. Porte A, Lutz F, Lund MR, Swartz ML, Cochran MA. Cavity designs for composite resins. Oper Dent 1984;9:50–55.

64. Qvist V, Strom C. 11-year assessment of Class III resin restorations completed with two restorative procedures. Acta Odontol Scand 1993;51:253–262.

65. Wilson NH, Wilson MA, Wastell DG, Smith GA. Performance of Occlusin in butt-joint and bevel-edged preparations: Five year results. Dent Mater 1991;7:92–98.

66. Ireland E, Xu X, Burgess JO. Microleakage of beveled and non-beveled Class 3 resin restorations [abstract 207]. J Dent Res 1998; 77(special issue):131.

67. Summitt JB, Chan DCN, Dutton FB. Retention of Class 3 composite restorations: Retention grooves versus enamel bonding. Oper Dent 1993;18:88–93.

68. van Dijken JW, Kieri C, Carlen M. Longevity of extensive Class II open-sandwich restorations with a resin-modified glass-ionomer cement. J Dent Res 1999;78:1319–1325.

69. Trushkowsky RD, Gwinnett AJ. Microleakage of Class V composite, resin sandwich, and resin-modified glass ionomers. Am J Dent 1996;9:96–99.

70. Vilkinis V Hörsted-Bindslev P, Baelum V. Two-year evaluation of Class II resin-modified glass ionomer cement/composite open sandwich and composite restorations. Clin Oral Invest 2000;4:133–139.

71. van Meerbeek B, Peumans M, Gladys S, Braem M, Lambrechts P, Vanherle G. Three-year clinical effectiveness of four total-etch dentinal adhesive systems in cervical lesions. Quintessence Int 1996; 27:775–784.

72. Espinosa HD. In vitro study of resin-supported internally etched enamel. J Prosthet Dent 1979;40:526–529.

73. Erickson RL, McComb D, Wood RE, et al. Caries inhibition by fluoride-releasing liners. Am J Dent 1992;5:293–295.

74. van Dijken JW. 3-year clinical evaluation of a compomer, a resin-modified glass-ionomer and a composite in Class III cavities. Am J Dent 1996;9:195–198.

75. Gutz DP. Fractured permanent incisors in a clinical population. J Dent Child 1971;38:94–95.

76. Black JB, Retief DH, Lemmons JE. Effect of cavity design on the retention of Class 4 composite resin restorations. J Am Dent Assoc 1981;103:42–46.

77. Bagheri J, Denehy GE. Effect of enamel bevel and restoration length on Class 4 acid-etch retained composite resin restorations. J Am Dent Assoc 1983;107:951–953.

78. Burke FJT. Reattachment of a fractured central incisor tooth fragment. Br Dent J 1991;170:223–225.

79. Croll TP. Emergency repair followed by complete-coronal restoration of a fractured mandibular incisor. Quintessence Int 1992;23: 817–822.

80. Simonsen RJ. Restoration of a fractured central incisor using the original tooth fragment. J Am Dent Assoc 1982;105:646–648.

81. Worthington RB, Murchison DF, Vandewalle KS. Incisal edge reattachment: The effect of preparation utilization and design. Quintessence Int 1999;30:637–643.

82. Andreasen FM, Noren JG, Andreasen JO, Engelhardtsen S, Lindh-Stromberg U. Long term survival of fragment bonding in the treatment of fractured crowns: A multicenter clinical study. Quintessence Int 1995;26:669–681.

83. Cavalleri G, Zerman N. Traumatic crown fractures in permanent incisors with immature roots: A follow-up study. Endod Dent Traumatol 1995;11:294–296.

84. Darveniza M. Cavity design for Class 4 composite resin restorations—A systematic approach. Aust Dent J 1987;32:270–275.

85. Neumeyer S, Gernet W, Kappert HF, Hellekes E, Botsch H. PCR pin-anchored anterior fracture restorations. Gen Dent 1992;40:200–202.

86. Cobb DS, Vargas MA, Fridich TA, Bouschlicher MR. Metal surface treatment: Characterization and effect on composite-to-metal bond strength. Oper Dent 2000;25:427–433.

87. Matinlinna JP, Lassila LV, Ozcan M, Yli-Urpo A, Vallittu PK. An introduction to silanes and their clinical applications in dentistry. Int J Prosthet Dent 2004;17:155–164.

88. Peumans M, van Meerbeek B, Lambrechts P, Vanherle G. Porcelain veneers: A review of the literature. J Dent 2000;28:163–177.

89. Grajower R, Fuss Z, Hirschfeld Z. Reflectance spectra of composite resins on liners. J Prosthet Dent 1979;41:650–656.

90. Levin JB. Esthetic diagnosis. Curr Opin Cosmet Dent 1995;1:9–17.

91. Weinstein AR. Esthetic applications of restorative materials and techniques in the anterior dentition. Dent Clin North Am 1993; 37:391–409.

92. Gillen RJ, Schwartz RS, Hilton TJ, Evans DB. Analysis of selected normative tooth proportions. Int J Prosthodont 1994;7:410–417.

93. Crigger LP, Foster CD, Young JM, Stockman TD. Visible-Light Curing Units. Aeromedical Review. San Antonio, TX: USAF School of Aerospace Medicine, 1984.

94. Young JM, Satrom KD, Berrong JM. Intraoral dental lights: Test and evaluation. J Prosthet Dent 1987;57:99–107.

95. Yap AUJ, Bhole S, Tan KBC. Shade match of tooth-colored restorative materials based on a commercial shade guide. Quintessence Int 1995;26:697–702.

96. Medlock JW, Zinck JH, Norling BK, Sisca RF. Composite resin porosity with hand and syringe insertion. J Prosthet Dent 1985;54:47–51.

97. Podshadley AG, Gullett G, Crim G. Interface seal of incremental placement of visible light-cured composite resins. J Prosthet Dent 1985;53:625–626.

98. Versluis A, Douglas WH, Cross M, Sakaguchi RL. Does an incremental filling technique reduce polymerization shrinkage stresses? J Dent Res 1996;75:871–878.

99. Ruyter IE. Unpolymerized surface layers on sealants. Acta Odontol Scand 1981;39:27–32.

100. Suh BI. Oxygen-inhibited layer in adhesion dentistry. J Esthet Rest Dent 2004;16:316–323.

101. Silverstone LM, Saxton CA, Dogon JL, Fejerskov O. Variation in the pattern of acid etching of human dental enamel examined by scanning electron microscopy. Caries Res 1975;9:373–387.

102. Zalkind M, Heling I. Composite resin layering: An esthetic technique for restoring fractured anterior teeth. J Prosthet Dent 1992;68:204–205.

103. Cook WD. Spectral distributions of dental photopolymerization sources. J Dent Res 1982;61:1436–1438.

104. Newman SM, Murray GA, Yates JL. Visible lights and visible light–activated composite resins. J Prosthet Dent 1983;50:31–35.

105. Friedman J. Variability of lamp characteristics in dental curing lights. J Esthet Dent 1990;1:189–190.

106. Blankenau RJ, Kelsey WP, Powell GL, Shearer GO, Barkmeier WW, Cavel WT. Degree of composite resin polymerization with visible light and argon laser. Am J Dent 1991;4:40–42.

107. Pratten DH, Johnson GH. An evaluation of finishing instruments for an anterior and posterior composite. J Prosthet Dent 1988;60:154–158.

108. Stoddard JW, Johnson GH. An evaluation of polishing agents for composite resins. J Prosthet Dent 1991;65:491–495.

109. Jeffries SR. The art and science of abrasive finishing and polishing in restorative dentistry. Dent Clin North Am 1998;42:613–627.

110. Leinfelder KF, Wilder AD, Teixeira AC. Wear rates of posterior composite resins. J Am Dent Assoc 1986;112:829–833.

111. Wu W, Toth EE, Ellison JA. Subsurface damage layer of in vivo worn dental composite restorations. J Dent Res 1984;63:675–680.

112. Ratanapridakul K, Leinfelder KF, Thomas J. Effect of finishing on the in vivo wear rate of a posterior composite resin. J Am Dent Assoc 1989;118:524–526.

113. Dickinson GL, Leinfelder KF. Assessing the long term effects of a surface penetrating sealant. J Am Dent Assoc 1993;124:68–72.

114. Boghosian AA, Randolph RG, Jekkals VJ. Rotary instrument finishing of microfilled and small-particle hybrid composite resins. J Am Dent Assoc 1987;115:299–301.

115. Berastegui E, Canalda C, Brau E, Miquel C. Surface roughness of finished composite resins. J Prosthet Dent 1992;68:742–790.

116. Dodge WW, Dale RA, Cooley RL, Duke ES. Comparison of wet and dry finishing of resin composites with aluminum oxide discs. Dent Mater 1991;7:18–20.

117. Christensen GJ. Overcoming challenges with resin in Class II situations. J Am Dent Assoc 1997;128:1579–1580.

118. Jordan RE. Esthetic Composite Bonding, ed 2. St. Louis: Mosby, 1993:48.

119. Albers HF. Tooth-Colored Restoratives, ed 8. Santa Rosa, CA: Alto, 1996.

120. Farah J, Powers J. Composite finishing and polishing. Dent Advisor 1998;15:3.

121. Goldstein RE. Finishing of composites and laminates. Dent Clin North Am 1989;33:305–318.

122. Heath JR, Jordan JH, Watts DC. The effect of time of trimming on the surface finish of anterior composite resins. J Oral Rehab 1993; 20:45–52.

123. Galan JR, Mondelli J, Coradazzi JL. Marginal leakage of two composite restorative systems. J Dent Res 1976;55:74–76.

124. Garman TA, Fairhurst CW, Heuer GA, Williams HA, Beglau DL. A comparison of glazing materials for composite restorations. J Am Dent Assoc 1977;95:950–956.

125. Gibson GB, Richardson AS, Patton RE, Waldman R. A clinical evaluation of occlusal composite and amalgam restorations: One-year and two-year results. J Am Dent Assoc 1992;104:335–337.

126. Kawai K, Leinfelder KF. Effect of surface-penetrating sealant on composite wear. Dent Mater 1993;9:108–113.

Direct Posterior Esthetic Restorations

Thomas J. Hilton
James C. Broome

The use of resin composite as a material for restoring posterior teeth has continued to increase. Patients are attracted to a restoration that matches the color of natural teeth.[1,2] Resin composite meets this demand and has become the most frequently used esthetic restorative material in dentistry.[3–5] In addition, resin composites avoid the mercury controversy, are thermally nonconductive,[1] and bond to tooth structure with the use of adhesives.[6–8] There are problems associated with using resin composite in posterior restorations, however, including shrinkage that occurs on setting,[9] occasional postoperative sensitivity,[10,11] and less-than-ideal resistance to wear.[12–14] Minimizing these negative aspects requires meticulous operative technique. Along with appropriate case selection, it is one of the most important variables governing the success of posterior resin composite restorations.[15–17]

Although some questions about longevity remain, there is increasing evidence that properly accomplished posterior resin composite restorations can be quite durable.[14,18] Tables 10-1 to 10-3 are compilations of clinical studies on posterior amalgam, cast-gold, and resin composite restorations, respectively. Because studies use different methods to assess restoration survival, an annual failure rate for each study has been computed to allow a means of comparison. As shown, study duration and the range of annual failure rates are comparable among the three materials. Considering that the materials used in the resin composite studies, particularly the studies of longer duration, are of earlier formulations and that materials have improved considerably in recent years, it is reasonable to conclude that resin composites can provide very successful posterior restorations. Long-term success of resin composite posterior restorations

depends on cavity size, restoration type, and tooth type.[30,35,36] Used properly, resin composite has demonstrated the ability to perform as well as amalgam in posterior restorations for up to 10 years.[25,35]

It is interesting to note the contrast in annual failure rates for amalgam, cast gold, and resin composite in a private practice setting (Fig 10-1) vs controlled clinical studies (Fig 10-2). As can be seen, there is a marked difference among material longevity in private practices, whereas the controlled clinical trials show relatively similar results among the materials. These findings have been reinforced by more recent extensive reviews of clinical trials investigating posterior restoration performance.[15,36,41] One such review,[15] presented in Table 10-4, shows that restorations placed as part of a controlled clinical trial typically last longer than restorations placed in private practice and evaluated as part of a cross-sectional study. An analysis of more than 300,000 amalgam and resin composite restorations placed in posterior teeth during a 7-year period in private practices revealed that a patient with a resin composite restoration had a 16.4% greater chance of restoration failure than those with an amalgam restoration at any time period in the analysis.[42] While this appears ominous for resin composite as a posterior restorative material, it should be noted that the probability of a posterior resin composite restoration surviving more than 5 years (93%) differed little from that of an amalgam restoration (94%).

There are a number of valuable lessons to be garnered from this discussion regarding the durability of posterior restorations. First, there are, without doubt, a variety of explanations for the different study results based on restorative material and type of

Table 10-1	Longevity of amalgam restorations		
Investigators	Study time (y)	No. of restorations	Annual failure rate (%)
Smales et al[19]	18	1,801	2.5
Smales et al[20]	18	1,680	1.5–6.0
Osborne et al[21]	14	320	0.9
Crabb[22]	10	407	6.3
Collins et al[23]	8	52	0.7
Letzel et al[24]	7	2,431	1.3–2.4
Fukushima et al[25]	5	73	0.8

Table 10-2	Longevity of cast-gold restorations		
Investigators	Study time (y)	No. of restorations	Annual failure rate (%)
Fritz et al[26]	1–30	2,717	3.0–4.0
Bentley and Drake[27]	1–25	1,207	0.9
Crabb[22]	10	86	5.9

Table 10-3	Longevity of posterior resin composite restorations		
Investigators	Study time (y)	No. of restorations	Annual failure rate (%)
Wilder et al[18]	17	60	1.3
Pallesen and Qvist[28]	10	93	1.6
Barnes et al[29]	8	28	2.9
Collins et al[23]	8	161	1.2–2.0
Wilson et al[30]	5	94	3.4
Fukushima et al[25]	5	432	1.0
Letzel[31]	4	696	1.5
Rowe[32]	4	266	1.5
Geurtsen et al[33]	4	1,214	3.0
Palleson and Qvist[34]	11	54	1.4
Gaengler et al[14]	10	194	2.6

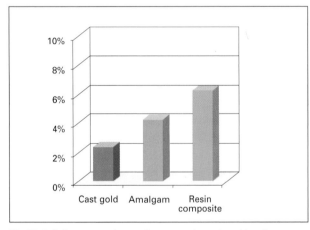

Fig 10-1 Failure rates of posterior restorations placed in private practices.[37]

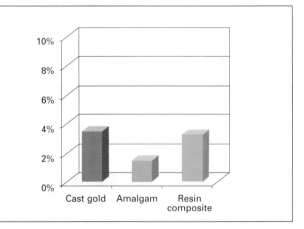

Fig 10-2 Median annual failure rate ranges for posterior restorations evaluated in 17 clinical studies.[18–25,27–33,38–40]

Table 10-4	Median annual failure rates based on restoration and study type[15]	
	Annual failure rate (%)	
Restoration type	Longitudinal studies	Cross-sectional studies
Amalgam	1.1	3.7
Resin composite (direct)	2.1	3.3
Cast gold	1.0	1.3

study, including patient selection, technique sensitivity, and differences in approach related to practice setting. Although the clinical studies are often accomplished in relatively controlled environments, they clearly demonstrate the materials' potential. Next, at the current stage of material development, it is not possible to say that resin composite is a true amalgam replacement, capable of providing clinical service to the same level of performance in all of the same clinical situations as amalgam. However, with appropriate case selection and clinical technique, posterior resin composite restorations can serve very acceptably. This chapter presents the factors that will lead to clinical success by examining the advantages, dis-

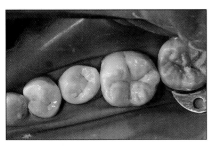

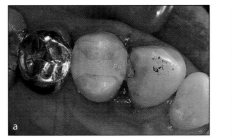

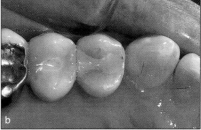

Fig 10-3 Modern resin composite materials can provide an esthetic restoration, such as the mesio-occlusal restoration in the mandibular first molar. (Courtesy of Dr Bill Dunn, United States Air Force Dental Corps.)

Figs 10-4a and 10-4b Heavily filled resin composite formulations tend to give the restoration a more opaque appearance.

advantages, indications, and placement procedures for resin composite as a posterior restorative material.

Advantages of Resin Composite as a Posterior Restorative Material

Esthetics

Manufacturers have developed sophisticated resin composite systems with multiple shades, tints, and opaque resins that allow the practitioner to place highly esthetic restorations (Fig 10-3). Clinical studies often report excellent color match of resin composite with tooth structure. One study found that 93% of posterior resin composite restorations provided an acceptable color match to adjacent tooth structure after 10 years,[14] while another study found that 94% of resin composite restorations still provided excellent color match at 17 years.[18] Visible-light–cured (VLC) resin composites have less amine content than the autocured systems, resulting in less yellowing of the restoration and greater color stability over time.[43] Microfilled resin composites have the smoothest surface finish of all the systems and tend to stain less than other types.[43] Because they are more heavily filled, hybrid resin composites tend to impart a more opaque appearance to restorations (Figs 10-4a and 10-4b).[44]

Conservation of Tooth Structure

In the past, it was recommended that preparation design for posterior resin composite restorations be patterned after the traditional amalgam preparation[17] as described by Dr G. V. Black. Researchers today recommend a more conservative approach.[45,46] The adhesive preparation has evolved to take advantage of resin composite's positive properties and to minimize its negative ones. The current design limits the removal of tooth structure to that needed to eliminate carious tooth structure and fragile enamel.[47]

The adhesive preparation for posterior Class 2 resin composite restorations differs from Black's traditional amalgam design in several ways[48]:

1. The preparation tends to be shallower. Because retention is provided through bonding to tooth structure rather than mechanical undercuts, there is no need to penetrate to dentin if the caries lesion does not. This conserves tooth structure and expands the area of enamel available for bonding (Fig 10-5a).
2. The preparation tends to have a narrower outline form, which allows less occlusal contact on the restoration and reduces wear.[29,30,32,49,50] A less bulky restoration helps to decrease the adverse effects of resin composite polymerization shrinkage, resulting in improved marginal integrity[47] and less cuspal deflection[51] (Fig 10-5b).
3. The preparation has rounded internal line angles; this conserves tooth structure, decreases stress concentration associated with sharp line angles,[43] and enhances resin adaptation during placement[52,53] (Fig 10-5c).
4. There is no "extension for prevention" (Fig 10-5d). The occlusal fissures are included in the preparation only if the presence of carious tooth structure dictates this need. Extending the Class 2 preparation through occlusal fissures does not make the restoration more resistant to fracture than the more conservative proximal-slot restoration.[45,54] In clinical studies, use of a proximal-slot preparation for posterior resin composite restorations showed no failures after more than 2 years of service[55] and 70% success after up to 10 years.[56] In this long-term study,[56] no restorations were lost due to loss of retention or to wear. This may be attributed to the study's requirement that there be an occlusal stop on enamel. Adjacent pits and fissures can be

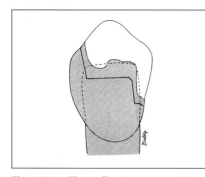

Fig 10-5a The adhesive preparation is extended only enough to provide access and to remove carious tooth structure. It may not penetrate the dentinoenamel junction *(upper solid line)*, unlike the traditional preparation *(lower solid line)*. The dotted line represents the dentinoenamel junction.

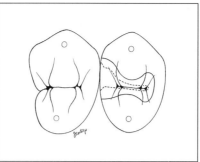

Fig 10-5b The more conservative outline form of the adhesive resin composite restoration *(dotted line)* compared to that of the traditional restoration *(solid line)*.

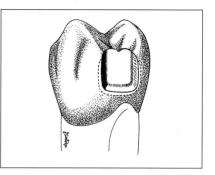

Fig 10-5c In the adhesive preparation, internal angles are rounded.

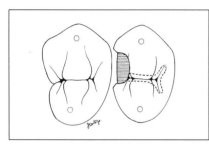

Fig 10-5d If there is no occlusal caries lesion, a Class 2 preparation for a resin composite restoration can be very conservative, similar to a Class 3 preparation. The occlusal fissures can be sealed *(dotted line)* after restoration placement.

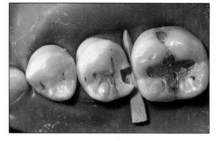

Figs 10-5e A conservative Class 2 preparation has been made. The occlusal fissures are stained but not carious.

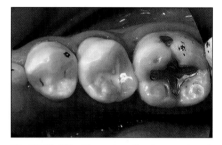

Fig 10-5f After the restoration is completed, a sealant is placed in the fissures.

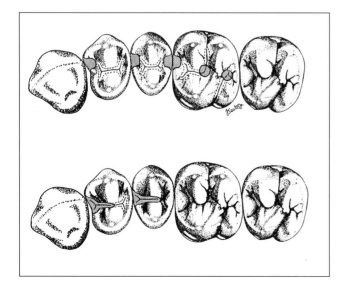

Fig 10-6 Outline of various Class 2 resin composite restorations. Access is limited to that required for removal of carious tooth structure and/or previous restoration(s), so outline form will vary based on the extent of carious lesions. Occlusal pits and fissures that are not carious may be treated with sealants. Deeply stained or demineralized fissures may be opened with a small bur (0.3- or 0.4-mm diameter) or air abrasion prior to sealing. (Dashed outlines indicate sealant; dotted areas indicate composite.)

treated with sealants to enhance caries prevention[43] (Figs 10-5e and 10-5f). Figure 10-6 shows some examples of outline form of posterior resin composite restorations; each is designed to treat the pathosis presented, and none has a "standard" shape.

Adhesion to Tooth Structure

The clinical success of bonded resin composite restorations is well documented.[14,18,34,57] The bond between resin composite and tooth structure achieved with bonding systems offers the potential to seal the margins of the restoration[58] and reinforce remaining tooth structure against fracture.[7,59] It has also been suggested that less cuspal flexure occurs with bonded resin composite restorations under subcatastrophic occlusal loads, providing protection against the propagation of cracks that can ultimately lead to fatigue failure.[60] However, not all studies have found that teeth with bonded restorations have an increased resistance to fracture.[60,61] The longevity of the bond is shortened by increased occlusal forces.[62] A recent study of nearly 11,000 posterior teeth found the prevalence of cusp fracture in posterior resin composite restorations to be no lower than in amalgam restorations.[63] This supports the fact that bonded posterior restorations cannot be relied upon to provide long-term reinforcement of tooth structure.

Low Thermal Conductivity

Because resin composites do not readily transmit temperature changes, there is an insulating effect may help to reduce postoperative temperature sensitivity.[7]

Elimination of Galvanic Currents

Resin composite does not contain metal and so will not initiate or conduct galvanic currents.[43]

Radiopacity

Radiopaque restorative materials are necessary to allow the practitioner to evaluate the contours and marginal adaptation of the restoration as well as to distinguish among the restoration, caries lesions, and sound tooth structure.[64,65] Studies have shown that the detection of voids and recurrent caries lesions adjacent to restorations is enhanced when the radiopacity of the restorative material is equal to, or slightly greater than, the radiopacity of enamel.[66–68]

Most, although not all, modern resin composites have a radiopacity in excess of that of enamel.[65,69,70] In order for manufacturers to claim that a material is radiopaque, the American Dental Association requires them to demonstrate that a composite has a radiopacity greater than that of an equal thickness of aluminum, which has a radiopacity approximately equal to dentin.[71]

Alternative to Amalgam

Amalgam, despite having a long track record of clinical success,[72–74] has declined in use as a restorative material primarily because of its unesthetic appearance, but also because of its mercury content. Concerns about mercury in amalgam are more psychological than scientific, as evidenced by a recent comprehensive literature review of 950 scientific and medical studies that found no correlation between dental amalgam and health problems.[75] Despite this, there is an increasing desire to find mercury-free alternatives to dental amalgam.[76] Patients are aware of indictments against amalgam, and some express concern about potential health hazards.[77] Amalgam is also less attractive to dental professionals as government agencies consider classifying it as hazardous waste[78] and requiring that dental offices install expensive systems to remove mercury from wastewater.[76,79] As a result, resin composite use in posterior restorations continues to gain popularity in the profession.[76]

Disadvantages of Resin Composite as a Posterior Restorative Material

Polymerization Shrinkage

Despite improvements in resin composite formulations over the years, modern systems are still based on variations of the bis-GMA molecule, which has been used for more than 30 years.[80] One of the major drawbacks of this material is the polymerization shrinkage that occurs during the setting reaction. Modern resin composites undergo volumetric polymerization shrinkage of 2.6% to 7.1%.[81]

Most of the problems associated with posterior resin composite restorations can be related directly or indirectly to polymerization shrinkage. During polymerization, resin composite may pull away from the least retentive cavity margins (usually those with little or no enamel on them), resulting in gap formation.[82–84] Tensile forces developed in enamel margins can result in marginal degradation from mastication.[85] Contraction forces on cusps can result in cuspal deformation,[86] enamel cracks and crazes[87] (Figs 10-7a and 10-7b), and, ultimately, decreased fracture resistance of the cusps.[88]

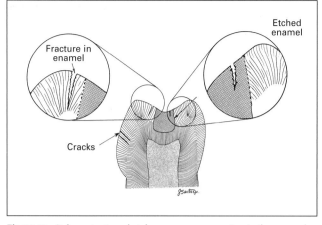

Fig 10-7a Polymerization shrinkage can cause crazing in the enamel or fractures within the resin composite.

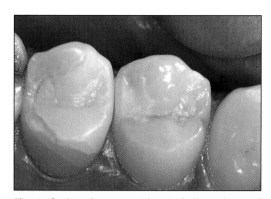

Fig 10-7b Craze lines are evident in the lingual cusp of the maxillary right second premolar bonded to a very large Class 2 resin composite restoration.

Polymerization shrinkage occurs regardless of the system used to initiate the setting reaction. For many years, it was believed that autocured resin composite polymerizes toward the center of the mass of the resin composite, while VLC resin composite polymerizes toward the light source.[9,84] Recent research has provided evidence that polymerization shrinkage occurs toward the walls of cavity preparations to which it is bonded most strongly, regardless of the initiator mode.[89,90]

A number of techniques have been suggested to decrease the adverse effects of polymerization shrinkage. The most commonly used technique is incremental placement of VLC resin composite, which decreases the effect of setting contraction by reducing the bulk of resin composite cured at a time.[84] In addition, incremental insertion reduces the ratio of bonded to unbonded surface area, which helps to relieve the stress developed at the bond between tooth and resin composite.[91] The incremental placement technique is discussed later in this chapter.

Beta-quartz inserts, which can be incorporated into the resin composite during insertion, have been developed to reduce the bulk of composite material and resultant polymerization shrinkage.[92] While little clinical evidence is available, in vitro studies have shown that inserts have not reduced cuspal strain[93] or marginal leakage.[94,95] One clinical trial showed relatively poor performance, with a 59% survival rate after 3 years.[96]

Autocured resin composites are sometimes recommended for posterior restorations because an autocured composite tends to induce less polymerization stress than does a comparable bulk of VLC composite. This is due in part to greater porosity being incorporated into the autocured resin compos-ite as a result of mixing. The incorporated oxygen inhibits the set of resin immediately adjacent to the voids and decreases the ratio of bonded to unbonded surface area.[97] The voids increase the free surface area for stress compensation by flow of the resin during the setting reaction.[98] In addition, because of a slower polymerization rate, autocured resin composites develop shrinkage stresses more slowly than do VLC materials. This allows for increased restorative-material flow during polymerization.[81,99] However, a number of problems associated with the use of autocured resin composite in posterior restorations argue against its use. These problems are discussed in subsequent sections.

Decreasing the rate of polymerization of VLC resin composite can be accomplished by varying the curing-light intensity. This has resulted in a form of curing for VLC resin composites variously referred to as *two-step* or *soft-start* polymerization. Some studies have shown that by reducing the initial irradiance to approximately 150 mW/cm^2, followed by high-level irradiance (650 mW/cm^2 or greater), the curing reaction is slowed, marginal integrity is enhanced, and physical properties are not adversely affected.[100–104] However, results with these reduced-irradiance curing regimens have been equivocal,[105] and it is difficult to assess whether or not the laboratory results will have any clinical impact. Recent research has demonstrated that a truly significant decrease in polymerization shrinkage stress may require clinically impractical curing regimens.[105]

The best hope for overcoming the problems of polymerization shrinkage lies in the future development of tooth-colored materials that do not contract during setting, an area of vigorous research.[106–108]

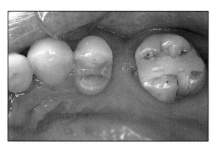

Fig 10-8a In these posterior resin composite restorations, the dark shadowing adjacent to the occlusal margins was caused by recurrent caries lesions.

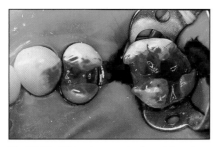

Fig 10-8b After placement of a rubber dam, the resin composite restorations are removed and caries-detecting solution is placed.

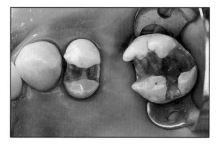

Fig 10-8c Stained areas confirm the presence of demineralized tooth structure.

Secondary Caries Lesions

Several clinical studies and reviews of clinical studies have demonstrated that secondary caries is a significant cause of failure of posterior resin composite restorations.[23,31,37,38,109–111] It is believed that the marginal gap formed at the gingival margin as a result of polymerization shrinkage allows the ingress of cariogenic bacteria[31] (Figs 10-8a to 10-8c). Because marginal degradation has been demonstrated to increase with time,[29,38,112,113] the risk of secondary caries also increases with time.

Studies have shown that levels of mutans streptococcus, the organism linked most closely to the production of dental caries lesions,[114] are significantly higher in the plaque adjacent to proximal surfaces of posterior resin composite restorations than in plaque adjacent to either amalgam or glass-ionomer restorations. A retrospective study by Qvist et al[109] revealed that less secondary caries occurred in all classes of amalgam restorations combined than in resin composite restorations. In addition, the organic acids of plaque have been found to soften bis-GMA polymers, and this in turn could have an adverse effect on wear and surface staining.[115] These facts emphasize the need for regular recall and close follow-up of patients with posterior resin composite restorations.

Postoperative Sensitivity

Postoperative sensitivity has been associated with the placement of posterior resin composite restorations. One clinical study noted that 29% of teeth exhibited sensitivity following placement of the restorations.[10] Reports of postoperative sensitivity have diminished somewhat with improvements in dentin adhesives.[110,116,117] However, studies continue to report postoperative sensitivity following the placement of even small posterior resin composite restorations.[55,116]

A number of reasons have been postulated for the occurrence of postoperative sensitivity, but the most commonly accepted theories relate to polymerization shrinkage. As previously discussed, polymerization shrinkage results in formation of a gap, which allows bacterial penetration and fluid flow within it. The bacteria or their noxious products may enter the dentinal tubules and cause pulpal inflammation and tooth sensitivity.[118] Gap formation also allows a slow, continuous outflow of dentinal fluid from the pulp through the tubules to the gap. Cold or other stimuli may cause a contraction of fluid in the gap, leading to a sudden, rapid outflow of tubular fluid that the pulp interprets as pain.[119]

Contraction forces of polymerization shrinkage may also result in cuspal deformation, with resultant cracking and crazing of remaining tooth structure (see Fig 10-7b), which can cause tooth sensitivity.[82] Flexure of resin composite under an occlusal load may cause hydraulic pressure in the tubular fluid to be transmitted to the odontoblastic processes, another possible cause of tooth sensitivity.[82,119]

Postoperative sensitivity can be a disturbing sequela for both patient and dentist. Obviously the discomfort associated with restoration placement is unpleasant for the patient. Likewise, it is often frustrating for the dentist to try to determine the cause and eliminate postoperative sensitivity. This frustration is increased with the awareness that patients who experience postoperative sensitivity within 1 month of posterior resin composite restoration placement are about twice as likely to have that restoration fail within 5 years as those who do not experience postoperative sensitivity. This risk increases as the size of the restoration increases.[11] Awareness of the potential for postoperative sensitivity allows the practitioner to forewarn the patient of this possibility. Careful adherence to the guidelines for case selection and restoration placement, including the rebonding procedure described later in this chapter, will help to reduce this problem.

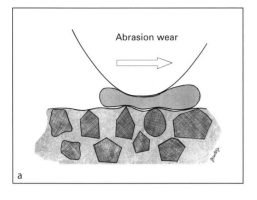

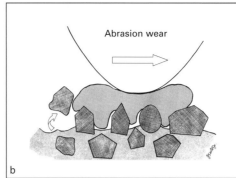

Fig 10-9 Abrasion wear occurs across the entire occlusal surface of the resin composite. *(a)* The softer resin is preferentially worn away, exposing the harder filler particles. *(b)* Eventually, enough of the filler particle is exposed so that it is "plucked" from the surface of the resin composite.

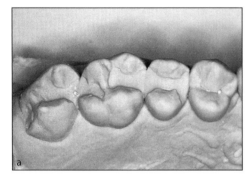

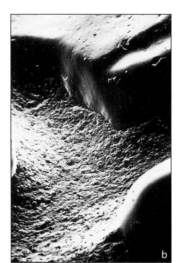

Fig 10-10 *(a)* Abrasion wear has traditionally been a problem with posterior resin composite restorations. A cast reveals generalized wear of the posterior resin composite restorations in the maxillary right first and second molars and second premolar. In addition, proximal wear has resulted in broad, flat contacts and loss of arch length. The material used was an early, larger-particle resin composite. *(b)* Scanning electron photomicrograph of a posterior tooth that, several years previously, had been restored with an early-generation (large-filler-particle) resin composite. Note the severe loss of restorative material.

Decreased Wear Resistance

The wear resistance of posterior resin composite restorations has been the subject of considerable attention. This characteristic has long been a concern for restoration longevity,[44,120] although it has improved as refinements in materials have occurred.[117] In reports of recent clinical studies, it has been noted that no posterior resin composite restorations were replaced as a result of excessive wear after 7 years[121] or 8 years,[23] and only one was replaced as a result of excessive wear in a 10-year study.[35]

Resin composite wear results from the combination of chemical damage to the surface of the material and mechanical breakdown.[122–125] Resin composites undergo wear by two different mechanisms. *Abrasion* is generalized wear that occurs across the entire occlusal surface of the resin composite as a result of the abrasive action of particles during mastication (Fig 10-9). This type of wear occurs in all areas of the restoration (Fig 10-10). *Attrition* is the loss of material that occurs as a result of direct contact with opposing tooth surfaces in the

occlusal contact areas of the restoration (Fig 10-11).[126] Generally, wear can be related to either material or clinical factors.

Material factors relate primarily to the resin composite's filler-particle content, size, and distribution.[127] Clinical studies have shown less heavily filled composites (less than 60% filled by volume) to exhibit unacceptable wear.[44,120] Because of their generally lower filler content (30% to 50%), microfilled composites are more subject to attrition[85] and marginal breakdown,[23,112,113,128] especially adjacent to occlusal contact areas.[85] However, they are more resistant to abrasion because of their smoother surfaces, decreased interparticle spacing, and lowered coefficient of friction.[129] The more heavily filled hybrid resin composites are more resistant to attrition than are the microfilled materials.[50,128] However, resin composites that have a larger mean particle size (greater than 3 µm) tend to have significantly higher abrasion wear.[44,49,50,108,120] This is due to the loss of the larger filler particles, leading to three-body wear and increased stress transfer from the filler particles to the resin matrix, which results in formation of cracks during mastication.[21,120]

Fig 10-11 Attrition wear occurs in occlusal contact areas. *(a)* Cracks occur in the resin matrix as a result of occlusal stress. *(b)* Eventually the cracks coalesce and result in loss of resin composite material from the surface.

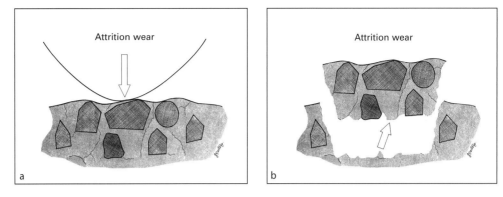

The rate of wear varies with particle size as well. As mean filler particle size decreases (below 1 μm), the wear rate tends to be linear with time. Conversely, composites with increased mean filler particle size tend to have more rapid wear initially but slower wear with time.[108,112,113,130,131]

Clinically relevant wear factors include the size of the restoration, its location in the arch, the occlusal load it must withstand, and how well the resin composite is cured. As the surface area and length of cavosurface margins increase, so does the exposure to occlusal forces, with a resultant increase in wear.[29,30,32,49,50] The more posterior a tooth, the greater the masticatory forces and the more rapid the wear of the restoration.[29,30,38,117,132] Fracture resistance decreases as a result of fatigue from chewing,[133] and increased chewing pressure will result in increased wear.[134] Finally, if the clinician does not properly cure the composite material, the degree of conversion of the composite will suffer and wear will increase.[128]

Proximal surfaces are subjected to the forces of abrasion during function as well, due to individual tooth movement during mastication that causes wear in the interproximal contact areas. Proximal surface wear of posterior resin composite restorations was found to be significantly greater than that of enamel proximal surfaces[29,38,135,136] (see Fig 10-10a). One study found proximal wear rates to be higher than occlusal wear rates in resin composite restorations,[137] possibly due to increased contact time between contacting surfaces, differences in cure, or different environments. However, recent studies do not indicate that proximal surface wear due to interproximal contact is a problem with current resin composites.[121,138,139]

Clinical studies show that resin composite formulations have acceptable wear characteristics for up to 17 years.[18,35,117] In fact, some studies have indicated that posterior resin composite restorations resist wear as well as amalgam restorations.[32,35,124] However, other studies report that resin composites have significantly higher wear rates than amalgam,[12,23,31,50,126,140] and no resin composite has been shown to exhibit less wear than amalgam.

Other Mechanical Properties

Generally, the more closely the mechanical properties of a restorative material simulate those of enamel and dentin, the better the restoration's longevity.[3,108,141] A number of the mechanical properties of resin composite are inferior to those of tooth structure and of other restorative materials. These inferior properties can have an adverse effect on the durability of the restoration.

Resin composite materials have low fracture toughness in comparison to metallic restorative materials.[31,83] Indeed, bulk fracture of posterior resin composite restorations has been noted as a significant cause of failure in many clinical studies.[23,28,33,111,117] Increased filler loading of resin composite leads to improved fracture toughness.[123,133] Research in altering resin composite formulations to increase fracture toughness is ongoing.[141]

Resin composite has a relatively high degree of elastic deformation (ie, a low modulus of elasticity) of six to eight times that of amalgam.[119] Failures of resin composite restorations associated with the high elastic deformation of the material have included bulk fracture,[83] microcrack formation,[123] and relatively low resistance to occlusal loading.[10] As with fracture resistance, more highly filled composites exhibit less elastic deformation than their less-filled counterparts.[108]

The coefficient of thermal expansion of resin composite is another property that differs significantly from that of tooth structure.[143,144] Because the coefficient of thermal expansion of resin composite is higher than that of tooth structure, composite tends to expand and contract more than enamel and dentin when subjected to variations in temperature. This can increase marginal gap formation and exacerbate the effects of polymerization shrinkage on cuspal deformation, and it may result in the fracture of composite or enamel.[83,141] It has been demonstrated that as the mismatch in thermal-expansion properties between restorative material and the tooth structure increases, so does marginal leakage.[145] As the filler con-

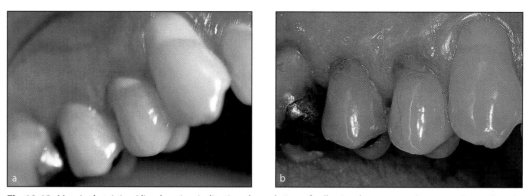

Fig 10-12 Marginal staining/discoloration indicating degradation of adhesion between resin composite and cavity preparation that occurs with aging. *(a)* Facial Class 5 resin composite restorations in the maxillary right first and second premolar. *(b)* The same restorations 3 years later. Discoloration is evident, particularly at the gingival (dentin) margins of the restorations.

tent of resin composite increases, however, the mismatch decreases.[143]

Water Sorption

Water sorption is another factor influencing the clinical performance of resin composites. Water is absorbed preferentially into the resin component of resin composite materials, and water content is therefore increased when resin content is increased.[80,83] Because of the swelling of the resin matrix from water sorption, the filler particle bond to resin is weakened. If the stress is greater than the bond strength, the resulting debond is referred to as *hydrolytic breakdown*.[83,146] Incompletely cured resin composite will exhibit more water sorption and greater hydrolytic degradation.[147]

It has been suggested that the swelling of resin composite caused by water sorption can be beneficial due to closing of the marginal gap caused by polymerization shrinkage. However, studies have shown that the swelling from moisture absorption usually is not enough to overcome the polymerization shrinkage gap.[85] Even if water sorption did result in a closed marginal gap, it would only provide a close adaptation, without adhesion between the resin composite and tooth structure.[148]

Variable Degree of Conversion

Analysis of the amount of cross-linking in polymerization, or degree of conversion, of resin composites reveals that certain characteristics of this material are at odds with one another. As the degree of conversion of a resin composite material increases, the mechanical properties improve.[80,97,129] Clinical research has clearly demonstrated that a reduced degree of

conversion causes significantly increased wear.[128] However, polymerization shrinkage also increases with more cross-linking.[149] Resins with decreased filler content exhibit decreased viscosity and improved diffusion of reactive groups during the polymerization reaction and, thereby, improved cure.[150] However, a decreased filler content also results in inferior mechanical properties[108,123,133,143] and poorer clinical performance.[10,50,85,112,113] Achieving the best balance among these factors is a challenge for both manufacturers and clinicians.

VLC composites have been shown to achieve a somewhat higher degree of conversion than autocured materials.[150,151] Several factors influence the extent of polymerization of VLC composites. Lighter shades cure more easily and in less time than darker shades.[9] Resin composites with larger filler particles tend to transmit light throughout the material more effectively than those with smaller filler particles.[152] The longer the composite is subjected to the curing light, the more effective the cure,[153] but the thickness of each increment should be limited to 2.0 mm.[9] The degree of conversion is inversely related to the distance of the light tip from the resin composite,[153] and tip distances greater than 6 mm from the surface of the increment can significantly decrease resin composite cure.[154] The condition of the curing unit can, of course, also impact the effectiveness of the cure.[39]

Inconsistent Dentin Adhesion (Marginal Leakage)

Polymerization shrinkage causes the resin composite to pull away from cavity margins, resulting in gap formation.[82–84] Despite advances in dentin adhesive systems, they still do not consistently and reliably achieve bond strengths to dentin and cementum that are high enough to prevent this occurrence (Fig 10-12; see also Fig 12-13).[155–157] This sometimes results in open margins, sensitivity, interfacial staining, and bacterial invasion.[158] In addition, the bond between adhesive and tooth structure has been shown to degrade with aging, both in vitro[159] and in vivo.[160–162]

Technique Sensitivity

Because of the negative aspects of using resin composite as a posterior restorative material described previously, one of the most important variables in clinical success is the placement technique.[44] There is little room for error.[16] Application technique has been shown to significantly affect adhesive bond strength.[163] Technique may also account for the great variability reported in clinical success rates for posterior resin composite restorations.[31] The meticulous operative procedures demanded for placing these restorations require increased chair time. Clinical research has shown that posterior resin composite restorations require significantly more time to place than do comparable amalgam restorations.[35]

Indications for Resin Composite as a Posterior Restorative Material

Results of clinical studies demonstrate that resin composite can serve adequately when used in posterior restorations. However, resin composite restorations placed in occlusal surfaces of molars fare worse than those in premolars; Class 2 restorations fare worse than Class 1 restorations; restorations subjected to high masticatory forces fare worse than those subjected to lesser forces; and large restorations fare worse than small to moderate-sized restorations.[36,111] Therefore, limiting the size of the outline form and ensuring that the occlusal forces are absorbed by tooth structure are important to the clinical success of these restorations.[30,32,164] Based on these facts and the previous discussion, several factors should be considered before a posterior resin composite restoration is recommended to a patient. The following circumstances would be considered *ideal* for using resin composite in a posterior restoration:

1. The patient should not be allergic or sensitive to resin-based materials.
2. The patient should exhibit acceptable oral hygiene. Secondary caries is a significant cause of posterior composite failure.[34,165]

3. Centric occlusal stops should be located primarily on tooth structure. Maintaining occlusal stops on enamel has been shown to promote low posterior resin composite wear.[56]
4. The patient should not exhibit excessive wear from clenching or grinding.[16] Posterior resin composite restorations have improved longevity when subjected to lower functional and nonfunctional stresses.[36]
5. The tooth should be amenable to rubber dam isolation.[16] Margins of Class 2 resin composite restorations placed without a rubber dam showed marginal leakage 4 to 6 weeks after placement.[166]
6. Esthetics should be a prime consideration.[46] Composites do not exhibit the same durability in posterior teeth as do other, less esthetic restorative materials such as amalgam and gold.[15,42]
7. The faciolingual width of the cavity preparation should be restricted to no more than one third of the intercuspal distance to reduce occlusal forces and wear.[16,30]
8. All cavosurface margins should be on enamel. Of particular importance is that the gingival cavosurface margin in Class 2 restorations should be located on intact enamel.[167,168] The bond of adhesives to dentin degrades with time,[162] placing an external cavosurface margin on dentin at increased risk for recurrent caries.

It should be emphasized that the above list contains ideal circumstances. A similar list could be constructed for the use of another restorative material. As more clinical research results of the performance of resin composites in posterior teeth are reported, particularly results from long-term studies, it becomes evident that current resin composites and bonding systems may be considered acceptable in less ideal situations.

Although it is ideal that the faciolingual width of a resin composite restoration be less than one third the intercuspal distance, a number of clinical trials have included restorations with faciolingual widths between one half and two thirds the intercuspal distance that have shown acceptable performance.[14,18,34–36] These restorations, with up to 17 years of service, showed annual failure rates between 0.7% and 3.1%, which is within the range demonstrated in Tables 10-3 and 10-4 and Figs 10-1 and 10-2.

Indeed, the remaining tooth structure should be judged to be self-supporting, ie, not relying on the bond of the restoration to weak, free-standing tooth structure to prevent its fracture. As has been stated previously, natural cusps bonded to resin composite restorations fracture at a rate similar to cusps adjacent to unbonded amalgam restorations.[63] The clear implication is that bonded resin composite restorations cannot be relied upon to provide long-term reinforcement of weakened tooth structure (Fig 10-13).

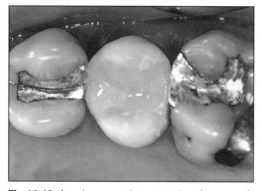

Fig 10-13 A resin composite restoration that exceeds one third of the intercuspal distance. This exposes more of the restoration to wear and fracture. Remaining tooth structure should be self-supporting.

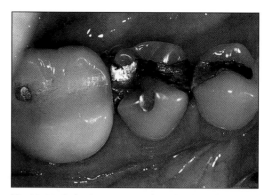

Fig 10-14 Defective mesio-occlusodistal amalgam restoration in the mandibular second premolar. Excessive width and need for cusp replacement precludes this amalgam restoration from being replaced with resin composite. A discolored fracture line and recurrent caries running from the MOD amalgam to the amalgam in the facial cusp tip would necessitate cuspal coverage with the replacement restoration.

Also, in regard to resin composite restorations with margins in thin enamel near the cementoenamel junction or on cementum or dentin, the use of a *bonded-base* or *open sandwich technique* has been shown to provide acceptable clinical performance,[169–172] providing significant protection of the tooth structure near the gingival margin against demineralization.[169] In the open sandwich technique, a restorative resin-modified glass ionomer (RMGI) is used in the portion of the restoration near the gingival margin. In a Class 2 restoration, that would be the gingival increment or material placed in the proximal box. When using this technique, however, it is important that the patient be at low risk of developing caries lesions. A clinical trial evaluating the use of this technique found that 67% of recurrent caries lesions adjacent to the RMGI portion of an open sandwich restoration occurred in subjects with poor oral hygiene.[171] For a description of the bonded-base technique, see the section on Class 2 resin composite restorations in this chapter.

Replacing cusps, particularly functional cusps, with resin composite is not supported by clinical research and therefore cannot be recommended at this time (Fig 10-14). Clinical studies have not yet been accomplished to establish that it is appropriate to use resin composite in cuspal-coverage restorations.[173,174]

Informed Consent

It is incumbent upon the dentist to provide the patient with appropriate information regarding the restorative procedures being recommended. This should include a description of the proposed procedures in lay language, any risks associated with the procedures, and other options the patient may wish to consider. In addition, the patient should be provided the opportunity to have his or her questions answered. This is sometimes referred to as the *PARQ process* (Procedures, Alternatives, Risks, Questions). Dlugokinski and Browning[175] surveyed dentists and patients regarding their respective attitudes and preferences toward informed consent. The survey focused on offering patients the alternatives of resin composite vs amalgam for direct-placement posterior restorations. Sixty percent of the dentists surveyed were aware of resin composite's shortcomings as a posterior restorative material when compared with amalgam. Despite this, these dentists believed that their materials and techniques would yield equivalent results. The survey also revealed that as a dentist performed more resin composite restorations compared to the number of amalgam restorations performed, the dentist was less likely to discuss the adverse aspects of resin composite.[175]

Conversely, the survey revealed some intriguing insights from the patient's perspective[175]:

- 100% of patients wanted the dentist to tell them about all aspects of alternative restorative materials.
- 75% of patients preferred a written explanation rather than simply an oral explanation.
- 82% of patients would *not* choose a posterior resin composite restoration to replace an adequate amalgam restoration.

• Patients were equivocal over cost as a factor for selecting amalgam vs resin composite; 43% would still choose a resin composite restoration even if it cost 50% more than an amalgam restoration and would not last as long (vs 36% preferring amalgam).

The results clearly show that patients do not want the dentist alone to decide which restoration will be placed. While most patients desire the dentist's recommendation, the ultimate decision is theirs, and they want to be fully informed to make the best choice for their particular situation. Most patients want information in writing. Several commercial companies and the American Dental Association (ADA) offer pamphlets that explain the indications, advantages, and disadvantages of various restorative materials. The ADA also provides a document with information on various restorative materials that can be downloaded at no charge.[176]

Autocured vs Light-Cured Resin Composites

Autocured resin composite restorative materials largely disappeared from clinical practice in the 1980s because of the popularity of the light-cured materials. Some clinicians have recommended the use of autocured resin composites, either alone or in combination with VLC resin composites, for posterior applications.[177–179] The primary advantage of an autocured material is that it can be placed in bulk, saving time compared to the incremental insertion technique used with VLC materials.

Although more time-consuming, use of VLC resin composites has a number of advantages over use of autocured resin composites. VLC composites achieve more complete polymerization,[151] resulting in superior mechanical properties,[80,87,154] and they exhibit better color stability.[180] Autocured composites tend to incorporate voids as a result of mixing two-paste systems,[98] and the increased porosity decreases tensile strength and surface smoothness,[181] accelerating wear.[182] Mixing interrupts the polymerization process and may compromise the size and configuration of the final polymer molecules, resulting in reduced strength and wear resistance.[183]

VLC composites should be used with an incremental placement technique to reduce polymerization shrinkage stress and achieve optimal polymerization in the final restoration.[184] This technique allows the practitioner to build up and

sculpt the restoration. Research has shown VLC composite increments to have adequate interfacial strength.[185] Perhaps most importantly, VLC resin composites performed better in clinical trials than autocured materials over 1 year[50] and 3 years.[135]

Direct Posterior Resin Composite Restorations

Preoperative Evaluation

The factors noted in the above list as indications should be considered in the preoperative evaluation. The occlusion should be marked with articulating paper as a guide to preparation design. It is helpful to apply copal varnish to the teeth prior to marking the occlusion with articulating paper. A thin layer of copal varnish helps the transfer of marks from the articulating paper to the teeth and also helps to retain the marks on the teeth throughout the operative procedure. The best type of resin composite for the restoration should be chosen. At present, the heavily filled hybrid composites are considered best suited for posterior use.[15,108,111]

For many posterior resin composite restorations, shade selection is not critical. In fact, some clinicians prefer a deliberate shade mismatch to aid in subsequent finishing and future evaluation procedures. But when shade is important, shade selection should be performed before isolation of the tooth, because isolated teeth become dehydrated and dehydration changes the shade of the enamel. A shade is chosen from the shade guide that accompanies the composite, and then a small portion of the composite is placed on the unprepared and unetched tooth and polymerized (Fig 10-15). The resin "test shade" can easily be removed because the tooth surface has not been etched or primed prior to its placement.

If the dentist is going to use a warm-composite placement technique, an appropriate amount of resin composite may be transferred to a syringe tip (Centrix) that is amber-colored or opaque to prevent premature polymerization. The Centrix syringe tip is then placed in a composite warming tray (Fig 10-16). Alternatively, the syringe tip may be placed in a sealed plastic bag (eg, a resealable sandwich bag) and placed in a warm water bath (60° to 68°C; 140° to 155°F). This will reduce the resin composite's viscosity and aid in subsequent placement. The rationale for this technique is discussed in the section on Class 2 resin composite restorations later in this chapter.

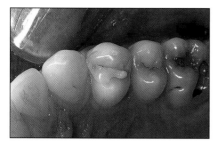

Fig 10-15 A small amount of resin composite is placed on the unprepared tooth to verify the shade prior to isolation with a rubber dam.

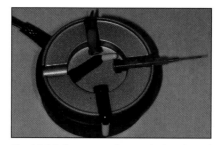

Fig 10-16 An appropriate resin is selected and placed into a light-protected syringe tip, and the protected syringe tip is put into a warmer (60° to 68°C; 140° to 155°F) to reduce viscosity.

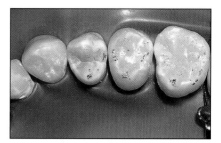

Fig 10-17 The occlusion is marked and rubber dam isolation achieved. The rubber dam has been inverted around the teeth to ensure moisture control.

Isolation

Securing and maintaining control of the operative field is essential to the success of the restoration. One clinical study has demonstrated no difference in the performance of posterior resin composite restorations whether or not a rubber dam was used during restoration placement.[186] However, in another clinical study, the margins of all Class 2 resin composite restorations placed without a rubber dam demonstrated marginal leakage 4 to 6 weeks after placement.[166] With the advent of adhesive systems that use more hydrophilic components, research has shown that contamination with moisture or saliva affects some adhesives but not others.[187–189] Blood contamination will adversely affect adhesion in all bonding systems.[188,189] In the authors' opinion, the most reliable method to accomplish field isolation is the placement of a rubber dam. The rubber dam prevents moisture contamination and protects gingival tissues from laceration (Fig 10-17).[166]

Sealants and Preventive Resin Restorations

Sealants

While not normally considered to be posterior resin composite restorations, fissure sealants have been in use as a preventive restorative procedure for several decades. Sealants provide an effective means of reducing the incidence of caries lesions in fissures. Compared to teeth with unsealed fissures, teeth with sealed fissures have demonstrated a 35% reduction in fissure-caries lesions during a 5-year period;[190] a 43%

reduction over 4 years;[191] and a 55% reduction over 7 years.[192] However, there are a number of factors that must be considered regarding fissure sealant effectiveness. Numerous clinical studies have demonstrated that sealants tend to fail at a rate of 5% to 10% per year.[40,193–196] This is significant because the caries rate for teeth in which sealants are partially or totally lost increases significantly, in many cases equaling the caries rate of unsealed teeth.[190–192,194,195] The key to sealant success in preventing caries lesions is total retention of the sealant.[190,192,195] Enhancing complete sealant retention will therefore enhance the caries reduction benefit. Some factors that affect sealant retention and effectiveness include the following:

1. Mandibular teeth show higher retention rates than maxillary teeth; premolars show higher retention rates than molars.[194,197]
2. Annual recall of patients and repair of partially or totally lost sealants improves effectiveness.[40,194,196]
3. Use of bonding agents prior to sealant placement helps to wet fissures,[198] improve sealant penetration into fissures,[199] increase bond strength,[200,201] improve sealant adhesion to saliva-contaminated enamel,[200–202] and improve clinical retention of sealants.[203–205]
4. Slight mechanical preparation of fissures with a very small bur (0.3- to 0.4-mm diameter, rounded tip) or air abrasion to provide sound, unstained enamel prior to etchant placement enhances sealant penetration and attachment, decreases bubble formation, improves marginal adaptation,[206,207] decreases marginal leakage,[208] improves microbial elimination,[209] and increases clinical retention compared to unprepared fissures.[207]

5. Clinical studies of RMGI sealants show good caries prevention but very poor mechanical retention compared to resin sealants. However, these studies are of very short duration, and the long-term effectiveness of RMGIs used as sealants remains unknown.[210,211]

6. Flowable resin composite materials have been shown to perform well as fissure sealants. One short-term clinical study demonstrated comparable performance of a flowable resin composite and a sealant,[212] while another showed improved performance of a flowable resin composite material when compared to a traditional resin sealant.[213]

7. The level of caries activity is critical to the cost-effectiveness of sealants; if a patient exhibits a low caries index, then the value of this procedure is low.[214] Clinical parameters including occlusal fissure morphology; number of decayed, missing, or filled surfaces (DMFS); and the clinician's subjective judgment are all significant predictors of future occlusal caries activity.[215,216] Therefore, sealant use should be based on a determination of the patient's disease level and his or her potential for future fissure-caries lesions; sealants should not be placed universally.

Preventive Resin Restorations

A restoration that maximizes the benefits of conservative, adhesive dentistry is the *preventive resin restoration* (PRR). Suggested by Ulvestad[217] in 1975 and popularized by Simonsen[218,219] and Simonsen and Stallard,[220] the PRR was developed to overcome problems associated with traditional "extension for prevention" in restorations necessitated by minimal occlusal caries lesions.

The PRR limits preparation to pits and fissures that are carious. Once the lesion is eliminated, no further preparation is performed. If the resultant preparation is restricted to a narrow and shallow opening of the fissure, a resin sealant (or flowable resin composite material) is placed. If additional tooth structure is removed, a posterior resin composite is placed in that area, and the remaining fissures and the surface of the resin composite restoration(s) are sealed with resin sealant material or flowable composite. A number of advantages have been ascribed to this technique, including the following:

1. Conservation of tooth structure: One 5-year clinical study determined that the average occlusal amalgam occupied 25% of the occlusal surface compared to just 5% for an average PRR.[221]

2. Enhanced esthetics: This is provided by the tooth-colored restorative material.[222]

3. Improved seal of restorative material to tooth structure: This is through the bond of resin composite to etched enamel with an adhesive resin.[223]

4. Minimal wear: This is due to restricted cavity-preparation size, so that occlusal contacts on the restoration are limited.[224]

5. No progression of sealed caries lesions: If a caries lesion is inadvertently allowed to remain in or at the base of a sealed fissure, it will not progress, because the seal prevents nutrients from supplying cariogenic bacteria.[225]

6. Good longevity: Clinical studies have demonstrated that PRRs are successful for periods of up to 10 years[222–226] and can equal[221] or exceed the performance of amalgam restorations.[225]

The same provisos concerning sealants must be applied to PRRs; that is, the sealants placed in association with PRRs will tend to be lost at a rate of 5% to 10% per year.[222,224,226] Therefore, these restorations must be monitored over time, and the sealants and/or restorations must be repaired or replaced as needed.[222]

Indications and Contraindications

A PRR is indicated when some areas of the fissure system of a tooth are associated with carious dentin and others are not. The extent of the anticipated restoration should be such that occlusal forces will be primarily limited to tooth structure.

Technique

The preoperative evaluation, marking of occlusion, shade selection, and rubber dam isolation should be accomplished first (Fig 10-18a). After the resin composite is selected, it may be used directly from a unit-dose ampule; if it is in a syringe, it should be placed into a light-protected syringe tip (see Fig 10-16). If desired, the viscosity of the resin composite may be further reduced by heating in a water bath or composite warming tray to enhance adaptation to the cavity preparation as described in the section on Class 2 restorations.

The conservative adhesive preparation eliminates demineralized dentin, overlying unsupported enamel, and associated demineralized enamel. The preparation should be initiated with the smallest instrument that will accomplish this limited preparation, such as a No. 1⁄16, 1⁄8, or 1⁄4 round bur (Figs 10-18b and 10-18c), fissurotomy bur (Fig 10-18d), or air abrasion (see Fig 11-4). Larger instrumentation is used only as the size of the caries lesion dictates. Any fragile or unsupported enamel remaining on the occlusal surface after removal of the demineralized dentin should be removed. No bevels should be placed on the occlusal margins of the preparation.

Typically, these restorations are limited in size and depth, so no pulpal protection is needed (Fig 10-18e), but a PRR is

Fig 10-18 Technique for placing preventive resin restorations.

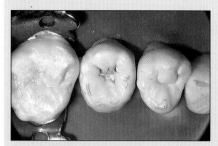

Fig 10-18a The occlusal surfaces of the maxillary first and second premolars exhibit demineralization of deep occlusal fissures. The rubber dam has been placed and inverted. The occlusion was marked prior to rubber dam placement.

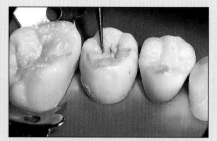

Fig 10-18b Preparation is initiated with a small (No. ¹/₈) round bur in a high-speed handpiece.

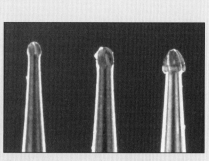

Fig 10-18c ¹/₁₆, ¹/₈, and ¹/₄ round burs (0.3, 0.4, and 0.5 mm in diameter, respectively) work well to open occlusal fissures.

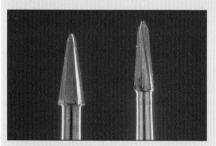

Fig 10-18d Alternatively, fissurotomy burs (SS White; designed by Dr Dan Boston, Temple University) can be used to open occlusal fissures.

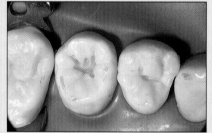

Fig 10-18e Completed preparations, which were limited to access for removal of carious tooth structure. The preparation of the first premolar was limited and mostly confined to fissure enameloplasty. Penetration to dentin was minimal in the second premolar, occurring in only limited locations.

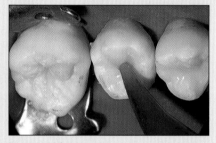

Fig 10-18f Restorative resin composite is syringed into the deeper (greater than 0.5 mm) areas of the preparation.

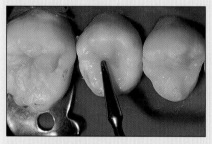

Fig 10-18g A hand instrument, such as the PKT3 shown, is used to develop occlusal anatomy in the final resin composite increment prior to curing.

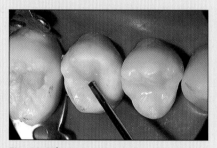

Fig 10-18h Occlusal sealant is placed over the resin composite and any remaining pits and fissures.

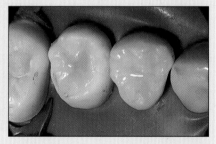

Fig 10-18i Completed occlusal preventive resin restorations.

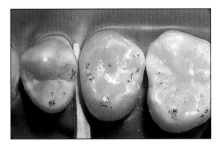

Fig 10-19 A wedge is placed before preparing the mesial surface of the maxillary second premolar; it provides tooth separation to help ensure adequate interproximal contact in the final restoration, and it helps prevent damage to the adjacent tooth, rubber dam, and gingival tissues.

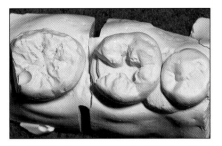

Fig 10-20a Stone cast made following Class 2 preparation involving the distal surface of a mandibular first molar.

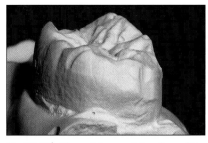

Fig 10-20b View of the mesial surface of the mandibular second molar shows the damage that resulted from inadequate protection during preparation of the distal surface of the first molar.

indicated even with a deep caries lesion when areas of the fissure system are not carious. Etching and application of an adhesive agent are the same as with other adhesive restorative procedures. Those areas of the preparation that have extended into dentin are filled with a highly filled restorative resin composite, which should be cured in increments no greater than 2 mm in thickness (Fig 10-18f). If the preparation is narrow and shallow, sealant material, flowable resin composite, or warmed resin composite may be used. Prior to curing the final increment, occlusal anatomy is sculpted with a hand instrument (Fig 10-18g). Occlusal sealant is then placed over the resin composite, through remaining prepared or unprepared etched fissures, and cured (Fig 10-18h). If, after curing the final increment, excess restorative material is present, the surface should be adjusted to provide desired contours and anatomy. The entire fissure system, including the resin composite and sealant, should be re-etched and a surface-sealing resin applied.[49,227]

After completion of the restoration (Fig 10-18i), the rubber dam is removed and correct occlusion verified or obtained.

Other Class 1 Resin Composite Restorations

When a Class 1 restoration is being placed due to initial caries lesion(s), the PRR is usually the technique of choice. If there was a previous restoration, the outline form and depth of the preparation will be determined by the previous restoration and any new pathosis. Margins of occlusal preparations for resin composite should not be beveled.[228] Lining and bonding techniques should be used as described for Class 2 restorations.

Class 2 Resin Composite Restorations

As with PRRs, Class 2 restorations should be limited to obtaining access to the carious dentin and removing the carious dentin and any overlying fragile or demineralized enamel.

Prewedging

Obtaining adequate interproximal contact in the final restoration starts at this stage of the restorative procedure, not at matrix placement or material insertion, as is the norm for amalgam restorations. Uncured resin composites, even the so-called packable composites, do not have the ability to hold the matrix band in close adaptation to an adjacent tooth.[229,230] This makes obtaining an adequate interproximal contact one of the more difficult aspects of placing a Class 2 resin composite restoration. Placement of an interproximal wedge at the start of the procedure is recommended to open the contact with the adjacent tooth and to compensate for the thickness of the matrix band. It has been demonstrated that multiple wedging, ie, inserting a wedge initially and then reapplying seating pressure several times during the course of the procedure, is more effective in opening the contact than is a single placement of a wedge.[136] In addition, the wedge can protect the rubber dam from damage and gingival tissues from laceration, thereby reducing leakage into the operative site.[46] Tooth separation obtained from prewedging promotes more conservative preparation and helps protect adjacent teeth from damage during preparation (Fig 10-19). Failure to take measures to protect adjacent teeth during proximal surface preparation with rotary instruments will usually result in damage to the adjacent teeth (Figs 10-20a and 10-20b).[231] Furthermore, this damage makes it significantly more likely

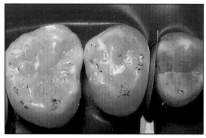

Fig 10-21a A small piece of matrix band is placed prior to a Class 2 preparation to protect the proximal surface of the adjacent tooth. A wooden wedge has been placed to help maintain the matrix in position and to gain separation to aid in obtaining an appropriate contact in the final restoration.

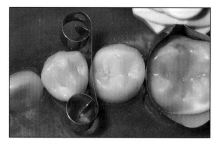

Fig 10-21b Alternate strategies for protecting the proximal surfaces of adjacent teeth during tooth preparation of the second premolar: (1) Interguard (Ultradent) is placed between the first and second premolars; (2) a circumferential metal matrix band is placed on the first molar.

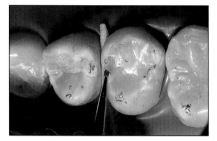

Fig 10-22a Preparation is initiated just inside the marginal ridge with a small round bur (No. ¼).

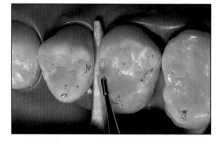

Fig 10-22b The preparation is extended with a No. 329 bur. Note that the proximal surface is left intact.

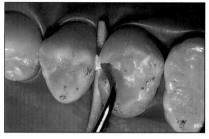

Fig 10-22c After the proximal surface is thinned, a spoon excavator is used to fracture and remove the thinned enamel.

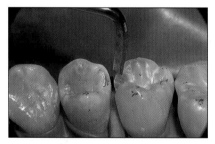

Fig 10-22d Bevels at the cavosurface margins of the proximal walls are placed with hand instruments.

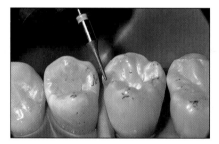

Fig 10-22e Alternatively, fine grit diamonds or carbide finishing burs can be used to place bevels.

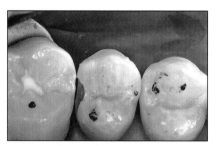

Fig 10-22f When a preparation exits the external tooth surface at an obtuse angle (greater than 90 degrees), no beveling of proximal walls is necessary.

that the damaged surface will require subsequent restoration.[232] Strategies for protecting adjacent proximal surfaces of adjacent teeth during preparation of a proximal area are presented in Figs 10-21a and 10-21b.

Preparation

As a general principle, preparation should be limited to eliminating carious tooth structure and providing access for res-

toration placement and finishing (Figs 10-22a to 10-22c). If there are one or more areas of fissure-caries lesions in the tooth, in addition to the proximal surface lesion(s), they should be treated separately, if possible, as described in the section on preventive resin restorations.

Bevel placement is a point of controversy with this preparation. When used in conjunction with adhesive agents and resin composites, bevels in enamel provide more area for acid etching and bonding. In addition, the bevel is designed to expose enamel rods transversely (cross cut or "end-on") to achieve a more effective etching pattern. Research has indicated that etching of transversely exposed enamel rods (ends of rods) results in a bond that is significantly stronger than that attained with etching of longitudinally cut enamel rods (sides of rods).[233] Clinical research has demonstrated favorable results with the use of acid-etched, beveled preparations in Class 3 resin composite restorations.[234]

Following are recommendations regarding bevel placement in Class 2 preparations for resin composite restorations.

Facial and Lingual Proximal Margins

Since enamel rods exit the tooth at approximately right angles to the external tooth surface, it is necessary for the cavity preparation to form an obtuse angle (greater than 90 degrees) with the external tooth surface to expose the ends of the enamel rods. If the external cavosurface margin forms a right angle with the tooth surface, conservative bevels (0.5 mm) should be placed at an approximately 45-degree angle to the surface, on the facial and lingual cavosurface margins of the proximal box preparation (Figs 10-22d and 10-22e). This will achieve the benefits of beveling, as well as aid in placing the margins in a more accessible location for finishing and polishing. Research has demonstrated that bevels on these margins significantly reduce marginal leakage.[235,236] If the preparation exits the tooth at an obtuse angle, no further beveling of the proximal walls is necessary (Fig 10-22f).

Gingival Margins

The decision to place a gingival margin bevel requires clinical judgment. The gingival margin should be beveled only if the margin is in enamel well away from the cementoenamel junction and an adequate band of enamel remains (Figs 10-5c and 10-23). When sufficient dentin-supported enamel remains for adequate bevel placement, resin composite adaptation is enhanced.[237] As the preparation nears the cementoenamel junction, the enamel layer is thinner than in other regions of the crown, and beveling the preparation increases the potential for removing the little enamel that remains. Because of the presence of prismless enamel in this region, acid etching is often less effective.[238] When a cavity preparation approaches within approximately 1 mm of the cementoenamel junction, adhesion is essentially no better than bonding to dentin (Fig 10-24).[167,168]

Use of an inverse or so-called internal bevel, leaving enamel that is not supported by dentin at the gingival cavosurface margin (Fig 10-25), has been shown to significantly reduce microleakage compared to a butt margin[239] (Fig 10-25b) and would be preferable to placing the gingival margin on or near the cementoenamel junction. This type of marginal configu-

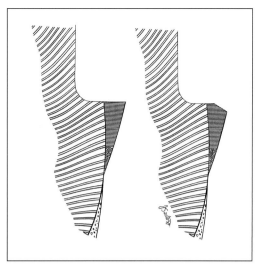

Fig 10-23 When enamel is adequate, a bevel is placed to enhance resin composite adaptation and seal.

ration should not be created intentionally with a bur, but if a lip of unsupported enamel remains after removal of demineralized dentin, it should be configured to an inverse bevel rather than planing the unsupported enamel off to form a butt margin in cementum or dentin.

Occlusal Margins

The use of occlusal cavosurface margin bevels is not indicated. Some clinicians have advocated the use of bevels on occlusal cavosurface margins to maximize the exposure of end-cut enamel rods.[238] However, it has been noted that a normal preparation in the occlusal surface will result in end-cut enamel rods because of the orientation of the enamel rods in cuspal inclines[182] (Fig 10-26). Avoidance of bevels on the occlusal surface prevents the loss of sound tooth structure, decreases the surface area of the final restoration, lessens the chance of occlusal contact on the restoration, eliminates a thin area of resin composite that would be more susceptible to fracture and wear, and presents a well-demarcated marginal periphery to which resin composite can be finished more precisely.[1,17,38,174]

Placement of occlusal bevels has demonstrated no benefit to the longevity of Class 2 resin composite restorations.[30] A clinical study demonstrated that posterior resin composite restorations placed in cavities with beveled occlusal margins had significantly greater wear than those placed with occlusal butt margins.[228] A significant factor predicting the survivability of posterior resin composite restorations is the proportion

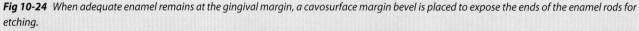

Fig 10-24 *When adequate enamel remains at the gingival margin, a cavosurface margin bevel is placed to expose the ends of the enamel rods for etching.*

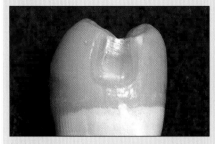

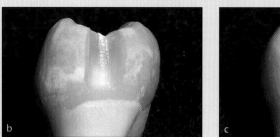

Fig 10-24a Appropriate proximal cavosurface margin bevels when the enamel is well above the cementoenamel junction. Gingival as well as facial and lingual vertical cavosurface margins are beveled.

Figs 10-24b and 10-24c As the gingival margin approaches 1 to 1.5 mm from the cementoenamel junction *(b)*, or is apical to the cementoenamel junction *(c)*, no gingival bevel is placed. Note that the facial and lingual vertical cavosurface margins are still beveled.

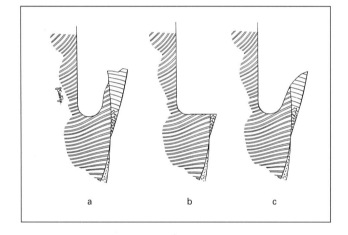

Fig 10-25 Excavation of a proximal caries lesion will sometimes result in a more gingival extent of the preparation in dentin than in enamel (a). If the preparation is extended straight out to the cavosurface margin, remaining enamel for bonding is compromised (b). Refining the preparation with a slow-speed round bur or a sharp hand instrument to eliminate very thin enamel and prepare an inverse bevel will expose enamel rods for etching on their internal ends and secure better adhesion to the gingival margin (c). Assuming removal of carious dentin created the situation shown in (a), the marginal configuration shown in (c) is preferable to that in (b).

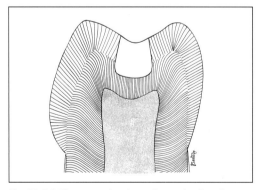

Fig 10-26 The enamel rods on the occlusal surface are oriented in such a way that the ends are exposed without beveling.

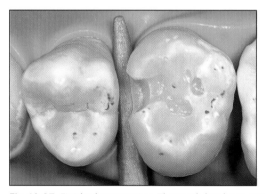

Fig 10-27 Finished preparation. The tooth has been prepared only in those areas where carious dentin was present. The preparation has not penetrated to dentin in other areas of the occlusal surface. Proximal facial, lingual, and gingival cavosurface margins have been beveled; occlusal cavosurface margins have not been beveled.

of the occlusal surface restored; this factor is increased by occlusal beveling.[30,240] Therefore, occlusal cavosurface margin bevels should be avoided (Fig 10-27).

It should be noted that occlusal enamel should not be left unsupported by dentin, particularly in an area of occlusal stress. Research has shown that unsupported occlusal enamel, even if the lost dentin has been replaced with glass ionomer, RMGI, or bonded composite, is significantly weaker than enamel supported by dentin.[241]

Use of Cavity Liners

If used, calcium-hydroxide liner should be limited to those areas of the preparation that are believed to be very close to the pulp, where there is the possibility of a minute pulpal exposure.[117] Placement of a calcium-hydroxide liner over an extensive area of dentin provides no benefit to the pulp and decreases the surface area of dentin available for adhesion. Dissolution of the liner during acid etching can interfere with a sound bond to enamel and dentin.[31] If the preparation is conservative in size, no liner is required in addition to adhesive agent. In deeper preparations and those in which the gingival margin approaches or extends beyond the cementoenamel junction, a glass-ionomer liner may be beneficial. Pulpal considerations are discussed in depth in chapter 5.

Glass-ionomer liners are reported to offer a number of potential advantages when used under posterior resin composite restorations. Glass-ionomer materials bond to both tooth structure and overlying resin composite,[242] and they introduce less polymerization stress into tooth structure than does resin composite.[81] Glass ionomer releases fluoride into adjacent tooth structure,[243] which may be advantageous because of the tendency for secondary caries lesions to occur adjacent to posterior resin composite restorations.[17] Use of a glass-ionomer liner has been demonstrated to improve marginal integrity[244] and decrease marginal leakage.[166,245,246] Less bulk of resin composite material is required to fill the preparation, reducing the amount of polymerization shrinkage[247] and improving marginal adaptation.[84] Glass-ionomer liners can reinforce the preparation walls by adhering to dentin and minimizing cuspal deformation under load.[247] Glass-ionomer liners also reduce the rise in pulpal temperature associated with application of the curing light during incremental insertion procedures.[248] With improvements in dentin adhesives, the use of glass ionomer under posterior resin composite restorations has been greatly reduced in recent years. However, use of a glass-ionomer liner on dentin cavity surfaces has been shown to significantly reduce postoperative sensitivity compared to use of a dentin adhesive alone.[249] Therefore, clinicians should consider use of a glass-ionomer liner even if an adequate band of enamel surrounds the entire preparation.

Bonded-Base Technique

If the gingival margin of a Class 2 preparation is in enamel but within 1 mm of the cementoenamel junction, or if it is in dentin, and an alternative restorative material cannot be used, an RMGI restorative material should be placed as the initial increment in the proximal box. This technique, known as the *bonded-base* or *open-sandwich technique*, has demonstrated a number of advantages when compared with use of an adhesive agent alone. There is considerable in vitro evidence that the bonded-base technique results in a reduction in marginal leakage.[250–256] Additionally, glass ionomers have demonstrated good antibacterial activity against microorganisms associated with dental caries.[257] Most importantly, the bonded-base technique has demonstrated good clinical performance. The first evaluation of the bonded-base technique used a conventional restorative glass ionomer as the initial increment in the proximal box. Unfortunately, this technique showed poor clinical longevity.[258] However, use of an RMGI restorative material for the initial increment in the proximal box has proven to be a viable technique. One clinical study showed that RMGI provided a significantly better cervical margin adaptation in Class 2 cavity preparations than did resin composite.[259] Several studies have shown that the bonded-base Class 2 restoration performs comparably to resin composite restorations using adhesive systems alone in most clinical parameters.[169–172] In addition, the bonded-base technique has demonstrated some important clinical advantages vs bonded Class 2 composite, including reduced postoperative sensitivity[172] and reduced in vivo demineralization adjacent to the gingival margin.[169] For these reasons, the bonded-base restoration should be considered whenever a posterior resin composite restoration will include a gingival margin in close proximity or apical to or below the cementoenamel junction.

The technique for accomplishing a bonded-base restoration is demonstrated in Figs 10-28a to 10-28e. After completion of the preparation, the matrix is applied and a wedge is placed. The gingival portion of the proximal box is treated with the RMGI conditioner. The RMGI is mixed, transferred to a light-protected Centrix syringe tip, and injected into the gingival aspect of the proximal box. Since glass ionomer does not have the same level of wear resistance as composite,[260,261] this increment of RMGI should remain apical to the proximal contact. The surface of the RMGI increment is smoothed and light cured. The entire cavity preparation, including the RMGI in the gingival portion of the proximal box, is etched, and the

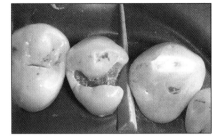

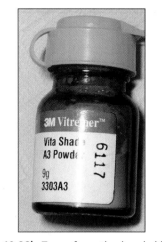

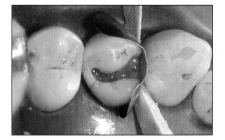

Fig 10-28a Following caries excavation, the gingival margin of the proximal box extends below the cementoenamel junction onto dentin. Note that the gingival margin extends to the fluted area of the root.

Fig 10-28b To perform the bonded-base technique, an RMGI restorative (vs a lining glass ionomer) is used. In this case Vitremer (3M/ESPE) was used.

Fig 10-28c Following treating the gingival portion of the proximal box with the RMGI conditioner, the RMGI restorative is mixed, placed into a Centrix syringe tip, injected into the gingival portion of the proximal box, smoothed, and cured. The RMGI should remain apical to the proximal contact. Note that two wedges have been used to contour the gingival margin of the matrix into the fluted area of the root.

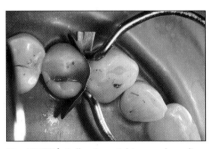

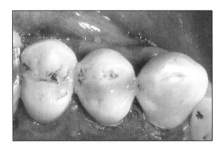

Fig 10-28d Following etching and application of the adhesive system to the RMGI and remaining aspects of the cavity preparation, the preparation is filled using an incremental placement technique.

Fig 10-28e The completed restoration.

adhesive system is applied according to the manufacturer's instructions. The preparation is filled and finished as described in the subsequent sections of this chapter.

Acid Etching

The walls of the preparation should be etched with 30% to 40% phosphoric acid for 15 seconds and rinsed.[262] A small piece of metal or clear plastic matrix band material is placed to protect the adjacent proximal surface from being etched. This will prevent inadvertent bonding to this surface in subsequent resin composite placement procedures (Fig 10-29). The enamel can be dried to examine for a frosted, matte appearance to confirm proper enamel etching (see Fig 10-46h). If this is done, the dentist must be aware that the dentin will

usually be dried as well; this can adversely affect dentin adhesion. If this occurs, the dentin should be rewetted prior to proceeding with resin adhesive system application (see chapter 8).

Application of Bonding Resin

The manufacturer's instructions for the particular bonding system should be followed. In most fourth-generation (multicomponent) adhesive systems, a primer is placed after etching and is followed by an adhesive resin. The primer is usually a hydrophilic resin contained in a volatile liquid carrier. After application of the primer, the carrier evaporates, leaving behind a very thin layer of resin. It is imperative that the solvent be thoroughly evaporated with air from an air syringe before

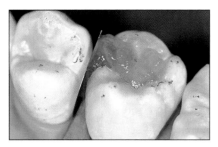

Fig 10-29 Acid etchant is placed over the entire preparation. A small piece of matrix has been placed to protect the adjacent proximal surface.

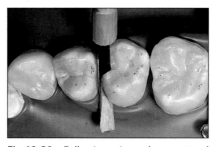

Fig 10-30a Following primer placement and solvent evaporation, adhesive resin is placed with a brush.

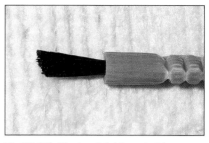

Fig 10-30b The brush is blotted with a gauze sponge to absorb excess adhesive resin from the preparation. Air thinning of the adhesive component of fourth-generation (multiple component) dentin bonding systems should be avoided.

adhesive placement; failure to do so will significantly impair the quality of adhesion, particularly to dentin.[263] The adhesive is then applied in a thin layer (Fig 10-30a) and thinned further with a blotted brush (Fig 10-30b). Care should be taken not to overly thin the adhesive layer. Research has demonstrated that increased adhesive resin thickness results in reduced polymerization shrinkage stress,[264] decreased gap formation,[265] and decreased microleakage.[266] An air stream should not be used to thin the adhesive resin because this has been shown to significantly reduce bond strength.[267] However, it is possible to leave adhesive layers that are too thick, which can also reduce bond strength.[268] In addition, layers of adhesive resin that are 42 μm thick or greater can be detected on bite-wing radiographs[265] and might be mistaken for a marginal defect or a caries lesion.

In fifth-generation, or "single-bottle," adhesive systems, in which the primer and adhesive components have been combined, a different placement technique is required. Air thinning is needed to ensure adequate evaporation of the solvent; however, the air stream also thins the adhesive resin component. Additional applications of these adhesive resins (double the number noted by the manufacturer) are recommended to maximize the bond to dentin.[269]

The sixth-generation systems, in which the conditioner and primer have been combined, and the seventh-generation, or "all-in-one" self-etch systems, in which all components are applied simultaneously, also utilize placement techniques unique to their formulations. These systems use a nonrinse application procedure. However, air thinning is still required to evaporate solvents.

If the preparation is etched and the bonding resin is placed before application of the matrix, visualization and access to all areas of the preparation are better, and it is easier to brush thin the adhesive and avoid pooling. A small piece of matrix band material, used to protect the adjacent proximal surface,

may be kept in place. However, the wedge either should not be replaced at this time or should be placed between the matrix material and the preparation. This gives the resin adhesive access to all areas of the preparation and provides an escape for the resin adhesive at the margin to prevent it from pooling. Placement of a matrix after applying the adhesive sometimes results in contamination of the preparation with blood or saliva, so the operator may prefer to place the matrix and wedge prior to etching and application of the adhesive. If so, special care must be taken to ensure the absence of pooling of the resin adjacent to the matrix. Enamel and dentin adhesives are discussed at length in chapter 8.

Matrix Application

Several useful matrices are available, including the clear plastic matrix, the ultrathin (0.001-inch) Tofflemire metal matrix (Fig 10-31), the thin (0.0015-inch) sectional matrix, and the Tofflemire metal matrix with photoetch-thinned (0.0005-inch) contact areas.

The clear matrix can be used in conjunction with a light-reflecting wedge (see Fig 10-31b) and offers the advantage of allowing penetration of the curing light from multiple directions. This allows the clinician to cure the increments of resin composite from the proximal and gingival directions, rather than from the occlusal aspect only, to ensure adequate polymerization of each increment. In addition, it has been reported that this technique allows more favorable direction of the polymerization shrinkage. One study showed enhanced gingival margin adaptation using this technique when the proximal box was prepared in enamel,[270] although another study failed to show a similar benefit when the gingival margin was in dentin.[168] However, the clear matrix is thicker than the thinnest metal matrices, and its lack of rigidity makes placement through tight interproximal contacts difficult.[38] In

Fig 10-31 Two common matrices for Class 2 resin composite restorations.

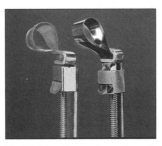

Fig 10-31a Clear and metal matrix bands are shown with Tofflemire retainers.

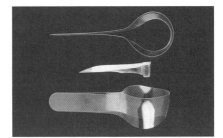

Fig 10-31b The clear matrix is usually used with a light-reflecting wedge.

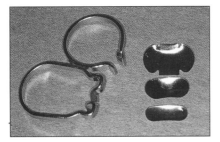

Fig 10-32a Palodent sectional matrix system (Dentsply).

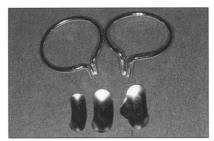

Fig 10-32b Composi-Tight sectional matrix system (Garrison Dental Solutions).

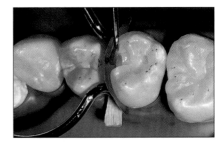

Fig 10-33 Sectional matrix and Composi-Tight ring in place. The matrix is burnished in the contact area to enhance proximal contour and contact.

addition, the rigidity and smoothness of the plastic, light-reflecting wedge makes it less effective than a wooden wedge in gaining the slight tooth separation needed to ensure adequate interproximal contact. Methods to compensate for this lack of separation are described later in this chapter. However, because of these drawbacks, most clinicians prefer metal matrices and wooden wedges.

Tight interproximal contacts are more easily developed with the ultrathin metal matrices than with the clear matrices because they are easier to place, maintain their shape better, and can be burnished against the adjacent tooth. One disadvantage of a metal matrix that wraps around the facial and lingual surfaces of the tooth is that increments must be initially cured only from the occlusal aspect. After removal of the matrix, the proximal resin composite may be further polymerized from the facial and lingual aspects. To avoid flat proximal-surface contours, precontoured matrices should be used or the metal matrices should be shaped or contoured by burnishing before or after they are placed.

Other devices that are helpful in developing adequate interproximal contacts are the sectional matrix systems, used with metal rings with springlike properties (Figs 10-32a and 10-32b). After the sectional matrix and wooden wedge are placed, the ring is placed using rubber dam clamp or similar forceps so that the vertical points of the ring are positioned in the facial and lingual embrasures adjacent to the box preparation. The ring holds the ends of the sectional matrix tightly against the tooth and exerts a continuous separating force between the teeth. The matrix should be burnished gently against the adjacent proximal contact (Fig 10-33). The sectional matrices in these systems are typically made of "dead soft" metal. Heavy burnishing will cause grooves to be formed in the matrix that will be replicated in the restoration. This makes for a rough, irregular contact that can tear and shred floss when the patient performs oral hygiene measures, so only light burnishing should be used.

These "ring" systems have a number of advantages: they provide wedging to ensure good interproximal contact; they provide better proximal contours for posterior resin composite restorations than traditional matrices; and they simplify matrix placement for single proximal-surface restorations compared to a circumferential band.[271,272] It should be recognized that the ring provides progressive tooth separation, so if it is left in place for a long period of time, excess separation can occur, resulting in a very tight contact.

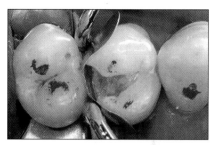

Fig 10-34a Conservative proximal preparation allows the ring for a sectional matrix system to be placed above (coronal to) the wedge. This placement provides a separating action and contours the matrix to provide correct proximal contours.

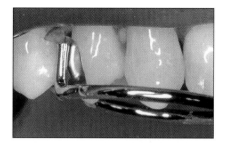

Fig 10-34b Facial view showing placement of the ring.

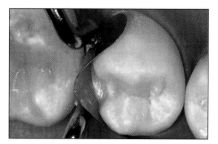

Fig 10-34c In this preparation, the lingual proximal wall extends onto the lingual surface. The ring has been placed above (coronal to) the wedge. However, the lingual tine has caused the matrix to partially collapse into the preparation, resulting in the matrix band covering a portion of the gingival floor of the preparation.

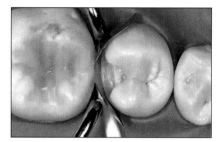

Fig 10-34d The ring has been repositioned between the wooden wedge and the adjacent tooth. This prevents the tines from collapsing the matrix into the preparation. It also causes the wedge to bend, enhancing the gingival seal of the matrix and wrapping the matrix around the tooth to develop appropriate proximal contour.

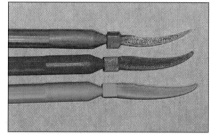

Fig 10-34e Plastic wedges are more flexible than wooden wedges and may be more useful when the ring must be placed between the wedge and the adjacent tooth (Wedge Wands, Garrison Dental Solutions).

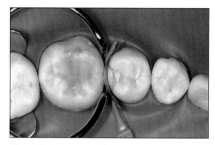

Fig 10-34f Ring placed between plastic wedge and adjacent tooth. Note the pronounced wrapping of the wedge at the gingival aspect of the preparation.

The placement of the ring relative to the prepared tooth and the wedge should vary based on the location of the proximal margins and the type of ring. Proper placement of the ring depends on facial and lingual extensions of the proximal box and the size and shape of the tines of the particular ring being used. Rings with wider tines (eg, the Palodent system) tend to limit the ability to place the ring in different locations relative to the wedge, whereas rings with narrower tines (eg, the Composi-Tight system) provide more flexibility in this regard. If the facial and lingual proximal extensions of the proximal box do not extend significantly onto the facial or lingual surfaces of the tooth, it is possible to place the ring with the tines occlusal to the wedge (Figs 10-34a and 10-34b) or between the wedge and enamel adjacent to the proximal surface being restored. However, if one or both of the proximal walls reach the facial or lingual surfaces of the tooth, placement of the tines of the ring in these locations may cause the

matrix to be deformed (Fig 10-34c). In this case, the tines may be placed between the wooden wedge and the proximal surface of the adjacent tooth. The ring will have enough tension to separate the teeth adequately and to cause the wedge to wrap slightly around the tooth, providing a tight gingival seal and wrapping of the sectional matrix around the tooth to form the proper proximal contour (Fig 10-34d). Plastic wedges have been developed that allow additional wrapping of the wedge and matrix when the ring is placed between the wedge and adjacent tooth surface (Figs 10-34e and 10-34f).

Yet another type of sectional matrix involves a short piece of thin, stainless steel matrix material that is contoured only occlusogingivally and does not surround the tooth at all (Fig 10-35). This allows some light curing from facial and lingual aspects. The contoured matrix is secured with a wooden wedge and lies passively against the adjacent tooth surface or is held there with an instrument during curing of the first

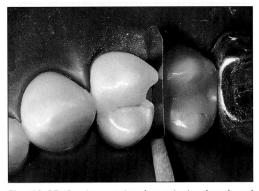

Fig 10-35 Passive sectional matrix is placed and wedged. Resin composite will be sculpted in facial and lingual embrasures with a thin instrument such as an interproximal carver.

increment. That increment then holds the matrix against the adjacent tooth during placement of succeeding increments. When this technique is used, resin composite in facial and lingual embrasures must be contoured or sculpted with a thin-bladed instrument, such as an interproximal carver (IPC), prior to curing.

Resin Composite Placement: Incremental Technique

VLC resin composite should be placed in successive, laminated increments to ensure proper curing and prevent excessive polymerization shrinkage.[16] Incremental curing decreases the effects of polymerization shrinkage, enhances marginal adaptation, decreases gap formation, reduces marginal leakage, decreases cuspal deformation, makes the cusps more resistant to subsequent fracture, and decreases postoperative sensitivity.[82,84,270,273,274]

One of the greatest benefits to the incremental fill technique may be its effect on cavity configuration, or *C-factor*. The C-factor is the ratio of bonded to unbonded restoration surface areas and has been shown to have a profound impact on polymerization shrinkage stress (see chapter 8). As the C-factor increases, that is, as the surface area of resin composite bonded to cavity walls increases relative to the surface area of unbonded resin composite, shrinkage stresses increase dramatically.[91,275,276] By placing and curing resin composite incrementally, the C-factor of each increment is reduced compared to bulk placement and cure.[277] As C-factor decreases, bond strength increases.[278] The end result is that the incrementally placed and cured restoration is bonded better to the cavity walls than if the preparation had been filled and the resin composite material cured in bulk.

First Increment

Some general guidelines should be followed for the placement of the resin composite. Proper handling of the bonding system and resin composite at the gingival margin is critical because of the tendency for microleakage to occur in that area.[246] A clinical study that assessed gingival margin quality in Class 2 resin composite restorations showed that only 27% were satisfactory.[279] Therefore, techniques must be used to enhance the bond and reduce the adverse effects of polymerization shrinkage. First, an increment no thicker than 1.0 mm is placed against the gingival wall.[280] A thin first layer will ensure proper light irradiation throughout the increment.

If a clear matrix and light-reflecting wedge are being used, the initial curing should be directed through the flat end of the wedge. The amount of light that a reflecting wedge will transmit varies in the literature. One study indicated that 90% to 95% of the incident light is transmitted,[270] while another showed that it could be as low as 66%.[281] Because of the possible attenuation of light through the wedge, exposure time should be increased by 50% (to 60 seconds when using a light with optimum output) to ensure adequate polymerization. It has been suggested that the light-reflecting wedge will direct the curing light to the gingival margin of the restoration and draw the polymerization shrinkage toward that margin. When the gingival margin is on enamel, this method has been shown to result in better marginal adaptation than curing from an occlusal direction.[84,270,282,283] However, when the gingival margin is on dentin, this technique failed to reduce gingival margin microleakage compared to other techniques.[168]

Because most plastic wedges are rigid and smooth, they may slip out of proper position easily and may not maintain the pressure necessary to ensure proper adaptation of the gingival aspect of the matrix band and separation from the adjacent tooth. Two suggestions may help to overcome this problem. After the plastic wedge is positioned, a wooden wedge may be inserted beside it on the side away from the tooth being restored. Alternatively, the plastic wedge can be maintained in proper position by applying pressure to its flat end with the light-curing tip during curing of the initial increment (Fig 10-36). After this is completed, the plastic wedge has accomplished its purpose and may be replaced with a wooden wedge for succeeding increments.

If a metal matrix that surrounds the tooth has been chosen, all increments must be cured from the occlusal aspect. The tip of the light should be positioned as close as possible to the resin being cured.[9] After the metal matrix is removed, all proximal areas of the restoration should receive additional curing with the light.

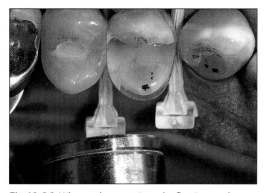

Fig 10-36 When a clear matrix and reflecting wedge are used, the initial cure for the gingival resin composite increment is through the wedge. The end of the light guide can be used to maintain pressure on the smooth plastic wedge during initial polymerization to help ensure interproximal contact. Due to loss of irradiance when curing through a wedge, cure times should be increased by one half.

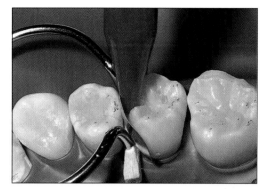

Fig 10-37 Previously warmed resin composite is syringed into the preparation via a Centrix placement tip to maximize adaptation to the cavity walls.

Resin composites that are marketed for posterior use vary widely in their viscosity.[284] This can have an impact on adaptation of resin composite to the walls of a cavity preparation.[285] Thicker-consistency resin composites have significantly increased cavity wall voids compared to medium- or thinner-viscosity materials.[284] Resin composites that are supplied in preloaded resin composite tips or ampules tend to have a higher viscosity than do composites that are supplied in syringes.[284] Placement technique can also determine how well the resin composite adapts to the cavity preparation walls. Use of a placement tip (Centrix) (Fig 10-37) for resin composite decreases the viscosity of the material[284] and significantly decreases voids adjacent to the preparation walls compared to either smearing the material into place with a plastic instrument or "condensing" it.[285]

Injecting a heavily filled composite through a narrow placement tip can be difficult, if not impossible. A technique that will further enhance the flow of the resin composite into a cavity preparation is to use resin composite that has been warmed prior to injecting. If a syringe of resin composite is used, the required amount is transferred into a Centrix syringe tip. The tip and composite can be warmed in a water bath or a commercial composite warmer to reduce the viscosity and improve flow.[286] If a water bath is used, the tip should be sealed in a small plastic bag prior to immersion to protect the resin composite material from moisture. The temperature to which the composite is warmed is based somewhat on individual preference, but typically will be in a range of 140° to 155°F (60° to 68°C) This material can then be syringed into place more easily, and the lowered viscosity enhances resin composite adaptation to the cavity walls (see Fig 10-37).

In addition to these advantages for warming and injecting resin composite of reduced viscosity and improved resin composite flow, other advantages have been demonstrated. Use of warmed resin composite has reduced marginal leakage in Class 2 resin composite restorations compared to using either room temperature resin composite or flowable composite.[287] Warmed resin composite has improved cure, as compared to room-temperature resin composite.[288] Since most temperature increase is due to reaction kinetics and heat from the curing unit, the warmed resin composite adds very little temperature increase to that which already occurs.[288] Resin composite does not polymerize in the warming unit, even if kept at 130°F (55° C) for 4 hours or 158°F (70°C) for 15 minutes.[288] Finally, prewarming of the resin composite does not adversely affect the material's strength.[289]

Flowable Resin Composites

Another method that has been suggested is the use of low-viscosity, or "flowable," resin composites for the first increment.[290] The rationale is that these materials flow more readily than standard hybrid formulations and will therefore easily and thoroughly adapt to all areas of the cavity preparation. Also, because of their lower filler content and reduced elastic modulus, it is theorized that these materials could act as "stress breakers" to absorb forces of polymerization shrinkage or cyclic loading.[291] However, the efficacy of this method has not been demonstrated.[291]

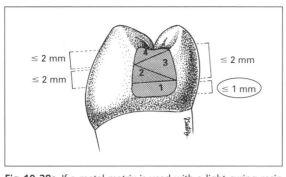

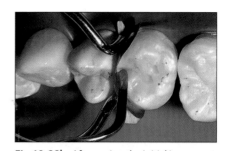

Fig 10-38a If a metal matrix is used with a light-curing resin composite, the minimal (1.0 mm) gingival increment is placed and cured. The material is then layered in alternating oblique increments. No increment exceeds 2.0 mm in thickness. To minimize cuspal deformation and polymerization stress, an oblique increment should not contact both facial and lingual cavity walls. This placement technique can also be used with a clear matrix and reflecting wedge.

Fig 10-38b After curing the initial increment, the next increment is syringed into place and "ramped" obliquely with a plastic instrument or interproximal carver. Here, the Composi-Tight matrix and ring are used, and an oblique increment is shaped with an interproximal carver.

There are a number of problems associated with these materials. Because of their higher resin content,[292] flowable resin composites demonstrate up to three times greater polymerization shrinkage than do standard hybrid resin composite formulations.[292,293] This generates significantly greater polymerization shrinkage forces that surpass any benefit that might be derived from the lower elastic modulus.[294] This adversely impacts the adhesion of the resin composite to the cavity preparation, as higher polymerization shrinkage[295] and polymerization shrinkage stress[278] have been shown to significantly decrease bond strength.

The use of a cured increment of a flowable resin composite in conjunction with Class 2 resin composite restorations has shown mixed results in studies of marginal leakage. Some studies have shown improved marginal seal,[296,297] and others have indicated worsened gingival seal.[298,299] However, the majority of studies show no benefit from using a cured portion of flowable composite as the initial increment in placement of a Class 2 resin composite restoration.[256,300–303] In addition, due to their lower filler loading, flowable resin composites have inferior mechanical properties compared to traditional resin composites.[291] This leads to concern that occlusal forces may introduce increased deflection of the overlying hybrid resin composite, which has a higher modulus of elasticity, due to the inability of the flowable resin composite to provide adequate support.[291] In fact, the use of a flowable resin liner in conjunction with a high-viscosity (packable) resin composite has been shown to weaken the strength of the polymerized packable material.[304]

The reduced viscosity of flowable resin composites improves adaptation to the preparation but may also result in undesirable effects. One study found that use of a flowable composite always led to increased incidence of gingival margin overhangs in beveled Class 2 cavity preparations.[305]

An additional concern with flowable resin composites pertains to their radiopacity. Detection of voids and recurrent caries lesions is maximized when a restorative material has the same radiopacity as, or slightly greater radiopacity than, enamel.[66–68] Many flowable resin composites have not met the standard of being at least as radiopaque as enamel.[69,70,306,307]

Clinical trials using flowable resin composite for the initial increments in posterior resin composite restorations have not demonstrated any difference in either postoperative sensitivity[308] or overall clinical performance[309] compared to the use of heavily filled resin composite alone.

A recent suggestion that may hold promise for the use of flowable composites in conjunction with posterior resin composite restorations has been called the *snowplow technique*.[310] In this technique, an initial thin increment of flowable composite is placed over the gingival and/or pulpal floors of the cavity preparation. This layer is not cured at this stage, but rather an initial increment of heavily filled restorative resin composite is syringed or pushed into the unset flowable resin composite. Most of the flowable resin composite is displaced by the restorative composite and is subsequently removed from the cavity preparation. As a result, most of the flowable composite, and therefore its potentially disadvantageous characteristics, is not present in the cavity preparation. Instead, there is only a small amount of flowable resin composite remaining in those areas of the cavity in which the higher viscosity resin composite did not completely adapt to the prepa-

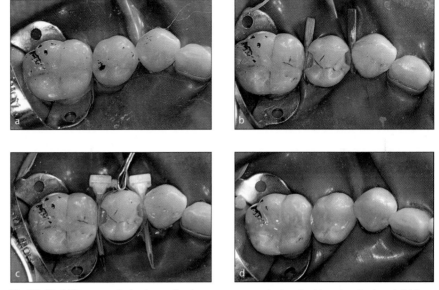

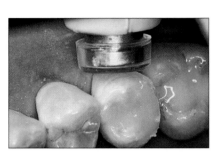

Fig 10-39 If a surrounding metal matrix was used, the restoration should be cured from the facial and lingual aspects after matrix removal.

Fig 10-40 *(a)* Preoperatively, the occlusal contacts are marked and rubber dam is placed. *(b)* Conservative mesio-occlusal and disto-occlusal preparations have been made in the mandibular left second premolar. Wooden wedges are in place for prewedging. *(c)* A clear matrix and reflecting wedges in place. *(d)* When the resin composite restorations are completed, a surface sealer is placed.

ration and that otherwise may have been voids. The combined increment of flowable resin composite and restorative resin composite is then cured. This technique has demonstrated significantly reduced void formation compared to placement of restorative composite alone.[310] It has also shown significantly decreased gingival margin leakage in Class 2 resin composite restorations when compared to use of a restorative resin composite alone or to placement of a cured increment of flowable resin composite prior to restorative resin composite placement.[256] It should be noted, however, that no clinical studies with this technique have been reported.

Additional Increments

Subsequent increments should be placed in thicknesses no greater than 2.0 mm. An oblique layering technique should be used whenever access allows (Figs 10-38a and 10-38b), and the restoration should be cured from the facial and lingual aspects after removal of the matrix (Fig 10-39). If a clear matrix is employed, the oblique technique (see Fig 10-38a) should be used, and additional curing from the facial and lingual aspects can be accomplished through the matrix to ensure thorough cure.

When the proximal boxes have been filled and the resin composite polymerized, the occlusal channel, if present, is filled and cured incrementally. Alternatively, after the proximal box has been filled to the level of the pulpal floor, the proximal box and occlusal preparations can be incrementally filled and cured simultaneously. With the exception of the initial increment in the gingival aspect of the proximal box, subsequent resin composite increments should not contact both the facial and lingual preparation walls simultaneously; this is to minimize polymerization shrinkage stress[311] and cuspal deformation.[93] Figure 10-40 presents posterior resin composite restorations placed using a clear matrix and light-reflecting wedges.

An alternative to the layering techniques is the use of a conical light-curing tip (Fig 10-41). The proximal box is filled with composite to just gingival to the contact area, and the conical tip is wedged into the resin composite. The cone is used to apply pressure to the matrix band and push it against the adjacent tooth during curing. Subsequent increments restore the cone-shaped gap formed by the tip. This technique is designed to ensure adequate interproximal contact and to minimize the thickness of resin composite that the light must penetrate. While the technique has not become particularly popular and is relatively untested, study results have shown some benefits, including formation of fewer marginal gaps than in the more traditional incremental techniques,[312] reduced cusp deflection,[313] improved hardness, and decreased porosity.[314]

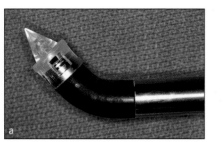

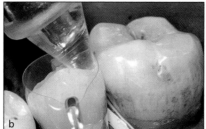

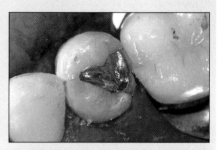

Fig 10-41 A conical light tip (a) can be placed into uncured resin composite increment (b) to provide curing while also pushing the matrix against the adjacent tooth to enhance proximal contact.

Fig 10-42 Examples of composite contact forming instruments.

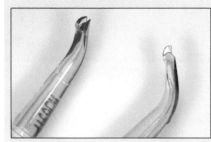

Fig 10-42a ContactPro (C. E. J Dental).

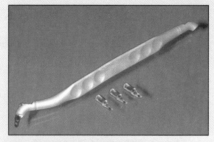

Fig 10-42b TriMax (AdDent; designed by Dr. Richard Trushkowsky, private practice, Staten Island, NY).

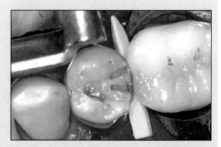

Fig 10-42c Preoperative photo of disto-occlusal amalgam restoration in a mandibular right second premolar to be removed due to a recurrent caries lesion.

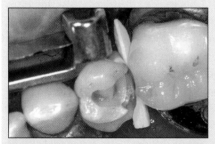

Fig 10-42d Completed preparation with matrix and wedge in place.

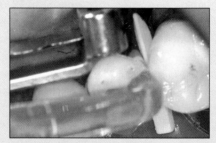

Fig 10-42e An initial increment of composite has been placed into the proximal portion of the cavity preparation. The ContactPro has been inserted into the unpolymerized composite and rotated and wedged against the mandibular right first molar. The composite will be cured while the ContactPro is held in this position.

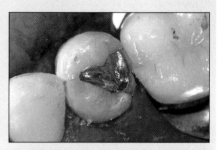

Fig 10-42f After removal of the Contact Pro. Note that the cured composite between the tines of the contact-forming instrument is maintaining a definite interproximal contact.

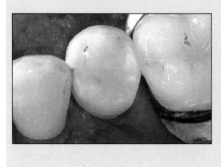

Fig 10-42g Final restoration with appropriate proximal contact.

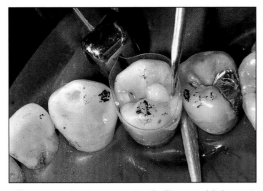

Fig 10-43 Use of a precured resin composite "ball" to establish proximal contact. A small amount of composite is placed on the tip of an instrument (such as the Hollenback No. ¹/₂ carver) and cured. It is then pushed into uncured resin composite material in the proximal box. While the precured ball is wedged tightly against the contact, the composite in the proximal box is cured.

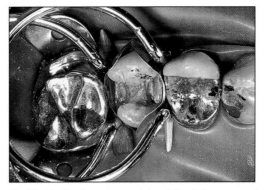

Fig 10-44 Simultaneous mesial and distal placement of sectional matrices and rings for a mesio-occlusodistal restoration.

A similar technique to help establish interproximal contact is to place the first increment into the proximal box, but instead of pushing the matrix with the conical tip, it is held against the adjacent tooth during the polymerization with a plastic instrument, condenser, or similar instrument. That increment, after it is hardened, will then hold the matrix against the tooth as successive increments are placed.

Some manufacturers have devised instruments that are precontoured to provide a wedging effect of a matrix band against the adjacent tooth. These instruments are designed to ensure good contact while maintaining proper occlusogingival contours. (See Fig 10-42 for examples.)

The use of balls of prepolymerized resin composite has also been suggested to aid in establishing interproximal contact. The normal incremental technique is used until the proximal box is filled to just gingival to the proximal contact. A small, slightly flattened ball of resin composite is precured on the tip of an instrument (eg, a Hollenback No. ¹/₂ carver). An additional increment of uncured resin composite is placed into the proximal box. The precured ball is pushed into this increment to wedge the matrix tightly against the adjacent tooth; then the resin composite is cured (Fig 10-43).[315]

If both the mesial and distal surfaces of a tooth are being restored with resin composite, it is sometimes difficult to obtain adequate interproximal separation for both proximal surfaces simultaneously. When mesio-occlusal and disto-occlusal restorations (or a mesio-occlusodistal restoration) are being placed, one proposed remedy is to remove the wedge from one interproximal area, reapply pressure to the remaining wedge to maximize separation, and incrementally place resin composite to fill that box only. The wedge is then removed from the interproximal area adjacent to the restored surface and inserted adjacent to the unrestored surface, and that box is incrementally filled. Sectional matrix systems with rings may be used in a similar manner, or simultaneously, on the mesial and distal aspects (Fig 10-44).

Final Increment

Careful control of the final increment will minimize the amount of finishing. A number of techniques are helpful in accomplishing this goal. A rounded, cone-shaped instrument (eg, PKT3), slightly moistened with resin adhesive or a low-viscosity resin specifically designed to prevent sticking of resin composite to the instrument, may be used to shape and form the occlusal surface before curing (Figs 10-18g and 10-45a). It is important that only a thin layer of low-viscosity resin be applied to the instrument to act as a lubricant. The best way to ensure this is to place a drop of resin in a gauze sponge and then wipe the end of the instrument with the gauze. A fine-bristled brush (eg, sable) can be very helpful in smoothing the composite surface and achieving intimate adaptation of the resin composite to the cavosurface margins (Fig 10-45b).

The use of an occlusal stent can reduce or even eliminate finishing of preventive resin or Class 1 resin composite restorations (Fig 10-46). This technique uses polyvinylsiloxane (PVS) impression material bonded to a tongue depressor.[316] With the advent of stiffer PVS occlusal registration materials, it is possible to eliminate the tongue depressor and use the PVS registration material alone.

Another method for replacing occlusal anatomy and reducing finishing is called the *successive cusp build-up technique*.[317] With this procedure, incremental resin composite placement is accomplished as described in the preceding sections. However, the clinician stops the oblique layer place-

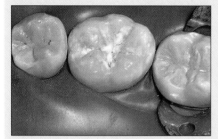

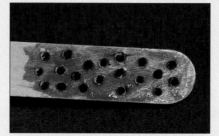

Fig 10-45 *(a)* A small condenser or burnisher, lightly moistened with adhesive, is used to establish preliminary occlusal contours in the final resin composite increment before light curing. *(b)* A sable brush is used to smooth the composite surface and ensure intimate adaptation of the restorative composite to the cavosurface margins.

Fig 10-46 *An alternative technique for placing preventive resin restorations.*

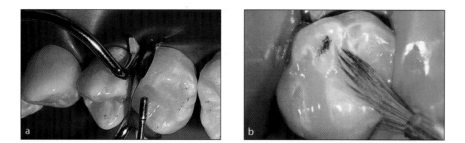

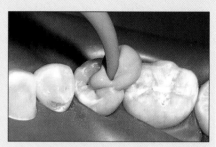

Fig 10-46a Extensively demineralized enamel in the fissures of the mandibular first molar.

Fig 10-46b Wooden tongue depressor perforated using a No. 8 round bur and coated with adhesive for PVS impression material.

Fig 10-46c PVS impression material syringed onto occlusal surfaces.

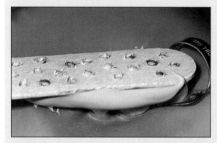

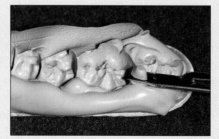

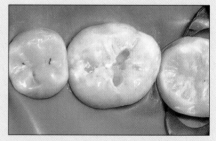

Fig 10-46d The perforated tongue depressor is covered with a layer of impression material and gently seated over the teeth.

Fig 10-46e Areas of the impression that might interfere with reseating are removed with a No. 15 scalpel blade.

Fig 10-46f Completed preparation. Only areas of demineralized dentin and overlying enamel were removed; where the dentin at the base of the fissures was not carious, the fissures were slightly opened to remove demineralized enamel and to leave sound enamel for bonding.

ment and cure at a point judged to be the base of the pit-and-fissure anatomy for the final restoration. The final increments of resin composite are positioned and adapted to replace the missing portions of the inner inclines of the cusps, one cusp at a time. Because of their stiffer viscosity, packable resin composites work well in this situation. The packable resin composite can be adapted and shaped without slumping prior to curing. As each cusp is replaced with resin com-

posite, it is briefly cured (5 seconds) to set the material in place. It is not necessary to fully cure each increment at this point, since the entire occlusal surface, and therefore all preceding increments, will be irradiated after the final cusp is replaced with resin composite and is irradiated for the full curing time. This technique has been shown to provide enhanced occlusal anatomy, thereby reducing subsequent finishing. Figure 10-47 demonstrates this technique.

Fig 10-46 (continued)

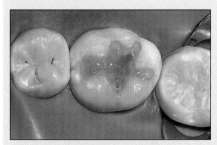

Fig 10-46g Etching the preparation.

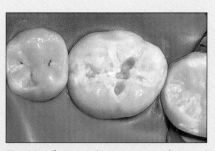

Fig 10-46h Frosted appearance of enamel confirms adequate etch.

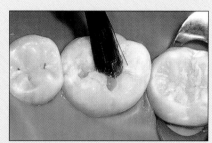

Fig 10-46i A dentin bonding system is used to bond resin composite in deeper portions of the preparation and to enhance adhesion of sealant (when used) in fissures.

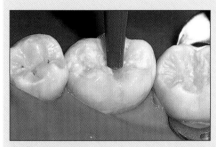

Fig 10-46j Warmed resin composite is syringed into deeper areas of the preparation.

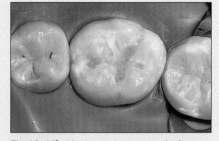

Fig 10-46k Maximum increment thickness is 2.0 mm; an initial increment is placed and cured in any area of the preparation deeper than 2.0 mm.

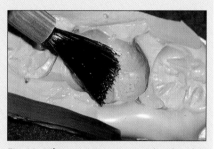

Fig 10-46l Impression is painted with a thin layer of adhesive resin. This layer is not cured.

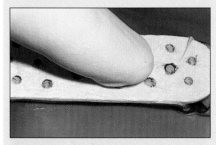

Fig 10-46m After the warmed resin composite is syringed into the remaining unfilled aspects of the preparation, the impression is repositioned on the teeth.

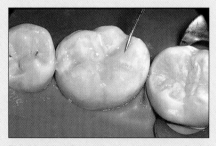

Fig 10-46n The impression is removed, and an explorer is used to remove excess resin composite material. With the flowability achieved by warming the resin composite and perfect adaptation of the impression to the teeth, all pits and fissures are filled with resin composite, making subsequent sealant placement unnecessary.

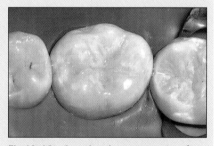

Fig 10-46o Completed restoration. A surface-penetrating sealant is placed and cured to ensure that all aspects of the occlusal surface are sealed. Close reproduction of the original occlusal surface with this technique often minimizes the need for occlusal adjustment.

Fig 10-47 The successive cusp build-up technique.

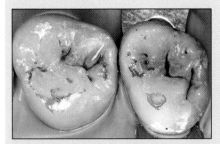

Fig 10-47a Preoperative view of maxillary left molars with occlusal caries. Note that the occlusal contacts have been marked prior to rubber dam placement.

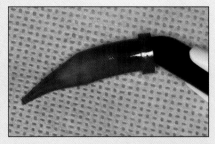

Fig 10-47b The appropriate resin composite shade is selected and transferred to a light-protected Centrix syringe tip.

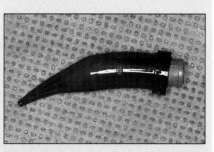

Fig 10-47c The rubber plug is placed into the Centrix syringe tip.

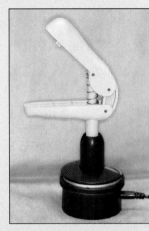

Fig 10-47d The Centrix syringe tip is placed into the placement syringe and transferred to the composite warmer (Calset, Addent).

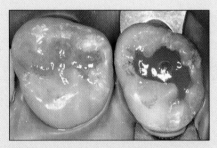

Fig 10-47e The completed preparations are etched.

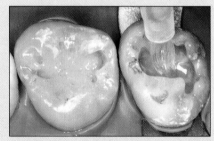

Fig 10-47f The adhesive system is applied according to the manufacturer's instructions.

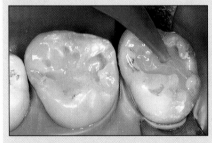

Fig 10-47g The warmed resin composite is injected into the preparations and cured in increments no thicker than 2 mm.

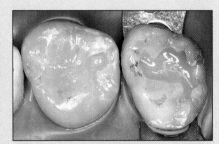

Fig 10-47h The initial warmed composite placement and cure is stopped at the anticipated level of the pits and fissures in the final restoration. Those aspects of the restoration that require little contouring for the final anatomy have been entirely filled with the warm composite (mesial/central portions of maxillary left first molar).

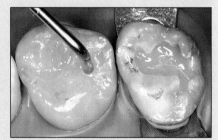

Fig 10-47i An increment of restorative composite (in this case, packable resin composite) is adapted to the lingual incline of the disto-facial cusp of the maxillary left first molar.

Fig 10-47 *(continued)*

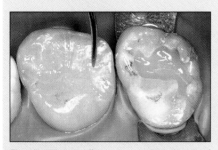

Fig 10-47j A small instrument (PKT1) is used to form the missing cuspal anatomy in resin composite. The remaining tooth structure is used as a guide to replace the cusp inclines to the level of the fissure. The facial cuspal incline of the distolingual cusp has already been completed.

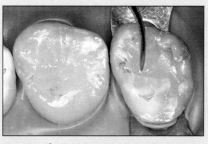

Fig 10-47k The lingual incline of the mesial facial cusp of the maxillary left second molar is formed in resin composite to the level of the fissure. This increment is briefly cured (5 seconds).

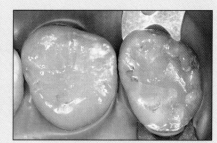

Fig 10-47l The lingual incline of the mesiofacial cusp has been replaced in resin composite.

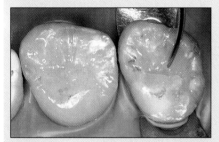

Fig 10-47m Each remaining cusp will be restored successively. Here the lingual incline of the distofacial cusp is being shaped with the PKT1. This increment will be cured for 5 seconds.

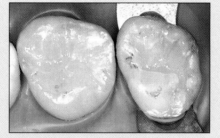

Fig 10-47n The completed lingual inclines of the facial cusps.

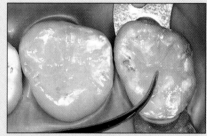

Fig 10-47o The facial incline of the lingual cusp is replaced in resin composite. Because this is the final resin composite increment, the entire occlusal surface will be light cured for the full irradition period.

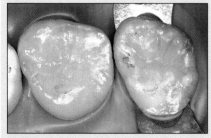

Fig 10-47p The completed occlusal anatomy using the successive cusp build-up technique. While this technique takes slightly longer during placement, it reduces finishing time.

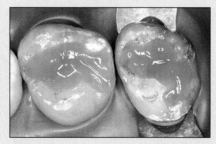

Fig 10-47q The restorations and adjacent enamel are re-etched.

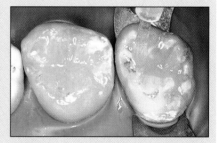

Fig 10-47r The restorations are sealed with a surface sealing resin (Fortify, Bisco).

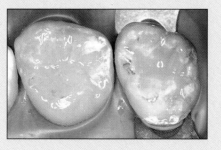

Fig 10-47s The completed restorations using the successive cusp build-up technique.

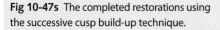

As a final step in resin composite placement and cure for Class 2 restorations, the wedge is removed and the matrix is wrapped against the adjacent tooth (Fig 10-48a). This allows access for the resin composite to be cured from the facial and lingual aspects to help ensure adequate polymerization throughout the entire restoration (see Fig 10-39). The matrix is allowed to remain in place to provide protection of the adjacent tooth during proximal-surface finishing (Fig 10-48b) and re-etching prior to sealing (Fig 10-48c).

Resin Composite Placement: Other Techniques

Materials other than VLC resin composites have been suggested for placement in the proximal box preparation. Autocured (or self-curing) resin composites are available for this purpose in both low- and high-viscosity formulations. It has been suggested that the portion of the autocured resin composite adjacent to the cavity preparation walls cures first, especially if used in conjunction with an autocured (or dual-cured) adhesive. The shrinkage of the autocured composite is said to be directed toward the cavity walls due to initiation of the curing reaction by the ongoing polymerization of the adhesive resin, and the reaction is said to be accelerated in that area by the higher temperature of the preparation walls due to body heat. This supposedly results in less polymerization shrinkage stress at the cavity margins,[177,178] thus improving marginal adaptation. However, research has failed to demonstrate either enhanced marginal adaptation[318] or reduced marginal leakage when this technique has been compared to VLC incremental placement techniques.[168]

Resin Composite Placement: Alternative Polymerization Techniques

A number of alternative techniques and devices have been introduced for curing VLC resin composites in recent years, including variable-curing-intensity halogen units, lasers, plasma arc high-intensity units, and light-emitting diode (LED) curing units (Figs 10-49a to 10-49d).

Argon laser units have demonstrated the ability to produce an increased degree of conversion of resin composite compared to standard halogen or tungsten-quartz-halogen light–curing units.[319] In addition, the depth of cure with the laser is improved,[319] and bond strength is less affected as the light guide is moved farther from the surface of the resin composite.[320] However, when the light guide is kept approximated to the composite increment, and increment depth is limited to 1.5 to 2 mm, no difference in bond strength is seen between that achieved with laser and standard halogen

lights.[320,321] Laser light is monochromatic,[320] with the bandwidth of the laser being much narrower than that of the halogen light and centered at approximately 470 nm, the maximal absorption wavelength for camphorquinone, the photoinitiator most commonly used in resin adhesives and resin composites.[319,322] However, some manufacturers are starting to use proprietary photoinitiators with absorption spectra differing from that of camphorquinone, making it possible that the argon laser curing unit would be less likely to initiate the polymerization reaction than would a halogen unit. The high price of these units, compared to other resin composite polymerization options, has limited their use in the profession.

Plasma arc curing (PAC) units generate notably higher irradiance levels than do standard halogen units. The purpose of this increased intensity is to increase the resin composite polymerization rate. Argon laser units also cure resin composite at a faster rate than do the halogen curing lights.[319] Considerable evidence has been accumulated to show that this increased rate of cure does not enhance adhesion of resin composite to cavity walls. Class 5 restorations cured with argon lasers or PAC units showed significantly increased microleakage[323] and poorer marginal adaptation[324] when compared to similar restorations cured with a standard halogen curing light. This is likely due to the fact that the rate at which the modulus of elasticity, or stiffness, of the setting composite develops has a significant impact on marginal integrity. Decreasing the polymerization reaction rate allows additional time for molecular conformational changes and material flow that can relieve polymerization shrinkage stress.[81,99] This has led to research in which the polymerization reaction rate is slowed even further by reducing the irradiance of halogen curing units. Lowering irradiance to 250 mW/cm² has been shown to significantly improve marginal adaptation in cavity preparations vs irradiating the resin composite in those same preparations at either 450 mW/cm² or 650 mW/cm².[100,325] There has been some concern, however, that simply reducing the irradiance to these levels, while enhancing marginal adaptation, might adversely affect physical properties.[325] This has led to the "two-step," "soft-start," or "ramped" curing technique. Regardless of the name, the underlying principle is the same: initial cure at diminished irradiance to initiate the polymerization reaction at a slower rate to minimize polymerization stress, followed by a period of higher irradiance to maximize degree of conversion and mechanical properties. In laboratory studies, this technique has proven to significantly enhance marginal adaptation without impairing mechanical properties.[102,103,324] However, recent research has demonstrated that resin composite factors such as shade, translucency, photoinitiator concentration, and

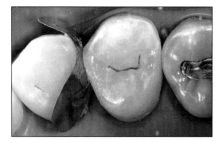

Fig 10-48a After the final resin composite increment has been placed and cured from the occlusal aspect, the wedge is removed and the matrix is wrapped against the adjacent tooth. This provides access for the proximal portion of the Class 2 restoration to be cured from the facial and lingual aspects to ensure maximal cure (see Fig 10-39).

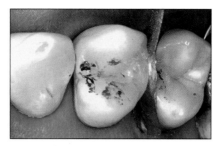

Fig 10-48b The matrix is allowed to remain in place during finishing to protect the adjacent tooth from inadvertent damage when finishing the proximal portion of the restoration.

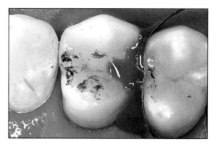

Fig 10-48c The matrix should also remain in place during re-etching and sealing to protect the adjacent tooth from being etched and bonded to the completed restoration.

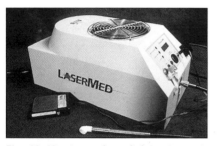

Fig 10-49a Argon laser light-curing unit (LaserMed).

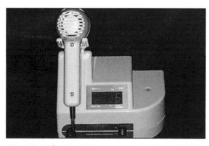

Fig 10-49b Variable-intensity halogen light-curing unit (Bisco).

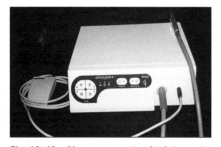

Fig 10-49c Plasma arc curing high-intensity light-curing unit (DMD).

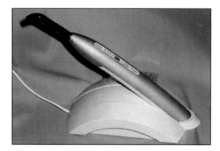

Fig 10-49d LED light-curing unit (3M/ESPE).

elastic modulus are more important in determining cure than a particular curing mode,[105,326] and that curing regimens that reduce polymerization shrinkage stress to a point that it is clinically significant are not feasible.[105]

Most recently developed are the LED curing units. These units have a number of advantages compared to other curing units, including a wavelength spectrum emission that is closely matched to camphorquinone. In addition, these units are more energy efficient, allowing them to be battery operated. The diodes have a life span that is approximately 1,000 times longer than the typical halogen bulb. While the earlier versions of LED curing units provided inadequate irradiance, the newer generation has overcome this deficiency. About the only disadvantage to these units is their narrow wavelength spectrum, limiting their usefulness in curing any materials that do not use camphorquinone as the photoinitiator.[327,328]

A 1999 evaluation of dental practices reported that 46% of the halogen visible light–curing units used in private practices provided inadequate output to cure resin composite.[329] More recent evaluations have shown an improvement in that percentage, but a large percentage of halogen units still have inadequate output.[330] It is important for the practitioner to

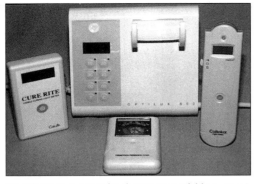

Fig 10-50 Commercial radiometers available to monitor adequacy of visible light–curing unit irradiance. (Courtesy of USAF Dental Evaluation and Consultation Service.)

ensure that the curing-light unit is in proper working condition and provides adequate and accurate irradiance. Testing of units can be conveniently accomplished with a radiometer (Fig 10-50).

Packable Resin Composites

"Condensable" or "packable" resin composites were specifically designed for posterior use. In these materials, the filler type, size, and/or particle distribution differ from those of conventional restorative hybrid and microfilled resin composite materials[331,332] in order to increase viscosity and impart a consistency that more closely mimics that of dental amalgam. Claims of enhanced clinical performance, reduced polymerization shrinkage, and enhanced wear characteristics have been made. The term *condensable* is not appropriate for these materials, since condensation, by definition, denotes an increase in density, as occurs when dental amalgam is condensed into a cavity preparation. Such a volume reduction does not occur with resin composites when they are pushed into a preparation.[331]

Considerable in vitro research has been accomplished to test these materials. In general, properties such as wear,[331,333–336] flexural modulus,[337,338] flexural strength,[337–339] fracture toughness,[337,340] and polymerization shrinkage[331] of the packable resin composites are comparable, but not superior, to those of other hybrid or reinforced microfilled resin composites currently available. One clinical study of a packable composite showed extreme and unacceptable wear.[341] Of particular concern with the packable resin composites is the claim by some manufacturers that these materials can be bulk-cured in thicknesses of 5 mm or greater. Independent research has clearly demonstrated that this is not the case, and adequate polymerization of the resin composite can be accomplished only in thicknesses of 2 mm or less.[229,340]

In general, practitioners can anticipate that the handling characteristics of the packable resin composite formulations may vary somewhat from other hybrid or microfilled materials. In particular, they may have a heavier consistency with a "drier" feel. Clinical trials of packable composites, mostly short-term, have demonstrated that, with proper technique, the clinical performance of these materials can be comparable to that of other resin composites.[342–344]

The decision to use these materials should be based on individual operator preference concerning handling characteristics and not on expectations of improved clinical performance.

Finishing

Placement procedures that minimize the need for finishing and polishing should be used. The smoothest surface that can be obtained is that of unfinished resin composite that has been cured against a smooth matrix.[345–348] Finishing and polishing procedures are inherently destructive to the restoration surface and may result in the formation of microcracks at and below the surface.[349,350] Because cracks may also be produced or exacerbated during mastication, the fracture toughness of the resin composite may be significantly reduced by destructive finishing techniques.[133]

Early finishing of resin composite (3 minutes after placement) has been shown to significantly increase microleakage.[351] Therefore, finishing should be delayed as long as is practical to minimize adverse effects. Delaying finishing for 10 to 15 minutes will allow approximately 70% of maximal polymerization to occur during the "dark-curing" phase following application of the curing light.[97,352]

A variation of the previously described soft-start technique for posterior resin composite restorations is the so-called pulse delay technique. With this technique, the final composite increment is cured for a brief period (3 to 5 seconds) at very low irradiance (150 mW/cm^2) to initiate the curing reaction at a reduced rate. After 3 to 5 minutes, the composite is again cured with a high level of irradiance. During the interim between the two curing periods, the occlusal surface is shaped and finished.[353] It should be noted, however, that the effects of manipulating this incompletely cured resin composite on physical properties and clinical performance have not been determined by independent research.

The finishing and polishing process for posterior resin composite restorations is similar to that used with other composites. A No. 12 or 12b scalpel blade, sharp No. 14L carver, Wedelstaedt chisel, or other thin, sharp-edged hand instrument is useful for removing flash from the proximal and gingival margins and for shaping proximal surfaces of resin composite (Figs 10-51a and 10-51b). The composite material can

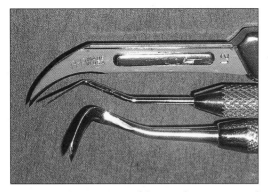

Fig 10-51a Instruments useful in initial contouring and removal of flash: *(top)* No. 12b scalpel blade; *(middle)* interproximal carver; *(bottom)* No. 14L carver.

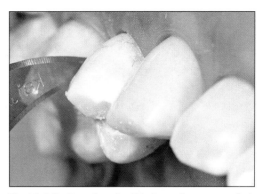

Fig 10-51b No. 12b scalpel blade used to remove flash from a resin composite restoration in the distal aspect of a maxillary first premolar.

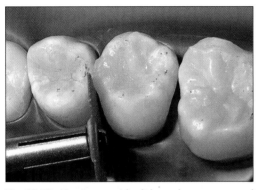

Fig 10-52 Aluminum oxide disk used to contour and polish the proximal surface of a resin composite restoration.

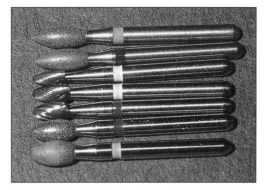

Fig 10-53 Fine diamonds and multifluted carbide burs for finishing resin composite restorations come in a variety of sizes, shapes, and grits.

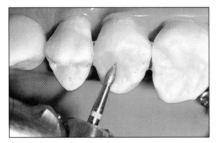

Fig 10-54a Finishing diamond used to refine occlusal anatomy in a resin composite restoration.

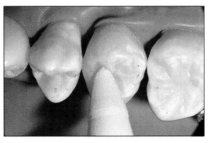

Fig 10-54b A flexible point impregnated with aluminum oxide is used for smoothing the occlusal surface of the restoration.

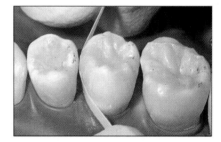

Fig 10-54c Aluminum oxide finishing strip for contouring/finishing/polishing the proximal surface gingival to the interproximal contact.

then be finished and blended to the tooth with successively finer grits of polishing points, cups, or disks. Aluminum oxide disks, used in series from coarse to very fine, tend to render some of the smoothest finishes to resin composite.[346,347,354] These work well for restoration contours that are relatively flat or convex, such as those in the facial and lingual proximal embrasure areas (Fig 10-52).

Abrasive disks are not practical for finishing occlusal surfaces. Shaping of these surfaces may be accomplished with multifluted carbide finishing burs or fine diamonds (Figs 10-53 and 10-54a). There is some controversy as to which of these instruments provides the smoothest surface and/or minimizes trauma-induced microleakage. Studies indicate that carbide finishing burs perform better,[354] finishing diamonds perform

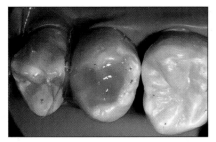

Fig 10-55a Etching the restoration margins prior to rebonding. Note the thin plastic shim placed interproximally to protect the adjacent tooth.

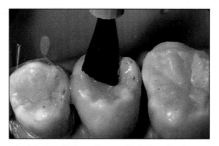

Fig 10-55b Rebonding resin is brushed onto the restoration surface and margins.

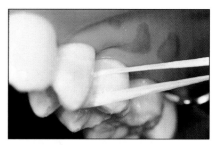

Fig 10-56 Proximal contact and contours are verified with dental floss. Floss is wrapped around the proximal contact to confirm appropriate contact area.

better,[355,356] or both perform equally well.[347,357] It is clear that the use of burs with 18 or fewer flutes leaves a significantly roughened surface, so these burs should not be the final rotary instruments used in the finishing process.[347] Rubber or silicone disks, points, cups, and brushes impregnated with aluminum oxide, silicon dioxide, or diamond particles have been found to provide very acceptable results[345–347,358,359] and can be used to smooth the resin composite surface after initial finishing (Fig 10-54b). Finishing strips coated with aluminum oxide particles can be used to finish proximal surfaces (Fig 10-54c). As with the disks, these strips should be used in series, from coarse to very fine grit. A final high polish may be accomplished using a rubber prophylaxis cup with aluminum oxide or diamond polishing pastes.

Rebonding and Final Cure

As previously mentioned, finishing procedures are destructive to the resin composite restoration and have been shown to adversely affect wear.[223] In addition, the composite surface that was closest to the light tip during curing, and therefore has the best mechanical properties, is removed during finishing procedures. Finishing procedures can also exacerbate the marginal gaps formed during polymerization.[82–84]

For these reasons, the occlusal surface and all accessible restoration margins should be rebonded with an unfilled VLC resin. The lower the viscosity of the rebonding resin, the more effective it will be in penetrating interfacial gaps and microcracks.[263,360] Several low-viscosity resins, called *surface sealers*, are available for use in rebonding. Rebonding, the application of a low-viscosity resin to the finished surface and margins of a restoration, has been shown to improve the marginal integrity of resin composite restorations in vitro[361] and in vivo,[226] significantly reduce microleakage in vitro,[360,362–364] and reduce marginal staining in vivo.[49] Rebonding has been demonstrated in clinical studies to significantly reduce wear and prolong marginal integrity.[49,226,361]

Although the need for etching before rebonding is somewhat controversial, phosphoric acid is usually applied to the marginal areas for 10 seconds (Fig 10-55a) and then rinsed off and the area thoroughly dried. The rebonding resin is placed, thinned with a blotted brush (Fig 10-55b) or applicator, and light cured for 20 to 40 seconds. This not only will polymerize the rebonding resin, but it may also provide additional polymerization of the resin composite.[129,152,154] To prevent the rebonding resin from joining the restored tooth to the adjacent tooth, a piece of matrix or other thin material may be placed interproximally prior to performing the rebonding procedure. Alternatively, floss is passed through the interproximal contact after the rebonding resin has been applied and before it is cured. After curing, any ledges of excess rebonding resin should be removed with a sharp-bladed instrument.

The proximal contact and contours are verified with dental floss (Fig 10-56). The rubber dam is removed, and the occlusion is checked. If further occlusal adjustment is required, rebonding resin should be reapplied in the areas that were adjusted.

The Tunnel Restoration

An alternative to the traditional approach for gaining access to proximal carious dentin has been termed the *tunnel preparation*. It was first suggested by Jinks[365] in 1963 as a method for placing a silver alloy mixed with sodium silicofluoride in the distal aspect of primary second molars to "inoculate" permanent first molars with fluoride as they erupted. Hunt[366] and Knight[367] later modified this procedure for use as a conservative technique for restoring teeth with small proximal caries lesions.

Advantages

Several advantages are claimed for this technique. The outer surface of the proximal enamel is removed only if cavitated by caries, so there is less potential for a restorative overhang. Overhangs have been shown to occur 25% to 76% of the time with traditional Class 2 restorations; this can lead to inflammation within periodontal tissues and bone loss.[368] With an occlusal approach, the marginal ridge is preserved, and destruction of tooth structure is minimized. A two-surface, Class 2 cavity preparation has been shown to reduce tooth stiffness by 46%; only a 20% reduction occurs with an occlusal preparation.[369] The perimeter of the restoration is reduced, decreasing the potential for microleakage.[370] Because minimal preparation is required interproximally, the potential for disturbance of the adjacent tooth is reduced. If the carious tooth structure is more extensive than originally thought and greater access is required, the preparation can easily be extended and converted into a more traditional Class 2 design.[371]

Disadvantages

Despite seemingly attractive benefits of the tunnel procedure, it remains largely unused in practice. It is a difficult procedure, demanding careful control of the preparation by the operator. The angulation of the bur for the preparation causes it to pass near the pulp. Studies have shown that the tunnel preparation often invades to within 1.0 mm of the pulp. A more traditional Class 2 preparation, in which penetration toward the pulp is determined by the depth of the caries lesion, tends to leave greater remaining dentinal thickness between the preparation and the pulp.[372,373] Because of the small entrance to the tunnel preparation, visibility is decreased, and removal of carious dentin is more uncertain.[366,371,374] In vitro studies on the effectiveness of caries lesion removal in the tunnel preparation have shown that there is a high rate of residual carious tooth structure after completion of the preparation.[373,375,376] For this reason, a caries-detecting solution should be used to disclose remaining carious tooth structure.

There is also concern that the marginal ridge is undermined and its strength reduced. As the diameter of the preparation increases, the marginal ridge strength decreases.[71,377,378] Although use of an adhesive restorative material has been shown to restore much of the strength of the marginal ridge,[71,377,378] this is not always the case,[372] and the degree to which marginal ridge strength is restored can depend on the size of the preparation.[377]

A number of clinical studies of tunnel restorations have been published (Table 10-5). Tunnel restorations tend to fail

Table 10-5 Longevity of tunnel restorations

Investigators	Study time (y)	No. of restorations	Annual failure rate (%)
Pilebro et al[379]	3	262	6.7
Strand et al[380]	3	161	10.0
Lumley and Fisher[381]	7	33	3.0
Hasselrot[382]	7	282	7.1

at a considerably higher rate than do other types of posterior restorations. Other problems noted in these studies include the fact that 34% to 41% of the restorations show either residual carious dentin or progression of enamel caries.[379,380] The most common causes of restoration failure are marginal ridge fracture and secondary caries. In an evaluation of tunnel restorations compared to slot amalgam restorations, 21% of tunnel restorations failed during a 7-year period compared to zero failures for the slot restorations.[381]

Indications and Contraindications

Tunnel restorations are rarely indicated. Consideration of the tunnel preparation should be limited to those patients with high esthetic demands and a low caries index who exhibit small, noncavitated proximal caries lesions that can be removed without penetrating the proximal surface.[380,382] This preparation should be avoided when large caries lesions are present, where access is particularly difficult, or when the overlying marginal ridge is subject to heavy occlusal loads or a crack in the marginal ridge is evident.

Preoperative Evaluation

The above factors must be assessed before the tunnel preparation is initiated. The occlusion should be marked with articulating tape.

Rubber Dam Isolation

For the reasons mentioned previously, use of a rubber dam is very important for this procedure.

Preparation

Access may be gained through the occlusal surface with a No. 2 round bur used in a high-speed handpiece and directed toward the caries lesion. The preparation should be started

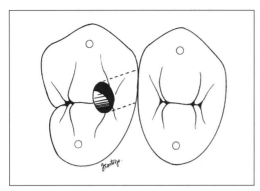

Figs 10-57a In the tunnel preparation, access is made in the occlusal fossa adjacent to the marginal ridge.

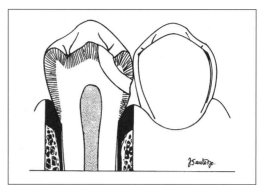

Fig 10-57b A "tunnel" is made under the marginal ridge to the carious dentin, usually just below the interproximal contact.

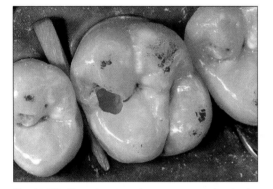

Fig 10-57c Tunnel preparation access opening in the maxillary first molar.

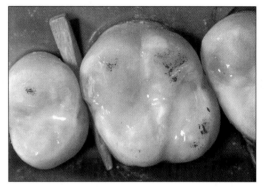

Fig 10-57d Tunnel restoration. Occlusal fissures have been sealed.

about 2.0 mm into the occlusal surface from the crest of the marginal ridge (Figs 10-57a and 10-57b). Removal of carious dentin can be accomplished with a No. 2 round bur in a low-speed handpiece. Because of the limited access, a caries-disclosing solution is needed to improve visualization of carious dentin.[371] Dentin stained with a caries-disclosing solution, unless very near the pulp, is removed.[383] Magnifying loupes help the clinician ascertain the completeness of removal of carious dentin.

After the carious dentin has been removed, the proximal enamel lesion is evaluated. If the proximal surface is intact, it is left alone.[371] The early enamel lesion is more resistant to caries attack than sound enamel[384] and should be left intact and allowed to remineralize. Tunnel restorations in which the proximal enamel is perforated, the so-called open tunnel restoration, tend to fail at a higher rate due to marginal ridge fracture.[380,382] If the clinician determines that the marginal ridge has been undermined, the tunnel preparation should be converted to a traditional Class 2 preparation.

Restoration

Glass ionomer was the original restorative material of choice. Cermet glass ionomers were originally used because of their radiopacity and fluoride release. Compared to amalgam, they have been shown to reduce occurrence of recurrent caries lesions around the restoration as well as in the adjacent tooth surface.[385] In addition, mutans streptococcus levels in plaque adjacent to proximal glass-ionomer restorations are lower than levels adjacent to either resin composite or amalgam restorations.[386,387] However, although one study showed good sealing in tunnel restorations with a glass-ionomer cermet,[388] another did not.[389] Another study showed that the use of cermet glass ionomer did not prevent lesion progression in many cases.[379]

RMGIs are the current materials of choice for this restoration. They are radiopaque and have been shown to prevent microleakage.[390] The glass ionomer should be placed in accordance with the manufacturer's recommendations, to approximately the level of the occlusal dentinoenamel junction.

Glass ionomer has shown a marked propensity to fail under occlusal stress.[391] Resin composites are more wear resistant than glass ionomers and may help to increase the fracture resistance of the restored tooth.[151] Therefore, the occlusal 1.5 to 2.0 mm of the preparation should be filled with a VLC resin composite, using the techniques previously described. Finishing and rebonding should be accomplished as described previously in this chapter. Figures 10-57c and 10-57d show a tunnel preparation and restoration.

References

1. Jordan RE, Suzuki M. Posterior composite restorations. Where and how they work best. J Am Dent Assoc 1991;122:30–37.
2. Leinfelder KF. Posterior composite resins. J Can Dent Assoc 1989; 55:34–39.
3. Leinfelder KF. Composite resin systems for posterior restorations. Pract Periodontics Aesthet Dent 1993;suppl 1:23–27.
4. American Dental Association. Survey of Dental Services Rendered. Chicago: American Dental Association, 1999.
5. American Dental Association. Distribution of Dentists in the U.S. by Region and State. Chicago: American Dental Association, 1999.
6. Eakle WS. Fracture resistance of teeth restored with Class II bonded composite resin. J Dent Res 1986;65:149–153.
7. Kasloff Z, Galan D, Williams PT. Cuspal deflection studies using an electronic probe [abstract 2264]. J Dent Res 1993;72:386.
8. Morin DL, Delong R, Douglas WH. Cusp reinforcement by the acid-etch technique. J Dent Res 1984;63:1075–1078.
9. Ferracane JL. Materials in Dentistry. Principles and Applications. Philadelphia: Lippincott, 1995:88–102.
10. Stangel I, Barolet RY. Clinical evaluation of two posterior composite resins: Two-year results. J Oral Rehabil 1990;17:257–268.
11. Hayashi M, Wilson NHF. Failure risk of posterior composites with post-operative sensitivity. Oper Dent 2003;28:681–688.
12. Kilpatrick NM. Durability of restorations in primary molars. J Dent 1993;21:67–73.
13. Van Dijken JW. Direct resin composite inlays/onlays: An 11 year follow-up. J Dent 2000;28:299–306.
14. Gaengler P, Hoyer I, Montag R. Clinical evaluation of posterior composite restorations: The 10-year report. J Adhes Dent 2001;3: 185–194.
15. Hickel R, Manhart R. Longevity of restorations in posterior teeth and reasons for failure. J Adhes Dent 2001;3:45–64.
16. Ferracane JL. Using posterior composites appropriately. J Am Dent Assoc 1992;123:53–58.
17. Leinfelder KF. Using a composite resin as a posterior restorative material. J Am Dent Assoc 1991;122:65–70.
18. Wilder AD Jr, May KN Jr, Bayne SC, Taylor DF, Leinfelder KF. Seventeen-year clinical study of ultraviolet-cured posterior composite Class I and II restorations. J Esthet Dent 1999;11:135–142.
19. Smales RJ, Webster DA, Leppard PI. Survival predictions of four types of dental restorative materials. J Dent 1991;19:278–282.
20. Smales RJ, Webster DA, Leppard PI. Survival predictions of amalgam restorations. J Dent 1991;19:272–277.
21. Osborne JW, Norman RD, Gale EN. A 14-year clinical assessment of 12 amalgam alloys. Quintessence Int 1991;22:857–864.
22. Crabb HSM. The survival of dental restorations in a teaching hospital. Br Dent J 1981;150:315–318.
23. Collins CJ, Bryant RW, Hodge KLV. A clinical evaluation of posterior composite resin restorations: 8-year findings. J Dent 1998;26: 311–317.
24. Letzel H, van't Hof MA, Vrijhoef MMA, Marshall GW Jr, Marshall SJ. A controlled clinical study of amalgam restorations: Survival, failures, and causes of failure. Dent Mater 1989;5:115–121.
25. Fukushima M, Setcos JC, Iwaku M. Posterior composite restoration failures in five-year clinical studies [abstract 792]. J Dent Res 1992; 71:204.
26. Fritz U, Fischbach H, Harke I. Langzeitverweildauer von Goldgussfüllungen. Deutsch Zahnärtzl Z 1992;47:714–716.
27. Bentley C, Drake CW. Longevity of restorations in a dental school clinic. J Dent Educ 1986;50:594–600.
28. Pallesen U, Qvist V. Clinical evaluation of three posterior composite resins: 10-year report [abstract 30]. J Dent Res 1995;74:404.
29. Barnes DM, Blank LW, Thompson VP, Holston AM, Gingell JC. A 5- and 8-year clinical evaluation of a posterior composite resin. Quintessence Int 1991;22:143–151.
30. Wilson NHF, Wilson MA, Wastell DG, Smith GA. Performance of Occlusin in butt-joint and bevel-edged preparations: Five-year results. Dent Mater 1991;7:92–98.
31. Letzel H. Survival rates and reasons for failure of posterior composite restorations in multicentre clinical trial. J Dent 1989;17:S10–S17.
32. Rowe AHR. A five year study of the clinical performance of a posterior composite resin restorative material. J Dent 1989;17:S6–S9.
33. Geurtsen W, Schoeler J, Layhausen G. 4-year retrospective clinical study of posterior hybrid composite fillings [abstract 629]. J Dent Res 1994;73:180.
34. Pallesen U, Qvist V. Composite resin fillings and inlays. An 11-year evaluation. Clin Oral Invest 2003;7:71–79.
35. Mair LH. Ten-year clinical assessment of three posterior resin composites and two amalgams. Quintessence Int 1998;29:483–490.
36. Manhart J, Garcia-Godoy F, Hickel R. Direct posterior restorations: Clinical results and new developments. Dent Clin North Am 2002; 46:303–339.
37. Jokstad A, Mjor IA, Qvist V. The age of restorations in situ. Acta Odontol Scand 1994;52:234–242.
38. Barnes DM, Holston AM, Strassler HE, Shires PJ. Evaluation of clinical performance of twelve posterior composite resins with a standardized placement technique. J Esthet Dent 1990;2:36–43.
39. Friedman J. Variability of lamp characteristics in dental curing lights. J Esthet Dent 1989;1:189–190.
40. Romcke RG, Lewis DW, Maze BD, Vickerson RA. Retention and maintenance of fissure sealants over 10 years. J Can Dent Assoc 1990;56:235–237.
41. Hickel R, Manhart J, Garcia-Godoy F. Clinical results and new developments of direct posterior restorations. Am J Dent 2000;13(spec. no.):41D–54D.
42. Bogacki R, Hunt R, del Aguila M, Smith W. Survival analysis of posterior restorations using an insurance claims database. Oper Dent 2002;27:488–492.
43. Wilson EG, Mandradjieff M, Brindock T. Controversies in posterior composite resin restorations. Dent Clin North Am 1990;34:27–44.
44. Willems G, Lambrechts P, Braem M, Vanherle G. Three-year follow-up of five posterior composites: In vivo wear. J Dent 1993;21:74–78.
45. Summit JB, Della Bona A, Burgess JO. The strength of Class II composite resin restorations as affected by preparation design. Quintessence Int 1994;25:251–257.

46. Warren JA, Clark NP. Posterior composite resin: Current trends in restorative techniques, part I. Pre-preparation considerations, preparation, dentin treatment, etching/bonding. Gen Dent 1987;35:368–372.

47. Hinoura K, Setcos JC, Phillips RW. Cavity design and placement techniques for Class 2 composites. Oper Dent 1988;13:12–19.

48. Black GV. A Work on Operative Dentistry. Chicago: Medico Dental Publishing, 1908.

49. Gibson GB, Richardson AS, Patton RE, Waldman R. A clinic evaluation of occlusal composite and amalgam restorations: One- and two-year results. J Am Dent Assoc 1982;104:335–337.

50. Lutz F, Phillips RW, Roulet JF, Setcos JC. In vivo and in vitro wear of potential posterior composites. J Dent Res 1984;63:914–920.

51. Suliman AA, Boyer DB, Lakes RS. Cusp movement in premolars resulting from composite polymerization shrinkage. Dent Mater 1993;9:6–10.

52. Douvitsas G. Effect of cavity design on gap formation in Class II composite resin restorations. J Prosthet Dent 1991;65:475–479.

53. Jacobsen PH. The restoration of Class II cavities by polymeric materials. J Dent 1984;12:47–52.

54. Castillo MD. Class II composite marginal ridge failure: Conventional vs. proximal box only preparation. J Clin Pediatr Dent 1999;23:131–136.

55. Kreulen CM, van Amerongen WE, Akerboom HB, Borgmeijer PJ. Two-year results with box-only resin composite restorations. ASDC J Dent Child 1995;62:395–400.

56. Nordbo H, Leirskar J, von der Fehr FR. Saucer-shaped cavity preparations for posterior approximal resin composite restorations: Observations up to 10 years. Quintessence Int 1998;29:5–11.

57. Busato AL, Loguercio AD, Reis A, de Oliveira Carrilho MR. Clinical evaluation of posterior composite restorations: 6-year results. Am J Dent 2001;14:304–308.

58. Manhart J, Chen HY, Mehl A, Weber K, Hickel R. Marginal quality and microleakage of adhesive Class V restorations. J Dent 2001;29:123–130.

59. Macpherson LC, Smith BG. Reinforcement of weakened cusps by adhesive restorative materials: An in-vitro study. Br Dent 1995;178:341–344.

60. Stamplia LL, Nicholls JI, Brudvik JS, Jones DW. Fracture resistance of teeth with resin-bonded restorations. J Prosthet Dent 1986;55:694–698.

61. Joynt RB, Wieczkowski G, Klockowski R, Davis EL. Effects of composite restorations on resistance to cuspal fracture in posterior teeth. J Prosthet Dent 1987;57:431.

62. Fissore B, Nicholls JI, Youdelis RA. Load fatigue of teeth restored by a dentin bonding agent and a posterior composite resin. J Prosthet Dent 1991;65:80–85.

63. Wahl M, Schmitt M, Overton D, Gordon M. Prevalence of cusp fractures in teeth restored with amalgam and with resin-based composite. J Am Dent Assoc 2004;135:1127–1132.

64. Espelid I, Tveit AB, Erickson RL, Keck SC, Glasspoole EA. Radiopacity of restorations and detection of secondary caries. Dent Mater 1991;7:114–117.

65. Toyooka H, Taira M, Wakasa K, Yamaki M, Fujita M, Wada T. Radiopacity of 12 visible-light-cured dental composite resins. J Oral Rehabil 1993;20:615–622.

66. Goshima T, Goshima Y. The optimum level of radiopacity in posterior composite resins. Dentomaxillofac Radiol 1989;18:19–21.

67. Goshima T, Goshima Y. Radiographic detection of recurrent carious lesions associated with composite restorations. Oral Surg Oral Med Oral Pathol 1990;70:236–239.

68. Curtis P, von Fraunhofer J, Farman A. The radiographic density of composite restorative resins. Oral Surg Oral Med Oral Pathol 1990;70:226–230.

69. Turgut M, Attar N, Önen A. Radiopacity of direct esthetic restorative materials. Oper Dent 2003;28:508–514.

70. Sabbagh J, Vreven J, Leloup G. Radiopacity of resin-based materials measured in film radiographs and storage phosphor plate (Digora). Oper Dent 2004;29:677–684.

71. Akerboom HBM, Dreulen CM, van Amerongen WE, Mol A. Radiopacity of posterior composite resins, composite resin luting cements, and glass ionomer lining cements. J Prosthet Dent 1993;70:351–355.

72. Dawson AS, Smales RJ. Restoration longevity in an Australian defence force population. Aust Dent J 1992;37(3):196–200.

73. Klausner LH, Green TG, Charbeneau GT. Placement and replacement of amalgam restorations. Oper Dent 1987;12:105–111.

74. Robbins JW, Summitt JB. Longevity of complex amalgam restorations. Oper Dent 1988;13:54–57.

75. Life Science Research Office. Review and Analysis of the Literature on the Potential Adverse Health Effects of Dental Amalgam. Available at: http://www.lsro.org/amalgam/frames_amalgam_home.html. Accessed 26 May 2005.

76. Bonner P. Advances in dental materials: An exclusive interview with Dr. Karl Leinfelder. Dent Today 1994;March:32–34.

77. Bryant RW. Direct posterior composite resin restorations: A review. 1. Factors influencing case selection. Aust Dent J 1992;37(2):81–87.

78. Douglas DD. Environmental cops hot on the trail of mercury discharge: Dentists avert mercury pollution rules. AGD Impact 1995;23:8–12.

79. FDI. Amalgam update. FDI Dent World 1992;14–15.

80. Bowen RL, Marjenhoff WA. Dental composites/glass ionomers: The materials. Adv Dent Res 1992;6:44–49.

81. Feilzer AJ, de Gee AJ, Davidson CL. Curing contraction of composites and glass-ionomer cements. J Prosthet Dent 1988;59:297–300.

82. Eick JD, Welch FH. Polymerization shrinkage of posterior composite resins and its possible influence on postoperative sensitivity. Quintessence Int 1986;17:103.

83. Lambrechts P, Braem M, Vanherle G. Evaluation of clinical performance for posterior composite resins and dentin adhesives. Oper Dent 1987;12:53–87.

84. Lutz F, Krejci I, Barbakow F. Quality and durability of marginal adaptation in bonded composite restorations. Dent Mater 1991;7:107–113.

85. Mazer RB, Leinfelder KF, Russell CM. Degradation of microfilled posterior composite. Dent Mater 1992;8(3):185–189.

86. Pearson GJ, Hegarty SM. Cusp movement of molar teeth with composite filling materials in conventional and modified MOD cavities. Br Dent J 1989;166:162–165.

87. Marzouk MA, Ross JA. Cervical enamel crazings associated with occluso-proximal composite restorations in posterior teeth. Am J Dent 1989;2:333–337.

88. Wieczkowski F, Joynt RB, Klockowski R, Davis EL. Effects of incremental versus bulk fill technique on resistance to cuspal fracture of teeth restored with posterior composites. J Prosthet Dent 1988;60:283–287.

89. Versluis A, Tantbirojn D, Douglas WH. Do dental composites always shrink toward the light? J Dent Res 1998;77:1435–1445.

90. Suh B, Wang Y. Determining the direction of shrinkage in dental composites by changes in surface contour for different bonding configurations. Am J Dent 2001;14:109–113.

91. Feilzer AJ, de Gee AJ, Davidson CL. Setting stress in composite resin in relation to configuration of the restoration. J Dent Res 1987;66: 1636–1639.

92. Eichmiller FC. Clinical use of beta-quartz glass-ceramic inserts. Compend Contin Educ Dent 1992;13(7):568–574.

93. Donly KJ, Wild TW, Bowen RL, Jensen ME. An in vitro investigation of the effects of glass inserts on the effective composite resin polymerization shrinkage. J Dent Res 1989;68:1234–1237.

94. Applequist EA, Meiers JC. Effect of bulk insertion, prepolymerized resin composite balls, and beta-quartz inserts on microleakage of Class V resin composite restorations. Quintessence Int 1996;27: 253–258.

95. Coli P, Derhami K, Brannstrom M. In vitro marginal leakage around Class II resin composite restorations with glass-ceramic inserts. Quintessence Int 1997;28:755–760.

96. Sjogren G, Hedlund SO, Jonsson C, Sandstrom A. A 3-year follow-up study of preformed beta-quartz glass-ceramic insert restorations. Quintessence Int 2000;31:25–31.

97. Alster D, Feilzer AJ, De Gee AJ, Mol A, Davidson CL. The dependence of shrinkage stress reduction on porosity concentration in thin resin layers. J Dent Res 1992;71:1619–1622 [erratum 1993;72:87].

98. Feilzer AJ, de Gee AJ, Davidson CL. Setting stresses in composites for two different curing modes. Dent Mater 1993;9:2–5.

99. Kemp-Scholte CM, Davidson CL. Marginal integrity related to bond strength and strain capacity of composite resin restorative systems. J Prosthet Dent 1990;64:658–664.

100. Feilzer AJ, Dooren LH, de Gee AJ, Davidson CL. Influence of light intensity on polymerization shrinkage and integrity of restoration-cavity interface. Eur J Oral Sci 1995;103:322–326.

101. Goracci G, Mori G, Casa de'Martinis L. Curing light intensity and marginal leakage of resin composite restorations. Quintessence Int 1996;27:355–362.

102. Koran P, Kurschner R. Effect of sequential versus continuous irradiation of a light-cured resin composite on shrinkage, viscosity, adhesion, and degree of polymerization. Am J Dent 1998;11:17–22.

103. Mehl A, Hickel R, Kunzelmann K-H. Physical properties and gap formation of light-cured composites with and without 'softstart-polymerization.' J Dent 1997;25:321–330.

104. Uno S, Asmussen E. Marginal adaptation of a restorative resin polymerized at reduced rate. Scand J Dent Res 1991;99:440–444.

105. Lim BS, Ferracane JL, Sakaguchi RL, Condon JR. Reduction of polymerization contraction stress for dental composites by two-step light-activation. Dent Mater 2002;18:436–444.

106. Eick J, Robinson S, Byerley TJ, Chappelow CC. Adhesives and non-shrinking dental resins of the future. Quintessence Int 1993;24: 632–640.

107. Glantz P-OJ, Nilner K, Jendresen MD, Sundberg H. Quality of fixed prosthodontics after 15 years. Acta Odontol Scand 1993;51:247–252.

108. Willems G, Lambrechts P, Braem M, Vanherle G. Composite resins of the 21st century. Quintessence Int 1993;24:641–658.

109. Qvist V, Qvist J, Mjor IA. Placement and longevity of tooth-colored restorations in Denmark. Acta Odontol Scand 1990;48:305–311.

110. Opdam N, Loomans B, Roeters F, Bronkhorst E. Five-year clinical performance of posterior resin composite restorations placed by dental students. J Dent 2004;32:379–383.

111. Brunthaler A, König F, Lucas T, Sperr W, Schedle A. Longevity of direct resin composite restorations in posterior teeth. Clin Oral Invest 2003;7:63–70.

112. Dickinson GL, Gerbo LR, Leinfelder KF. Clinical evaluation of a highly wear resistant composite. Am J Dent 1993;6:85–87.

113. Wendt SL Jr, Leinfelder KR. Clinical evaluation of a posterior resin composite: 3-year results. Am J Dent 1994;7:207–211.

114. Zickert I, Emilson C-G, Krasse B. Correlation of level and duration of streptococcus mutans infection with incidence of dental caries. Infect Immun 1983;39:982–985.

115. Asmussen E. Softening of BISGMA-based polymers by ethanol and by organic acids of plaque. Scand J Dent Res 1984;92:257–261.

116. Perdigao J, Geraldeli S, Hodges JS. Total-etch versus self-etch adhesive: Effect on postoperative sensitivity. J Am Dent Assoc 2003; 134:1621–1629.

117. Bayne SC, Heymann HO, Swift EJ Jr. Update on dental composite restorations. J Am Dent Assoc 1994;125:687–701.

118. Brannstrom M. Infection beneath composite resin restorations: Can it be avoided? Oper Dent 1987;12:158–163.

119. Bryant RW, Mahler DB. Modulus of elasticity in bending of composites and amalgams. J Prosthet Dent 1986;56:243–248.

120. Willems G, Lambrechts P, Lesaffre E, Braem M, Vanherle G. Three-year follow-up of five posterior composites: SEM study of differential wear. J Dent 1993;21:79–86.

121. Türkün L, Aktener B, Ates M. Clinical evaluation of different posterior resin composite materials: A 7-year report. Quintessence Int 2003;34:418–426.

122. Bailey SJ, Swift EJ Jr. Effects of home bleaching products on composite resins. Quintessence Int 1992;23:489–494.

123. Ferracane JL, Marker VA. Solvent degradation and reduced fracture toughness in aged composites. J Dent Res 1992;71:13–19.

124. Hengchang X, Tong W, Vingerling PA, Shiqing S. A study of surfaces developed on composite resins in vivo during 45 years; observations by SEM. J Oral Rehabil 1989;16:407–416.

125. Wu W, Toth EE, Ellison JA. Subsurface damage layer of in vivo worn dental composite restorations. J Dent Res 1984;63:675–680.

126. Mair LH, Vowles RW, Cunningham J, Williams DF. The clinical wear of three posterior composites. Br Dent J 1990;169:355–360.

127. Johnson WW, Dhuru VB, Brantley WA. Composite microfiller content and its effect on fracture toughness and diametral tensile strength. Dent Mater 1993;9:95–98.

128. Ferracane JL, Mitchem JC, Condon JR, Todd R. Wear and marginal breakdown of composites with various degrees of cure. J Dent Res 1997;76:1508–1516.

129. Bayne SC, Taylor DF, Heymann HO. Protection hypothesis for composite wear. Dent Mater 1992;8:305–309.

130. Gerbo L, Leinfelder KF, Mueninghoff L, Russell C. Use of optical standards for determining wear of posterior composite resins. J Esthet Dent 1990;2:148–152.

131. Mitchem JC, Gronas DG. In vivo evaluation of the wear of restorative resin. J Am Dent Assoc 1982;104:333–335.

132. Lambrechts P, Braem M, Vuylsteke-Wauters M, Vanherle G. Quantitative in vivo wear of human enamel. J Dent Res 1989;68: 1752–1754.

133. Ferracane JL, Antonio R, Matsumoto H. Variables affecting the fracture toughness of dental composites. J Dent Res 1987;66: 1140–1145.

134. Lutz F, Krejci I, Barbakow F. Chewing pressure vs. wear of composites and opposing enamel cusps. J Dent Res 1992;71:1525–1529.

135. Cunningham J, Mair LH, Foster MA, Ireland RS. Clinical evaluation of three posterior composite and two amalgam restorative materials: 3-year results. Br Dent J 1990;169:319–323.

136. Wang J-C, Charbeneau GT, Gregory WA, Dennison JB. Quantitative evaluation of approximal contacts in Class 2 composite resin restorations: A clinical study. Oper Dent 1989;14:193–202.

137. Wendt S, Ziemiecki T, Leinfelder K. Proximal wear rates by tooth position of resin composite restorations. J Dent 1996;24:33–39.

333

138. Baratieri L, Ritter A. Four-year clinical evaluation of posterior resin-based composite restorations placed using the total-etch technique. J Esthet Restor Dent 2001;13:50–57.

139. Wilson M, Cowan A, Randall R, Crisp R, Wilson N. A practice-based, randomized, controlled clinical trial of a new resin composite restorative: One-year results. Oper Dent 2002;27:423–429.

140. Hendriks FHJ, Letzel H, Vrijhoef MMA. Composite versus amalgam restorations: A three-year clinical evaluation. J Oral Rehabil 1986; 13:401–411.

141. Wilson HJ. Resin-based restoratives. Br Dent J 1988;164:326–330.

142. Hilton TJ, Ferracane JL, Condon JR. The effect of collodial silica surface treatment on composite wear [abstract 2741]. J Dent Res 1999;78:448.

143. Craig RG, ed. Dental Restorative Materials. St Louis: Mosby, 1989.

144. Versluis A, Douglas WH, Sakaguchi RL. Thermal expansion coefficient of dental composites measured with strain gauges. Dent Mater 1996;12:290–294.

145. Bullard RH, Leinfelder KF, Russell CM. Effect of coefficient of thermal expansion on microleakage. J Am Dent Assoc 1988;116: 871–874.

146. Söderholm KJ, Zigan M, Ragan M, Fischlschweiger W, Bergman M. Hydrolytic degradation of dental composites. J Dent Res 1984;63: 1248–1254.

147. Mitchem JC. The use and abuse of aesthetic materials in posterior teeth. Int Dent J 1988;38:119–125.

148. Koike T, Hasegawa T, Manabe A, Itoh K, Wakumoto S. Effect of water sorption and thermal stress on cavity adaptation of dental composites. Dent Mater 1990;6:178–180.

149. Venhoven BA, DeGee AJ, Davidson C. Polymerization contraction and conversion of light-curing BisGMA-based methacrylate resins. Biomaterials 1993;14:871–874.

150. Ferracane J, Greener E. Fourier transform infrared analysis of degree of polymerization in unfilled resins—Methods comparison. Dent Res 1984;63:1093–1095.

151. Asmussen E. Factors affecting the quantity of remaining double bonds in restorative resin polymers. Scand J Dent Res 1982;90: 490–496.

152. Rueggeberg FA, Caughman WF, Curtis JW Jr, Davis HC. Factors affecting cure at depths within light-activated resin composites. Am J Dent 1993;6:91–95.

153. Pires JAF, Cvitko E, Denehy GE, Swift EJ. Effects of curing tip distance on light intensity and composite resin microhardness. Quintessence Int 1993;24:517–521.

154. Rueggeberg FA, Jordan DM. Effect of light-tip distance on polymerization of resin composite. Int J Prosthodont 1993;6:364–370.

155. Retief DH, Mandras RS, Russell CM. Shear bond strength required to prevent microleakage at the dentin/restoration interface. Am J Dent 1994;7:43–46.

156. Sorensen JA, Dixit NV, White SN, Avera SP. In vitro microleakage of dentin adhesives. J Am Dent Assoc 1991;4:213–218.

157. Tyas MJ. Clinical evaluation of five adhesive systems. Am J Dent 1994;7:77–80.

158. Coli P, Brannstrom M. The marginal adaptation of four different bonding agents in Class II composite resin restorations applied in bulk or in two increments. Quintessence Int 1993;24:583–591.

159. Watanabe I, Nakabayashi N. Bonding durability of photocured phenyl-P in TEGDMA to smear layer-retained bovine dentin. Quintessence Int 1993;24:335–342.

160. Hansen EK. In vivo cusp fracture of endodontically treated premolars restored with MOD amalgam or MOD resin fillings. Dent Mater 1988;4:169–173.

161. Schwartz R, Murchison D, Hermesch C, et al. Three year clinical evaluation of three dentin treatments [abstract 1188]. J Dent Res 1997;76:162.

162. Hashimoto M, Ohno H, Kaga M, Endo K, Sano H, Oguchi H. In vivo degradation of resin-dentin bonds in humans over 1 to 3 years. J Dent Res 2000;79:1385–1391.

163. Frankenberger R, Kramer N, Petschelt A. Technique sensitivity of dentin bonding: Effect of application mistakes on bond strength and marginal adaptation. Oper Dent 2000;25:324–330.

164. Mair LH. Wear patterns in two amalgams and three posterior composites after 5 years' clinical service. J Dent 1995;23:107–112.

165. Mjor IA, Jokstad A. Five-year study of Class II restorations in permanent teeth using amalgam, glass polyalkenoate (ionomer) cerment and resin-based composite materials. J Dent 1993;21:338–343.

166. Abdalla AI, Davidson CL. Comparison of the marginal integrity of in vivo and in vitro Class II composite restorations. J Dent 1993;21: 158–162.

167. Ferrari M, Mannocci F, Kugel G, Garcia-Godoy F. Standardized microscopic evaluation of the bonding mechanism of NRC/Prime & Bond NT. Am J Dent 1999;12:77–83.

168. Hilton TJ, Schwartz RS, Ferracane JL. Microleakage of four Class II resin composite insertion techniques at intraoral temperature. Quintessence Int 1997;28:135–144.

169. Burgess JO, Summit JB, Robbins JW, et al. Clinical evaluation of base, sandwich and bonded Class 2 composite restorations [abstract 3405]. J Dent Res 1999;78:531.

170. Hubel S, Mejare I. Conventional versus resin-modified glass-ionomer cement for Class II restorations in primary molars. A 3-year clinical study. Int J Paediatr Dent 2003;13:2–8.

171. van Dijken J, Kieri C, Carlen M. Longevity of extensive Class II open-sandwich restorations with a resin-modified glass-ionomer cement. J Dent Rest 1999;78:1319–1325.

172. Vilkinis V, Horsted-Bindslev P, Baelum V. Two-year evaluation of Class II resin-modifed glass ionomer cement/composite open sandwich and composite restorations. Clin Oral Invest 2000;4:133–139.

173. Statement on posterior resin-based composites. ADA Council on Scientific Affairs; ADA Council on Dental Benefit Programs. J Am Dent Assoc 1998;129:1627–1628.

174. Williams PT, Johnson LN. Composite resin restoratives revisited. J Can Dent Assoc 1993;59:538–543.

175. Dlugokinski M, Browning WD. Informed consent: Direct posterior composite versus amalgam. J Am Coll Dent 2001;68:31–40.

176. American Dental Association. Dental Filling Options. Available at: http://www.ada.org/public/topics/fillings.asp. Accessed 27 May 2005.

177. Bertolotti RL. Posterior composite technique utilizing directed polymerization shrinkage and a novel matrix. Pract Periodontics Aesthet Dent 1991;3(4):53–58.

178. Fusayama T. Indications for self-cured and light-cured adhesive composite resins. J Prosthet Dent 1992;67:46–51.

179. Fusayama T. Biologic problems of the light-cured composite resin. Quintessence Int 1993;24:225–226.

180. Tyas MJ. Colour stability of composite resins: A clinical comparison. Aust Dent J 1992;37(2):88–90.

181. DeGee AJ. Some aspects of vacuum mixing of composite resins and its effects on porosity. Quintessence Int 1979;10:69–75.

182. Leinfelder KF. Composite resins. Dent Clin North Am 1985;29: 359–371.

183. Wilder AD, May KN, Leinfelder KF. Three-year clinical study of UV-cured composite resins in posterior teeth. J Prosthet Dent 1983; 50:26–30.

184. Tjan AHL, Bergh BH, Lidner C. Effect of various incremental techniques on the marginal adaptation of Class II composite resin restorations. J Prosthet Dent 1992;67:62–66.

185. Podshadley AG, Gullett CE, Binkley TK. Interface strength of incremental placement of visible light-cured composites. J Am Dent Assoc 1985;110:932–934.

186. Raskin A, Setcos J, Vreven J, Wilson N. Influence of the isolation method on the 10-year clinical behaviour of posterior resin composite restorations. Clin Oral Investig 2000;4:148–152.

187. Fritz U, Finger W, Stean H. Salivary contamination during bonding procedures with a one-bottle adhesive system. Quintessence Int 1998;29:567–572.

188. Abdalla A, Davidson C. Bonding efficiency and interfacial morphology of one-bottle adhesives to contaminated dentin surfaces. Am J Dent 1998;11:281–285.

189. van Schalkwyk J, Botha F, van der Vyver P, de Wet F, Botha S. Effect of biological contamination on dentine bond strength of adhesive resins. SADJ 2003;58:143–147.

190. Horowitz HS, Heifetz SB, Poulsen S. Retention and effectiveness of a single application of an adhesive sealant in preventing occlusal caries: Final report after five years of a study in Kalispell, Montana. J Am Dent Assoc 1977;95:1133–1139.

191. Going RE, Haugh LD, Grainger DA, Conti AJ. Four-year clinical evaluation of a pit and fissure sealant. J Am Dent Assoc 1977;95: 972–981.

192. Mertz-Fairhurst EJ, Fairhurst CW, Williams JE, Della-Giustina VE, Brooks JD. A comparative clinical study of two pit and fissure sealants: 7-year results in Augusta, GA. J Am Dent Assoc 1984; 109:252–255.

193. Barrie AM, Stephen KW, Kay EJ. Fissure sealant retention: A comparison of three sealant types under field conditions. Community Dent Health 1990;7:273–277.

194. Chestnutt IG, Schafer F, Jacobson APM, Stephen KW. The prevalence and effectiveness of fissure sealants in Scottish adolescents. Br Dent J 1994;177:125–129.

195. Shapira J, Fuks A, Chosack A, Houpt M, Eidelman E. A comparative clinical study of autopolymerized and light-polymerized fissure sealants: Five-year results. Pediatr Dent 1990;12:168–169.

196. Wendt LK, Koch G. Fissure sealant in permanent first molars after 10 years. Swed Dent J 1988;12:181–185.

197. Eklund SA, Ismail AI. Time of development of occlusal and proximal lesions: Implications for fissure sealants. J Public Health Dent 1986; 46:114–121.

198. Davenport S, Feigal R. Contact angle and penetrativity of bonding agents effective in wet-bonding. J Dent Res 1997;76:67.

199. Symons AL, Chu C-Y, Meyers IA. The effect of fissure morphology and pretreatment of the enamel surface on penetration and adhesion of fissure sealants. J Oral Rehabil 1996;23:791–798.

200. Hitt JC, Feigal RJ. Use of a bonding agent to reduce sealant sensitivity to moisture contamination: An in vitro study. Pediatr Dent 1992;14:41–46.

201. Tulunoglu O, Bodur H, Uctasli M, Alacam A. The effect of bonding agents on the microleakage and bond strength of sealant in primary teeth. J Oral Rehabil 1999;26:436–441.

202. Choi JW, Drummond JL, Dooley R, Punwani I, Soh JM. The efficacy of primer on sealant shear bond strength. Pediatr Dent 1997; 19:286–288.

203. Feigal RJ, Hitt J, Splieth C. Retaining sealant on salivary contaminated enamel. J Am Dent Assoc 1993;124:88–96.

204. Levy MP, Feigal RJ. Intermediate bonding agents increase clinical success of occlusal sealants on newly-erupted molars. J Dent Res 1996;75:179.

205. Feigal R, Musherure P, Gillespie B, Levy-Polack M, Quelhas I, Hebling J. Improved sealant retention with bonding agents: A clinical study of two-bottle and single-bottle systems. J Dent Res 2000;79:1850–1856.

206. Brocklehurst PR, Joshi RI, Northeast SE. The effect of air-polishing occlusal surfaces on the penetration of fissures by a sealant. Int J Paediatr Dent 1992;2:157–162.

207. Shapira J, Eidelman E. Six-year clinical evaluation of fissure sealants placed after mechanical preparation: A matched pair study. Pediatr Dent 1986;8:204–205.

208. Hatibovic-Kofman S, Wright GZ, Braverman I. Microleakage of sealants after conventional, bur, and air-abrasion preparation of pits and fissures. Pediatr Dent 1998;20:173–176.

209. Kramer PF, Zelante F, Simionato MR. The immediate and long-term effects of invasive and noninvasive pit and fissure sealing techniques on the microflora in occlusal fissures of human teeth. Pediatr Dent 1993;15:108–112.

210. Pereira AC, Basting RT, Pinelli C, de Castro Meneghim M, Werner CW. Retention and caries prevention of Vitremer and Ketac-bond used as occlusal sealants. Am J Dent 1999;12:62–64.

211. Smales RJ, Wong KC. 2-year clinical performance of a resin-modified glass ionomer sealant. Am J Dent 1999;12:59–61.

212. Autio-Gold JT. Clinical evaluation of a medium-filled flowable restorative material as a pit and fissure sealant. Oper Dent 2002;27: 325–329.

213. Boksman L, Carson B. Two-year retention and caries rates of Ultra-Seal XT and FluoroShield light-cured pit and fissure sealants. Gen Dent 1998;46:184–187.

214. Eklund SA. Factors affecting the cost of fissure sealants: A dental insurer's perspective. J Public Health Dent 1986;46:133–140.

215. Bader JD, Graves RC, Disney JA, et al. Identifying children who will experience high caries increments. Community Dent Oral Epidemiol 1986;14:198–201.

216. Disney JA, Graves RC, Stamm JW, Bohannan HM, Abernathy JR, Zack DD. The University of North Carolina Caries Risk Assessment study: Further developments in caries risk prediction. Community Dent Oral Epidemiol 1992;20:64–75.

217. Ulvestad H. Clinical trials with fissure sealant materials in Scandinavia. In: Silverstone LM, Dogon IL (eds). Proceedings of an International Symposium on the Acid Etch Technique. St Paul, MN: North Central Publishing, 1975:165–174.

218. Simonsen RJ. Preventive resin restorations (I). Quintessence Int 1978;9:69–76.

219. Simonsen RJ. Preventive resin restorations (II). Quintessence Int 1978;9:95–102.

220. Simonsen RJ, Stallard RE. Sealant-restorations utilizing a diluted filled composite resin: One year results. Quintessence Int 1977; 8(6):77–84.

221. Welbury RR, Walls AWG, Murray JJ, McCabe JF. The management of occlusal caries in permanent molars. A 5-year clinical trial comparing a minimal composite with an amalgam restoration. Br Dent J 1990;169:361–366.

222. Stadtler P. A 3-year clinical study of a hybrid composite resin as fissure sealant and as restorative material for Class I restorations. Quintessence Int 1992;23:759–762.

223. King NM, Yung LKM, Holmgren CJ. Clinical performance of preventive resin restorations placed in a hospital environment. Quintessence Int 1996;27:627–632.

224. Houpt M, Fukus A, Eidelman E. The preventive resin (composite resin/sealant) restoration: Nine-year results. Quintessence Int 1994; 25:155–159.

225. Mertz-Fairhurst EJ, Curtis JW Jr, Ergle JW, Rueggeberg FA, Adair SM. Ultraconservative and cariostatic sealed restorations: Results at year 10. J Am Dent Assoc 1998;129:55–66.

226. Granath L, Schroder U, Sundin B. Clinical evaluation of preventive and Class-I composite resin restorations. Acta Odontol Scand 1992; 50:359–364.

227. Kawai K, Leinfelder KF. Effect of surface-penetrating sealant on composite wear. Dent Mater 1993;9:108–113.

228. Lang LA, Burgess JO, Lang BR, Wang R-F. Wear of composite resin restorations in beveled and nonbeveled preparations [abstract 1226]. J Dent Res 1995;74(special issue):165.

229. Charlton D. SureFil high density posterior restorative. USAF Dental Items of Significance 1999;58:11.

230. Hilton T. Solitaire. USAF Dental Items of Significance 1999;56:16.

231. Lussi A, Gygax M. Iatrogenic damage to adjacent teeth during classical approximal box preparation. J Dent 1998;26:435–441.

232. Qvist V, Johannessen L, Brunn M. Progression of approximal caries in relation to iatrogenic preparation damage. J Dent Res 1992; 71(7):1370–1373.

233. Munechika T, Suzuki K, Nishiyama M, Ohashi M, Horie K. A comparison of the tensile bond strengths of composite resins to longitudinal and transverse sections of enamel prisms in human teeth. J Dent Res 1984;63:1079–1082.

234. Qvist V, Strom C. 11-year assessment of Class-III resin restorations completed with two restorative procedures. Acta Odontol Scand 1993;51:253–262.

235. Opdam NJ, Roeters JJ, Kuijs R, Burgersdijk RC. Necessity of bevels for box only Class II composite restorations. J Prosthet Dent 1998; 80(3):274–279.

236. Opdam NJM, Roeters JJM, Burgersdijk RCW. Microleakage of Class II box-type composite restorations. Am J Dent 1998;11:160–164.

237. Dietschi D, Scampa U, Campanile G, Holz J. Marginal adaptation and seal of direct and indirect Class II composite resin restorations: An in vitro evaluation. Quintessence Int 1995;26:127–138.

238. Martin FE, Bryant RW. Acid-etching of enamel cavity walls. Aust Dent J 1984;29:308–314.

239. Holan G, Eidelman E, Wright GZ. The effect of internal bevel on marginal leakage at the approximal surface of Class 2 composite restorations. Oper Dent 1997;22(5):217–221.

240. Isenberg BP, Leinfelder KF. Efficacy of beveling posterior composite resin preparations. J Esthet Dent 1990;2:70–73.

241. Grisanti LP 2nd, Troendle KB, Summitt JB. Support of occlusal enamel provided by bonded restorations. Oper Dent 2004;29:49–53.

242. Hinoura K, Moore BK, Phillips RW. Tensile bond strength between glass ionomer cement and composite resin. J Am Dent Assoc 1987; 114:167–172.

243. Yamamoto H, Iwami Y, Unezake T, Tomii Y, Tuchitani Y. Fluoride uptake around cavity walls; two-dimensional mapping by electron probe microanalysis (EPMA-WDX) method. Oper Dent 2000;25: 104–112.

244. Kemp-Scholte CM, Davidson CL. Complete marginal seal of Class V resin composite restorations effected by increased flexibility. J Dent Res 1990;69:1240–1243.

245. Hembree JH Jr. Microleakage at the gingival margin of Class II composite restorations with glass-ionomer liner. J Prosthet Dent 1989; 61:28–30.

246. Prati C. Early marginal microleakage in Class II resin composite restorations. Dent Mater 1989;5:392–398.

247. Krejci I, Lutz F, Krejci D. The influence of different base materials on marginal adaptation and wear of conventional Class II composite resin restorations. Quintessence Int 1988;19:191–198.

248. Goodis HE, White JM, Marshall SJ, Koshrovi P, Watanabe LG, Marshall GW Jr. The effect of glass ionomer liners in lowering pulp temperatures during composite placement, in vitro. Dent Mater 1993; 9:146–150.

249. Akpata ES, Sadiq W. Post-operative sensitivity in glass-ionomer versus adhesive resin-lined posterior composites. Am J Dent 2001;14: 34–38.

250. Aboushala A, Kugel G, Hurley E. Class II composite resin restorations using glass-ionomer liners: Microleakage studies. J Clin Pediatr Dent 1996;21:67–71.

251. Miller MB, Castellanos ER, Vargas MA, Denehy GE. Effect of restorative materials on microleakage of Class II composites. J Esthet Dent 1996;8:107–113.

252. Loguercio AD, Alessandra R, Mazzocco KC, et al. Microleakage in Class II composite resin restorations: Total bonding and open sandwich technique. J Adhes Dent 2002;4:137–144.

253. Wibowo G, Stockton L. Microleakage of Class II composite restorations. Am J Dent 2001;14:177–185.

254. Hagge M, Lindemuth J, Mason J, Simon J. Effect of four intermediate layer treatments on microleakage of Class II composite restorations. Gen Dent 2001;49:489–495.

255. Retief D, McCaghren R, Russell C. Microleakage of Vitrebond/P-50 Class II restorations. Am J Dent 1992;5:130–132.

256. Hilton T, Quinn R. Marginal leakage of Class 2 composite/flowable restorations with varied cure technique [abstract 502]. J Dent Res 2001;80:589.

257. Herrera M, Castillo A, Bravo M, Liebana J, Carrion P. Antibacterial activity of resin adhesives, glass ionomer and resin-modified glass ionomer cements and a compomer in contact with dentin caries samples. Oper Dent 2000;25:265–269.

258. van Dijken J. A 6-year evaluation of a direct composite resin inlay/ onlay system and glass ionomer cement-composite resin sandwich restorations. Acta Odontol Scand 1994;5:368–376.

259. Andersson-Wenckert I, van Dijken J, Horstedt P. Modified Class II open-sandwich restorations: Evaluation of interfacial adaptation and influence of different restorative techniques. Eur J Oral Sci 2002;110:270–275.

260. Braga RR, Condon JR, Ferracane JL. In vitro wear simulation measurements of composite versus resin-modified glass ionomer luting cements for all-ceramic restorations. J Esthet Restor Dent 2002; 14:368–376.

261. Shabanian M, Richards LC. In vitro wear rates of materials under different loads and varying pH. J Prosthet Dent 2002;87:650–656.

262. Walshaw PR, McComb D. Microscopic features of clinically successful dentine bonding. Dent Update 1998;25:281–286.

263. Tay FR, Gwinnett AJ, Pang KM, Wei SHY. Variability in microleakage observed in a total-etch wet-bonding technique under different handling conditions. J Dent Res 1995;74:1168–1178.

264. Moon PC, Chang YH. Effect of DBA layer thickness on composite resin shrinkage stress [abstract 1375]. J Dent Res 1992;71:275.

265. Opdam NJM, Roeters FJM, Verdonschot EH. Adaptation and radiographic evaluation of four adhesive systems. J Dent 1997;25: 391–397.

266. Swift EJ, Triolo PT, Barkmeier WW, Bird JL. Effect of low-viscosity resins on the performance of dental adhesives. Am J Dent 1996; 9:100–104.

267. Hilton TJ, Schwartz RS. The effect of air thinning on dentin adhesive bond strength. Oper Dent 1995;20:133–137.

268. Langdon RS, Moon PC, Barnes RF. Effect of dentin bonding adhesive thickness on bond strength [abstract 244]. J Dent Res 1994; 73:132.

269. Hilton TJ, Schwartz RS, Ferracane JL. Fifth generation bonding application technique effects on bond strength [abstract 214]. J Dent Res 1998;77(special issue):132.

270. Lutz F, Krejci I, Luescher B, Oldenburg TR. Improved proximal margin adaptation of Class II composite resin restorations by use of light-reflecting wedges. Quintessence Int 1986;17:659–664.

271. Hilton T. Composi-Tight sectional matrix system. USAF Dental Items of Significance 1999;56:15.

272. Hilton T. Palodent sectional matrix system. USAF Dental Items of Significance 1999;56:14.

273. Crim GA. Microleakage of three resin placement techniques. Am J Dent 1991;4:69–72.

274. Opdam NJ, Feilzer AJ, Roeters JJ, Smale I. Class I occlusal composite resin restorations: In vivo post-operative sensitivity, wall adaptation, and microleakage. Am J Dent 1998;11:229–234.

275. Feilzer AJ, De Gee AJ, Davidson CL. Quantitative determination of stress reduction by flow in composite restorations. Dent Mater 1990;6:167–171.

276. Davidson CL, de Gee AJ, Feilzer A. The competition between the composite-dentin bond strength and the polymerization contraction stress. J Dent Res 1984;63:1396–1399.

277. Dauvillier B, Aarnts M, Feilzer A. Developments in shrinkage control of adhesive restoratives. J Esthet Dent 2000;12:291–299.

278. Yoshikawa T, Sano H, Burrow MF, Tagami J, Pashley DH. Effects of dentin depth and cavity configuration on bond strength. J Dent Res 1999;78:898–905.

279. Opdam NJM, Roeters FJ, Feilzer AJ, Smale I. A radiographic and scanning electron microscopic study of approximal margins of Class II resin composite restorations placed in vivo. J Dent 1998;26:319–327.

280. Bryant RW. Direct posterior composite resin restorations: A review. 2. Clinical technique. Aust Dent J 1992;37(3):161–171.

281. Ciamponi AL, Del Portillo Lujan VA, Santos JFF. Effectiveness of reflective wedges on the polymerization of composite resins. Quintessence Int 1994;25:599–602.

282. Lutz F, Krejci I, Barbakow F. Restoration quality in relation to wedge-mediated light channeling. Quintessence Int 1992;23:763–767.

283. Lutz E, Krejci I, Oldenburg TR. Elimination of polymerization stresses at the margins of posterior composite resin restorations: A new restorative technique. Quintessence Int 1986;17:777–784.

284. Opdam NJM, Roeters JJM, Peters TCRB, Burgersdijk RC, Kuijs RH. Consistency of resin composites for posterior use. Dent Mater 1996;12:350–354.

285. Opdam NJM, Roeters JJM, Peters TCRB, Burgersdijk RC, Teunis M. Cavity wall adaptation and voids in adhesive Class I resin composite restorations. Dent Mater 1996;12:230–235.

286. Holmes R, Blalock J, Rueggeberg F. Composite film thickness at various temperatures [abstract 3265]. J Dent Res 2004;81.

287. Aksu M, Neme A, Walker S, Pink F, Linger J, Wagner W. Effect of preheating composite on microleakage in Class II restorations [abstract 498]. J Dent Res 2004;81.

288. Trujillo M, Newman S, Stansbury J. Use of near-IR to monitor the influence of external heating on dental composite photopolymerization. Dent Mater 2004;20:766–777.

289. Li J, Nicander I, von Beetzen M, Sundstrom F. Influence of paste temperature at curing on conversion rate and bending strength of light-cured dental composites. J Oral Rehabil 1996;23:298–301.

290. Behle C. Flowable composites: Properties and applications. Pract Periodontics Aesthet Dent 1998;10:347, 350–351.

291. Bayne SC, Thompson JY, Swift EJ Jr, Stamatiades P, Wilkerson M. A characterization of first-generation flowable composites. J Am Dent Assoc 1998;129:567–577.

292. Labella R, Lambrechts P, Van Meerbeek B, Vanherle G. Polymerization shrinkage and elasticity of flowable composites and filled adhesives. Dent Mater 1999;15:128–137.

293. Tolidis K, Setcos JC. Initial degree of polymerization shrinkage exhibited by flowable composite resins [abstract 3015]. J Dent Res 1999;78:482.

294. Braga R, Hilton T, Ferracane J. Contraction stress of flowable composite materials and their efficacy as stress-relieving layers. J Am Dent Assoc 2003;134:721–728.

295. Oberholzer TG, Pameijer CH, Grobler SR, Rossouw RJ. The effect of different power densities and method of exposure on the marginal adaptation of four light-cured dental restorative materials. Biomaterials 2003;24:3593–3598.

296. Olmez A, Oztas N, Bodur H. The effect of flowable resin composite on microleakage and internal voids in Class II composite restorations. Oper Dent 2004;29:713–719.

297. Attar N, Turgut M, Gungor HC. The effect of flowable resin composites as gingival increments on the microleakage of posterior resin composites. Oper Dent 2004;29:162–167.

298. Chuang SF, Jin YT, Lin TS, Chang CH, Garcia-Godoy F. Effects of lining materials on microleakage and internal voids of Class II resin-based composite restorations. Am J Dent 2003;16:84–90.

299. Amin Parsa M, Kunzelmann K-H. Effect of the "lining technique" on marginal adaptation [abstract 1684]. J Dent Res 2000;79:354.

300. Russell RR, Mazer RB. Microleakage of Class II restorations using a flowable composite as a liner [abstract 203]. J Dent Res 1998;77:131.

301. Walshaw PR, McComb D. Microleakage in Class 2 resin composites with low-modulus, intermediate materials [abstract 204]. J Dent Res 1998;77:131.

302. Neme A, Maxson B, Pink F, Aksu M. Microleakage of Class II packable resin composites lined with flowables: An in vitro study. Oper Dent 2002;27:600–605.

303. Sensi LG, Marson FC, Monteiro S Jr, Baratieri LN, Caldeira de Andrada MA. Flowable composites as "filled adhesives:" A microleakage study. J Contemp Dent Pract 2004;5:32–41.

304. Rashid R, Ricks J, Monaghan P. Strengths of condensable composite resins with flowable liners [abstract 403]. J Dent Res 1999;78:156.

305. Frankenberger R, Kramer N, Pelka M, Petschelt A. Internal adaptation and overhang formation of direct Class II resin composite restorations. Clin Oral Investig 1999;3:208–215.

306. Murchison DF, Charlton DG, Moore WS. Comparative radiopacity of flowable resin composites. Quintessence Int 1999;30:179–184.

307. Bouschlicher M, Cobb D, Boyer D. Radiopacity of compomers, flowable and conventional resin composites for posterior restorations. Oper Dent 1999;24:20–25.

308. Perdigao J, Anauate-Netto C, Carmo A, et al. The effect of adhesive and flowable composite on postoperative sensitivity: 2-week results. Quintessence Int 2004;35:777–784.

309. Ernst C, Canbek K, Aksogan K, Willeshausen B. Two-year clinical performance of a packable posterior composite with and without a flowable composite liner. Clin Oral Investig 2003;7:129–134.

310. Opdam N, Roeters J, Deborri T, Peschier D, Bronkhorst E. Voids inside restored micropreparations using various resin composites and application techniques [abstract 3132]. J Dent Res 2002;81:A-389.

311. Jedrychowski JR, Bleier RG, Caputo AA. Shrinkage stresses associated with incremental composite filling techniques in conservative Class II restorations. ASDC J Dent Child 2001;68:161–167.

312. Ericson D, Derand T. Reduction of cervical gaps in Class II composite resin restorations. J Prosthet Dent 1991;65:33–37.

313. Ericson D, Paulsson L, Sowiak H, Derand T. Reduction of cusp deflection resulting from composite polymerization shrinkage, using a light-transmitting cone. Scand J Dent Res 1994;102:244–248.

314. von Beetzen M, Li J, Nicander I, Sundstrom F. Microhardness and porosity of Class 2 light-cured composite restorations cured with a transparent cone attached to the light-curing wand. Oper Dent 1993;18:103–109.

315. Warren JA, Clark NP. Posterior composite resin: Current trends in restorative techniques. Part 2: Insertion, finishing, and polishing. Gen Dent 1987;35:497–499.

316. Vandewalle KS, Munro GA, Gureckis KM. Esthetic occlusal composite resin restorations. J Esthet Dent 1994;6:73–76.

317. Liebenberg W. Successive cusp build-up: An improved placement technique for posterior direct resin restorations. J Can Dent Assoc 1996;62:501–507.

318. van Dijken JW, Horstedt P, Waern R. Directed polymerization shrinkage versus a horizontal incremental filling technique: Interfacial adaptation in vivo in Class II cavities. Am J Dent 1998;11:165–172.

319. Tarle Z, Meniga A, Ristic M, Sutalo J, Pichler G, Davidson CL. The effect of the photopolymerization method on the quality of composite resin samples. J Oral Rehabil 1998;25:436–442.

320. Hinoura K, Miyazaki M, Onose H. Influence of argon laser curing on resin bond strength. Am J Dent 1993;6:69–71.

321. Shanthala BM, Munshi AK. Laser vs visible-light cured composite resin: An in vitro shear bond study. J Clin Pediatr Dent 1995;19:121–125.

322. Bouschlicher MR, Vargas MA, Boyer DB. Effect of composite type, light intensity, configuration factor and laser polymerization on polymerization contraction forces. Am J Dent 1997;10:88–96.

323. Puppala R, Hegde A, Munshi AK. Laser and light cured composite resin restorations: In-vitro comparison of isotope and dye penetrations. J Clin Pediatr Dent 1996;20:213–218.

324. Burgess JO, DeGoes M, Walker R, Ripps AH. An evaluation of four light-curing units comparing soft and hard curing. Pract Periodontics Aesthet Dent 1999;11:125–132.

325. Unterbrink GL, Muessner R. Influence of light intensity on two restorative systems. J Dent 1995;23:183–189.

326. Sakaguchi R, Ferracane J. Effect of light power density on development of elastic modulus of a model light-activated composite during polymerization. J Esthet Restor Dent 2001;13:121–130.

327. Hammesfahr PD, O'Connor MT, Wang X. Light-curing technology: Past, present, and future. Compend Contin Educ Dent 2002 Sep;23(9 suppl 1):18–24.

328. Caughman W, Rueggeberg F. Shedding new light on composite polymerization. Oper Dent 2002;27:636–638.

329. Pilo R, Oelgiesser D, Cardash HS. A survey of output intensity and potential for depth of cure among light-curing units in clinical use. J Dent 1999;27:235–241.

330. Pham TA, Barghi N. Revisiting the intensity output of curing lights in private practices [abstract 3108]. J Dent Res 2005;84(special issue A).

331. Choi KK, Ferracane JL, Hilton TJ, Charlton D. Properties of packable dental composites. J Esthet Dent 2000;12:224–234.

332. Tabassian M, Moon PC. Filler particle characterization in flowable and condensible composite resins [abstract 3022]. J Dent Res 1999;78:483.

333. Barkmeier WW, Wilwerding TM, Latta MA, Blake SM. In vitro wear assessment of high density composite resins [abstract 2737]. J Dent Res 1999;78:448.

334. Dang HM, Sarrett DC. Wear behavior of flowable and condensable composite resins [abstract 2736]. J Dent Res 1999;78:447.

335. Knoblach L, Kerby R, Seghi R. Wear resistance of posterior condensable composite resins [abstract 2735]. J Dent Res 1999;78:447.

336. Suzuki S. In vitro wear of condensable resin composite restoratives [abstract 2734]. J Dent Res 1999;78:447.

337. Kelsey WP, Latta MA, Barkmeier WW. Physical properties of high density composite restorative materials [abstract 810]. J Dent Res 1999;78:207.

338. Ruddell DE, Thompson JY, Stamatiades PJ, et al. Mechanical properties and wear behavior of condensable composites [abstract 407]. J Dent Res 1999;78:156.

339. MacGregor KM, Cobb DS, Vargas MA. Physical properties of condensable versus conventional composites [abstract 411]. J Dent Res 1999;78:157.

340. Kerby R, Lee J, Knobloch L, Seghi R. Hardness and degree of conversion of posterior condensable composite resins [abstract 414]. J Dent Res 1999;78:157.

341. Flessa H-P, Simoncic B, Kunzelmann K-H, et al. Quantitative 3D wear analysis of composite fillings in vivo [abstract 1051]. J Dent Res 1998;78:237.

342. Yip K, Poon B, Chu F, Poon E, Kong F, Smales R. Clinical evaluation of packable and conventional hybrid resin-based composites for posterior restorations in permanent teeth: Results at 12 months. J Am Dent Assoc 2003;134:1581–1589.

343. Lopes L, Cefaly D, Franco E, Mondelli R, Lauris J, Navarro M. Clinical evaluation of two "packable" posterior composite resins: Two-year results. Clin Oral Investig 2003;7:123–128.

344. Turkun LS, Turkun M, Ozata F. Two-year clinical evaluation of a packable resin-based composite. J Am Dent Assoc 2003;134:1205–1212.

345. Chung KH. Effects of finishing and polishing procedures on the surface texture of resin composites. Dent Mater 1994;10:325–330.

346. Hoelscher DC, Neme AML, Pink FE, Hughes PJ. The effect of three finishing systems on four esthetic restorative materials. Oper Dent 1998;23:36–42.

347. Hondrum SO, Fernandez RJ. Contouring, finishing and polishing Class 5 restorative materials. Oper Dent 1997;22:30–36.

348. Pratten DH, Johnson GH. An evaluation of finishing instruments for an anterior and a posterior composite. J Prosthet Dent 1988;60:154–158.

349. Leinfelder KF, Wilder AD, Teixeira ER. Wear rates of posterior composite resins. J Am Dent Assoc 1986;112:829–833.

350. Wu W, Cobb EN. A silver staining technique for investigating wear of restorative dental composites. J Biomed Mater Res 1981;15:343–348.

351. Fusayama A, Kohno A. Marginal closure of composite restorations with the gingival wall in cementum/dentin. J Prosthet Dent 1989;61:293.

352. Albers HE. Direct composite restoratives. Adept Report 1991;2:53–64.

353. Kanca IJ, Suh B, Vinson W. Pulse activation of resin composite: Reducing stresses at cavosurface interfaces [abstract 678]. J Dent Res 1998;77:190.

354. Berastegui E, Canalda C, Brau E, Miquel C. Surface roughness of finished composite resins. J Prosthet Dent 1992;68:742–749.

355. Ashe MJ, Tripp GA, Eichmiller FC, George LA, Meiers JC. Surface roughness of glass-ceramic insert-composite restorations: Assessing several polishing techniques. J Am Dent Assoc 1996;127:1495–1500.

356. Kaplan BA, Goldstein GR, Vijayaraghavan TV, Nelson IK. The effect of three polishing systems on the surface roughness of four hybrid composites: A profilometric and scanning electron microscopy study. J Prosthet Dent 1996;76:34–38.

357. Brackett WW, Gilpatrick RO, Gunnin TD. Effect of finishing method on the microleakage of Class V resin composite restorations. Am J Dent 1997;10:189–191.

358. Yap A, Yap S, Teo C, Ng J. Finishing/polishing of composite and compomer restoratives: Effectiveness of one-step systems. Oper Dent 2004;29:275–279.

359. Reis A, Giannini M, Lovadino J, Ambrosano G. Effects of various finishing systems on the surface roughness and staining susceptibility of packable composite resins. Dent Mater 2003;19:12–18.

360. Reid JS, Saunders WP, Chen YY. The effect of bonding agent and fissure sealant on microleakage of composite resin restorations. Quintessence Int 1991;22:295–298.

361. Dickinson GL, Leinfelder KF. Assessing the long-term effect of a surface penetrating sealant. J Am Dent Assoc 1993;124:68–72.

362. Garcia-Godoy F. Microleakage of posterior composite restorations after rebonding. Compend Contin Educ Dent 1987;8:606–609.

363. Tjan AHL, Tan DE. Microleakage at gingival margins of Class V composite resin restorations rebonded with various low-viscosity resin systems. Quintessence Int 1991;22:565–573.

364. Torstenson B, Brannstrom M. A new method for sealing composite resin contraction gaps in lined cavities. J Am Dent Assoc 1985;64:450–453.

365. Jinks GM. Fluoride-impregnated cements and their effect on the activity of interproximal caries. J Dent Child 1963;30:87–92.

366. Hunt PR. A modified Class II cavity preparation for glass ionomer restorative materials. Quintessence Int 1984;15:1011–1018.

367. Knight GM. The use of adhesive materials in the conservative restoration of selected posterior teeth. Aust Dent J 1984;29:324–331.

368. Brunsvold MA, Lane JJ. The prevalence of overhanging dental restorations and their relationship to periodontal disease. J Clin Periodontol 1990;17:67–72.

369. Reeh ES, Messer HH, Douglas WH. Reduction in tooth stiffness as a result of endodontic and restorative procedures. J Endod 1989;15:512–516.

370. Papa J, Wilson PR, Tyas MJ. Tunnel restorations: A review. Quintessence Int 1992;4:4–9.

371. Hunt PR. Microconservative restorations for approximal carious lesions. J Am Dent Assoc 1990;120:37–40.

372. Papa J, Cain C, Messer HH, Wilson PR. Tunnel restorations versus Class II restorations for small proximal lesions: A comparison of tooth strengths. Quintessence Int 1993;24:93–98.

373. Strand GV, Tveit AB. Effectiveness of caries removal by the partial tunnel preparation. Scand J Dent Res 1993;101:270–273.

374. Zenkner J, Baratieri LN, Monteiro SJ, et al. Clinical and radiographic evaluation of cement tunnel restorations on primary molars. Quintessence Int 1993;24:783–791.

375. Papa J, Cain C, Messer HH. Efficacy of tunnel restorations in the removal of caries. Quintessence Int 1993;24:715–719.

376. Strand GV, Tveit AB, Espelid I. Variations among operators in the performance of tunnel preparations in vitro. Scand J Dent Res 1994;102:151–155.

377. Fasbinder DJ, Davis RD, Burgess JO. Marginal ridge strength in Class II tunnel restorations. Am J Dent 1991;4:77–82.

378. Hill FJ, Halaseh FJ. A laboratory investigation of tunnel restorations in premolar teeth. Br Dent J 1988;165:364–367.

379. Pilebro CE, van Dijken JWV, Stenberg R. Durability of tunnel restorations in general practice: A three-year multicenter study. Acta Odontol Scand 1999;57:35–39.

380. Strand GV, Nordbo H, Tveit AB, Espelid I, Wikstrand K, Eide GE. A 3-year clinical study of tunnel restorations. Eur J Oral Sci 1996;104:384–389.

381. Lumley PJ, Fisher FJ. Tunnel restorations: A long-term pilot study over a minimum of five years. J Dent 1995;23:213–215.

382. Hasselrot L. Tunnel restorations in permanent teeth. A 7 year follow up study. Swed Dent J 1998;22:1–7.

383. Sato Y, Fusayama T. Removal of dentin by fuchsin staining. Dent Res 1976;55:678–683.

384. Kidd EA, Joyston-Bechal S. Susceptibility of natural carious lesions in enamel to an artificial caries-like attack in vitro. Br Dent J 1986;160:345–348.

385. Svanberg M. Class II amalgam restorations, glass-ionomer tunnel restorations, and caries development on adjacent tooth surfaces: A 3-year clinical study. Caries Res 1992;26:315–318.

386. Svanberg M, Krasse B, Ornerfeldt HO. Mutans streptococci in interproximal plaque from amalgam and glass ionomer restorations. Caries Res 1990;24:133–136.

387. Svanberg M, Mjor IA, Orstavik D. Mutans streptococci in plaque from margins of amalgam, composite, and glass-ionomer restorations. J Dent Res 1990;69:861–864.

388. Garcia-Godoy F, Marshall TD, Mount GJ. Microleakage of glass ionomer tunnel restorations. Am J Dent 1988;1:53–56.

389. Robbins JW, Cooley RL. Microleakage of Ketac silver in the tunnel preparation. Oper Dent 1988;13:8–11.

390. Doerr CL, Hilton TJ, Hermesch CB. Effect of thermocycling on the microleakage of conventional and resin-modified glass ionomers. Am J Dent 1996;9:19–21.

391. Wilkie R, Lidums A, Smales R. Class II glass ionomer cermet tunnel, resin sandwich and amalgam restorations over 2 years. Am J Dent 1993;6:181–184.

Amalgam Restorations

J. D. Overton
James B. Summitt
John W. Osborne

The word *amalgam* means an alloy of mercury with another metal or metals.[1] This type of alloying is called *amalgamation*.[2] In dentistry, before these metals are combined with mercury to make dental amalgam, they are known as *dental amalgam alloys*. Prior to the development of high-copper amalgam alloys, dental amalgam alloys contained at least 65 wt% silver, 29 wt% tin, and less than 6 wt% copper. The high-copper amalgam alloys[3,4] contain between 12 wt% and 30 wt% copper and at least 40 wt% silver.[5] This higher level of copper has resulted in the elimination of the highly corrodible and weak gamma 2 (tin-mercury) phase that existed in the low-copper dental amalgams.[6–8]

Zinc is added to amalgam to enhance its mechanical properties,[9] reduce marginal fracture,[10,11] and prolong the service of the restoration.[11,12] When moisture is incorporated during condensation of a zinc-containing low-copper amalgam, delayed expansion will occur.[13] Zinc-containing high-copper amalgams do not exhibit the phenomenon of delayed expansion,[14–16] but isolation to prevent any moisture contamination is important for both zinc-containing and zinc-free amalgam restorations.[14] Contamination of dental amalgam with moisture will create porosity in the restoration, which will decrease strength and increase both corrosion and creep.[14,16]

Amalgam is made by mixing mercury with a powder of amalgam alloy. This process is called *trituration*.[17] The powder may be of the lathe-cut variety (Fig 11-1a), which is made by milling an ingot of the alloy, or of the spherical type (Fig 11-1b), which is made by atomizing liquid alloy.[18] The spherical particles usually are not true spheres but take on various

rounded shapes. Some dental amalgam alloys contain only lathe-cut particles, called *filings*; others contain only spheres, and some contain both spheres and filings. Those containing only filings are called *conventional* or *lathe-cut* amalgam alloys, those containing only spheres are called *spherical alloys*, and those containing both filings and spheres are called *admixtures*[5] (Fig 11-1c).

Dental amalgam continues to be one of the most-used restorative materials.[19,20] It has served as a dental restorative for more than 175 years; it was used as early as 1820 in Europe, and, by the mid-1830s, it was in use in the United States.[21,22] At times, its use has been controversial.[22] The most recent controversy is related to amalgam's release of mercury. There is considerable evidence of the safety of dental amalgam.[23–28] To date, there is no confirmed evidence to indicate that the mercury in dental amalgam is related to any disease.[29–32] Research reveals that no toxic effect has been linked to the level of mercury released from amalgam, even when amalgam restorations are removed.[33,34] Several agencies, including the World Health Organization,[35] the US Public Health Service,[36] the National Institutes of Health,[37] and the Swedish Medical Research Council[38] have reaffirmed their positions that there are no data to compel a change in the current use of dental amalgam.[21,39]

Dental amalgam is a metallic compound that is approximately 50% mercury, and some people worry about mercury, known to be toxic in high doses of certain forms, being present in the mouth. Mercury in amalgam is bound in the core-matrix complex, and the bonds are very stable and exhibit very high strength characteristics. The covalent, ionic, and/or

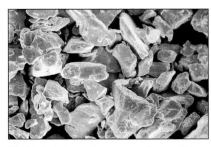
Fig 11-1a Lathe-cut amalgam alloy particles.

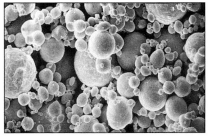
Fig 11-1b Spherical amalgam alloy particles.

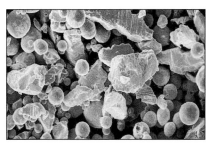
Fig 11-1c Admixed amalgam alloy particles.

intermetallic bonds in amalgam are very difficult to break, and only very heavy pressure or high heat can potentially cause the bonds in the restoration to come apart. During mastication, pressures of 30,000 psi or higher are common, and this force, with friction, can generate heat in small areas. It has been theorized[28] that this heat could cause amalgam to release small amounts of mercury during the lifetime of a restoration.[40] If a patient had 12 amalgam restorations in his or her mouth, the amount of metallic mercury released per day would be in the range of 1.7 µg, an extremely small amount.[41]

Any component of amalgam or any other restorative material can elicit an allergic reaction, but hypersensitivity to mercury is extremely rare. Of those who have an established allergy to mercury, fewer than 1% demonstrate clinically observable reactions to mercury in dental amalgam restorations.[22]

Advantages and Disadvantages

Dental amalgam has many advantages as a restorative material. It is strong, durable, and relatively easy to use. It wears at a rate similar to that of tooth structure. Over time, amalgam has the ability to bring about, through formation of corrosion products, reduced microleakage at its interface with tooth structure.[6,42] Resin composite placed at and below the gingival crest has been found to alter the subgingival microflora in favor of a more pathogenic mix.[43] In the same study, subgingival amalgam margins did not significantly alter the bacterial biofilm.[43] A review of insurance claim data indicated that molars restored with amalgam restorations required endodontic therapy much less frequently than those restored with resin composite;[44] however, this review was done prior to current bonding systems, so future reviews may have different findings. When replacing restorations, it is much easier to avoid enlarging the cavity preparation during removal of amalgam than it is when removing resin composite, because of the contrast between the color of tooth structure and amalgam.[45–47] In contrast, removal of resin composite materials consistently results in a larger preparation than the original. Of the long-term restorative materials, dental amalgam is the least time-consuming to place and has the lowest cost.

Clinical research does not support the often-made claim that dental amalgam causes cuspal fracture. Wahl et al[48] have presented data showing that teeth restored with amalgam do not fracture any more frequently than teeth restored with resin composite. Weakening of tooth structure by large restorative tooth preparations is a likelier cause of fracture in tooth structure adjacent to restorations.

Dental amalgam also has disadvantages. Its primary disadvantage is that it is not tooth-colored. In addition, it does not, on its own, bond to tooth structure, although amalgam bonding systems have been proven to provide a fairly reliable mechanical attachment of amalgam to enamel and dentin.[49] Amalgam contains mercury, which must be handled properly or the vapor can create a safety hazard for the dental staff. Despite its disadvantages, dental amalgam is an economical and reliable direct restorative material that is still used in a majority of dental practices. When placed properly in well-designed tooth preparations, it will serve well for long periods of time.[12,50,51] Many studies have demonstrated the excellent longevity of dental amalgam.[11,50,52,53]

This chapter addresses Class 1 and 2 preparations and placement techniques for dental amalgam. Complex restorations involving the replacement of cusps with dental amalgam are also described.

Resistance Form

One of G.V. Black's steps in tooth preparation is obtaining resistance form. There are two considerations in resistance form when a tooth is being prepared to receive an amalgam restoration. First, resistance form should be developed for the restoration; the restoration must be of adequate thickness and have a marginal design that will allow it to bear the forces of mastication without fracture or deformation. In that regard, the restoration must have adequate occlusogingival depth to resist fracture in function or parafunction (bruxing or clenching). Second, the remaining tooth structure must be left in such a state that it, too, will resist the forces of mastication. As much sound tooth structure as possible must be maintained. If adequate resistance form cannot be maintained in the tooth to resist masticatory forces, the weak portion of the occlusal surface should be cut away and replaced with amalgam or another strong restorative material.[54]

To maximize resistance form for tooth structure, minimum sound tooth structure should be removed when teeth are prepared for Class 1 or Class 2 amalgam restorations. Several studies[55–59] have demonstrated that, as an amalgam restoration becomes wider faciolingually, the tooth is more subject to fracture and the integrity of the restoration is less likely to be maintained. An increase in the depth of the occlusal portion of an amalgam preparation has also been linked to a decrease in resistance to fracture of the tooth.[56] Class 2 restorations that are confined to the marginal ridge areas (proximal slot restorations) may minimize the severity of tooth fracture compared to Class 2 restorations that extend through occlusal grooves.[60,61] Based on this knowledge, the following goals should guide the preparation and restoration of teeth: *(1)* removal of carious tooth structure, *(2)* preservation of the integrity of the tooth and periodontium, and *(3)* maximization of the life of the restored tooth.[51,62]

The Class 1 Preparation

Indications

Occlusal Caries

The indication for an initial Class 1 amalgam restoration is carious tooth structure in the occlusal fissures (or in facial or lingual pits in posterior teeth) detected clinically and with bite-wing radiographs. The objectives of treatment are to eliminate caries lesions, to remove any enamel that has been undermined by the caries process, to preserve as much sound tooth structure as possible, and to create a strong restoration that mimics the original sound tooth structure and allows little or no marginal leakage.

For the purpose of this chapter, it is necessary to review the definitions of the terms *groove*, *fissure*, and *pit*.[63] A groove, or a developmental groove, is a linear channel on the surface of a tooth, usually at the junction of dental lobes (cusps or ridges). A fissure is a developmental linear cleft, the result of incomplete fusion of the enamel of adjoining dental lobes. A pit is a pinpoint fissure or the junction of several fissures.

The presence of deep or stained fissures alone does not justify placement of a restoration. When there is concern that dentin at the base of a deep fissure may become carious, the fissure should be sealed with a resin fissure sealant or flowable resin composite material. In a tooth that has been determined to have a localized fissure caries lesion or lesions, the carious tooth structure should be removed and one or more occlusal restorations placed, with the number of restorations determined by the number of areas in which carious tooth structure was removed. Remaining fissures that are considered to be susceptible to caries should then be sealed with a resin sealant (Fig 11-2).

If deep fissures that are to be sealed exhibit enamel demineralization or heavy stains, they may benefit from being prepared with a small bur (No. $1/16$ or $1/8$) to a width and depth of approximately 0.4 mm before they are acid etched and sealed with a resin fissure sealant[64–66] (Fig 11-3). Alternatively, these fissures may be opened or cleaned with an air-abrasive instrument or an air-polishing prophylaxis unit[67–71] (Fig 11-4).

Traditionally, in a Class 1 amalgam preparation, occlusal fissures, or at least those in the developmental grooves, have been included in the preparation even when areas of the fissure system have not been carious. The justification for this has been that carious dentin, although not evident visually or radiographically, may be lurking at the base of one of those fissures. There is strong evidence that carious dentin inadvertently left at the base of a sealed fissure does not progress[72–76] and that the sealing of fissures associated with occlusal amalgam restorations is an extremely effective treatment.[77–80] Therefore, the routine extension of cavity preparations through fissures not known to be carious cannot be justified. Additionally, extension of cavity preparations through grooves in which there are no fissures is contraindicated.

Defective Restorations and Recurrent Caries

Another indication for a Class 1 restoration is the replacement of a restoration that is defective beyond repair or associated with a recurrent caries lesion. A recurrent caries lesion is one that occurs adjacent to an existing restoration. Optimally, the margins of a restoration are sealed or leakproof. In reality, most restorations exhibit some leakage at their margins, although it is minimal in most cases. When the leakage becomes greater, usually because of a defective restoration or flexure of tooth structure, plaque can form in the space between the tooth and the restoration, which can produce demineralization to form a caries lesion. There is some evidence that cleaning, etching, and sealing leaky amalgam margins with a resin sealant can prolong the life of a restoration.[81]

Fig 11-2 Amalgam should be used as a restorative material only in areas where actual carious tooth structure has been removed; remaining noncarious fissures and amalgam restoration margins are etched and sealed with resin fissure sealant.

Fig 11-2a This drawing shows the extent of carious dentin as if it could be seen through the occlusal enamel.

Fig 11-2b An amalgam restoration has been placed in the area where carious dentin and unsupported enamel were removed; the remaining fissures were sealed.

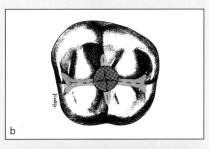

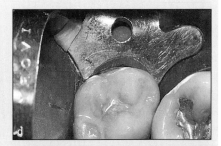

Figs 11-2c and 11-2d Maxillary second molar preparation, sealed restoration, and sealed fissures.

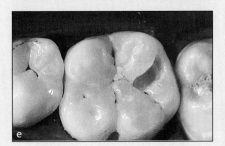

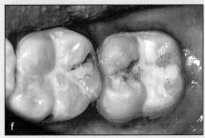

Figs 11-2e and 11-2f Mandibular first molar preparation, sealed restoration, and sealed fissures.

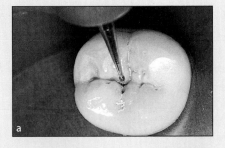

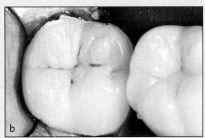

Fig 11-3 Fissures can be opened with a small round bur for sealing.

Fig 11-3a A No. ¹⁄₁₆ bur (0.3-mm diameter), ¹⁄₈ bur (0.4-mm diameter), or a ¹⁄₄ bur (0.5-mm diameter) is used to open the fissures.

Fig 11-3b The fissure system of a mandibular second molar is shown pretreatment.

Fig 11-3c The fissures have been opened for sealing.

Fig 11-3d Scanning electron photomicrograph of fissures prepared with a small round bur.

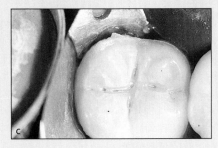

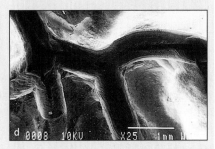

Fig 11-4 *Fissures can be opened with an air-abrasion unit (KCP FlexiJet, American Medical Technologies).*

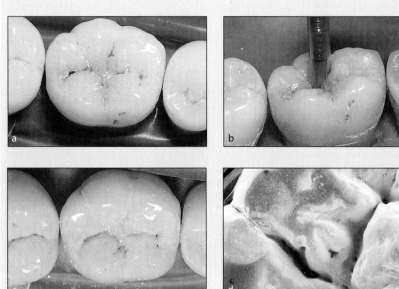

Fig 11-4a The fissure system of a mandibular molar is shown prior to air abrasion.

Fig 11-4b Fifty-micron alumina powder is projected into the fissure.

Fig 11-4c The fissures are shown after air abrasion.

Fig 11-4d Scanning electron photomicrograph of fissures opened with air abrasion.

Outline Form

When an occlusal restoration must be placed because of initial caries lesions, two guidelines should be applied in establishing the outline form: *(1)* carious tooth structure should be eliminated, and *(2)* margins should be placed on sound tooth structure. The enamel at the margin of the preparation should be supported by sound dentin. Any enamel that has been undermined by the removal of carious dentin should be removed. If a noncarious fissure is evident in the wall of a preparation, the preparation should not be extended solely to include the fissure; the fissure should, instead, be sealed after the amalgam has been placed.

If there is no cavitation in the area of the lesion, a bur such as a No. 329 or 330 is used to cut through enamel to gain access to the carious dentin. The preparation is widened to give access to all carious dentin and to remove any enamel not supported by sound dentin. The preparation should be widened only enough to obtain enamel walls supported by sound dentin.

Although the outline form should not contain sharp angles, sound tooth structure should not be removed simply to obtain wide, smooth curves in the outline form. The outline form should be smooth to facilitate the uncovering of the margins during carving of amalgam. That is, the margins of the preparation should not be jagged or rough, because it is difficult for the dentist to know whether a restoration margin appears to be irregular because the enamel margin is rough or

because amalgam extends past the margins onto the surface of the tooth (overextended amalgam or amalgam flash).

When replacing a defective restoration or a restoration associated with a recurrent caries lesion, the outline form will be determined by several factors. First, the outline form of the old restoration will have a major influence. Also, the outline form may have to be extended because of additional pathosis. Finally, the resistance form for the tooth structure or restoration may have to be improved, and that will affect the outline form.

Resistance and Retention Form

To provide retention form for the amalgam, opposing walls of Class 1 occlusal restorations should be parallel to each other or should converge occlusally. Enamel rods in most areas of the occlusal surface are directed roughly parallel to the long axis of the tooth,[82] a factor that should be considered when the angulation of the margin of the amalgam preparation is designed. To enhance their ability to resist fracture, enamel margins should be prepared at a slight obtuse angle (90 degrees or greater); enamel margins of less than 90 degrees are much more subject to fracture (Fig 11-5).

For resistance form in the amalgam restoration, amalgam margins should be approximately 90 degrees. Although many amalgam restorations will have amalgam margins that are significantly less than 90 degrees on the occlusal surface, very acute amalgam margins are much more subject to fracture

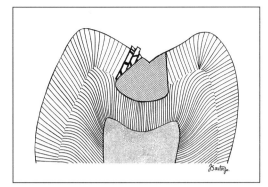

Fig 11-5 An acute cavosurface margin of enamel has the potential for fracture; a 90-degree enamel margin on the occlusal surface will withstand occlusion.

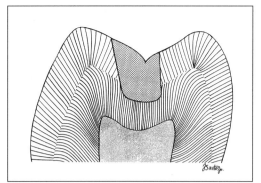

Fig 11-6 The left margin exhibits an acute "fin" of amalgam, which has a greater propensity for fracture, depending on the load applied to it during mastication. The right marginal configuration allows nearly a 90-degree angle for amalgam, imparting greater strength.

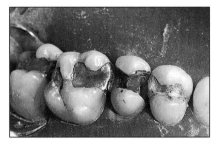

Fig 11-7a The mesio-occlusodistal preparation in the premolar, after removal of a defective restoration, is greater than one third the intercuspal distance; therefore, the cusps ideally should be protected by reduction and coverage with a restoration, or they should be cross splinted (see Fig 11-40).

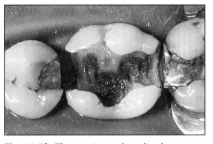

Fig 11-7b The mesio-occlusodistal preparation in the molar leaves cusps much too thin to resist occlusal loading; they must be reduced and protected with a complete occlusal coverage restoration.

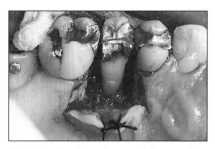

Fig 11-7c The lingual cusp of the maxillary premolar, which was not protected or reinforced during restoration, has fractured.

(Fig 11-6). Marginal fracture will usually cause marginal gaps, or ditches, between the amalgam and the enamel.

If the faciolingual width of the preparation exceeds one third of the distance between the tips of the facial and lingual cusps (intercuspal distance), the remaining cusps themselves should be carefully evaluated. Even in narrower preparations, cusps should be evaluated for cracks that could lead to fracture, and the functional loading to which they will be exposed should be assessed. If a cusp is too weak to withstand function (Figs 11-7a to 11-7c), it should be reduced for coverage with amalgam or attached in some way to the amalgam to provide cuspal reinforcement (described in the section on complex amalgam restorations).

Occlusal amalgam restorations should have an occlusogingival thickness of at least 1.5 mm, and preferably 2.0 mm, to resist fracture during function (resistance form for the restora-

tion). When carious dentin and the overlying enamel are removed, the preparation will be at least that depth and usually deeper.

Figure 11-8a shows a diagram of a cross section of the crown of a posterior tooth with carious dentin at the base of the fissure. Figure 11-8b shows a cross section of the amalgam restoration that is indicated because of that caries lesion. Figure 11-9 shows the outline form of several occlusal amalgam restorations; the outline form was determined by the extent of the demineralized dentin at the base of the fissures. Again, fissures not known to be carious, in a surface receiving an amalgam restoration due to fissure caries, should be sealed with a resin fissure sealant.

If an occlusal caries lesion encroaches on the enamel of the proximal surface so that, when the carious dentin is removed, the proximal enamel has no dentinal support, consideration

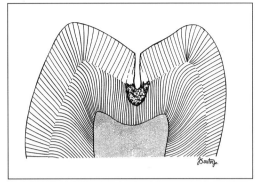

Fig 11-8a Fissure-caries lesion in this tooth involves demineralization of the enamel at the depth of the fissure and advance of the lesion into dentin.

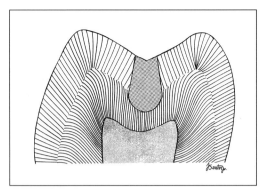

Fig 11-8b Tooth preparation involves removal of the carious dentin and of the enamel not supported by sound dentin. Only the diseased dentin is removed; additional dentin is not removed simply to create a flat pulpal floor for the preparation.

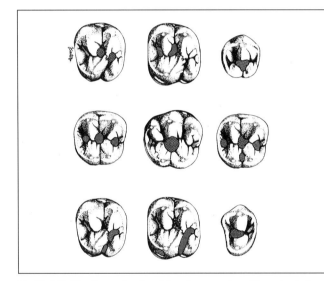

Fig 11-9 Outline form of various Class 1 preparations. The extent of carious demineralization is the determinant of outline form, so outline form will vary in every situation involving caries. Fissures not known to be carious should be sealed with a resin fissure sealant; fissures may be opened with a small bur to a depth of approximately 0.4 mm prior to sealing to ensure sound enamel for bonding.

The Class 2 Preparation

Indications

An initial Class 2 restoration is usually placed because a caries lesion is present on a proximal surface of a molar or premolar. Proximal caries lesions can sometimes be detected visually during a clinical examination, but they are usually detected with bite-wing radiographs. The depth of the penetration of demineralization in enamel and dentin is actually greater than it appears to be in a bite-wing radiograph. A caries lesion that appears radiographically to have penetrated about two thirds of the way through the proximal enamel has actually penetrated the dentinoenamel junction (DEJ). However, even if the lesion has slightly penetrated the DEJ, the tooth still has the potential for remineralization if the etiologic conditions are changed.[83,84] Each patient must be individually evaluated for improved oral hygiene, alteration of diet, and reduction in cariogenic bacteria before the decision is made to surgically remove a minimally deep caries lesion. In most cases, a restorative procedure should not be undertaken to treat a proximal caries lesion unless there is radiographic evidence of at least slight penetration of the lesion into dentin toward the pulp.[84]

If a minimally deep dentinal caries lesion, initiated through demineralization of enamel in a proximal surface, necessitates a restoration, it may be treated with what is referred to as a *tunnel restoration*. One clinical study compared the longevity of glass-ionomer and cermet tunnel restorations to small Class 2 slot amalgam restorations (defined below). That clinical trial, however, demonstrated a relatively high rate of failure for tunnel restorations after 3 years of service, with no

should be given to converting the Class 1 preparation to a Class 2 preparation. An important part of this consideration should be the determination of the forces to which the marginal ridge will be exposed. If there is direct occlusal contact between the opposing tooth and the weakened marginal ridge, the marginal ridge should be removed and replaced with amalgam.

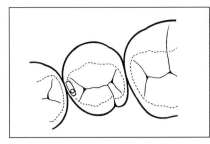

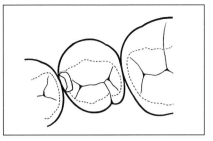

Fig 11-10a For a Class 2 preparation to treat an initial proximal surface caries lesion, an initial cut is made through the marginal ridge with a narrow bur to penetrate to carious dentin; then the slot is widened faciolingually.

Fig 11-10b The mesial and distal aspects of the proximal enamel plate are thinned to facilitate its fracture and removal.

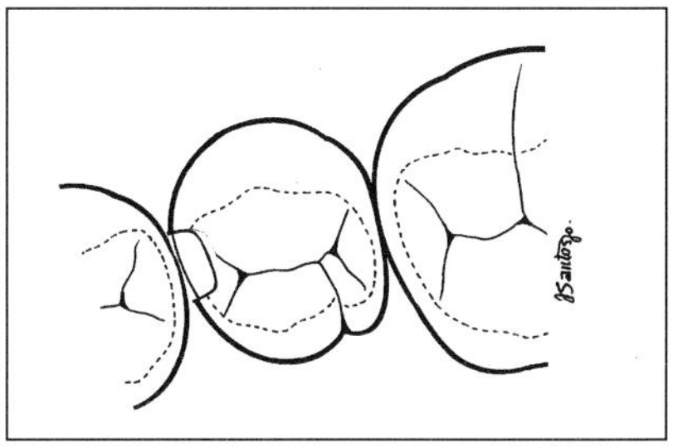

Fig 11-10c The final preparation outline will be determined after all carious tooth structure is removed. It should provide for at least minimal separation of margins from the adjacent tooth.

failures of the slot amalgam restorations.[85] Because the tunnel restoration does not usually involve the use of dental amalgam, it is discussed in the chapter on direct posterior esthetic restorations (chapter 10).

Outline Form

As with Class 1 restorations, Class 2 restorations that leave as much sound tooth structure as possible will contribute to resistance to fracture of the tooth. Tooth preparation necessitated by a caries lesion on a proximal surface should, when possible, avoid extension of the occlusal outline more than is necessary to allow access to the proximal lesion, to remove demineralized enamel and dentin, and to remove enamel not supported by sound dentin. If an occlusal caries lesion is present, it should be treated with a separate occlusal restoration. If the preparation necessitated by the occlusal caries lesion is in close proximity to the occlusal outline of the proximal preparation, so that there is minimal or no sound tooth structure separating the two preparations, they should be joined. As when Class 1 occlusal restorations are placed, fissures not known to be carious but believed to be susceptible to caries should be sealed with a resin fissure sealant.[80] Fissures that contact the outline of a Class 1 or Class 2 preparation should be sealed. Retention form for the proximal restoration should be attained within the proximal preparation; the preparation should not be extended further into a sound occlusal surface to provide retention of the proximal restoration, because this will weaken the tooth's resistance to fracture.

Access to the proximal caries lesion is usually made by preparation through the marginal ridge. The proximal preparation begins with the creation of a slot, cut with a small bur in the center (mesiodistally) of the crest of the marginal ridge and occlusal to the caries lesion (Fig 11-10a). The slot is deepened gingivally until the bur "falls" into the soft carious dentin, which has little resistance to the advance of the bur.

The preparation is widened facially and lingually to eliminate all demineralized tooth structure at the DEJ and to remove enamel that is not supported by sound dentin. Demineralized enamel should usually be removed as well. However, if demineralization is superficial (less than halfway through the enamel), and there is evidence that the patient will reduce his or her caries risk status, consideration should be given to stopping the extension of the preparation short of removing some superficial demineralized enamel. After the amalgam restoration has been placed, the demineralized enamel can be treated with fluoride to enhance remineralization, or it can be acid etched and coated with light-cured resin for at least short-term protection from further demineralization.[86] Alternatively, the demineralized enamel can be removed with a round bur or hand instrument; then the sound enamel walls of the dished-out area can be etched and the area can be restored to contour with bonded resin composite.

The Class 2 restoration necessitated only because of a proximal caries lesion and having an occlusal outline limited to the marginal ridge area will be referred to in this chapter and others as a *slot restoration*. If it involves the distal surface with access from the occlusal surface, it will be called a *disto-occlusal slot restoration* (Fig 11-11).

When the proximal slot restoration is prepared, a shell of enamel should be left between the preparation and the adjacent tooth (Figs 11-10b and 11-12a to 11-12c). This will prevent accidental nicking, scarring, or other damage to the adjacent tooth. One study[87] found that proximal surfaces of adjacent teeth were damaged during Class 2 preparation 69% of the time and that these damaged surfaces were almost three times as likely to become carious as were undamaged surfaces. Special care to avoid damage to the adjacent tooth is warranted. Any nicking or scarring of an adjacent tooth should be polished away before the restoration is placed.

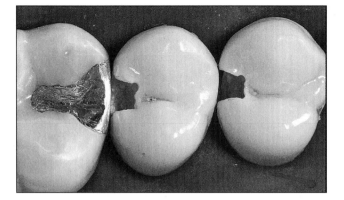

Fig 11-11 In the disto-occlusal slot preparations in the maxillary first and second premolars, the preparations have been opened facially and lingually so that contact is just broken to allow for carving and burnishing.

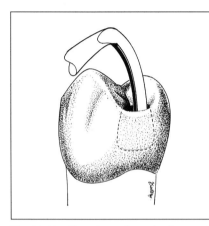

Fig 11-12a The plate of proximal enamel should be fractured with a hand instrument to prevent damage to the adjacent tooth by a bur. The instrument is placed in the slot.

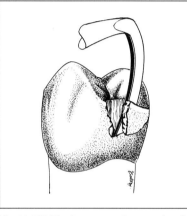

Fig 11-12b The instrument is rotated to fracture the plate.

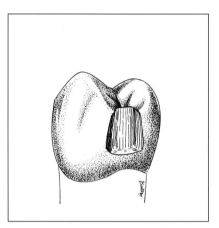

Fig 11-12c The fractured margins have been planed with a gingival margin trimmer or hatchet.

The proximal surface margins of a Class 2 amalgam preparation should not usually be in contact with the adjacent tooth (Fig 11-10c). Breaking contact slightly will allow the amalgam at those margins to be carved and burnished (with a very thin carver, such as the interproximal carver) during the restoration placement procedure. However, if a significant amount of sound enamel that is supported by sound dentin would have to be cut away to eliminate contact with the adjacent tooth, consideration should be given to allowing contact to remain.

During the removal of carious dentin, the demineralized dentin in the periphery of the preparation (at or near the DEJ) should be removed and the outline form should be extended to ensure that the enamel at the margins of the preparation is supported by sound dentin. Carious dentin should be removed with the largest round bur that will fit into the area. After the periphery of the preparation is clear of demineralized tooth structure, the carious dentin near the pulp should be removed. The bur should be rotated very slowly in a low-speed handpiece; the rotation should be so slow that the individual blades of the bur can be seen as it rotates. The blades of the slowly rotating bur are like multiple spoon excavator blades, but the depth that a blade can penetrate into the carious dentin is limited by the edge angle of the bur and by the depth of each bur blade toward the center of the bur, so the bur will remove only a limited depth of carious dentin during each rotation. During removal of deep carious dentin, this procedure is less likely to result in a pulpal exposure than is the use of a spoon excavator.

Resistance and Retention Form

After the shape of the preparation is roughed out with a bur, hand instruments such as a gingival margin trimmer (11-80-8-14 or 11-95-8-14) may be used to fracture away the shell of enamel; to shape the facial, lingual, and gingival walls and margins; and to scrape away any fragile enamel from the margins (Figs 11-13a to 11-13h). The facial and lingual walls

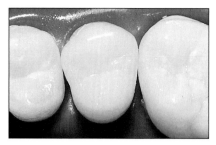

Fig 11-13a A disto-occlusal slot amalgam preparation will be made because an initial caries lesion is present.

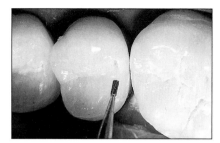

Fig 11-13b A small bur is used to cut a slot, beginning at the crest of the marginal ridge and extending gingivally to "fall" into carious tooth structure. A thin plate of enamel separates the bur from the adjacent tooth to prevent damage to the adjacent tooth.

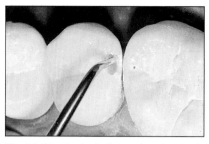

Fig 11-13c A gingival margin trimmer is placed into the slot created by the bur and rotated to apply pressure to the thin plate of proximal enamel.

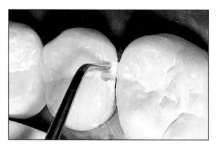

Fig 11-13d The thin plate is fractured.

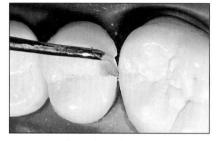

Fig 11-13e The walls and margins are planed with the margin trimmer to smooth them and to eliminate any remaining fragile enamel.

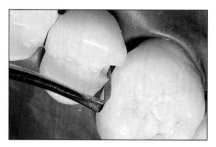

Fig 11-13f There is enough separation of the margins from the adjacent tooth to allow access for a thin carver (IPC) to carve and burnish the margins.

Fig 11-13g Retention grooves are placed with a No. 1/8 or 1/4 bur.

Fig 11-13h The preparation is completed.

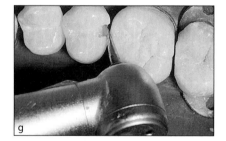

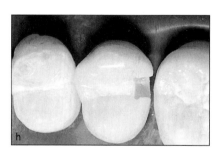

of a Class 2 slot preparation should converge slightly toward the occlusal surface to provide retention form for the restoration (Fig 11-14).

To provide resistance form for the Class 2 amalgam restoration, the proximal preparation should have a mesiodistal dimension of about 1.5 mm or more. If there is sound dentin supporting occlusal enamel in the fossa adjacent to the marginal ridge, that dentin and enamel should be left intact. If the caries lesion extends from the proximal DEJ deeper into dentin, the demineralized dentin should be removed completely, especially in the areas near the DEJ, and sound dentin should be left in place.

The gingival floor of the proximal preparation may be flat and approximately perpendicular to the long axis of the tooth, or it may be curved and/or slanted faciolingually, as determined by the extent and configuration of the caries lesion that necessitated the restoration. The location of the gingival floor, therefore, should be determined by the gingival extent of the carious lesion and/or by the level necessary to provide separation of the gingival margin from the adjacent tooth. The gingival wall, like the facial and lingual walls of the proximal preparation, should form an angle of approximately 90 degrees with the surface of the tooth. This provides strength to both the amalgam and enamel and prevents

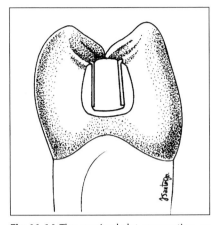

Fig 11-14 The proximal slot preparation, or the proximal box of a Class 2 preparation, should have walls that meet the proximal surface of the tooth at 90 degrees and converge occlusally to provide resistance and retention form.

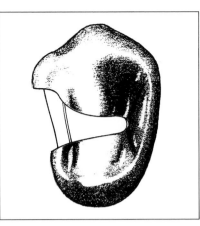

Fig 11-15a Although extension of a Class 2 preparation into occlusal grooves is not usually necessitated by carious tooth structure, if such an extension is already present from a previous restoration of the tooth, it will provide some resistance form for the proximal portion.

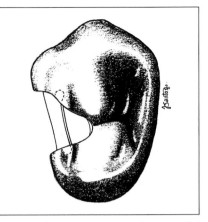

Fig 11-15b An extension without parallel cavosurface margins, however, will not provide the resistance form needed to prevent displacement of the proximal amalgam during mastication, so retention grooves (dotted lines) should be added.

enamel not supported by sound dentin from being left at the margins of the restoration.

Convergence toward the occlusal surface of the facial and lingual walls of the proximal slot preparation gives retention form to the restoration to keep it from dislodging occlusally. Although, with initial proximal surface caries lesions, it is not often necessary to extend the Class 2 preparation into occlusal grooves, the operator will frequently need to replace an existing restoration that was prepared with an occlusal extension. If the restoration is extended into occlusal grooves, this extension will provide resistance to displacement of the restoration proximally (that is, toward the adjacent tooth). To provide enough resistance, however, the extension into the occlusal surface must have a faciolingual dimension of at least one fourth of the distance between the facial and lingual cusp tips[88] (intercuspal distance), and the facial and lingual margins of the occlusal extension must be approximately parallel to each other in a mesiodistal direction (Fig 11-15a).

Undercuts

If the extension into the occlusal surface is narrower, or if there is no extension into the occlusal surface, as with the proximal slot restoration, retentive undercuts (retention grooves or points) must be cut into the dentin of the facial and lingual walls of the proximal box (Fig 11-15b). Use of a No. ¼ (ISO 005) round bur, with a head diameter of 0.5 mm,[88–90] or a No. ⅛ (ISO 004) round bur, with a head diameter of 0.4 mm, is recommended for preparation of retention

grooves and points for Class 2 amalgam restorations (see Fig 11-13g). For a proximal slot restoration, retentive undercuts should be very distinct (at least 0.5 mm deep) and should oppose each other to form a dovetail effect in the dentin. Long grooves, extending from the gingival floor to the occlusal surface, are recommended for a proximal slot restoration[90,91] (Fig 11-16a). If the occlusal extension is narrow, short retention grooves, or retentive points, should be prepared in the dentin of the facial and lingual walls to supplement the resistance form provided by the occlusal extension[89] (Fig 11-16b). If there is a bulky extension of amalgam into the occlusal surface of the tooth, retentive undercuts should not be necessary[88] (Fig 11-16c). For preparing any retentive undercuts with a bur, it is advisable to use a handpiece at low speed, without water spray, and to use magnification to enable visualization, because the location and direction of the undercuts are critical to the success of the restoration.

Retentive undercuts in the dentin of the facial and lingual walls should be completely in dentin and not at the proximal DEJ; this obviates the removal of the dentinal support for the proximal enamel adjacent to the restoration. The undercuts should not, however, be placed so far away from the DEJ that the pulp chamber could be penetrated. A good rule is to place a retentive undercut so that there is approximately 0.25 to 0.5 mm of dentin between the groove and the DEJ and so that the groove is approximately 0.5 mm deep and 0.5 mm wide. Again, the 0.5-mm diameter of the No. ¼ round bur, or the 0.4-mm diameter of the No. ⅛ bur, is ideal as a gauge of

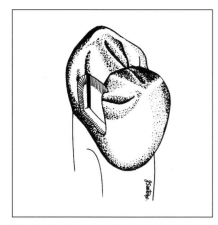

Fig 11-16a In a proximal slot or proximal box–only preparation, retention grooves should be long and very distinct.

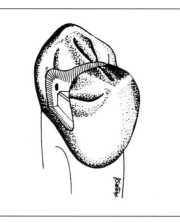

Fig 11-16b In preparations with narrow occlusal extensions, short (0.5- to 1.0-mm) retention grooves or points are placed in facial and lingual walls just gingival to the occlusal DEJ.

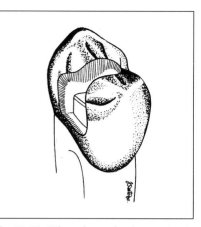

Fig 11-16c When the occlusal extension is wide (1.5 mm or more faciolingually) and has parallel walls, retention points or grooves are not necessary.

dimension. So that retentive undercuts do not penetrate through the dentin to the DEJ when they are placed in the facial and lingual walls, they should be cut parallel faciolingually to the DEJ and to the external surface of the tooth (Fig 11-17).

When retentive undercuts are necessary, they must be actual undercuts in the facial and lingual dentin that oppose each other (see Fig 11-17). This is especially important in proximal slot restorations, in which the undercuts are the only feature that will prevent dislodgment of the restoration proximally. In the preparation with a deep proximal box the retention grooves should be in the proximal walls just inside the DEJ and not in the corners of the box (Fig 11-18). Without correctly located, distinct retention grooves, a proximal slot restoration is doomed to failure.

When well designed, the proximal slot restoration can last indefinitely. Figure 11-19 shows two Class 2 slot amalgam restorations; one has been in function for more than 58 years and the other for more than 20 years.

Mechanical Retention

If a proximal box or slot is so wide that retentive undercuts will not oppose each other (Fig 11-20a), another type of retention and resistance method, such as amalgam bonding or a self-threading pin, placed horizontally or vertically, should be used (Fig 11-20b). Amalgam bonding and the use of pins are discussed later in this chapter.

Because the outline form of Class 2 amalgam restorations is always determined by the pathologic problem being treat-

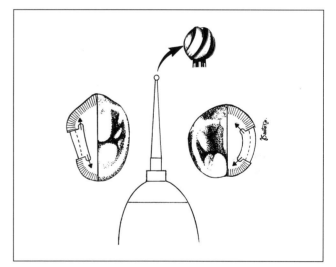

Fig 11-17 Location and direction of retentive undercuts (retention grooves) for the proximal portion of a Class 2 restoration. The illustrated grooves are approximately 0.5 mm wide and 0.5 mm deep (No. 1/4 bur head is shown) and are directed approximately parallel to the DEJ (and the external surface of the tooth). *(left)* For a fairly flat surface, such as the proximal surface of a maxillary premolar, the grooves are directed almost in the facial and lingual directions. *(right)* For a convex proximal surface, such as in a mandibular premolar, their direction is considerably vectored.

ed, there are an infinite number of variations in occlusal outline form. Figure 11-21 illustrates the outline form of some typical Class 2 restorations that would be placed to treat initial caries lesions.

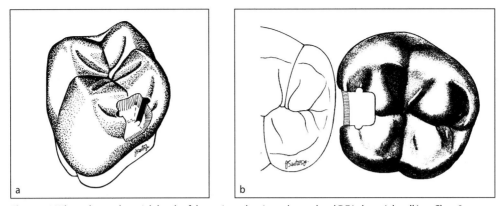

Fig 11-18 When, due to the axial depth of the carious dentin at the occlusal DEJ, the axial wall in a Class 2 preparation must be deeper pulpally than approximately 1 mm inside the DEJ, retention grooves (or points) should be placed so that they are just inside the proximal DEJ, not at the line angles of the deep preparation. *(a)* Proximal view of an axially deep Class 2 preparation showing retention grooves in dentin near the proximal DEJ and extending occlusally through the occlusal enamel; *(b)* occlusal view.

Fig 11-19 *Proximal slot restorations placed by Dr Miles Markley; photographed in 1992.*

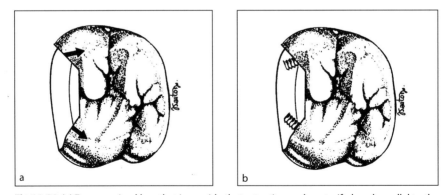

Fig 11-19a The mesio-occlusal slot restoration in the maxillary first molar has served for more than 58 years.

Fig 11-19b This mesio-occlusal slot restoration is more than 20 years old.

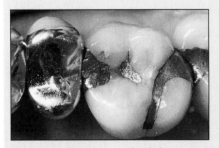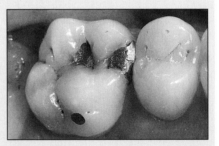

Fig 11-20 *(a)* For a proximal box that is so wide that retentive undercuts, if placed parallel to the adjacent DEJ, would not oppose each other to provide needed undercut retention, undercuts (retention grooves) should not be placed. *(b)* Instead, other types of resistance and retention features, such as these horizontal self-threading pins, should be employed.

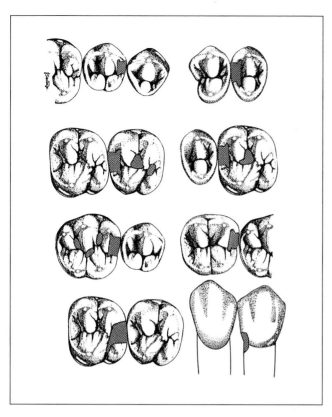

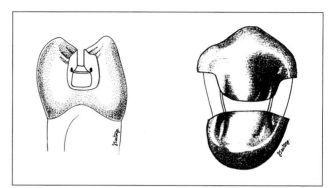

Fig 11-21 Typical outline forms of Class 2 restorations placed to treat initial caries lesions. Because outline form is determined by the pathosis present and the morphology and position of the tooth, there are an infinite number of variations. The bottom right-hand restoration represents a facial slot or keyhole restoration to treat root caries, or caries at the cementoenamel junction.

Fig 11-22 When extension through occlusal fissures or grooves cannot be avoided, such as when an old, defective amalgam restoration is being replaced, the faciolingual width of the occlusal portion of the preparation should be kept as narrow as possible to maintain tooth strength. *(left)* Proximal view; *(right)* occlusal view of mesio-occlusodistal preparation.

Facial and Lingual Access

Most Class 2 amalgam restorations have occlusal access, as already discussed. If a proximal caries lesion is at or apical to the cementoenamel junction, however, it is often more conservative to use facial, and occasionally lingual, access.[92] The preparation for a Class 2 amalgam restoration with facial or lingual access, sometimes referred to as a *keyhole preparation* or a *facial* or *lingual slot preparation*, is similar to a slot preparation with occlusal access. The entire preparation is apical to the proximal contact. The location and configuration of the carious tooth structure and the access preparation determine the outline form of the keyhole preparation (see Fig 11-21, bottom right). Its margins, which are at least partly on cementum or dentin, should provide for cavosurface angles of approximately 90 degrees. Groove retention, similar to that recommended for a proximal slot preparation with occlusal access, is indicated and can usually be placed with a No. ¼ or No. ⅛ bur in the dentin of the occlusal and gingival walls; occasionally, grooves must be placed with a hand instrument, such as a gingival margin trimmer.

Replacement of Restorations with Occlusal Extensions

Patients commonly will have existing Class 2 amalgam restorations that have extensions of the preparation through occlusal fissures and even through nonfissured grooves. Although this preparation outline form should not currently be advocated, existing restorations of this type will need to be replaced from time to time. Therefore, some design concepts to promote their longevity must be discussed. First, the narrower (faciolingually) the extension through the occlusal surface, the less marginal breakdown will occur[55,58] (Fig 11-22). Second, the junction of the proximal portion and the occlusal extension of the Class 2 amalgam preparation must have adequate depth (1.5 to 2.0 mm). The occlusal outline form at the junction of the proximal and occlusal components should not be sharp or jagged, but no more than a very small amount of sound cuspal enamel should be sacrificed to make the junction slightly rounded instead of sharp.

353

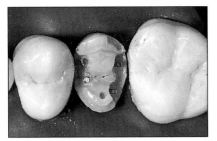

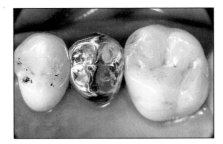

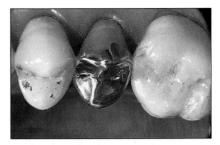

Fig 11-23a Because of a diagnosis of incomplete tooth fracture, the maxillary premolar has been prepared for a complex amalgam restoration.

Fig 11-23b The tooth has been restored with a complex amalgam restoration that protects the entire occlusal surface.

Fig 11-23c The occlusal height of the mesial aspect of the nonfunctioning facial cusp was only reduced 1.5 mm to preserve facial enamel for esthetics.

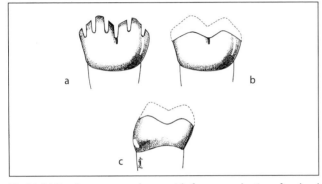

Fig 11-24 Depth cuts are used to provide for even reduction of occlusal tooth structure of a mandibular molar and consistent thickness of amalgam. (a) Depth cuts 2.5 mm deep; (b) cuspal reduction viewed from the facial aspect; (c) cuspal reduction viewed from the mesial aspect.

Complex Preparations

Historically, the term *complex amalgam restoration* referred to one that involved three or more surfaces of a tooth. The term has been redefined in recent years[52] to refer to an amalgam restoration that replaces one or more cusps.

When a metal cuspal-coverage restoration is indicated, a gold casting is considered the restoration of choice. Gold has wear characteristics similar to those of enamel and has the ability to maintain a stable occlusion. However, for various reasons, a gold casting cannot always be chosen as the definitive restoration. In these situations, amalgam is an excellent alternative restorative material.

The efficacy of the amalgam cuspal-coverage restoration has been shown in both laboratory and clinical studies.[52,53,93,94] The key to the successful placement of cuspal-coverage restorations is a thorough understanding of the underlying engineering principles. Preparations for amalgam

restorations have traditionally been designed to provide adequate retention form. Retention has been defined as prevention of dislodgment of the restoration along the path of insertion (with tensile forces). Resistance is defined as prevention of dislodgment or fracture by oblique or compressive forces. Although retention form is important in the complex amalgam restoration, more emphasis should be placed on the resistance of both the restoration and the remaining tooth structure. Retention and resistance form can be obtained through the use of metal threaded pins, nonpin mechanical features, and amalgam bonding, all of which will be described.

Cuspal-Coverage Preparations

Often, individuals seek treatment because of a fractured cusp or cusps in posterior teeth. If the treatment option agreed on for the tooth is a complex amalgam restoration, the tooth preparation will usually include removal of any existing amalgam restoration, removal of any carious tooth structure and fragile enamel and/or dentin, and preparation of margins to provide a cavosurface angle of approximately 90 degrees in all areas. In addition, weak cusps that have not fractured should be reduced for coverage and protection with amalgam.

The thickness of amalgam needed for cuspal protection will vary, depending on the functional load to which the cusp will be exposed. A good guideline for amalgam thickness in centric holding cusps (stamp cusps) of molars and premolars is 2.5 mm. In a facial cusp of a maxillary premolar, occasionally a reduced thickness of amalgam is acceptable to allow a maximum amount of facial enamel to remain for esthetics (Figs 11-23a to 11-23c).

When cusps are reduced for coverage, the occlusal tooth structure should be reduced anatomically to provide for an adequate and consistent occlusal amalgam thickness. To facilitate consistent reduction, depth cuts are recommended. Figure 11-24 illustrates the use of depth cuts to ensure consis-

Fig 11-25 Reduction of weak cusps of a mandibular molar for coverage.

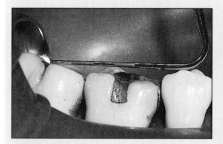

Fig 11-25a An instrument is placed so that it touches cusp tips of the adjacent teeth. A note can be made of the position of the cusps to be reduced so they can be rebuilt in amalgam and carved to approximately the correct height before the rubber dam is removed.

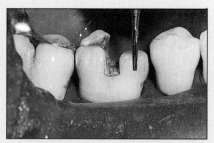

Fig 11-25b Half the 5.5-mm length of a No. 169L bur head is used to make depth cuts approximately 2.5 mm deep in the cusps.

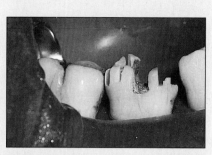

Fig 11-25c The depth cuts are completed.

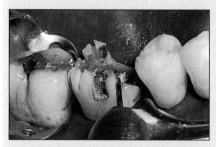

Fig 11-25d The head of the handpiece is rotated so that the 169L bur can be used to reduce the cuspal structure between the depth cuts.

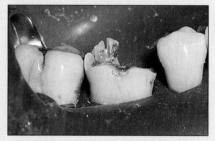

Fig 11-25e Facial cusps are reduced.

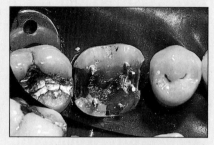

Fig 11-25f All cusps are reduced, and resistance features are placed.

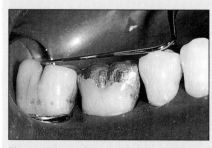

Fig 11-25g Amalgam is placed, carved, and smoothed. The instrument is replaced to ensure that cuspal height is similar to preoperative cuspal height.

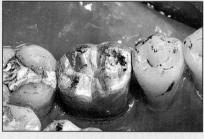

Fig 11-25h Completed restoration.

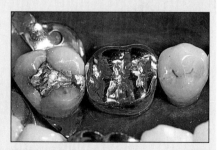

Fig 11-25i Polished restoration.

tent reduction of occlusal tooth structure for coverage. Figure 11-25 shows a clinical case in which depth cuts provided consistent reduction.

The length of the head of the bur that is used for depth cuts must be known. Because head lengths vary from manu-facturer to manufacturer, and even among burs of a single manufacturer, it is good practice to measure the length of a bur head prior to preparation of depth cuts (Fig 11-26). A periodontal probe should be available for measuring the length of bur heads.

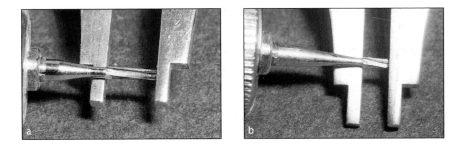

Fig 11-26 *(a)* A Boley gauge is used to measure a No. 56 bur head (4.0 mm in this case). *(b)* A Boley gauge is used to measure a No. 330 bur head (2.0 mm in this case). The periodontal probe is a handy instrument for measuring bur head length.

Fig 11-27 *Preoperative registration of the height of cusps to be reduced and restored with amalgam.*

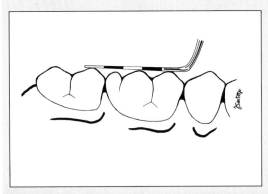

Fig 11-27a The midfacial and distofacial cusps are to be reduced for coverage. A periodontal probe is placed along the facial cusp tips of the tooth to be restored and the adjacent teeth, and the relationships of the cusp tips to the probe are remembered or drawn.

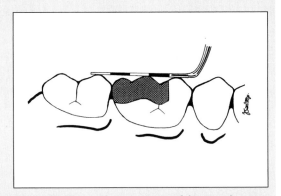

Fig 11-27b The amalgam cusp tips of the carved restoration are seen to have a similar relationship to the probe.

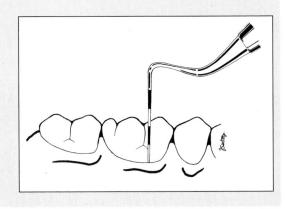

Fig 11-27c If there are no adjacent teeth or cusp tips to guide the height of amalgam cusp tips, the distance from a landmark (such as the cervical line) may be measured with a periodontal probe.

Consistent reduction of cusps provides anatomic reduction rather than flat reduction. Anatomic reduction imparts adequate strength to the amalgam while preserving and protecting as much natural tooth structure as possible. Some operators reduce to a flat surface perpendicular to the long axis of the tooth; no scientific justification for this practice can be found in the literature.

A time-saver in practice is to take note of cuspal height and cusp tip location, or even to make a drawing, prior to cuspal reduction, so that cusps may be built and carved back to their original height prior to removal of the rubber dam (Fig 11-27).

Resistance and Retention Methods

For amalgam restorations that do not replace cusps, or at least large portions of cusps, the walls of the preparation provide retention and resistance form. Retention form is provided by convergent walls and undercuts placed in dentin. When a large amount of cuspal tooth structure is lost or removed, the walls, or portions of them, which provide resistance and retention for the amalgam, are lost. For this reason, it is necessary to add features or adhesives to the preparation that will provide adequate resistance and retention for the restora-

Fig 11-28 *Scanning electron micrographs of self-threading pins. (Courtesy of Dr John O. Burgess.)*

Fig 11-28 *Scanning electron micrographs of self-threading pins. (Courtesy of Dr John O. Burgess.)*

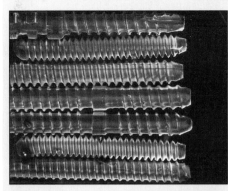

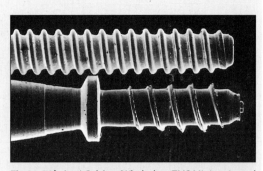

Fig 11-28a *(top to bottom)* Brasseler PPS (titanium alloy); Denovo Denlok (stainless steel); Vivadent Filpin (titanium); Coltène/Whaledent TMS (Thread Mate System) Link Plus (titanium alloy); Coltène/Whaledent TMS Link Plus (stainless steel); Coltène/Whaledent TMS Minim (stainless steel); Fairfax Dental Stabilok (stainless steel).

Fig 11-28b *(top)* Coltène/Whaledent TMS Minim pin and *(bottom)* Max pin (with threads more widely separated to allow for greater thickness of dentinal threads).

tion. Several methods of obtaining resistance and retention for complex amalgam restorations are discussed.

Pins

Although pins were first described in the 19th century,[95,96] Markley popularized the concept of cemented stainless steel pins.[97–99] Later, stainless steel pins, which were malleted into slightly undersized channels in dentin (friction-locked pins),[100] and threaded stainless steel pins, which were screwed into channels in dentin,[101] were developed. Laboratory studies have since investigated the properties of these three types of pins (cemented, friction-locked, and self-threading), and, because of these studies, the self-threading pins are the primary pins in current use (Fig 11-28). In a study by Dilts and coworkers,[102] self-threading pins were found to be more retentive in dentin than cemented or friction-locked pins. The authors also recommended a depth in dentin of 2.0 to 3.0 mm as optimum for self-threading pins. Moffa and others[103] found that a pin length of approximately 2.0 mm into amalgam provides optimum retention. The relationship between retention and the diameter of the pin has also been investigated. As would be expected, larger-diameter pins are more retentive.[102–104]

Self-threading pins are manufactured in a variety of configurations. Some are self-shearing and some have heads. Figure 11-28a shows several pins from various manufacturers. In one study of self-threading pins,[105] pins manufactured by Coltène/Whaledent and Brasseler demonstrated superior resistance and retention.

Most currently marketed pins have the metal threads separated to provide thicker, bulkier dentinal threads. When a pin is pulled from a pin channel, it is the dentinal threads that shear and not the metal threads. The pin design with wider dentinal threads is retained well in dentin (see Fig 11-28b). Another feature of many of the currently available pins is a shoulder stop. The purpose of this feature is to prevent the end of the pin from putting stress on the dentin at the end of the pin channel; the PPS pin (Brasseler) and the Max pin (Coltène/Whaledent) have an effective shoulder stop incorporated into their design. A shoulder is a part of the design of the Link Plus pin (Coltène/Whaledent), but its diameter is similar to that of the threads, so it does not provide an effective stop.[106] Although a definite shoulder stop is theoretically beneficial, there is no evidence of problems associated with pins that lack effective shoulder stops.

Coltène/Whaledent pins and pin-channel (or twist) drills in Regular, Minim, and Minikin sizes are shown in Fig 11-29; a smaller size (Minuta, 0.0135-mm diameter pin channel drill; 0.015-mm diameter pin) is available, but we have been unable to find a practical use for it. The gold-plated stainless steel TMS Regular and Minim pins (see Figs 11-34b and 11-34c) are also available as self-shearing pins, and in double-shear (two pins in one) form as well as single-shear form. All TMS Link and Link Plus (with shoulder) pins are self-shearing;

Fig 11-29 Color-coded pin channel (twist) drills and pins of various diameters and lengths (Coltène/Whaledent TMS).

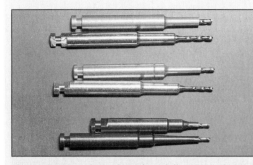

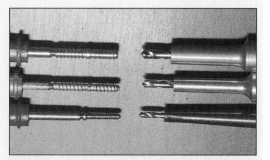

Fig 11-29a Pin channel (Kodex) drills: *(top to bottom)* Regular (gold, 0.027-inch [0.675-mm] diameter, 2.0- and 5.0-mm lengths); Minim (silver, 0.021-inch [0.525-mm] diameter, 2.0- and 5.0-mm lengths); Minikin (red, 0.017-inch [0.425-mm] diameter, 1.5-mm length).

Fig 11-29b Pins with corresponding pin channel drills: *(top to bottom)* Regular (0.031-inch diameter) gold-plated stainless steel Link Plus pin with Regular (0.027-inch diameter) pin channel drill (2.0-mm depth-limiting); Minim (0.024-inch diameter) titanium alloy Link Plus pin with Minim (0.021-inch diameter) pin channel drill (2.0-mm depth-limiting); Minikin (0.019-inch diameter) titanium alloy Link Series pin with Minikin (0.017-inch diameter) pin channel drill (1.5-mm depth-limiting).

Link Plus Regular and Minim pins are also available in the two-in-one (double-shear) form. The Link and Link Plus pins are available in either gold-plated stainless steel or titanium alloy; these may be inserted manually or with any low-speed, latch-type handpiece. The bulk TMS pins are available only in gold-plated stainless steel and are usually inserted manually. Selection among these pins should be based on operator preference; they all have performed well in laboratory studies.

Number to use. It is difficult to develop a guideline that would determine the appropriate number of pins for all situations. Although it has been demonstrated that as the size and number of pins increase, the amount of resistance form imparted by the pins increases[107]; the number of pins used will vary with the size of pin, the amount of remaining tooth structure, other mechanical resistance features used, the use of amalgam bonding systems, and the expected functional requirements of the final restoration.

Channel preparation. A rubber dam should be in place when pin channels are prepared and when pins are placed to protect the patient from aspiration and to prevent contamination by saliva in case there is pulpal perforation during pin channel preparation.

Because the tips of pin channel drills tend to move around on the cut dentin surface, when the rotating tip is placed against the surface, it is usually helpful to place an indenta-

tion or starting point in the dentin at the desired location for the initiation of the pin channel. The starting point may be placed with a small bur, such as a No. ¼ or No. ⅛ bur.

Various lengths and diameters of pin channel drills are available for preparation of pin channels (see Fig 11-29). The most popular pin channel drills have depth-limiting shoulders, which ensure that the optimum pin channel depth is not exceeded. To avoid perforation of either the pulp or the external surface of the tooth, location of the pin channel is critical. The channel should usually be prepared parallel to the nearest external tooth surface. Before channel preparation is initiated, approximately 2.0 mm of the end of the pin channel drill should be placed against the external surface of the tooth. If that much of the side of the tooth is exposed above the rubber dam, alignment is facilitated. Frequently, however, adjacent soft tissue under the rubber dam obscures visualization of the tooth surface in the area adjacent to the desired pin location. For alignment, the drill is placed against the external tooth surface, and the angulation of the drill is changed until the drill separates from the margin of the preparation; it is then rotated back until it just contacts the margin (Figs 11-30a to 11-30c).

Pin channels should be initiated at least 0.5 mm from the DEJ if the nearby preparation margin is coronal to the cementoenamel junction; a 1.0-mm distance from the DEJ is preferable.[102] If the nearby margin is apical to the cementoenamel

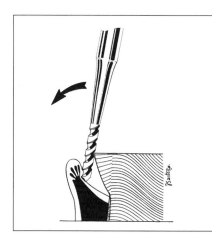

Fig 11-30a To align the pin channel drill with the side of the tooth when the external tooth surface is obscured, the drill is placed in the sulcus so that the drill is touching the preparation margin; the drill is then rotated *(arrow)*.

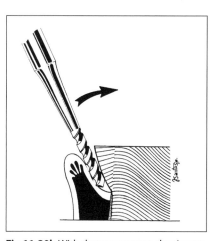

Fig 11-30b With that movement, the tip contacts the external surface and the portion of the drill that was in contact with the margin is rotated slightly away from it; then the length of the drill is rotated *(arrow)*.

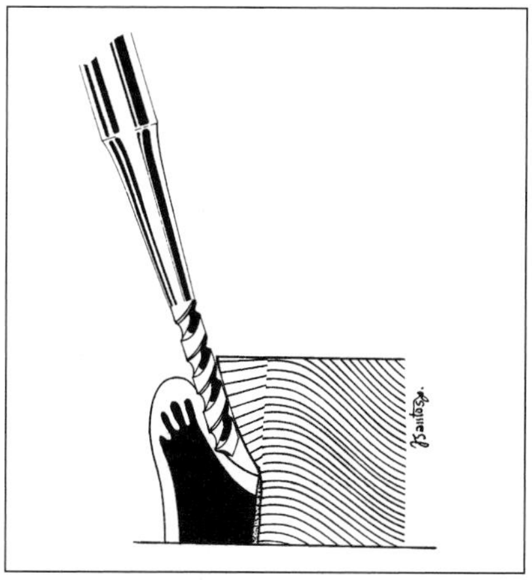

Fig 11-30c With that rotation, the drill returns just to touch the margin. It is now aligned parallel to the external surface.

junction, there should be at least 1.0 mm of dentin between the channel and the external surface of the tooth.

The most common location for pins is at the line angles of the tooth because of the greater thickness of dentin between the external surface and the pulp and the decreased risk of perforation. The risk of perforation is especially increased in furcation areas. Figure 11-31 illustrates the preferable locations for pins.[108] Areas to be avoided in posterior teeth include proximal areas and tooth structure that lies over furcations or concavities in the root. Wherever the pin is to be located, the external surface of the tooth should be assessed and the pin channel drill aligned parallel to it (Figs 11-32a to 11-32c).

Pins should be located so that the channels enter the dentin at an approximately 90-degree angle to the prepared dentin surface. If a depth-limiting pin channel drill is used, the drill will not be able to achieve optimum pin channel depth if the surface of dentin adjacent to the entrance of the channel is at an angle to the drill. In addition, a pin should not be located immediately adjacent to a wall of the preparation; there should be access to condense amalgam around the full circumference of the pin. If a pin is located an optimal distance from the DEJ and a dentinal wall is adjacent to the pin, a small "cove" may be cut in the dentin to provide adequate space for amalgam (Fig 11-33).

To provide maximum cutting efficiency, the pin channel drill must be sharp so that it will be efficient at low speeds. A drill loses cutting efficiency with extended use and steam autoclaving.[109,110] Pin channel drills should be sterilized with dry heat, chemical vapor, or immersion in glutaraldehyde rather than in the steam autoclave. Drills should be discarded when a diminished cutting efficiency is sensed by the operator.[111,112] If preparation of a pin channel is difficult, it is likely that the flutes of the drill are obstructed by debris, the drill is dull, the handpiece is running in reverse, or the tip of the drill is in contact with enamel rather than dentin.

The correctly prepared pin channel will be slightly smaller in diameter than the pin; this size difference is called the *pin–to–pin-channel mismatch*. The mismatch must be small to ensure that excessive stresses are not exerted on the dentin during insertion of the pin and that the pin will be retained by the dentin.

During preparation of a pin channel to a depth of 2.0 mm or more, it is advisable to withdraw the drill from the channel at least once to allow dentinal cuttings to be cleared from the flutes of the drill; this allows more efficient pin channel preparation and less heat generation. Care must be taken, however, to avoid overenlargement of the channel with multiple entries and withdrawals.

If an amalgam bonding material is used in addition to pins, it is applied after the pins have been inserted so that amalgam can be condensed immediately after placement of the bonding material.

Insertion. The insertion of self-threading pins may be accomplished in more than one way. They may be inserted by hand, using a small pin wrench (Figs 11-34a and 11-34b) or with a low-speed or finger-driven handpiece[113] (Figs 11-34c, 11-35, and 11-36). Placement by hand is preferred by some dentists because *(1)* it allows the operator to feel the insertion and to reverse the pin one quarter turn once the tip has contacted

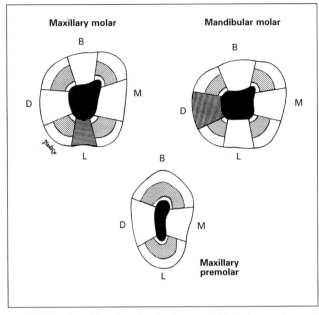

Fig 11-31 Preferred locations for pin placement. *(dotted areas)* The most preferred locations—at the line angles; *(white areas)* areas to avoid because of concavities, furcations, or thin dentin; *(lined areas on the molars)* areas where pins may be placed with added caution because the angulation of the root in relation to the crown is frequently severe.[108]

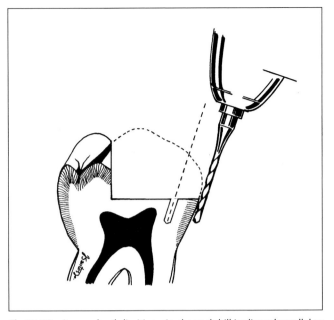

Fig 11-32a A non–depth-limiting pin channel drill is aligned parallel to the external surface.

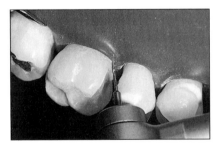

Fig 11-32b A pin channel drill is aligned with the mesial surface of the maxillary molar before it is carried into the preparation.

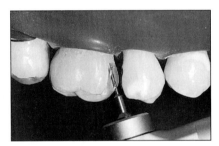

Fig 11-32c The drill is used to cut the pin channel to the same alignment.

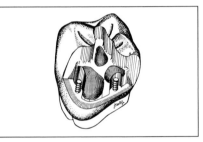

Fig 11-33 There should be adequate space around the full circumference of a pin for amalgam. If a pin is located adjacent to a dentinal wall, a small cove may be cut in the wall to provide adequate space for condensation of amalgam.

the end of the channel, thus avoiding excessive stresses in the dentin; and *(2)* stripping of the dentinal threads created by the self-threading pin is less likely. Insertion of pins with a low-speed handpiece is preferred by many because it is much more time efficient. The thread design of some pins (such as the Link Plus series) provides for wider dentinal threads; dentinal stripping is less frequent when such designs are used.

Because the portion of a pin that will extend into the amalgam usually is only 2.0 mm long or less, the pin is aligned parallel to the external surface of the tooth, and the channel

entrance is about 1.0 mm inside the DEJ, a pin rarely needs to be bent. The only reason for bending a pin is to keep it well within the bulk of the planned amalgam restoration. If bending should be needed, it may be accomplished with a small, fork-shaped pin bender (Fig 11-37a) or a small hemostat (Fig 11-37b) before the pin is shortened.

Shortening. The portion of a pin extending from the pin channel is often longer than desired, so it will need to be shortened after insertion. The pin may be efficiently and safe-

Fig 11-34 Pins and pin drivers (or wrenches) (TMS system).

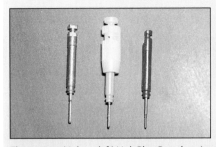

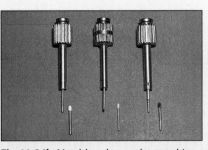

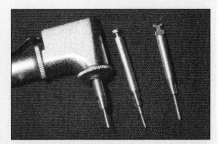

Fig 11-34a *(right to left)* Link Plus Regular pin, Link Plus Minim pin, and Link Series Minikin pin. A plastic Universal Hand Driver (for Link Plus and Link Series pins) is shown on the Link Plus Minim pin.

Fig 11-34b Metal hand wrenches or drivers with individual TMS gold-plated stainless steel pins: *(left to right)* Regular, Minim, and Minikin. The hand driver with the band around the handle is for Minim pins; the nonbanded hand driver is for Regular and Minikin pins.

Fig 11-34c Pin drivers for insertion into a motorized or hand-operated handpiece to place individual gold-plated stainless steel pins (shown installed in drivers).

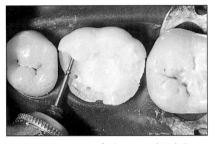

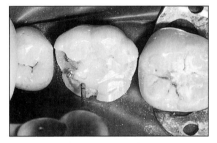

Fig 11-35 Insertion of a horizontal Link Series Minikin pin in a facial cusp of a mandibular molar.

Fig 11-36 A low-speed handpiece is used to insert a vertical Link Plus Minim pin.

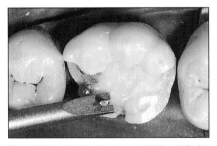

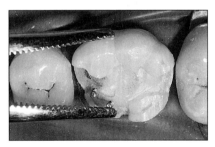

Fig 11-37a To bend pins, a Coltène/Whaledent pin bender can be used.

Fig 11-37b If a hemostat is used to bend a pin, the jaw of the hemostat should contact the pin at its tip, and very controlled pressure should be used in bending the pin.

ly cut by gently brushing the pin with either a thin fissure bur or a diamond bur in a high-speed handpiece. The small segment of pin that is sectioned is a potential projectile that should be controlled with an instrument when possible. Both the bur and the diamond should be used with air or water coolant to prevent the pin, and therefore the surrounding tooth structure, from being overheated during the operation.

If a bur is used, it must be sharp. If the bur approaches from an oblique angle, the clockwise rotation of the bur can cause counterclockwise rotation of the pin so that it is unscrewed. Therefore, if the pin cannot be approached perpendicularly by the bur (Fig 11-38a), it should be grasped with the pin wrench, cotton forceps, or a hemostat to stabilize it during the cutting process (Fig 11-38b), or, minimally, an instrument

Fig 11-38 *Shortening a pin. A light, brushing stroke and air or water coolant should be used while a pin is cut.*

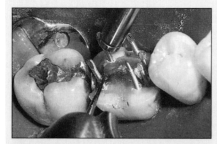

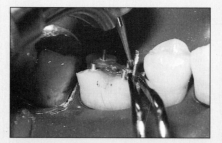

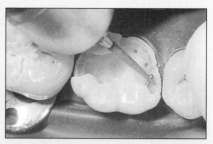

Fig 11-38a When a No. 169L tapered fissure bur is used to approach the pin at approximately 90 degrees, no stabilization is necessary.

Fig 11-38b When a No. 35 inverted cone bur is approaching the pin obliquely, the pin is stabilized to prevent it from being unscrewed from the pin channel.

Fig 11-38c This needle-shaped diamond is approaching the pin at approximately 90 degrees.

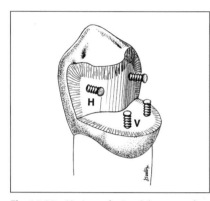

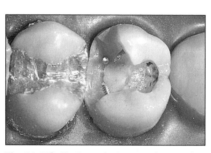

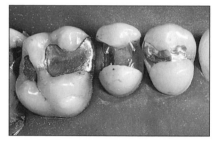

Fig 11-39a Horizontal pins (H) are used to attach the wall of a cusp to the amalgam restoration. Vertical pins (V) attach the restoration to the radicular portion of the tooth.

Fig 11-39b Horizontal pins can be used in conjunction with vertical pins. In this clinical situation, a proximal box had to be extended significantly facially to eliminate caries and unsupported enamel.

Fig 11-40 Horizontal pins are used to cross splint the cusps of a maxillary premolar.

should be pressed against the pin during the process to dampen vibration from the bur, which tends to initiate the unscrewing. A long, narrow diamond is preferred by many operators for cutting pins, because it causes less vibration and is less likely to "catch" in the metal of the pin to initiate reverse rotation (Fig 11-38c).

Horizontal Pins

Studies[114,115] have demonstrated the efficacy of using pins oriented horizontally, that is, inserted into the dentin of a vertical wall of a preparation (Figs 11-39a and 11-39b). Burgess[114] found two horizontal self-threading pins (Coltène/Whaledent TMS Minim and Minikin) placed into a free-standing facial cusp of a maxillary premolar to be effective in reinforcing the cusp (see Fig 11-39a). Other investigators[115] have found that horizontal pins, used to cross splint cusps of maxillary premolars, reinforce and strengthen the cusps (Fig 11-40).

Adequate dentin must be present for horizontal pins to be employed. When the channels for horizontal pins are prepared, they should be initiated in dentin 0.5 to 1.0 mm from the DEJ. They should be directed approximately parallel to the adjacent DEJ (and external surface of the tooth). But, because of their horizontal orientation, such pin channels, prepared only 1.5 to 2.0 mm deep, will often contact enamel. When the pin channel drill, in its progress through dentin, seems to stop its penetration short of reaching its depth-limiting shoulder, it is probably because it has reached enamel. Further deepening of the channel should not be attempted; even 1.0 mm of depth will impart some retention for a pin, and attempts to deepen the channel into enamel will result in an enlarged dentinal channel and increased potential for enamel fracture.

Horizontal pins should be positioned fairly near to the occlusal surface in the dentin of a vertical wall, 0.5 mm to 1.0 mm gingival to the occlusal DEJ, so that their mechanical

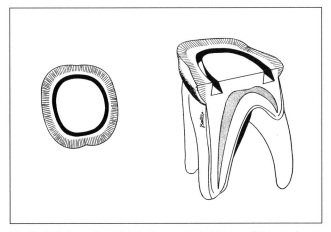

Fig 11-41 A circumferential slot is prepared with a small, inverted cone bur, such as a No. 33½.

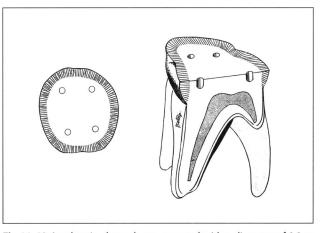

Fig 11-42 Amalgapin channels are prepared with a diameter of 0.8 to 1.0 mm, such as that of a No. 330 bur, to a depth of approximately 1.5 mm.

advantage is enhanced for reinforcement of the cusp. A horizontal pin should be oriented so that it will not be near the anticipated surface of the amalgam and so that amalgam may be condensed around the entire circumference of the pin.

Perforation During Pin Channel Preparation

Perforations during pin channel preparation should be avoided through careful design and placement of the channel. However, if a perforation does occur, it is important to determine what has been perforated, the external surface of the tooth or the pulp chamber. When the pulp chamber with a vital pulp has been perforated, the channel should be covered with calcium hydroxide, and another pin channel should be placed in a new location. Alternatively, a different type of resistance feature should be used. A perforation of the external surface of the tooth may be more problematic. If the perforation is located above the epithelial attachment, the channel should be filled with amalgam. If the pin is inserted and the tip protruding on the external surface is cut even with the surface and polished, the pin will not totally obturate the perforation, and leakage will occur.[116] If the perforation occurs below the epithelial attachment, the channel may be obturated with mineral trioxide aggregate (MTA) or with amalgam.

Nonpin Mechanical Resistance and Retention Features

Birtcil and Venton[117] suggested that more attention be directed toward using the available tooth structure to provide retention and resistance form in complex amalgam restorations. They recommended parallelism in all walls of the preparation, proximal box form, retention grooves in the proximal

line angles, box form in buccal and lingual groove areas of molars, dovetails, rectangular boxes in areas other than proximal surfaces, and reduction of undermined cusps for coverage with amalgam. In recent years, several additional nonpin resistance and retention methods have been described and investigated. These include the circumferential slot and the amalgapin, as well as adhesive bonding (described in the Amalgam Bonding section and in Chapter 8).

Circumferential slots. Outhwaite and others,[118] who introduced the circumferential slot prepared with a No. 33½ inverted cone bur (Fig 11-41), compared it to four pins (TMS Minim) in an in vitro study and found no significant differences between the resistance provided by the two techniques. They also reported that the pin restorations had a greater tendency to slip on their bases before failure, whereas slippage did not occur with circumferential slots. However, slot-retained restorations are more sensitive to displacement during matrix removal than are pin-retained restorations.

Amalgapins. Seng and others[119] tested circular chambers that they cut vertically into dentin to provide resistance and retention form for the restoration; they called these features *amalgam inserts.* Preparations for the inserts were made with a No. 35 inverted cone bur and were approximately 1.4 mm in diameter and depth. In their study, amalgam inserts provided resistance to displacement similar to that provided by self-threading pins. Shavell[120] described a variation of the amalgam insert, which he termed the *amalgapin* (Fig 11-42). The amalgapin channel described by Shavell was prepared with a No. 1157 or No. 1156 bur and had a depth of 3.0 mm. Lab-

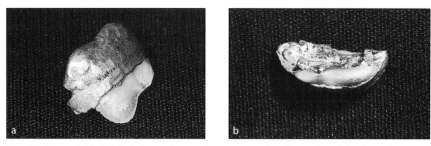

Figs 11-43a and 11-43b Failed complex amalgam restoration that replaced the lingual cusps of a mandibular molar. Note the fin of cervical tooth structure that fractured.

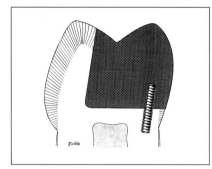

Fig 11-43c The dentin lingual to the pin was the only tooth structure that was opposing a lingually directed load on the restoration.

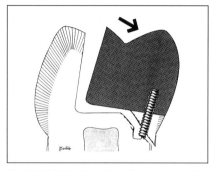

Fig 11-43d A load pushing the restoration lingually caused failure. Failure can be attributed to a lack of distribution of resistance and retention features.

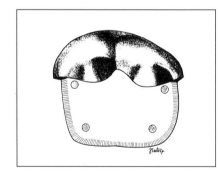

Fig 11-43e Alternatively, had two of the four pins been placed vertically in the facial aspect of the preparation, this could have reduced the likelihood of failure.

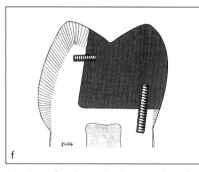

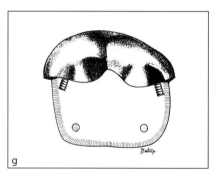

Figs 11-43f and 11-43g Had two of the four pins been located horizontally, failure would likely have been averted.

oratory studies of the amalgapin[121,122] have demonstrated that the resistance to displacement provided by amalgapins is similar to that provided by pins. It has been demonstrated[122] that a depth of 1.5 to 2.0 mm is adequate for amalgapins and that an amalgapin with a diameter of 0.8 mm provides resistance similar to that of an amalgapin with a diameter of 1.0 mm. In addition to the burs advocated by Shavell (No. 1156 and No. 1157), others with similar diameters (such as the No.

330 and No. 56) also function well in creating amalgapin channels.[122]

Efficacy of Resistance and Retention Methods

For the most part, the resistance form provided by various resistance and retention methods has been tested in flattened molars, as described by Buikema and others,[107] with 4.0-mm-high restorations retained by given macromechanical resistance features or amalgam bonding. These teeth were mounted at a 45-degree angle and were loaded in compression; the mean loads at the time of failure were calculated. Although this method of testing is not as enlightening as long-term clinical tests, it probably provides a good indicator of how well a resistance feature will perform in a clinical situation. It has been shown, however, that if these standard resistance-test restorations are loaded at a 90-degree angle instead of a 45-degree angle, the stainless steel pins provide significantly more resistance than amalgam inserts.[123,124] Few forces in the mouth are directed at a 90-degree angle to the long axis of the tooth, however, and few restorations are placed on preparations that are totally flat, without any walls or irregularities in the dentin.

One of the most telling studies pertaining to resistance form for complex amalgam restorations was reported by Plasmans and coworkers.[125] This group created preparations for complex amalgam restorations that combined the use of boxes, shelves, and amalgapins as resistance and retention features. They then loaded specimens at 45 degrees, as in most previous studies of resistance form, but they loaded half of the restorations from one side and half from the other. Their finding was, generally, that more load was required to cause failure of a restoration when the resistance and retention features (walls, boxes, and amalgapin channels) that opposed the direction of the load were increased.

It is important to distribute mechanical resistance features into all areas of the preparation and not to cluster them in any one area.[124–126] Figures 11-43a to 11-43d show a restoration that originally replaced two missing cusps of a mandibular molar. The probable cause of failure was that the resistance features (pins) were clustered in the lingual aspect of the cavity preparation. In function, there was nothing to attach the facial aspect of the restoration to the tooth. If two of the four vertical pins had been placed in the facial portion of the preparation (Fig 11-43e), or if two horizontal pins had been placed in the facial cusps (Figs 11-43f and 11-43g), the restoration would, in all likelihood, have had adequate resistance to withstand its load in function.

When the technical requirements for placement of vertical pins can be met, vertical pins provide excellent retention and resistance form. However, risks are involved with pin placement: crazing of tooth structure, perforation into the pulp or periodontium, and weakening of the amalgam restoration over pins.[127] Additionally, the use of both vertical and horizontal pins may be limited by inadequate access; in these cases, alternative resistance and retention methods should be employed. When a cusp has been reduced, and increased resistance form is needed, adhesive bonding, an amalgapin, or a segment of a circumferential slot may be indicated.

Amalgam Bonding

The use of adhesive resins to increase the retention, resistance, and marginal seal of amalgam restorations has gained a strong foothold in restorative dentistry. There is now more than adequate evidence that properly bonded amalgam restorations will be as successful as pin-retained amalgam restorations. Several clinical studies have demonstrated success after several years of service.[94,128–131] In one clinical study of complex amalgam restorations,[128] all bonded and pin-retained restorations were classified as successful at 2 years. Six-year results were reported for another clinical study[94] in which 32 bonded (Amalgambond Plus with HPA powder, Parkell) and 28 pin-retained (TMS pins) amalgam restorations were compared; each restoration replaced at least one cusp and, in some of the restorations, the only sources of retention were the pins or the adhesive bonding (see example in Fig 11-78). After 5 years, seven of the pin-retained and two of the bonded restorations had failed (n = 46). Failures of bonded restorations involved loss of another cusp. None of the bonded amalgam restorations had debonded. At 6 years, the results continued to demonstrate that bonded amalgam restorations performed as well as pin-retained amalgam restorations, with failure of one from each category in the 6th year (n = 27). The number and length of clinical studies[132] is now sufficient to indicate that bonded amalgam restorations can perform as well as restorations using mechanical resistance and retention features when the bonding technique is accomplished properly.

Pins and bonding can have an additive effect in which the resistance to displacement is superior to either technique alone.[133–136] In one in vitro study,[133] the mean resistance to dislodgment provided by a filled amalgam-bonding material combined with self-threading pins was approximately equal to the sum of the mean resistance produced by pins alone and the mean resistance produced by bonding alone.

For use of bonding resins in amalgam restorations, current research suggests the improved efficacy of filled resins compared with unfilled or minimally filled resins.[136–139] The method of incorporation of the filler varies from manufacturer to manufacturer. One system (Amalgambond Plus, Parkell) uses very fine methyl methacrylate powder, added to the liquid resin, as the filler.[140] Another system (All-Bond 2 and Liner F, Bisco) uses a filled flowable resin composite liner to provide the filled resin. With both types of system, the amalgam is condensed into the filled resin while the resin is in a viscous liquid form. Microscopic "fingers" of resin are incorporated into the amalgam at the interface. When hardened, these provide the attachment of amalgam to resin. Because light cannot penetrate to the resin underlying amalgam restorations, it is important to use a self-curing or chemically activated bonding resin. The bonding resin of an amalgam bonding system is supplied in two parts that are to be mixed. Either chemically cured resins or dual-cured (chemical and light initiation) resins may be effective. The attachment of resin to tooth structure when amalgam bonding systems are used is accomplished as with other dental bonding systems, as described in chapter 8.

There is ample evidence of decreased leakage of fluids when an amalgam bonding system is used compared with noncoated or varnish-coated amalgam cavity walls.[141–146] Many dentists have reported that amalgam bonding systems have reduced the incidence of postoperative tooth sensitivity, but most research has not supported these observations. Clinical studies[147,148] comparing postoperative sensitivity in bonded and nonbonded restorations have reported no significant difference. One study[149] involving 40 teeth with symptoms of cracked-tooth syndrome prior to restoration found no difference in thermal sensitivity between pin-retained and bonded restorations at 2 weeks but found less thermal sensitivity in teeth with bonded restorations at 3 and 12 months.

For reinforcing cusps in posterior teeth weakened by significant pathosis or large restorations, there is in vitro evidence that amalgam bonding can result in some strengthening of teeth.[150–153] However, much of this effect may be lost with time.[154–156] At present, it is still advisable to reduce severely weakened cusps for replacement and protection with a strong restorative material.[127] The use of amalgam for this purpose is described in this chapter. Other types of occlusal-coverage restorations are described in chapters 18 and 19.

Evidence from clinical and laboratory studies supports the contributions to resistance to displacement that come from the various resistance features and methods (cavity form, threaded pins, slots, grooves, amalgapins, and filled adhesives). The resistance mechanisms used in any restoration should be selected based on the functional load to which the restoration is expected to be exposed. Amalgam bonding probably should not be used as the sole means of retaining an amalgam restoration, but it may be effective for supplementing mechanical resistance features in large, complex amalgam restorations, especially those replacing cusps. Most preparations have some box form and surface irregularities that, when combined with resin bonding, can provide long-term retention of the restoration. A filled amalgam bonding system should be used. Amalgam bonding should be used when an improved initial seal is needed, such as after a direct or indirect pulp capping procedure in the tooth being restored. Adequate moisture control and meticulous attention to product instructions are necessary to duplicate the success that has been demonstrated in clinical trials.

Matrices

To confine the amalgam and allow adequate pressure for optimum condensation, the preparation must be boxlike, that is, with confining walls and floors. A Class 1 occlusal preparation provides these by virtue of its location and definition. Whenever an amalgam preparation extends from one surface of the tooth to another, some form of matrix is needed to confine the amalgam for condensation. If a matrix is not used, condensation forces will tend to push the amalgam out of the preparation rather than condensing the amalgam.

The simplest and fastest method of adequately providing a matrix should be used. Occasionally, as with the occlusolingual restoration of the maxillary molar, the blade of a hand instrument placed on the lingual surface of the molar and held in place during condensation may be adequate (Fig 11-44). In most cases, a matrix system, such as a Tofflemire matrix, is indicated. Rarely, a customized matrix will be necessary for a particular situation. A matrix system is needed in almost every case for multisurface Class 2 amalgam restorations.

There are myriad types of matrix systems; most involve a thin piece of stainless steel that is contoured and placed adjacent to the proximal portions of Class 2 preparations. The purpose of the matrix is to:

1. Confine the amalgam so that adequate condensation forces can be applied.
2. Allow re-establishment of contact with the adjacent tooth.
3. Restrict extrusion of the amalgam and the formation of an overhang at a hidden margin, such as the proximal gingival margin.
4. Provide for adequate physiologic contour for the proximal surface of the restoration.
5. Impart an acceptable surface texture to the proximal surface, especially in the area of the contact that cannot be carved and burnished.

Tofflemire Matrix

Probably the most commonly used type of matrix system in the United States is the Tofflemire system. The system consists of a matrix band and retainer (Figs 11-45a to 11-45j). The Tofflemire retainer consists of four parts (see Fig 11-45b).

Parts
Head. This is the part that has the open side. In the U-shaped head, there are two slots in the open side. These slots are used to position the matrix band. The open side of the head should be held facing upward while the band is installed. The open side of the head faces gingivally when the band is

placed around the tooth. There are two types of Tofflemire retainers based on the angulation of the head (see Fig 11-45g).

Slide. This element has a diagonal slot. The round ends of the band, when installed, extend at least 1.0 or 2.0 mm beyond the slot in the side of the slide. The amount of the band extending beyond the slot in the side of the slide will depend on the size of the tooth being treated. More of the band should extend from the slide for premolars than for molars. The slide is positioned near the head for installation of the band in the retainer and for placement of the band around the tooth.

Rotating spindle. This is used to adjust the distance between the slide and the head. The retainer is held with the thumb and forefinger of one hand (contacting both the head and slide) while the rotating spindle is turned with the other hand, clockwise and counterclockwise, to advance and retract the slide. This movement adjusts the size of the loop of the matrix band.

Set-screw. The threaded shaft of the set-screw locks and unlocks the matrix band in the slide.

Types

The types of Tofflemire bands include flat bands of multiple shapes, precontoured bands, and bands with and without memory (dead-soft metal).

Flat bands. Bands for the Tofflemire system come in several shapes (see Fig 11-45c) and in three thicknesses: 0.0010, 0.0015, and 0.0020 inches. The thicker band is stiffer to resist deformation during condensation; the thinner bands are often used to help ensure a tight contact in Class 2 restorations. Any of the three thicknesses can be used to achieve excellent results, and selection is primarily a matter of operator preference.

By far the most frequently used shape is the No. 1, or Universal, band. The No. 2 (so-called MOD) band has two extensions projecting at its gingival edge to allow matrix application in teeth with very deep gingival margins in the proximal aspects of the tooth. In most cases, there will be only one deep area, so one of the extensions is usually cut off with scissors (see Fig 11-45f). The No. 3 band also has projections for deeper gingival margins, but the band is narrower than the No. 2 band. The No. 3 band is ordinarily considered suitable for premolars and the No. 2 band for molars, but the size that best suits the situation should be used.

Because these bands are flat, they should be contoured so that they will impart physiologic contours to the restorations.

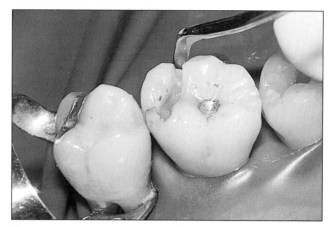

Fig 11-44 An instrument is held in place to act as a matrix for a small occlusolingual Class 1 restoration in a maxillary molar.

A flat band may be contoured before it is placed in the retainer. The band is laid on a paper pad or other compressible surface, and the area to be contoured is heavily rubbed with an ovoid burnisher, a beavertail burnisher, the convex back of the blade of a spoon excavator, or a convex side of the cotton forceps. A band may also be contoured after it has been applied to the tooth. The area to be contoured is rubbed with the back of the blade of the spoon excavator or other thin, convex instrument (Fig 11-46a). Contact with the adjacent tooth should be more than a pinpoint touch (Fig 11-46b).

Precontoured bands. Precontoured Tofflemire matrix bands are also available. One such band is the contour matrix band or Dixieland Band (Waterpik Technologies) developed by Dr Wilmer Eames (see Fig 11-45d). When these bands are removed from interproximal contacts, the contour must be considered, and the band must be rotated in such a way that the trailing edge does not break or alter the shape of the marginal ridge as the band is being removed.

Placement

Assembly. When the matrix retainer and band are assembled, the two ends of the matrix band must be even as they protrude from the diagonal slot of the slide. The loop can extend from the retainer in three different ways: straight, to the left, or to the right (see Fig 11-45h). The straight assembly is for restorations near the front of the mouth where the rubber dam–covered cheek will not get in the way if the retainer protrudes perpendicularly from the line of teeth. The right and left assemblies allow the retainer to be aligned parallel or tangent to the line of teeth in more posterior areas. The band should be placed in the retainer so that the loop extends from the appropriate side of the retainer and the set-screw knob is directed toward the front of the mouth.

Fig 11-45a to 11-45j Tofflemire matrix system.

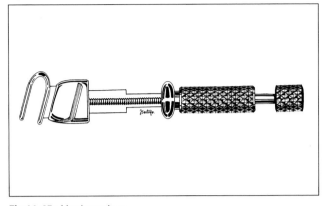

Fig 11-45a Matrix retainer.

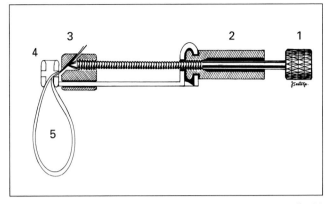

Fig 11-45b Parts of the assembly: (1) set-screw; (2) rotating spindle; (3) slide; (4) head; (5) band.

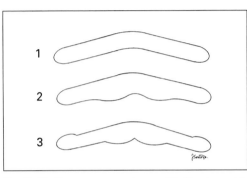

Fig 11-45c Three common shapes of Tofflemire matrix flat bands (No. 1 is also called a Universal band; No. 2 and No. 3 are also called MOD bands).

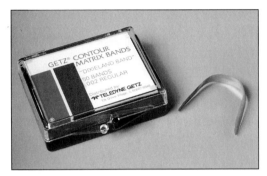

Fig 11-45d Precontoured Dixieland Bands.

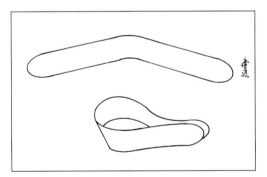

Fig 11-45e The matrix band is folded for insertion into the retainer.

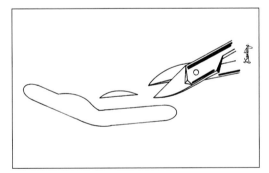

Fig 11-45f One of the projections of a No. 2 or 3 band may be cut off if there is only one deep proximal area of the preparation.

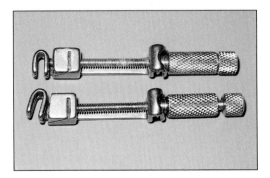

Fig 11-45g Two types of Tofflemire retainer: *(top)* straight; *(bottom)* contra-angled.

Fig 11-45 (continued)

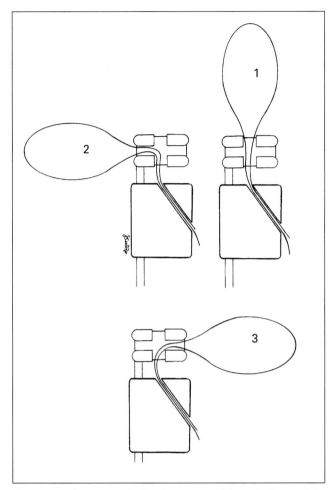

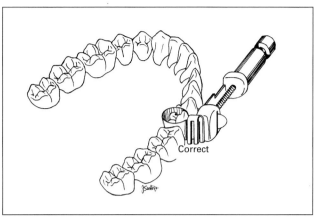

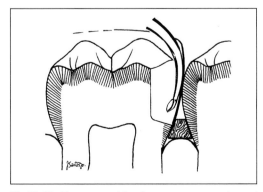

Fig 11-45h The loop of the band may extend from the head of the retainer in one of three directions: (1) straight; (2) left; (3) right.

Fig 11-45i The matrix must be assembled with the slots in the head directed gingivally.

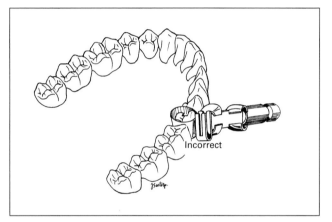

Fig 11-45j The slots in the head of the matrix should not be directed occlusally.

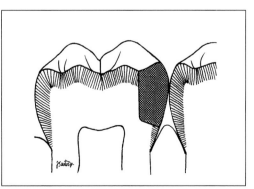

Fig 11-46a The convex side of a spoon excavator is used to impart a convex contour to the matrix band.

Fig 11-46b This will help to achieve a contact area, as opposed to a pinpoint contact, with the adjacent tooth.

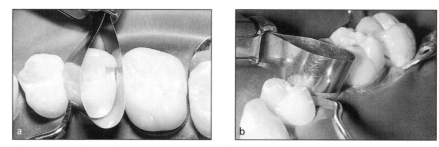

Figs 11-47a and 11-47b The blade of a plastic filling instrument has been placed into the gingival embrasure and is being slightly rotated (torqued) to provide enough separation to allow the matrix band to slip through the contact.

Because of the shape of the Tofflemire matrix band, when it is placed in the retainer, one opening of the loop has a greater diameter than the other (see Fig 11-45e). In other words, the loop will be shaped somewhat like a funnel. The wider opening is oriented toward the occlusal aspect. The short knob of the set-screw is tightened so that the matrix band is held securely.

Application. The matrix is applied to the tooth to be restored. The matrix band will slide easily through the interproximal contact area when the preparation has opened the contact. It will often slide through an intact contact as well (for example, the mesial contact when there is a disto-occlusal preparation). If it will not slide through the intact contact, a bladed plastic filling instrument (such as the No. 1-2, shown in Figs 11-47a and 11-47b) may be used to open the contact slightly to allow the band through. For this slight tooth separation, the blade of the instrument is placed in the gingival embrasure (gingival to the contact), moved occlusally until it is stopped by the contact, and torqued very slightly. At the same time, the matrix band is slipped through the contact. When the matrix is around the tooth, it should be tightened snugly, but not too tightly because a very tight matrix will deform the tooth.[157–159]

Wedging. Wooden wedges may be placed from either the facial or the lingual aspect. A wedge should usually be inserted from the side with the widest embrasure. For example, between the first and second premolars, the largest embrasure is usually the lingual embrasure. The wedge should be inserted tightly to enable development of an adequate contact despite the thickness of the matrix material.

Wedges are available in a variety of shapes and sizes. Figure 11-48a shows Wizard wedges (Waterpik Technologies), which are triangular and available in four sizes. Figures 11-48b and 11-48c show Sycamore wedges (Premier), which are shaped to aid the establishment of physiologic proximal con-

tours. The Premier wedges, with seven color-coded sizes, are recommended for amalgam restorations.

The matrix band must extend gingival to the gingival margin of the proximal box of a Class 2 restoration, and the wedge must be positioned so that its base is also gingival to the gingival margin. If the wedge cannot be placed so that its base is gingival to the preparation margin, a concavity will be created in the matrix just occlusal to the gingival margin, and this concavity will be transferred to the amalgam. Occasionally, the gingival papilla will need to be surgically reflected from the interproximal area to allow the wedge to be positioned apical to the gingival margin. Another option is to use a rigid bladed instrument to hold the matrix against the gingival margin during condensation. Custom wedges may be made for special situations; the wedge in Fig 11-48d was fabricated from a wooden tongue blade.

Contouring. The band should be burnished and contoured to impart the desired proximal contours to the restoration. This can be accomplished with the back (convex side) of a spoon excavator (see Fig 11-46a). The wedged matrix should be in solid contact with the adjacent tooth in the desired contact area. It should be possible to feel the convexity of the proximal surface of the adjacent tooth with an instrument through the matrix as the matrix is burnished.

Removal

In a multiple surface restoration, amalgam is condensed in the preparation after matrix placement. Amalgam condensation is discussed in the next section.

When amalgam placement using a Tofflemire matrix has been completed and preliminary carving of the occlusal aspect accomplished, first the slide and then the set-screw of the matrix retainer is loosened. A finger or thumb is placed on the loop of the matrix band to keep it in place on the tooth, and the retainer is pulled occlusally to remove it. The distal end of the matrix band is grasped and pulled occlusally and

Fig 11-48 *Wooden interproximal wedges.*

Fig 11-48a Wizard wedges have a triangular shape.

Fig 11-48b Premier Sycamore wedges are shaped to impart a more physiologic contour to the matrix. There is a larger selection of sizes, and they are color coded for easy selection.

Fig 11-48c Note the anatomic shape of the Premier Sycamore wedges. The snow-sled point helps to prevent catching of the rubber dam during insertion.

Fig 11-48d A custom-made wooden wedge may also be used. This one was made from a tongue blade.

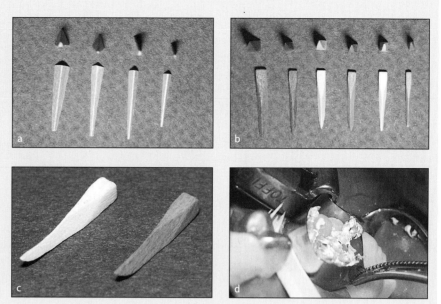

lingually (if the free ends are on the facial aspect) and out of the distal contact of the tooth. The mesial end is then grasped and pulled facially and occlusally until the band is out of the contact. The matrix band can be grasped with fingers, cotton forceps, or a hemostat. There are a few techniques that may help the dentist remove the Tofflemire matrix without breaking the marginal ridge:

1. As the matrix edge is coming out of the contact, the matrix can be tipped so that the edge will not "flip" the newly carved marginal ridge and break it.
2. A condenser can be held against the marginal ridge to support it and prevent it from breaking as the matrix is removed.
3. The movement of the band should be primarily to the facial or lingual aspect as the band slips occlusally out of the contact.
4. The band may be cut close to the teeth on the lingual aspect and then pulled facially from the contact.

The matrix band should be used only once and then discarded.

Other Matrix Systems

Many matrix systems other than Tofflemire matrices are available (Figs 11-49 to 11-53). Each has its own advantages and disadvantages. In addition, stainless steel matrix material may be spot-welded to provide a custom matrix for any situation.

One commercial system (Denovo) has prewelded bands in various sizes (see Figs 11-49a and 11-49b). To remove a spot-welded matrix from a tooth after the restoration is placed, a small bur in a high-speed handpiece is used to cut through the welds and allow the two ends of the matrix to separate. The absence of a matrix retainer in the Denovo system is a distinct advantage.

T-bands have long been used in dentistry and provide a very simple and inexpensive matrix system (see Fig 11-50). The AutoMatrix system has a built-in matrix retainer that is much smaller than the Tofflemire matrix retainer, which is an advantage (see Figs 11-51a and 11-51b). The Palodent matrix (Dentsply) system provides small, precontoured matrices that are placed, wedged, and held in place by a flexible metal Bitine ring. A major advantage of this system is that, for a restoration involving only one proximal surface, there is no need for the matrix to be placed in the other contact (see Figs 11-52a to 11-52c). The Omni-Matrix is basically a disposable Tofflemire retainer and band that is preassembled and has a head that moves from side to side (see Fig 11-53). Because there is no assembly time, this system takes less time to use than a Tofflemire matrix, but it is more expensive.

Reinforcing Matrices with Modeling Compound

Among the desirable qualities of a matrix are adequate rigidity and ability to maintain the shape established by the operator to impart the desired contour to the restoration. When a

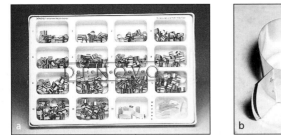
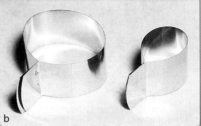

Figs 11-49a and 11-49b Denovo matrix system.

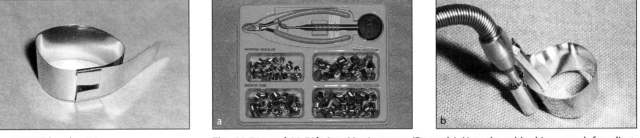

Figs 11-50 T-band matrix.

Figs 11-51a and 11-51b AutoMatrix system (Dentsply). Note the cable-drive wrench for adjusting the size of the loop.

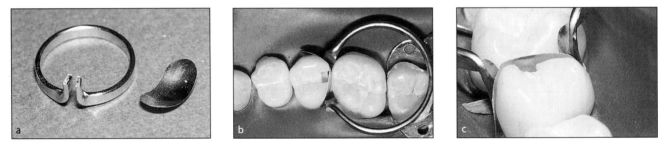

Figs 11-52a to 11-52c Palodent matrix system. Note the metal ring for holding the ends of the matrix snugly against the facial and lingual enamel. It will also provide some tooth separation.

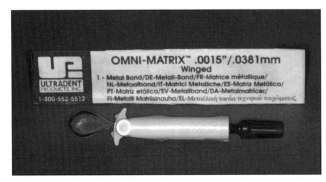

Fig 11-53 The Omni-Matrix (Ultradent) is basically a preassembled Tofflemire retainer and band that is intended for one-time use and then disposal. It is available with 0.0010- and 0.0015-inch-thick metal matrix band material, with "wings" (as shown) or without.

Class 2 preparation has only proximal boxes that are adjacent to other teeth, and when the preparation does not, to any significant degree, extend to facial and lingual surfaces, the stainless steel matrix is usually well supported by the adjacent tooth or teeth. In these cases, no reinforcement is necessary. In larger restorations that involve surfaces not supported by adjacent teeth, it is often desirable to reinforce or support the matrix in some way in these areas to maintain the rigidity and shape of the matrix.

Occasionally, a single unsupported area of a matrix may be reinforced during condensation by the operator, who places a finger or holds an instrument against the matrix in a facial or lingual area. For large unsupported areas, however, modeling compound may be used (Figs 11-54a to 11-54j).

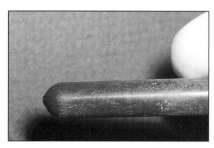

Fig 11-54a Modeling compound can be used to support a matrix.

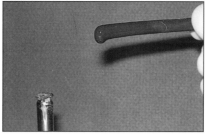

Fig 11-54b The compound stick is heated over an alcohol flame, then removed from the flame to allow warmth to diffuse to the core of the stick.

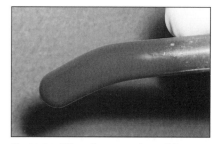

Fig 11-54c When the warmed tip of the compound stick begins to droop, softness is uniform throughout, and the compound is ready for use.

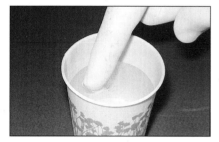

Fig 11-54d A finger is dampened in water to prevent the glove from sticking to the softened compound.

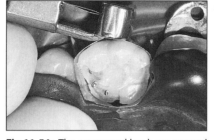

Fig 11-54e The compound has been pressed into place. It will be cooled with air to reharden it.

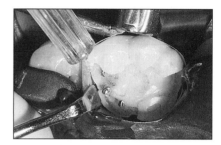

Fig 11-54f The matrix may be recontoured after application of the compound. A warmed instrument is used to soften the compound and reshape the matrix.

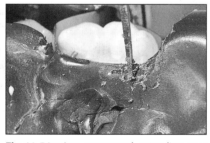

Fig 11-54g Any compound extending past the edge of the matrix should be trimmed to prevent chipping during amalgam condensation.

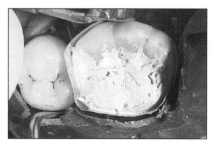

Fig 11-54h The compound is removed after amalgam condensation and initial carving.

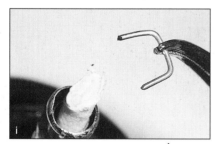

Figs 11-54i and 11-54j Staples can be used to hold compound segments in place.

There are various ways of applying compound to support a metal matrix. Probably the simplest is to employ a stick of compound (see Fig 11-54a). Approximately 1 inch of one end of the compound stick is heated over an alcohol burner. The stick is moved back and forth, while being rotated, over the tip of the flame (see Fig 11-54b). After 5 to 10 seconds, the stick is removed from the flame and held for a few seconds until the heat has diffused through the radius of the stick to its center, as indicated by its starting to droop or sag (see Fig 11-54c). At that point, the 1-inch end is soft enough to carry to the matrix and press into place with a dampened, gloved finger (see Figs 11-54d and 11-54e). If adhesion of the compound to the matrix and adjacent teeth is desired, the softened end of the stick should be passed through the flame again just before it is carried to the mouth; this will provide a tacky surface that will impart some adhesion.

After the compound is pressed into place (see Fig 11-54e), it is cooled and hardened with air from a three-way syringe. The matrix may be recontoured after compound application. A warmed instrument may be used inside the matrix to soften the compound and exert pressure on the matrix to give it the shape that will allow the restoration contours and shape to be similar to the original shape of the tooth (see Fig 11-54f). Again, the compound should be cooled with air after reshaping with a warmed instrument. If modeling compound extends occlusal to the occlusal edge of the matrix band, it should be trimmed back with a sharp instrument (see Fig 11-54g), or pieces of compound could chip off during amalgam condensation and contaminate the amalgam.

If condensation forces dislodge the compound, matrix reinforcement will be lost; steps should be taken, therefore, to ensure that the compound does not dislodge. While it is soft, a portion of it may be pushed onto the cusps of an adjacent tooth to provide retention, or, when compound is present on both the facial and lingual aspects, a staple-shaped piece of metal, made from a paper clip or other wire, may be warmed in the flame (see Fig 11-54i) and placed to hold the facial and lingual segments of compound together (see Fig 11-54j). When it is time to remove the staple, the tips of a hemostat are warmed in the flame, the staple is grasped, and the heat is allowed to diffuse into the compound surrounding the staple so that it is softened. The compound can usually be pried away from the adjacent teeth and matrix with an instrument such as a Hollenback carver or enamel hatchet (see Fig 11-54h). After the compound is removed, the matrix may be removed as previously described.

Matrices for Bonded Amalgam Restorations

If a hydrophilic resin or bonding system is used to coat the walls of the preparation, the material should be applied before the matrix is placed, or care should be taken to prevent or minimize resin application to the matrix. If resin is applied to the matrix, it may cause the matrix to stick to the amalgam. This sticking can lead to fracture of the amalgam during removal of the matrix. Attachment of the matrix to the amalgam is most significant when amalgam bonding materials are used. Because amalgam must be inserted immediately after placement of the adhesive, the bonding material cannot be placed before matrix application; the best solution at present is to avoid, as much as possible, getting the bonding material on the matrix. A very small applicator should be used to apply the resin to the preparation walls so that it may be kept away from the matrix. It is advisable to try to stop the resin approximately 1 mm short of the cavosurface margins that are adjacent to the margins. Unless the set of the material is too advanced by the time the amalgam is placed, it will be pushed to the margin in a thin coat as the amalgam is condensed.

Because matrices that resist the bonding materials are not yet available, the application of a very thin coat of wax, with a wax pencil or crayon or with a piece of inlay wax or boxing wax, may be helpful. The wax is rubbed onto the inner surface of the matrix band, and excess is rubbed off with a gloved finger.

Placement of Amalgam

The technique for amalgam placement is basically the same regardless of the type or classification of the preparation. Amalgam is mixed (triturated), carried to the cavity preparation, and condensed into the preparation so that voids are eliminated and all areas of the preparation are filled. The amalgam is then carved to reproduce the portion of the tooth that is missing.

Spherical alloys produce an amalgam that requires a lower mercury-alloy ratio and less condensation force. However, the direction of the condensing force is extremely important for spherical amalgams. They do not adapt to the cavity walls as well as lathe-cut or admixture amalgams.[160] Spherical amalgams are said to be less condensable, and lateral condensation is even more important when spherical amalgams are

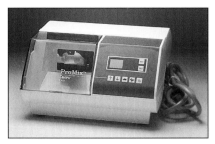

Fig 11-55a Pro-Mix amalgamator (Caulk/Dentsply).

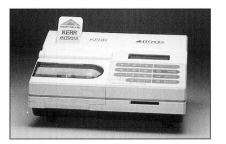

Fig 11-55b Automix amalgamator (Kerr/Sybron).

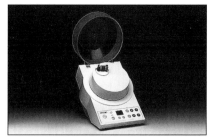

Fig 11-55c RotoMix centrifugal capsule mixer (3M ESPE).

used than when conventional or admixture amalgams are used. It is also somewhat more difficult to obtain good interproximal contacts in Class 2 amalgam restorations with spherical amalgams than with lathe-cut amalgams or admixtures. It has been demonstrated, however, that spherical amalgams are less sensitive to variations in condensation pressure than the amalgams containing nonspherical particles.[161] In addition, the spherical materials generally have a shorter working time and demonstrate a faster set than the admixtures.

Trituration

The trituration process includes the combining or mixing of liquid mercury with dry amalgam alloy powder. Electric amalgam mixers (also called *amalgamators* and *amalgam triturators*) are used for the trituration process (Figs 11-55a to 11-55c). The objective is to remove the oxide coating and wet each particle of alloy with mercury.[8] This begins the reaction that will produce a solid mass. Although amalgam alloy pellets and bottled mercury are still available separately, the use of precapsulated amalgam alloy, that is, a weighed, standardized amount of amalgam powder and mercury sealed into a capsule, is strongly recommended. The precapsulated products are not only ready for trituration, but they provide more consistent mixes of amalgam and virtually eliminate the possibility of mercury spills in the dental office.

The duration and speed of trituration should be just enough to coat all alloy particles with mercury, produce the amalgam matrix, and provide a plastic mix. Excessive trituration should be avoided because it generates heat and creates excess matrix in the microstructure of the resulting set material. In addition, an overtriturated mix of amalgam will set prematurely after trituration, and this will prevent adequate condensation and adaptation to the walls of the preparation, resulting in a weakened product. A mix of amalgam that is too plastic due to excess mercury, or, as is more frequently the case, is not plastic enough, must be discarded. A good mix of amalgam is plastic enough to condense well. If the mix is too

hard, brittle, or hot, reduction of the mixing time and/or the mixing speed is indicated.

Condensation

Condensation is the process of compressing and directing the dental amalgam into the tooth preparation with amalgam-condensing instruments (called *condensers* or *pluggers*) until the preparation is completely filled, and then overfilled, with a dense mass of amalgam. Proper condensation promotes adaptation of the amalgam to the walls of the preparation, and it compacts the material, eliminating voids and reducing the amount of residual mercury in the restoration. Both voids and increased residual mercury have been associated with a weakened amalgam product, so effective condensation continues trituration[162] and increases the strength[161,162] and serviceability[12] of the restoration.

Adequate condensation technique requires that a significant amount of force be applied to the condenser.[163] The force should be 2 to 5 kg (5 to 10 lbs) for a condensable amalgam (admixture or conventional); the condensation force required for spherical amalgams will be considerably less,[161,162] because heavy forces with the condenser tend to push the spherical particles to the side and cause the condenser to "punch through" the amalgam mass. The size of the condenser nib (end) determines the amount of pressure actually transferred from the operator's hand to the amalgam mass; the larger the nib, the less force per unit area (pressure) is applied to the mass for a given force from the operator's hand. In other words, when a larger-faced condenser is used, the operator must exert more force on the condenser to deliver adequate condensation pressure. Larger condensers should be used for spherical amalgam, rather than for admixtures, to allow adequate force to be applied without displacement of the spherical amalgam to the side.

When amalgam bonding systems are used, amalgam must be condensed into the bonding resin on all walls of the preparation before filling of the preparation is begun.

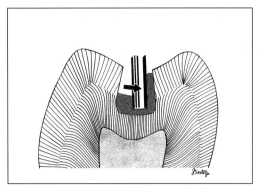

Fig 11-56a Lateral condensation toward all walls and toward the adjacent tooth in a Class 2 restoration will improve adaptation to walls and ensure a contact area with the adjacent tooth.

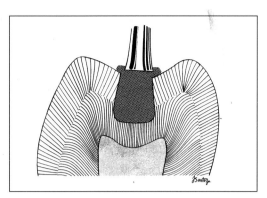

Fig 11-56b Overfill should be condensed with a large condenser.

Adequate condensation force will cause a slight movement of the patient's mandible or head, and often this movement will need to be stabilized by the dentist or assistant. A secure finger rest will enable the operator to perform more controlled, forceful strokes, using arm as well as finger pressure. The condensers are held with the pen grasp or a modification. Many operators use a finger or thumb of the hand that is not holding the condenser to apply additional condensation force. It has been demonstrated that dentists tend to use less condensation pressure during the later stages of amalgam placement; investigators[163] have emphasized the need for maintaining condensation pressures for both admixed and spherical amalgams throughout the condensation process.

After the preparation has been made ready to receive the amalgam, the amalgam alloy and mercury should be mixed (triturated) to give a plastic and moldable mass of amalgam. For most restorations, an amalgam carrier (see Fig 6-36) is valuable for delivering the amalgam to the preparation. For small restorations and for placing amalgam in proximal box preparations, care must be exercised to ensure increments of amalgam are small enough. If increments are too large, the condensing force cannot be adequate to adapt the amalgam material at the deepest area of the increment. For very large complex amalgam preparations, the entire mix may be carried to the preparation, or the mix may be divided in half and one half at a time carried to the preparation with cotton forceps. No matter how the amalgam is carried, it should be spread in the preparation so that the increment is thin for optimum condensation. Each portion of amalgam carried to the preparation should result in an increment thickness of 1.0 mm or thinner to ensure maximum condensation effectiveness.

Condensers that fit into all areas of the preparation should be used. Flat-faced, round condensers are generally consid-

ered to allow maximum condensation pressure. Convex-ended condensers are also available, as are flat-ended condensers with diamond, rectangular, and triangular shapes. When spherical amalgams are used, the largest condenser that will fit into the area of the preparation where the amalgam is being condensed should be used. For all amalgams, a large condenser should be used for the overfilling of the preparation.

Amalgam must be condensed into the preparation as soon as trituration is completed. One increment of amalgam should not be allowed to set significantly before the next increment is added. Amalgam should be condensed both vertically and horizontally or laterally (toward the walls of the preparation). This will promote a close adaptation of the amalgam to the walls as well as to the floor of the preparation. Lateral condensation, whether or not an amalgam bonding system is being used, can be achieved in more than one way. One is to alter the direction of the face (end) of the condenser so that the face is pushed toward the walls. Another method is to place the condenser into the preparation vertically, then to move it laterally toward the walls so that the side of the condenser condenses the amalgam against the walls (Fig 11-56a). Lateral condensation is especially important for spherical amalgams because, paradoxically, it is more difficult to adapt these materials to cavity walls.

When amalgam is condensed, mercury tends to be brought to the surface, creating a mercury-rich amalgam on the surface. To reduce the amount of mercury left in the restoration (residual mercury), the preparation is overfilled (Fig 11-56b) and the mercury-rich excess is carved off. The lower the residual mercury in the carved restoration, the greater its strength[17] and the better the expected longevity of the restoration.

Condensation when Amalgam Bonding Resins Are Used

As with the use of the matrix, there are some additional considerations and slightly altered techniques when amalgam bonding systems are used. Because the polymerization of amalgam bonding resins is chemically initiated, the amalgam must be ready to place when the two parts of the bonding resin are mixed to initiate polymerization. Although all walls of the cavity preparation should be coated, caution should be exercised to minimize the amount of bonding resin placed on the walls. One problem resulting from excess bonding resin is the reduction of the amalgam strength by incorporation of large amounts of resin into the bulk of the amalgam.[164] Another is the increased probability of transferring the bonding resin to the metal matrix during condensation, as described earlier. Another potential problem is the creation of voids in the proximal amalgam due to excess resin being pulled from the restoration while removing the matrix.

After the bonding resin has been applied to the walls of the preparation, the amalgam is placed in the preparation and condensed against all walls. After amalgam has been condensed into the resin on all walls, it should be added in increments as described for nonbonded amalgam restorations.

Precarve Burnishing

After it is condensed with amalgam condensers, the amalgam may be further condensed and shaping of occlusal anatomy begun with a large burnisher, such as an ovoid (football) burnisher (see Fig 11-64h). This is called *precarve burnishing*, and it should take place immediately after completion of condensation. The burnisher should be used with heavy strokes, made in the mesiodistal and faciolingual directions, that pinch much of the amalgam off as the burnisher contacts the cusp inclines and, in some places, the margins of the preparation. It has been shown that precarve burnishing produces denser amalgam at the margins of restorations.[165] In addition to aiding condensation, precarve burnishing is the first step in shaping the occlusal surface of the restoration.

Carving

Amalgam may be carved with any bladed dental instrument that has a sharp edge. Numerous carvers are available, and each has its own merit. Recommended amalgam carvers that satisfy most amalgam carving needs are a small cleoid-discoid carver; a Walls No. 3 (or Tanner No. 5) carver; a Hollenback No. ½ carver; an interproximal carver (developed by Baum); and a No. 14L sickle-shaped carver (see Fig 6-39). In addition, some cutting instruments, such as a small spoon excavator

and hoe, make excellent amalgam carvers, especially for carving occlusal anatomy in large restorations. The carving instruments selected should allow the operator to create contours and occlusion that reproduce, or occasionally make improvements to, the missing tooth structure.

Carving may begin immediately after condensation and precarve burnishing. Before the setting of the amalgam is very advanced, it carves very easily, but it is also easy to miscarve or overcarve, so care must be taken. As the setting of the amalgam advances, it does not carve as easily, but it remains carvable with sharp carvers for a long time. In fact, amalgam that has been in the mouth for many years can still be carved with sharp carvers.

The need for sharp carvers cannot be overemphasized, and it is advisable to have a sterilized sharpening stone available during placement of a large amalgam restoration. Amalgam seems to cause rapid dulling of carvers, possibly because of the effect of the mercury in penetrating and imparting brittleness to the steel.

Most occlusal carving is performed with pulling strokes, but the pushing stroke can also be advantageous in developing occlusal anatomy. Smaller occlusal and Class 2 restorations should be carved with the enamel tooth surface as a guide (Fig 11-57). The carver should rest on the enamel adjacent to the preparation and be pulled in a direction parallel to the margin of the preparation. When a stroke that is perpendicular to the margin of the preparation is needed, the carver should be pulled from enamel to amalgam. If it is pulled from amalgam to enamel, it will be more likely to carve the surface of the amalgam to a level that is below the surface of the enamel. It is desirable that the two surfaces be even (at the same level) so that there is no "step down" from the enamel to the amalgam.

It is good to register a mental picture of the outline of the preparation before the amalgam is placed so that the outline can be visualized after carving. Amalgam preparations should have enamel margins that are not jagged or rough; if the margins of a carved restoration appear ragged, it will be due to thin amalgam flash that extends outside of the preparation onto the adjacent enamel surface. This flash is more difficult to remove when amalgam bonding resins are used. A sharp carver is even more necessary for effective removal of this flash.

Amalgam should not be overcarved such that groove anatomy is deep, leaving thin fins of amalgam adjacent to the preparation margins. The operator should try to develop margins of amalgam that will leave a 75- to 90-degree angle at the margin of occlusal amalgam. Acute angles (fins) of amalgam at the margins on an occlusal surface are subject to fracture during function.

Fig 11-57 The enamel margin is used as a guide for carving smaller restorations.

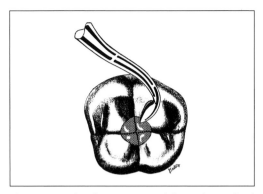

Fig 11-57a Cleoid carver viewed from the occlusal aspect.

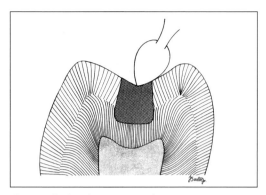

Fig 11-57b Cleoid carver viewed in cross section.

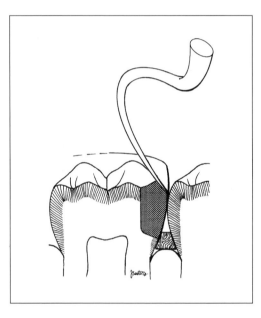

Fig 11-58 The tip of the No. 23 explorer is used at a 45-degree angle to the matrix to begin shaping the occlusal embrasure.

For Class 2 restorations, while the matrix is in place (Fig 11-58), the marginal ridge should be carved very nearly to the height of the adjacent marginal ridge (see Fig 11-64i). Development of the occlusal embrasure of the marginal ridge is begun with the tip of an explorer angled at approximately a 45-degree angle to the long axis of the tooth and touching the matrix band (see Figs 11-58 and 11-64j). The explorer tip should be moved from the facial enamel, past the margin of the box, to the center of the marginal ridge, and then from the lingual enamel, past the margin of the box, to the center. The explorer should not be moved from the amalgam toward the margin, because this movement could easily result in over-carving, leaving the marginal ridge with a deficient contour.

Most carving will be accomplished while the rubber dam is in place. For Class 2 restorations, after the matrix is removed, amalgam flash on proximal surfaces should be removed and the proximal contours should be refined. A thin carver, such as the interproximal carver, is useful for both removing flash and refining proximal contours (Fig 11-59; also see Figs 11-64w to 11-64y). Because the proximal contour is so crucial for periodontal health,[166] removal of the matrix is strongly advocated early in the carving process. While the amalgam is still soft, proper contours, as well as removal of excess amalgam from proximal margins, can readily be achieved. As previously stated, if a bonding system has been used, it is important to minimize the amount of bonding resin at proximal

Fig 11-59 *An interproximal carver is used to remove flash and to contour and burnish the amalgam in interproximal areas.*

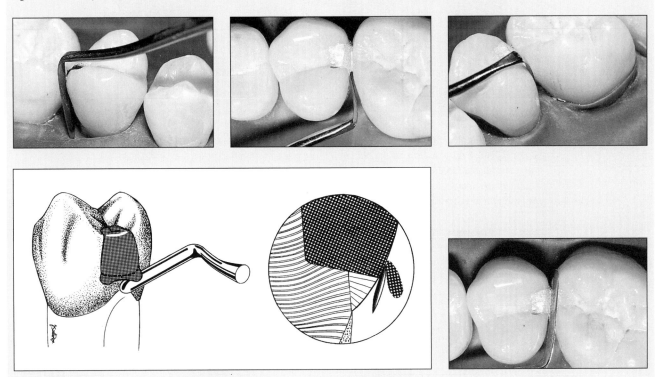

margins to prevent marginal voids that can be produced if the resin at margins is pulled out during carving. A very sharp carver will slice this incompletely set resin instead of catching and dislodging it.

Adjusting the Occlusion

When the carving appears to be correct, the dam is removed, and the occlusion is checked. This is accomplished with articulating ribbon, which marks the points of contact when the mandibular and maxillary teeth are brought together (Figs 11-60a and 11-60b). It is wise not to ask the patient to close, because, if the amalgam has not been carved adequately, it will be "high" in occlusion so that it contacts first, prior to any other tooth contact. The masseter muscles are very strong, and when the proprioceptive innervation relates to the patient's brain that there is something between the maxillary and mandibular teeth, it is reflex action for the patient to attempt to masticate it. In the case of a high amalgam restoration, disaster can result; the amalgam will usually be fractured, and the operator will have to remove the remaining amalgam and begin again.

It is best, therefore, for the operator to perform the tapping of the teeth by grasping the patient's chin, having the patient close to very near contact, and then, by hand, manipulating the mandible so that mandibular and maxillary teeth are tapped together in maximum intercuspation position (MIP) (centric occlusion). The dentist's arm, no matter how strong, will be unable to impart nearly as much force in mandibular closure as the masseter muscles are capable of achieving. An alternative to this tapping by the dentist is to instruct the patient to "very, very gently, tap the back teeth together."

The amalgam must be carved until contacts on the restoration occur simultaneously with other occlusal MIP contacts on that tooth and adjacent teeth. These can be seen as marks made by articulating ribbon, but they should also be felt by the dentist with 0.0005-inch (12-µm) thick shimstock (Artus) (Figs 11-61a and 11-61b). To do this, the patient should be instructed to close in maximum intercuspation position ("bite the back teeth together") while shimstock is in place on the tooth being restored. With the teeth in maximum intercuspation, the shimstock should be held securely in place. The same test should be performed with the shimstock on adjacent teeth, and it should again be held securely (assuming that those teeth held shimstock prior to the restorative procedure). If the adjacent teeth do not hold the shimstock, the newly placed restoration is probably in hyperocclusion and needs additional carving.

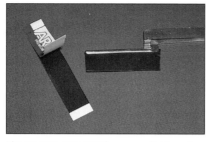

Fig 11-60a For initial gross adjustment, a piece of articulating paper with a thickness of 20 μm (0.0008 inch) or more is useful. When articulating paper forceps are used, the total length of the piece of articulating tape or paper should be supported by the forceps.

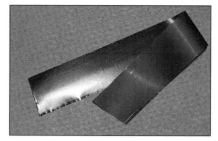

Fig 11-60b For refining occlusion, especially in complex amalgam restorations, an articulating tape with a thickness of 15 μm (0.0006 inch) or less is advantageous.

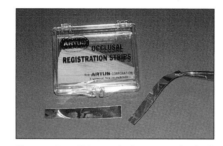

Fig 11-61a Shimstock (0.0005-inch thick Mylar) is supplied in books with paper separators between pieces of silver-colored shimstock. It may be held in the fingers or with a hemostat (as shown at right).

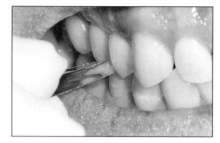

Fig 11-61b Shimstock is used to "feel" contacts between maxillary and mandibular teeth.

When the restoration occlusion is correct in maximum intercuspation, it must be checked to ensure that no interferences are caused by the restoration in excursive movements (laterotrusive, mediotrusive [right or left], or protrusive movements) of the mandible. This may also be evaluated with the use of the shimstock. Two colors of articulating ribbon (preferably ribbons that do not easily cause smudge marks), one color for latero-/mediotrusive and protrusive excursions, followed by the other to mark maximum intercuspation occlusal contacts, are used. To eliminate excursive contacts in the amalgam, the amalgam marked with the color used to register the excursions should be carved, and the amalgam marked with the centric marks should be preserved. For complex amalgam restorations, it should be ensured that the restoration does not cause interference in the slide between centric relation occlusion and maximum intercuspation.

Postcarve Burnishing

Postcarve burnishing is the light rubbing of the surface of a carved amalgam restoration with a burnisher, such as the PKT3 (P. K. Thomas). Heavy forces should not be used, and postcarve burnishing should be avoided near the margins of restorations of fast-setting amalgam.[167] The purpose of postcarve burnishing is to smooth the surface of the restoration.

After completion of carving and postcarve burnishing, if the carving time was short and the amalgam is still fairly soft, the surface may be wiped over with a dry or water-damp cotton ball or cotton roll to provide additional smoothing. If the set of the amalgam is advanced, so that the cotton will not smooth the surface, a rubber prophylaxis cup with damp flour of pumice or prophylaxis paste will smooth the amalgam (see the section on finishing and polishing). If the cup is used, it should be rotating at a very low speed and should be kept moving at all times; if the cup is allowed to rotate in one place, it will groove the recently carved amalgam.

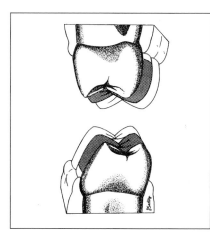

Fig 11-62 Facial and lingual contours are noted by looking down the line of teeth in a quadrant. The contour of the restoration must harmonize with natural tooth contours in the quadrant.

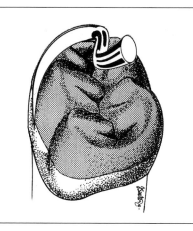

Fig 11-63a A No. 14L sickle-shaped carver will carve a very convex surface if it approaches the surface to be carved at just less than a 90-degree angle.

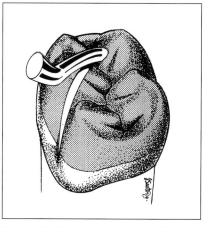

Fig 11-63b The same instrument will carve a surface with less convexity if it is rotated so that it approaches the surface at an angle of much less than 90 degrees.

Placement of Amalgam in Complex Preparations

Several special considerations for placing complex amalgam restorations, such as the possible need for reinforcement of matrices with compound, have already been discussed. Following are some other considerations that may help the operator to successfully place complex amalgam restorations:

1. Visualize the finished product, and shape the matrix to allow for that product.
2. In addition to visualizing the height of the cusp tips before making the tooth preparation and building cusps back to that height, make a mental picture of facial and lingual contours before cutting away natural tooth structure so that you can reproduce the natural contours in amalgam as closely as possible. Note the contours by viewing down the line of teeth from the facial and/or lingual aspect. Make sure that the final contours harmonize with the contours of other teeth in the quadrant (Fig 11-62; see also Fig 11-64ee).

3. Place larger increments of amalgam, for instance, the entire two-spill (600-mg) mix, when replacing the entire occlusal surface of a molar, or a half mix for less extensive restorations.
4. Consider the use of carvers that contribute to proper contours, such as the No. 14L carver, which simplifies the carving of convex axial contours (Figs 11-63a and 11-63b).
5. Because carving of large amalgam restorations involves the carving of more surface area, consider sharpening the carvers during the procedure to allow more efficient carving.
6. Smooth the carved amalgam with a water slurry of flour of pumice or with a prophylaxis paste.

A series showing the insertion of a complex amalgam restoration, beginning with matrix application and ending just before rubber dam removal, is shown in Figs 11-64a to 11-64ee. Several amalgam preparations and restorations are shown in Figs 11-65 to 11-78.

Figs 11-64a to 11-64ee Condensation and carving of a complex amalgam restoration.

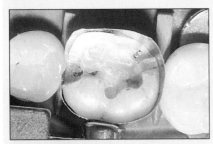

Fig 11-64a A Tofflemire matrix is placed and shaped to provide desired contours.

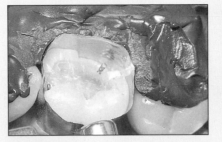

Fig 11-64b The matrix is stabilized with modeling compound.

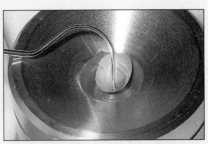

Fig 11-64c A two-spill mix of amalgam is halved.

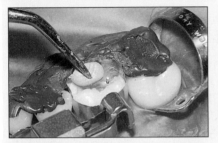

Fig 11-64d Half of the mix of amalgam is carried to the preparation.

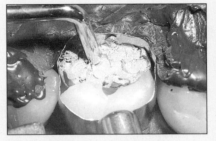

Fig 11-64e Amalgam is spread over the entire preparation floor and condensed.

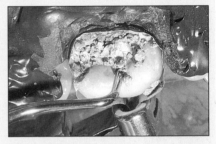

Fig 11-64f A small condenser is used to condense amalgam into the amalgapin channel. It should also be used to condense amalgam into internal line angles and at corners created by the matrix band at cavosurface margins.

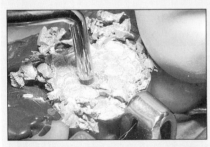

Fig 11-64g Amalgam increments are added in 1.0-mm thicknesses until the preparation is overfilled.

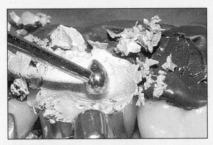

Fig 11-64h Amalgam shaping is begun with a large ovoid burnisher used to pinch excess amalgam off against the enamel (precarved burnishing).

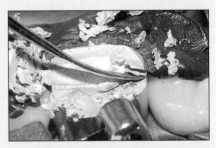

Fig 11-64i Marginal ridge shaping is begun by reducing amalgam in the area to the approximate desired height of the marginal ridge.

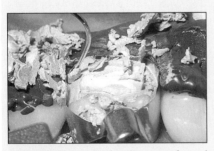

Fig 11-64j The occlusal embrasure is formed with an explorer tip.

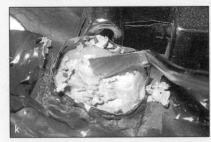

Figs 11-64k and 11-64l A chisel-shaped carver (Walls No. 3) is used to begin shaping cusps and grooves while the matrix is still in place.

Fig 11-64 *(continued)*

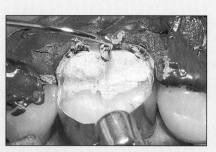

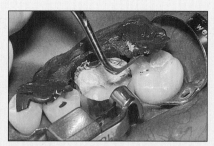

Fig 11-64m An explorer tip is used to begin shaping the lingual contour inside the matrix.

Fig 11-64n The compound and matrix are removed.

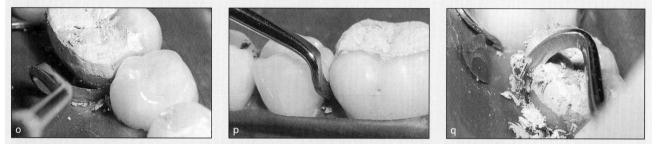

Figs 11-64o to 11-64q A sickle-shaped carver (No.14L) is used to remove gingival flash, shape proximal surfaces, and shape lingual contour.

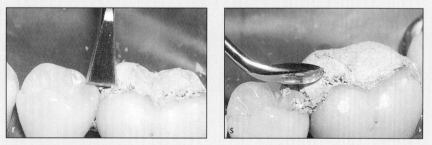

Figs 11-64r and 11-64s The marginal ridge is adjusted to height by resting the carver (Walls No. 3) on the adjacent marginal ridges during carving.

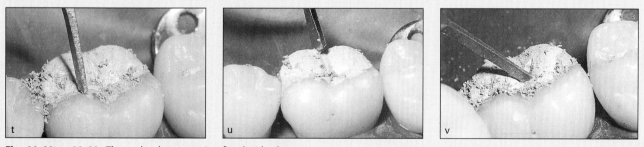

Figs 11-64t to 11-64v The occlusal anatomy is refined with a hoe.

Fig 11-64 *(continued)*

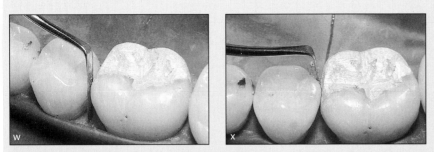

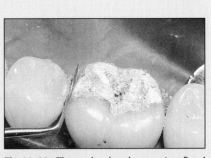

Figs 11-64w and 11-64x The proximal contours and contact position are refined with a very thin interproximal carver.

Fig 11-64y The occlusal embrasure is refined with an interproximal carver, which is rested on the adjacent enamel to guide the marginal ridge contour.

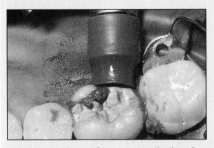

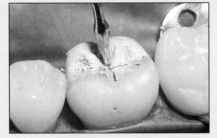

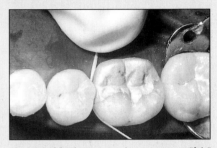

Fig 11-64z The surface is smoothed with a medium-grit prophylaxis paste in a rubber cup.

Fig 11-64aa The bases of the grooves are smoothed with a burnisher (PKT 3).

Fig 11-64bb The proximal contours are "felt" with floss to ensure smoothness and to clear any amalgam carvings from the contact.

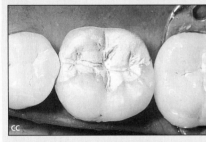

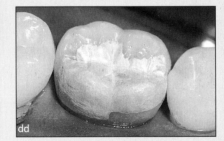

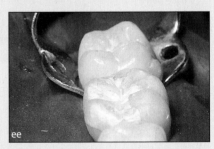

Figs 11-64cc to 11-64ee Carving is completed. Note that the lingual contour harmonizes with the contours of the adjacent teeth. The rubber dam is then removed, the occlusion is refined, and the surface is resmoothed with pumice or a prophylaxis paste.

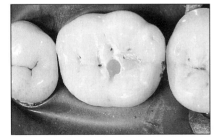

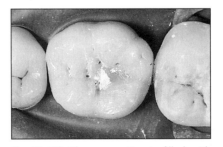

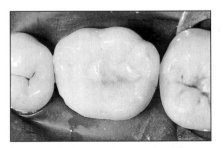

Fig 11-65a A small area of carious dentin and overlying unsupported enamel has been removed to complete the occlusal amalgam preparation.

Fig 11-65b The preparation is filled with amalgam.

Fig 11-65c The remaining occlusal fissures were opened with a No. ¼ bur to a depth of 0.5 mm, etched, and sealed with resin fissure sealant.

Fig 11-66a Mesio-occlusal slot preparation.

Fig 11-66b Slot restoration. There was no treatment of occlusal fissures. (Note that the distal contour of the amalgam should have been corrected as part of the procedure.)

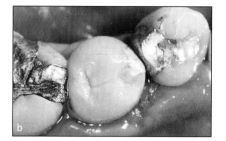

Fig 11-67a Disto-occlusal slot preparation.

Fig 11-67b Slot restoration. There was no treatment of occlusal fissures.

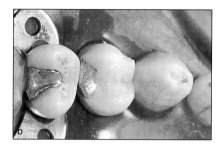

Fig 11-68a Mesio-occlusal preparation.

Fig 11-68b Restoration with conservative extension through the occlusal fissures. Avoiding the extension of the amalgam preparation and, instead, using a fissure sealant would have been a more conservative approach.

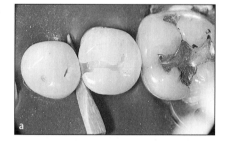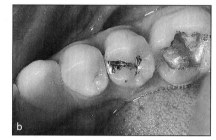

Fig 11-69a Disto-occlusal slot preparations.

Fig 11-69b Slot restorations. The occlusal fissures were sealed without being opened.

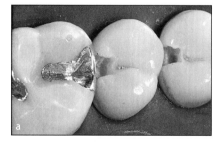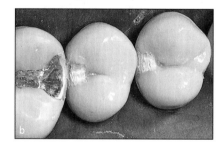

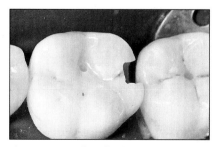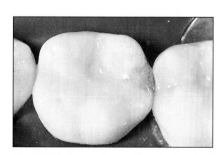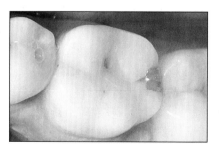

Fig 11-70a Small occlusal and disto-occlusal slot amalgam preparations.

Fig 11-70b Restorations with sealed occlusal fissures.

Fig 11-70c Restorations at 2 years.

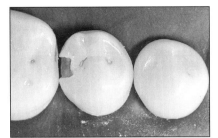

Fig 11-71a Disto-occlusal slot preparation.

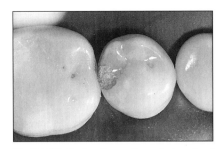

Fig 11-71b Restoration with sealed occlusal fissures.

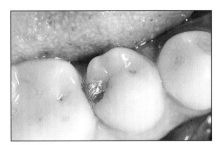

Fig 11-71c Restoration at 2 years.

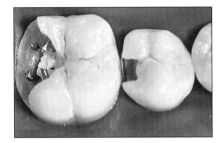

Fig 11-72a Complex amalgam preparation with vertical and horizontal pins in the molar and a disto-occlusal slot preparation in the premolar.

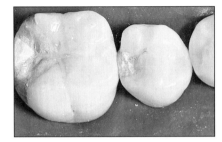

Fig 11-72b Restorations with sealed occlusal fissures.

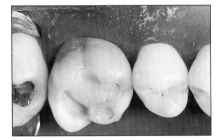

Fig 11-73a Old resin composite restoration with recurrent caries.

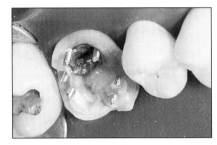

Fig 11-73b Complex amalgam preparation with six vertical pins.

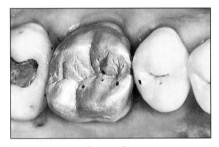

Fig 11-73c Complex amalgam restoration.

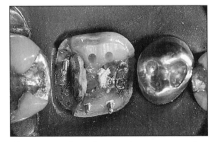

Fig 11-74a Complex amalgam preparation with pins, boxes, and amalgapins.

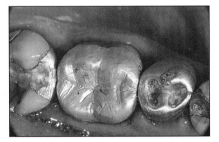

Fig 11-74b Complex amalgam restoration.

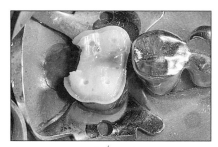

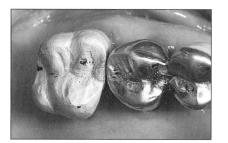

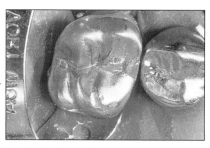

Fig 11-75a Complex amalgam preparation with boxes, amalgapins, and a shelf.

Fig 11-75b Complex amalgam restoration.

Fig 11-75c Restoration at 3 years.

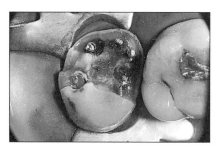

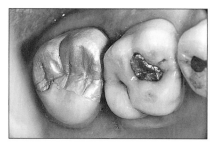

Fig 11-76a Complex amalgam preparation that used horizontal and vertical pins.

Fig 11-76b Complex amalgam restoration.

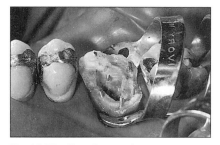

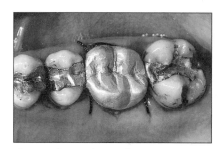

Fig 11-77a Complex amalgam preparation for a severely broken-down, endodontically treated molar, utilizing the chamber plus horizontal and vertical pins.

Fig 11-77b Complex amalgam restoration.

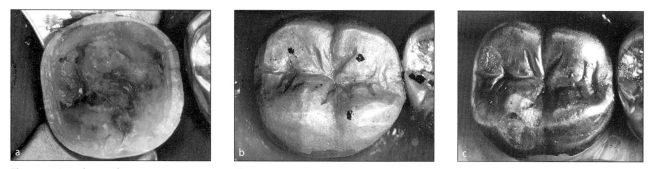

Fig 11-78 Complex amalgam restoration covering all cusps, with no mechanical retention form prepared; this restoration was bonded with a resin bonding system (Amalgambond Plus with HPA powder): *(a)* preparation; *(b)* completed restoration, immediately after placement; *(c)* restoration at 6-year recall.

Fig 11-80 Abrasive disks, manufactured for polishing resin composite restorations, are also useful for polishing amalgam.

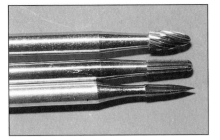

Fig 11-79 Finishing burs for a friction-grip handpiece: *(top to bottom)* No. 7404 (bud or egg shaped), No. 7803 (bullet shaped), No. 7901 (needle shaped).

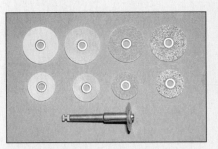

Fig 11-80a Brown-yellow series of Sof-Lex disks and the pop-on mandrel (3M). Also available is the thicker, but more flexible, black-blue series of Sof-Lex disks.

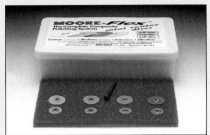

Fig 11-80b Moore-Flex disks (EC Moore) are similar to the Sof-Lex disks.

Finishing and Polishing Amalgam Restorations

Finishing of an amalgam restoration includes evaluating the restoration for problems and correcting them, ensuring that the margins are even and that the contours and occlusion are correct, and smoothing the restoration. Polishing is defined as smoothing the surface to a point of high gloss or luster. It has been demonstrated that polishing a high-copper amalgam restoration does not enhance its clinical performance,[168] but finishing is an important part of restoration placement. Finishing is usually accomplished at the placement appointment, but it may be refined at succeeding appointments.

Despite the lack of evidence that longevity is increased or performance improved when an amalgam restoration is polished, a high luster is often more comfortable to the patient's tongue than an unpolished surface, so polishing is sometimes desirable. There are no contraindications to polishing a restoration, but care must be taken not to create excessive heat during the polishing procedure. Excessive heat generation may be injurious to the pulp of a vital tooth.

After placement of a restoration, its surface should be rubbed with a burnisher or with cotton until it is smooth. For amalgam with a more advanced set, a rubber cup with wet pumice or a prophylaxis paste may be used to smooth the restoration. Polishing of an amalgam restoration should be accomplished at a succeeding appointment, or at least some time after placement of the restoration. If an amalgam is adequately smoothed immediately after placement, imparting a high luster is usually a very simple and quick procedure.[169] If the restoration is not made smooth at placement, more time is required for polishing.

If, at the time of polishing, the restoration surface is not smooth, it should be smoothed. Gross smoothing of set amalgam can be accomplished with sharp amalgam carvers and finishing burs (Fig 11-79). For polishing convex surfaces (facial, lingual, and proximal), a series of progressively finer disks may be used (Fig 11-80). Alternatives for smoothing and polishing convex surfaces are the abrasive-impregnated rubber cups, first the coarser cups, and then the finer cups (Fig 11-81). Abrasive-impregnated rubber points are useful for smoothing and polishing concave surfaces such as the occlusal surface. It is especially important that rubber polishers and abrasive disks are used with an abundance of air coolant and intermittent contact with the amalgam to prevent excessive generation of heat.

Although the disks and rubber polishers are more convenient, a less expensive, time-tested alternative method is the use of a prophylaxis cup, first with pumice in a water carrier as the "prepolishing" step, and then with tin oxide in a water or alcohol carrier for a high shine. One study[169] showed the pumice and tin oxide polishing procedure to be faster, but the investigator concluded that the impregnated points and cups are more desirable because they do not produce splatter.

A highly polished amalgam restoration is often more pleasing to the dentist than to the patient. A high polish can make a posterior amalgam restoration more noticeable, and this can be esthetically unpleasant to the patient. If this should occur, air abrasion with 50-μm aluminum oxide (Microetcher, Danville Engineering) or abrasion with pumice and a prophylaxis cup may be used to eliminate the high shine without making the restoration noticeably rough to the patient's tongue.

Fig 11-81 Abrasive-impregnated rubber cups and points.

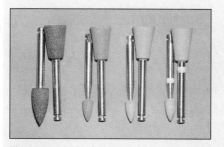

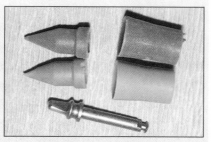

Fig 11-81a Brasseler cups and points: *(left to right)* coarsest (black), prepolish (brown), high shine (gray), and super high shine (yellow band).

Fig 11-81b Min-Identoflex polishers (Centrix): brown (prepolish) point and cup; green (final polish) point and cup. These polishers snap onto the mandrel shown.

Repair of Amalgam Restorations

When an amalgam restoration has a defective area but the remainder of the restoration is adequate, a repair procedure may be the most appropriate treatment. For instance, if a cusp that was left in place adjacent to an amalgam restoration has fractured but the remaining amalgam restoration is serviceable, it might be appropriate to simply build a new cusp with amalgam. Or, if an amalgam fracture has occurred in the mesial box portion of a mesio-occlusodistal restoration, but the remaining disto-occlusal portion involves a very gingivally deep distal margin, the most conservative and simplest treatment might be to replace only the mesio-occlusal portion of the restoration.

Attachment of new amalgam to old can be achieved, but the attachment strength is only 30% to 60% of unrepaired amalgam.[72,170,171] Additional mechanical retention or amalgam bonding should be considered.

References

1. Webster's Unabridged Dictionary of the English Language. New York: Portland House, 1989.
2. Anusavice KJ. Phillips' Science of Dental Materials, ed 10. Philadelphia: Saunders, 1996.
3. Innes DBK, Youdelis WV. Dispersion strengthened amalgam. J Can Dent Assoc 1963;29:587–593.
4. Mahler DB. Discovery! The high-copper dental amalgam alloys. J Dent Res 1997;76:537–541.
5. Craig RG. Restorative Dental Materials, ed 9. St Louis: Mosby-Year Book, 1993.
6. Guthrom CE, Johnson LD, Lawless KR. Corrosion of dental amalgam and its phases. J Dent Res 1983;62:1372–1381.
7. Marek M, Okabe T, Butts MB, Fairhurst CW. Corrosion of the eta'(Cu-Sn) phase in dental amalgam. J Biomed Mater Res 1983; 17:921–929.
8. Mitchell RJ, Okabe T. Setting reactions in dental amalgam. Part 1. Phases and microstructures between one hour and one week. Crit Rev Oral Biol Med 1996;7:12–22.
9. Sarkar NK, Park JR. Mechanism of improved corrosion resistance of Zn-containing dental amalgams. J Dent Res 1988;67:1312–1316.
10. Osborne JW, Berry TG. Zinc containing high copper amalgam: A three-year clinical evaluation. Am J Dent 1992;5:43–45.
11. Osborne JW, Norman RD. 13-year clinical assessment of 10 amalgam alloys. Dent Mater 1990;6:189–194.
12. Letzel H, van't Hof MA, Marshall GW, Marshall SJ. The influence of amalgam alloy on the survival of amalgam restorations: A secondary analysis of multiple controlled trials. J Dent Res 1997;76: 1787–1798.
13. Schoonover IC, Souder W, Beall JR. Excessive expansion of dental amalgam. J Am Dent Assoc 1942;29:1825–1832.
14. Osborne JW, Howell ML. Effects of water contamination on certain properties of high copper amalgams. Am J Dent 1994;7:337–341.
15. Osborne JW. Expansion of contaminated dental amalgams assessed by photoelastic resin [abstract 2556]. J Dent Res 1998;77(special issue B):951.
16. Yamada T, Fusayama T. Effect of moisture contamination on high copper amalgam. J Dent Res 1981;60:716–723.
17. Pashley EL, Galloway SE, Pashley DH. Protective effects of cavity liners on dentin. Oper Dent 1990;15:11–17.
18. Demaree NC, Taylor DF. Properties of dental amalgams made from spherical alloy particles. J Dent Res 1962;41:890–896.
19. Leinfelder KF. Dental amalgam alloys. Curr Opin Dent 1991;1: 214–217.
20. Use survey—1990. Clin Res Assoc Newsletter 1990;14(12):1.
21. Berry TG, Nicholson J, Troendle K. Almost two centuries with amalgam: Where are we today? J Am Dent Assoc 1994;125:392–399.

22. Miller A, Okabe T, DePaola DP, Cole JS. Amalgam and mercury toxicity: An update. Tex Dent J 1991;108:25–29.

23. Ahlquist M, Bergtsson C, Furnes B. Number of amalgam fillings in relation to cardiovascular disease, diabetes, cancer, and early death in Swedish women. Community Dent Oral Epidemiol 1988;16:227–231.

24. Björkman L, Pedersen NA, Lichtenstein P. Physical and mental health related to dental amalgam fillings in Swedish twins. Community Dent Oral Epidemiol 1996;24:260–267.

25. Henningsson M, Sundbom E. Defensive characteristics in individuals with amalgam illness as measured by the percept-genetic method Defense Mechanism Test. Acta Odontol Scand 1996;54:176–181.

26. Kingman A, Albertini T, Brown LJ. Mercury concentration in urine and whole blood associated with amalgam exposure in a US military population. J Dent Res 1998;77:461–471.

27. Osborne JW, Albino JE. Psychological and medical effects of intake of mercury from dental amalgams. A status report for the American Journal of Dentistry. Am J Dent 1999;12:151–156.

28. Osborne JW. Safety of dental amalgam. J Esthet Restor Dent 2004;16:377–388.

29. Anneroth G, Ericson T, Johansson I, et al. Comprehensive medical examination of a group of patients with alleged adverse effects from dental amalgams. Acta Odontol Scand 1992;50:101–111.

30. Bagedahl-Strindlund M, Ilie M, Furhoff AK, et al. A multidisciplinary clinical study of patents suffering from illness associated with mercury released from dental restorations: Psychiatric aspects. Acta Psychiatr Scand 1997;96:475–482.

31. Bratel J, Haraldson T, Ottosson JO. Potential side effects of dental amalgam restorations: No relation between mercury levels in the body and mental disorders. Eur J Oral Sci 1997;105:244–250.

32. Mackert JR, Berglund A. Mercury exposure from dental amalgam fillings: Absorbed dose and the potential for adverse health effects. Crit Rev Oral Biol Med 1997;8:411–436.

33. Molin M, Bergman B, Marklund SL, Schutz A, Skerfving S. Mercury, selenium, and glutathione peroxidase before and after amalgam removal in man. Acta Odontol Scand 1990;48:189–202.

34. Sandborgh-Englund G, Elinder CG, Langworth S, Schutz A, Ekstrand J. Mercury in biological fluids after amalgam removal. J Dent Res 1998;77:615–626.

35. WHO consensus statement on dental amalgam. FDI World Dental Federation. FDI World 1997;6:9.

36. US Department of Health and Human Services, Public Health Service. Dental Amalgam: A Scientific Review and Recommended Public Health Service Strategy for Research, Education, and Regulation. Washington, DC: US Department of Health and Human Services, Public Health Service, Jan 1993.

37. National Institutes of Health. Technology Assessment Conference. Effects and Side-Effects of Dental Restorative Materials. Bethesda, MD: US Department of Health and Human Services, 1991.

38. Bergman B, Bostrom H. Larsson KS, Loe H (eds). Potential Biological Consequences of Mercury Released from Dental Amalgam. A State of the Art Conference in Stockholm, April 1992. Stockholm: Swedish Medical Research Council, 1992.

39. Corbin SB, Kohn WG. The benefits and risks of dental amalgam: Current findings reviewed. J Am Dent Assoc 1994;125:381–388.

40. Dodes JE. The amalgam controversy. An evidence-based analysis. J Am Dent Assoc 2001;132:348–356.

41. Berglund A. Estimation by a 24-hour study of the daily dose of intra-oral mercury vapor inhaled after release from dental amalgam. J Dent Res 1990;69:1646–1651.

42. Swartz ML, Phillips RW. In vitro studies on the marginal leakage of restorative materials. J Am Dent Assoc 1961;62:141–151.

43. Paolantonio M, D'ercole S, Perinetti G, et al. Clinical and microbiological effects of different restorative materials on the periodontal tissues adjacent to subgingival Class V restorations. J Clin Periodontol 2004;31:200–207.

44. Bogacki RE, Hunt RJ, del Aguila M, Smith WR. Survival analysis of posterior restorations using an insurance claims database. Oper Dent 2002;27:488–492.

45. Szep S, Barm C, Alamouti C, Schmidt D, Gerhard T, Heidemann D. Removal of amalgam, glass-ionomer cement and compomer restorations: Changes in cavity dimensions and duration of the procedure. Oper Dent 2002;17:613–620.

46. Gordan VV, Mondragon E, Shen C. Replacement of resin-based composite: Evaluation of cavity design, cavity depth, and shade matching. Quintessence Int 2002;33:273–278.

47. Mjör IA, Reep RL, Kubilis PS, Mondragon BE. Change in size of replaced amalgam restorations: A methodological study. Oper Dent 1998;23:272–277.

48. Wahl MJ, Schmitt MM, Overton DA, Gordon MK. Prevalence of cusp fractures in teeth restored with amalgam and with resin-based composite. J Am Dent Assoc 2004;135:1127–1132.

49. Nakabayashi N, Watanabe A, Gendusa NJ. Dentin adhesion of "modified" 4-META/MMA-TBB resin: Function of HEMA. Dent Mater 1992;8:259–264.

50. Mjör IA, Jokstad A, Qvist V. Longevity of posterior restorations. Int Dent J 1990;40:11–17.

51. Osborne JW, Norman RD, Gale EN. A 14-year clinical assessment of 12 amalgam alloys. Quintessence Int 1991;22:857–864.

52. Robbins JW, Summitt JB. Longevity of complex amalgam restorations. Oper Dent 1988;13:54–57.

53. Smales RJ. Longevity of cusp-covered amalgams: Survivals after 15 years. Oper Dent 1991;16:17–20.

54. Osborne JW, Summitt JB. Extension for prevention: Is it relevant today? Am J Dent 1998;11:189–196.

55. Berry TG, Laswell HR, Osborne JW, Gale EN. Width of isthmus and marginal failure of restorations of amalgam. Oper Dent 1981;6:55–58.

56. Blaser PK, Lund MR, Cochran MA, Potter RH. Effects of designs of Class 2 preparations on resistance of teeth to fracture. Oper Dent 1983;8:6–10.

57. Larson TD, Douglas WH, Geisfeld RE. Effect of prepared cavities on the strength of teeth. Oper Dent 1981;6:2–5.

58. Osborne JW, Gale EN. Relationship of restoration width, tooth position, and alloy to fracture at the margins of 13- to 14-year-old amalgams. J Dent Res 1990;69:1599–1601.

59. Vale WA. Cavity preparation. Irish Dent Rev 1956;2:33–41.

60. Caron GA, Murchison DF, Broom JC, Cohen RB. Resistance to fracture of teeth with various preparations for amalgam [abstract 208]. J Dent Res 1994;73:127.

61. El-Mowafy OM. Fracture strength and fracture patterns of maxillary premolars with approximal slot cavities. Oper Dent 1993;18:160–166.

62. Summitt JB, Osborne JW. Initial preparations for amalgam restorations. J Am Dent Assoc 1992;123:67–72.

63. Glossary of Operative Dentistry Terms. Washington DC: Academy of Operative Dentistry, 1983.

64. Dachi SF, Stigers RW. Reduction of pulpal inflammation and thermal sensitivity in amalgam-restored teeth treated with copal varnish. J Am Dent Assoc 1967;74:1281–1285.

65. Kramer PF, Zelante F, Simionato MRL. The immediate and long-term effects of invasive and noninvasive pit and fissure sealing techniques on the microflora in occlusal fissures of human dentin. Pediatr Dent 1993;16:108–112.

66. Shapira J, Eidelman E. The influence of mechanical preparation of enamel prior to etching on the retention of sealants: Three-year follow-up. J Pedod 1984;8:272–277.

67. Brocklehurst PR, Joshi RI, Northeast SE. The effect of air-polishing occlusal surfaces on the penetration of fissures by a sealant. Int J Paediatr Dent 1992;2:157–162.

68. DeCraene LGP, Martens LC, Dermaut LR, Surmont PAS. A clinical evaluation of a light-cured fissure sealant (Helioseal). J Dent Child 1989;56:97–102.

69. Garcia-Godoy F, Medlock JW. An SEM study of the effects of air-polishing on fissure surfaces. Quintessence Int 1988;19:465–467.

70. Goldstein RE, Parkins FM. Using air-abrasive technology to diagnose and restore pit and fissure caries. J Am Dent Assoc 1995;126:761–766.

71. Vesterhus Strand G, Raadal M. The efficiency of cleaning fissures with an air-polishing instrument. Acta Odontol Scand 1988;46:113–117.

72. Jeronimus DJ Jr, Till MJ, Sveen OB. Reduced viability of microorganisms under dental sealants. ASDC J Dent Child 1975;42:275–280.

73. Handelman SL, Washburn F, Wopperer P. Two-year report of sealant effect on bacteria in dental caries. J Am Dent Assoc 1976;93:967–970.

74. Handelman SL, Leverett DH, Iker HP. Longitudinal radiographic evaluation of the progress of caries under sealants. J Pedod 1985;9:119–126.

75. Mertz-Fairhurst EJ, Schuster GS, Williams JE, Fairhurst CW. Clinical progress of sealed and unsealed caries. Part I: Depth changes and bacterial counts. J Prosthet Dent 1979;42:521–526.

76. Swift EJ. The effect of sealants on dental caries: A review. J Am Dent Assoc 1988;116:700–704.

77. Going RE, Loesche WJ, Grainger DA, Syed SA. The viability of microorganisms in carious lesions five years after covering with a fissure sealant. J Am Dent Assoc 1978;97:455–462.

78. Jensen ME, Handelman SL. Effect of an autopolymerizing sealant on viability of microflora in occlusal dental caries. Scand J Dent Res 1980;88:382–388.

79. Mertz-Fairhurst E, Smith CD, Williams JE, et al. Cariostatic and ultra-conservative sealed restorations: Six-year results. Quintessence Int 1992;23:827–838.

80. Mertz-Fairhurst E, Curtis JW, Ergle JW, Rueggeberg FA, Adair SM. Ultraconservative and cariostatic sealed restorations: Results at year 10. J Am Dent Assoc 1998;129:55–66.

81. Cassin AM, Pearson GJ, Picton DCA. Fissure sealants as a means of prolonging longevity of amalgam restorations—An in-vitro feasibility study. Clin Mater 1991;7:203–207.

82. Fernandes DP, Chevitarese O. The orientation and direction of rods in dental enamel. J Prosthet Dent 1991;65:793–800.

83. Anderson MH, Bales DJ, Omnell KA. Modern management of dental caries: The cutting edge is not the dental bur. J Am Dent Assoc 1993;124:37–44.

84. Anusavice KJ. Treatment regimens in preventive and restorative dentistry. J Am Dent Assoc 1995;126:727–743.

85. Lumley PJ, Fisher FJ. Tunnel restorations: A long-term pilot study over a minimum of five years. J Dent 1995;23:213–215.

86. Garcia-Godoy F, Summitt J, Donly K, Buikema D. Resistance to further demineralization of white spot lesions by sealing [abstract 1643]. J Dent Res 1993;72:309.

87. Qvist V, Johannessen L, Bruun M. Progression of approximal caries in relation of iatrogenic preparation damage. J Dent Res 1992;71:1370–1373.

88. Summitt JB, Osborne JW, Burgess JO, Howell ML. Effect of grooves on resistance form of Class 2 amalgams with wide occlusal preparations. Oper Dent 1993;18:42–47.

89. Summitt JB, Howell ML, Burgess JO, Dutton FB, Osborne JW. Effect of grooves on resistance form of conservative Class 2 amalgams. Oper Dent 1992;17:50–56.

90. Summitt JB, Osborne JW, Burgess JO. Effect of grooves on resistance/retention form of Class 2 approximal slot amalgam restorations. Oper Dent 1993;18:209–213.

91. Sturdevant JR, Taylor DF, Leonard RH, Straka WF, Roberson TM, Wilder AD. Conservative preparation designs for Class II amalgam restorations. Dent Mater 1987;3:144–148.

92. Battock RD, Rhoades J, Lund MR. Management of proximal caries on the roots of posterior teeth. Oper Dent 1979;4:108–112.

93. Liberman R, Judes H, Cohen E, Eli I. Restoration of posterior pulpless teeth: Amalgam overlay versus cast gold onlay restorations. J Prosthet Dent 1987;57:540–543.

94. Summitt JB, Burgess JO, Berry TG, Robbins JW, Osborne JW, Haveman CW. Six-year clinical evaluation of bonded and pin-retained complex amalgam restorations. Oper Dent 2004;29:269–276.

95. Dwinelle WH. Crystalline gold, its varieties, properties, and use. Am J Dent Sci 1855;5:249–297.

96. How WS. Bright metal screw posts and copper amalgam. Dent Cosmos 1839;31:237–238.

97. Markley MR. Pin reinforcement and retention of amalgam foundations. J Am Dent Assoc 1958;56:675–679.

98. Markley MR. Pin-retained and pin-reinforced amalgam. J Am Dent Assoc 1966;73:1295–1300.

99. Markley MR. Pin retained and reinforced restorations and foundations. Dent Clin North Am 1967;3:229–244.

100. Goldstein PM. Retention pins are friction-locked without use of cement. J Am Dent Assoc 1966;73:1103–1106.

101. Going RE. Pin-retained amalgam. J Am Dent Assoc 1966;73:619–624.

102. Dilts WE, Welk DA, Stovall J. Retentive properties of pin materials in pin-retained silver amalgam restorations. J Am Dent Assoc 1968;77:1085–1089.

103. Moffa JP, Razzano MR, Doyle MG. Pins—A comparison of their retentive properties. J Am Dent Assoc 1969;78:529–535.

104. Dilts WE, Duncanson MG, Collard EW, Parmley LE. Retention of self-threading pins. J Can Dent Assoc 1981;47:119–120.

105. Burgess JO, Summitt JB. Retention and resistance provided by nine self-threading pins. Oper Dent 1991;16:55–60.

106. Marshall TD, Porter KH, Re GJ. In vitro evaluation of the shoulder stop in a self-threading pin. J Prosthet Dent 1986;56:428–430.

107. Buikema DJ, Mayhew RB, Voss JE, Bales DJ. Pins and their relation to cavity resistance form for amalgam. Quintessence Int 1985;16:187–190.

108. Gourley JV. Favorable locations for pins in molars. Oper Dent 1980;5:2–6.

109. Cooley RL, Marshall TD, Young JM, Huddleston AM. Effect of sterilization on the strength and cutting efficiency of twist drills. Quintessence Int 1990;21:919–923.

110. Ulusoy N, Denli N, Atakul F, Nayyar A. Thermal response to multiple use of a twist drill. J Prosthet Dent 1992;67:450–453.

111. Marshall TD, Cooley RL. Evaluation of the Max titanium alloy retentive pins. Am J Dent 1989;2:349–353.

112. Newitter DA, Gwinnett AJ, Caputo L. The dulling of twist drills during pin channel placement. Am J Dent 1989;2:81–85.

113. Podshadley AG, Chambers MS. A new instrument for placement of self-threading retention pins. J Prosthet Dent 1994;71:429.

114. Burgess JO. Horizontal pins: A study of tooth reinforcement. J Prosthet Dent 1985;53:317–322.

115. Lambert RL, Robinson FB, Lindemuth JS. Coronal reinforcement with cross-splinted pin-amalgam restorations. J Prosthet Dent 1985;54:346–349.

116. Collins JF, Antonson DE. Treatment of external pin perforations. J Acad Gen Dent 1987;35:200–202.

117. Birtcil RF, Venton EA. Extracoronal amalgam restorations utilizing available tooth structure for retention. J Prosthet Dent 1976;35:171–178.

118. Outhwaite WC, Garman TA, Pashley DH. Pin vs. slot retention in extensive amalgam restorations. J Prosthet Dent 1979;41:396–400.

119. Seng GF, Rupell OL, Nance GL, Pompura JP. Placement of retentive amalgam inserts in tooth structure for supplemental retention. J Acad Gen Dent 1980;28:62–66.

120. Shavell HM. The amalgapin technique for complex amalgam restorations. J Calif Dent Assoc 1980;8:48–55.

121. Davis SP, Summitt JB, Mayhew RB, Hawley RJ. Self-threading pins and amalgapins compared in resistance form for complex amalgam restorations. Oper Dent 1983;8:88–93.

122. Roddy WC, Blank LW, Rupp NW, Pelleu GB. Channel depth and diameter effects on transverse strength of amalgapin-retained restorations. Oper Dent 1987;12:2–9.

123. Leach CD, Martinoff JT, Lee CV. A second look at the amalgapin technique. J Calif Dent Assoc 1983;11:43–49.

124. Summitt JB, Rindler EA, Robbins JW, Burgess JO. Effect of distribution of resistance features in complex amalgam restorations. Oper Dent 1994;19:53–58.

125. Plasmans PJ, Kusters ST, Thissen AM, Van'T Hof MA, Vrijhoef MM. Effects of preparation design on the resistance for extensive amalgam restorations. Oper Dent 1987;12:42–47.

126. Certosimo AJ, House RC, Anderson MH. The effect of cross-sectional area on transverse strength of amalgapin-retained restorations. Oper Dent 1991;18:70–76.

127. Burgess JO, Hartsfield C, Jordan T. Strength of amalgam with varying amalgam thickness covering the pins [abstract 549]. J Dent Res 1990;69:177.

128. Belcher MA, Stewart GP. Two-year clinical evaluation of an amalgam adhesive. J Am Dent Assoc 1997;128:309–314.

129. Mach Z, Ruzickova T, Staninec M, Setcos JC. Bonded amalgam restorations: Three year clinical results [abstract 3106]. J Dent Res 1998;77(special issue B):1020.

130. Setcos JC, Staninec M, Wilson NHF. Clinical evaluation of bonded amalgam restorations over two years [abstract 2589]. J Dent Res 1998;77(special issue B):955.

131. Staninec M, Marshall GW, Lowe A, Ruzickova T. Clinical research on bonded amalgam restorations. Part 1: SEM study of in vivo bonded amalgam restorations. Gen Dent 1997;45:356–360, 362.

132. Smales RJ, Wetherell JD. Review of bonded amalgam restorations and assessment in a general practice over five years. Oper Dent 2000;25:374–381.

133. Burgess JO, Alvarez AN, Summitt JB. Fracture resistance of complex amalgams. Oper Dent 1997;22:128–132.

134. Imbery TA, Burgess JO, Batzer RC. Comparing the resistance of dentin bonding agents and pins in amalgam restorations. J Am Dent Assoc 1995;126:753–758.

135. Imbery TA, Hilton TJ, Reagan SE. Retention of complex amalgam restorations using self-threading pins, amalgapins, and Amalgambond. Am J Dent 1995;8:117–121.

136. Lo CS, Millstein PL, Nathanson D. In vitro shear strength of bonded amalgam cores with and without pins. J Prosthet Dent 1995;74:385–391.

137. Diefenderfer KE, Reinhardt JW. Shear bond strengths of ten adhesive resin/amalgam combinations. Oper Dent 1997;22:50–56.

138. Ruzickova T, Staninec M, Marshall GW. SEM analysis of resin-amalgam adhesion after debonding [abstract 2289]. J Dent Res 1994;73(special issue):388.

139. Summitt JB, Miller B, Buikema DJ, Chan DCN. Shear bond strength of Amalgambond Plus cold and at room temperature [abstract 1345]. J Dent Res 1998;77(special issue A):274.

140. Miller B, Chan DC, Cardenas HL, Summitt JB. Powder additive effect on shear bond strengths of bonded amalgam [abstract 1346]. J Dent Res 1998;77(special issue A):274.

141. Ben-Amar A, Liberman R, Judes H, Nordenberg D. Long-term use of dentine adhesive as an interfacial sealer under Class II amalgam restorations. J Oral Rehabil 1990;17:37–42.

142. Berry FA, Tjan AHL. Microleakage of amalgam restorations lined with dentin adhesives. Am J Dent 1994;7:333–336.

143. Charlton DG, Moore BK, Swartz ML. In vitro evaluation of the use of resin liners to reduce microleakage and improve retention of amalgam restorations. Oper Dent 1992;17:112–119.

144. Dutton FB, Summitt JB, Chan DCN, Garcia-Godoy F. Effect of a resin lining and rebonding on the marginal leakage of amalgam restorations. J Dent 1993;21:52–56.

145. Korale ME, Meiers JC. Microleakage of dentin bonding systems used with spherical and admixed amalgams. Am J Dent 1996;9:249–252.

146. Tangsgoolwatana J, Cochran MA, Moore BK, Li Y. Microleakage evaluation of bonded amalgam restorations: Confocal microscopy versus radioisotope. Quintessence Int 1997;28:467–477.

147. Browning WD, Johnson WW, Gregory PN. Postoperative pain following bonded amalgam restorations. Oper Dent 1997;22:66–71.

148. Kennington B, Davis RD, Murchison DF. Short-term clinical evaluation of post-operative sensitivity with bonded amalgams. Am J Dent 1998;11:177–180.

149. Davis R, Overton JD. Efficacy of bonded and nonbonded amalgam in the treatment of teeth with incomplete fractures. J Am Dent Assoc 2000;131:469–478.

150. Boyer DB, Roth L. Fracture resistance of teeth with bonded amalgams. Am J Dent 1994;7:91–94.

151. Eakle WS, Staninec M, Lacy AM. Effect of bonded amalgam on the fracture resistance of teeth. J Prosthet Dent 1992;68:257–260.

152. Oliveira JP, Cochran MA, Moore BK. Influence of bonded amalgam restorations on the fracture strength of teeth. Oper Dent 1996;21:111–115.

153. Pilo R, Brosh T, Chweidan H. Cusp reinforcement by bonding of amalgam restorations. J Dent 1998;26:467–472.

154. Bonilla E, White SN. Fatigue of resin-bonded amalgam restorations. Oper Dent 1996;21:122–126.

155. Gwinnett AJ, Yu S. Effect of long-term water storage on dentin bonding. Am J Dent 1995;8:109–111.

156. Santos AC, Meiers JC. Fracture resistance of premolars with MOD amalgam restorations lined with Amalgambond. Oper Dent 1994;19:2–6.

157. Bell JG. An elementary study of deformation of molar teeth during amalgam restorative procedures. Aust Dent J 1977;22:177–181.

158. Powell GL, Nicholls JI, Shurtz DE. Deformation of human teeth under the action of an amalgam matrix band. Oper Dent 1977;2:64–69.

159. Powell GL, Nicholls JI, Molvar MP. Influence of matrix bands, dehydration, and amalgam condensation on deformation of teeth. Oper Dent 1980;5:95–101.

160. Mahler DB. The amalgam-tooth interface. Oper Dent 1996;21:230–236.

161. Brown IH, Miller DR. Alloy particle shape and sensitivity of high-copper amalgams to manipulative variables. Am J Dent 1993;6:248–254.

162. Osborne JW, Phillips RW, Norman RD, Swartz ML. Influence of certain manipulative variables upon the static creep of amalgam. J Dent Res 1977;56:616–621.

163. Brown IH, Maiolo C, Miller DR. Variation in condensation pressure during clinical packing of amalgam restorations. Am J Dent 1993;6:255–259.

164. Charlton DG, Murchison DF, Moor BK. Incorporation of adhesive liners in amalgam: Effect on compressive strength and creep. Am J Dent 1991;4:184–188.

165. Kanai S. Structure studies of amalgam. II. Effect of burnishing on the margins of occlusal amalgam fillings. Acta Odontol Scand 1966;24:47–53.

166. Hazen SP, Osborne JW. Relationship of operative dentistry to periodontal health. Dent Clin North Am 1967;Mar:245–254.

167. Woods PW, Marker VA, McKinney TW, Miller BH, Okabe T. Determining amalgam marginal quality: Effect of occlusal surface condition. J Am Dent Assoc 1993;124:60–65.

168. Mayhew RB, Schmeltzer LD, Pierson WP. Effect of polishing on the marginal integrity of high-copper amalgams. Oper Dent 1986;11:8–13.

169. Eames WB. A clinical view of dental amalgam. Dent Clin North Am 1976;20:385–395.

170. Diefenderfer KE, Reinhardt JW, Brown SB. Surface treatment effects on amalgam repair strength. Am J Dent 1997;10:9–14.

171. Jessip JP, Vandervalle KS, Hermesch CB, Buikema DS. Effects of surface treatments on amalgam repair. Oper Dent 1998;23:15–20.

Diagnosis and Treatment of Root Caries

Michael A. Cochran
Bruce A. Matis

Evidence indicates that root caries was the major dental problem in ancient civilizations.[1,2] Today, demographic predictors suggest that root caries is likely to become one of the more significant patient management issues of the future.[3–9] Greater life expectancies coupled with improved dental care have resulted in an increasing number of patients who retain most of their dentition into old age. Almost 80% of the US population between the ages of 55 and 64 years are dentate (mean, 19.3 teeth) while 56.8% of people 75 years or older retain a mean of 16.1 teeth.[7,10] With age, the occurrence of root surfaces exposed to the oral environment increases, predisposing the affected teeth to loss of cervical structure, cervical hypersensitivity, and root caries.[11] In a study assessing the periodontal status in the United States,[12] gingival recession of 1 mm or more was reported in 11.5% of 18- to 24-year-olds, 46.3% of 35- to 44-year-olds, 78.3% of 55- to 64-year-olds, and 86.5% of people 65 or older. Consequently, root caries is a problem of increasing importance in the elderly, dentate patient.[8,13–18]

Definition, Clinical Appearance, and Location of Root Caries Lesions

The prevalent definition in the dental literature for a root caries lesion is "a soft, irregularly shaped lesion either *(1)* totally confined to the root surface or *(2)* involving the undermining of enamel at the cemento-enamel junction, but clinically indicating that the lesion initiated on the root surface."[19] A root caries lesion can be initiated only if the root surface is first exposed to the oral environment.[7,10,12,20]

A root caries lesion appears as a softening and/or cavitation in the root surface with no initial involvement of the adjacent enamel (Fig 12-1). These lesions generally begin at or slightly occlusal to the free gingival margin but can extend into the gingival sulcus and/or undermine the coronal enamel as the lesion progresses (Fig 12-2). Lesions also begin at the margins of restorations that have their cervical interfaces on root structure. Two reports by Mjör[21,22] indicate that secondary caries lesions occur more frequently at cervical margins because many restorations terminate on root surfaces in areas where access and isolation are most difficult. An active root caries lesion usually spreads laterally and may encircle the tooth if left untreated[23] (Fig 12-3).

Early-stage lesions can be difficult to diagnose by appearance, as color changes are frequently not obvious until some progression of the caries activity has occurred. New lesions may appear as small, well-defined areas of a yellowish to light brown color. On probing, the dentin in an active lesion is softer than adjacent, unaffected cementum. As the lesion progresses, its surface frequently has a leathery consistency that can easily be peeled away with a sharp excavator. Advanced lesions appear darker brown to black and, if arrested, may be as hard or harder than the normal root surface. There has been an attempt by researchers to categorize lesions based on color (lighter lesions more active, darker lesions inactive)

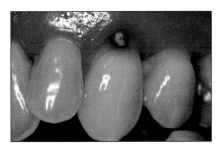

Fig 12-1 Root caries lesion on a tooth with gingival recession.

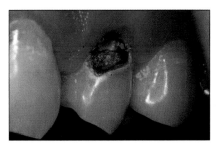

Fig 12-2 Root caries lesion undermining coronal enamel.

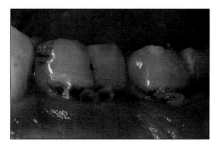

Fig 12-3 Active root caries lesion extending laterally.

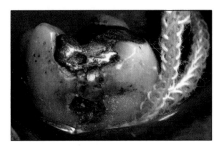

Fig 12-4 Proximal root caries lesion on a second molar.

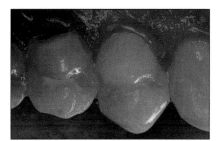

Fig 12-5 Caries lesion on the lingual aspect of a second premolar.

and/or texture (the harder the lesion, the less active).[24–27] While there has been some relation shown between color, texture, and dominant microorganism, the data have been conflicting and the link remains tenuous.[28] Currently, color is not considered a reliable indicator of caries activity.[17,29–31]

Caries lesions may occur on any exposed root surface, but initial lesions on the facial and proximal surfaces are most common.[32] Some studies have suggested that 50% to 75% of root caries lesions begin proximally (Fig 12-4).[33,34] Lingual/palatal locations are seen much less frequently as isolated lesions (Fig 12-5). In the mandible, molars appear to be the most susceptible to root caries, followed by premolars, canines, and incisors; in the maxilla, the order is reversed.[32,35,36] It is common for many of these lesions to be obscured by plaque, food debris, and calculus, so accurate detection is best accomplished after thorough debridement and prophylaxis.

Histochemistry, Histopathology, and Microbiology

The caries process on root surfaces is very similar to that in coronal caries. Plaque bacteria capable of metabolizing dietary carbohydrates into acids produce a drop in pH that initiates demineralization of the tooth structure. Root surfaces are more vulnerable to chemical dissolution than enamel surfaces.[37] The drop in pH necessary for demineralization in cementum and dentin (pH 6.2 to 6.7) is less than that required for enamel (pH 5.4 to 5.5).[38,39] This means that, given the proper environment, both the initiation and progression of root surface caries lesions will occur more rapidly in dentin than in an enamel surface.[40] Once cementum is lost, denaturation of collagen by collagenase-producing microorganisms, as well as degradation by nonspecific proteases, may accelerate the problem.[41] In addition, acid challenges can occur more readily and may continue for an extended period of time.[42] Any alteration in the delicate balance between the rates of demineralization and remineralization can result in the initiation of the caries process.[43–45]

While we tend to think of root surfaces as being covered with cementum, some studies[46] suggest that the cementum and enamel are not confluent in as many as 30% of teeth. For patients receiving periodontal therapy, the cementum on accessible root surfaces is often partially removed during scaling and root planing procedures. Therefore, root caries lesions commonly begins on a dentin interface. Regardless of the surface, the creation of an acidic environment by cariogenic bacteria initiates the caries process. Cemental clefts can form due to physical and chemical changes, allowing infiltration of bacteria into the dentinal tubules. Surface dissolution continues,

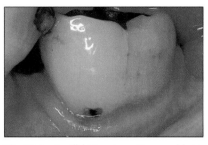

Fig 12-6a Small lesion in a 45-year-old patient. At this stage, if the lesion is active (soft), with cavitation, a restoration should be placed to prevent circumferential spread, and a preventive regimen should be initiated.

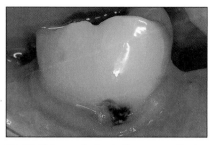

Fig 12-6b Larger lesion in the same patient.

followed by further demineralization and destruction of the collagen matrix.[47,48] Early microcavitation enlarges and produces the characteristic circumferential spreading seen with these lesions[48,49] (Figs 12-6a and 12-6b).

Some lesions become arrested. As demineralization progresses, there is a reactive sclerosing of the tubules and crystal formation, resulting in hypermineralization of the dentinal tubules.[50] This sclerosis is believed to be a result of the pulp's reaction to the stimulus of the caries process. The sclerotic appearance of many advanced lesions is probably related to the differences in mineral content found between the peritubular and intertubular dentin.[50,51] Various preventive regimens can lead to the arrest of root surface lesions. Arrested lesions frequently appear very dark and are hard on tactile examination.

Many studies attempting to identify the etiology of root caries have used selective culture techniques that focus on the identification of a limited number of bacterial species.[52,53] Unfortunately, this type of culturing often excludes some species that are directly or indirectly related. Studies of the predominant cultivable microflora, while more time and labor intensive, appear to be more useful in delineating the group of oral bacteria associated with the root caries process.[44,54,55]

Currently, no specific microorganisms have been conclusively proven to cause root surface caries. Early studies[27,56,57] pointed to *Actinomyces viscosus* as a prime suspect. More recent studies, however, have questioned the dominant role of *Actinomyces* while emphasizing the importance of *Streptococcus mutans* and *Lactobacillus*.[24,28,58–64] Lynch[28] and Zambon and Kasprzak[44] point out that, based on extensive research, *S mutans* and *Lactobacillus* spp both fulfill the criteria for implicating bacteria in the etiology of a mixed infection. They also suggest that virulence factors of specific species probably play an important role in both the formation and progress of root surface lesions. Work by Lundgren et al indicates that individuals harboring both *S sobrinus* and *S mutans*

had higher counts of *S mutans* than those who had *S mutans* alone.[65,66] It is likely that root caries is a continuous, destructive process involving a succession of bacterial populations that vary depending on the condition of the substrate and the depth of the lesion.[54,64] Modern molecular biology techniques, involving ribosomal RNA sequencing and DNA and RNA probes, may offer solutions to defining both species and virulence factors associated with root caries.[67]

Prevalence and Incidence

Because root caries lesions can be initiated only when root surfaces are exposed to the oral environment, the population presumed to be most at risk is older adults. However, younger patients with periodontal problems are susceptible as well. One epidemiologic study in Great Britain[68] found gingival recession in 60% of the population between 25 and 34 years of age. In addition, the most recent National Health and Nutrition Examination Survey for the United States reported gingival recession in all age groups 18 years and older.[12] It should also be noted that root surface exposure does not mean that caries activity is inevitable.

The actual prevalence of root caries is difficult to assess.[17,30,69] Interpretation of data from prevalence and incidence studies is complicated due to differences in diagnostic criteria, treatment decisions, and lack of homogeneity of the observed populations.[70] Numerous studies have reported the prevalence of root caries and its relationship to increasing age,[14,32,71–73] while international surveys have estimated that the disease affects 60% to 90% of adults.[11,26,74–76] In addition, it has been suggested that approximately one in nine root surfaces is at risk of becoming carious.[32] The extent of root caries appears to have a negative correlation with the number of teeth present. Because more mandibular teeth are retained in older individuals, these teeth have a higher incidence of root caries lesions than do maxillary teeth.[32,73,78,79] Other studies[32,74,80–83] suggest that approximately 15% to 20% of all teeth with gingival recession are affected by root caries, and the mean number of teeth affected per person is about 2.8.[37,75,84,86] It has also been stated that if root caries prevalence is based on the presence of active, restored, and arrested lesions, virtually every dentate American older than 65 years of age is at risk.[86]

Incidence data have been derived primarily from studies conducted on selected populations such as the chronically ill or nursing home residents. These studies[36,72,87–90] vary in duration from 1 to 8 years and report root caries/root restoration experience ranging from 19% to 69% depending on the population observed. Two studies on noninstitutionalized adults older than 65 years of age have reported similar incidences of root caries, 44%[91] and 37%.[35] The attack rates (mean surfaces per mouth) calculated for exposed root surfaces in the latter two studies ranged from 3.869 to 5.446 over a 3-year period.

Despite the variability of available data, there is general agreement that the prevalence of root caries will increase in the dentate older population. The prevalence of untreated caries, in general, has been found to be constant with age.[11,68] Statistically, however, as the number of teeth decreases with age, the ratio of caries lesions per tooth at risk increases, and root caries is a component of this. Thus, the ongoing loss of teeth with age is likely to produce an underestimation of the prevalence of root caries.[14] In the United States, it has been predicted that the dentate population older than 65 years of age will reach 85% or higher by 2020.[14]

Risk Factors and Assessment

The risk factors associated with root caries are provided in the box. It is of critical importance that clinicians identify at-risk patients early in the root caries process, ideally before the disease is clinically apparent. Early detection permits preventive and chemotherapeutic intervention to potentially enhance treatment outcome.

Because exposure of the root surface to the oral environment is a prerequisite for root surface caries, any patient with attachment loss, gingival recession, and/or periodontal pocketing is at risk for initiation of the disease process.[92] Patients in this category who are frequently overlooked are patients with cervical and proximal restorations that terminate on cemental surfaces. Even though the root surface may not be readily visible, the need for and placement of these restorations has met the primary risk criteria.

Risk Factors for Root Caries

Exposure of root surfaces
  Attachment loss
  Gingival recession
  Periodontal pocketing
Inadequate oral hygiene
  Low priority to patient
  Physical impairment
  Cognitive impairment
Cariogenic diet
Diminished salivary flow and/or buffering capacity
  Chronic medical conditions
  Medications
  Surgical/radiation therapy
  Physiologic aging
Previous caries lesions/restorations
Lack of access to and/or interest in dental services
  Low socioeconomic status
  Low educational level
Removable prosthesis
Advanced age
Eight or more missing teeth
Male gender
Smoking, alcoholism, drug use
Possibly ethnicity

All normal risk factors for caries lesion development are applicable to root caries, including inadequate oral hygiene, cariogenic diet, and poor utilization of routine dental services.[93,94] Past caries/restorative experience has also been shown to have a strong correlation and generally indicates the presence of conditions/behaviors that support caries activity (Fig 12-7).[35,85,95–102] Unfortunately, the effect of these conditions may be magnified in the root caries process as well as impacted by the myriad changes associated with aging and related health problems and treatments.[30,103]

In relation to caries activity, salivary flow rate is considered the most important of the nonmicrobial salivary parameters[104–106] since the cariostatic activity or efficacy of other salivary parameters is dependent on the flow rate.[107] Unstimulated flow rate has been shown to have a greater effect on salivary clearance time than stimulated flow[108,109] and is more affected by conditions producing hypofunction of the salivary glands.[110] A loss or significant reduction of unstimulated sali-

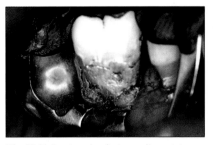

Fig 12-7 Root caries lesion adjacent to an amalgam margin.

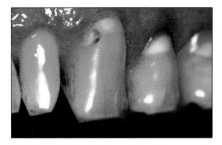

Fig 12-8 Caries lesion adjacent to a resin restoration in a xerostomic patient. Glass-ionomer restorations in the same patient did not exhibit recurrent caries lesions for the duration of the 5-year study.[75]

vary flow results in xerostomia, or "dry mouth," and is positively correlated with a number of adverse oral conditions, including rapidly progressive caries lesions and periodontal disease (Fig 12-8).[111,112] While there is debate as to the amount of saliva necessary to maintain oral health, an unstimulated flow rate of less than 0.2 mL/min is considered to be below normal.[110,111,113]

Xerostomia can be caused by a variety of factors,[13,38,111] including radiation therapy of the head and neck, immuno-suppressive therapy, radioactive iodine therapy, autoimmune diseases, HIV infection, and a myriad of commonly prescribed medications (see box). Basic management of xerostomic patients involves finding ways to reduce their oral dryness. If functioning salivary gland tissue is present, stimulation of natural flow is preferable to saliva substitutes. Pilocarpine (Salagen, MGI Pharma) and cevimeline (Evoxac, Daiichi Pharmaceutical) can be extremely effective salivary gland stimulants.[114] However, they have numerous side effects, contraindications, and drug interactions that make consultation with the patient's primary care physician preferable before prescribing them. Oral moisturizers are sometimes the only option for relieving the symptoms of xerostomia. These saliva substitutes can be used on a regular basis, but some commercial products have been found to have a pH below the demineralization point of enamel[55] and should be avoided.

The use of removable partial dentures has also been noted as a risk factor in this disease.[115,116] The position of retentive clasps and lingual/palatal connectors can contribute to retention of food debris and gingival recession. While the initial design may have been appropriate, prolonged wear and alterations of the clasps can produce physical stripping of the gingiva and abrasion of the tooth surface.

Medications that Induce Xerostomic Changes

Anorexiants
Antiasthmatics
Anticholinergics
Anticonvulsants
Antidepressants
Antiemetics
Antihistamines
Antihypertensives
Anti-inflammatories
Antinauseants
Antiparkinsonians
Antipruritics
Antispasmodics
Appetite suppressants
Cold medications
Decongestants
Diuretics
Expectorants
Muscle relaxants
Neuroleptics
Psychotropic drugs
    Central nervous system depressants
    Dibenzoxazepine derivatives
    Monoamine oxidase inhibitors
    Phenothiazine derivatives
    Tranquilizers
Sedatives
Sympathomimetics

Other factors that contribute to the potential for root caries include previous caries and restorative experience. Studies have indicated that individuals who have coronal caries lesions are 2 to 3.5 times more likely to develop root caries lesions.[117,118] Root caries is generally more prevalent and severe among males than females.[11] Smoking has also been implicated as a risk factor in both periodontal disease[119] and root caries.[120] Ethnicity is a relatively new variable in caries studies because of the difficulty in obtaining appropriate sample population sizes.[121,122] While there have been some indications that Asians[121,123] and blacks[35,124] exhibit a higher incidence of root caries, these data are not consistent between available studies, and the trends may be associated with socioeconomic factors, behavioral variables, and/or past caries experience and not directly related to race.[125]

Diagnosis

Although clinicians detect root caries lesions by judging changes in color (yellow, brown, black), texture (soft, hard), and surface contour (regular, irregular), examination strategies should focus on patients at risk for root caries. Therefore, the first step in the diagnosis of root caries is early identification of contributory factors and oral hygiene practices. Because plaque and debris often severely limit the visibility of root surfaces, a thorough dental prophylaxis should precede any clinical examination of patients at risk for root caries. Gentle tissue displacement with an air syringe and retraction with hand instruments can offer a better view of subgingival and interproximal areas, while the use of transillumination and/or lighted mirrors as well as intraoral cameras can also enhance visibility and improve diagnostic capability.

Lynch[28] found texture to be the best predictor of microbiologic activity in root caries lesions. Tactile exploration should be done carefully with only moderate pressure since the root surface is inherently softer than enamel. The gradient in tactile sensation between sound and carious cementum/dentin is much less than that between sound and carious enamel.[19] Active lesions may or may not display obvious cavitation and are generally described as "tacky" or "leathery" to tactile exploration while offering some resistance to removal of the explorer tip. One study demonstrated that an alteration in the explorer tip (producing a 30-degree angle at the tip of the explorer) increased the ability of the operator to detect root caries lesions.[126]

Radiographs can be useful in identifying early proximal root lesions, but can occasionally be prone to misinterpretation because of cervical "burnout" artifacts. Vertical bite-wing radiographs permit better evaluation of the proximal root surfaces in persons with significant loss of attachment.[127]

Newer diagnostic tools and techniques, such as dye-enhanced laser fluorescence (DELF) and quantitative laser fluorescence (QLF), have shown promise in in vitro[128,129] and in vivo[85,130,131] studies in enamel. This type of diagnostic aid should eventually be helpful in differentiating between active and inactive lesions by finding a correlation between lesion severity and degree of mineral loss. Clarification is needed since the current system of classification of root caries lesions is generally considered unsatisfactory[132] and many of the new technologies have not been evaluated on root surfaces in vivo.

Preventive and Chemotherapeutic Strategies

Clinical observations suggest that root caries lesions can be arrested, obviating restorative therapy.[133–135] The majority of evidence relating to demineralization and remineralization in root caries lesions comes from in vitro research.[136,137] However, in vivo[54,138] and in situ[95,139,140] studies have demonstrated success in preventing and/or arresting root caries through plaque removal, diet modification, topical fluoride application, and use of antimicrobials.[141,142]

Plaque removal alone has been shown to play an important role in arresting active root caries.[134] In situ studies have confirmed that both plaque thickness and acidogenic response to sucrose exposure are significantly reduced when lesions become inactive.[140,143] A 0.12% chlorhexidine rinse (Peridex, Zila; Periogard, Colgate) can also be used in treating root caries. While chlorhexidine has been used primarily as an antimicrobial treatment for gingivitis and periodontal disease, it is very effective in eliminating cariogenic bacteria (primarily mutans streptococci). The recent National Institutes of Health Consensus Conference suggests the data on the use of chlorhexidine rinses for caries prevention and management is not as strong as that for chlorhexidine varnishes and gels, which are not currently available in the United States but probably will be soon.

Topical fluoride is accepted as an appropriate chemotherapeutic agent in the management of root caries. Prevention/arrest of root surface lesions has been demonstrated in both in situ and clinical studies using fluoridated water,[144–146] fluoride solutions,[147] fluoride gels,[25] fluoride mouth rinses,[148] fluoride dentifrices,[87,149] fluoride varnishes,[133,150] fluoride chewing

Treatment Protocol for Patients at Risk for Root Caries

Eliminate active infection

For cavitated lesions (both coronal and root surface), treat restoratively

Seal deep, retentive pits and fissures

Implement preventive measures

Increase patient awareness of potential problems

Survey diet; recommend modifications as necessary

Instruct on prophylaxis and oral hygiene

Provide periodontal therapy as needed

Evaluate salivary flow rate

Provide in-office fluoride

- Gels: 1.23% acidulated phosphate fluoride or 2% neutral sodium fluoride; 4-minute tray technique, 4 applications over 2 to 4 weeks
- Varnishes: Duraflor (Pharmascience), Duraphat (Colgate), Cavity-Shield (Omni), Fluor Protector (Vivadent); isolate each quadrant with cotton rolls, apply to teeth, repeat in 3 to 6 months

Home fluoride: fluoride-containing dentifrices, gels, rinses (preferably at least 3 fluoride exposures daily)

Xylitol chewing gum: advise patient to chew 2 pieces for 5 minutes, 3 times daily (preferably within 5 minutes after each meal)

Prescribe antibacterial mouth rinses (after active caries lesions are eliminated)

- Chlorhexidine gluconate (0.12%): rinse with $\frac{1}{2}$ oz for 30 seconds, morning and night for 2 weeks

Examine at 3-month recall

Monitor and reinforce preventive measures

Monitor sealant retention

Perform bacterial testing (*S mutans* test)*

- If scores are 0 or 1, continue home fluoride administration and recall in 3 months
- If scores are 2 or 3, repeat program

*Possible reasons for persistently high *S mutans* levels
- Patient maintaining diet high in refined carbohydrates
- Lack of patient compliance with program
- Undetected caries lesions still present
- Possible inoculation from another individual (eg, spouse)

---

gums,[151] and intraoral fluoride-releasing devices.[151,152] A synergistic, beneficial effect of argon laser irradiation and acidulated phosphate fluoride (APF) gels on root lesions in vitro has also been demonstrated.[153] However, the optimum delivery system of fluoride for protection against root caries has yet to be determined.[136]

A large number of studies have shown the benefits of substituting dietary polyols for sucrose in chewable dietary items. Xylitol, a 5-carbon sugar alcohol, has been under investigation since the early 1970s and has been found to be a safe and effective dietary supplement in humans (it was approved by the FDA in 1963 for special dietary purposes). Xylitol is not metabolized by *S mutans* and has been shown to have an anticariogenic effect,[154,155] decrease plaque formation,[156] increase plaque pH,[157] and possibly enhance remineralization.[158] Extensive research over the past 25 years has demonstrated that consuming 5 to 10 g of xylitol daily in the form of chewing gum can result in a 30% to 85% reduction in dental caries.[159,160]

The use of calcium phosphate has also been investigated as a mechanism for arresting root caries,[161] and many new preventive strategies are on the horizon.[162] The goal of the dental practitioner should be to initiate preventive and remineralization therapies that will inhibit or eliminate the dis-

ease process before tissue destruction occurs. The excavation of actively carious tooth structure and placement of restorative materials is, at best, a repair of the damages inflicted by the disease process and does not address the control of the disease itself. An effective preventive/remineralization regimen for the treatment of patients at risk for root caries is outlined above (see box).

Restorative Treatment

Clearly, many teeth with root caries lesions do not need restorative treatment. Accessible, shallow lesions can be made caries free and easy to clean through debridement with hand instruments, finishing burs, and/or polishing disks.[25,163] Arrested lesions with a hard to leathery surface are often amenable to treatment with topical fluorides in combination with a chlorhexidine rinse.[24]

When a root caries lesion has progressed such that restoration of lost structure is necessary, the dentist faces difficulties that differ considerably from those posed by many coronal lesions. The challenges to the restorative dentist include impaired visibility, difficult access, moisture control, pulpal proximity, and the nature of the dentinal substrate itself.

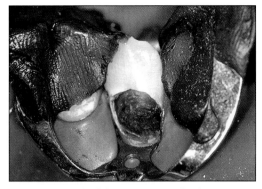

Fig 12-9 Because of the importance of a dry operating field, unobstructed access, and good visibility for treatment of root caries lesions, isolation is key to long-term success.

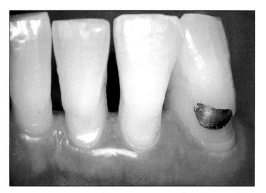

Fig 12-10 Direct gold restoration performing well 43 years after placement.

These factors tend to compromise the ideal restoration, which should conserve remaining tooth structure and provide long-term integrity of marginal seal. There is general agreement today that, when possible, adhesive fluoride-releasing restorative materials are preferred.[164]

Isolation is the key to long-term success in root surface restorations. Inability to obtain a dry operating field, unobstructed access, and visibility frequently results in a compromised restoration. The use of rubber dam and retractors, retraction cord, and/or surgical exposure will usually satisfy the necessary criteria. At times, the isolation may take more time than the actual preparation and restoration to obtain a satisfactory result (Fig 12-9).

Preparation design for cervical restorations and the properties of dental materials are described in chapters 11, 13, and 14. Preparation should involve removal of demineralized tooth structure with only minimal removal of sound tooth tissue for access and retention.

Direct Filling Gold

When properly placed and maintained in the right oral environment, gold foil restorations provide unequaled durability and longevity (Fig 12-10). Unfortunately, due to their perceived technique sensitivity and placement time, they are offered by a diminishing number of practitioners. Cavity preparation for direct gold placement requires removal of sound tooth structure for mechanical retention, and gold offers no chemotherapeutic benefit. However, these restorations are extremely well tolerated by supporting tissues and have demonstrated excellent longevity. For the xerostomic patient, this would not be the restorative material of choice because of cost, lack of chemotherapeutic effect, and likelihood of failure.

Silver Amalgam

Amalgam has the longest clinical history of the direct restorative materials with the exception of the direct filling golds. It has excellent wear characteristics, increasing marginal seal over time, and some bacteriostatic properties (Fig 12-11). Amalgam is relatively easy to place and is less sensitive to variations in handling than many other materials. Like direct gold, amalgam must be mechanically retained and does not offer significant chemotherapeutic benefit. With the introduction of adhesive fluoride-releasing materials and the current demand for tooth-colored restorations, the use of amalgam in cervical lesions has declined. While not recommended for use in xerostomic patients, it may still be the material of choice when isolation is a problem.

Resin Composite

With the advent of relatively reliable dentin bonding systems, resin composite materials, including compomers (polyacid-modified resins) and flowable composites, have become extremely popular with dental practitioners (Fig 12-12). Unfortunately, all of these materials exhibit a degree of polymerization shrinkage that can severely stress the adhesive interface provided by dentin bonding systems. When this is combined with the difference in coefficient of thermal expansion between these materials and tooth structure, the result is often a loss of marginal seal and microleakage (Figs 12-13a and 12-13b). Fluoride release is less than that of glass ionomer, and these materials do not currently offer any fluoride uptake. They are primarily indicated in root caries situations in which esthetics is of major importance. Microfilled or hybrid resin composites appear to offer advantages over compomers and flowable composites.

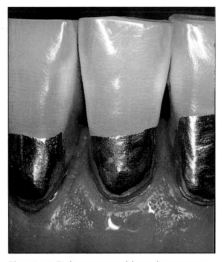

Fig 12-11 Eighteen-year-old amalgam restorations in mandibular incisors.

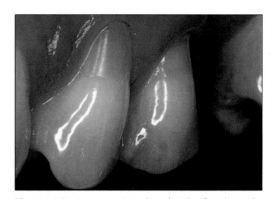

Fig 12-12 Resin composites placed with a fourth-generation bonding system.

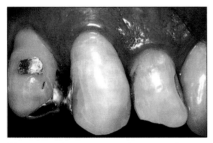

Fig 12-13a A resin composite restoration immediately after placement.

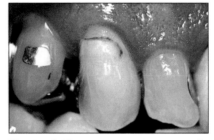

Fig 12-13b The same restoration 18 months later, showing leakage at the restoration-cementum interface.

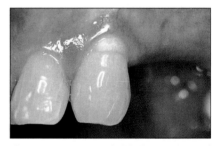

Fig 12-14 A Ketac-Fil (ESPE) conventional glass-ionomer restoration placed 10 years earlier.

Glass-Ionomer Cement/Resin-Modified Glass-Ionomer Cement

Glass-ionomer cement is the material of choice for most root caries lesions (see chapter 13). The material offers adhesive bonding, long-term fluoride release, and the ability to "recharge" or take up fluoride when exposed to an external source (eg, topical application, mouth rinse). Clinical studies have demonstrated successful 10-year longevity[165] (Fig 12-14) as well as reasonable success in xerostomic patients.[166–168]

Conclusion

Dental caries is a bacterial infectious disease associated with diet[1,169] and should be treated as such. Extensive research has moved our concept of caries from the early "worm theory" to a better understanding of the multifactorial, chronic nature of the disease. For this reason, modern dentistry has experienced a paradigm shift, with a move from complete reliance on the traditional surgical (restorative) approach to an acceptance of the fact that treatment of dental caries is not complete until the infection and contributing factors are controlled. This concept should guide the management of both coronal and root surface caries.

References

1. Katz RV. Development of an index for the prevalence of root caries. J Dent Res 1984;63:814–818.

2. Hardwick JL. The incidence and distribution of caries throughout the ages in relation to the Englishman's diet. Br Dent J 1960;108:9–17.

3. Douglass CW, Furino A. Balancing dental service requirements and supplies: Epidemiologic and demographic evidence. J Am Dent Assoc 1990;121:587–592.

4. Fedele DJ, Sheets CG. Issues in the treatment of root caries in older adults. J Esthet Dent 1998;10:243–252.

5. National Institutes of Health. Technology Assessment Conference. Effects and side effects of dental restorative materials. Bethesda, MD: US Department of Health and Human Services, 1991.

6. Brown L, Winn D, White B. Dental caries, restorations and tooth conditions in US adults, 1988–1991. J Am Dent Assoc 1996;127:1315–1325.

7. Winn DM, Brunelle JA, Selwitz RH, et al. Coronal and root caries in the dentition of adults in the United States, 1998–1991. J Dent Res 1996;75(special issue):642–651.

8. Warren JJ, Cowen HJ, Watkins CM, Hand JS. Dental caries prevalence and dental care utilization among the very old. J Am Dent Assoc 2000;131:1571–1579.

9. Anusavice KJ. Dental caries: Risk assessment and treatment solutions for an elderly population. Compend Contin Dent Educ 2002;23(10 suppl):12–20.

10. Drury TF, Brown LJ, Zion GR. Tooth retention and tooth loss in the permanent dentition of adults: 1988–1991. J Dent Res 1996;75(special issue):684–695.

11. Miller AJ, Brunell JA, Carlos JD, et al. Oral Health of United States Adults (NIH Publication no. 87-2868). Bethesda, MD: US Department of Health and Human Services, 1987.

12. Brown LJ, Brunelle JA, Kingman A. Periodontal status in the United States, 1988–1991: Prevalence, extent, and demographic variation. J Dent Res 1996;75(special issue):672–683.

13. Astroth JD. Caring for the elderly adult: How to prevent, manage root surface caries. Dent Teamwork 1996;9:15–19.

14. Beck JD. The epidemiology of root caries: North American studies. Adv Dent Res 1993;7:42–51.

15. Christensen GJ. A new challenge—root caries in mature people. J Am Dent Assoc 1996;127:379–380.

16. Shay K. Root caries in the elderly: An update for the next century. J Indiana Dent Assoc 1997–98;76:37,39–43.

17. Leake JL. Clinical decision-making for caries management in root surfaces. J Dent Educ 2001;65:1147–1153.

18. Ettinger RL, Hand JS. Factors influencing the future need for treatment of root surfaces. Am J Dent 1994;7:256–260.

19. Katz RV. The clinical diagnosis of root caries: Issues for the clinician and researcher. Am J Dent 1995;8:335–341.

20. Katz R. The RCI revisited after 15 years: Used, reinvented, modified, debated, and natural logged. J Pub Health Dent 1999;56:28–34.

21. Mjör IA. Placement and replacement of restorations. Oper Dent 1981;6:49–54.

22. Mjör IA. Frequency of secondary caries at various anatomical locations. Oper Dent 1985;10:88–92.

23. Banting DW. The diagnosis of root caries. J Dent Educ 2001;65:991–996.

24. Beighton D, Lynch E, Heath MR. A microbiological study of primary root-caries lesions with different treatment needs. J Dent Res 1993;72:623–629.

25. Billings RJ, Brown LR, Kaster AG. Contemporary treatment strategies for root surface dental caries. Gerodontology 1985;1:20–27.

26. Fejerskov O, Luan WM, Nyvad B, Budtz-Jorgensen E, Holm-Pedersen P. Active and inactive root surface caries lesions in a selected group of 60- to 80-year-old Danes. Caries Res 1991;25:385–391.

27. Syed SA, Loesche WJ, Pape HL Jr, Grenier E. Predominant cultivable flora isolated from human root surface caries plaque. Infect Immun 1975;11:727–731.

28. Lynch E. Relationship between clinical criteria and microflora of primary root caries. In: Stookey GK (ed). Early Detection of Dental Caries. Cincinnati, OH: Sidney Printing Works, 1996:195–242.

29. Hellyer P, Lynch E. The diagnosis of root caries—A review. Gerodontology 1990;9:95–102.

30. Galan D, Lynch E. Epidemiology of root caries. Gerodontology 1993;10:59–71.

31. Lynch E, Beighton D. A comparison of primary root caries lesions classified according to color. Caries Res 1994;28:233–238.

32. Katz RV, Hazen SP, Chilton NW, Mumma RD Jr. Prevalence and intraoral distribution of root caries in an adult population. Caries Res 1982;16:265–271.

33. Hals E, Selvig KA. Correlated electron probe microanalysis and microradiography of carious and normal dental cementum. Caries Res 1977;11:62–75.

34. Wag BJ. Root surface caries: A review. Community Dent Health 1984;1:11–20.

35. Lawrence HP, Hunt RJ, Beck JD. Three-year root caries incidence and risk modeling in older adults in North Carolina. J Public Health Dent 1995;55:69–78.

36. Leske GS, Ripa LW. Three-year root caries increments: An analysis of teeth and surfaces at risk. Gerodontology 1989;8:17–21.

37. Nyvad B, Fejerskov O. Root surface caries: Clinical, histopathological and microbiological features and clinical implications. Int Dent J 1982;32:312–326.

38. Atkinson JC, Wu AJ. Salivary gland dysfunction: Causes, symptoms, treatment. J Am Dent Assoc 1994;125:409–416.

39. Hoppenbrouwers PMM, Driessens FCM, Borggreven JMPM. The mineral solubility of human tooth roots. Arch Oral Biol 1987;32:319–322.

40. Dung TS-Z, Liu AH-H. Molecular pathogenesis of root dentin caries. Oral Dis 1999;5:92–99.

41. Schupbach P, Lutz F, Guggenheim B. Human root caries: Histopathology of arrested lesions. Caries Res 1992;26:153–164.

42. Erickson RL. Root surface treatment with glass ionomers and resin composites. Am J Dent 1994;7:279–285.

43. Park KK, Zitterbart PA, Christen AG. Preventive management of root caries: State of the art. Indiana Dent Assoc J 1987;66:11–19.

44. Zambon J, Kasprzak SA. Microbiology and histopathology of human root caries. Am J Dent 1995;6:323–328.

45. Wefel JS. Root caries histopathology and chemistry. Am J Dent 1994;5:261–265.

46. Ramsey DJ, Ripa LW. Enamel prism orientation and enamel cementum relationship in the cervical region of premolars. Br Dent J 1969;126:165–167.

47. Johansen E. Electron microscopic and chemical studies of carious lesions with reference to the organic phase of affected tissues. Ann N Y Acad Sci 1965;131:776–785.

48. McIntyre JM, Featherstone JD, Fu J. Studies of dental root surface caries. 2: the role of cementum in root surface caries [comment]. Aust Dent J 2000;3:215.

49. Dietz W, Kraft U, Hoyer I, Klingberg G. Influence of cementum on the demineralization and remineralization process of root surface caries in vitro. Acta Odontol Scand 2002;60:241–247.

50. Love RM, Jenkinson HF. Invasion of dentinal tubules by oral bacteria. Crit Rev Oral Biol Med 2002;13:171–183.

51. Weber DF. Human dentin sclerosis: A microradiographic survey. Arch Oral Biol 1974;19:163–169.

52. Beighton D, Lynch E. Comparison of selected microflora of plaque and underlying carious dentine associated with primary root caries lesions. Caries Res 1995;29:154–158.

53. van Houte J, Lopman J, Kent R. The predominant cultivable flora of sound and carious human root surfaces. J Dent Res 1994;73:727–734.

54. Schupbach P, Osterwalder V, Guggenheim B. Human root caries: Microbiota of a limited number of root caries lesions. Caries Res 1996;30:52–64.

55. Brailsford SR, Shah B, Simons D, et al. The predominant aciduric microflora of root-caries lesions. J Dent Res 2001;80:1828–1833.

56. Jordan HV, Hammond BF. Filamentous bacteria isolated from human root caries. Arch Oral Biol 1972;17:1333–1342.

57. Socransky SS, Hubersak C, Propas D. Introduction of periodontal destruction in gnotobiotic rats by a human oral strain of Actimomyces naeslundii. Arch Oral Biol 1970;15:993–995.

58. Beighton D, Hellyer PH, Lynch EJ, Heath MR. Salivary levels of mutans streptococci, lactobacilli, yeasts, and root caries prevalence in non-institutionalized elderly dental patients. Community Dent Oral Epidemiol 1991;219:302–307.

59. Brown LR, Billings RJ, Kaster AG. Quantitative comparisons of potentially cariogenic microorganisms cultured from noncarious and carious root and coronal tooth surfaces. Infect Immun 1986;51:765–770.

60. Emilson CG, Klock B, Sanford CB. Microbial flora associated with presence of root surface caries in periodontally treated patients. Scand J Dent Res 1988;96:40–49.

61. Fure S, Romaniec M, Emilson CG, Krasse B. Proportions of Streptococcus mutans, lactobacilli and Actinomyces spp in root surface plaque. Scand J Dent Res 1987;95:119–123.

62. Keltjens HM, Schaeken MJ, van der Hoeven JS, Hendrilos JC. Microflora of plaque from sound and carious root surfaces. Caries Res 1987;21:193–199.

63. Ravald N, Birkhed D. Factors associated with active and inactive root caries in patients with periodontal disease. Caries Res 1991;25:377–384.

64. van Strijp AJ, van Steenbergen TJ, Ten Cate JM. Bacterial colonization of mineralized and completely demineralized dentine in situ. Caries Res 1997;31:349–355.

65. Lundgren M, Emilson CG, Osterberg T. Caries prevalence and salivary and microbial conditions in 88-year-old Swedish dentate people. Acta Odontol Scand 1996;54:193–199.

66. Lundgren M, Emilson CG, Osterberg T. Root caries and some related factors in 88-year-old carriers and non-carriers of Streptococcus sobrinus in saliva. Caries Res 1998;32:93–99.

67. Moore MA, Gregory RL, Switalski LM, Hakki ZW, Gfell LE, Kowolik MJ. Differential activation of human neutrophils by Streptococcus mutans isolates from root surface lesions and caries-free and caries-active subjects. Oral Microbiol Immunol 1998;13:41–46.

68. Todd JE, Lader D. Adult Dental Health 1988. United Kingdom. London: HMSO, 1991:114.

69. Burt BA, Ismail AI, Edlund SA. Root caries in an optimally fluoridated and high-fluoride community. J Dent Res 1986;65:1154–1158.

70. Clarkson JE. Epidemiology of root caries. Am J Dent 1995;8:329–334.

71. Banting DW, Ellen RP, Fillery ED. Prevalence of root surface caries among institutional older persons. Community Dent Oral Epidemiol 1980;8:84–88.

72. Banting DW, Ellen RP, Fillery ED. A longitudinal study of root caries: Baseline and incidence data. J Dent Res 1985;64:1141–1144.

73. Lohse W, Carter H, Brunelle J. The prevalence of root surface caries in a military population. Mil Med 1977;142:700–703.

74. Hellyer PH, Beighton D, Heath MR, Lynch EJ. Root caries in older people attending a general dental practice in East Sussex. Br Dent J 1990;169:201–206.

75. Katz RV. Root caries—Is it the problem of the future? J Can Dent Assoc 1985;51:511–514.

76. Locker D, Slade GD, Leake JL. Prevalence of and factors associated with root decay in older adults in Canada. J Dent Res 1989;68:768–772.

77. Luan WM, Boelum V, Chen X. Dental caries in adult and elderly Chinese. J Dent Res 1989;68:1771–1776.

78. Hix JO, O'Leary TJ. The relationship between cemental caries, oral hygiene status and fermentable carbohydrate levels. J Periodontol 1976;47:398–404.

79. Sumney DL, Jordan HV, Englander HR. The prevalence of root surface caries in selected populations. J Periodontol 1973;44:500–504.

80. Fure S, Zickert I. Prevalence of root surface caries in 55, 65, and 75-year-old Swedish individuals. Community Dent Oral Epidemiol 1990;18:100–105.

81. Gustavsen F, Clive JM, Tveit AF. Root caries prevalence in a Norwegian adult dental population. Gerodontics 1988;18:100–105.

82. Kalsbeek H, Truin GJ, Burgersdijk R, van't Hof M. Tooth loss and dental caries in Dutch adults. Community Dent Oral Epidemiol 1991;19:201–204.

83. Whelton HP, Holland TJ, O'Mullane DM. The prevalence of root surface caries amongst Irish adults. Gerodontology 1993;10:72–75.

84. Al-Khateeb S, Angma-Mansson B, DeJosselin E. In vivo quantification of changes in caries lesions in orthodontic patients [abstract]. J Dent Res 1996;75:127.

85. Beck JD, Kohout F, Hunt RJ. Identification of high caries risk adults: Attitudes, social factors and diseases. Int Dent J 1988;38:231–238.

86. Fejerskov O. Recent advancements in the treatment of root surface caries. Int Dent J 1994;44:139.

87. Jensen ME, Kohout F. The effect of a fluoride dentifrice on root and coronal caries in an older adult population. J Am Dent Assoc 1988;117:829–832.

88. Ravald N, Hamp SE, Birkhed D. Long-term evaluation of root surface caries in periodontally treated patients. J Clin Periodontol 1986;13:758–767.

89. Ripa LW, Leske GS, Forte F. Effect of a 0.05% neutral NaF mouthrinse on coronal and root caries of adults. Gerodontology 1987;6:131–136.

90. Wallace MC, Retief DH, Bradley EL. Incidence of root caries in older adults [abstract 272]. J Dent Res 1988;67:147.

91. Hand JS, Hunt RJ, Beck JD. Coronal and root caries in older Iowans: 36-month incidence. Gerodontics 1988;4:136–139.

92. El-Hadary ME, Ramadan AE, Kamar AA, Nour ZM. A study of the incidence of and distribution of root surface caries and its relation to periodontal disease. Egypt Dent J 1975;21:43–52.

93. Vehkalahti MM, Vrbic VL, Peric LM, Matvoz ES. Oral hygiene and root caries occurrence in Slovenian adults. Int Dent J 1997;47:26–31.

94. Nyvad B, ten Cate JM, Fejerskov O. Arrest of root caries in situ. J Dent Res 1997;76:1845–1853.

95. Joshi A, Papas AS, Giunta J. Root caries incidence and associated risk factors in middle-aged and older adults. Gerodontology 1993; 10:83–89.

96. Locker D. Incidence of root caries in an older Canadian population. Community Dent Oral Epidemiol 1996;24:403–407.

97. MacEntee MI, Clark DC, Glick N. Predictors of caries in old age. Gerodontology 1993;10:90–97.

98. Powell LV, Mancl LA, Senft GD. Exploration of prediction models for caries risk assessment of the geriatric population. Community Dent Oral Epidemiol 1991;19:291–295.

99. Scheinin A, Pienihakkinen K, Tiekso J, Holmberg S. Multifactorial modeling for root caries prediction. Community Dent Oral Epidemiol 1992;20:35–37.

100. Kitamura M, Kiyak HA, Mulligan K. Predictors of root caries in the elderly. Community Dent Oral Epidemiol 1986;14:34–38.

101. DePaola PF, Soparkar PM, Tavares M, Kent RL. The clinical profiles of individuals with and without root surface caries. Gerodontology 1989;8:9–15.

102. Fure S. Five-year incidence of caries, salivary and microbial conditions in 60-, 70-, and 80-year-old Swedish individuals. Caries Res 1998;32:166–174.

103. Beck JD, Kohout FJ, Hunt RJ, Heckert DA. Root caries: Physical, medical and psychosocial correlates in an elderly population. Gerodontics 1986;3:242–247.

104. Dawes C. A mathematical model of salivary clearance of sugar from the oral cavity. Caries Res 1983;17:321–324.

105. Younger H, Harrison T, Streckfus C. Relationship among stimulated whole glandular salivary flow rates and root caries prevalence in an elderly population: A preliminary study. Spec Care Dentist 1998;18: 156–163.

106. Diaz-Arnold AM, Marek CA. The impact of saliva on patient care: A literature review. J Prosthet Dent 2002;88:337–343.

107. Tenovuo J. Salivary parameters of relevance in assessing caries activity in individuals and populations. Community Dent Oral Epidemiol 1997;25:82–86.

108. Lagerlöf F, Dawes R, Dawes C. Salivary clearance of sugar and its effects on pH changes by *Streptococcus mitior* in an artificial mouth. J Dent Res 1984;63:1266–1270.

109. Lagerlöf F, Dawes C. The effect of swallowing frequency on oral sugar clearance and pH changes by *Streptococcus mitior* in vivo after sucrose ingestion. J Dent Res 1985;64:1229–1232.

110. Dodds M, Suddick R. Caries risk assessment for determination of focus and intensity of prevention in a dental school clinic. J Dent Educ 1995;59:945–956.

111. Haveman CW, Redding SW. Dental management and treatment of xerostomic patients. Texas Dent J 1998;115:43–56.

112. Ravald N, Hamp SE. Prediction of root surface caries in patients treated for advanced periodontal disease. J Clin Periodontol 1981;8: 400–414.

113. Bardow A, Nyvad B, Nauntofte B. Relationships between medication intake, complaints of dry mouth, salivary flow rate and composition, and the rate of tooth demineralization in situ. Arch Oral Biol 2001;46:413–423.

114. Ferguson MM. Pilocarpine and other cholinergic drugs in the management of salivary gland dysfunction. Oral Surg Oral Med Oral Pathol 1993;75:186–191.

115. Shay K. Dental management considerations for institutionalized geriatric dental patients. J Prosthet Dent 1994;72:510–516.

116. Steele JG, Sheiham A, Marcenes W, Fay N, Walls AW. Clinical and behavioural risk indicators for root caries in older people. Gerodontology 2001;18:95–101.

117. Hand JS, Hunt RJ, Beck JD. Incidence of coronal and root caries in an older adult. J Public Health Dent 1988;48:14–19.

118. Pappas A, Koski A, Guinta J. Prevalence and intraoral distribution of coronal and root caries in middle-aged and older adults. Caries Res 1992;26:459–465.

119. Tonetti MS. Cigarette smoking and periodontal diseases: Etiology and management of disease. Ann Periodontol 1998;3:88–101.

120. Ravald N, Birkhed D. Prediction of root caries in periodontally treated patients maintained with different fluoride programmes. Caries Res 1992;26:450–458.

121. Powell LV, Leroux BG, Persson RE, Kiyak HA. Factors associated with caries incidence in an elderly population. Community Dent Oral Epidemiol 1998;26:170–176.

122. Ravald N, Birkhed D, Hamp SE. Root caries susceptibility in periodontally treated patients. Results after 12 years. J Clin Periodontol 1993;20:124–129.

123. Persson RE, Persson GR, Powell LV, Kiyak HA. Periodontal effects of a biobehavioral prevention program. J Clin Periodontol 1999;25: 322–329.

124. Drake CW, Hunt RJ, Beck JD, Koch GG. Eighteen-month coronal caries incidence in North Carolina older adults. J Public Health Dent 1994;54:24–30.

125. Lawrence HP, Hunt RJ, Beck JD, Davies GM. Five-year incidence and intraoral distribution of root caries among community-dwelling older adults. Caries Res 1996;30:169–179.

126. Newitter DA, Katz RV, Clive JM. Detection of root caries: Sensitivity and specificity of a modified explorer. Gerodontics 1985;1:65–67.

127. Jones JA. Root caries: Prevention and chemotherapy. Am J Dent 1995;8:352–357.

128. Ando M, Analoui M, Schemehorn BR. Comparison of lesion analysis by microradiography and confocal microscopy [abstract 209]. J Dent Res 1995;74:48.

129. Ferreira AG, Analoui M, Ando M. Using dye enhanced QLF for analyzing incipient lesions [abstract 1446]. J Dent Res 1995;74:192.

130. de Josselin de Jong E, Sundstrom F, Angmar-Mansson B, Ten Bosch JJ. QLF-vision: Reproducibility of in vivo quantification of enamel mineral loss [abstract]. J Dent Res 1994;73:200.

131. de Josselin de Jong E, Sundstrom F, Westerling H, Tranaeus S, ten Bosch JJ, Angmar-Mansson B. A new method for in vivo quantification of changes in initial enamel caries with laser fluorescence. Caries Res 1995;29:2–7.

132. van der Veen MH, Tsuda H, Arends J, ten Bosch JJ. Evaluation of sodium fluorescein for quantitative diagnosis of root caries. J Dent Res 1996;75:588–593.

133. De Paola PF. Caries in our aging populations: What are we learning? In: Bowen WH, Tabak LA (eds). Cariology for the Nineties. Rochester, NY: University of Rochester Press, 1993:25–35.

134. Emilson CG, Ravald N, Birkhed D. Effects of a 12-month prophylactic programme on selected oral bacterial populations on root surfaces with active and inactive carious lesions. Caries Res 1993;27:195–200.

135. Burgess JO, Gallo JR. Treating root-surface caries. Dent Clin North Am 2002;46:385–404.

136. Featherstone JDB. Fluoride, remineralization and root caries. Am J Dent 1994;7:271–274.

137. Hicks MJ, Flaitz CM, Garcia-Godoy F. Root-surface caries formation: Effect of in vitro APF treatment. J Am Dent Assoc 1998;129:449–453.

138. Nyvad B, Fejerskov O. Active root-surface caries converted into inactive caries as a response to oral hygiene. Scand J Dent Res 1986;94:281–284.

139. Nyvad B, ten Cate JM, Fejerskov O. Microradiography of experimental root-surface caries in man. Caries Res 1989;23:218–224.

140. Nyvad B, Larsen MJ. Effect of daily plaque removal on Stephan pH response of active root caries lesions in situ. Caries Res 1992;26:227–228.

141. Lynch E. Antimicrobial management of primary root carious lesions: A review. Gerodontology 1996;13:118–129.

142. Brailsford SR, Fiske J, Gilbert S, Clark D, Beighton D. The effects of the combination of chlorhexidine/thymol- and fluoride-containing varnishes on the severity of root caries lesions in frail institutionalised elderly people. J Dent 2002;30:319–324.

143. Nyvad B, Fejerskov O. Effect of tooth cleaning on microbial invasion of experimental root surface caries [abstract 78]. Caries Res 1993;27:229.

144. Brustman B. Impact of exposure to fluoride-adequate water on root surface caries in the elderly. Gerodontics 1986;2:203–207.

145. Hunt RJ, Eldredge JB, Beck JD. Effect of residence in a fluoridated community on the incidence of coronal and root caries in an older adult population. J Public Health Dent 1989;49:138–141.

146. Stamm JW, Banting DW, Imrey PB. Adult root caries survey of two similar communities with contrasting natural water fluoride levels. J Am Dent Assoc 1990;120:143–149.

147. Mukai Y, Lagerweij MD, ten Cate JM. Effect of a solution with high fluoride concentration on remineralization of shallow and deep root surface caries in vitro. Caries Res 2001;35:317–324.

148. Teranaka T, Koulourides T. Effect of 100 ppm fluoride mouthrinse on experimental root caries in human. Caries Res 1987;21:326–332.

149. Baysan A, Lynch E, Ellwood R, Davies R, Petersson L, Borsboom P. Reversal of primary root caries using dentifrices containing 5,000 and 1,100 ppm fluoride. Caries Res 2001;35:41–46.

150. Arends J, Duschner H, Ruben JL. Penetration of varnishes into demineralized root dentine in vitro. Caries Res 1997;31:201–205.

151. De Los Santos R, Lin YT, Corpron RE, Beltran ED, Strachan DS, Landry PA. In situ remineralization of root surface lesions using a fluoride chewing gum or a fluoride releasing device. Caries Res 1994;28:441–446.

152. Mirth DB, Shern RJ, Emilson CG, et al. Clinical evaluation of an intraoral device for controlled release of fluoride. J Am Dent Assoc 1982;105:791–797.

153. Hicks MJ, Westerman GH, Flaitz CM, Blankenau RJ, Powell GL, Berg JH. Effects of argon laser irradiation and acidulated phosphate fluoride on root caries. Am J Dent 1995;8:10–14.

154. Nuuja T, Meurman JH, Torkko H. Xylitol and the bactericidal effect of chlorhexidine and fluoride on Streptococcus mutans and Streptococcus sanguis. Acta Odontol Scand 1993;51:109–114.

155. Trahan L. Xylitol: A review of its action on mutans streptococci and dental plaque—Its clinical significance. Int Dent J 1995;45(suppl 1):77–92.

156. Isotupa KP, Gunn S, Chen CY, Lopatin D, Makinen KK. Effect of polyol gums on dental plaque in orthodontic patients. Am J Orthod Dentofac Orthop 1995;107:497–504.

157. Aguirre-Zero O, Zero DT, Proskin HM. Effect of chewing xylitol chewing gum on salivary flow rate and the acidogenic potential of dental plaque. Caries Res 1993;27:55–59.

158. Wennerholm K, Arends J, Birkhed D, Ruben J, Emilson CG, Dijkman AG. Effect of xylitol and sorbitol in chewing-gums on mutans streptococci, plaque pH and mineral loss of enamel. Caries Res 1994;28:48–54.

159. Mäkinen KK, Bennett CA, Hujoel PP, et al. Xylitol chewing gums and caries rates: A 40-month cohort study. J Dent Res 1995;74:1904–1913.

160. Mäkinen KK, Mäkinen PL, Pape HR Jr. Stabilisation of rampant caries: Polyol gums and arrest of dentine caries in two long-term cohort studies in young subjects. Int Dent J 1995;45(suppl 1):93–107.

161. Chow LC, Takagi S. Remineralization of root lesions with concentrated calcium and phosphate solutions. Dent Mater J 1995;14:131–136.

162. Westerman GH, Hicks MJ, Flaitz CM, Blankenau RJ, Powell GL. Argon laser irradiation effects on sound root surfaces: In vitro scanning electron microscopic observations. J Clin Laser Med Surg 1998;16:111–115.

163. Wallace MC, Retief DH, Bradley EL. The 48-month increment of root caries in an urban population of older adults participating in a preventive dental program. J Public Health Dent 1993;43:133–137.

164. Burgess JO. Dental materials for the restoration of root surface caries. Am J Dent 1995;8:342–351.

165. Matis BA, Cochran MA, Carlson TJ. Longevity of glass-ionomer restorative materials: Results of a 10-year evaluation. Quintessence Int 1996;27:373–382.

166. Haveman CW, Burgess JO, Summitt JB. A clinical comparison of restorative materials for caries in xerostomic patients [abstract 1441]. J Dent Res 1999;78:286.

167. Hara AT, Turssi CP, Serra MC, Nogueira MCS. Extent of the cariostatic effect on root dentin provided by fluoride-containing restorative materials. Oper Dent 2002;27:480–487.

168. Haveman CW, Summitt JB, Burgess JO, Carlson K. Three restorative materials and topical fluoride gel used in xerostomic patients: A clinical comparison. J Am Dent Assoc 2003;134:177–184.

169. van Houte J, Jordan HV, Laraway R, Kent R, Soparkar PM, DePaola PF. Association of the microbial flora of dental plaque and saliva with human root surface caries. J Dent Res 1990;69:1463–1468.

Fluoride-Releasing Materials

John O. Burgess
Xiaoming Xu

Fluorides are an important adjunct in the prevention of caries. It has been known for years that benefits can be gained through the use of systemic and topically applied fluoride. More recently, a variety of fluoride-releasing dental materials have become available. This chapter discusses fluoride-releasing materials, their effectiveness in inhibiting recurrent caries lesions, and their clinical longevity. The caries process and methods of caries management are discussed in chapter 4. Root caries and its prevention and treatment are discussed in chapter 12.

Caries is a multifactoral disease caused by bacteria.[1] Since the bacteria producing this disease are introduced into the oral cavity by transfer from an infected host, the best method for preventing the disease is by blocking the transfer. However, once established in the oral biofilm, caries-causing bacteria are not easily removed. The effects of caries are produced by bacteria that metabolize sucrose or other cariogenic sugars and secrete organic acids (lactic, propionic, and formic) that cause the loss of mineral ions (calcium and phosphates) from the tooth (demineralization).[2] Mineral lost by this method can be replaced during periods of neutral pH (remineralization) from calcium and phosphates in the saliva. Remineralization is facilitated by fluoride and can arrest carious demineralization in enamel by the formation of a hard outer surface. Periods of demineralization and remineralization make up a continuous cycle by which minerals in tooth structure are removed and replaced. If the balance is tipped toward demineralization, caries lesions develop.

The effect of the caries process in dentin is similar to its effects on enamel, except that dentin demineralization begins at a higher pH (6.4, compared to 5.5 for enamel) and proceeds about twice as rapidly; this is because dentin has only half the mineral content of enamel. Low fluoride levels are insufficient to initiate dentin remineralization but are adequate to facilitate enamel remineralization.[3] Fluoride-ion concentration in saliva is low, averaging about 0.03 ppm (1.6 µmol/L) in the normal subject.[4] In enamel, at fluoride levels around 3 ppm, the balance of mineral uptake and loss is shifted from net demineralization to net remineralization.[5] Because root structure is primarily composed of dentin and because root-surface caries lesions require significantly greater amounts of fluoride than enamel caries lesions to promote remineralization, restorative materials that release fluoride are often recommended for root surfaces.

Individuals with high-caries-risk profiles are those with frequent carbohydrate intake, reduced salivary flow, increased plaque retention, low fluoride exposure during tooth formation, and high bacteria counts. A normal unstimulated salivary flow rate is approximately 0.3 mL/min, while stimulated salivary flow ranges from 1.5 to 2.5 mL/min.[4] Low salivary flow is often associated with (1) medications such as antihypertensives, antidepressants, and anticholinergics; (2) a history of head and neck irradiation; or (3) Sjögren syndrome.[6,7] Low salivary flow reduces the bicarbonate, calcium, and phosphate ions that are provided with normal salivary flow rates. This reduces the buffering ability of the saliva, which, in turn, reduces the ability of the saliva to induce remineralization of demineralized tooth structure. Fluorides are most effective in inducing remineralization on smooth surfaces of teeth.

Exposure to high levels of fluoride during tooth formation produces fluorapatite crystals in tooth

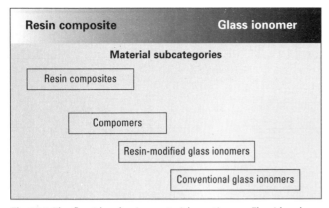

Fig 13-1 The fluoride-releasing materials continuum. Fluoride release and recharge increase from left to right among the materials. Locations on the continuum are characterized by compositional variants, curing mechanisms, and mechanical and physical properties.

structure. Fluorapatite crystals have a critical pH of 4.5, allowing fluorapatite to resist acid demineralization significantly better than hydroxyapatite.

It is clear that fluoride plays a significant role in caries prevention. Unfortunately, compliance in caries-control programs is often poor and requires significant effort from the caries-prone individual. Fluoride-releasing materials supply levels of fluoride from restorations that provide a measure of caries prevention; this fluoride source does not require patient compliance. Therefore, fluoride-releasing materials are an essential element in treating the patient who is at high risk for developing caries lesions.

The Fluoride-Releasing Materials Continuum

The first popular fluoride-releasing tooth-colored restorative material was silicate cement. This material had poor bonding properties, high solubility, and poor mechanical properties and did not survive well in the oral environment. However, recurrent caries lesions associated with these restorations were rare. This anticaries effect was associated with the fluoride released from the silicate cement. Current fluoride-releasing materials have coupled the fluoride release with significantly improved physical properties.

Fluoride-releasing materials may be classified into four categories[6-8] based on similarities in physical, mechanical, and setting properties. These include resin composite, compomer, resin-modified glass ionomer, and traditional glass ionomer (Fig 13-1). Fluoride-releasing resin composites are on one end

of the continuum and release the least fluoride, while conventional glass ionomers are on the other end and demonstrate the highest levels of fluoride release. Compomers are more similar to resin composites, and resin-modified glass ionomers are more similar to conventional glass ionomers.

Table 13-1 compares the mechanical and physical properties of the four different categories of fluoride-releasing materials. Table 13-2 describes the water content, form in which supplied, and setting mechanism (acid-base reaction or free-radical polymerization) for these materials. Materials that are powder-liquid must have the powder mixed with the liquid to initiate set; paste-paste materials must have the two pastes mixed to initiate set; visible-light–cured (VLC) materials must be exposed to a curing light. Table 13-3 lists representative products in each category of the continuum.

Resin Composites

Fluoride-releasing resin composites have better mechanical properties, no inherent adhesive properties, greater thermal expansion coefficients, and better wear resistance compared to other materials in the continuum. However, they also have the smallest amount of fluoride release and provide almost no long-term fluoride release through recharge.

Glass Ionomers

Conventional glass ionomers are adhesive, release comparatively high levels of fluoride, and have thermal-expansion coefficients similar to those of tooth structure. Early brand-name glass ionomers that are still widely used today have poor mechanical properties and wear resistance. A newer generation of high-viscosity glass ionomers (Ketac-Molar and Fuji IX) have improved mechanical properties and provide higher levels of fluoride release compared to traditional glass ionomers[8,9] (Table 13-3 and Fig 13-2). Although wear resistance is improved, these materials do not have wear resistance similar to resin composites and should not be used to restore load-bearing areas in the permanent dentition. Walls and Mather[9] reported a 1-year wear rate of 73 µm, which is significantly greater than the 10 to 20 µm/y wear reported for resin composites.

Resin-Modified Glass Ionomers

Resin-modified glass ionomers contain elements of conventional glass ionomers and light-cured resins and have properties similar to each of those materials. Resin-modified glass ionomers have been modified in several ways since the fluoride-releasing materials continuum was proposed.

Table 13-1	Mechanical properties of materials in the fluoride-releasing materials continuum[60]			
	Material class			
	Glass ionomer	Resin-modified glass ionomer	Compomer	Resin composite
Flexural strength (MPa)	15–25	35–70	60–94	85–97
Compressive strength (MPa)	170–200*	180–210	190–250	230–270
Diametral tensile strength (MPa)	22–25	35–40	45–47	40–60
Shear bond strength (MPa)	3–7	7–16	14–22	24–28
Fluoride release	High	High	Moderate	Low
Fluoride recharge	High	High	Moderate	Low

*Ultimate compressive strength. Glass ionomers may achieve this after several weeks' storage prior to testing; early strengths are significantly lower.

Table 13-2	Composition, form supplied, and setting reaction of the materials in the fluoride-releasing materials continuum		
Glass ionomer	Resin-modified glass ionomer	Compomer	Resin composite
Contains water	Contains water	No water	No water
Powder-liquid only	Powder-liquid or paste-paste	VLC paste	VLC paste or paste-paste
Acid-base only	Acid-base and radical	Radical only	Radical only

Table 13-3	Representative products in each category of the fluoride-releasing materials continuum		
Glass ionomer	Resin-modified glass ionomer	Compomer	Resin composite
Ketac-Fil*	Photac-Fil*	Dyract AP[†]	Heliomolar[‡]
Fuji II[§]	Fuji II LC[§]	Hytac*	Tetric[‡]
Ketac-Molar*	Vitremer*	Compoglass[‡]	Solitaire[∥]
Fuji IX[§]		F 2000*	SureFil[†]

*3M ESPE
[†]Caulk Dentsply
[‡]Ivoclar Vivadent
[§]GC America
[∥]Heraeus Kulzer

Fig 13-2 Compressive strengths of some fluoride-releasing restorative materials at different setting times.

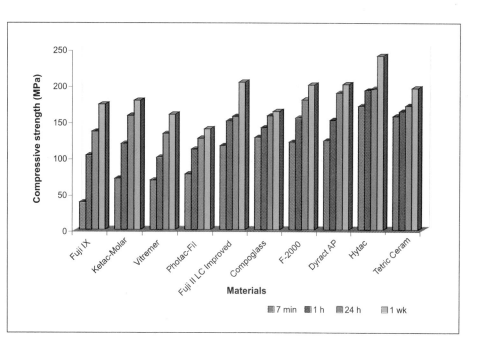

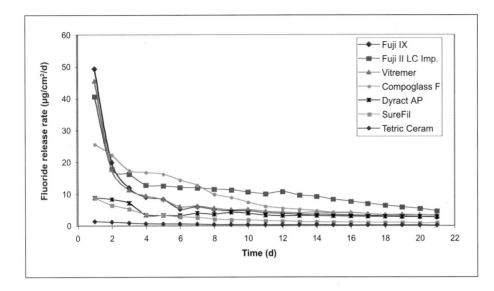

Fig 13-3 Fluoride release profiles of some fluoride-releasing materials over 21 days.

Improved manufacturing has led to smaller filler particles, resulting in a smoother restoration surface and increased fluoride release.[10] Recently, paste-paste resin-modified glass ionomers (those supplied as two pastes that are to be mixed together) have been marketed as luting cements. A paste-paste restorative material is also being developed. Paste materials are easier to mix and place than resin-modified glass ionomers supplied in powder-liquid form. The paste-paste systems will have mechanical and physical properties similar to those of the powder-liquid systems. Resin-modified glass ionomers, like conventional glass ionomers, should not be used for restorations in occlusal load–bearing areas.

Compomers

Compomers are also blends of resin composite and glass ionomer. However, they incorporate more resin than the resin-modified glass ionomers, and their physical and mechanical properties are more similar to those of the fluoride-releasing resin composites. Compomers require a bonding system and acid etching of tooth structure to achieve a clinically usable bond.[11,12] These materials release more fluoride than resin composites but less than conventional glass ionomers or resin-modified glass ionomers. Their abrasion resistance is intermediate between resin-modified glass ionomers and resin composites. Compomer restorative materials and cements have undergone considerable improvements since their introduction. These improvements have produced materials with increased fluoride release and better mechanical properties. Expansion due to water sorption was an early problem with compomers, but this problem is less severe in currently available products.[13]

Fluoride Release

Several researchers have reported that fluoride released from restorative materials affects tooth structure. Decreased recurrent caries rates around silicate restorations have been associated with their fluoride release. Early in vivo work by Hals and Norderval[14] examined recurrent caries around Class 5 restorations and reported a lower occurrence of caries lesions around the silicate restorations. In 1957 Phillips and Swartz[15] examined the effect of fluoride-releasing restorative materials on enamel solubility. Since the influence of water fluoridation in reducing enamel solubility was already well established, it was postulated that fluoride released from dental restorative materials could be incorporated into the tooth structure around the restorations and would contribute to reduced enamel solubility. This study demonstrated that fluoride present in silicate cements reduced the solubility of the adjacent enamel and suggested that fluoride in low concentrations could be added to dental materials to reduce enamel solubility.

In 1960, Norman et al[16] reported the results of a study in which they measured the fluoride content of powdered enamel exposed to fluoride released from porcelain, resin with added sodium fluoride, zinc phosphate cement, zinc phosphate cement with added 10% calcium fluoride, 2% sodium fluoride, and silicate cements. Silicates released large amounts of fluoride for the first 24 hours, but the levels decreased with time. The enamel specimens exposed to the silicates had the greatest fluoride uptake (495% increase). The results of this study suggested that materials releasing high levels of fluoride produced significant fluoride uptake by enamel. Furthermore, whenever large amounts of fluoride ion were present in solution, only a small percentage of the available fluoride ion (eg, 18% in the case of enamel exposed to silicate cement) was actually absorbed by the enamel. With smaller amounts of fluoride ion in solution, a larger percentage was absorbed by the enamel. This demonstrates that low levels of fluoride can be absorbed and that the long-term low release rate is most important.

Subsequent research by Norman et al[17] examined fluoride uptake by enamel slabs exposed to the same dental materials. The data from powdered enamel and intact enamel were generally in agreement. Most of the materials tested produced some measurable increase in enamel fluoride content, and fluoride increases correlated with reduced acid solubility of the intact enamel.

Norman et al[18] expanded their research to examine the effects of restorative materials on bacterial plaque. They compared plaque composition associated with amalgam, gold foil, cast gold (inlay), methyl methacrylate resin, and silicate cement restorations. They reported that comparable plaque developed on all tested materials with the exception of the silicate cement. Based on this research, it appeared that the fluoride component of the silicate cement somehow altered the composition of the plaque, both at the margin of the restoration and on the tooth surface. Although silicate cement released fluoride, it was a poor restorative material, and silicate-cement restorations failed due to their high degree of solubility and poor mechanical properties.

The common denominator in this early research on the effects of various restorative materials on plaque and caries activity appeared to be the presence of fluoride. Since fluoride was present in, and leached from, silicate cements, subsequent research was devoted to finding other materials with improved physical properties that might release fluoride in a more predictable and ultimately more successful manner. This preliminary work led to the development of glass-ionomer cement.

There are significant numbers of in vitro and in vivo studies that demonstrate the fluoride-releasing capability of glass ionomers.[13,19] Researchers have measured the fluoride release from four glass-ionomer cements and reported that the greatest release occurred on the first day; subsequently, it decreased sharply the second day and gradually diminished over 3 weeks to a low-level, long-term release. After 1 year, all specimens were still releasing fluoride with daily concentrations of at least 0.5 ppm. Other studies have also shown a "burst" of fluoride release, with high early release for 1 to 2 days, followed by a rapid decline.[20–31]

Xu and others[10] measured the compressive strength and the fluoride-release and fluoride-recharge profiles of 14 fluoride-releasing materials. The fluoride-release profiles of some of these materials are shown in Fig 13-3. The study demonstrated a negative (reverse) correlation between fluoride release and compressive strength. Materials that have a high level of fluoride release generally have lower strengths than materials with a low level of fluoride release.

In a recent study, Hsu et al[30] measured the fluoride released from a resin-modified glass ionomer (Vitremer) and a high-viscosity conventional glass ionomer (Fuji IX). Using a continuous flow apparatus with the flow rate adjusted to 20 mL/h, they reported that Vitremer released more fluoride than Fuji IX over an 8-hour period. In addition, the fluoride release rate decreased rapidly after recharging, and most of the fluoride was released within 6 hours. This is clinically significant because it indicates that the fluoride-releasing materials should be recharged with external neutral sodium fluoride daily to increase their fluoride release and remineralizing potential (see Fig 13-3).

In a comprehensive study of fluoride-releasing materials, Cranfield et al[22] reported that fluoride release is influenced by the shape of the specimen used in the study. Specimens with larger surface areas released more fluoride. They also reported that pH influenced fluoride release. Storage media with a lower pH produced higher fluoride release, probably due to erosion of the glass-ionomer surface.

The release from a restoration of fluoride that can be incorporated into tooth structure and into the walls of the cavity preparation is perhaps the most important benefit of glass ionomer.[15,32,33] However, the fluoride release can be inhibited by the injudicious use of bonding agents beneath and/or covering the restoration. Interestingly, some authors and manufacturers continue to recommend the use of these resins with glass ionomers.[34]

Fluoride released from glass-ionomer restorations has been collected in whole saliva.[35] In vivo research by Hatibovic-Kofman and Koch[35] and by Hattab et al[36] found significant increases of fluoride in saliva following the placement of glass-ionomer restorations. In one study,[35] salivary fluoride concentrations remained elevated even 1 year after placement of glass-ionomer restorations (0.3 ppm after placement, 0.04 ppm 1 year later). In the other study,[36] subjects wore maxillary appliances with four glass-ionomer (Ketac-Fil) restorations every night. The unstimulated salivary fluoride content was measured before insertion of the device and after overnight wear. In all subjects, salivary fluoride increased after wearing the appliance.[36]

Fluoride released from these materials is incorporated into bacteria[4] and inhibits bacterial acid production.[5] However, the fluoride in plaque on teeth adjacent to or several teeth distant from a glass-ionomer restoration is not increased. Protection provided by fluoride-releasing materials is probably confined

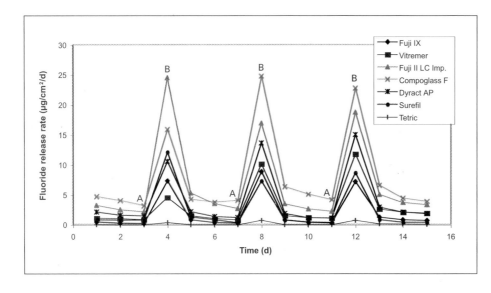

Fig 13-4 Fluoride recharge profiles of some fluoride-releasing restorative materials. (A) Baseline amount of fluoride release prior to application of topical fluoride; (B) amount of fluoride release 1 day after recharge.

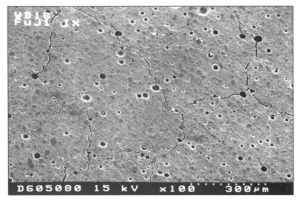

Fig 13-5 Photomicrograph of porosity in Fuji IX that allows fluoride-rich materials to be absorbed and released.

to tooth structure immediately adjacent to the restoration. One study demonstrated that fluoride released from restorative materials has an effective zone of about 1 mm from the restoration's margins.[37]

Fluoride Recharging

Perhaps the most important variable in fluoride release is not the amount of fluoride released from the material initially after placement, since this declines rapidly with time (see Fig 13-3), but the ability of the material to be recharged with fluoride from external sources (Fig 13-4). Forsten evaluated fluoride release[26] and uptake[38] by traditional glass ionomers to determine whether glass-ionomer materials could not only release fluoride but also take up fluoride from a fluoride-rich solution applied to the glass ionomer. He reported that after

an initial high rate of fluoride release, a constant level of release occurred at about 3 weeks and that topical fluoride applications could recharge glass-ionomer restorations. Forsten[38] also reported a constant release rate of approximately 0.5 to 1.0 µg/mL for all glass ionomers except cermets (glass ionomers containing silver particles) during the second year. Other investigators[35,39,40] have confirmed the recharge phenomenon when high-fluoride-content solutions are applied to glass ionomers. Regardless of the units used to express the recharge, increased fluoride uptake occurs when glass ionomers are exposed to fluoride-containing solutions.

Compomers and resin-modified glass ionomers can be recharged as well.[41] Resin-modified glass ionomers (Photac-Fil, Vitremer, and Fuji II LC) and conventional glass ionomers (Fuji IX and Ketac-Molar) demonstrate the greatest fluoride recharge capacity. Fluoride-releasing resin composites such as Heliomolar and Tetric Ceram release little additional fluoride after being exposed to a fluoride-rich solution. The compomers, such as Dyract AP and Compoglass, have a recharge capacity between that of resin-modified glass ionomers and resin composites but more similar to that of resin-modified glass ionomers. For those materials demonstrating recharge capability, the fluoride release remains at increased levels for only 1 day. This recharge capability may be due to the microporosities present in glass ionomers (Fig 13-5) and resin-modified glass ionomers.

Glass-ionomer restorative materials, then, are fluoride reservoirs; once the fluoride is depleted, it may be replenished from other fluoride sources such as toothpastes, mouth rinses, or topical fluoride solutions. Concentrated fluoride solutions such as gels applied to fluoride-releasing materials produce a greater fluoride recharge than toothpastes and rinses. The release after recharge is short, and recharge must be accomplished daily to maintain an elevated level. In a study by Xu and others,[10] the resin-modified glass ionomers, as a group, had the greatest recharge; compomers were intermediate, followed by traditional glass ionomers; and fluoride-releasing resin composites had the least recharge (see Fig 13-4).

The pH of the topical fluoride[42–44] used to recharge glass-ionomer restorations is important. Studies have reported that acidic topical fluoride solutions such as acidulated phosphate fluoride solutions and other acidified fluoride preparations cause degradation of glass-ionomer materials and should therefore be avoided. Resin-modified glass ionomers are more resistant to surface degradation than conventional glass ionomers but still degrade when exposed to acids.[44] Resin composites are degraded by frequent applications of acidic fluoride solutions, producing filler dislodgment and destruction of the resin matrix interface.[45]

Antibacterial Effects of Fluoride

The high fluoride levels released from glass-ionomer restorative materials in the first few days after placement may be beneficial because of antibacterial effects. Initial microleakage often occurs after placement, before the hygroscopic expansion of the restorative material results in an improved seal. Fluoride has three effects on bacteria: inhibition of metabolism, inhibition of growth, and bacterial death. Fluoride is bactericidal in concentrations greater than 200 ppm, which is more than the amount released by fluoride-releasing materials. Thus, a direct bactericidal effect probably does not occur from fluoride released by restorative materials because the amount released is too low. Fluoride levels produced by fluoride-releasing materials probably affect bacterial metabolism. By reducing bacterial acid production and altering the environment, this effectively changes the succession of bacteria necessary for acid production. This subtle mechanism is difficult to measure but may profoundly reduce acid production and tooth demineralization by cariogenic bacteria.

Norman et al[18] observed that plaque composition was similar on surfaces of amalgam, gold foil, cast gold, and resin but was reduced around silicate-cement restorations. They speculated that fluoride released from the silicate cement altered plaque composition, both at the margins of the restoration and on the tooth surface. Loyola-Rodriguez et al[46] observed similar inhibition of Streptococcus mutans by resin-modified and conventional glass-ionomer restorative materials. Forss et al[47,48] demonstrated a higher level of fluoride in plaque growing on glass ionomer than in plaque growing on resin composite restorations, with a significant reduction of S mutans near the glass-ionomer restorations.

In an in vitro study, Palenik et al[49] measured the inhibition of microbial adherence and growth of five different bacteria typical in human plaque (Actinomyces viscosus, Streptococcus mitis, S mutans, Lactobacillus casei, and Streptococcus sanguis) by six different glass-ionomer materials. All materials inhibited growth and/or adherence to some degree. The extent of inhibition varied according to the material used and the specific bacterium. Growth inhibition was directly related to the amount of fluoride ion released; materials with a higher rate of release had a greater effect. McComb and Ericson[50] demonstrated that a pH of 2.6 was produced with freshly mixed glass ionomer; the pH rose to 7.4 during the setting reaction. These investigators proposed that both the low pH and the fluoride release were responsible for the antibacterial effects. DeSchepper et al[51,52] used an agar-diffusion-assay method to determine the inhibitory effects on S mutans of 11 glass-ionomer cements and their powder and liquid components. They measured the zone of inhibition of bacterial growth and the fluoride levels in the surrounding agar. Since glass-ionomer liquids (polyacids) were acidic, they inhibited bacterial growth. The mixed materials released significant amounts of fluoride. Inhibition zones correlated well with fluoride levels; high fluoride-releasing materials had greater zones of inhibition than low fluoride-releasing materials. However, in a subsequent study[53] measuring the antibacterial effects of light-cured glass ionomers, a neutral sodium fluoride control was included. Although Vitrebond (3M ESPE) and XR Ionomer (Kerr) produced significant inhibition zones, the neutral sodium fluoride produced no inhibition zone. When the pH of the tested materials was adjusted to 5 by adding sodium hydroxide, none had antibacterial effects. The authors concluded that the mechanism of action for bacterial inhibition was probably a combination of fluoride release and low pH.

Bacteria in plaque located on glass-ionomer restorations are affected less as the age of the restoration increases. Bacterial composition of plaque on glass-ionomer restorations, up to a month after placement,[47] generally shows a strong positive correlation between fluoride release and reduced S mutans counts. However, older restorations, which release less fluoride, do not reduce bacterial counts. Studies by Svanberg et al[54] and van Dijken et al[55] found a more prolonged antibacterial effect. Perhaps the difference between these studies occurred when oral hygiene measures were discontinued to allow plaque to accumulate. By removing the recharge from fluoride-containing toothpaste, less antibacterial effects would be seen. An in vitro investigation by Seppä et al[5] established a dose-response relationship between fluoride release, bacterial acid production, and, quite possibly, caries.

Because fluoride release from all materials declines rapidly with time, the materials must be recharged to provide the fluoride levels necessary to remineralize tooth structure. Application of fluoride gel to aged glass-ionomer samples reestablishes the fluoride-releasing properties of the materials. Because the fluoride release and antibacterial properties of all fluoride-releasing materials appear to be short-lived, supplemental fluoride from topical fluoride gels, fluoride-containing toothpastes, and/or fluoride-containing mouth rinses should be used daily to augment the fluoride output of the fluoride-releasing materials.

Do Fluoride-Releasing Materials Inhibit Caries?

Several mechanisms have been suggested for the anticaries effect of fluorides. These include the formation of fluorapatite, which is more acid resistant than hydroxyapatite; the enhancement of remineralization; the interference of ionic bonding during pellicle and plaque formation; and the inhibition of microbial growth and metabolism.[56] Fluoride released from restorative materials can inhibit development of caries lesions through all of these mechanisms, although it seems likely that enhancement of remineralization is the most important mechanism of action for fluoride released from restorative materials. Evidence for the caries-inhibiting effect of fluoride-releasing materials comes from studies of the incidence of caries lesions adjacent to orthodontic bands and brackets, direct filling materials in patients at high risk for caries, and areas around atraumatic restorative technique (ART) restorations.

Enamel demineralization frequently occurs adjacent to fixed orthodontic appliances. White spot lesions appear within a few weeks after appliance placement, particularly with ill-fitting bands.[57–59] An increased cariogenic challenge is introduced around orthodontic bands and brackets due to markedly higher plaque retention levels caused by food retention and hindered patient oral hygiene efforts. A rise in the numbers of cariogenic bacteria (S mutans and Lactobacillus spp) has been documented following placement of orthodontic appliances.[60] The overall occurrence of white-spot formation during orthodontic therapy is 11% to 12%, with little difference between bonded brackets and zinc phosphate–cemented bands. A daily rinse of 0.2% sodium fluoride retards lesion development but does not completely inhibit lesion formation. Unfortunately, patients most in need of significant preventive intervention are often least compliant.

Fluoride-releasing resin composites and resin-modified glass-ionomer cements have been proposed for inhibiting demineralization adjacent to orthodontic bands and brackets. Zinc phosphate cement traditionally has been used to cement orthodontic bands. However, bands cemented with glass-ionomer cements have increased retention with less demineralization compared to bands cemented with zinc phosphate.[61–63] An added advantage of glass-ionomer cements is their tendency, unlike zinc phosphate, to remain on the enamel surface should a band loosen, providing some physical protection for the tooth. Although resin-modified glass ionomers have been recommended as bracket-bonding cements, little fluoride is released from brackets bonded with resin-modified glass ionomer because only a film of glass ionomer is present at the bracket-tooth interface. Decreased enamel demineralization under orthodontic bands retained with conventional glass-ionomer cements in vivo has been reported.[64–68]

Three prospective in vivo studies describe fluoride-releasing restorative materials used in high-caries-risk patients. Wood et al[68] placed 54 pairs of Class 5 conventional glass-ionomer (Ketac-Fil) and amalgam (Sybralloy, Kerr) restorations in xerostomic patients who had been treated with radiation for head-and-neck cancer. When topical fluoride was not used, glass-ionomer restorations had longer survival times than amalgam restorations. When a topical sodium fluoride solution (pH 5.8) was used, amalgam restorations had a longer survival time than the glass-ionomer restorations, but recurrent caries was reduced in both groups. This study demonstrated that a fluoride-releasing material, when used without a topical fluoride gel, was effective in inhibiting recurrent caries and that acidic fluoride solutions degrade glass-ionomer restorations. It clearly demonstrates the effectiveness of fluoride-releasing materials in noncompliant patients.

Haveman et al[69] used a similar population to measure the effectiveness of fluoride-releasing materials in high-caries-risk patients. In this study, Class 5 restorations were placed using conventional glass ionomer (Ketac-Fil), resin-modified glass ionomer (Vitremer), and amalgam (Tytin, Kerr). At the 2-year recall, 15% of the glass-ionomer restorations, 12% of the resin-modified glass-ionomer restorations, and 44% of the amalgam restorations had recurrent caries lesions at the margins. Restorations with fluoride-releasing materials had significantly fewer recurrent caries lesions associated with them than did amalgam restorations.

McComb et al[70] reported that fluoride-releasing materials reduced the incidence of recurrent caries lesions in 45 patients who had received head-and-neck radiation therapy. After removal of carious tooth structure, the investigators placed Class 5 glass-ionomer (Ketac-Fil), resin-modified glass-ionomer (Vitremer), and resin composite restorations. At the end of the 2-year clinical trial, subjects were classified as daily fluoride users if they used topical fluoride in trays more than 50%

of the time. Topical fluoride users had no recurrent caries lesions associated with these restorations. Nonusers had an 80% reduction in recurrent caries lesions adjacent to fluoride-releasing restorations compared to the non–fluoride-releasing materials. This evidence demonstrates that if a patient uses tray-delivered supplemental fluoride, a significant reduction in caries lesions can be expected because the concentration of fluoride in the tray materials is greater than that released from the restorative material. However, if the patient does not use supplemental fluoride, then the fluoride release from the restorations still provides some level of protection for the high-caries-risk patient.

These three studies suggest that fluoride-releasing materials are somewhat effective in preventing recurrent caries lesions. However, recurrent caries lesions occurred around fluoride-releasing materials in each study, demonstrating quite clearly that the remineralizing effects of fluoride released from restorations can be overwhelmed if the acid challenge is great enough.

Possibly the greatest proof for the success of fluoride-releasing materials comes from a recent meta-analysis of clinical studies in which glass-ionomer restorative materials were placed, under primitive operating conditions, in the permanent dentition using the ART.[71] In the ART, carious tooth structure is removed with hand instruments without rubber-dam isolation. The glass-ionomer restorative material is inserted with finger pressure into the cavity and allowed to cure. Frencken et al[71] divided the clinical studies using the ART into two groups. In the first group, low-strength traditional glass ionomers, such as Ketac-Fil and Fuji II, were used, and in the second group, high-viscosity glass ionomers, such as Fuji IX and Ketac-Molar, were used. Single-surface restorations were the focus of the analysis. At 3-year recalls, the high-viscosity glass ionomers had success rates that equaled those of amalgam restorations evaluated in some of the studies in the analysis. Low-viscosity glass ionomers had significantly poorer results, demonstrating that the finger-pressure insertion technique combined with the stronger materials provided better results.

Not all studies on recurrent caries inhibition demonstrate a clear benefit from fluoride release, however. Tyas[72] found no significant difference in recurrent caries in teeth restored with resin composite (Silux, 3M) or glass ionomer (Fuji II) in a population at low risk for caries. In two other clinical studies[73,74] involving almost 7,000 restorations, recurrent caries lesions developed within 10 years for amalgam restorations, 8 years for resin composite restorations, and 5 years for glass-ionomer restorations. Recurrent caries lesions led to the replacement of almost half the glass-ionomer restorations. In these populations, fluoride released from glass-ionomer restorations did not provide protection against primary or recurrent caries. Mjör et al[75] reported that in 9,805 replacement restorations made by 243 Norwegian dentists in general practice, glass ionomers provided little protection. Unfortunately, these retrospective studies may show that clinicians used glass ionomers in patients at high risk for caries and other materials in patients at lower risk for caries. The results in both of these clinical studies may be due in part to the lack of randomization of patients into the study groups. Fluoride-releasing materials do not eliminate recurrent caries but should be viewed as one part of a complete program to reduce caries incidence.

How Much Fluoride Is Enough?

The question remains: how much fluoride release from restorative materials is enough to inhibit recurrent or secondary caries? DeSchepper et al[52] reported that all antibacterial activity from glass ionomers was lost when the pH of the glass-ionomer liquid was adjusted to 5. A minimum inhibitory concentration of 100 to 200 µg/mL of sodium fluoride is required to inhibit the growth of oral streptococci,[41] while 30 times that concentration is required to be bactericidal. Naturally occurring fluoride at concentrations as high as 21 µg/mL does not produce any obvious effect on the composition of supragingival plaque. No glass ionomer maintains its acidity longer than 48 hours. Because fluoride-releasing materials release reduced amounts of fluoride and other ions with time, bacterial plaque accumulates on glass-ionomer restorations. Therefore, the direct bactericidal effect of fluoride released from restorative materials is very limited and is due to the combination of fluoride and acidity. Although the fluoride levels in bacteria associated with glass-ionomer restorations are elevated, the effect of fluoride on reducing bacterial acid production, metabolism, and division has yet to be clarified.

High levels of fluoride release produce remineralization of enamel and dentin. One study[76] demonstrated that enamel demineralization decreased as fluoride release from a resin composite restorative material increased. By extrapolating data, the authors concluded that a resin composite releasing 200 to 300 µg/cm^2 of fluoride over a 1-month period would completely inhibit secondary caries. Unfortunately, this is approximately 40 to 50 times more fluoride than is released by current fluoride-releasing resin composites. Eichmiller and Marjenhoff[23] authored an excellent review of fluoride-releasing materials and noted that caries inhibition and tooth remineralization potential have been shown in vitro by all fluoride-releasing materials when release rates were approximately 1 µg/mL. Resin-modified glass ionomers and conventional glass ionomers have similar fluoride release and recharge rates.[13]

The remineralization of dentin is more complex than that of enamel. Active dentinal caries destroys collagen matrix as well as demineralizing apatite crystals. Remineralization of dentin may be affected by the remaining mineral, the remaining collagen, or the ultrastructure of the dentin. Collagen matrix devoid of mineral does not support remineralization.[77] The difficulty in protecting root surfaces with fluoride-releasing materials may be due to the higher concentrations of fluoride needed to remineralize root surfaces compared to enamel surfaces. Wefel[77] reported that demineralized dentin, with its exposed organic matrix, did not act as a suitable matrix for remineralization, but that remineralization did occur on any remaining apatite crystals. It seems clear that increased fluoride is required to remineralize dentin and that the degree of remineralization that can occur in dentin may be controlled by the amount of remaining mineral content.

Based on the previous studies, it is recommended that materials with a long-term fluoride release rate of at least 2 to 3 μg/mL/d be used. With present materials, this rate of release can only be maintained when supplemental fluorides are used to recharge fluoride-releasing restorations.

Clinical Considerations for Fluoride-Releasing Materials

Although the recurrent caries inhibition effect of fluoride-releasing materials is evident, their clinical effectiveness has been questioned based on the durability of the materials. Even in primary teeth, these materials should be used selectively, and the time that the material will be expected to survive (how long the tooth will remain in the oral cavity) should be evaluated against its strength and wear resistance. One report[78] describes the wear resistance of a compomer (Dyract, Dentsply) and shows that this material has lower wear resistance than resin composite. At 1 year in a clinical evaluation of 91 Dyract restorations in conservative Class 1 and 2 restorations in primary teeth, the mean wear of Dyract was 190 μm, compared to approximately 10 μm with a wear-resistant resin composite. Another study[79] measuring marginal adaptation of Class 2 restorations in the permanent dentition reported that compomers showed such poor adaptation after 6 months of clinical wear that they should not be used as definitive restorations in load-bearing areas. Although the absolute numbers may vary, the typical compomer undergoes greater wear than the typical resin composite. Therefore, compomers should not be used in Class 1 or 2 load-bearing areas in the permanent dentition. However, the wear resist-

ance and fluoride recharge of compomer restorative materials continue to improve, and it is now apparent that they can be used with success in both Class 5 and Class 2 open sandwich restorations. Three in vivo studies[53,80,81] have reported the clinical success of Dyract as a Class 5 restorative material in noncarious cervical lesions. In these studies, Dyract was clinically acceptable at the end of 3 years[53] and was superior to resin-modified glass ionomers.[80,81] Compomers continue to improve as new versions are introduced. However, much clinical testing is necessary to document their clinical performance before they can be endorsed.

Treating the high-caries-risk patient requires special selection of restorative materials. Resin-modified glass ionomers and compomers are recommended as the esthetic restorative materials of choice in Class 5 restorations in xerostomic patients and other patients at high risk for caries. This is due to the fluoride release and fluoride recharge capabilities of these materials. Because resin-modified glass ionomers and compomers have poorer wear resistance than resin composites, a resin composite should be used for restorations in load-bearing areas.

Another strategy for Class 2 restorations that extend gingivally below the cementoenamel junction is the "open sandwich" technique. In this technique, the fluoride-releasing material is placed into the proximal box of a preparation when the gingival margin extends to cementum or dentin (see chapter 10). The resin-modified glass ionomer or compomer is cured, and resin composite is placed in increments to restore the occlusal surface for adequate wear resistance. The open sandwich technique was successful at the 5-year recall in a report of a recent clinical trial[82] in which Class 2 composite restorations were placed in patients with moderate to high caries risk. A resin-modified glass ionomer (Vitremer) was placed in the gingival portion of the proximal box and covered with a resin composite (Z100, 3M ESPE). Conventional glass ionomers are less successful in the open sandwich technique.[83] The open sandwich technique in Class 2 restorations combines the wear resistance of a resin composite with the fluoride release and recharge potential of resin-modified glass ionomers or compomers.

As dental restorative materials continue to proliferate, it becomes increasingly difficult to choose the appropriate material for a particular clinical situation. Fluoride-releasing materials are no exception, and clinicians need guidelines to select and use these materials. Today, there is modest but growing evidence from clinical trials that fluoride-releasing materials, especially resin-modified and conventional glass ionomers, reduce recurrent caries. There is also evidence of a dose-response relationship between fluoride release and decreased caries. While materials with higher fluoride-releasing capability have a greater caries-inhibiting effect, these materials are not panaceas. The physical limitations of glass ionomers and compomers, especially poor wear resistance, contribute markedly to restoration failure. Evidence suggests that resin-modified glass-ionomer materials may provide an improved combination of physical integrity and caries inhibition.

Fluoride-releasing materials should be used in high-caries-risk patients as one component of their overall treatment. High-caries-risk patients also require oral hygiene counseling, diet modification, and specific application of chemicals like chlorhexidine and xylitol to inhibit caries activity. An absolute requirement for these patients is a neutral sodium fluoride supplement for nightly use. In addition, fluoride varnishes are effective. Generally a 5% sodium fluoride–containing varnish should be used in hard-to-clean areas. For patients with low salivary output, a regimen of Recaldent (Recaldent Pty), an amorphous calcium phosphate–containing paste, is also recommended to increase levels of calcium and phosphate in the saliva and promote remineralization. These recommendations, combined with frequent oral hygiene checks and reinforcement, should provide maximum care for the individual who is at high risk for caries.

References

1. Loesche WJ, Hockett, RN, Syed SA. The predominant cultivable flora of tooth surface plaque removed from institutionalized subjects. Arch Oral Biol 1973;17:1311–1325.

2. Featherstone JD. The caries balance: Contributing factors and early detection. J Calif Dent Assoc 2003;31:129–133.

3. ten Cate JM, Buijs MJ, Damen JJM. pH-cycling of enamel and dentin lesions in the presence of low concentrations of fluoride. Eur J Oral Sci 1995;103:362–367.

4. McIntyre J. Preservation and Restoration of Tooth Structure. London: Mosby, 1998:20–23.

5. Seppä L, Korhonen A, Nuutinen A. Inhibitory effect on *S. mutans* by fluoride-treated conventional and resin-reinforced glass ionomer cements. Eur J Oral Sci 1995;103:182–185.

6. Bardow A, Nyvad B, Nauntofte B. Relationships between medication intake, complaints of dry mouth, salivary flow rate and composition, and the rate of tooth demineralization in situ. Arch Oral Biol 2001;46:413–423.

7. Billings RJ, Proskin HM, Moss ME. Xerostomia and associated factors in a community-dwelling adult population. Community Dent Oral Epidemiol 1996;24:312–316.

8. Yip HK, Smales RJ, Ngo HC, Tay FR, Chu FC. Selection of restorative materials for the atraumatic restorative treatment (Art) approach: A review. Spec Care Dentist 2001;21:216–221.

9. Walls AWG, Mather E. Fuji restorations in occlusal cavities of molar teeth, 12-month data [abstract 1443]. J Dent Res 1999;78:286.

10. Xu X, Burgess JO. Compressive strength, fluoride release and recharge of fluoride-releasing materials. Biomaterials 2003;24: 2451–2461.

11. Elderton RJ, Aboush YEY, Vowles RW, et al. Retention of cervical Dyract compomer restorations after two years [abstract 49]. J Dent Res 1996;75:24.

12. Gallo JR, Burgess JO, Ripps AH, et al. Three-year clinical evaluation of a compomer and a resin composite as Class V filling materials. Oper Dent 2005;30:275–281.

13. Hermesch CB , Wall BS, McEntire JF. Dimensional stability of dental restorative materials and cements over four years. Gen Dent 2003;51:518–523.

14. Hals E, Norderval IT. Histopathology of experimental in vivo caries around silicate fillings. Acta Odont Scand 1973;31:357–367.

15. Phillips RW, Swartz ML. Effect of certain restorative materials on solubility of enamel. J Am Dent Assoc 1957;54:623–636.

16. Norman RD, Phillips RW, Swartz ML. Fluoride uptake by enamel from certain dental materials. J Dent Res 1960;39:11–16.

17. Norman RD, Platt JR, Phillips RW, Swartz ML. Additional studies on fluoride uptake by enamel from certain dental materials. J Dent Res 1961;40:529–537.

18. Norman RD, Mehra RV, Swartz ML, Phillips RW. Effects of restorative materials on plaque composition. J Dent Res 1972;51:1596–1601.

19. Perrin C, Persin M, Sarrazin J. A comparison of fluoride release from four glass ionomer cements. Quintessence Int 1994;25:603–608.

20. Alvarez AN, Burgess JO, Chan DCN. Short term fluoride release of six ionomers—recharged, coated and abraded [abstract 260]. J Dent Res 1994;73:134.

21. Burkett L, Burgess JO, Chan DCN, Norling BK. Fluoride release of glass ionomers coated and not coated with adhesive [abstract 1242]. J Dent Res 1993;72:258.

22. Cranfield M, Kuhn A, Winter GB. Factors relating to the rate of fluoride-ion release from glass-ionomer cement. J Dent 1982;10: 333–341.

23. Eichmiller FC, Marjenhoff WA. Fluoride-releasing dental restorative materials. Oper Dent 1998;23:218–228.

24. Forsten L, Paunio IK. Fluoride release by silicate cements and resin composites. Scand J Dent Res 1972;80:515–519.

25. Forsten L. Fluoride release of glass ionomers. J Esthet Dent 1994;6: 216–222.

26. Forsten L. Short- and long-term fluoride release from glass ionomers and other fluoride-containing filling materials in vitro. Scand J Dent Res 1990;98:179–185.

27. Forsten L. Fluoride release from a glass ionomer cement. Scand J Dent Res 1977;85:503–504.

28. McKnight-Hanes C, Whitford GM. Fluoride release from three glass ionomer materials and the effects of varnishing with or without finishing. Caries Res 1992;26:345–350.

29. Mitra SB. In vitro fluoride release from a light-cured glass-ionomer liner/base. J Dent Res 1991;70:75–78.

30. Hsu HM, Huang GF, Chang HH, Wang YL, Guo MK. A continuous flow system for assessing fluoride release/uptake of fluoride-containing restorative materials. Dent Mater 2004;20:740–749.

31. Woolford MJ, Grieve AR. Release of fluoride from glass polyalkenoate (ionomer) cement subjected to radiant heat. J Dent 1995; 23:233–237.

32. Halgren A, Oliveby A, Twetman S. Fluoride concentration in plaque adjacent to orthodontic appliances retained with glass ionomer cement. Caries Res 1993;27:51–54.

33. Forsten L, Rytomaa I, Anttila A, Keinonen J. Fluoride uptake from restorative dental materials by human enamel. Scand J Dent Res 1976;84:391–395.

34. Besnault C, Attal JP, Ruse D, Degrange M. Self-etching adhesives improve the shear bond strength of a resin-modified glass-ionomer cement to dentin. J Adhes Dent 2004;6:55–59.

35. Hatibovic-Kofman S, Koch G. Fluoride release from glass ionomer cement in vivo and in vitro. Swed Dent J 1991;15:253–258.

36. Hattab FN, el-Mowafy OM, Salem NS, el-Badrawy WA. An in vivo study on the release of fluoride from glass-ionomer cement. Quintessence Int 1991;22:221–224.

37. Tantbirojn D, Douglas WH, Versluis A. Inhibitive effect of a resin-modified glass ionomer cement on remote artificial caries. Caries Res 1997;31:275–280.

38. Forsten L. Fluoride release and uptake by glass ionomers. Scand J Dent Res 1991;99:241–245.

39. Damen JJM, Buijs MJ, ten Cate JM. Uptake and release of fluoride by saliva-coated glass ionomer cement. Caries Res 1996;30:454–457.

40. Diaz-Arnold AM, Holmes DC, Wistrom DW, Swift EJ. Short-term fluoride release/uptake of glass ionomer restoratives. Dent Mater 1995;11:96–101.

41. Ekstrand J, Fejerskov O, Silverstone LM. Fluoride in Dentistry. Copenhagen: Munksgaard, 1988:76.

42. Burgess JO, Cardenas HL. Surface roughness of topical fluoride treated glass ionomers [abstract 775]. J Dent Res 1995;74:108.

43. Diaz-Arnold AM, Wistrom DW, Swift EJ. Topical fluoride and glass ionomer microhardness. Am J Dent 1995;8:134–136.

44. El-Badrawy WA, McComb D. Effect of home-use fluoride gels on resin-modified glass-ionomer cements. Oper Dent 1998;23:2–9.

45. Papagiannoulis L, Tzoutzas J, Eliades G. Effect of topical fluoride agents on the morphologic characteristics and composition of resin composite restorative materials. J Prosthet Dent 1997;77:405–413.

46. Loyola-Rodriguez JP, Garcia-Godoy F, Lindquist R. Growth inhibition of glass ionomer cements on mutans streptococci. Pediatr Dent 1994;16:346–349.

47. Forss H, Jokinen J, Spets-Happonen S, et al. Fluoride and mutans streptococci in plaque growing on glass ionomer and composite. Caries Res 1991;25:454–458.

48. Forss H, Nase L, Seppa L. Fluoride and caries associated microflora in plaque on old GIC fillings [abstract 2468]. J Dent Res 1994;73:410.

49. Palenik CJ, Behnen MJ, Setcos JC, Miller CH. Inhibition of microbial adherence and growth by various glass ionomers in vitro. Dent Mater 1992;8:16–20.

50. McComb D, Ericson D. Antimicrobial action of new, proprietary lining cements. J Dent Res 1987;66:1025–1028.

51. DeSchepper ED, Thrasher MR, Thurmond BA. Antibacterial effects of light-cured liners. Am J Dent 1989;2:74–76.

52. DeSchepper ED, White RR, von der Lehr W. Antibacterial effects of glass ionomers. Am J Dent 1989;2:51–56.

53. Jedynakiewicz NM, Martin N, Fletcher JM. A three year evaluation of a compomer restorative [abstract 1189]. J Dent Res 1997;76:162.

54. Svanberg M, Mjör IA, Orstavik D. Mutans streptococci in plaque from margins of amalgam, composite, and glass-ionomer restorations. J Dent Res 1990;69:861–864.

55. van Dijken JW, Kalfas S, Litra V, Oliveby A. Fluoride and mutans streptococci levels in plaque on aged restorations of resin-modified glass ionomer cement, compomer and resin composite. Caries Res 1997;31:379–383.

56. Niessen LC, Gibson G. Oral health for a lifetime: Preventive strategies for the older adult. Quintessence Int 1997;28:626–630.

57. O'Reilly MM, Featherstone JDB. Demineralization and re-mineralization around orthodontic appliances: An in vivo study. Am J Orthod Dentofac Orthop 1987;92:33–40.

58. Øgaard B, Rölla G, Arends J, ten Cate JM. Orthodontic appliances and enamel demineralization. Part 2. Prevention and treatment of lesions. Am J Orthod Dentofac Orthop 1988;94:123–128.

59. Rezk-Lega F, Øgaard B, Rölla G. Availability of fluoride from glass-ionomer luting cements in human saliva. Scand J Dent Res 1991;99:60–63.

60. Lundstrom F, Krasse B. Streptococcus mutans and Lactobacillus frequency in orthodontic patients: The effect of chlorhexidine treatments. Eur J Orthod 1987;2:27–39.

61. Fricker JP, McLachlan MD. Clinical studies of glass ionomer cements—Part 2, a two year clinical study comparing glass ionomer cement with zinc phosphate cement. Aust Orthod J 1987;10:12–14.

62. Norris DS, McInnes-Ledoux P, Schwanginger B, Weinberg R. Retention of orthodontic bands with new fluoride-releasing cements. Am J Orthod 1986;89:206–211.

63. Stirrups DR. A comparative clinical trial of a glass ionomer and a zinc phosphate cement for securing orthodontic bands. Br J Orthod 1991;18:15–20.

64. Kvam E, Broch J, Nissen-Meyer IH. Comparison between a zinc phosphate cement and a glass ionomer cement for cementation of orthodontic bands. Eur J Orthod 1983;5:307–313.

65. Marcusson A, Norevall L, Persson M. White spot reduction when using glass ionomer cement for bonding in orthodontics: A longitudinal and comparative study. Eur J Orthod 1997;19:233–242.

66. Ortendahl T, Thilander B, Svanberg M. Mutans streptococci and incipient caries adjacent to glass ionomer cement or resin-based composite in orthodontics. Am J Orthod Dentofac Orthop 1997;112:271–274.

67. Seeholzer HW, Dasch W. Bonding with a glass ionomer cement. J Clin Orthod 1986;22:165–169.

68. Wood RE, Maxymiw WG, McComb D. A clinical comparison of glass ionomer (polyalkenoate) and silver amalgam restorations in the treatment of Class 5 caries in xerostomic head and neck cancer patients. Oper Dent 1993;18:94–102.

69. Haveman C, Burgess J, Summitt JB. A clinical comparison of restorative materials for caries in xerostomic patients [abstract 1441]. J Dent Res 1999;78:286.

70. McComb D, Ericson RL, Maxymiw WG, Wood RE. A clinical comparison of glass-ionomer, resin-modified glass ionomer and resin-composite restorations in the treatment of cervical caries in xerostomic head and neck radiation patients. Oper Dent 2002;27:430–437.

71. Frencken JE, van't Hof MA, van Amerongen WE, Holmgren CJ. Effectiveness of single-surface ART restorations in the permanent dentition: A meta-analysis. J Dent Res 2004;83:120–123.

72. Tyas MJ. Cariostatic effect of glass ionomer cement: A five year study. Aust Dent J 1991;36:236–239.

73. Mjör IA, Jokstadt A. Five-year study of Class II restorations in permanent teeth using amalgam, glass polyalkenoate (ionomer) cermet and resin-based composite materials. J Dent 1993;21:338–343.

74. Mjör IA. Glass-ionomer cement restorations and secondary caries: A preliminary report. Quintessence Int 1996;27:171–174.

75. Mjör IA, Moorhead JE, Dahl JE. Reasons for replacement of restorations in permanent teeth in general dental practice. Int Dent J 2000;50:361–366.

76. Dijkman GEHM, Arends J. Long-term fluoride release of visible light-activated composites in vitro: A correlation with in situ demineralization data. Caries Res 1993;27:117–123.

77. Wefel JS. Root caries histopathology and chemistry. Am J Dent 1994;7:261–265.

78. Peters TCRB, Roeters JJM, Frankenmolen FWA. Clinical evaluation of Dyract in primary molars: 1-year results. Am J Dent 1996;9:83–87.

79. Kersten S, Besek MJ, Lutz F. Marginal adaptation in Class II compomer restorations in vivo [abstract 2286]. J Dent Res 1999;78:391.

80. Abdalla AI, Alhadainy HA, Garcia-Godoy F. Clinical evaluation of glass ionomers and compomers in Class 5 carious lesions. Am J Dent 1997;10:18–20.

81. Loher C, Kunzelman RH, Hickel R. Clinical evaluation of glass ionomer cements (LC), compomer and composite restorations in Class V cavities—Two year results [abstract 1190]. J Dent Res 1997;76:162.

82. Burgess JO, Summitt JB, Robbins JW, et al. Clinical evaluation of base, sandwich and bonded Class 2 resin composite restorations [abstract 304]. J Dent Res 1999;78:531.

83. Welbury RR, Murray JJ. A clinical trial of the glass ionomer cement–composite resin "sandwich" technique in Class II cavities in permanent premolar and molar teeth. Quintessence Int 1990;21:507–512.

Class 5 Restorations

J. D. Overton
Mark L. LittleStar
Clifford B. Starr

Class 5 lesions are those carious and noncarious defects found in the gingival third of facial and lingual tooth surfaces. As described in chapter 4, Class 5 caries lesions are produced by bacterial plaque attaching to the surface of teeth and producing acids that cause demineralization. A Class 5 lesion resulting from factors other than dental caries is known as a *noncarious cervical lesion* (NCCL). Chapter 12 contains an excellent discussion of the treatment of caries-damaged root surfaces that is applicable to the treatment of caries lesions in cervical areas. This chapter focuses mainly on the unique etiology, diagnosis, and restorative treatment of noncarious cervical lesions. For restorative treatment in cervical areas, procedures are similar for both caries lesions and noncarious lesions except that carious dentin is removed in restorative treatment of caries lesions (Figs 14-1 to 14-5).

Caries Lesions

Tooth color is not a good predictor of root caries damage. A root surface may be discolored and still have a hard, sclerotic surface that would not warrant preparation and placement of a restoration unless the discoloration presented an esthetic problem for the patient. In contrast, some root caries lesions will have the color of healthy tooth structure but will be soft when tested with a dental instrument. Caries-disclosing dyes may be inconsistent in identifying demineralized cementum/dentin on root surfaces. The best correlation to date for clinical detection of caries lesions on root surfaces is the softness of the surface as evaluated with a dental instrument.

Noncarious Cervical Lesions

Incidence

It appears that NCCLs are unique to modern man. In an anthropologic study of the skulls of humans living in the Copper Age and Middle Age (2050–2080 BC and 1100–1400 AD), no NCCLs were found in 3,927 teeth from 259 individuals.[1] Today, NCCLs can be found in the teeth of children as well as adult teeth. Prevalence in varying patient and population groups ranges from "rare" to 89%.[2] Several studies show incidence increasing with age.[2,3] One study[3] involved examination of 1,753 children at 12 years of age and then again at 14 years of age. Erosion was present in 56.3% of the children at 12 years of age and 64.1% of the same children at 14 years of age.[3] Another study[4] looked at 1,002 adult inhabitants of Rijeka, Croatia, chosen at random from four dental practices. After excluding restored facial surfaces, 18% of the teeth had evidence of facial tooth wear. In this study, only 5% of subjects younger than 26 years of age were identified with cervical wear. With every 10-year increase in patient age, the lesions became more common. Cervical wear was identified in 48% of subjects older than 65 years of age.[4]

Etiology

The entire etiology of noncarious cervical lesions has not been determined. While the various possible causes and their degree of involvement may be controversial, there is overwhelming evidence that the cause is multifactorial.[5] *Erosion*, the loss of tooth

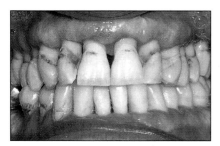

Fig 14-1a Numerous stained Class 5 caries lesions.

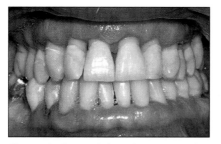

Fig 14-1b The teeth have been restored to meet the patient's esthetic demands.

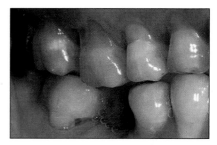

Fig 14-2 Cupped, saucer-shaped noncarious cervical lesions consistent with erosion.

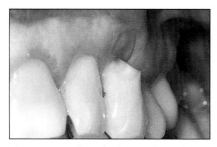

Fig 14-3 A moderately deep, V-shaped cervical notch in a maxillary canine.

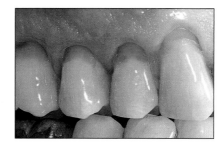

Fig 14-4 Multiple adjacent defects that fit the description of abfraction lesions.

structure from chemical dissolution, *abrasion*, the loss of tooth structure by mechanical or frictional forces, and *abfraction* or *stress corrosion*, the loss of cervical tooth structure due to occlusal forces, have all been implicated in the formation of NCCLs. Patients should be informed of the possible etiologies, implications of the presence of lesions, prevention methods, treatment alternatives, and expected outcomes. Failure to appropriately prevent and treat NCCLs can result in progression of tooth structure loss; tooth sensitivity; the need for endodontic therapy; tooth loss; and the occurrence of additional lesions.[6]

The ability of ions in saliva to induce remineralization of demineralized tooth structure should be considered an important factor in the inhibition of NCCLs as well as in the inhibition of caries. Caries lesions and noncarious lesions are more common on facial surfaces of teeth than on lingual surfaces because of differences in the chemistry and character of saliva in lingual and facial areas, which bring about differences in remineralization of tooth structure and the dilution and buffering of acids.[7,8] The effects of xerostomia on oral health are well documented[9–11] and are discussed in chapter 12. However, even in the healthy patient, dehydration from perspiration with physical activity can create impaired salivary flow and inhibit buffering of oral acids in the oral cavity.[12,13]

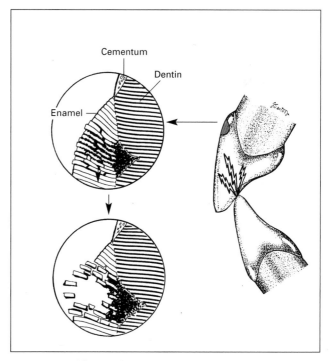

Fig 14-5 The abfraction theory holds that tooth flexure causes loosening of enamel rods, which initiates the cervical lesions.

In addition to in vivo studies, laboratory studies have contributed to the knowledge base about NCCLs. Finite-element analysis has predicted that occlusal loads could cause stress fractures or stress corrosion in the cervical areas of teeth.[14,15] Litonjua et al[16] found that without any acids present, occlusal loading had no effect in creating NCCLs in recently extracted teeth subjected to a toothpaste slurry and tooth brushing at the cervical margins. Brushing with the toothpaste slurry caused similar cervical wear patterns regardless of whether the tooth was loaded.[16] In contrast, Palamara et al[17] found that enamel dissolution increased significantly when teeth were subjected to cyclic tensile load while immersed in 1% lactic acid (pH 4.5). The acidic environment and loading made the teeth more susceptible to cervical tissue loss. Volumetric loss was greater in the cervical third than in the middle third and much greater in the mesiobuccal segment (under tension) than in the distobuccal segment (under compression).[17] These findings could offer some explanation for the differences in size, shape, and location of NCCLs.

The morphologic presentation of NCCLs, such as a "wedge" or a "saucer" shape, can perhaps aid the practitioner in discovering their etiology, but the ability to differentiate etiologies based on lesion shape has yet to be adequately supported with evidence. Whitehead et al, studying stress corrosion of enamel at low pH, found that axial loading of extracted premolar teeth in an acid solution resulted in macroscopic and microscopic features similar to those observed in NCCLs in vivo.[18] Changes occurring only in the presence of acids would be consistent with the anthropology samples that did not have NCCLs despite showing evidence of heavy occlusal wear.[1] It appears that liquid acid, frequently found in modern diets, may be necessary to make occlusal loading a significant factor in the formation of cervical lesions.

Diet and Noncarious Cervical Lesions

Dietary (extrinsic) acids from foods such as soft drinks, wines, and fruits and fruit juices, and gastric (intrinsic) acids that result from gastric reflux, bulimia, and other disorders are both capable of causing tooth dissolution. It is well established in the literature that acids cause dissolution of tooth structure.[6] Soft drinks, which contain citric and/or phosphoric acids, are probably the most frequent source for liquid dietary acids in the US population. Orange juice has also been shown in several studies to cause erosive loss of dentin and enamel.[19,20] When the pH of citric acid and phosphoric acid solutions was adjusted to be similar, citric acid caused more erosion of both enamel and dentin samples than did phosphoric acid.[21]

Toothbrush Abrasion and Noncarious Cervical Lesions

When a tooth is softened by acid dissolution, the effects of any mechanical wear are greatly accelerated. The effect of the acid on enamel and dentin makes the tooth more susceptible to abrasion and attrition (occlusal wear).[22] A study by Attin and others[23] confirmed previous studies[22,24] that showed that eroded enamel is extraordinarily sensitive to mechanical impacts such as tooth brushing performed immediately after demineralization. The fact that a demineralized tooth surface can be remineralized if not exposed to brushing or other mechanical insult after it has been softened by demineralization is critical in understanding the etiology, prevention, and treatment of NCCLs. Tooth structure can be remineralized after a period of exposure to saliva.[25] These findings are contrary to past, and sometimes current, recommendations by dentists that brushing immediately after a meal or other acid challenge should be routine. On the contrary, tooth structure loss as a result of abrasion can be minimized by delaying brushing by at least 1 hour.[23] In addition, patients with NCCLs should be encouraged to use a minimal amount of dentifrice and light forces when brushing. Anecdotal claims that the majority of toothbrush abrasion lesions appear on the opposite arch from the dominant hand have not been verified with clinical studies.[26] While it is agreed that tooth brushing is a significant factor in the initiation and progress of NCCLs, the degree to which tooth brushing is the cause of these lesions has not been defined. Piotrowski et al[27] attributed 85% of lesion occurrence to the toothbrush, and Oginni et al[26] found 62% to be associated with toothbrush abrasion.

Occlusion and Noncarious Cervical Lesions

Of all the possible etiologies for noncarious cervical lesions, occlusal stress forces have received the most attention in recent years. Dentin and enamel have different tensile strengths. With occlusal loading, stress concentration occurs in the cervical area.[28,29] The abfraction theory, also known as the occlusal stress or stress corrosion theory, maintains that tooth flexure in the cervical area results in microfractures of the crystalline structure of the enamel and dentin in that area. The lesion, in theory, would continue to enlarge as the bending and flexing is repeated. Associating wear facets (attrition) with NCCLs is an important component in this theory. Occlusal wear facets appear in combination with many NCCLs. Studies have found both occlusal wear and NCCLs to occur in the same teeth, but the degree to which this association has been found has varied from 15%[27] to 38%[26] to 95%.[30,31]

The lack of consistency of findings among studies could be due to variations in the definition of wear facets, differences in the populations studied, or differences in the exclusion criteria applied. While the studies differ on the significance that occlusal forces play in the etiology of NCCLs, they do agree that the cause is multifactorial.

Determination of Probable Etiology of Noncarious Cervical Lesions

Before any treatment is performed for a patient with one or more noncarious cervical lesions, a careful examination and determination of possible causes for the lesions should be made. Considering that there is a general consensus in the literature that the etiology is multifactorial, the practitioner's initial approach should not be based on an assumed cause. The mere presence of occlusal wear facets accompanying NCCLs does not indicate that the cause is unifactorial, that is, that the lesion is the result of occlusal forces only. Likewise, for a patient with a known history of gastric reflux, it should not be assumed that the patient's NCCLs are the sole result of a constant intrinsic acid challenge that is causing cervical erosion. While there may be a primary etiology, other contributing factors must also be considered. In all cases of NCCLs, the dentist should obtain a careful health history and provide a thorough dental examination that includes, but is certainly not limited to, an occlusal analysis. The patient's oral hygiene habits should be discussed and evaluated, and a dietary analysis should be considered. Only after determining the probable causes should any treatment commence.[32]

Treatment of Noncarious Cervical Lesions

The first goal of any treatment is to remove the primary cause or causes of the noncarious cervical lesion. Once the etiologic factors for a patient are understood, the dentist can begin to help the patient to understand them and to change those that are under his or her control. If a patient is experiencing acute sensitivity associated with one or more lesions, treatment to alleviate the sensitivity should be accomplished. This treatment could involve desensitizing the tooth, restoring the tooth, or possibly performing a periodontal procedure, such as a connective tissue graft, to cover and protect the affected area.[33–40]

Because of the location of Class 5 lesions, access for restorative treatment is often troublesome, moisture control can be exceedingly difficult to obtain and maintain, and soft tissue surgical approaches may be required. Due to the sclerotic nature of the tooth structure in a cervical lesion and to the physical properties of restorative materials, long-term retention of the restoration presents a unique challenge. If a decision is made to place a restoration, some lesions can be treated without cavity preparation, and others require preparation to obtain adequate retention of the restoration.

Shallow lesions that lead to thermal sensitivity or sensitivity to touch should first be treated with bonding resins or desensitizing agents. These treatments are low risk and have reasonable potential for success. Long-term cervical sensitivity studies are very difficult to standardize. Over the course of time some teeth will become symptom free without treatment.[41] Some of the self-etch dentin bonding systems show good promise for controlling cervical sensitivity without requiring any habit changes, such as tooth brushing changes and diet modification.[42] Desensitizing toothpaste and fluoride gel formulations are effective for treating cervical sensitivity; these require continuation of use for weeks or months, or longer, to maintain the therapeutic effect.[43] The use of fluoride desensitization solutions have proven effective in many situations.[44,45]

The decision to place a restoration because of a Class 5 lesion is not always easily made. Certainly, if active caries is present, treatment should be initiated to control the active disease and to prevent disease progression. Treatment decisions relating to NCCLs or arrested caries lesions, however, are more difficult. It is generally believed that NCCLs should be treated to protect remaining tooth structure if the amount of tooth structure lost is extensive or progressing, if esthetics is compromised, or to control sensitivity not relieved by·less invasive procedures.[46–51] In contrast, a few clinicians believe that all noncarious Class 5 lesions require restorative treatment and describe many reasons for doing so.[48] In an attempt to aid clinicians in the sometimes-difficult treatment decisions and provide objective guidelines, the Academy of Operative Dentistry has published recommendations for the treatment of NCCLs.[6] Their recommendations state that the decision to restore a tooth affected with a NCCL should depend upon the following factors:

1. Inability to eliminate or greatly reduce the rate of lesion progression through elimination of etiologic factors
2. Esthetic unacceptability of the lesion to the patient
3. Significant sensitivity of exposed dentin to cold liquids, food, and air
4. Threat to the strength of the tooth and integrity of the coronal-radicular unit because of the lesion's depth

Of course the preferred treatment for a minimal lesion is to eliminate the causes and stop lesion progression. This pre-

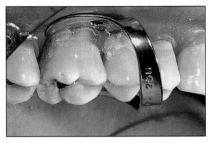

Fig 14-6 An additional rubber dam clamp is sometimes helpful to retract the rubber dam and soft tissue.

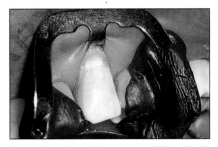

Fig 14-7a A No. 212SA clamp stabilized with modeling compound.

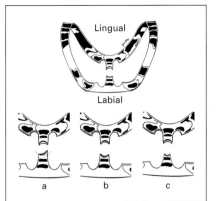

Fig 14-7b Modifications to the No. 212SA clamp are sometimes necessary for proper adaptation to the tooth.

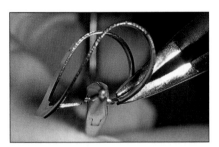

Fig 14-7c With two sets of pliers, the lingual jaw of the No. 212SA clamp is bent incisally/occlusally so that it rests on lingual tooth structure, avoiding damage to gingival tissues.

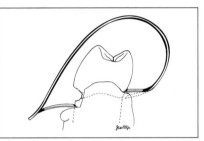

Fig 14-7d Modified *(solid line)* and unmodified *(dotted line)* No. 212SA clamp.

vents initiation of the "re-restoration cycle," that is, the repetitious replacement of lost or defective restorations with increasingly larger ones.[52,53]

Access and Isolation

When cervical lesions occur supragingivally, access to the area for preparation and restoration is often easily obtained. But if the lesion has progressed to or below the free gingival margin, isolation for complete caries removal, tooth preparation, restoration placement, and finishing can be difficult. If a restoration is placed without obtaining complete access to sound tooth structure on all margins, carious tooth structure may remain and the restoration may fail. Even in noncarious lesions, inability to gain sufficient access to the gingival margin may result in a poor restoration-tooth interface, increased microleakage, and premature loss of the restoration.

Nonsurgical Retraction

While a rubber dam is the ideal method of field isolation and moisture control for all direct-placement restorations, many Class 5 lesions can be adequately treated using retraction cord, cotton rolls, and other materials to isolate the lesion and absorb or evacuate moisture. If the lesion extends to or below the gingival margin, a rubber dam is useful to retract the tissue. Often a rubber dam retracting clamp placed directly on the tooth to be restored will provide additional gingival retraction (Fig 14-6). A No. 212SA clamp is effective for this purpose (Fig 14-7a), but modifications to the clamp may be necessary to provide adequate retraction (Figs 14-7b to 14-7d; see also chapter 7).

The clamp must be stabilized to keep it from moving and possibly damaging the restoration or the tooth surface during the operative procedure. Modeling compound is the traditional stabilizing material used (see Figs 14-7a and 7-21b). If lesions in two adjacent teeth are to be treated, modified No. 212SA clamps can be used to provide field isolation (see Figs 14-10d, 7-21c, and 7-21d).

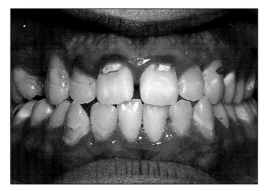

Fig 14-8a Carious Class 5 lesions on the maxillary central incisors requiring surgical access.

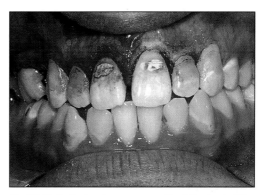

Fig 14-8b A gingivectomy exposes the full extent of the clinical crowns and provides access to the lesions.

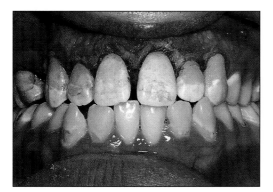

Fig 14-8c Maxillary central incisors after placement of restorations.

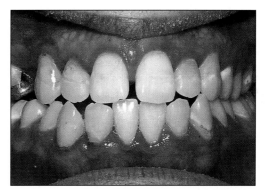

Fig 14-8d Restorations and soft tissue after 2 weeks of healing.

Surgical Retraction

Gingivoplasty

When the rubber dam clamp cannot be positioned to provide complete visualization and access to the entire lesion without causing excess trauma to gingival tissue, a surgical approach must be used. First, the width of attached gingiva is determined by subtracting the probing depth from the width of keratinized tissue. If an adequate amount of attached, keratinized gingiva will remain after surgery, a gingivoplasty may be useful in providing access as long as the lesion to be treated will be fully exposed and the biologic width will not be violated[54,55] (Figs 14-8a to 14-8d). If gingivoplasty would result in less than 3 mm of attached gingiva adjacent to the restoration, an apically positioned flap or graft procedure may be necessary to preserve or increase the zone of attached gingiva.[56] An inadequate zone of attached gingiva is an absolute contraindication for gingivoplasty.

Miniflap

As described in chapter 7, the use of miniflaps can often provide sufficient access to subgingival lesions.[54,55] One or two small incisions are made in gingival tissue, not including the papilla, beginning at the gingival margin at the mesial and/or distal aspect of the lesion (Figs 14-9a to 14-9e; see also Fig 7-47). Each incision is first directed at a right angle to the gingival margin and extended approximately a millimeter; the scalpel is then turned so that the remainder of the incision is vertical, approximately parallel with the long axis of the tooth. It is essential that the entire lesion be exposed, including all demineralized tooth structure. The incision(s) should not be extended past the mucogingival junction. This will allow the small flap of keratinized tissue to be reflected for access, then replaced to the same position after completion of the restoration. Sutures are usually not necessary. If the flap extends past the mucogingival junction, sutures may be required after the restorative procedure has been completed.

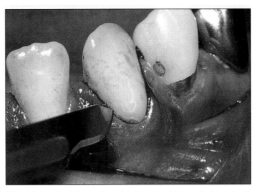

Fig 14-9a Position of scalpel for making miniflap incision.

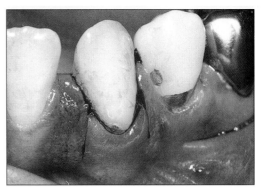

Fig 14-9b Mesial and distal miniflap incisions.

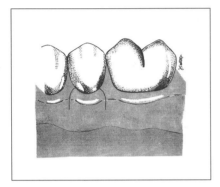

Fig 14-9c Short vertical incisions are made within the keratinized tissue at the line angles of the tooth. This allows additional tissue retraction with minimal trauma to the tissue or attachment apparatus.

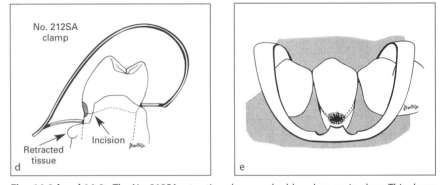

Figs 14-9d and 14-9e The No. 212SA retracting clamp and rubber dam are in place. This clamp should always be stabilized with modeling compound or similar material.

Conventional Flap Surgery

On occasion, a miniflap would provide insufficient access, and a larger mucoperiosteal flap is required for a cervical restoration.[41,57–60] If restorations on two adjacent teeth are to be placed simultaneously and both require a surgical procedure for adequate access, a miniflap cannot be used; instead, a mucoperiosteal flap is necessary (Figs 14-10a to 14-10j). Surgical crown lengthening with ostectomy may be necessary to provide sufficient access to the lesion and to reestablish dimension for a healthy connective tissue and junctional epithelial attachment[61] (Figs 14-11a and 14-11b). A mucoperiosteal flap should be reflected and ostectomy performed as needed. In some cases, repositioning the envelope flap to its original location will provide the optimal result for esthetics and function. In other cases, the flap will need to be apically positioned. It is important to remember that the flap will not reattach to the newly placed restoration. If the margin of the flap is placed 3 mm occlusal or incisal to the gingival margin of the restoration, the tooth will immediately have a 3-mm pocket adjacent to the restoration. After healing, a 3-mm pocket will remain, or the gingival margin will recede until it reaches a stable position.

Timing of Surgery

A combined surgical-restorative procedure provides better access to the restorative site than a two-step procedure, in which crown-lengthening surgery is accomplished several weeks prior to the restorative procedure. This is because, with the combined procedure, the soft tissue flap is reflected away from the area while the restoration is being placed (Figs 14-12a to 14-12e). Moisture and hemorrhage control can best be provided with a well-placed rubber dam. Two interdependent goals are accomplished with a combined surgical procedure: the source of the gingival inflammation is eliminated, and the

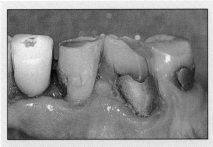

Fig 14-10a Defective Class 5 restorations in the mandibular left canine and first premolar with subgingival margins.

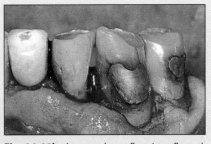

Fig 14-10b An envelope flap is reflected, revealing larger defects than were originally evident.

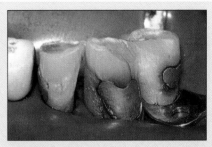

Fig 14-10c The rubber dam provides good control of bleeding and moisture but insufficient isolation of the mandibular left canine.

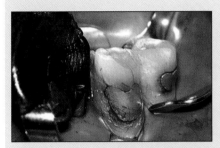

Fig 14-10d A modified No. 212SA clamp or a Schultz clamp, stabilized with modeling compound, provides additional retraction and isolation.

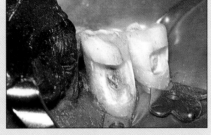

Fig 14-10e The final preparations.

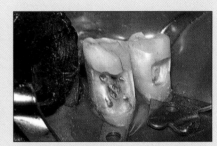

Fig 14-10f Pins were placed in the mandibular left canine for additional retention.

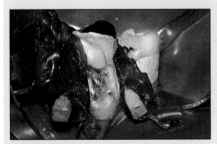

Fig 14-10g A custom matrix, stabilized with wedges and compound, provides lateral walls and support for amalgam placement.

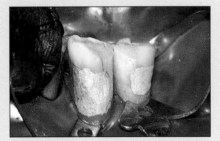

Fig 14-10h The completed restorations.

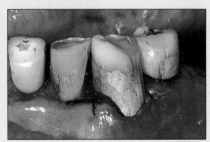

Fig 14-10i The envelope flap is returned to place and sutured.

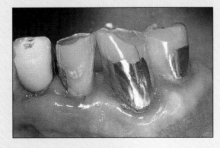

Fig 14-10j The final, polished restorations after 2 weeks of soft tissue healing.

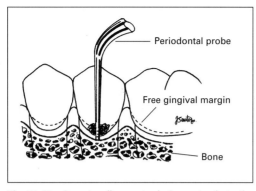

Fig 14-11a Occasionally a caries lesion extends to the base of the sulcus, making restoration difficult. Sounding with the periodontal probe shows that the restoration is likely to encroach on the biologic width. Therefore, crown lengthening is indicated.

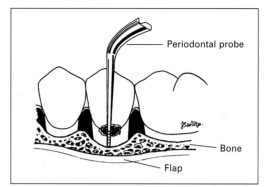

Fig 14-11b A full-thickness mucogingival flap is reflected and bone is removed so that 3 mm of root surface separate the bone and the caries lesion. The restoration can be placed prior to suturing, or restorative procedures can be delayed while the tissue heals.

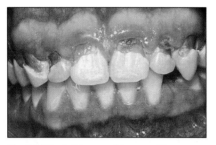

Fig 14-12a A 24-year-old man with numerous Class 5 caries lesions extending subgingivally.

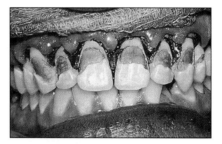

Fig 14-12b An envelope flap provides access to the caries lesions.

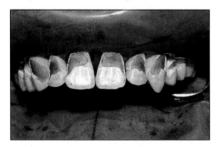

Fig 14-12c After the flap is reflected, a rubber dam is placed. Bleeding is well controlled.

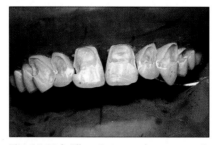

Fig 14-12d All carious tooth structure is removed, and provisional restorations are placed for caries control. The flap is apically repositioned.

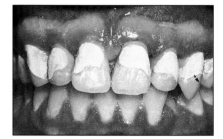

Fig 14-12e One week postoperatively, the tissues are healing and the provisional restorations are coronal to the tissue.

lost tooth structure is restored. In a broad sense, the tooth and the environment are restored simultaneously.

If surgical crown lengthening is to be done prior to tooth restoration due to carious root lesions, at least 6 weeks must elapse after surgery in order to obtain maturation of the altered periodontium.[56] In esthetic areas, a longer healing period is often required to allow the gingival margin to stabilize before restoration placement.

Restorations in the Cervical Area

Restorative Materials, Design, and Retention

Once the decision to place a restoration is made, the dentist must select a restorative material (see box) and design the cavity preparation. For any Class 5 restoration, the expected extent of the restoration should be determined by the extent of the lesion.

Class 5 Restorative Materials

Nonesthetic materials
Amalgam
Gold foil (direct) (not widely used)
Gold inlay (not widely used)

Esthetic materials
Resin composite (with dentin bonding system)
Resin composite (with glass-ionomer liner—sandwich technique)
Flowable resin composite
Glass ionomer
Resin-modified glass ionomer
Compomer
Porcelain inlay (not widely used)

Amalgam

Amalgam preparations will be the same whether the lesion requiring the placement of the restoration is carious or noncarious. For noncarious cervical lesions, preparation requires the removal of sound tooth structure to create a box form for amalgam bulk and retention, so adhesive materials are usually preferred.

For treating caries lesions, the preparation should be extended only enough to provide removal of carious tooth structure and unsupported enamel (Figs 14-13a to 14-13c). There is no need to make sharp internal line angles or to remove sound dentin for axial depth greater than 1 mm. The cavosurface margins should be as close to 90 degrees as possible. Cavosurface bevels are contraindicated in preparations for amalgam because of its low edge strength. With this design, the walls of the Class 5 preparation often diverge because of the curvature of the tooth surface. For nonbonded amalgam restorations, grooves should be placed in the dentin of both the occlusal and gingival walls to help retain the amalgam. In large preparations, pins or other retentive devices may also be beneficial. Amalgam bonding studies of Class 5 restorations have not been accomplished, but clinical studies of restorations that are subjected to considerably more load than Class 5 restorations have been reported.[62–67] These studies indicate that bonding is an excellent method to retain amalgam. This should be considered evidence of predicted success of bonded amalgam in the cervical area.

If the mesial and distal walls are flared so that the amalgam has no lateral walls to confine it for condensation, a custom matrix may be used to facilitate restoration placement and condensation. The simplest method for a facial Class 5 amalgam restoration is to use a hand instrument (Fig 14-14). If the preparation wraps well into the proximal areas, this method may not suffice. Another simple method utilizes a metal matrix band cut to a length that wraps around the lingual aspect of the tooth and extends slightly facial to the interproximal contacts (see Fig 14-10g). Interproximal wedges are placed to support and stabilize the matrix, and modeling compound may be softened and pressed interproximally if further support is needed.

After the amalgam has been carved to proper contours, a smoother surface may be attained with burnishing and then smoothing with a rubber cup and a fine abrasive paste. Although polishing has been shown to have no long-term benefit,[68] a smooth surface tends to be less plaque retentive.

Bonded Tooth-Colored Restorations

Many techniques and materials have been developed in an attempt to obtain long-term retention for esthetic materials placed in cervical locations. Polymerization shrinkage can cause resin composite to pull away from the tooth-restoration interface, leaving an open margin and pathway for microleakage to occur.[69] For moderate-sized to large restorations, incremental resin composite placement is recommended to decrease the effects of polymerization shrinkage[60,70–73] (Fig 14-15).

If the margins of the restoration will be completely on enamel, the retention of bonded restorations should be predictably successful. Beveling of enamel margins is recommended when it would improve esthetic blending of the resin with the tooth structure.[70] Beveling the gingival margin that ends on cementum is not recommended.[74]

The role tooth flexure plays in the premature loss of cervical restorations is well supported.[60,61,75] As lateral forces are placed on the buccal or lingual cusp of the tooth, the cusp may deflect. These forces may result in dislodgment of a Class 5 restoration that does not have sufficient retention form or adequate bond to tooth structure. If the restoration is retained, the flexural forces at the gingival margin may increase leakage at that site. Cusp flexure can be even greater if there is a Class 2 restoration in the tooth, allowing greater flexure in the cervical area.[76]

An often-overlooked treatment that may be important to successful restoration longevity is occlusal adjustment to

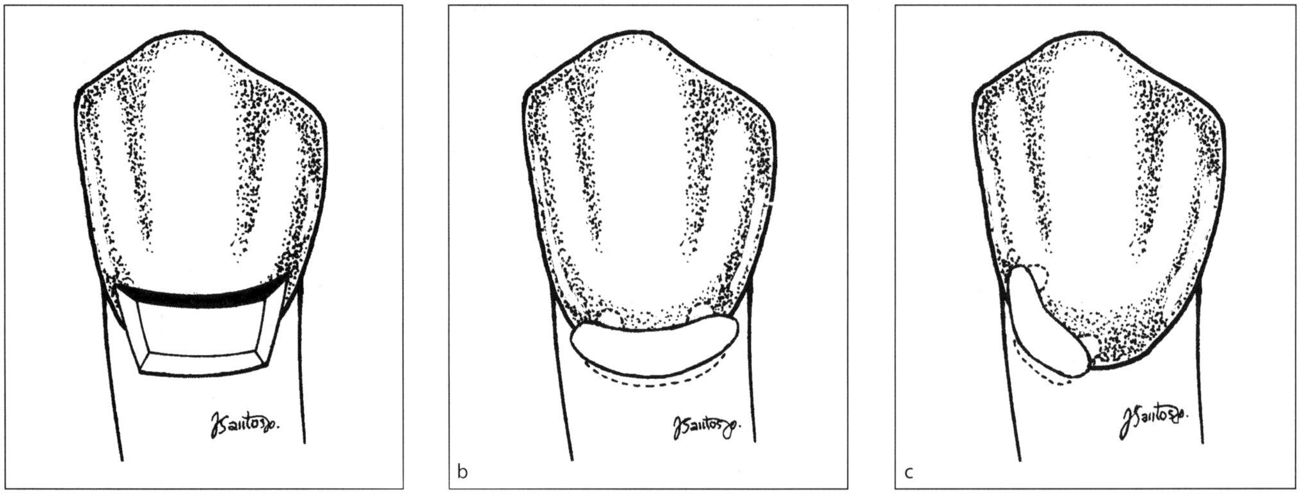

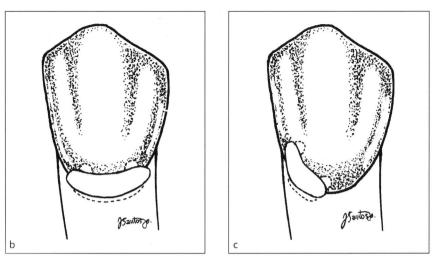

Fig 14-13a The traditional preparation for a Class 5 direct gold restoration had a trapezoidal outline form that required removal of sound, as well as carious, tooth structure.

Figs 14-13b and 14-13c The outline form currently recommended for all restorative materials includes removal of carious tooth structure and unsupported enamel. The dotted lines indicate retentive undercuts for amalgam restorations. Undercuts are not required when adhesive restorations are placed.

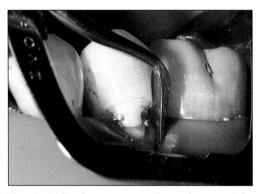

Fig 14-14 A hand instrument may be used as a matrix for Class 5 amalgam restorations.

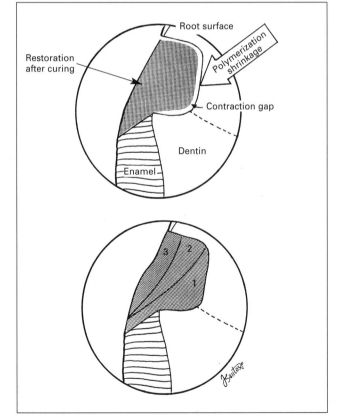

Fig 14-15 If the restoration is large, the resin composite should be placed in at least two increments to compensate for polymerization shrinkage.

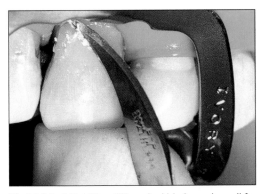

Fig 14-16a A No. 12 or 12b scalpel blade works well for removing flash.

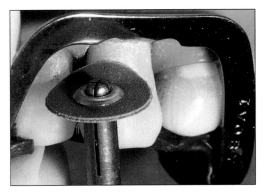

Fig 14-16b Finishing disks may be used to contour and polish Class 5 restorations.

reduce eccentric loading of the tooth with the Class 5 restoration.[71] Occlusal adjustment could decrease the dislodging forces placed on the cervical restoration during tooth flexure.

Resin Composite

The extent and depth of the lesion should determine the outline and depth of the preparation for resin composite, whether the lesion is carious or noncarious. For noncarious cervical lesions, little or no preparation is required. Retention of a resin composite restoration is primarily due to the bond, so the bonding system must be used meticulously. Although roughening the surface of a noncarious lesion has been thought to enhance the bond by removing some sclerotic dentin, one clinical trial found no increase in retention when sclerotic lesions were roughened with a bur.[77] Laboratory data have suggested that perhaps an increase in etch time for some fourth-generation, total-etch dentin bonding systems improves the bond to sclerotic dentin.[78,79] The current self-etch adhesive systems appear to have inferior bonds to sclerotic dentin when matched against dentin bonding systems that require washing away of the etching gel.[80,81]

Failure to meticulously apply the components of the bonding system could lead to early failure of the restoration. This includes the use of multiple coats if necessary, the use or non-use of the air syringe for drying, and all other product-specific instructions. For small restorations, the resin composite may be inserted and cured in one increment unless esthetic considerations call for layering. For restorations that are moderate to large in size, the first increment of resin composite should be placed from about the midpoint of the gingival floor to the incisal or occlusal cavosurface margin and light polymerized. The second increment can then fill the remainder of the preparation. Larger preparations may require more

than two increments. Resin composite should be placed in increments no thicker than 2 mm to ensure adequate penetration of light for polymerization.[82] In order to preserve the cementum or dentin at the gingival margin, careful finishing with a No. 12 or 12b scalpel blade is recommended (Fig 14-16a). Diamond burs, carbide finishing burs, or aluminum oxide disks may be used for contouring (Fig 14-16b). Polishing may be performed with progressively finer-grit disks (see Fig 14-16b) or impregnated rubber points or cups. The highest luster may be achieved with microfilled materials, but most of the current generations of hybrid composites also polish well. One study's recommendation[75] to use microfilled composites instead of hybrids in Class 5 restorations due to their lower modulus of elasticity appears to have been refuted. In a more recent study, Browning and others[57] concluded that there are no differences in retention rates between microfilled and hybrid resin composites. As with the placement of any resin composite restoration, careful technique is critical to long-term success. Rebonding, as discussed in chapter 10, is recommended for Class 5 restorations.

Flowable Resin Composite

Flowable resin composites have reduced filler particle loading, a lower elastic modulus, significantly higher polymerization shrinkage, a higher coefficient of thermal expansion, and lower fracture toughness relative to traditional resin composites.[14] Flowable resin composites have been recommended for Class 5 restorations with the suggestion that, like microfilled resin composites, as the tooth flexes, the less rigid restoration might be able to accommodate the change in cavity shape and therefore be more difficult to dislodge.[14] The theoretical advantages to more flexible materials in cervical restorations have not been confirmed in clinical trials. Stiff

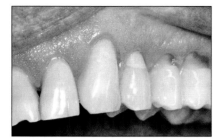

Fig 14-17a Multiple adjacent Class 5 lesions in the mandibular left canine through the second molar and more posterior teeth.

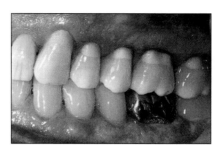

Fig 14-17b The teeth were restored with conventional glass ionomer, which is opaque and relatively unesthetic.

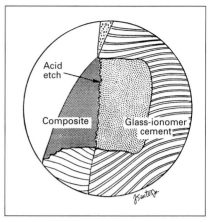

Fig 14-18 The sandwich technique combines a glass-ionomer base with a veneer of resin composite.

restorations have performed as well or better than the flexible resin composites in long-term clinical trials. The use of a flowable resin composite as a liner has not been shown to improve clinical performance.[57,83,84]

Glass Ionomer and Resin-Modified Glass Ionomer

Glass ionomer has been used successfully in Class 5 restorations for many years. One clinical study reported an 80% retention rate of restorations placed without mechanical retention at 10 years.[85] Traditional glass-ionomer materials suffer surface degradation rather rapidly, especially in the presence of acidic foods. Resin-modified glass ionomers (RMGIs) appear to offer high fluoride release and excellent recharge capacity. Patients at high risk for caries would probably be best served with RMGI restorations on root surfaces (see chapters 4, 12, and 13).

The preparation for glass-ionomer restorations is similar to that for resin composite. Cavosurface bevels are not recommended for the preparation because glass ionomer is a brittle material that requires bulk. After placement of RMGI material into the preparation, it is light polymerized in a manner similar to photocuring resin composite. The use of a clear cervical matrix is optional. The restoration may be contoured and polished immediately with the same techniques described for resin composite. Retention rates of 93%[86] and 99%[87] after 2 years have been reported for Class 5 RMGI restorations placed in preparations without mechanical undercuts.

Glass-Ionomer Sandwich Technique. Because autocured glass-ionomer materials often provide less-than-optimal esthetics[27] (Figs 14-17a and 14-17b), many clinicians use the sandwich technique. Glass ionomer is used to replace the missing dentin, reduce microleakage,[86,87] and increase retention, while a veneer of resin composite is placed to enhance esthetics and polishability and to increase abrasion resistance[58,88] (Fig 14-18). In one clinical study using the sandwich technique, a 100% retention rate was reported after 3 years.[61] Another clinical trial resulted in a 96% survival rate of sandwich restorations at 5 years, demonstrating the success rates attainable with this type of restoration.[89]

Compomer

Compomer materials are polyacid-modified resin composites (see chapter 13). They are recommended to restore teeth that have carious and noncarious cervical lesions.[48,49,79] On the continuum of fluoride-releasing materials, compomer materials fall between resin composites and RMGI materials but are much more like resin composites. They require acid etching of both enamel and dentin and the use of a dentin bonding system. Most physical properties of compomers are inferior to those of conventional resin composites. Compomers have very favorable handling characteristics. Specifically, their lack of "stickiness" has brought them ready acceptance in the marketplace. In clinical trials, properly bonded compomers appear to survive similarly to other tooth-colored filling materials. However, the marginal integrity of compomers has been worse than resin composites in long-term clinical trials.[90–103]

Dentinal Sensitivity

Dentinal sensitivity, a problem reported to affect approximately one in seven people,[104] is often associated with gingival recession and noncarious cervical lesions.[61] A survey of new patients found that, of 780 patients, 32% reported sensitivity but only 5% had sought professional help.[105] Tooth sensitivity was the chief complaint in 60% of the referrals to a periodontal specialty clinic.[106] Sensitivity is caused by exposure of dentinal tubules that communicate between the pulp and the oral cavity; the degree of sensitivity is influenced by the number and size of the open tubules.[3,80] The hydrodynamic theory[107] is the most widely accepted explanation of dentinal sensitivity. Changes in the direction of fluid movement within open dentinal tubules are perceived as pain by mechanoreceptors near the pulp. Tactile, thermal, or osmotic stimuli can induce changes in fluid flow and elicit a pain response.

Traditionally, most dentists have treated NCCLs only with restorative methods, for example, resin composite restorations. However, in many cases, a periodontal or a combined restorative/periodontal approach provides a better esthetic and functional result.[108] In teeth with shallow lesions and those in which esthetic prerequisites are met, a connective tissue graft, pedicle graft, double-papilla procedure, or coronally positioned flap may be used to cover the exposed cervical area and protect the tooth from further tooth structure loss.[33–40] However, periodontal surgery is not always a treatment option. Therefore, other methods of treating dentin hypersensitivity may be necessary.

In a clinical study, caries-free teeth that were planned for extraction were stimulated to determine if exposed dentin was hypersensitive. Microscopic analysis of the teeth found that the teeth that were hypersensitive had eight times more tubules per unit area, and the tubules in the sensitive teeth were twice as wide.[109]

Treatment or prevention of hypersensitivity is usually accomplished by the use of some method to occlude the open dentinal tubules.[110–112] Dentin adhesives provide at least short-term relief.[113–115] Stannous fluorides have also been used with positive results.[44,116] A study found that 10% strontium chloride solution, 2% sodium fluoride solution, and 40% formalin solution significantly reduced dentin hypersensitivity, whereas a 5% solution of potassium nitrate did not.[117] A potassium chloride–containing chewing gum was found to be effective in the treatment of hypersensitive teeth.[118]

No treatment to date has been effective for every patient every time. The variety of treatments available would suggest that, by using proper diagnostic and clinical skills, the dentist should be able to help most patients who have sensitive teeth.

Summary

The preponderance of evidence supports the conclusion that the loss of cervical enamel, cementum, and dentin is due to a combination of many factors. These may include intake of acidic foods, reflux of gastric acids into the oral cavity, bacteria-produced acids, inadequate buffering ability of saliva, inadequate salivary flow rate, and mechanical abrasion. While not completely understood, occlusal forces inducing stresses in the cervical areas of teeth may play an important role in the development of cervical lesions. For treatment of a caries lesion, after the carious tooth structure has been removed, the treatment protocol is very similar to that for a NCCL. When the etiologic factors have been reduced or eliminated and all other conservative management of cervical lesions has been attempted, there may still be a need to restore areas where there has been significant cervical tooth loss. The decision to restore should be tempered by the certainty that restorations are not permanent.

References

1. Aubry M, Mafart B, Donat B, Brau JJ. Brief communication: Study of noncarious cervical tooth lesions in samples of prehistoric, historic, and modern populations from the South of France. Am J Phys Anthropol 2003;121(1):10–14.
2. Li P, Li J, Zhang Q. Investigations on the incidence of dental wedge-shaped defects and abrasion in 501 elderly population and their correlation. Zhonghua Kou Qiang Yi Xue Za Zhi 1998;33:227–229.
3. Dugmore CR, Rock WP. The progression of tooth erosion in a cohort of adolescents of mixed ethnicity. Int J Paediatr Dent 2003; 13:295–303.
4. Borcic J, Anic I, Urek MM, Ferreri S. The prevalence of non-carious cervical lesions in permanent dentition. J Oral Rehab 2004;31: 117–123.
5. Bader JD, McClure F, Scurria MS, Shugars DA, Heymann HO. Case-control study of non-carious cervical lesions. Community Dent Oral Epidemiol 1996;24:286–291.
6. Academy of Operative Dentistry. Non-carious cervical lesions. Recommendations for clinical practice. Oper Dent 2003;28:109–113.
7. Dawes C. Physiological factors affecting salivary flow rate, oral sugar clearance and the sensation of dry mouth in man. J Dent Res 1987;66:648–653.
8. Young WG. Anthropology, tooth wear, and occlusion ab origine. J Dent Res 1998;77:1860–1863.
9. Astroth JD. Caring for the elderly adult: How to prevent, manage root surface caries. Dent Teamwork 1996;9:15–19.
10. Atkinson JC, Wu AJ. Salivary gland dysfunction: Causes, symptoms, treatment. J Am Dent Assoc 1994;125:409–416.
11. Haveman CW, Redding SW. Dental management and treatment of xerostomic patients. Tex Dent J 1998;115:43–56.
12. Young WG, Khan F. Sites of dental erosion are saliva-dependent. J Oral Rehabil 2002;29:35–43.

13. Khan F, Young WG, Daley TJ. Dental erosion and bruxism. A tooth wear analysis from south east Queensland. Aust Dent J 1998;43: 117–127.

14. Rees JS. The effect of variation in occlusal loading on the development of abfraction lesions: A finite element study. J Oral Rehabil 2002;29:188–193.

15. Geramy A, Sharafoddin F. Abfraction: 3D analysis by means of the finite element method. Quintessence Int 2003;34:526–533.

16. Litonjua LA, Bush PJ, Andreana S, Tobias TS, Cohen RE. Effects of occlusal load on cervical lesions. J Oral Rehabil 2004;31:225–232.

17. Palamara JE, Palamara D, Messer HH. Effect of stress on acid dissolution of enamel. Dent Mater 2001;17:109–115.

18. Whitehead SA, Wilson NH, Watts DC. Development of noncarious cervical notch lesion in vitro. J Esthet Dent 1999;11:332–337.

19. Hughes JA, Jandt KD, Baker N, et al. Further modification to soft drinks to minimise erosion. A study in situ. Caries Res 2002;36: 70–74.

20. Absi EG, Addy M, Adams D. Dentine hypersensitivity—The effect of toothbrushing and dietary compounds on dentine in vitro: An SEM study. J Oral Rehabil 1992;19:101–110.

21. West NX, Hughes JA, Addy M. The effect of pH on the erosion of dentine and enamel by dietary acids in vitro. J Oral Rehabil 2001; 28:860–864.

22. Attin T, Koidl U, Buchalla W, Schaller HG, Kielbass AM, Hellwig E. Correlation of microhardness and wear in differently eroded bovine dental enamel. Arch Oral Biol 1997;42:243–250.

23. Attin T, Buchalla W, Gollner M, Hellwig E. Use of variable remineralization periods to improve the abrasion resistance of previously eroded enamel. Caries Res 2000;34:48–52.

24. Davis WB, Winter PJ. The effect of abrasion on enamel and dentine after exposure to dietary acid. Br Dent J 1980;148:253–256.

25. Jaeggi T, Lussi A. Toothbrush abrasion of erosively altered enamel after intraoral exposure to saliva: An in situ study. Caries Res 1999; 33:455–461.

26. Oginni AO, Olusile AO, Udoye CI. Non-carious cervical lesions in a Nigerian population: Abrasion or abfraction? Int Dent J 2003;53: 275–279.

27. Piotrowski BT, Gillette WB, Hancock EB. Examining the prevalence and characteristics of abfractionlike cervical lesions in a population of U.S. veterans. J Am Dent Assoc 2001;132:1694–1701.

28. Palamara D, Palamara JE, Tyas MJ, Messer HH. Strain patterns in cervical enamel of teeth subjected to occlusal loading. Dent Mater 2000;16:412–419.

29. Kuroe T, Hidemi I, Caputo AA, Konuma M. Biomechanics of cervical tooth structure lesions and their restoration. Quintessence Int 2000;31:267–274.

30. Miller N, Penaud J, Ambrosini P, Bisson-Boutelliez C, Briancon S. Analysis of etiologic factors and periodontal conditions involved with 309 abfractions. J Clin Periodontol 2003;30:828–832.

31. Mayhew RB, Jessee SA, Martin RE. Association of occlusal, periodontal, and dietary factors with the presence of non-carious cervical dental lesions. Am J Dent 1998;11:29–32.

32. LittleStar ML, Summitt JB. Non-carious cervical lesions: An evidenced-based approach to their diagnosis. Tex Dent J 2003;120:972–980.

33. Majzoub Z, Landi L, Grusovin MG, Cordioli G. Histology of connective tissue graft. A case report. J Periodontol 2001;72:1607–1615.

34. Saletta D, Pini Prato G, Pagliaro U, Baldi C, Mauri M, Nieri M. Coronally advanced flap procedure: Is the interdental papilla a prognostic factor for root coverage? J Periodontol 2001;72:760–766.

35. Ito K, Murai S. Adjacent gingival recession treated with expanded polytetrafluoroethylene membranes: A report of two cases. J Periodontol 1996;67:443–450.

36. Cordioli G, Mortarino C, Chierico A, Grusovin MG, Majzoub Z.. Comparison of 2 techniques of subepithelial connective tissue graft in the treatment of gingival recessions. J Periodontol 2001;72: 1470–1476.

37. Novaes AB Jr, Grisi DC, Molina GO, Souza SL, Taba M Jr, Grisi MF. Comparative 6-month clinical study of a subepithelial connective tissue graft and acellular dermal matrix graft for the treatment of gingival recession. J Periodontol 2001;72:1477–1484.

38. Rosetti EP, Marcantonio RA, Rossa C Jr, Chaves ES, Goissis G, Marcantonio E Jr. Treatment of gingival recession: Comparative study between subepithelial connective tissue graft and guided tissue regeneration. J Periodontol 2000;71:1441–1447.

39. Tozum TF, Dini FM. Treatment of adjacent gingival recessions with subepithelial connective tissue grafts and the modified tunnel technique. Quintessence Int 2003;34:7–13.

40. Harris RJ. Connective tissue grafts combined with either double pedicle grafts or coronally positioned pedicle grafts: Results of 266 consecutively treated defects in 200 patients. Int J Periodontics Restorative Dent 2002;22:463–471.

41. Morris MF, Davis RD, Richardson BW. Clinical efficacy of two dentin desensitizing agents. Am J Dent 1999;12:72–76.

42. Baysan A, Lynch E, Treatment of cervical sensitivity with a root sealant. Am J Dent 2003;16:135–138.

43. Schiff T, Zhang YP, DeVizio W, et al. A randomized clinical trial of the desensitizing efficacy of three dentifrices. Compend Contin Educ Dent Suppl 2000;27:4–10.

44. Thrash WJ, Dodds MW, Jones DL. The effect of stannous fluoride on dentinal hypersensitivity. Int Dent J 1994;44(1 suppl 1):107–118.

45. Thrash WJ, Jones DL, Dodds WJ. Effect of a fluoride solution on dentinal hypersensitivity. Am J Dent 1992;5:299–302.

46. Baum LG, Phillips RW, Lund MR. Textbook of Operative Dentistry, ed 3. Philadelphia: Saunders, 1995:210–212, 262.

47. Crispin BJ. Contemporary Esthetic Dentistry: Practice Fundamentals. Chicago: Quintessence, 1994:112.

48. Grippo JO. Noncarious cervical lesions: The decision to ignore or restore. J Esthet Dent 1992;4(suppl):55–64.

49. Levitch LC, Bader JD, Shugars DA, Heymann HO. Non-carious cervical lesions. J Dent 1994;22:195–207.

50. Powell LV, Gordon GE, Johnson GH. Sensitivity of restored Class 5 abrasion/erosion lesions. J Am Dent Assoc 1990;121:694–696.

51. Sturdevant CM, Robeson TM, Heymann HO, Sturdevant JR. The Art and Science of Operative Dentistry, ed 3. St Louis: Mosby, 1995: 486–499.

52. Brantley CF, Bader JD, Shugars DA, Nesbit SP. Does the cycle of re-restoration lead to larger restorations? J Am Dent Assoc 1995;126: 1407–1413.

53. Fontana M, Gonzalez-Cabezas C. Secondary caries and restoration replacement: An unresolved problem. Compend Contin Educ Dent 2000;21:15–18, 21–24, 26 passim.

54. Reagan SE. Periodontal access techniques for restorative dentistry. Gen Dent 1989;37:117–121.

55. Starr CB. Management of periodontal tissues for restorative dentistry. J Esthet Dent 1991;3:195–208.

56. Maynard JG, Wilson RDK. Physiologic dimensions of the periodontium significant to the restorative dentist. J Periodontol 1979;50:170–174.

57. Browning WD, Brackett WW, Gilpatrick RO. Two-year clinical comparison of a microfilled and a hybrid resin-based composite in non-carious Class V lesions. Oper Dent 2000;25:46–50.

58. Suzuki M, Jordan RE. Glass ionomer-composite sandwich technique. J Am Dent Assoc 1990;120:55–57.

59. Vandewalle KS, Vigil G. Guidelines for the restoration of Class 5 lesions. Gen Dent 1997;45:254–260.

60. McCoy RB, Anderson MH, Lepe X, Johnson GH. Clinical success of Class 5 composite resin restorations without mechanical retention. J Am Dent Assoc 1998;129:593–599.

61. Powell LV, Johnson GH, Gordon GE. Factors associated with clinical success of cervical abrasion/erosion restorations. Oper Dent 1995;20:7–13.

62. Belcher MA, Stewart GP. Two-year clinical evaluation of an amalgam adhesive. J Am Dent Assoc 1997;128:309–314.

63. Summitt JB, Burgess JO, Berry TG, Robbins JW, Osborne JW, Haveman CW. Six-year evaluation of Amalgabond Plus and pin-retained amalgam restorations. Oper Dent 2004;29(3):261–268.

64. Evans DB, Neme AML. Shear bond strength of composite resin and amalgam adhesive systems to dentin. Am J Dent 1999;12:19–25.

65. Gorucu J, Tiritoglu M, Ozgunaltay G. Effects of preparation designs and adhesive systems on retention of Class II amalgam restorations. J Prosthet Dent 1997;78:250–254.

66. Oliveira JP, Cochran MA, Moore BK. Influence of bonded amalgam restorations on the fracture strength of teeth. Oper Dent 1996;21:110–115.

67. Staninec M, Marshall GW, Lowe A, Ruzickova T. Clinical research on bonded amalgam restorations. Gen Dent 1997;45:356–362.

68. Mayhew RB, Schmeltzer LD, Pierson WP. Effect of polishing on the marginal integrity of high copper amalgam. Oper Dent 1986;11:8–13.

69. Carvalho RM, Pereira JC, Yoshiyama M, Pashley DH. A review of polymerization contraction: The influence of stress development versus stress relief. Oper Dent 1996;21:17–24.

70. Albers H. Tooth Colored Restorations, ed 8. Santa Rosa, CA: Alto Books, 1996:8c1–8c6.

71. Leinfelder KF. Restoration of abfracted lesions. Compend Contin Educ Dent 1994;15:1396–1400.

72. Lutz F, Krejci I, Oldenburg TR. Elimination of polymerization stresses at the margins of posterior resin composite restorations: A new restorative technique. Quintessence Int 1986;17:777–784.

73. Tjan AHL, Bergh BH, Lidner C. Effect of various incremental techniques on marginal adaptation of Class II resin composite restorations. J Prosthet Dent 1992;67:62–66.

74. Owens BM, Halter TK, Brown DM. Microleakage of tooth colored restorations with a beveled gingival margin. Quintessence Int 1998;29:356–361.

75. Heymann HO, Sturdevant JR, Bayne S, Wilder AD, Sluder TB, Brunson WD. Examining tooth flexure effects on cervical restorations: A two-year clinical study. J Am Dent Assoc 1991;122:41–47.

76. Assif D, Marshak B, Pilo R. Cuspal flexure associated with amalgam restorations. J Prosthet Dent 1990;60:258–262.

77. van Dijken JW. Clinical evaluation of three adhesive systems in Class V non-carious lesions. Dent Mater 2000;16:285–291.

78. Lopes GC, Baratieri CM, Baratieri LN, Monteiro S Jr, Cardoso Vieira LC. Bonding to cervical sclerotic dentin: Effect of acid etching time. J Adhes Dent 2004;6:19–23.

79. Lopes GC, Vieira LC, Monteiro S Jr, Caldeira de Andrada MA, Baratieri CM. Dentin bonding: Effect of degree of mineralization and acid etching time. Oper Dent 2003;28:429–439.

80. Kwong SM, Cheung GS, Kei LH, et al. Micro-tensile bond strengths to sclerotic dentin using a self-etching and a total-etching technique. Dent Mater 2002;18:359–369.

81. Tay FR, Kwong SM, Itthagarun A, et al. Bonding of a self-etching primer to non-carious cervical sclerotic dentin: Interfacial ultrastructure and microtensile bond strength evaluation. J Adhes Dent 2000;2:9–28.

82. Jensen ME, Chan DCN. Polymerization shrinkage and microleakage. In: Vanherle G, Smith DC (eds). Posterior Resin Composite Dental Restorative Materials. Utrecht, The Netherlands: Szulc, 1985:243–262.

83. Ernst CP, Buhtz C, Rissing C, Willershausen B. Clinical performance of resin composite restorations after 2 years. Compend Contin Educ Dent 2002;23:711–714, 716–717, 720 passim.

84. Tyas MJ, Burrow MF. Three-year clinical evaluation of One-Step in non-carious cervical lesions. Am J Dent 2002;15:309–311.

85. Matis BA, Cochran M, Carlson T. Longevity of glass ionomer restorative materials: Results of a 10-year evaluation. Quintessence Int 1996;27:373–382.

86. Brackett WW, Gilpatrick RO, Browning WD, Gregory PN. Two-year clinical performance of a resin modified glass ionomer restorative material. Oper Dent 1999;24:9–13.

87. Abdalla AI, Alhadainy HA. Clinical evaluation of hybrid ionomer restoratives in Class V abrasion lesions: Two-year results. Quintessence Int 1997;28:255–258.

88. Frazier KB, Rueggeberg FA, Mettenburg DJ. Comparison of wear-resistance of Class 5 restorative materials. J Esthet Dent 1998;10:309–314.

89. Tyas MJ, Burrow MF. Clinical evaluation of a resin-modified glass ionomer adhesive system: Results at five years. Oper Dent 2002;27:438–441.

90. van Dijken JW. 3-year clinical evaluation of a compomer, a resin-modified glass ionomer and a resin composite in Class III restorations. Am J Dent 1996;9:195–198.

91. Huth KC, Manhart J, Selbertinger A, et al. 4-year clinical performance and survival analysis of Class I and II compomer restorations in permanent teeth. Am J Dent 2004:17:51–55.

92. Hse KM, Wei SH. Clinical evaluation of compomer in primary teeth: 1-year results. J Am Dent Assoc 1997;128:1088–1096.

93. Andersson-Wenckert IE, Folkesson UH, van Dijken JW. Durability of a polyacid-modified composite resin (compomer) in primary molars. A multicenter study. Acta Odontol Scand 1997;55:255–260.

94. Roeters JJ, Frankenmolen F, Burgersdijk RC, Peters TC. Clinical evaluation of Dyract in primary molars: 3-year results. Am J Dent 1998;11:143–148.

95. Prati C, Chersoni S, Cretti L, Montanari G. Retention and marginal adaptation of a compomer placed in non–stress-bearing areas used with the total-etch technique: A 3-year retrospective study. Clin Oral Investig 1998;2:168–173.

96. Papagiannoulis L, Kakaboura A, Pantaleon F, Kavvadia K. Clinical evaluation of a polyacid-modified resin composite (compomer) in Class II restorations of primary teeth: A two-year follow-up study. Pediatr Dent 1999;21:231–234.

97. Di Lenarda R, Cadenaro M, De Stefano Dorigo E. Cervical compomer restorations: The role of cavity etching in a 48-month clinical evaluation. Oper Dent 2000;25:382–387.

98. van Dijken JW. Durability of new restorative materials in Class III cavities. J Adhes Dent 2001;3:65–70.

99. Abdalla AI, Mahallawy SE, Davidson CL, et al. Clinical and SEM evaluations of three compomer systems in Class V carious lesions. J Oral Rehabil 2002;29:714–719.

100. Folwaczny M, Mehl A, Kunzelmann KH, Hickel R. Clinical performance of a resin-modified glass-ionomer and a compomer in restoring non-carious cervical lesions. 5-year results. Am J Dent 2001;14:153–156.

101. Wucher M, Grobler SR, Senekal PJ. A 3-year clinical evaluation of a compomer, a composite and a compomer/composite (sandwich) in Class II restorations. Am J Dent 2002;15:274–278.

102. Huth KC, Manhard J, Hickel R, Kunzelmann KH. Three-year clinical performance of a compomer in stress-bearing restorations in permanent posterior teeth. Am J Dent 2003;16(4):255–259.

103. Qvist V, Laurberg L, Poulsen A, Teglers PT. Class II restorations in primary teeth: 7-year study on three resin-modified glass ionomer cements and a compomer. Eur J Oral Sci 2004;112:188–196.

104. Krauser JT. Hypersensitive teeth. Part 1. Etiology. J Prosthet Dent 1986;56:153–156.

105. Liu HC, Lan WH, Hsieh CC. Prevalence and distribution of cervical dentin hypersensitivity in a population in Taipei, Taiwan. J Endod 1998;24:45–47.

106. Taani SD, Awartani F. Clinical evaluation of cervical dentin sensitivity (CDS) in patients attending general dental clinics (GDC) and periodontal specialty clinics (PSC). J Clin Periodontol 2002;29:118–122.

107. Brannstrom M. The hydrodynamics of the dentinal tubule and of pulp fluid. A discussion of its significance in relation to dentinal sensitivity. Caries Res 1976;1:310–322.

108. Terry DA, McGuire MK, McLaren E, Fulton R, Swift EJ Jr. Perioesthetic approach to the diagnosis and treatment of carious and non-carious cervical lesions: Part I. J Esthet Restor Dent 2003;15:217–232.

109. Absi EG, Addy M, Adams D. Dentin hypersensitivity. A study of the patency of dentinal tubules in sensitive and non-sensitive cervical dentin. J Clin Periodontol 1987;14:280–284.

110. Hodosh M, Hodosh SH, Hodosh AJ. About dentinal hypersensitivity. Compendium 1994;15:658, 660, 662 passim.

111. Pashley DH, Muzzin K. Clinical Management of Dentin Hypersensitivity. Philadelphia: Lippincott, 1990.

112. Trowbridge HO, Silver DR. A review of current approaches to in-office management of tooth hypersensitivity. Dent Clin North Am 1990;34:561–581.

113. Dondi dall'Orologio G, Malferrari S. Desensitizing effects of Gluma and Gluma 2000 on hypersensitive dentin. Am J Dent 1993;6:283–286.

114. Watanabe T, Sano M, Itoh K, Wakumoto S. The effects of primers on the sensitivity of dentin. Dent Mater 1991;7:148–150.

115. Swift EJ Jr, May KN Jr, Mitchell S. Clinical evaluation of Prime & Bond 2.1 for treating cervical dentin hypersensitivity. Am J Dent 2001;14:13–16.

116. Tarbet WJ, Silverman G, Fratarcangelo PA, Kanapka JA. Home treatment for dentinal hypersensitivity: A comparative study. J Am Dent Assoc 1982;105:227–230.

117. Kishore A, Mehrotra KK, Saimbi CS. Effectiveness of desensitizing agents. J Endod 2002;28:34–35.

118. Krahwinkel T, Theiss P, Willershausen B. Clinical effectiveness of a potassium chloride containing chewing gum in the treatment of hypersensitive teeth. Eur J Med Res 2001;6(11):483–487.

Natural Tooth Bleaching

Van B. Haywood
Thomas G. Berry

For well over a century, bleaching has been used to achieve a lighter and more desirable tooth color. Dental journals in the last half of the 19th century frequently contained articles on the efficacy of bleaching teeth.[1–3] The safety of the procedure was well investigated and the chemistry understood; most of the bleaching agents were considered to be safe by the standards of the time. Although the process was thought to be time-consuming and relapse was considered a consistent problem, bleaching was well accepted by many dentists.[4–6] By the mid-1800s, the bleaching agent of choice for nonvital teeth was chloride of lime.[7–9] Around that time, Truman[5] introduced chlorine from a calcium hydroxide and acetic acid solution for bleaching nonvital teeth; this was supplied commercially as a liquid chloride of soda. Other agents used in the 1800s for nonvital tooth bleaching included aluminum chloride,[10] oxalic acid,[3,11] Pyrozone (ether peroxide) (McKesson and Robbins),[2] hydrogen dioxide (hydrogen peroxide or perhydrol),[12] sodium peroxide,[12] sodium hypophosphate,[8] and cyanide of potassium. The active ingredient common to all of these was an oxidizing agent that acted either directly or indirectly on the organic portion of the tooth. Sulfurous acid, in contrast, achieved results as a reducing agent.[13,14] Generally, the most effective yet safe bleaching agents were direct oxidizers or an indirect oxidizer such as a chlorine derivative.[6,15] However, the choice of bleaching agent depended primarily on the stain being removed. Iron stains were removed with oxalic acid, silver and copper stains with chlorine, and iodine stains with ammonia.[16–18] Metallic stains (such as those from amalgam) were considered the most resistant to bleaching. Concern about the effect of some of these bleaching agents on the teeth, tissues, and health of the patient was raised because some agents used, such as cyanide of potassium, were very poisonous.[12] Other bleaching agents were caustic.

The early emphasis was on bleaching nonvital teeth. However, as early as the 1890s, a 3% solution of Pyrozone was used safely as a mouthwash by both children and adults. It reduced caries and whitened the teeth.[19] A 5% solution proved to be safe and effective, but a 25% solution was caustic, causing tissue burns.[19] By 1910, an in-office bleaching technique similar to techniques used today, using high concentrations of hydrogen peroxide activated by heat or light, was well established. Over the next few decades, the bleaching agents varied. By the 1940s, hydrogen peroxide and ether were used for vital teeth,[20] while, by the late 1950s, Pyrozone and sodium perborate were used for nonvital teeth.[21,22]

The current home bleaching technique, employing a custom-fit tray containing 10% carbamide peroxide solution, was first used by Klusmier in the late 1960s.[23] However, the profession did not embrace the concept until it was described in a 1989 article,[24] the publication of which coincided with the market introduction of carbamide peroxide as a bleaching agent.[25,26] This ushered in the current technique for at-home bleaching. Various chemical combinations have been tried. The effective ones all release oxidizing agents, whether supplied as hydrogen peroxide, carbamide peroxide, sodium percarbonate, or some other compound.[27]

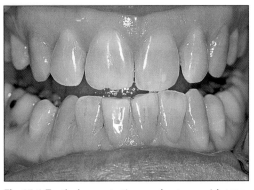

Fig 15-1 Teeth demonstrating moderate, grayish tetracycline stain.

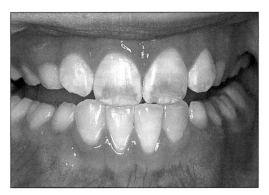

Fig 15-2 Fluorosis stain produces brownish areas surrounded by whiter areas.

Types and Nature of Stains/Discolorations

Many types of color problems affect the appearance of the teeth. The cause of these problems varies, so the speed with which they may be removed also varies. Discolorations may be extrinsic or intrinsic. Extrinsic stains are located on the surface of the tooth and are most easily removed by external cleaning. Intrinsic stains are located within the tooth and are accessible only by bleaching. Some extrinsic stains that remain on the tooth for a long time become intrinsic. Extrinsic color changes may be due to poor oral hygiene, ingestion of chromatogenic foods and drinks, and tobacco use. Intrinsic color changes may be caused by aging, ingestion of chromatogenic foods and drinks, tobacco usage, microcracks in the enamel, tetracycline medication, excessive fluoride ingestion, severe jaundice in infancy, porphyria, dental caries, restorations, and the thinning of the enamel layer. Other, less common, medical situations and conditions may also cause the loss of desirable tooth color.

The causes of staining need to be assessed carefully to better predict the rate and degree to which bleaching will improve tooth color, since some stains are more responsive to the process than others.[24,28] For instance, the yellow discoloration of aging responds quickly to bleaching in most cases,[29] whereas a blue-gray tetracycline stain is tenacious.[26] In general, tetracycline-stained teeth are the slowest to respond to bleaching; brown-fluoresced teeth are moderately responsive; and teeth discolored by age, genetics, smoking, or coffee are the fastest to respond.[30–32] White spots are not removed by bleaching but may be less noticeable when the remainder of the tooth is lighter.[33] By recognizing the likely cause of the stain, the dentist can better tell the patient the rate at which the teeth may lighten in color and the limits on the amount of improvement that can be expected.

Discoloration from drug ingestion may occur either before or after the tooth is fully formed. Tetracycline is incorporated into the dentin sometime during tooth calcification (Fig 15-1), probably through chelation with calcium, forming tetracycline orthophosphate.[34–36] There are several variations of tetracycline, and each derivative produces a different color in the tooth. Some teeth may be "banded" from the ingestion of different derivatives of tetracycline. When the teeth are exposed to sunlight, they become darker, with a distinct gray/blue-gray tinge. The teeth not exposed to the sunlight (eg, molars) do not darken to the same degree but remain more yellow in color. Tetracycline has also been reported to discolor fully formed, erupted permanent teeth. This discoloration is most often associated with minocycline, a drug commonly used in the treatment of acne.[37,38] The primary route of deposition is thought to be in the secondary dentin, although some reports suggest a staining similar to iron deposition. Other antibiotics may also interact with calcium, iron, or other elements to form insoluble complexes that stain teeth.[39]

Excessive fluoride in drinking water, greater than 1 to 2 ppm, can cause metabolic alteration in the ameloblasts, resulting in a defective matrix and improper calcification of teeth.[40,41] An affected tooth shows a hypomineralized, porous subsurface enamel and a well-mineralized surface layer. These teeth have a glazed surface and may be very white except for areas of yellow, brown (Fig 15-2), or even black shading.

Some systemic conditions can cause tooth discoloration. Severe jaundice leads to staining by bilirubin. Erythroblastosis fetalis may also stain the teeth by the destruction of red blood cells. Porphyria, a rare condition, manifests with purplish-brown teeth.

Aging is a common cause of discoloration. Over time, the underlying dentin tends to darken from the formation of secondary dentin, which is darker and more opaque than the original dentin. This occurs while the overlying enamel becomes thinner, a combination that often produces distinctly darker teeth.

Dental caries produces varying stains during its process. Examples of caries-induced discolorations include an opaque white "halo," a grayish tinge, or a brown-to-black stain. These stains arise from the bacterial degradation of food debris. Metallic restorations, most notably dental amalgam, may cause a distinct staining of the tooth in addition to the shadow they may cast through adjacent enamel walls.

Current Bleaching Modalities

Mode of Action

The bleaching process is designed to enable the oxidizing agent to reach sites within the enamel and dentin to allow a chemical reaction to occur. No matter the bleaching technique or specific bleaching action, the intention is to deliver the active ingredient to the discolored segments of the tooth to dislodge or decolor the chromatic particles.

Hydrogen peroxide diffuses through the organic matrix of the enamel and dentin because of its low molecular weight.[42–46] One current theory of whitening is that the free radicals attack organic molecules to achieve stability; this releases other radicals. These radicals can react with other unsaturated bonds, disrupting the electron conjugation and providing a change in the absorption energy of the organic molecules in the enamel. The simpler molecules formed reflect less light, so the tooth appears lighter in shade.[47] In the early stages of this process, bleaching opens the more highly pigmented carbon-ring compounds and converts them to chains that are lighter in color. The carbon double-bond compounds (yellow in color) are converted to hydroxyl groups (essentially colorless). The bleaching process continues to the extent that all the original pigment is rendered essentially colorless.[48] At this point, lightening of the teeth reaches a plateau with regard to the speed at which it progresses. The continuation of the bleaching process is not beneficial beyond this point. Further research is needed to determine what gives the tooth its baseline color and, in turn, the oxidation reaction of bleaching that changes the tooth color.

The chemistry of carbamide peroxide used in at-home bleaching is thought to be a bit different from hydrogen peroxide, although the final stages do involve the reaction of hydrogen peroxide with the compounds within the tooth. When introduced into the mouth, the agent breaks down into urea and hydrogen peroxide, both of which access the internal portions of the tooth in minutes. In addition, bleach-

ing not only removes discoloration from within the tooth, it also alters/brightens the inherent color of the dentin itself.[49]

Types of Bleaching Therapy

Generally, bleaching can first be categorized into treatment for either endodontically treated teeth or vital teeth. Furthermore, endodontically treated teeth can be bleached in the office or outside of the office. Outside-the-office (at-home) treatment consists of applying a material inside or outside the tooth that actively lightens the tooth while the patient is away from the office. The in-office technique accomplishes all lightening during treatment in the office. Vital tooth bleaching also offers a choice between an in-office technique or an at-home technique. In-office techniques include the application of a bleaching material to teeth isolated by a rubber dam and may include activation of the process by heat or light. At-home bleaching uses a different bleaching agent applied in a custom-fit tray that the patient wears at home, usually while sleeping.

Factors Affecting Both the In-Office and At-Home Bleaching Processes

Several factors must be considered carefully before bleaching is begun and then controlled during the process to ensure maximum benefit.

Surface Cleanliness

All surface debris must be removed to distinguish intrinsic stains from extrinsic staining and to ensure that the agent has maximum contact with the tooth surface. However, bleaching should be delayed for several days after dental prophylaxis to allow any gingival or tooth sensitivity related to the prophylaxis to abate.

Concentration of Peroxide

The higher the concentration of peroxide, the more rapid the lightening effect, although the effect is not linear (ie, 20% is not twice as fast as 10%).[50,51] In-office bleaching materials are usually supplied in concentrations of 35% hydrogen peroxide, although some concentrations may be as high as 50%. The caustic nature of 35% to 50% hydrogen peroxide mandates that the soft tissues be isolated from any possible contact with the bleaching material. Tissue contact results in an immediate chemical burn (Fig 15-3).[46] The usual concentration of the at-home bleaching agents is 10% carbamide peroxide (equal to approximately 3.4% hydrogen peroxide), which is relatively safe in contact with soft tissue. The range of concentrations of carbamide peroxide may vary from 5%

to 35%. When evaluating concentrations of peroxide for appropriate bleaching techniques, it is important to distinguish hydrogen peroxide from carbamide peroxide because of their radically different safety indices and effects on tissue. In addition, carbamide peroxide is much more stable than hydrogen peroxide; it has a shelf life of 1 to 2 years compared to only a few weeks for hydrogen peroxide. A 10% solution of carbamide peroxide is approximately 3.4% hydrogen peroxide and 6.5% urea. Concentrations higher than 10% carbamide peroxide may cause increased tooth sensitivity, tissue irritation, or increased tooth surface alterations.[52]

Temperature (In-Office Bleaching)

The higher the temperature, the faster the rate of oxygen release and, therefore, the faster the rate of the reaction. An increase of 10°C doubles the rate of chemical reaction.[53–56] However, this does not necessarily alter the rate of the color change.[48] Additionally, temperatures elevated to an uncomfortable level may result in tooth sensitivity or even irreversible pulpal inflammation. Bleaching materials are always applied without anesthesia to avoid overheating the tooth. Nonvital teeth should not be heated to a temperature higher than one acceptable for a vital tooth.

pH

Hydrogen peroxide may have an acidic pH to help preserve its potency during shipping and storage. The optimum pH for hydrogen peroxide in bleaching is 9.5 to 10.8. A pH of 10.8 produces a 50% faster rate of bleaching than a pH of 9.5.[50,57] Most carbamide peroxide materials approved by the American Dental Association have a pH of approximately 7. Materials with a significantly lower pH can cause tooth surface alterations by their acidic nature. However, carbamide peroxide breaks down quickly into hydrogen peroxide and urea when applied. Urea is primarily responsible for raising the pH in the oral cavity above 8 for a number of hours.

Time

In addition to the concentration, the degree of bleaching is directly related to the amount of time that the bleaching agent is in contact with the tooth. The longer the contact, the more lightening will occur (until the plateau is reached); however, the longer the bleaching agent is in contact with the teeth, the greater the likelihood of tooth sensitivity.[57,58]

Sealed Environment

The bleaching efficiency of hydrogen peroxide is apparently increased when it is in a sealed environment. This is important for the nonvital tooth bleaching technique.[59]

Additives

Many of the peroxides have additives to alter the handling characteristics or patient acceptability of the product. Materials may be added to liquid hydrogen peroxide to form a gel for easier handling and safety, but this may also reduce the efficacy of the material. Carbamide peroxide may also have various ingredients added to promote thickness, stickiness, or viscosity. Carbamide peroxide can have many different base vehicles, including variations of glycerin, glycol, and toothpaste-like materials. Additionally, it is manufactured in many flavors, and some of the flavoring additives can cause mild adverse responses in certain patients.

Techniques for bleaching both vital and endodontically treated teeth are well accepted and have a good safety record.[29,60,61] Although the specific techniques for bleaching endodontically treated teeth vary from those for bleaching vital teeth, the principle remains essentially the same. Both rely on oxidation of the organic chromatic components. The techniques can be divided into the general categories of nonvital bleaching and vital bleaching.

Nonvital Bleaching

Endodontically treated teeth are especially susceptible to discolorations from blood products caused by trauma or endodontic therapy. A classic bleaching method uses 30% hydrogen peroxide applied to the pulp chamber in one of two techniques (Fig 15-4). The thermocatalytic technique uses heat applied several times during a 30-minute period to activate the solution in the pulp chamber, after which the solution is rinsed from the chamber. The alternative method, called a *walking bleach*, uses a mixture of 30% hydrogen peroxide and sodium perborate to make a paste that is sealed into the chamber to permit activation of the solution over several days. The two techniques are equally effective.[62] Internal bleaching by either method has been shown to return teeth to their desired color in 83% to 91% of cases.[63,64] Other options include the use of sodium perborate alone or 10% carbamide peroxide sealed in the pulp chamber.

The effect brought about by internal bleaching is not long term in most cases, however. Within 1 to 5 years, only 35% to 50% of the teeth maintain their esthetically pleasing appearance.[63–65] Therefore, the process must be repeated periodically. Unfortunately, re-bleaching presents a problem for a tooth in which the access preparation was filled with resin composite. Attempting to re-bleach would require removal of the previously bonded resin composite restoration. This removal generally results in additional loss of tooth structure, which weakens the tooth. A better treatment option once the tooth has been bleached internally and restored with

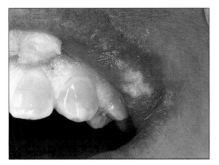

Fig 15-3 A high concentration of hydrogen peroxide can produce a chemical burn, as shown on this patient's lip.

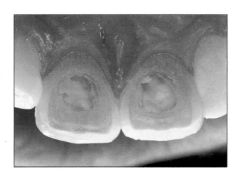

Fig 15-4 The access opening allows placement of bleaching agent directly into the pulp chamber.

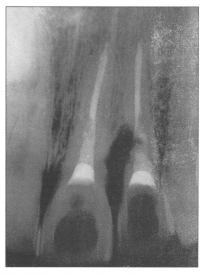

Fig 15-5 A radiograph reveals severe external root resorption in the lateral incisor. (Courtesy of Dr Sandra Madison.)

resin composite is to bleach the tooth externally using the same techniques used for vital teeth.

A more serious problem that affects about 7% of the teeth that have undergone internal bleaching is the occurrence of external root resorption[65–67] (Fig 15-5), which often causes tooth loss.[65,68–70] While the causes of root resorption are not fully known, a review of the literature indicates a number of possible causes. The patients in which root resorption occurred tended to be younger than 25 years old, and most had had traumatic injury. Some underwent bleaching with the application of heat and some did not, but heat does appear to be a causative factor. Animal studies have shown a cause-and-effect relationship between internal bleaching with 30% hydrogen peroxide and resorption, with a resorption incidence of 18% to 25% when heat was applied[71,72] and 0% to 6% without heat application.[71,73] Any one of several factors may also need to be present for resorption to occur, including: *(1)* deficiency in the cementum, exposing the cervical dentin to the oral cavity (normally affecting approximately 10% of the population); *(2)* injury to the periodontal ligament, triggering an inflammatory response (trauma); *(3)* infection, sustaining the inflammation; *(4)* lack of a seal over the gutta-percha; *(5)* high heat; and *(6)* high concentration of hydrogen peroxide.

Cementum deficiencies expose permeable dentin that can allow toxic substances and bacteria from within the chamber and root canals to emerge at the root surface, where they may cause an inflammatory process in the periodontal ligament.[74] A 30% solution of hydrogen peroxide is caustic enough to alter the chemical structure of cementum and dentin,[75] decrease their microhardness[76] and resorbability,[77] and enhance transtubular movement of bacteria.[78] The solution diffuses through the radicular dentinal tubules at an enhanced rate if cementum deficiencies are present[79] and when heat is applied.[80] These data indicate that internal bleaching with 30% hydrogen peroxide is not as safe as originally believed. However, in addition to cementum defects, a history of trauma and marked overheating are major factors in resorption.

Research has been conducted to determine if a protective restorative material can be placed in the cervical portion of the tooth to prevent this problem (Fig 15-6). Unfortunately, this barrier layer reduces the diffusion but does not prevent it[72,81] and does not necessarily protect the tooth against root resorption.[82] However, most of the teeth reported with cervical resorption did not have a barrier placed over the gutta-percha. It is not prudent to use heat or high concentrations of peroxide, and a barrier layer should be placed over the gutta-percha.

An alternative to hydrogen peroxide is sodium perborate used alone. The results of an in vitro study[83] demonstrated that after three applications, there was no difference in the efficacy of sodium perborate mixed with water and sodium perborate mixed with either 5% or 30% hydrogen peroxide. Another study[84] showed no root resorption after 3 years using sodium perborate, with a 90% esthetic success rate initially and a 49% esthetic success rate after 3 years. A newer technique involves the placement of 10% carbamide peroxide

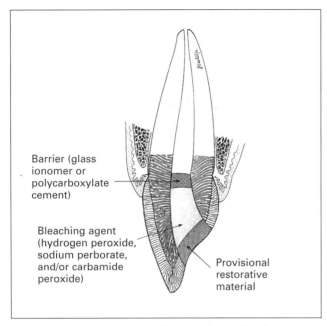

Barrier (glass ionomer or polycarboxylate cement)

Bleaching agent (hydrogen peroxide, sodium perborate, and/or carbamide peroxide)

Provisional restorative material

Fig 15-6 The restorative material blocking the canal at the cemento-enamel junction decreases dispersion of the bleaching agent through the root dentin.

sealed into the chamber. This lower concentration of peroxide also provides a large safety margin.

Another technique, which has limited application, is the practice of preparing the tooth as for the walking bleach technique combined with the at-home tray technique. The pulp chamber is left open, allowing the patient to place 10% carbamide peroxide inside the chamber and, at the same time, apply it externally with the tray. This technique, called *inside-outside bleaching*, is very effective.[85] However, it is best suited for patients who are very responsible and capable of applying the solution intraorally. With this technique, a barrier layer should be placed over the gutta-percha to prevent contamination of the root canal.

The initial esthetic success rate of internal bleaching is limited and may be temporary. Satisfactory results, when achieved, usually persist for 1 to 3 years, although they may be permanent. For the best combination of safety and effectiveness, the recommended treatment for internal bleaching is sodium perborate mixed with water or 10% carbamide peroxide, used after the placement of a protective barrier material in the cervical area.

Vital Bleaching

Vital bleaching may be accomplished by either of two techniques, each with some variations. The in-office technique currently is not as popular as the at-home technique, but it has historically met with success, and there are some definite indications for its use (Fig 15-7).

In-Office Technique

In-office bleaching of vital teeth generally uses a 35% hydrogen peroxide solution placed directly on the teeth and may involve application of light and/or heat to activate or enhance the peroxide release.[15,86] Because the hydrogen peroxide concentration is so high, soft tissues must be very well protected to prevent injury (Fig 15-8).[46] This technique is intended to produce the bleaching effect with limited need for patient compliance. It is indicated for achieving more rapid results or for patients who may have difficulty following the regimen for the at-home technique. There are several potential disadvantages, however. The fee is usually higher because more chair time is required; there is a possibility of tissue injury from the more potent agent used; and the results may not be as good as with the slower at-home method. It may require more than one treatment visit to achieve the desired results.[87] In fact, manufacturers of in-office bleaching systems usually recommend at-home bleaching after the in-office treatment is completed.[88] With in-office bleaching, a portion of the whitening effect is temporary and is due to dehydration of teeth from the isolation technique. Dehydration alone has been shown to cause a transient 3- to 12-shade change (on a Vita Classic shade guide), or an E of 6.7, after 1 hour.[66,89] The effects of in-office bleaching using rubber dam isolation must be evaluated after 1 to 2 weeks to allow rehydration of the teeth to a stable shade.

Dentist-Supervised At-Home Technique

At-home bleaching is the more commonly used bleaching process because it is easy to perform and is usually less expensive for the patient. It uses a custom-fit tray (Fig 15-9) with a 10% solution of carbamide peroxide (approximately equal to a 3.4% solution of hydrogen peroxide). Although the process requires longer contact time compared to the in-office bleaching technique,[90] it is safe, and the results are generally excellent. Products carrying the "ADA accepted" label have passed a rigorous set of safety and efficacy standards.[60,91–94] Manufacturers have offered carbamide peroxide in a variety of concentrations, ranging from 10% to 20% or higher, but the best combination of safety, limited side effects, and speed of action is obtained with a 10% solution. A survey indicated that 90% of the dentists surveyed used a 10% carbamide peroxide for at-home bleaching of vital teeth.[95]

More recently hydrogen peroxide products have been introduced for day wear of trays. Hydrogen peroxide is very unstable and is generally only active for 30 to 60 minutes. Hence, instructions for hydrogen peroxide products typically

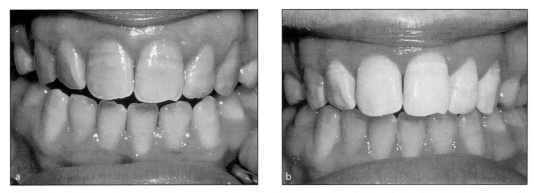

Fig 15-7 In-office bleaching can produce very good results quickly. (Courtesy of Dr Sandra Madison.) *(a)* Prior to bleaching. *(b)* After one bleaching session.

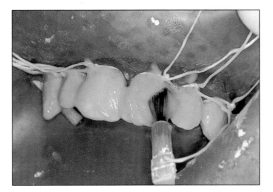

Fig 15-8 The rubber dam protects the soft tissues from the hydrogen peroxide bleach during an in-office bleaching procedure.

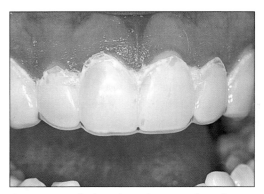

Fig 15-9 A well-adapted tray better confines the carbamide peroxide to the target teeth in the at-home technique.

recommend use for 1 hour or less per application.[96] Carbamide peroxide is active for up to 10 hours, with about 50% of the active agent being used in the first 2 hours.[2,97] Carbamide peroxide is designed for night application to achieve the maximum benefit.[19,98,99]

Safety Factors

Safety concerns include the potential for tooth/pulpal problems, irritation of periodontal or other oral tissues, and systemic effects.

Tooth and Pulpal Problems

Short-term pulpal response varies from patient to patient and even from tooth to tooth. Peroxide does penetrate through the tooth to the pulp in a matter of minutes.[100] Therefore, it can produce sensitivity,[29] but the pulp remains healthy and the sensitivity is completely reversible.[53,56,100] It is important that the process be carefully monitored to avoid creating

great sensitivity in the teeth. The patient should not be anesthetized for an in-office procedure, so that he or she will be able to detect any onset of discomfort. Patients undergoing at-home bleaching must also be informed that minor sensitivity occurs in as many as 2 in 3 patients. Double-blind studies have reported sensitivity in 25% to 70% of patients. However, these studies also show that 20% to 30% of the patients report sensitivity when a placebo is used and 18% report sensitivity just from wearing the bleaching tray without any gel.[33]

If sensitivity occurs, there are a number of approaches that can involve either passive treatment or active treatment. Passive treatment involves shortening the duration or frequency of treatment or interrupting the process for a day or more to allow the teeth to recover. The procedure can then be resumed. Active treatment involves the application of medicaments using the same bleaching tray. Historically, fluoride has been applied for sensitivity. Fluoride acts as a tubule blocker to limit the fluid flow to the pulp.[101] Even fluoride treatment prior to initiating bleaching may reduce sensitivity. A more

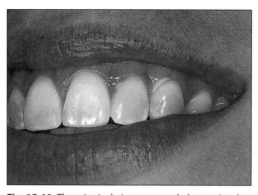

Fig 15-10 The gingival tissue around the canine has been chemically burned by contact with 35% hydrogen peroxide.

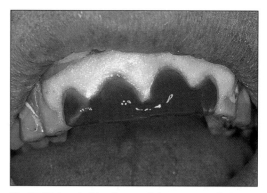

Fig 15-11 A resin "dam" around the target teeth. A 35% hydrogen peroxide bleach has been applied.

direct treatment is the application of 3% to 5% potassium nitrate gel in the tray. Potassium nitrate preparations are available from several bleaching agent manufacturers. Potassium nitrate penetrates the tooth to the pulp and has a numbing or calming effect on nerve transmission.[102,103] Potassium nitrate is found in many desensitizing toothpastes but generally takes 2 weeks to be effective via tooth brushing. However, application of a potassium nitrate preparation in the tray for 10 to 30 minutes before or after bleaching can reduce or eliminate sensitivity in many patients. Often treatment for sensitivity is a combination approach involving alteration of duration or frequency of treatment and use of medications, including anti-inflammatory medications, desensitizing toothpastes, and desensitizing medicaments applied in the tray. A combination of potassium nitrate and fluoride may be used in the tray to optimize the results.[104–106]

Questions have been raised about the effect of bleaching on the structure of the tooth itself. Recent studies have shown that low-pH solutions can produce a detectable loss of calcium from the surface enamel, along with a slight loss in surface hardness to a depth of approximately 25 μm.[27,107–109] However, this loss has not been shown to be significant because the surface quickly remineralizes after the procedure is completed.[110–114] In fact, there is less change in the calcium content of the tooth and surface hardness from 6 hours of bleaching with 10% carbamide peroxide than when a carbonated drink is consumed in a 2- to 3-minute period. No noticeable change in the surface luster and topography is seen clinically.

Soft Tissue Response

The more powerful in-office bleaching agents (30% to 35% hydrogen peroxide) can easily produce tissue burns, turning the tissue white (Fig 15-10).[115–117] If the exposure is limited in

time and quantity, it is quickly reversible with no long-term consequences. Rehydration and application of an antiseptic ointment (eg, Orabase B, Colgate Oral Pharmaceutical) quickly return the color to the tissue, reassuring the patient that the problem is not permanent.[118] Nevertheless, it can cause significant temporary discomfort and some alarm when first seen. It is important to protect soft tissues with a rubber dam or other means to avoid tissue burns (Fig 15-11).

Although soft tissue irritation during at-home bleaching has been reported,[119] the irritation is most likely the result of an ill-fitting tray rather than the agent itself.[120] Reports of harmful effects to soft tissues from hydrogen peroxide indicate that the effects resulted from dosages and exposure times that greatly exceeded those prescribed in any at-home bleaching technique. At-home agents containing 10% carbamide peroxide are not potent enough to produce significant or long-lasting effects on the soft tissues.[121]

Studies have indicated that approximately one third of patients experience no detectable side effects after bleaching, and the other two thirds experience only minor transitory tooth sensitivity and/or tissue irritation of short duration.[31,82] When examined at the cellular level, these effects on the soft tissue are less than or equal to those produced by commonly accepted dental medicaments such as eugenol and endodontic sealers.[122] The toxicity and mutagenicity of hydrogen peroxide are dose related. Concentrations used in the at-home bleaching technique are not sufficient to be of concern. A low dose of hydrogen or carbamide peroxide over a long time actually allows the cells of the oral tissues to adjust to the dosage even if it is increased beyond the original tolerable dosage. In the long history of these materials involving tissue contact in patients ranging in age from infancy[123,124] to old age, there has been no demonstrated problem.

Systemic Effects and Responses

There is more concern about possible adverse effects of at-home bleaching agents, although their concentrations are far less than those of the in-office bleaches. In-office bleach is carefully controlled and placed on the teeth only, avoiding contact with soft tissues. The patient swallows no solution. Very little, if any, of the agent is absorbed systemically. The at-home bleach, applied in the tray, unavoidably contacts soft tissues in many areas over several hours each day. Additionally, it is likely that the patient swallows small amounts of very dilute hydrogen peroxide during the bleaching procedure.[94] This has not proven to be a problem, however. Although very high concentrations of some forms of peroxide are mutagenic,[125,126] physiologic mechanisms quickly repair any limited damage that might occur.[127] Low levels of hydrogen peroxide do not cause real problems.[128] In fact, hydrogen peroxide has been approved as safe for use as a human food additive. The Food and Drug Administration recognizes 3% hydrogen peroxide and 10% to 15% carbamide peroxide as GRAS (generally recognized as safe) for oral use. Carbamide peroxide is also used for the treatment of candidiasis in newborn infants.[123] The conclusion, after decades of use and extensive research, is that the use of low concentrations of hydrogen peroxide in bleaching teeth is safe.[114,129–132]

Indications for Bleaching

The primary indication for bleaching is patient dissatisfaction with tooth color. While the source of the discoloration affects the degree of success and the rapidity with which it can be eliminated or minimized, it has been shown that even the most persistent discolorations can be lightened if the treatment is sufficiently extended. Bleaching may be done in lieu of bonded resin composite restorations, porcelain veneers, or crowns to improve the tooth color. Patients may be satisfied with the results of bleaching such that more invasive treatment is not needed. Even if laminate veneers are to be placed, the lighter color of the bleached teeth allows lighter and more translucent veneers, enhancing the natural appearance. Other indications include extending the esthetic life of existing crowns that are lighter than the natural teeth by returning the color of the natural teeth to the shade of the crown, or whitening a single dark tooth to the desired shade.

Contraindications for Bleaching

Although bleaching is a safe and effective aid in improving the appearance of the teeth, not every discolored tooth requires bleaching. Superficial or extrinsic stains may be completely removed by a rubber cup with prophylaxis paste or by light abrasion with a rotary polishing device. The removal of discolored carious tooth structure and/or a dark restoration and placement of a tooth-colored material may well make a marked improvement in the appearance of a tooth. Patients with hypersensitive teeth are generally not good candidates for bleaching, although management of the sensitivity may allow successful bleaching of their teeth. In-office bleaching advocates do not use bleaching for children with large pulps or teeth with cracks. At-home bleaching is generally not indicated for pregnant women or patients allergic to the ingredients in the carbamide peroxide preparations. Roots of teeth do not bleach as well as anatomic crowns, so patients with gingival recession that exposes roots will display yellow tooth structure in those areas.

There are few contraindications to bleaching. Because there is some evidence that peroxides may enhance the effect of known carcinogens, it may be prudent to have the patient forego tobacco use during the period of the bleaching process.[30,133,134] Although there is no evidence that bleaching is harmful to the fetus or to infants, it has been recommended that pregnant and lactating women do not undergo bleaching because of the increased potential for gingival irritation.[93,135] Patients with existing esthetic restorations must be warned that when bleaching lightens the natural tooth color, restorations may appear relatively dark and unattractive. The need for new restorations that are lighter in shade should be discussed with the patient prior to bleaching.

Contraindications for in-office bleaching with high concentrations of hydrogen peroxide include teeth with extremely large pulps, exposed root surfaces, or severe enamel loss. In one study of at-home bleaching, Nathanson and Parra[136] determined that there was no noticeable difference in the sensitivity reported by young patients compared to sensitivity reported by older patients, so larger pulp size may not be a factor. In a study of at-home bleaching with carbamide peroxide, Leonard and Bentley[33] determined that there were no predictors of individuals who would experience sensitivity other than a history of sensitive teeth and more than one bleach application per day.[137] All other delineators, such as pulp size, exposed dentin, cracks, gingival recession, caries, gender or age of the patient, or other physical characteristics, were not predictive of tooth sensitivity. Because bleaching tends to produce some sensitivity under ordinary circumstances, patients with preexisting tooth sensitivity must be cautioned that increased sensitivity, albeit transitory, will occur. If this is likely to be a problem, the placement of a desensitizing solution containing fluoride or potassium nitrate can be alternated with the bleaching solution.[138,139] This will increase the time needed to achieve the desired lightness of the teeth.

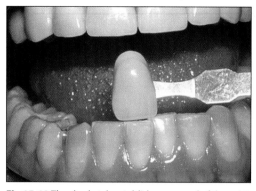

Fig 15-12 The shade tab establishes a record of the existing color.

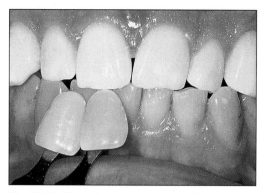

Fig 15-13 Note the strong contrast between the bleached maxillary teeth and the unbleached mandibular teeth (which match the shade tab).

Patients with a history of temporomandibular disorder (TMD) may not be good candidates for at-home bleaching or may need to wear the tray during waking hours only. A special tray design that covers only the facial surfaces of the teeth may also be helpful.[140] Bruxers also may have to alter wear times for at-home treatment or have several trays fabricated during treatment.

Bleaching does interfere with the bonding process because it results in a very high oxygen concentration in the enamel and dentin, which hinders polymerization of the resin composite.[118,141,142] A delay of 7 to 10 days after bleaching allows dissipation of the excess oxygen from the tooth structure so that there is no interference with the polymerization reaction.[143] Waiting 1 to 2 weeks is also important in resin bonding to allow the shade of the bleached teeth to stabilize.

Bleaching agents have the beneficial side effects of being both bacteriostatic and anticariogenic. They also discourage plaque formation. The bleaching process can begin prior to removal of caries lesions and can be performed at the same time as treatment of gingivitis.[144,145]

Treatment Planning and Patient Education

A basic understanding of the cause(s) of discoloration is necessary to better predict the course and duration of the treatment as well as the final outcome. Whether to use at-home or in-office bleaching is based on the patient's preference, financial situation, and ability and willingness to comply with the treatment protocol. Patients who are unwilling or unable to comply with the protocol for the at-home technique, or who are eager to finish bleaching in a very short period of time regardless of cost, are good candidates for in-office bleaching. Subsequent treatment procedures should be planned so that limits of the bleaching treatment are discussed in the context of solving the patient's other dental problems. The patient should be informed that the shade of any restoration placed previously will not be altered by bleaching, so bleaching should be performed before any esthetic restorative procedures. Information concerning the decision to bleach or not, as well as the rationale and costs for choosing a particular method, must be recorded to verify that the dentist and patient agree on the procedures and their predicted outcomes.

Shade Selection and Record Collection

A shade guide identifies the existing tooth color to establish the baseline (Fig 15-12). If the shade guide does not have a match for the tooth color, it should be estimated. It is important that the patient agree that the shade tab is the closest match to the current shade of the teeth. This shade should be recorded in the chart with the patient observing the entry. The patient may have difficulty recalling the original shade and, therefore, may be disappointed in the outcome because he or she may not believe that significant change has occurred. The patient should see the shade tab that represents the predicted target shade. The contrast between the tab representing the original shade and one showing the shade to be achieved may lead to more realistic patient expectations, especially if the patient already has light teeth. The best way to ensure patient awareness of the effect of bleaching is to bleach one arch at a time. In addition to minimizing the potential for TMD problems, it preserves one arch for an ongoing comparison of progress. Another reason for treating one arch at a time is to enable determination of the effectiveness of the bleaching procedure before the patient commits to bleaching of the second arch. If the first arch is deemed a success by the patient, the opposing arch can be bleached for an additional fee (Fig 15-13).

Impressions for diagnostic casts are necessary if bleaching trays are to be used for the at-home technique. For added documentation, close-up photographs of the patient's teeth and a full-face photograph of the patient with a full smile should be kept as part of the patient's record. The photographs may be helpful in treatment planning, in reminding the patient of the original appearance of the teeth, and as a record for a ceramist fabricating any restorations. Photographs should be taken at a consistent magnification and pose. Placing the incisal edges of the teeth in the bleached arch against the incisal edges of the teeth in the unbleached arch enables the best comparison of the before and after shades, emphasizing the effect of bleaching.

Patient Education

The patient should be well informed about the bleaching procedure. Information explaining the process, precautions, possible side effects, number of applications or appointments, anticipated total time for bleaching, and likely results should be provided. The dentist should also explain why the particular technique has been chosen. The steps of the procedure and consequences for not following them should be outlined. For the at-home technique, loading and insertion of the bleaching tray should be demonstrated and the length for each wear session outlined. Any questions the patient might have should be answered at this appointment. The patient should sign a consent form indicating that he or she has been informed about the procedure, its expected outcome, and any potential side effects. The consent form should also list other treatment options for this condition and state that those remain if the bleaching is not successful.

Bleaching Techniques

In-Office Technique for Vital Teeth

In-office bleaching utilizes a much more potent agent (usually a 35% solution of hydrogen peroxide, as opposed to a 10% solution of carbamide peroxide for the at-home technique). This powerful agent (10 times as powerful as a 10% carbamide peroxide) is necessary to produce the rapid improvement expected of an in-office procedure (Figs 15-14a and 15-14b).

The oral/perioral structures must be protected during the procedure. Generally, this is best accomplished with a well-placed rubber dam tightly adapted around the cervical areas of the teeth.[146,147] For the single isolated tooth, it may be possible to protect the gingiva with cotton rolls and a "liquid rubber dam" (light-polymerized resin). The light-polymerized resin is ejected onto the gingival tissues surrounding the target teeth and then light cured to form a flexible protective shield that can be removed easily. Any material covering the teeth should be trimmed to the proper extension to allow the bleach to reach that area. Cotton rolls and cheek retractors may be needed to protect the lips and tongue.

The teeth should not be anesthetized. This allows the patient to note any developing discomfort so the dentist can avoid overtreating the teeth during the several applications of the solution occurring in the appointment. The patient becomes the "control" for the number of applications that should be placed; he or she should be questioned after each application about any tooth discomfort or tingling in the gingiva, indicating a gap beginning between the teeth and the rubber dam. If any tooth discomfort is experienced, the treatment should be interrupted and continued at a future appointment to allow the teeth to recover. If the patient reports a tingling of the gingival tissues, the procedure should be immediately aborted, the dam removed, and the tissues rinsed with water (with or without baking soda) to neutralize the peroxide and avoid severe tissue burns.

Manufacturers provide their bleaching agents in various forms. Some are very watery, others are in a gel form. Some are packaged as a powder-liquid combination that is mixed to activate and then placed on the teeth (Fig 15-15), while others are provided as a ready-to-place solution in a syringe for direct placement. The solution is applied to the facial and proximal areas of the teeth for the prescribed time interval. If access is limited on the facial aspect because of the presence of restorations, the solution can be placed on the lingual surface. In such cases, the improvement of color, as observed from the facial surface, will take longer to occur. Etching of the enamel is not indicated. Heat treatment is optional. Heat releases the oxygen more rapidly.[148] If heat is to be used to speed the chemical reaction, it should be from a dental curing light or equipment specially fabricated for bleaching procedures.

In-office bleaching generally takes one to six appointments of 45 minutes to 1 hour each, with an average of three to four appointments to reach maximum lightness.[87] To achieve the optimal effect, the bleaching solution should be left on the teeth for the time recommended by the manufacturer. One product signals when the maximum effect of the application has occurred by altering its color (Hi-Light, Shofu).[149] The solution is rinsed off the teeth, and the tooth color evaluated to determine any improvement. The patient must be asked if any tooth sensitivity is occurring. The number of applications to bring about the desired result is not necessarily predictable, although some discolorations (eg, tetracycline stains) are known to be more tenacious. Development of

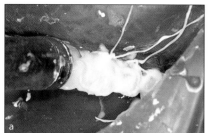

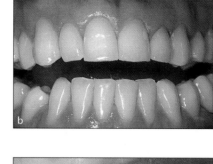

Fig 15-14a The rubber dam is in place, the teeth have been covered with the bleaching agent, and heat is being applied with a curing light.

Fig 15-14b The teeth reveal significant lightening after one session.

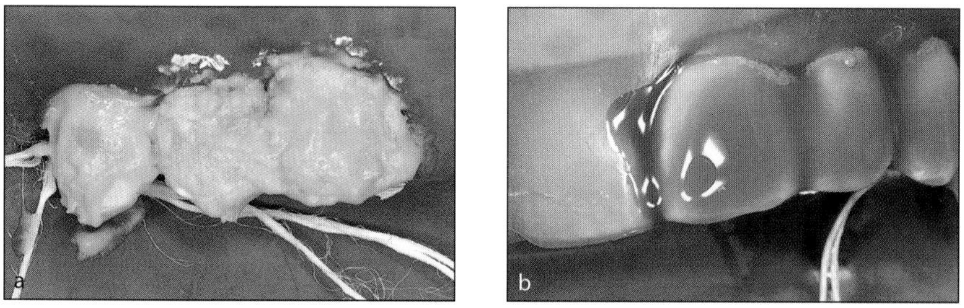

Fig 15-15 In-office bleach can be supplied in two forms: *(a)* a powder-liquid paste or *(b)* a viscous liquid.

discomfort is the single most important limitation to the number of applications per appointment. Appointments for subsequent treatment are scheduled 1 week apart to allow sensitivity to abate. Because the number of appointments necessary to achieve the desired whiteness is variable, the patient should be so informed and the fee per appointment set in advance. Generally, it is recommended that in-office bleaching be followed by at-home bleaching to enhance the effect and to minimize rebound.[88,150]

Laser- or Light-Assisted In-Office Bleaching

Dental lasers and other powerful light sources have been advocated by manufacturers for use in bleaching. It is claimed that they provide a powerful energy source to enhance the action of the hydrogen peroxide by promoting a more rapid release of the bleaching agent. Some concern has been raised over the safety of this use of lasers. Effects on hard tissues depend on the type of laser used, as well as the exposure time.[149] The temperatures created by high-energy light sources, which are influenced by the absorptive properties of enamel and dentin, can be great. The temperature level is also a product of the type of laser used. The argon laser, used appropriately, generates very little temperature rise in the pulp.[151,152]

One manufacturer recommends use of an argon laser with a wavelength of 488 nm for 30 seconds to accelerate the activity of the bleaching gel.[152] The gel is left on the tooth for 3 minutes and then removed. This is repeated four to six times. Another technique uses a CO_2 laser, after the procedure with the argon laser, to encourage deeper penetration of peroxide into the tooth structure.[153] Anecdotal reports have indicated that moderate to severe postprocedural pain and

sensitivity may occur.[153] Pulpal irritation or even necrosis has been demonstrated following CO_2 laser use.[154,155] The ADA does not recommend CO_2 laser use for bleaching. Studies of laser bleaching to date have not indicated any better results than with other in-office techniques, and the results are possibly not as good as those obtained with at-home bleaching.

The argon laser can be used in place of a conventional curing light if the manufacturer's directions are carefully followed. It is important to remember that the hydrogen peroxide performs the bleaching, not the laser.[153] In assessing shade changes produced by an in-office treatment visit, it must be recognized that the rubber dam isolation dehydrates the tooth so it appears lighter in color. Additionally, heat from the bleaching light source also dehydrates the tooth. Changes up to several shades may occur. The tooth then darkens as it rehydrates.[52,89] The laser merely serves as a heat source to activate the bleaching agent in the same way that a conventional curing light does. Its only potential advantage is its faster rate of supplying heat. Its disadvantages are the cost of the laser itself, which translates to higher patient fees, and the potential for damage to pulpal tissues and the surrounding periodontal tissues.

Other manufacturers have made claims about the use of high-intensity lights and their role in tooth whitening. The preponderance of evidence at this time does not support their efficacy in producing a superior result.[156–158]

At-Home Technique

At-home bleaching requires a proper dental and medical history, clinical examination, radiographs of the teeth to be

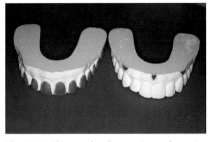

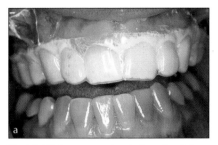

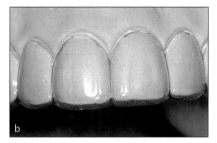

Fig 15-16 The cast has been trimmed to minimize bulk to aid in adapting the tray. Relief areas (for reservoirs) have been added to the cast on the left but not to the one on the right.

Fig 15-17 The tray can be designed as *(a)* nonscalloped, extending up onto the soft tissue, or *(b)* scalloped to the tissue contours around the teeth.

treated, and impressions for tray construction. After tray fabrication, an insertion appointment is required, unless the tray can be fabricated during the first appointment while the patient waits. Some dentists like to see the patient at weekly recall visits to assess progress and compliance, while others see the patient at the completion of treatment. As previously stated, initial treatment of only one arch has advantages. Plans for treatment of sensitivity and determination of total treatment time should be communicated to the patient during the first visit.

Tray Fabrication

Accurate impressions are critical to produce casts on which accurate vacuum-formed trays can be made. Casts should be altered for tray fabrication; this alteration often renders them unsuitable for other purposes. The initial alginate impression, properly handled, may be double-poured to provide an additional cast for other treatment needs.[159] The cast for the bleaching tray should be trimmed to the thinnest and narrowest dimensions possible without damaging surfaces representing the teeth or periodontal structures. Using a model trimmer, the cast is trimmed from the base rather than from the sides, until the vestibule is eliminated. The base of the cast should be as thin as 0.5 inch or trimmed to a horseshoe shape, leaving only the maxillary or mandibular teeth and periodontal tissues remaining, with no palatal or tongue section included. The base should be flat, with the central incisors perpendicular to it (Fig 15-16). This makes it easier to adapt the vacuum-formed tray material around the teeth and avoids the development of folds and wrinkles during fabrication. If the palate or tongue section remains, it is helpful to drill a hole through that section so that the vacuum better adapts tray material in all areas of the cast.

A number of materials have been used in tray fabrication, including materials used in fabricating orthodontic positioners, athletic mouthguards, provisional splints, and anti-snoring

devices. The original nightguard vital bleaching article[24,25] proposed a thick, semirigid material. The newer materials are thinner, softer, and easier to shape and trim and have reduced gingival and occlusal side effects. One system uses a tray supplied by the manufacturer that is custom-fitted to the patient using heat. An alginate impression is not needed. This thermoplastic technique results in a tray formed in the patient's mouth at the first appointment.[160]

Decisions to be made about tray design include whether to scallop the tray and whether to add reservoirs. Some advocates of at-home bleaching were concerned that the agent would harm gingival tissues over time. They recommended a scalloped tray border, positioned 1 mm incisal/occlusal to the soft tissue, to avoid contact of the tray or bleaching agent with the tissue (Fig 15-17).[79,161] This practice is not necessary for successful bleaching but may help in seating the tray when using highly viscous materials, to avoid pressure on the teeth and resulting sensitivity, or when gingival tissues are very delicate.[162–164] Scalloping may be indicated for sticky, non–water-soluble materials, as they tend to adhere to the gingiva and may produce localized irritation. However, scalloping may be counterproductive if a water-soluble material is being applied, as the material is more rapidly washed out of this type of tray by saliva. Additionally, scalloping can be annoying to the tongue or lips, depending on the patient and the teeth-to-tissue relationships. When tissue irritation during an at-home bleaching regimen has been reported, it often resulted from poor adaptation of a rigid tray and because the tongue, lips, and/or cheek rubbed against an edge of the tray.[165]

When using a viscous bleaching agent, it is not necessary to extend the tray to gingival tissue to ensure bleaching in the cervical portions of teeth. However, the tray may contact or even cover gingival tissue with no adverse effect. Watery solutions require tissue contact by the tray in order to maintain the bleaching material inside the tray. If tissue contact is preferred, the tray should not extend into tissue undercuts or be tight enough to blanch tissue. The tray borders should be smooth.

Foam liners for the tray have been advocated to hold the bleaching agent evenly against the teeth by preventing flow of the agent to more dependent areas of the tray. Despite manufacturers' claims that the inclusion of foam liners gives a more rapid bleaching effect, research has failed to demonstrate an advantage.[166] Some techniques incorporate a reservoir on the facial intaglio surface of the tray to hold a greater volume of the agent in the target areas of the teeth to enhance the process[148,167] or to allow bleaching gel to flow from areas of high concentration to areas of reduced concentration.[168] The theory seems sound, but there is little evidence that the creation of reservoirs actually improves bleaching efficacy. It is assumed that the solution, whether in greater volume in a reservoir or in lesser volume because of no reservoir, degrades at the same rate. Some clinicians do not advocate placement of reservoirs in the tray.[26,119,137,169] There may be some benefit to having the extra space provided by the reservoirs, to help in seating the tray and to avoid pressure on the teeth, especially if a very viscous solution is used. One study, however, has indicated no difference in patient comfort with or without tray reservoirs.[170]

Reservoir spaces are formed by using a manufacturer-supplied, light-polymerized resin, placed 0.5 to 1.0 mm thick, on the facial surfaces of the teeth of the cast. The resin spacer should terminate 1.0 mm short of the gingival area and should not extend into the embrasures. Nail polish, die spacer, or tinfoil may also be used to form reservoir spaces. The reservoir design should allow tray borders to contact the tooth. Spacers should not be placed in areas of occlusion (such as incisal aspects of mandibular anterior teeth or lingual aspects of maxillary anterior teeth), since the contact of the opposing teeth will displace the material from the tray.

Patient Instructions for At-Home Bleaching

Patient instructions should address expectations and course of treatment, technique for applying the bleaching agent, frequency and length of time for wearing the tray, tooth sensitivity/tissue irritation problems, interim appointments, and variations in total fee related to course of treatment.

It is critical that the patient understands the process and can make appropriate adjustments in the protocol (eg, discontinuing tray wear for 1 or 2 days if sensitivity begins to develop). The patient must recognize any developing problems early and inform the dentist. While this is a supervised procedure, most of the process occurs away from the dentist, so the patient becomes the progress monitor. The patient should be instructed to place enough bleaching agent into the tray to cover the facial surfaces of the target teeth. This includes the most posterior tooth visible when the patient smiles, laughs, or talks. Seating and removing the tray should be demonstrated to ensure that the patient is able to do so without undue difficulty or harm to the tray or the oral structures. To avoid tissue injury, the tray should be "peeled" from the second molar area rather than being "dug out with fingernails" in the canine region.

Instructions for Tray Wear. The patient should understand that he or she is to wear the tray for 4 or more hours per day or night, but that the specific consecutive 4-hour period is discretionary. Wear for fewer than 4 hours is a waste of agent because it retains its potency for several hours. One study demonstrated that 60% of the active agent remained after 4 hours.[171] The best option is probably for the patient to wear the tray during sleeping hours. Although the agent has lost most of its potency after 5 hours, compliance is much better when the bleaching treatment becomes part of a regular routine. If sensitivity is not a problem, the patient can even have two wearing periods per day. While this speeds the process, it is also likely to provoke tooth sensitivity. The patient should be informed of the potential for this to occur and of the need to reduce time and frequency of bleaching if it does. After the loaded tray is seated, the patient should use a damp cloth or finger to wipe the areas adjacent to the tray borders to remove any excess bleaching agent so that it won't be swallowed. The patient should be reminded to rinse and gently brush the tray after each session before storing it in a cool or room-temperature environment until the next bleaching session.

The bleaching process varies in the amount of time required. Some readily discernible improvement may occur within 2 to 14 days, or it may take as long as 6 to 12 months.[165] The time depends on the type of discoloration, patient compliance, and whether or not any tooth sensitivity occurs. It may be helpful to recall the patient after 5 to 7 days to check progress. The changes may occur somewhat slowly, albeit steadily, so the patient may forget the original shade. The patient can be shown the shade tab representing the original color to contrast it with the new whiteness of the teeth, or the patient can compare the treated maxillary arch with the untreated mandibular arch. At an interim appointment, tray adjustments may be made if necessary. The protocol can be reviewed to ensure that the patient is following it correctly. Alterations in protocol can be made to eliminate or minimize any problems or to speed the process. Some teeth may respond to bleaching more rapidly than others. More severely discolored and less responsive teeth may need more sessions of bleaching than others.[93,172] When isolated problem teeth exist, one approach is to begin treatment of those teeth

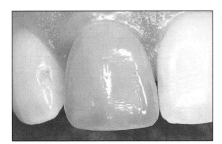

Fig 15-18a The single discolored tooth may require a unique tray design.

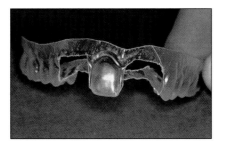

Fig 15-18b The tray is trimmed to fit around the discolored tooth only.

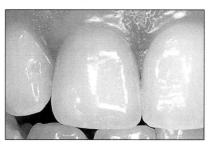

Fig 15-18c The discolored tooth is whitened; other teeth are not affected.

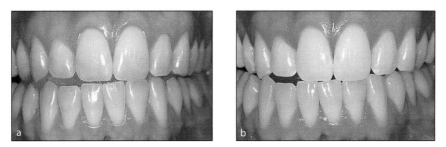

Fig 15-19 Yellow-brown stains usually respond quickly to at-home bleaching. *(a)* Prior to bleaching. *(b)* After 1 month of bleaching the maxillary teeth.

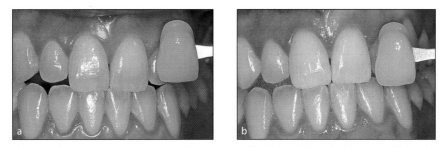

Fig 15-20 Many gray stains respond well to at-home bleaching. *(a)* Prior to bleaching. *(b)* Results after 4+ weeks of bleaching the maxillary teeth.

before bleaching the other teeth (Fig 15-18a to 15-18c). Place the bleaching solution in the area(s) of the tray corresponding to the problem area(s) for a few days before treating all the teeth. The patient should be informed that extra bleaching time for certain teeth may be necessary and that the problem tooth or teeth may become even more noticeable for a short time because the other teeth have whitened more rapidly.

Some teeth exhibit a splotchy look as different portions of the tooth respond at different rates. The patient should be encouraged to continue treatment until the remainder of the tooth achieves the same color. The splotchy areas tend to abate on completion of treatment. Considerable whitening of the teeth is routinely predictable (Figs 15-19 to 15-24).

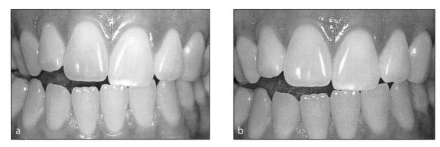

Fig 15-21 White spots become less noticeable when the teeth are whitened. *(a)* Prior to bleaching. *(b)* After bleaching the maxillary teeth. Note that the white spot is unchanged.

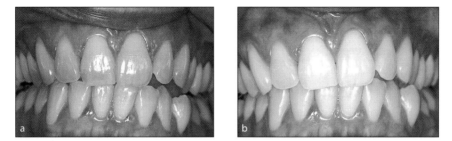

Fig 15-22 Yellow-brown stains can be removed easily with at-home bleaching. *(a)* Prior to bleaching. *(b)* After bleaching.

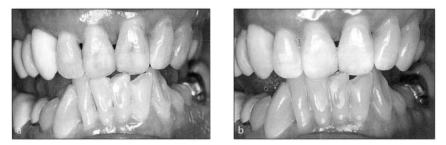

Fig 15-23 Yellow stains can be removed more readily from the coronal portion than from the root of the tooth. *(a)* Prior to bleaching. *(b)* After bleaching the maxillary teeth. The roots retain their yellowish coloration.

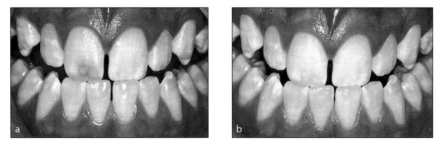

Fig 15-24 Fluorosis stains can be whitened. *(a)* Prior to bleaching. *(b)* After bleaching.

Patient-Managed Home Bleaching Methods

Over-the-counter (OTC) products are available in the form of tray systems, trayless systems, and paint-on products. The fundamental problem with OTC products is that there is no examination and diagnosis of the cause of discoloration. Hence, any effective bleaching treatment may mask symptoms of another problem. Discolored teeth could be caused by abscessed or nonvital teeth, dental caries, internal resorption, dark restorations, stained restorations, or discolored restorations. It is advisable for patients considering bleaching to have a proper examination and radiographs by a dentist, even if they are considering using OTC products.

In the past, OTC bleaching agents did not prove very effective. Although the initial cost of the agent or system was distinctly lower than dentist-prescribed methods, its ineffectiveness led to repeated purchases of the product, so that the final cost was significant and the results often unsatisfactory. Additionally, early reports cited detrimental effects of erosion to tooth structure from overuse of poorly manufactured or formulated solutions.

Recently introduced products have proven to be much more effective in whitening teeth. While the specific mode of application varies among the products, the manufacturers have made the products relatively easy for the patient to apply. One whitening system utilizes adhesive strips containing a relatively high concentration (approximately 6% to 14%) of hydrogen peroxide. The adhesive strips are designed to hold the peroxide against the teeth to allow it to effectively bleach the teeth. Patients are instructed to wear the strips for 30 minutes twice a day for maximum benefit. Studies have shown the whitening strips to be effective[173,174] without significant tooth sensitivity or tissue irritation. They are relatively convenient and less expensive than dentist-supervised at-home techniques. The strips may be difficult for some patients to adapt to the target teeth, especially if the teeth are malaligned. In addition, the strips do not extend past the canines in many people's mouths, so posterior teeth are not whitened. The result may not be pleasing in patients with a broad smile. Few studies have compared strips with daytime tray bleaching and nighttime tray bleaching using the same color measurement criteria as was used in previous tray-bleaching research. However, one study did show that day wear of hydrogen peroxide in the tray was equivalent to strips, but night wear of carbamide peroxide was more efficacious.[143] There continues to be great difficulty in measuring tooth color to assess bleaching changes. Shade guides are nonlinear and are intended for crown shade determination rather than for measuring color changes.[175] Other color-measuring techniques have limitations that cause difficulty in accurately assessing minor color changes.[9,175–178]

The second type of OTC product introduced recently uses a whitening gel applied to teeth with a brush applicator. These products use an anhydrous solution containing 19% sodium percarbonate or 18% carbamide peroxide.[179] The solution has a silicone polymer designed to form a substantive film that will cling to the enamel for an extended period of time. The film is applied to relatively dry and clean tooth surfaces and is worn overnight. Early clinical studies have indicated that these products produce results comparable to or slightly better than those produced by whitening toothpastes.[8,27,173]

A myriad of other OTC products, from toothpastes to chewing gums, claim tooth whitening with little or no research to support their claims. A great many of these products produce whitening by removing extrinsic or surface stains (with abrasives or peroxides), preventing staining (with chemicals), or merely physically removing food debris from already-white teeth (chewing gums).

Manufacturers continue to develop new OTC products. Although new chemistry may be introduced, their focus has been primarily on delivery systems that are easier and faster for the patient to apply.

Techniques for Tetracycline-Stained Teeth

Patients whose teeth have been stained by tetracycline ingestion present a great esthetic challenge. Tetracycline can be deposited in fetal tooth buds if ingested by an expectant mother in the third trimester of pregnancy or by a child during the tooth-formation years, between the ages of 3 to 4 months and 7 to 8 years.[180,181] Tetracycline may also be deposited in the teeth in early adult years if it is taken on a long-term basis for skin conditions (acne), especially during the formation of secondary dentin, during growth periods, and after trauma.[37,38]

Tetracycline has several different analogs (eg, tetracycline, doxycycline, oxytetracycline, minocycline, chlortetracycline, demeclocycline) that may produce several basic colors in the teeth. Colors may include various intensities of gray, blue, brown, and yellow. If seemingly normal yellow teeth are not responsive to the conventional 2 weeks of bleaching treatment, they may, in fact, be tetracycline stained.

Recent research has shown that tetracycline-stained teeth may respond to bleaching treatments, but at a rate different from teeth stained by other agents (Figs 15-25 and 15-26).[182,183] Whereas the normal bleaching time is 2 to 6 weeks, some tetracycline-stained teeth may require 2 to 12 months of

Fig 15-25 *Tetracycline stains are tenacious; results come much more slowly than with other types of stains.*

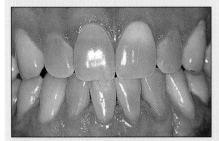

Fig 15-25a Prior to bleaching.

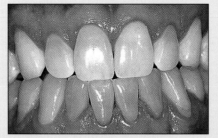

Fig 15-25b Treatment midpoint.

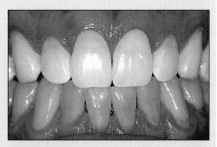

Fig 15-25c After approximately 7 months of at-home bleaching.

Fig 15-26 *A generalized tetracycline stain.*

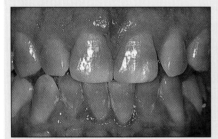

Fig 15-26a Prior to bleaching.

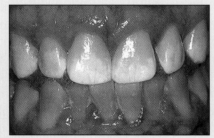

Fig 15-26b After several weeks.

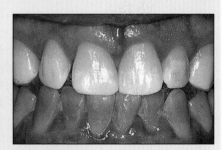

Fig 15-26c After more than 8 months of at-home bleaching.

daily treatment to achieve a significant improvement.[32,184] Tetracycline-stained teeth do not generally lose all discoloration. Although the tooth color is often much improved, teeth may retain some grayish-blue tint.

Research on the longevity of color change achieved indicates that most patients will have some degree of lightening and that 8 in 10 patients can expect to retain that lightening for at least 1 year. Even those patients who experience some regression indicate that they were glad they bleached their teeth and would do it again. A follow-up study showed a very high patient satisfaction rate at 7.5 years after completion of bleaching.[32]

There are several factors to consider when bleaching tetracycline-stained teeth for extended periods of time.[146] First, the location of the stained area has a great impact on the prognosis for success. A tooth generally lightens from the incisal to the gingival area because the tooth gets progressively thicker from incisal to gingival. Teeth heavily stained in the gingival third have the poorest prognosis for complete lightening. The further toward the incisal edge the stain resides, the better the prognosis. In any situation, absolute predictions of success are unrealistic. Patients must understand that each discoloration responds differently and that they may not see results in the first few months.

Extended treatment may increase the potential for tooth sensitivity, although most sensitivity still occurs in the first 2 weeks of treatment. To avoid or mitigate sensitivity, patients may have to titrate their exposure time (from overnight to 2 to 4 hours daily) or frequency (from every night to every second or third night). As with short-term bleaching, the presence of pretreatment sensitivity and the frequency of solution application are the only predictors of possible sensitivity. In extended-treatment situations, sensitivity may be sporadic and subside with no treatment. If it is chronic, patients may wish to apply fluoride or potassium nitrate solutions in the bleaching tray for 30 minutes either as needed or before the application of the bleaching solution. Desensitizing toothpastes containing potassium nitrate, used before the application of the bleaching agent, may also provide some relief or even help prevent sensitivity. A reduction in the concentration of carbamide peroxide may also help.

A practical consideration is the amount of bleaching material necessary for extended treatment and the appropriate fee for service. Practitioners may choose to either increase the total fee or use the initial fee for normal bleaching treatment with a monthly fee for each additional month of treatment. Patients can then pay as they go for extended treatment if there is continued, albeit slow, improvement.

Generally, teeth severely stained in gingival areas are candidates for porcelain veneers or crowns, but it is generally best to attempt bleaching first. Bleaching may achieve adequate results and eliminate the need for veneers, even if the result is not as esthetic as with veneers. The bleaching may have only a limited lightening effect, but it can reduce the amount of opacity necessary in the veneer for masking. This is especially important if the teeth are malaligned, since the preparation may be extended into the darker dentin. Even if the bleaching treatment is ineffective, the patient is aware that the most conservative avenues have been attempted first and is assured that porcelain veneers or porcelain-fused-to-metal or all-ceramic crowns are the best remaining options.

Dentists and physicians are well aware of the effect of tetracycline ingestion on dental esthetics,[25,34,35] although the results of tetracycline absorption in teenagers treated for acne has only recently been reported. Despite this awareness, tetracycline-stained teeth will continue to be seen. Tetracycline is still the drug of choice for outpatient treatment of Rocky Mountain spotted fever and is the most widely prescribed drug for acne. Dentists should consider bleaching a reasonable treatment option for the discoloration resulting from this treatment if the patient is willing to comply with extended treatment and does not expect total elimination of the stain.

Other Considerations

Effect on Restorations

Bleaching has little or no effect on most of the common restorative materials.[90,107] Perhaps its most significant effect is that it lightens teeth enough that previously placed restorations may appear comparatively dark, leading to the question of replacement. Bleaching has no effect on porcelain. It does encourage the release of mercury from some types of amalgam restorations.[185,186] The clinical significance of this is not known.[187] The surface of some types of resin composite is roughened slightly, and the hardness may be very slightly

increased, but neither is clinically significant.[44,63,188–192] Bleaching does affect methacrylate provisional restorative materials, causing them to yellow slightly.[193] Although bleaching releases much oxygen into the tooth, the bond of existing restorations is not weakened. There are no contraindications for bleaching in the presence of existing bonded restorations. However, as previously stated, the oxygen-rich tooth structure does not provide a good surface for bonding new restorations. The oxygen released hinders the polymerization of the resin.[103,154] There may also be changes in the surface morphology that affects the bonding.[54,109,122,194] A delay of a week or more following the bleaching process allows this effect to dissipate so that bonding can effectively be performed.[101] This also allows the tooth shade to stabilize before selection of the restorative material shade. A drying agent, such as acetone, can be used to diminish the oxygen in the outer layers of the tooth if there is concern that oxygen has been retained in the surface.[118]

Alternatives to Bleaching

The alternatives to bleaching are more aggressive in relation to the tooth structure and/or to the gingival tissues. These procedures include microabrasion, macroabrasion, bonded resin composite veneering, porcelain veneers, and porcelain or metal-ceramic crowns. Although all of these are legitimate treatment techniques with proven efficacy, they rely on the removal of tooth structure and/or the addition of materials that have finite replacement life cycles.

Microabrasion and Macroabrasion

One decision in the esthetic treatment planning for a patient is whether to remove discoloration by bleaching or by removal of tooth structure. *Microabrasion* is a process in which the tooth surface is subjected to a combination of an acid and an abrasive (Fig 15-27).[195–197] The acid removes mineral content, leaving the outer 22 to 27 µm weakened enough that the abrasive, with which the acid is mixed, quickly removes the stained outer surface of the tooth. Although the amount of enamel removed is very limited, this abrasive technique alters the outer surface of the enamel as the undesirable coloration is removed or at least modified. The abrasive, usually suspended in a water-soluble gel containing a low concentration of hydrochloric acid, is applied with a rubber cup or stiff bristle brush for 20 to 30 seconds to the enamel.[196] Superficial discolorations can usually be removed from the enamel surface, but it is not possible to know in advance whether the discoloration is superficial. Should the discoloration extend to the dentin or become more visible, a resin composite restoration will need to be placed to seal the defect and restore

Fig 15-27 *Microabrasion represents an alternative method of stain removal or modification.*

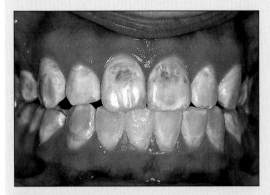

Fig 15-27a Original stains.

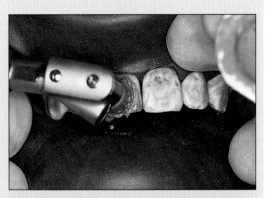

Fig 15-27b Application of acid/abrasive paste.

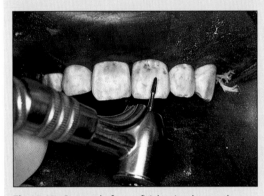

Fig 15-27c Removal of superficial stained enamel.

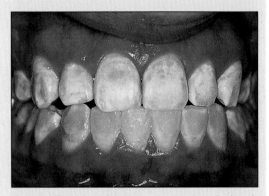

Fig 15-27d Final results. Resin composite can be bonded to conceal remaining discoloration.

contour. The choice of resin composite poses a shade-selection dilemma as to whether the material should match the original tooth color or the color the tooth will be. It is best to bleach first unless the tooth enamel is of a chalky texture. Then when abrasive techniques are initiated, the tooth shade is already established should a resin composite restoration be required. Bleaching has been estimated to remove 80% of brown discolorations.[24] White discolorations are not removed but may be much less noticeable when the surrounding area of the tooth is lightened. If bleaching is unsuccessful, then the more aggressive techniques can be initiated. The patient should be informed of the treatment options (bleaching, abrasion, bonding composite or porcelain) before treatment and should understand the different fees for these procedures. A combination of microabrasion or macroabrasion (described below) and bleaching may be sufficient to bring about the desired result.[105,197]

Another form of abrasion is *macroabrasion*. In this technique, the abrasion can be achieved by applying a fine diamond or carbide-finishing bur to the enamel at relatively low speeds and very light pressure. Some of the same instruments that are used to contour and polish composite restorations may also be used on enamel.[198] The effect is much the same as with the acid/abrasive technique. When using a high-speed handpiece, water should be applied to maintain the coloration of the teeth. As some teeth dehydrate, more subsurface defects may become visible; for these, treatment is not indicated. Air abrasive techniques can also be used quite effectively for microabrasion or macroabrasion. Only fine abrasive particles should be used to avoid overreduction of the tooth. Overreduction can be corrected by adding resin composite to the undercontoured areas.

All three techniques (diamond-stone surface alteration, chemical-physical microabrasion, and kinetic-energy prepara-

Fig 15-28 *Porcelain veneers on tetracycline-stained teeth often do not completely mask the discoloration. Bleaching of exposed enamel surfaces may lighten the teeth as seen through the veneers.*

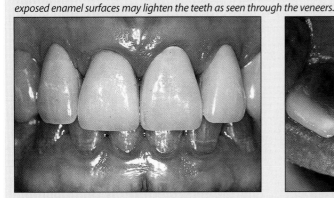

Fig 15-28a Gray stain shows through the porcelain.

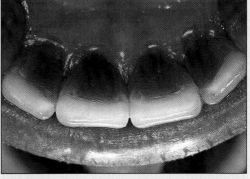

Fig 15-28b Palatal view of the teeth. Note the dark shadow of the teeth under the porcelain.

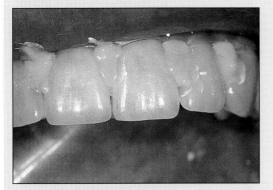

Fig 15-28c Hydrogen peroxide (35%) applied to lingual and proximal surfaces.

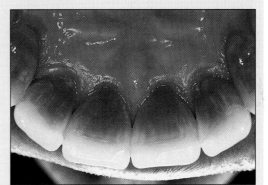

Fig 15-28d Teeth lightened after one appointment.

tion [air abrasion]) rely on the selective reduction of the outer surface of the tooth. While they may be very effective in removing a relatively shallow discolored area, they are not intended to eliminate overall discoloration, especially if it involves the underlying dentin. However, they are valuable techniques for treating limited areas and for supplementing tooth bleaching.[198] For patients with a limited demand for esthetic improvement in the color of the teeth, abrasion alone may satisfy the patient's needs. If abrasion techniques do not produce completely satisfactory results, more extravagant procedures may be performed.

Bleaching Before and After Placement of Veneers

Discolored teeth may be treated with bonded restorations to cover or disguise the underlying stain. It may be possible to place the material with little or no tooth reduction. The esthetic material, such as resin composite or porcelain (see chapter 16), is bonded to the tooth to provide good color and form. However, the natural appearance of the veneered surface depends strongly on some light reflecting from the underlying tooth structure. If the tooth structure is stained too darkly, the discoloration will show through the translucent resin composite or ceramic veneer. The only solution is to make the veneering material thicker and less translucent. To avoid overcontouring the tooth/restoration, it is necessary to remove more of the facial and proximal tooth structure to achieve the esthetic and functional objectives. Successful bleaching therapy eliminates the need for a thicker veneer and more tooth reduction.

Bleaching is possible even for teeth that have already received veneers. Bleach applied to the lingual surface can alter the apparent color of the translucent restoration on the facial surface (Figs 15-28 and 15-29), thereby improving esthetics.[8,9]

Fig 15-29 *Another example of bleaching tetracycline-stained teeth that have porcelain veneers.*

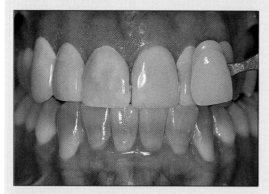

Fig 15-29a Prior to bleaching.

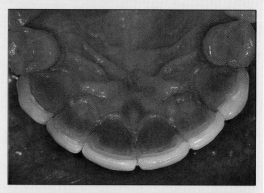

Fig 15-29b Palatal view prior to bleaching. The gray tetracycline stain is obvious.

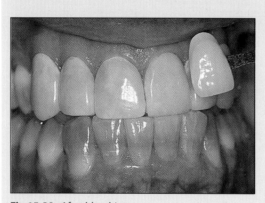

Fig 15-29c After bleaching.

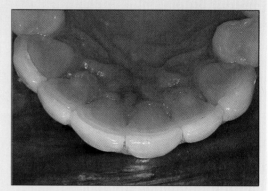

Fig 15-29d Palatal view after bleaching. The bleaching process has lightened the teeth noticeably.

References

1. How WS. Esthetic dentistry. Dent Cosmos 1886;28:741–745.
2. Atkinson CB. Fancies and some facts. Dent Cosmos 1861;3:57–60.
3. M'Quillen JH. Elongation and discoloration of a superior central incisor. Dent Cosmos 1868;10:225–227.
4. Burchard HH. A Textbook of Dental Pathology and Therapeutics. Philadelphia: Lea & Febiger, 1898.
5. Kirk EC. Chemical principles involved in tooth discoloration. Dent Cosmos 1906;48:947–954.
6. Marshall JS. Principles and Practice of Operative Dentistry. Philadelphia: Lippincott, 1901:464–476.
7. Dwinelle WW. Ninth Annual Meeting of American Society of Dental Surgeons, Article X. Am J Dent Sci 1850;1:57–61.
8. Harlan AW. The dental pulp, its destruction, and methods of treatment of teeth discolored by its retention in the pulp chamber or canals. Dent Cosmos 1891;31:137–141.
9. Barker GT. The causes and treatment of discolored teeth. Dent Cosmos 1861;3:305–311.
10. Harlan AW. Proceedings of the American Dental Association—Twenty-third Annual Session. Dent Cosmos 1884;26:97–98.
11. Bogue EA. Bleaching teeth. Dent Cosmos 1872;14:1–3.
12. Kirk EC. Hints, queries, and comments: Sodium peroxide. Dent Cosmos 1893;35:1265–1267.
13. Kirk EC. The chemical bleaching of teeth. Dent Cosmos 1889;31:273–283.
14. Stillwagen TC. Bleaching teeth. Dent Cosmos 1870;12:625–627.
15. Fein RA, Goldstein RE, Garber DA. Bleaching Teeth. Chicago: Quintessence, 1987.
16. Atkinson WH. Bleaching teeth, when discolored from loss of vitality: Means for preventing their discoloration and ulceration. Dent Cosmos 1862;3:74–77.
17. Kirk EC. An American Textbook of Operative Dentistry, ed 2. Philadelphia: Lea Brothers, 1890:540–560.
18. Spalding M, De Assis L, De Assis GF. Scanning electron microscopy study of dental enamel surface exposed to 35% hydrogen peroxide alone, with saliva, and with 10% carbamide peroxide. J Esthet Restor Dent 2003;15:154–165.

19. Atkinson CB. Hints, queries, and comments: Pyrozone. Dent Cosmos 1893;35:330–332.

20. Smith MS, McInnes JW. Further studies on methods of removing brown stains from mottled teeth. J Am Dent Assoc 1942;29:571.

21. Pearson HH. Bleaching of the discolored pulpless tooth. J Am Dent Assoc 1958;56:64–65.

22. Spasser JF. A simple bleaching technique using sodium perborate. N Y Dent J 1961;27:332–334.

23. Haywood VB, Drake M. Research on whitening teeth makes news. N C Dent Rev 1990;7(2):9.

24. Haywood VB, Heymann HO. Nightguard vital bleaching. Quintessence Int 1989;20:173–176.

25. Goldstein FW. New "at-home" bleaching technique introduced. Cosmetic Dent GP 1989;June:6–7.

26. Haywood VB. Overview and status of mouthguard bleaching. J Esthet Dent 1991;3(5):157–161.

27. Slezak B, Petron I, Bagley D, Li Y. Safety profile of a new liquid whitening gel. Compend Contin Educ Dent 2002;23:4–11.

28. Jordan RE, Boksman L. Conservative vital bleaching treatment of discolored dentition. Compend Contin Educ Dent 1984;5:803–805, 807.

29. Haywood VB. Current status of nightguard vital bleaching. Compend Contin Educ Dent 2000;21(suppl 28):S10–S17.

30. Haywood VB. Nightguard vital bleaching: Information and consent form. Esthet Dent Update 1995;6(5):130–132.

31. Haywood VB, Leonard RH, Nelson CF, Brunson WD. Effectiveness, side effects and long-term status of nightguard vital bleaching. J Am Dent Assoc 1994;125:1219–1226.

32. Leonard RH, Haywood VB, Caplan DJ, Tart ND. Nightguard vital bleaching of tetracycline-stained teeth 90 months post-treatment. J Esthet Restor Dent 2003;15:142–153.

33. Leonard RH Jr, Bentley C, Eagle JC, Garland GE, Knight MC, Phillips C. Nightguard vital bleaching: A long-term study on efficacy, shade retention, side effects, and patients' perceptions. J Esthet Restor Dent 2001;13:357–369.

34. Mello HS. The mechanism of tetracycline staining in primary and permanent teeth. J Dent Child 1967;34:478–487.

35. Milch RA, Rall DP, Tobie JE. Bone localization of the tetracyclines. J Natl Cancer Inst 1957;19:87–93.

36. Fein RA. Reviewing vital bleaching and chemical alterations. J Am Dent Assoc 1991;2:55–56.

37. Parkins FM, Furnish G, Bernstein M. Minocycline use discolors teeth. J Am Dent Assoc 1992;123:87–89.

38. Poliak SC, DiGiovanna JJ, Gross EG, Gantt G, Peck GL. Minocycline-associated tooth discoloration in young adults. JAMA 1985;254:2930–2932.

39. Chung HY, Bowles WH. Oxidative changes in minocycline leading to intrinsic dental staining [abstract A1855]. J Dent Res 1989;68(special issue):413.

40. Black GV, McKay FS. Mottled teeth: An endemic developmental imperfection of the enamel of the teeth heretofore unknown in the literature of dentistry. Dent Cosmos 1916;58:129.

41. Dodson DL, Bowles WH. Production of minocyclines pigment by tissue extracts [abstract A1267]. J Dent Res 1991;70(special issue):424.

42. Bowles WH, Thompson LR. Vital bleaching: The effect of heat and hydrogen peroxide on pulpal enzymes. J Endod 1986;12:108–112.

43. Bowles WH, Ugwuneri Z. Pulp chamber penetration by hydrogen peroxide following vital bleaching procedures. J Endod 1987;13:375–377.

44. Cooper JS, Bokmeyer TJ, Bowles WH. Penetration of the pulp chamber by carbamide peroxide bleaching agents. J Endod 1992;18(7):315–317.

45. Haywood VB. Current concepts: Bleaching of vital teeth. Quintessence Int 1997;28:424–425.

46. Haywood VB. Comparison of at-home and in-office bleaching. Dent Today 2000;19(4):44–53.

47. Frysh H. Chemistry of bleaching. In: Goldstein RE, Garber DA (eds). Complete Dental Bleaching. Chicago: Quintessence, 1995.

48. Albers H. Lightening natural teeth. ADEPT Report 1991;2:1–24.

49. McCaslin AJ, Haywood VB, Potter BJ, Dickinson GL, Russell CM. Assessing dentin color changes from nightguard vital bleaching. J Am Dent Assoc 1999;130:1485–1490.

50. Zaragoza VMT. Bleaching teeth: Technique. EstoModeo 1984;9:7–30.

51. Matis BA, Wang Y, Jiang T, Eckert GJ. Extended at-home bleaching of tetracycline-stained teeth with concentrations of carbamide peroxide. Quintessence Int 2002;33:645–655.

52. Nathoo S, Santana E 3rd, Zhang YP, et al. Comparative seven-day clinical evaluation of two tooth whitening products. Compend Cont Educ Dent 2001;22:599–604, 606.

53. Cohen SC. Human pulpal response to bleaching procedures on vital teeth. J Endod 1979;5(5):134–138.

54. Fasanaro TS. Bleaching teeth: History, chemicals, and methods used for common tooth discolorations. J Esthet Dent 1992;4(3):71–78.

55. Robertson WD, Melfi RC. Pulpal response to vital bleaching procedures. J Endod 1980;6:645–649.

56. Seale NS, McIntosh JE, Taylor AN. Pulpal reaction to bleaching of teeth in dogs. J Dent Res 1981;60:948–953.

57. Frysh H, Bowles WH, Baker F, Rivera-Hidalgo G. Effect of pH on bleaching efficiency [abstract A2248]. J Dent Res 1993;72(special issue):384.

58. Dickinson GL. Efficacy of six months of nightguard vital bleaching of tetracycline-stained teeth. J Esthet Dent 1997;9:13–19.

59. Trotman ER. Dyeing and chemical technology of treatable fibers. In: Encyclopedia of Science and Technology, vol 2, ed 6. New York: McGraw-Hill, 1987.

60. Li Y. Peroxide-containing tooth whiteners: An update on safety. Compend Contin Educ Dent Suppl 2000;(18):S4–S9.

61. Ritter AV, Leonard RH Jr, St Georges AJ, Caplan DJ, Haywood VB. Nightguard vital bleaching: 9 to 12 years post-treatment. J Esthet Restor Dent 2002;14:275–285.

62. Freccia WF, Peters DD, Lorton L, Bernier WE. An in vitro comparison of nonvital bleaching techniques in the discolored tooth. J Endod 1982;8(2):70–77.

63. Brown G. Factors influencing successful bleaching of the discolored root-filled tooth. Oral Surg Oral Med Oral Pathol 1965;20:238–244.

64. Howell RA. The prognosis of bleached root-filled teeth. Int Endod J 1981;14(1):22–26.

65. Friedman S, Rotstein I, Libfeld H, et al. Incidence of external root resorption and esthetic results in 58 bleached pulpless teeth. Endod Dent Traumatol 1988;4(1):23–26.

66. al-Nazhan S. External root resorption after bleaching: A case report. Oral Surg Oral Med Oral Pathol 1991;72:607–609.

67. Rotstein I, Torek Y, Misgav R. Effect of cementum defects on radicular penetration of 30% H_2O_2 during intracoronal bleaching. J Endod 1991;17(5):230–233.

68. Gimlin DR, Schindler WG. The management of postbleaching cervical resorption. J Endod 1990;16(6):292–297.

69. Harrington GW, Natkin E. External resorption associated with bleaching of pulpless teeth. J Endod 1979;5(11):344–348.

70. Lado EA, Stanley HR, Weisman MI. Cervical resorption in bleached teeth. Oral Surg Oral Med Oral Pathol 1983;55:78–80.

71. Madison S, Walton R. Cervical root resorption following bleaching of endodontically treated teeth. J Endod 1990;16(12):570–574.

72. Rotstein I, Friedman S, Mor C, et al. Histological characterization of bleaching-induced external root resorption in dogs. J Endod 1991;17(9):436–441.

73. Heller D, Skribner J, Lin LM. Effect of intracoronal bleaching on external cervical root resorption. J Endod 1992;18(4):145–148.

74. Friedman S. Internal bleaching: Long-term outcomes and complications. J Am Dent Assoc 1997;128(suppl):51S–55S.

75. Rotstein I, Dankner E, Goldman A, et al. Histochemical analysis of dental hard tissues following bleaching. J Endod 1996;22(1):23–26.

76. Lewinstein I, Hirschfeld Z, Stabholz A, Rotstein I. Effect of hydrogen peroxide and sodium perborate on the microhardness of human enamel and dentin. J Endod 1994;20(2):61–63.

77. Rotstein I, Lehr Z, Gedalia I. Effect of bleaching agents on inorganic components of human dentin and cementum. J Endod 1992; 18(6):290–293.

78. Heling I, Parson A, Rotstein I. Effect of bleaching agents on dentin permeability to Streptococcus faecalis. J Endod 1995;21(11):540–542.

79. Russell CM, Dickinson GL, Johnson MH, et al. Dentist-supervised home bleaching with ten percent carbamide peroxide gel: A six-month study. J Esthet Dent 1996;8(4):177–182.

80. Rotstein I, Torek Y, Lewinstein I. Effect of bleaching time and temperature on the radicular penetration of hydrogen peroxide. Endod Dent Traumatol 1991;7(5):196–198.

81. Brighton DM, Harrington GW, Nicholls JI. Intracanal isolating barriers as they relate to bleaching. J Endod 1994;20:228–232.

82. Costas FL, Wong M. Intracoronal isolating barriers: Effect of location on root leakage and effectiveness of bleaching agents. J Endod 1991;17(8):365–368.

83. Rotstein I, Zalkind M, Mor C, Tarabeah A, Friedman S. In vitro efficacy of sodium perborate preparations used for intracoronal bleaching of discolored non-vital teeth. Endod Dent Traumatol 1991; 7(4):177–180.

84. Holmstrup G, Palm AM, Lambjerg-Hansen H. Bleaching of discoloured root-filled teeth. Endod Dent Traumatol 1988;4(5):197–201.

85. Settembrini L, Gultz J, Kaim J, Scherer W. A technique for bleaching nonvital teeth: Inside/outside bleaching. J Am Dent Assoc 1997; 128:1283–1284.

86. Goldstein RE. Bleaching teeth: New materials—new role. J Am Dent Assoc 1987;115(special issue):44E–52E [erratum 1988;116:156].

87. Goldstein C. In Practice. Contemp Esthetics Restorative Pract 2002;7:12–17.

88. Miller MB. Power bleaching—Does it work or is it marketing hype? Prac Proced Aesthet Dent 2002;14:636.

89. Russell MD, Gulfraz M, Moss B. In vivo measurement of colour changes in natural teeth. J Oral Rehabil 2000;27:786–792.

90. Haywood VB. Nightguard vital bleaching: Current information and research. Esthet Dent Update 1990;1(2):20–25.

91. Haywood VB, Heymann HO. Nightguard vital bleaching: How safe is it? Quintessence Int 1991;22:515–523.

92. Howard WR. Patient-applied tooth whiteners: Are they safe, effective with supervision? J Am Dent Assoc 1992;123:57–60.

93. Haywood VB. Commonly asked questions about nightguard vital bleaching. J Indiana Dent Assoc 1993;72(5):28–33.

94. Haywood VB. History, safety, and effectiveness of current bleaching techniques and applications of the nightguard vital bleaching technique. Quintessence Int 1992;23:471–488.

95. Christensen GJ. Home-use bleaching survey—1991. Clin Res Assoc Newsletter 1991;15(10):2.

96. Cochran MA, Eckert GJ, Matis BA, Mokhlis GR. A clinical evaluation of carbamide peroxide and hydrogen peroxide whitening agents during daytime use. J Am Dent Assoc 2000;131:1269–1277.

97. Matis BA. Tray whitening: What the evidence shows. Compend Contin Educ Dent 2003;24(4A):354–362.

98. Gaiao U, Matis BA, Cochran MA, Blackman D, Schultz F. Clinical study of 10% carbamide peroxide degradation in bleaching trays [abstract 235]. J Dent Res 1998;77:135.

99. Blackman D, Eckert GJ, Gaiao U, Matis BA, Schults FA. In vivo degradation of bleaching gel used in whitening teeth. J Am Dent Assoc 1999;130:227–235.

100. Thitinanthapan W, Satmanont P, Vongsa VN. In vitro penetration of the pulp chamber by three brands of carbamide peroxide. J Esthet Dent 1999;11:259–264.

101. Gaffar A. Treating hypersensitivity with fluoride varnishes. Compend Contin Educ Dent 1998;19:1088–1097.

102. Hodosh M. A superior desensitizer—Potassium nitrate. J Am Dent Assoc 1974;88:831–832.

103. Markowitz K. Tooth sensitivity: Mechanisms and management. Compend Contin Educ Dent 1993;14:1032–1046.

104. Tam L. Effect of potassium nitrate and fluoride on carbamide peroxide bleaching. Quintessence Int 2001;32:766–770.

105. Haywood VB, Caughman WF, Frazier KB, Myers ML. Tray delivery of potassium nitrate–fluoride to reduce bleaching sensitivity. Quintessence Int 2001;32:105–109.

106. Jerome CE. Acute care for unusual cases of dentinal hypersensitivity. Quintessence Int 1995;26:715–716.

107. Hunsaker KJ, Christensen GJ, Christensen RP. Tooth bleaching and chemicals—Influence on teeth and restorations [abstract A1558]. J Dent Res 1990;69(special issue):303.

108. Swift EJ Jr, Perdigaoa J. Effects of bleaching on teeth and restorations. Compend Contin Educ Dent 1998;19:815–820.

109. Tong LS, Pang MK, Mok NY, King NM, Wei SH. The effects of etching, micro-abrasion, and bleaching on surface enamel. J Dent Res 1993;72:67–71.

110. Ben-Amar L, Liberman R, Gorfil C, Bernstein Y. Effect of mouthguard bleaching on enamel surface. Am J Dent 1995;8:29–32.

111. Leonard RH, Eagle JC, Garland GE, Matthews KP, Rudd AL, Phillips C. Nightguard vital bleaching and its effect on enamel surface morphology. J Esthet Restor Dent 2001;13:132–139.

112. Ernst CP, Marroquin BB, Willershausen-Zonnchen B. Effect of hydrogen peroxide–containing bleaching agents on the morphology of human enamel. Quintessence Int 1996;27:53–56.

113. Shannon H, Spence P, Gross K, Tira D. Characterization of enamel exposed to 10% carbamide peroxide bleaching agents Quintessence Int 1993;24:39–44.

114. Stindt DJ, Quenette L. An overview of Gly-Oxide liquid in control and prevention of dental disease. Compend Contin Educ Dent 1989;10:514–519.

115. Barghi N, Morgan J. Bleaching following porcelain veneers: Clinical cases. Am J Dent 1997;10:254–256.

116. Dorman HL, Bishop JG. Production of experimental edema in dog tongue with dilute hydrogen peroxide. Oral Surg Oral Med Oral Pathol 1970;29(1):38–43.

117. Martin JH, Bishop JG, Guentherman RH, Dorman HL. Cellular response of gingiva to prolonged application of dilute hydrogen peroxide. J Periodontol 1968;39:208–210.

118. Barghi N. Making a clinical decision for vital tooth bleaching: At-home or in-office. Compend Contin Educ Dent 1998;19:831–838.

119. Small BW. Bleaching with 10 percent carbamide peroxide: An 18-month study. Gen Dent 1994;42(2):142–146.

120. Li Y. Toxicological considerations of tooth bleaching using peroxide-containing agents. J Am Dent Assoc 1997;128(suppl):31S–36S.

121. Woolverton CJ, Haywood VB, Heymann HO. Toxicity of two carbamide peroxide products used in nightguard vital bleaching. Am J Dent 1993;6(6):310–314.

122. Yu D, Powell GL, Higuchi WI, Fox JL. Comparison of three lasers on dental pulp chamber temperature. J Clin Laser Med Surg 1993;11:119–122.

123. Dickstein B. Neonatal oral candidiasis: Evaluation of a new chemotherapeutic agent. Clin Pediatr (Phila) 1964;3:485–488.

124. Franchi GJ. A practical technique for bleaching discolored crowns of young permanent incisors. J Dent Child 1953;20:68–69.

125. Abu-Shakra A, Zeiger E. Effects of *Salmonella* genotypes and testing protocols on H_2O_2-induced mutation. Mutagenesis 1990;5:469–473.

126. Zeigler-Skylakakis K, Andrae U. Mutagenicity of hydrogen peroxide in V79 Chinese hamster cells. Mutat Res 1987;192(1):65–67.

127. Cantoni O, Murray D, Meyn RE. Effect of 3-aminobenzamide on DNA strand-break rejoining and cytotoxicity in CHO cells treated with hydrogen peroxide. Biochim Biophys Acta 1986;867:135–143.

128. White WE Jr, Pruitt KM, Mansson-Rahemtulla B. Peroxidase-thiocyanate-peroxide antibacterial system does not damage DNA. Antimicrob Agents Chemother 1983;23:267–272.

129. Freedman GA. Safety of tooth whitening. Dent Today 1990;9(3):32–33.

130. Reddy J, Salkin LM. The effect of a urea peroxide rinse on dental plaque and gingivitis. J Periodontol 1976;47:607–610.

131. Shipman B, Cohen E, Kaslick RS. The effect of a urea peroxide gel on plaque deposits and gingival status. J Periodontol 1971;42(5):283–285.

132. Tartakow DJ, Smith RS, Spinelli JA. Urea peroxide solution in the treatment of gingivitis in orthodontics. Am J Orthod 1978;73:560–567.

133. Berry JH. What about whiteners? Safety concerns explored. J Am Dent Assoc 1990;121:222–225.

134. Pieroli DA, Navarro MFL, Coradazzi JL, Consolaro A. Evaluation of carcinogenic potential of bleaching agents in DMBA-induction model [abstract A2149]. J Dent Res 1996;75(special issue):332.

135. Goldstein RE, Garber DA. Complete Dental Bleaching. Chicago: Quintessence, 1995.

136. Nathanson D, Parra C. Bleaching vital teeth: A review and clinical study. Compend Contin Educ Dent 1987;8:490–497.

137. Leonard RH Jr, Haywood VB, Phillips C. Risk factors for developing tooth sensitivity and gingival irritation associated with nightguard vital bleaching. Quintessence Int 1997;28:527–534.

138. Carrillo A, Arredondo Trevino MV, Haywood VB. Simultaneous bleaching of vital teeth and an open-chamber non-vital tooth with 10% carbamide peroxide. Quintessence Int 1998;29:643–648.

139. Leonard RH Jr. Efficacy, longevity, side effects, and patient perceptions of nightguard vital bleaching. Compend Contin Educ Dent 1998;19:766–774.

140. Robinson FG, Haywood VB. Bleaching and temporomandibular disorder using a half tray design: A clinical report. J Prosthet Dent 2000;83:501–503.

141. McGuckin RS, Thurmond BA, Osovitz S. In vitro enamel shear bond strengths following vital bleaching [abstract A892]. J Dent Res 1991;70(special issue):377.

142. Titley KC, Torneck CD, Smith DC, Adibfar A. Adhesion of composite resin to bleached and unbleached bovine enamel. J Dent Res 1988;67:1523–1528 [erratum 1989;68:inside back cov].

143. Barghi N, Godwin JM. Reducing the adverse effect of bleaching on composite-enamel bond. J Esthet Dent 1994;6:157–161.

144. Leonard RH, Austin SM, Haywood VB, Bentley CD. Change in pH of plaque and 10% carbamide peroxide during nightguard vital bleaching. Quintessence Int 1994;25:819–823.

145. Leonard RH, Bentley CD, Haywood VB. Salivary pH changes during 10% carbamide peroxide bleaching. Quintessence Int 1994;25:547–550.

146. Goldstein RE. In-office bleaching: Where we came from, where we are today. J Am Dent Assoc 1997;128(suppl):11S–15S.

147. Haywood VB. Bleaching of vital and nonvital teeth. Curr Opin Dent 1992;2:142–149.

148. Frazier KB. Nightguard bleaching to lighten a restored, nonvital discolored tooth. Compend Contin Educ Dent 1998;19:810–813 [erratum 1998;19:864].

149. Yamaguchi R, Katoh Y. A photocolorimetic study of vital bleaching with Shofu Hi-Lite [abstract 2441]. J Dent Res 2002;81(special issue):308.

150. Papathanasiou A, Kastali S, Perry R, Kugel G. Clinical evaluation of a 35% hydrogen peroxide in-office whitening system. Compend Contin Educ Dent 2002;23:335–338, 340, 343–344 passim.

151. Anic I, Pavelic B, Matsumoto K. In vitro pulp chamber temperature rises associated with the argon laser polymerization of composite resin. Lasers Surg Med 1996;19:438–444.

152. Powell GL, Morton TH, Whisenant BK. Argon laser oral safety parameters for teeth. Lasers Surg Med 1993;13:548–552.

153. ADA Council on Scientific Affairs. Laser-assisted bleaching: An update. J Am Dent Assoc 1998;129:1484–1487.

154. Haywood VB, Robinson FG. Vital tooth bleaching with nightguard vital bleaching. Curr Opin Cosmet Dent 1997;4:45–52.

155. Melcer J, Chaumette MT, Zeboulon S, et al. Preliminary report on the effect of the CO_2 laser beam on the dental pulp of the *Macaca mulatta* primate and the beagle dog. J Endod 1985;11(1):1–5.

156. Hein DK, Ploeger BJ, Hartup JK, Wagstaff RS, Palmer TM, Hansen LD. In-office vital tooth bleaching—What do lights add? Comp Contin Educ Dent 2003;24(4A):340–352.

157. Jones AH, Diaz-Arnold AM, Vargas MA, Cobb DS. Colorimetric assessment of laser and home bleaching techniques. J Esthet Dent 1999;11:87–94.

158. CRA News (Serial online) Why curing lights don't increase tooth whitening 2000;August. www.cranews.com.

159. Haywood VB, Powe A. Using double-poured alginate impressions to fabricate bleaching trays. Oper Dent 1998;23:128–131.

160. Haywood VB, Caughman WF, Frazier KB, Myers ML. Fabrication of immediate direct thermoplastic whitening trays. Contemp Esthet Restorative Pract 2001;9:2–3.

161. Reinhardt JW, Eivins SE, Swift EJ Jr, Denehy GE. A clinical study of nightguard vital bleaching. Quintessence Int 1993;24:379–384.

162. Curtis JW, Dickinson GL, Downey MC, et al. Assessing the effects of 10 percent carbamide peroxide on oral soft tissues. J Am Dent Assoc 1996;127:1218–1223.

163. Scherer W, Palat M, Hittelman E, Putter H, Cooper H. At-home bleaching system: Effect on gingival tissue. J Esthet Dent 1992;4(3):86–89.

164. Schulte JR, Morrissette DB, Gasior EJ, Czajewski MV. Clinical changes in the gingiva as a result of at-home bleaching. Compend Contin Educ Dent 1993;14:1362–1372.

165. Haywood VB, Leonard RH, Dickinson GL. Efficacy of six months of nightguard vital bleaching of tetracycline-stained teeth. J Esthet Dent 1997;9:13–19.

166. Haywood VB, Leonard RH Jr, Nelson CF. Efficacy of foam liner in 10% carbamide peroxide bleaching technique. Quintessence Int 1993;24:663–666.

167. Dunn JR. Dentist-prescribed home bleaching: Current status. Compend Contin Educ Dent 1998;19:760–764.

168. Matis BA, Gaiao U, Blackman D, Schultz FA, Eckert GJ. In vivo degradation of bleaching gel used in whitening teeth. J Am Dent Assoc 1999;130:227–235.

169. Javaheri DS, Janis JN. The efficacy of reservoirs in bleaching trays. Oper Dent 2000;25(3):149–151.

170. Miller MB, Castellanos IR, Rieger MS. Efficacy of home bleaching systems with and without tray reservoirs. Prac Periodontics Aesthet Dent 2000;12:611–614.

171. Nathoo SA, Richter R, Smith S, Zhang YP. Kinetics of carbamide peroxide degradation in bleaching trays [abstract A2149]. J Dent Res 1996;75(special issue):286.

172. Haywood VB. Nightguard vital bleaching and in-office bleaching. Contemp Esthet Rest Prac 1998;July/Aug:78–81.

173. Gerlach RW. Shifting paradigms in whitening: Introduction of a novel system for vital tooth bleaching. Compend Contin Educ Dent 2000;21(suppl):S4–S9.

174. Gerlach RW, Bibb RD, Sagel P. Initial color change and color retention with a hydrogen peroxide bleaching strip. Am J Dent 2002;15(1):3–7.

175. Browning WD. Use of shade guides for color measurement in tooth-bleaching studies. J Esthet Restor Dent 2003;15(suppl 1):S13–S20.

176. Westland S. Review of the CIE system of colorimetry and its use in dentistry. J Esthet Restor Dent 2003;15(suppl 1):S5–S12.

177. Bengel WM. Digital photography and the assessment of therapeutic results after bleaching procedures. J Esthet Restor Dent 2003;15(suppl 1):S21–S32.

178. Li Y. Tooth color measurement using Chroma Meter: Techniques, advantages, and disadvantages. J Esthet Restor Dent 2003;15(suppl 1):S33–S41.

179. Gerlach RW. Placebo-controlled clinical trial of a 19% sodium percarbonate whitening film: Initial and sustained whitening. Am J Dent 2003;16(special issue):12B–16B.

180. Moffitt JM, Cooley RO, Olsen NH, Hefferren JJ. Prediction of tetracycline-induced tooth discoloration. J Am Dent Assoc 1974;88:547–552.

181. Mull MM. The tetracyclines and the teeth. Dent Abstr 1967;12:346–350.

182. Haywood VB, Leonard RH. Six- and 12-month color stability after 6 months bleaching tetracycline teeth [abstract 2891]. J Dent Res 1996;75(special issue):379.

183. Haywood VB. Extended bleaching of tetracycline-stained teeth: A case report. Contemp Esthet Restorative Pract 1997;1:14–21.

184. Leonard RH, Haywood VB, Eagle JC, et al. Nightguard vital bleaching of tetracycline stained teeth: 54 months post-treatment. J Esthet Dent 1999;11:265–277.

185. Robertello FJ, Dishman MV, Sarrett DC, Elpperly AC. Effect of home bleaching products on mercury release from an admixed amalgam. Am J Dent 1999;12:227–230.

186. Rotstein I, Mor C, Arwaz JR. Changes in surface levels of mercury, silver, tin, and copper of dental amalgam treated with carbamide peroxide and hydrogen in vitro. Oral Surg Oral Med Oral Pathol Oral Radiol Endod 1997;83:506–509.

187. Hummert TW, Osborne JW, Norling BK, Cardenas HL. Mercury in solution following exposure of various amalgams to carbamide peroxides. Am J Dent 1993;6:305–309.

188. Elkhatib H, Nakajima M, Hiraishi N, Kitasako Y, Tagami J, Nomura S. Surface pH and bond strength of a self-etching primer/adhesive system to intracoronal dentin after application of hydrogen peroxide bleach with sodium perborate. Oper Dent 2003;28:591–597.

189. Bailey SJ, Swift EJ. Effects of home bleaching products on composite resin. Quintessence Int 1992;23:489–494.

190. Souyias J, Hoelscher DC, Neme AL. Effect of bleaching on posterior composite materials [abstract 1072]. J Dent Res 2000;79(special issue):278.

191. Cooley RL, Burger KM. Effect of carbamide peroxide on composite resins. Quintessence Int 1991;22:817–821.

192. Friend GW, Jones JE, Wamble SH, Covington JS. Carbamide peroxide tooth bleaching: Changes to composite resins after prolonged exposure [abstract A2432]. J Dent Res 1991;70(special issue):570.

193. Karpinia KA, Magnusson I, Barker ML, Gerlach RW. Placebo-controlled clinical trial of a 19% sodium percarbonate whitening film: Initial and sustained whitening. Am J Dent 2003;16(special issue):12B–16B.

194. Zalkind M, Arwaz J, Goldman A, Rotstein I. Surface morphology changes in human enamel, dentin, and cementum following bleaching: A scanning electron microscopy study. Endod Dent Traumatol 1996;12:82–88.

195. Croll TP, Bullock GA. Enamel microabrasion for removal of smooth surface decalcification lesions. J Clin Orthod 1994;28:365–370.

196. Croll TP, Segura A, Donly KJ. Enamel microabrasion: New considerations in 1993. Pract Periodont Aesthet Dent 1993;5:19–29.

197. Croll TP. Enamel microabrasion: Observations after 10 years. J Am Dent Assoc 1997;128(suppl):45S–50S.

198. Bodden KM, Haywood VB. Treatment of endemic fluorosis and tetracycline staining with microabrasion and nightguard vital bleaching: A case report. Quintessence Int 2003;34:87–91.

199. Haywood VB, Parker MH. Nightguard vital bleaching beneath existing porcelain veneers: A case report. Quintessence Int 1999;30:743–747.

Porcelain Veneers

Jeffrey S. Rouse
J. William Robbins

The porcelain veneer has gained wide acceptance in recent years as a primary restoration in esthetic dentistry. Since its introduction in the early 1980s, it has undergone an evolution in both techniques and materials. A significant number of long-term clinical studies confirm the excellent durability of the porcelain veneer restoration.[1–8]

Indications and Limitations

Because of their conservative preparation and beautiful esthetics, porcelain veneers have become the treatment of choice for restoration of the anterior dentition.[9] Porcelain veneers may be used to modify a tooth's color, shape, length, and/or alignment; to close space; and to restore fractured and endodontically treated teeth. The patient should be informed, however, of the possible morbidity associated with a specific indication, as well as the generally accepted limitations. Informed consent should include, but not be limited to, the following possible complications: *(1)* postoperative sensitivity; *(2)* marginal discoloration; *(3)* fracture; *(4)* debonding; and *(5)* wear of opposing teeth.

Treatment Planning

The patient's self-image must be considered during the initial patient interview.[10] A key element in the diagnostic phase is a clarification of the patient's expectations. If it can be determined initially that the patient's expectations are unrealistic, future grief may be avoided.

Assessment of the Face

When a treatment plan is being developed that includes restoration of teeth in the esthetic zone, attention must be directed not only to the shape and color of the teeth, but also to the shape of the face, the lips, the maxillary and mandibular lip lines, and the skin color. The teeth can be used to accentuate a positive feature or de-emphasize a negative feature. For example, a patient with a narrow face may desire longer and narrower teeth to emphasize the facial shape or shorter, rounded teeth to soften the narrowness of the face.

It is also important to evaluate skin color, especially if there is a possibility that it will change over time. For example, if porcelain veneers are being planned for a Caucasian patient with a dark tan, a determination must be made regarding the longevity of the tan prior to shade selection. If the dark tan is transient and skin color will revert to a lighter tone, this will significantly affect the decision on the color of the porcelain veneers. Veneers that appear to be bright and high in value against the tanned skin will look more yellow and lower in value as the skin tone becomes lighter. All of these parameters must be consciously considered during the diagnostic phase if consistently excellent results are to be obtained.

Assessment of the Smile

After the facial features have been considered, attention must be directed to the smile and its components. During the initial interview, the dentist should pay close attention to the overall appearance of the patient's mouth as he or she speaks and is in repose.

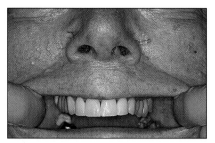

Fig 16-1 Pulling the upper lip parallel with the interpupillary line to examine the incisal plane. Note the sigmoid curve of the incisal plane.

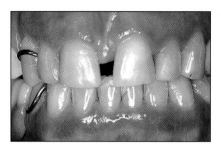

Fig 16-2a Diastema.

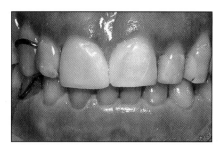

Fig 16-2b Diagnostic intraoral mock-up of diastema closure.

The dentist should note the maxillary incisal edge position in relation to the lower lip, the relationship of the maxillary incisal plane to the horizon, the amount of gingival display during smiling and speaking, the relationship of the anterior and posterior segments, and the overall quality of the smile. If the interpupillary line is parallel to the horizon, it may be used in evaluation of the incisal plane. The dentist pulls the upper lip parallel to the interpupillary line and then uses the lip to evaluate the incisal plane for a cant (Fig 16-1). The acceptability of the incisal plane must be determined during the diagnostic phase, or discrepancies may be incorporated into the final restorations. (See chapter 3 for a more complete discussion of esthetic diagnosis.)

Diagnostic Aids

Mock-ups

With an understanding of esthetic diagnostic parameters, the dentist can use several diagnostic methods to develop a treatment plan that will predictably result in success. Preparation and waxing on a diagnostic cast are sometimes helpful to the dentist, especially when the veneers are intended to lengthen teeth, close spaces, or correct malaligned teeth. However, a diagnostic waxup is not especially helpful in giving the patient a preview of the expected esthetic outcome. This can be accomplished better by one of the intraoral techniques.

A mock-up of the desired result can be accomplished with direct placement of composite in the patient's mouth to simulate the desired outcome (Figs 16-2a and 16-2b). Because the teeth are not acid etched before the intraoral mock-up, the composite can easily be removed from the tooth. This technique is especially helpful for simple procedures, such as diastema closure.

However, when major changes are being considered, such as lengthening several teeth, direct mock-up is time-consum-

ing. In this situation, a diagnostic waxup is done on a preoperative cast and duplicated, and a clear matrix is made. Resin composite material is placed in the clear matrix, which is placed over the teeth intraorally, and light cured. Once the excess flash of composite is cleaned from the teeth, the patient may preview the projected outcome. At this point, changes can be made (eg, shortening or lengthening of the teeth) until the patient is comfortable and satisfied. An impression can then be made of the corrected mock-up in the mouth, and the subsequent cast will serve as a reference cast for the laboratory technician. Because intraoral mock-up can be time-consuming, a more cost-effective method is to construct a resin composite shell or overlay on a diagnostic cast. The shell is placed intraorally to allow the patient to visualize the projected result. This is an especially helpful diagnostic tool for the patient with excessive gingival display. The composite shell can extend over the gingiva to demonstrate the esthetic effect of surgically lengthening the clinical crowns (Figs 16-3a to 16-3e).

Commonly, a preview of the projected outcome is achieved with the provisional restorations (Figs 16-4a to 16-4e). A diagnostic waxup is accomplished and a stent is fabricated. After the preparations are completed and the final impression is made, the provisional restorations are constructed using the stent. Once the patient is satisfied with the provisional restorations, a cast of the arch, with the provisional restorations in place, is made and sent to the laboratory to serve as a blueprint for the final restorations.

Computer Imaging

Another diagnostic method involves computer imaging of the patient's smile and making the desired esthetic changes on the screen. This provides both the patient and the dentist with a realistic preview of the expected result. However, imaging is limited because it does not allow for a dynamic evaluation in the same way that an intraoral mock-up allows the patient to

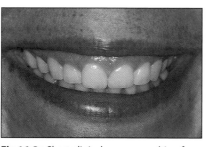

Fig 16-3a Short clinical crowns resulting from excess gingival coverage.

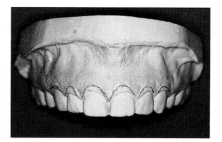

Fig 16-3b Preoperative study cast with lines drawn to aid in the fabrication of a diagnostic resin composite overlay.

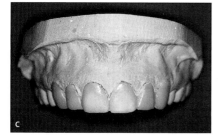

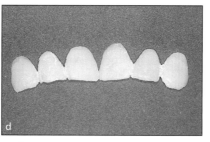

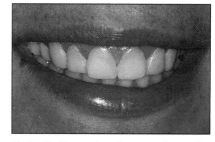

Figs 16-3c and 16-3d Diagnostic resin composite overlay.

Fig 16-3e Diagnostic resin composite overlay demonstrating the benefit of crown lengthening of the anterior teeth.

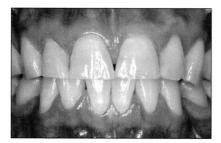

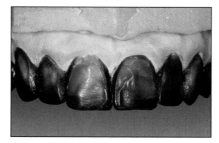

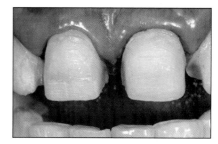

Fig 16-4a Patient preoperative presentation.

Fig 16-4b Diagnostic waxup.

Fig 16-4c Full veneer preparations.

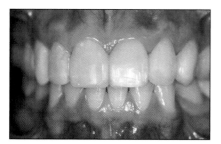

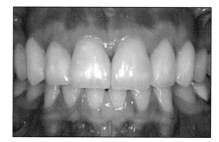

Fig 16-4d Composite provisional restorations fabricated from a stent made from the diagnostic waxup. The provisional restorations have been in service for 4 weeks.

Fig 16-4e Final porcelain veneer restorations. (Porcelain veneers created by Steve McGowan, CDT, Arcus Laboratory.)

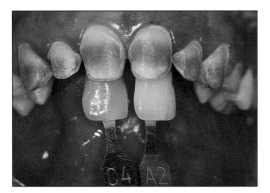

Fig 16-5 Shade tabs held under the incisal edges of the prepared teeth. Preparations of tetracycline-stained teeth are routinely extended interproximally through the contact area. In this patient, more interproximal tooth structure was removed because of existing Class 3 restorations.

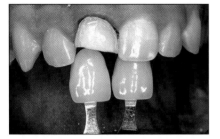

Fig 16-6a Preparation of a single fractured central incisor for a porcelain veneer with shade tabs for laboratory communication.

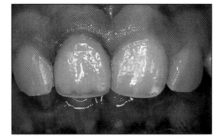

Fig 16-6b Single veneer on the right central incisor immediately after placement. (Porcelain veneer created by Steve McGowan, CDT, Arcus Laboratory.)

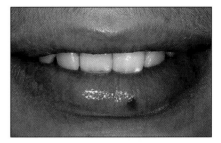

Fig 16-6c Final porcelain veneer restoration of the right central incisor.

experience the projected changes. Because many dentists do not have the in-office capability for computer imaging, the patient or a photograph or slide of the patient may be sent to a location that offers the service.

Photographs

Preoperative photographs offer another important diagnostic aid; they document the preoperative condition and aid the technician in the fabrication of the veneers. The series should include a full-face smile; a retracted frontal image of maxillary and mandibular teeth in occlusion; a retracted frontal view with a shade tab held directly beneath the incisal edges of the maxillary incisors; a retracted close-up view of the teeth to be veneered, with and without a shade tab; and a postpreparation view of the teeth to be veneered, with a shade tab (Fig 16-5). In addition, other photographs, such as a profile or a view of the intraoral diagnostic mock-up, should be included if they can benefit the laboratory technician.

Single Veneer

Perhaps the most difficult procedure in esthetic restorative dentistry is to perfectly match a full-coverage restoration to an adjacent natural central incisor. Commonly, the porcelain veneer is the restoration of choice in this situation. If the tooth

to be restored is not significantly discolored, the porcelain veneer is an excellent restorative option. The major advantage of the single porcelain veneer restoration is the dentist's ability to increase or decrease the value of the restoration with the bonding resin cement (Figs 16-6a to 16-6c).

Multiple Veneers

When the clinician has the option of veneering multiple anterior teeth, the problem of shade matching is minimized. It is easier to deal in even numbers when veneers are placed on anterior teeth. It is much simpler to veneer two central incisors than to attempt to match a veneer to a natural tooth. Therefore, the chances of obtaining an optimally esthetic result are enhanced when two, four, six, or eight veneers are placed.

An option that is commonly chosen is the placement of six veneers from canine to canine. In Fig 16-7, the anterior teeth are brighter and bolder, while the buccal corridor appears to become darker. This accentuates the anterior teeth and commonly creates the unpleasant illusion that the anterior teeth are larger and longer as well as brighter. This does not usually occur when only the four incisors are veneered (Figs 16-8a and 16-8b). Therefore, when veneers are planned for the incisors but there is no esthetic or functional requirement for canine veneers, the esthetic result is enhanced when the

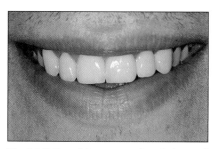

Fig 16-7 Porcelain veneers bonded on all maxillary anterior teeth. Note the apparent separation of anterior and posterior segments of the mouth because of the boldness of the porcelain veneers.

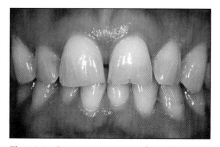

Fig 16-8a Preoperative view of maxillary central and lateral incisors.

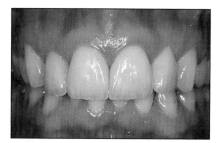

Fig 16-8b Porcelain veneers bonded on the maxillary central and lateral incisors to blend esthetically with the maxillary canines. (Porcelain veneers created by Steve McGowan, CDT, Arcus Laboratory.)

canines are left unrestored. However, when all six anterior teeth require veneers, consideration should be given to veneering one or more posterior teeth on each side, depending on the posterior extent of the smile and the maxillary arch form.

Tooth Preparation

The preparation of teeth for porcelain veneers is usually uncomplicated when the basic principles are understood and followed. Historically, veneers were placed on unprepared teeth, making the technique conservative and reversible. This led to overcontoured restorations, gingival irritation, and high failure rates (Fig 16-9).[5,11] The stress concentration is less severe on veneers fitted to prepared teeth.[12] In addition, the preparation removes the aprismatic and hypermineralized enamel layers, which can be resistant to acid etching.[13] Today, practitioners should focus on maintaining the preparation completely in enamel to maximize the resin bond strength and decrease the tensile stresses in the porcelain.[14–16] Even with the newest-generation bonding agents, the bond strength of porcelain to enamel is far superior to the bond strength of porcelain to dentin. Fractures, microleakage, and debonding are all failures that can be linked to preparations situated in dentin.[17]

Anterior Teeth

Gingival Finish Lines
When preparing teeth for porcelain veneers, it is essential to remember that the strongest and most predictable bond is to enamel. The more dentin that is exposed during the preparation, the poorer the bond of the veneer and the poorer the ultimate stress distribution during function.[14] For maxillary

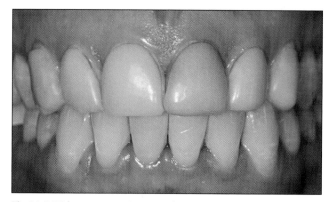

Fig 16-9 Without preparation, porcelain veneers can become overcontoured. The risk of microleakage and fracture increase due to the poor bonding substrate.

porcelain veneers, the gingival margin of the veneer should routinely be placed at the gingival crest or slightly subgingivally. A primary goal of the preparation is to have all margins on sound enamel, because the stress distribution in the veneer is much improved when all margins are bonded to enamel. The amount of exposed dentin in the central portion of the veneer preparation becomes much less important when all of the margins are bonded to enamel.[14] Because the enamel is only approximately 0.3 mm thick at 0.5 mm from the cementoenamel junction,[18,19] it is difficult to obtain adequate preparation depth while preserving the enamel. In a routine preparation, the facial enamel reduction must be exquisitely controlled. This can only be accomplished with depth cut burs, which are available from several manufacturers (Fig 16-10).[20–22] After the depth cuts are made, the enamel is uniformly removed with a round-ended, cylinder diamond. Unless the teeth to be veneered are dark (low value), the gingival preparation should not routinely extend more than minimally into the gingival sulcus. In the midfacial area,

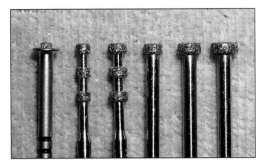

Fig 16-10 Depth cut burs of different designs and depths.

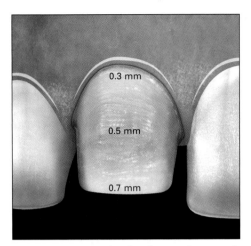

Fig 16-11 Average facial reduction for enamel-bonded veneer. (Illustrations for chapter 16 by John Bonfardeci, Studio Giovanni.)

the enamel thickness ranges from 0.8 to 0.9 mm on average. The preparation should deepen in the midfacial and taper into the incisal (Fig 16-11). This allows the technician to effectively disguise the transition from supported to unsupported porcelain.

When mandibular anterior teeth are prepared for porcelain veneers, the considerations are different from those for maxillary teeth. In most patients, the gingival half of the mandibular incisors remains covered by the lower lip at all times, resulting in no esthetic display. In addition, the marginal gingiva of the mandibular anterior teeth is commonly thin, and the gingival sulcus is narrow and shallow, making the placement of gingival retraction cord very difficult. For these reasons, the gingival margins of the preparations for mandibular anterior teeth is ideally placed at least 1.0 mm incisal to the marginal gingiva (see Figs 16-16 and 16-27a).

Interproximal Contact Area

For the purposes of veneer fabrication and placement, it is important that the preparation not be finished in the interproximal contact area. When the margin is stopped in the interproximal contact area, it is difficult to accurately capture the margin in the final impression. Additionally, veneer fabrication is more difficult for the laboratory technician, and bonding and finishing procedures are more difficult for the dentist. For these reasons, the preparation must either stop facial to the interproximal contact area (Fig 16-12a) or extend completely through the contact area to the lingual surface (Fig 16-12b).[19,23]

A major long-term problem with porcelain veneers is marginal staining.[4,6] This staining is most apparent at the proximal margins. Therefore, the current trend is to extend the preparation through the interproximal contacts (Fig 16-12c) from the mesial aspect of the canine to the mesial aspect of the contralateral canine. There is no esthetic need to extend the preparation through the contact areas on the distal surfaces of the canine teeth. With extension of the preparation through interproximal contacts in areas other than the distal contacts of canines, any proximal marginal staining is concealed. With dark teeth (eg, tetracycline-stained teeth), it is imperative that the preparation extend completely through the interproximal contact area to the lingual surface (see Fig 16-5). This decreases the risk of dark shadows appearing around the periphery of the veneer.

Incisal Edge

There is ongoing debate regarding the need to cover the incisal edge of a maxillary tooth with the porcelain veneer. If there is no esthetic requirement to change the incisal shape or length, and there is adequate remaining incisal tooth structure after facial reduction, the incisal margin may be terminated at the facio-incisal line angle (Fig 16-13a). This preparation is most commonly indicated for linguoverted teeth. An alternative is the "window preparation" (Fig 16-13b). This preparation provides the most protection for the veneer during function; however, it results in a visible composite-veneer interface at the facio-incisal margin. This preparation is most commonly indicated for the maxillary canine that has the correct length and incisal edge configuration and has a large lingual wear facet extending to the incisal edge. Because it is preferable not to place a veneer margin in a wear facet, the window preparation is appropriate. Neither of these preparations can

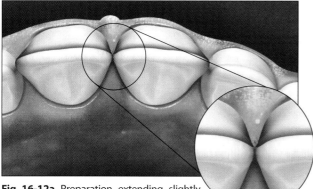

Fig 16-12a Preparation extending slightly facial to the interproximal contact area.

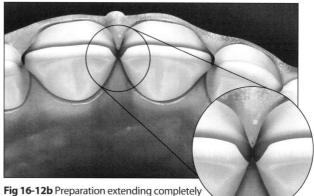

Fig 16-12b Preparation extending completely through the interproximal contact area to the palatal surface.

be used, however, when the tooth is being lengthened incisally with the porcelain veneer.

When the maxillary incisal edge is not reduced during the preparation, the veneer is inevitably thicker, and the incisal edge is too round buccolingually, lacking a more natural, sharp facio-incisal line angle. Additionally, veneers that do not cover the incisal edge are significantly more difficult to orient correctly during bonding.

The most universally applicable preparation, which allows the technician to incorporate the natural incisal translucency into the veneer, requires incisal edge reduction. If the incisal edge of the maxillary tooth is to be covered with the veneer, there must be room for at least 1 mm of porcelain over the incisal edge. However, a 1.5- to 2-mm incisal edge reduction from the final incisal edge position (Fig 16-14) allows the laboratory technician to provide maximum esthetics in the incisal third of the veneer. Therefore, a preoperative determination of the ideal incisal edge position must be made before preparing the tooth. A diagnostic waxup can be helpful in this evaluation. In the case of a worn or fractured tooth, more incisal porcelain length is acceptable if the veneer remains bonded to enamel and the fit will provide a cement thickness of 100 μm or less.[24,25]

Traditionally, the lingual finish line configuration was a chamfer. This placed the thin veneer in a high tensile stress area of the tooth, significantly weakening the restoration.[26] Today, the incisal edge should be flattened, leaving a butt finish line configuration on the lingual surface.[25,26] It is important to round the sharp facio-incisal line angle of the preparation to prevent stress concentration in the bonded veneer and to allow for an undetectable transition from unsupported to supported porcelain. If the practitioner chooses to maintain the interproximal contact, the proximal portion of the prepa-

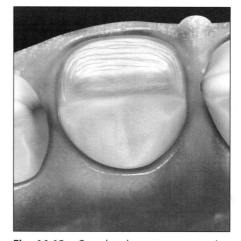

Fig 16-12c Completed veneer preparation through the interproximal contacts. This preparation is commonly referred to as a *full veneer*.

ration should follow the papilla and extend slightly under the interproximal contact to ensure coverage of the tooth in this area (Fig 16-15). This extension is called an *elbow preparation*. If the tooth is not prepared in this manner or extended through the contact, the darker, unprepared triangle of natural tooth structure results in less-than-optimal esthetics.

The incisal edges of mandibular anterior teeth should be routinely covered with porcelain of at least 1.5 to 2.0 mm thickness (Fig 16-16). Incisal edge flattening with a resultant lingual butt margin is also recommended for mandibular anterior teeth. Again, the facio-incisal line angle of the preparation must be rounded.

When multiple teeth are being prepared, incisal reduction should be symmetric (eg, both prepared lateral incisors should be the same length) for more uniform esthetics in the final

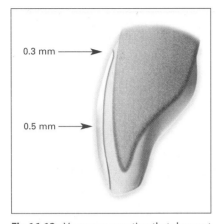

Fig 16-13a Veneer preparation that does not cover the incisal edge of the maxillary anterior tooth.

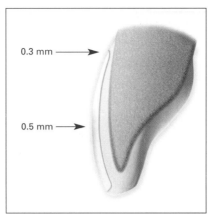

Fig 16-13b Window preparation on a maxillary anterior tooth.

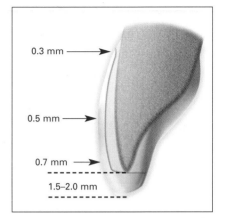

Fig 16-14 Standard veneer preparation for maxillary anterior teeth. Incisal reduction is 1.5 to 2.0 mm.

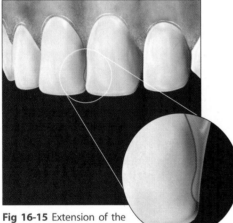

Fig 16-15 Extension of the veneer preparation into the subcontact area for improved esthetics.

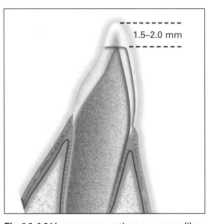

Fig 16-16 Veneer preparation on a mandibular incisor. There is at least 1.5 to 2.0 mm of incisal reduction, and the gingival margin is at least 1.0 mm incisal to the gingival crest.

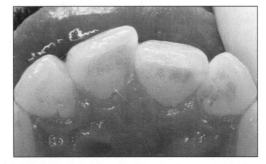

Fig 16-17a Correction of mild to moderate overlapping requires preparation through the contact to allow contour alteration.

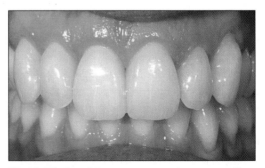

Fig 16-17b Porcelain veneer restorations on maxillary anteriors. (Porcelain veneers created by Gary Nunakowa, CDT, LeBeau Dental Laboratory.)

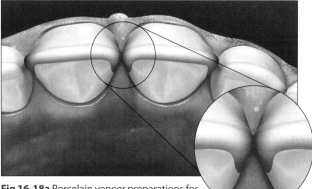

Fig 16-18a Porcelain veneer preparations for closing a small to moderate diastema.

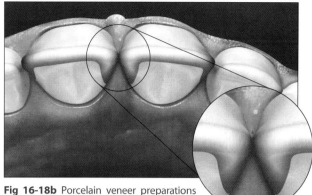

Fig 16-18b Porcelain veneer preparations for closing a large diastema. The preparations involve more of the lingual surfaces of the central incisors to develop adequate lingual contours.

restorations. After completion of all veneer preparations, the dentist should stand in front of the patient, retract the patient's lips, and confirm that the preparations are symmetric and the incisal edges parallel to the horizon.

Overlapping Teeth

When overlapping teeth are being prepared, the paths of insertion of the veneers must be considered. Where there is significant misalignment of the teeth, it is usually impossible to develop paths of insertion for the veneers without extending the preparations completely through the interproximal contact areas. In addition, significant alteration of the interproximal contact position and straightening of the facial surfaces is usually facilitated when the teeth are prepared through the contact (Figs 16-17a and 16-17b).

Space Closure

Preparation of teeth for space closure presents a unique situation. To obtain smooth lingual contours, the proximal finish lines adjacent to the space must be made more lingual. The wider the space to be closed, the more lingually the tooth must be prepared (Figs 16-18a and 16-18b). Also, the proximal margins adjacent to the space must be positioned subgingivally so that the gingival contours of the veneers minimize the black triangle between the bottom of the interproximal contact area and the tip of the papilla. However, the gingival margin of the veneer should be no closer than 2.5 mm to the crest of the alveolar bone.[27] As teeth separate, the scallop of the interproximal bone lessens, resulting in a wide, flat papilla. Extending the preparation subgingivally and lingually enables the technician to alter the interproximal contour of the veneers and reshape the papilla (Fig 16-19).

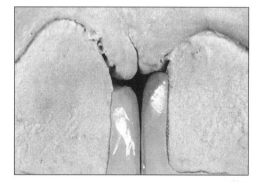

Fig 16-19 Overcontouring the veneers allows alteration of the interproximal tissue contour.

Premolars

The considerations for preparing maxillary premolars are similar to those for anterior teeth. The veneer preparation of the maxillary premolar may end on the facial surface of the tooth if the functional and esthetic requirements are met (Fig 16-20). Ideally, the occlusal margin should be placed so that it is not in an occlusal contact area and so that the opposing cusp does not function across it. If the anterior guidance immediately discludes the posterior teeth in mandibular excursive movements, the occlusal margin can be placed anywhere on the lingual incline of the buccal cusp, as long as there is no occlusal stop directly on the margin (Fig 16-21). However, when group-function occlusion is present, it may be necessary to extend the occlusal margin to the central groove. In this circumstance, occlusal reduction must be adequate to allow for an onlay of at least a 2-mm thickness of porcelain

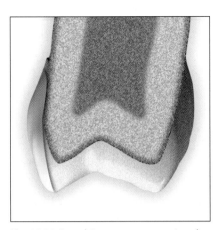

Fig 16-20 Porcelain veneer preparation that does not cover the buccal cusp of the maxillary premolar.

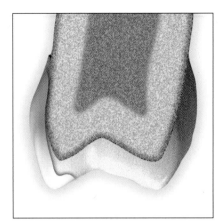

Fig 16-21 Veneer preparation overlapping the buccal cusp. There should be no occlusal stop directly on the veneer margin.

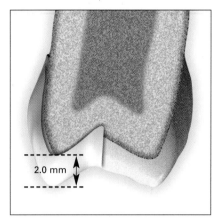

Fig 16-22 Porcelain veneer preparation that covers the buccal cusp of the maxillary premolar. Note the 2.0 mm of occlusal reduction on the buccal cusp.

over the buccal cusp, blending to the 0.3- to 0.5-mm reduction of the facial surface (Fig 16-22). In mandibular premolars, because the esthetic cusp is also the functional cusp, the tooth must generally be prepared for a porcelain onlay rather than simply for a buccal porcelain veneer (see chapter 18).

Existing Restorations

Existing resin composite restorations can complicate the veneer preparation. Ideally, no margins should be finished on an existing resin composite restoration. One clinical study reported a significantly higher failure rate for porcelain veneers placed over existing resin composite restorations.[5] Bonding effectively to an existing restoration is questionable, particularly if it has been in place for any period of time. Water sorption, unsilanated surfaces of filler particles, and limited unpolymerized resin in the set composite lead to a significant decrease in bond strength.[15,20] The resin composite restoration should be removed during tooth preparation for the veneer, and the missing tooth structure should be replaced as part of the porcelain veneer[28] (Figs 16-23a to 16-23c). Small areas of resin composite can remain centrally in the preparation to serve as an undercut block-out material.

Fractured Incisal Edge

A unique indication for the porcelain veneer is the restoration of the fractured incisal edge of an incisor (Figs 16-24a to 16-24c). Although there is little clinical data to support the

use of veneers for this purpose, laboratory data[28] are favorable.[24] The limits for the amount of missing tooth structure that can be replaced with a porcelain veneer are not known. However, anecdotal evidence seems to indicate that approximately 50% of the clinical crown can be replaced with a porcelain veneer when the preparation on the remaining tooth structure is in enamel. Because the veneered tooth does not require endodontic treatment for restorative reasons or the placement of a post and core, it is a highly desirable alternative to previous methods of restoring the fractured tooth. The preparation for this type of veneer extends to near the gingival crest on both the facial and lingual surfaces.

Noncarious Cervical Lesions

Noncarious cervical lesions, caused by erosion, abrasion, and/or abfraction, provide a poor substrate for bonding due to the sclerotic nature of the dentin.[29,30] Therefore, the best treatment solution is to surgically cover these areas with connective tissue grafting.[31] This results in more natural gingival architecture and allows the gingival margin of the veneer preparation to end on enamel. However, if the surgical option is not chosen and the esthetic demands require that the root be covered with a veneer, the preparation must extend onto the root surface. In this situation, a dentin bonding agent must be used in the bonding process. In addition, the patient should be advised that the risks of staining, microleakage, and/or veneer fracture in the gingival third are much greater due to the poor bonding substrate (Figs 16-25a and 16-25b).[14]

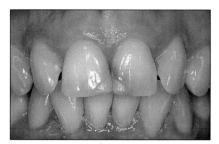

Fig 16-23a Maxillary central incisors with large Class 4 resin composite restorations.

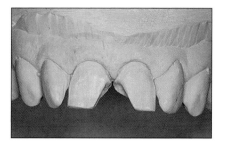

Fig 16-23b Stone cast with preparations of the maxillary central incisors for porcelain veneers. The resin composite is removed, and the missing tooth structure is replaced with the porcelain veneers.

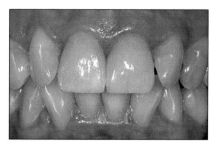

Fig 16-23c Porcelain veneer restorations on maxillary central incisors. (Porcelain veneers created by Steve McGowan, CDT, Arcus Laboratory.)

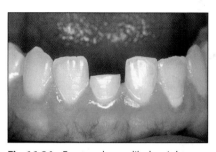

Fig 16-24a Fractured mandibular right central incisor.

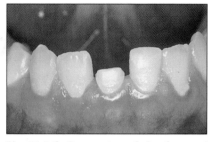

Fig 16-24b Preparation of the fractured mandibular right central incisor for a porcelain veneer.

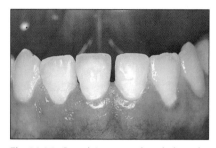

Fig 16-24c Porcelain veneer bonded on the mandibular right central incisor. (Porcelain veneers created by Gilbert Young, CDT, GNS Laboratory.)

Fig 16-25a Exposed dentin surfaces provide a poor bonding substrate for veneers, increasing the risk of fracture.

Fig 16-25b Adhesive failure of dentin bonded veneer.

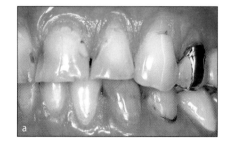

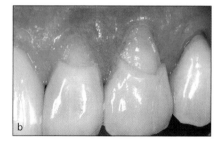

Impressions

When an impression is made of the maxillary teeth, retraction cord is placed to expose all gingival margins. This step is generally not necessary with mandibular teeth because the preparations are at least 1.0 mm incisal to the marginal gingiva. An accurate impression material, such as polyvinyl siloxane, polyether, or reversible hydrocolloid, is then used to make the final impression.

Provisional Restorations

The placement of provisional restorations over veneer preparations is an integral step in the predictable placement of porcelain veneers. Provisional restorations not only improve interim esthetics and decrease sensitivity, but they also provide essential diagnostic information, including veneer color, shape, length, and incisal edge configuration, that cannot be obtained in any other way.[32] When provisional restorations are being placed on one or two teeth, the procedure is best accomplished with freehand placement of composite. A small area in the incisal third of each tooth is etched with phosphoric acid for 15 seconds, washed, and dried. Adhesive resin is placed over the entire preparation and light cured. A large increment of resin composite is then patted into place with correct contours, the gingival margins are smoothed with an explorer tip or other fine-tipped instrument, and the provisional restoration is light cured. There should be no overhanging resin composite at the margins, and the provisional restoration should require virtually no adjustment.

When provisional restorations are being placed on multiple teeth, it is preferable to use a clear matrix made on a preoperative diagnostic cast. A diagnostic waxup is commonly required to change tooth length, alignment, and/or incisal edge configuration (Figs 16-26a and 16-26b). The diagnostic waxup is duplicated, and the clear matrix is fabricated (Fig 16-26c). The clear matrix may be made of a plastic stent material or a clear polyvinyl siloxane bite-registration material. The teeth are spot etched with 30% to 40% phosphoric acid in the incisal third (Fig 16-26d), washed, and air dried. The entire preparation is covered with adhesive resin, which is then light cured (Fig 16-26e). A self-etching primer system should not be used because the provisionals will be bonded to the entire preparation and are difficult to remove without altering the preparations. The facial and incisal areas in the clear matrix are filled with resin composite (Fig 16-26f), and the matrix is placed over the prepared teeth (Fig 16-26g). The gingival two thirds of the matrix is shielded from the polymerization light, and the incisal one third is polymerized with the light for 10 seconds per tooth (Fig 16-26h). The gingival two thirds is then lightly cured for 0.5 to 1 second per tooth (Fig 16-26i). The matrix is gently teased away from the tooth at the gingival margin to ensure that the resin composite does not stick to the matrix (Fig 16-26j). If the resin composite sticks to the matrix, the matrix is returned to place and the gingival two thirds is polymerized again for 0.5 second per tooth. The matrix is removed, and the excess partially cured resin composite is first removed proximally and lingually with a No. 12 scalpel blade (Fig 16-26k). Floss and a floss threader are then used in each gingival embrasure to ensure patency and that there are no overhangs (Fig 16-26l). The gingival margins are then carved with the No. 12 scalpel blade. If small areas of resin composite are chipped during the finishing process, adding additional resin composite easily repairs these areas. The incisal and facial embrasures are opened with a thin separating disk (Fig 16-26m), the occlusion is adjusted, and the provisional restorations are smoothed and polished (Figs 16-26n to 16-26p). Finally, the provisional restorations are coated with an adhesive (Fig 16-26q), and the entire restoration is light cured for 30 seconds per tooth (Figs 16-26r and 16-26s).

At the appointment for placement of the definitive veneers, the provisional restorations are removed. The resin composite over the small area of etched enamel in the incisal third of the facial surface is lightly removed with a diamond bur, cutting dry. If water is used, it is very difficult to determine the interface between the provisional composite and the tooth structure. The remaining resin composite is flicked off with a spoon excavator. If a veneer does not seat during the try-in, there is probably resin composite from the provisional restoration remaining in the etched area. The preparation should be closely inspected to ensure that all of the resin composite has been removed.

Alternatively, the provisional restoration may be made in the laboratory. After the veneer preparations are completed, an impression is made and poured in fast-setting die stone (Snap-Stone, Whip Mix). The cast is separated from the impression in 5 minutes and covered with a separating medium; the provisional restoration is constructed with the same matrix technique as previously described. The provisional restoration, which is constructed from either acrylic or resin composite, can then be cemented with polycarboxylate cement or temporarily bonded with a resin composite as previously described (Figs 16-27a to 16-27d).

Placement

The anatomy of a porcelain veneer is illustrated in Fig 16-28. The inner surface of the veneer must be etched with hydrofluoric acid or another ceramic etchant. This step is usually accomplished in the laboratory. The etching time must be followed closely. In addition to the microporosities that assist in micromechanical retention, microcracks are increased as etching time increases. These microcracks decrease the flexural strength of the porcelain and weaken the veneer.[15] (For a detailed description of the steps in veneer placement, see the Procedures for Porcelain Veneers box at the end of this chapter. The veneers are first tried in individually for marginal fit. They are then tried in together to ensure that interproximal contacts are correct. Finally, one veneer (or more) is filled with resin composite luting cement or try-in paste and taken to the mouth for the color try-in. The value of the veneer is almost always lower with the try-in resin or paste, because the natural color of the underlying tooth is transmitted through the veneer to the surface. If the color is acceptable to the patient, the dentist proceeds with the bonding procedure as outlined in the Procedures for Porcelain Veneers box.

Figs 16-26a to 16-26s *Fabrication of provisional restorations.*

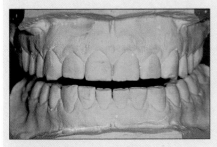

Fig 16-26a Preoperative casts.

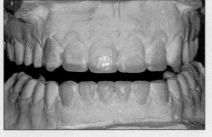

Fig 16-26b Diagnostic waxup.

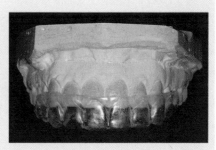

Fig 16-26c Clear stent made from duplicate cast of diagnostic waxup.

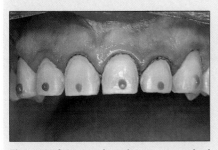

Fig 16-26d Prepared teeth are spot etched with 30% phosphoric acid on the incisal third.

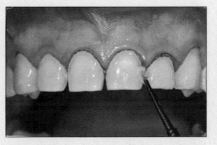

Fig 16-26e The entire surface of each prepared tooth is coated with resin adhesive and light cured.

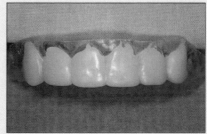

Fig 16-26f The facial and incisal areas of the clear matrix are filled with resin composite.

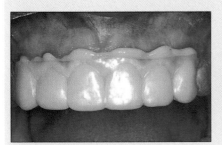

Fig 16-26g The filled matrix is placed over the prepared teeth.

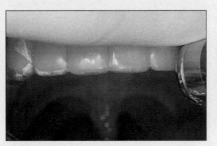

Fig 16-26h The gingival two thirds of the matrix is covered with a finger, while the incisal third is light cured for 10 seconds per tooth.

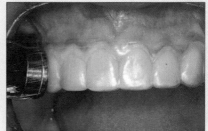

Fig 16-26i The gingival two thirds is lightly cured for 0.5 to 1 second per tooth.

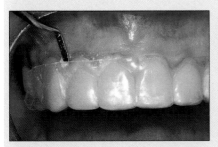

Fig 16-26j The matrix is gently teased away from the preparations to ensure that the resin composite does not stick to the matrix.

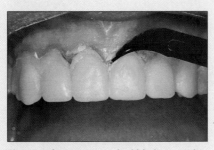

Fig 16-26k A No. 12 scalpel blade is used to remove the partially cured resin composite from proximal and lingual surfaces.

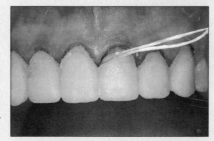

Fig 16-26l Floss and a floss threader are used in each gingival embrasure to ensure patency and overhang-free margins.

Fig 16-26 (continued)

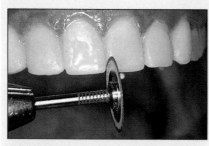

Fig 16-26m Facial and incisal embrasures are refined with a thin diamond disk.

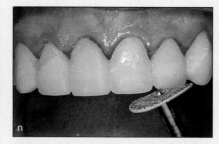
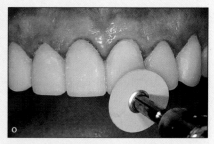

Figs 16-26n and 16-26o A series of composite finishing disks are used to finish the facial surfaces.

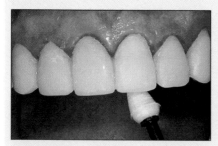

Fig 16-26p A composite polishing point is used to smooth and polish the lingual surfaces.

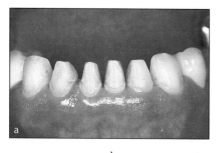
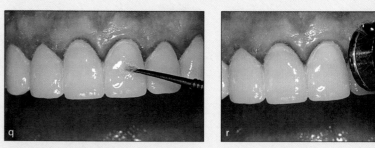

Figs 16-26q and 16-26r The facial surfaces of the provisional restorations are coated with an adhesive resin and light cured.

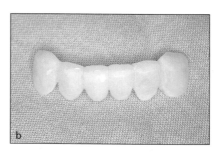

Fig 16-26s Completed provisional restorations.

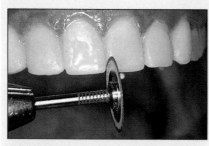

Fig 16-27a Porcelain veneer preparations on the mandibular anterior teeth. The gingival margins are located 1.0 mm above the gingival crests.

Fig 16-27b Laboratory-fabricated provisional restoration.

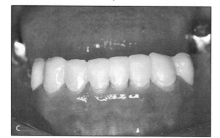
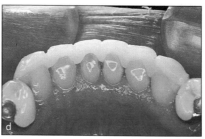

Figs 16-27c and 16-27d Provisional restoration in place.

Fig 16-28 Anatomy of a porcelain veneer.

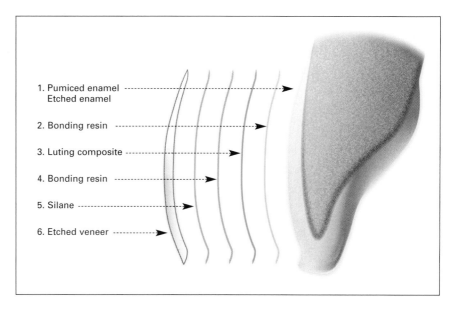

1. Pumiced enamel
   Etched enamel

2. Bonding resin

3. Luting composite

4. Bonding resin

5. Silane

6. Etched veneer

There are many resin luting cement kits available with differing degrees of translucency and viscosity (Figs 16-29a and 16-29b). Translucent cements are indicated as the standard material for veneer bonding. The more opaque cements tend to block the natural tooth color, resulting in a veneer with a less natural appearance. The opaque cements are more commonly used to help block the darkness of discolored teeth. However, the use of these cements can result in a monochromatic appearance and an opaque line at the thin gingival margin of the veneer (Figs 16-30a and 16-30b). It is preferable to block the darkness of discolored teeth with a layer of masking dentin, and/or with porcelain modifiers, in the body of the veneer rather than with opaque cement (Fig 16-31).

The second major difference in veneer luting cements is their viscosity. Initially, most resin cements had a low viscosity so that the veneers could be placed with minimal pressure, thereby decreasing the risk of fracture.[34] However, the low-viscosity resins have some disadvantages: (1) Because of their honeylike consistency, it is more difficult to ensure correct veneer placement, especially when the veneers have no positive stop, ie, no incisal overlap; (2) cleanup of excess resin is more difficult; and (3) at least theoretically, the physical properties are compromised because of the increased proportion of resin matrix. The major indication for the low-viscosity luting resin is the all-ceramic crown or a veneer that covers most of the tooth surfaces. Because of friction, high-viscosity luting resins will not allow complete seating of these restorations. Recently, interest in the higher-viscosity luting resins has increased because they overcome most of the disadvantages of the low-viscosity luting resins.

Friedman[35] has described a technique for using the highly filled resin composite from a standard restorative resin composite kit. The material is brought to room temperature and placed into the veneer in a thin layer through a ribbon tip. The thixotropic properties of the resin composite allow the highly filled material to flow under moderate seating pressure. However, placing the ampule of composite in a hot water bath (160°F) before ejecting the composite is a more effective method of improving the flow characteristics of the resin composite. With this technique, the seating of the veneers can be more accurately controlled, and cleanup is simplified (see the Procedures for Porcelain Veneers box).

The third difference between luting agents is in the chemical mechanism by which curing is initiated. The preferred method for bonding porcelain veneers is a light-cured luting composite. Light curing allows a longer working time, shorter finishing time, and superior color stability as compared to dual-cured or chemically cured material. If, however, the porcelain thickness is greater than 0.7 mm, the light-cured composites do not reach their maximum hardness.[36] In these situations, a dual-cured composite system is recommended. Dual-curing materials contain the initiation systems for both chemical-curing and light-curing composites. A strong bond can be obtained because of their high degree of polymerization with or without light curing.

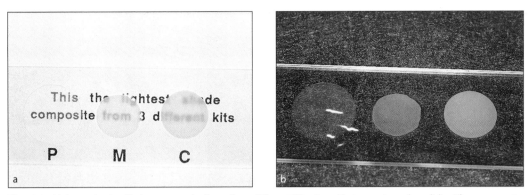

Fig 16-29 Lightest shade of luting composite from three different kits placed between two glass slides. The same materials are shown against two different backgrounds. Note the differences in translucency. (Fig 16-29a from Robbins.[33] Reprinted with permission.)

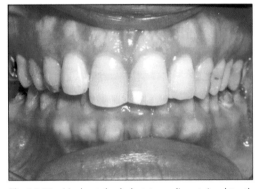

Fig 16-30a Moderately dark, tetracycline-stained teeth prior to veneer preparation.

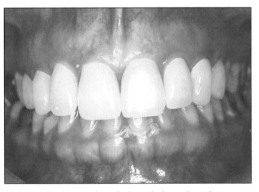

Fig 16-30b Veneers bonded on dark teeth with opaque resin cement. Note the opaque gingival margins on the right and left canines.

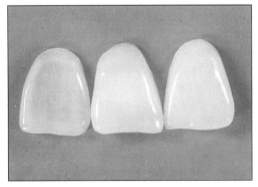

Fig 16-31 Veneers displaying different amounts of translucency. The left veneer is made from a very translucent porcelain and allows most of the underlying tooth color to show through. The center veneer has a base layer of masking dentin porcelain, which is used to block dark underlying tooth color yet maintain some degree of polychromicity. The right veneer has a layer of opaque resin cement bonded to the inner surface of the veneer. The opaque resin is very reflective and results in a displeasing, monochromatic appearance.

Color Management and Characterization

A common problem with porcelain veneer is the lack of color differentiation between the gingival and incisal portions of the restoration. Several methods of color characterization can be used to correct the monochromism.[33,37,38] The best and most basic method makes the color changes in the porcelain itself. A color diagram that outlines the desired shade and color changes and any other special characterization, such as hypocalcified or hyperchromatic areas, can be given to the technician. However, the most effective method of communicating color to the laboratory technician is with photographs (see Fig 16-6a). When characterization is incorporated into the veneer, it is there to stay. If the esthetic result is not satisfactory during the try-in, it is difficult, if not impossible, to successfully modify the veneer.

A second commonly used method involves the modification of the color with the underlying luting composite. All

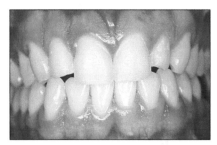

Fig 16-32a Veneer preparations on the maxillary central and lateral incisors. (From Robbins.[38] Reprinted with permission.)

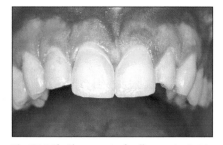

Fig 16-32b Placement of yellow resin tint in the gingival third and blue resin tint in the incisal third. (From Robbins.[38] Reprinted with permission.)

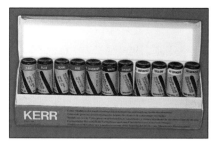

Fig 16-32c Kit of resin tints and opaques. (From Robbins.[38] Reprinted with permission.)

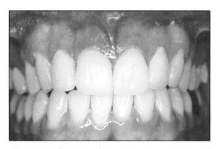

Fig 16-32d Monochromatic appearance of veneers tried in with try-in paste but without the use of resin tints. (From Robbins.[38] Reprinted with permission.)

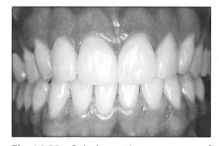

Fig 16-32e Polychromatic appearance of bonded veneers after the placement of resin tints. (From Robbins.[38] Reprinted with permission.)

porcelain veneer kits have several different shades of luting composite. If an appropriate shade of luting cement is not available, resin tints can be added to the luting composite to effect virtually any desired color.

A third and less commonly used method of characterization involves the direct placement of the resin tints on the tooth before placement of the veneer (Figs 16-32a to 16-32e). During the try-in, the desired resin tints are placed on the tooth and light cured. The chosen base shade of luting composite is placed in the veneer, and the veneer is placed on the tooth. A determination is then made regarding the esthetic result. The veneer can be removed, and the cured resin tint on the tooth can easily be scraped off with an explorer, because the enamel was not etched. If the esthetic result is acceptable, the dentist can proceed with the bonding, using the tints that were used during the try-in.

The final restoration will not always exhibit the same color displayed at the try-in. This occurs because the luting composite becomes more translucent when it is cured, allowing more of the underlying tooth color to show through.[39] Although not usually a problem, this color-change phenomenon will occasionally result in a disappointing esthetic result, espe-

cially when the dentist is attempting to match a single veneer to an adjacent natural tooth.

Discolored Teeth

Darkly discolored teeth present the greatest challenge for porcelain veneers. There are many causes of tooth discoloration, including extrinsic staining, fluorosis, pulpal injury, drugs (eg, tetracycline), and previous restorations. The ideal method of dealing with stain is to remove it, when possible. Extrinsic stains are easily removed during tooth preparation. Because fluoride predominantly affects the enamel, the discoloration of fluorosis is also commonly diminished by tooth preparation.

However, the by-products of pulpal injury, tetracycline, and previous restorations are found predominantly in the dentin, making their removal more difficult. The restoration of the high-chroma, low-value tetracycline-stained tooth with a porcelain veneer is perhaps the most difficult treatment situation. Instinctively, practitioners prepare the discolored teeth more deeply to allow more room for porcelain. However, as more enamel is removed, the underlying color becomes

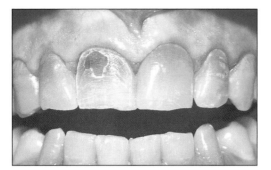

Fig 16-33 Preparation on the severely tetracycline-stained maxillary central incisor, which demonstrates increased darkness with increased depth of preparation.

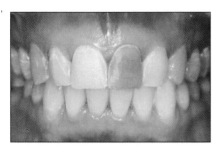

Fig 16-34a Removal of bonded resin composite veneers demonstrates significant discoloration of maxillary right canine and left central incisor.

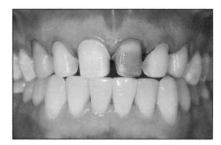

Fig 16-34b Final conservative full veneer preparations.

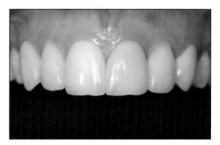

Fig 16-34c Porcelain veneers bonded with translucent resin demonstrating significant color correction with contemporary porcelains.

darker (Fig 16-33). Herein lies the major difficulty in placing porcelain veneers on tetracycline-stained teeth. Additional tooth structure should only be removed in the areas of discoloration, not over the entire preparation. Tetracycline-stained teeth are often severely discolored in the middle third of the tooth, with other areas having an acceptable or easily modified color. Ideally the preparation should stay within the enamel in the gingival and incisal thirds and only deepen in the middle third. The amount of reduction required depends on the color of the preparation and the desired chroma/value of the final restoration.

Ceramic Buildup

The evolution of contemporary porcelain materials and sophisticated fabrication techniques has allowed laboratory technicians to block out significant discolorations with ultra-thin veneers (Fig 16-34a to 16-34c). The color of the prepared tooth is used for the development of natural color. It is important that clinicians provide the laboratory with a photograph of the final preparation at a 1:1 magnification. With this photograph, the tooth can be measured by the technician and the maverick colors or discolorations located. Once blemishes have been identified, masking agents can be added selectively to the restoration. Color characteristic stains are routinely used to create optical effects and conceal discolorations in conservative veneer restorations. These stains are

opaque metal oxides that are painted into wet porcelains. The stains are used to mask discoloration or further characterize the appearance of the veneer and are subsequently covered with a thin layer of opalescent or fluorescent porcelain prior to firing. It is possible to modify the color of the tooth by one to two shades for every 0.2 mm of tooth reduction.

Masking

It is difficult to mask out dark underlying tooth color with a natural-appearing porcelain veneer (Figs 16-35a and 16-35b). If the luting cement is sufficiently opaque to mask the dark color, the final restoration commonly appears lifeless and monochromatic. Conversely, if the veneer and/or cement contains no opaque element, the darkness of the underlying tooth structure will be visible through the porcelain. As previously stated, it is preferable to incorporate the opaque elements into the porcelain rather than to attempt to mask the darkness with opaque resin composite. This requires excellent communication between the laboratory technician and the dentist. Postpreparation photographs with a shade tab for color comparison are very helpful to the technician when porcelain veneers are being fabricated for discolored teeth (see Fig 16-5). The photographs illustrate both the intensity of the darkness and the position of the bands of darkness.

Several methods of masking dark underlying tooth color with resin composite have been proposed. Friedman[35] report-

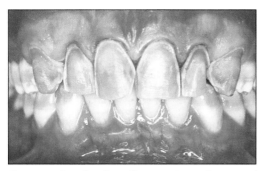

Fig 16-35a Discolored maxillary anterior teeth prepared for porcelain veneers. (From Robbins.[39] Reprinted with permisssion.)

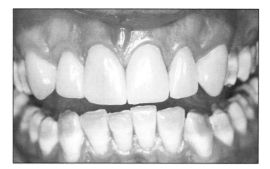

Fig 16-35b Discolored maxillary anterior teeth with bonded porcelain veneers. (From Robbins.[39] Reprinted with permisssion.)

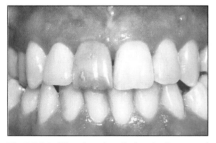

Fig 16-36a Discolored endodontically treated maxillary right central incisor. (From Robbins.[33] Reprinted with permission.)

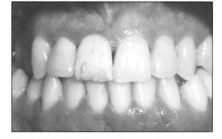

Fig 16-36b Maxillary right central incisor after completion of walking bleach procedure. (From Robbins.[33] Reprinted with permission.)

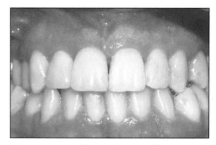

Fig 16-36c Maxillary right central incisor with a porcelain veneer bonded in place. (From Robbins.[33] Reprinted with permission.) (Porcelain veneer created by Danny Diebel, CDT, Dental Arts Studio.)

ed successful use of a standard highly filled restorative resin composite as the luting cement. Reid[37] discussed the use of complementary colors to mask underlying dark tooth color. For example, if the tooth is predominantly yellow, a violet tint is placed and light cured. This neutralizes the high-chroma yellow to a low-value gray. Opaque resin tint is then placed over the violet tint and light cured to increase the value, and the veneer is bonded in the routine manner. Although theoretically appealing, this technique has not proven to be of practical benefit.

When discoloration is localized rather than generalized, it can be removed mechanically with a bur and replaced with the appropriate shade of glass ionomer or resin composite. This is usually done after the veneer preparation is completed but before the final impression is made; however, it can be done immediately before cementation of the veneer.

Composite luting resin can be used to block underlying darkness to a limited degree. However, most of the masking must be accomplished with body modifiers that are incorporated into the porcelain veneer. Depending on the degree of darkness being masked, the technician must place 50 to 100 μm of die spacer on the refractory die prior to veneer fabrication. This allows space for an additional thickness of the lut-

ing composite, which aids in the masking of the underlying darkness. Although the appearance of discolored teeth can usually be improved with porcelain veneers, the patient must understand the limitations of the restoration.

Bleaching

When a discolored tooth can be lightened before veneer placement, the final result is routinely improved. This can be accomplished in endodontically treated teeth with a "walking bleach" technique[40] (Figs 16-36a to 16-36c) (see also chapter 15). A 2.0-mm-thick base of glass-ionomer cement is placed in the base of the pulp chamber to protect the cervix from bleach. A paste mixture of sodium perborate and water is placed in the pulp chamber, which is sealed with a temporary cement for 3 to 5 days. This can be repeated for several treatments until the desired result is attained. The mixture is ultimately removed, and the access area is restored with a resin composite restoration. At this point, the tooth is prepared for the porcelain veneer restoration. If the darkness returns in future years, the walking bleach can be accomplished again through the lingual access without disturbing the porcelain veneer restoration.

The success of bleaching vital teeth before veneer placement is not as clear-cut. It is known that vital teeth that have been bleached have the potential to revert toward their original color with time.[41] However, the effect that the placement of porcelain veneers has on this relapse is not known. If color relapse does occur, the veneer restorations will also get darker. There has been reported success in bleaching teeth that have veneers bonded to them (see chapter 15).

Bleaching teeth with 35% hydrogen peroxide[42] or carbamide peroxide[43] immediately before the bonding procedure has a catastrophic effect on the resultant bond strength. Any bonding procedure should be delayed at least 1 week after the completion of bleaching. It is hoped that future research will clarify the effects of bleaching on the success of porcelain veneers.

Crown and Veneer Combinations

When a combination of veneers and crowns is placed, all restorations must be tried in individually and then simultaneously for fit. They must also be tried in for color evaluation with a try-in medium. The final color of the veneers may be modified with the choice of the resin cement. For this reason, the full crowns are bonded first, because it is easier to make minor modifications in the color of the veneers with the veneer luting resin to match the crowns than to surface stain the all-ceramic crowns to match the bonded veneers.

Failure

The most common cause of failure of porcelain veneers is fracture.[8,16,18] Clinical studies report a modest 0% to 5% failure rate due to fracture. Higher fracture rates (7% to 14%)[15] were noted in cases with unfavorable occlusion, significant parafunction, large dentin-bonding surfaces, and bonding to existing restorations. In a 15-year review, Friedman[17] classified the fractures into three categories: static, cohesive, and adhesive. When a segment of a veneer fractures but remains intact, it is defined as a static fracture (Fig 16-37a). These failures are caused by excessive loading or polymerization shrinkage. The key factors are the internal fit of the ceramic restoration and the amount of unsupported porcelain. The crack propensity is inversely proportional to the internal fit of the veneer. An internal fit discrepancy of 100 μm or less will minimize internal stress and prevent static fracture.[25,44] Cohesive fractures occur within the body of porcelain due to tensile loads from excessive functional or parafunctional loading (Fig 16-37b). Enamel imparts stiffness to the tooth much like a metal coping does for a metal-ceramic crown. Removal of the enamel negatively affects the stress-strain distribution of the subsequent veneer. This leads to an increase in flexure under load and, ultimately, cohesive fracture.[44] The most important areas in which to maintain enamel are the incisal and cervical areas. Lack of adhesion in those areas produces higher fringe-order stress on loading and increased risk of cohesive fracture.[14,16] Finally, an adhesive fracture is due to a failure of the bonding interface between the porcelain/luting composite and the tooth structure (see Figs 16-25a and 16-25b). It is a result of a weak bond or severe occlusal loading. Friedman[17] reports that 86% of the adhesive fractures occurred at a resin-dentin interface.

On rare occasions, a porcelain veneer will debond. When this happens, it is important to determine at which bonded interface the failure occurred. If the luting composite remains on the tooth, the failure is likely due to either inadequate etching of the veneer or the use of old silane (Fig 16-38a). The stated shelf life of silane is approximately 1 year when it is refrigerated, but it is known that silane efficacy decreases with time.

If the luting composite remains on the inside of the veneer, then there was a problem with either the bonding materials, the placement technique, or the bonding substrate (Fig 16-38b). Veneers that are bonded to a predominantly dentinal substrate have a significantly greater likelihood of debonding than veneers that are predominantly bonded to enamel.[14]

When the luting composite remains on the inner surface of the veneer, it must be removed before the veneer can be rebonded. The veneer is placed in a glazing oven, and the temperature is slowly increased to 600°C and held for 10 minutes to ensure burnout of the luting composite. After the veneer is removed from the oven and cooled to room temperature, it is cleaned with acetone and re-etched with 9.5% hydrofluoric acid for 4 minutes. If 9.5% hydrofluoric acid is not available, 1.23% acidulated phosphate fluoride can be used to etch the porcelain; however, this requires a 10-minute etching time. The veneer is then washed, dried, silanated,[45] and rebonded. The patient must know that there is a significant risk of veneer fracture during removal of the luting composite.

A small percentage of veneers will fracture.[3–5] It is possible to repair fractured porcelain. First, the porcelain fracture site is etched with 9.5% hydrofluoric acid for 4 minutes. After the veneer is washed and dried, silane is placed and dried. The repair is then accomplished with conventional bonded resin composite. Because the hydrofluoric acid should not be allowed to contact natural tooth structure or soft tissue, this etching procedure should be performed with rubber dam isolation. Alternatively, the porcelain can be prepared with 1.23% acidulated phosphate fluoride or by air abrasion with 50-μm aluminum oxide.

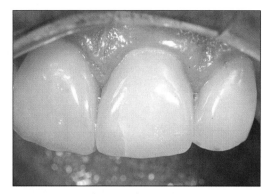

Fig 16-37a Static fracture of a porcelain veneer.

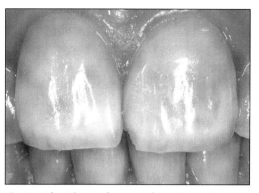

Fig 16-37b Cohesive fracture of maxillary left central incisor veneer due to excessive force.

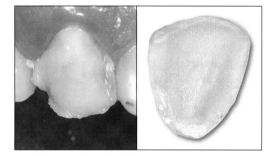

Fig 16-38a Debonding of the veneer leaving resin composite bonded to the tooth is a result of inadequate porcelain etching or contaminated silane.

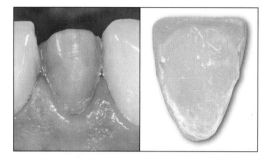

Fig 16-38b Resin composite attached to the debonded veneer indicates a predominantly dentinal substrate.

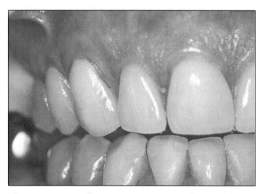

Fig 16-39 Minimally penetrating stain at the mesial margin of the maxillary right canine.

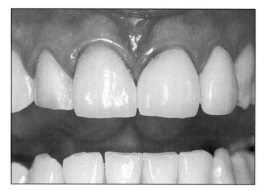

Fig 16-40 Deeply penetrating stain under the porcelain veneer on the right central incisor.

Marginal staining and leakage are common causes of failure of porcelain veneers.[4,6] The staining is caused by an influx of oral fluids containing chromogenic bacteria or organic stains. The composite-tooth interface is the primary site for the leakage. It has been noted that these areas of microleakage are always devoid of enamel.[17] If the marginal stain is superficial, it can be removed by tray bleaching with 10% carbamide peroxide for several days. After the stain has been removed, the margin can be etched with 30% to 40% phosphoric acid and sealed with a dentin bonding agent. If the stain is slightly penetrating at the margin (Fig 16-39), it can be mechanically removed with a small bur and the area restored with conventional bonded resin composite. When there is significant penetration of stain under the veneer, the entire veneer must be removed (Fig 16-40).

Fig 16-41 *Veneer removal.*

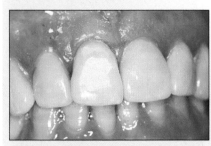 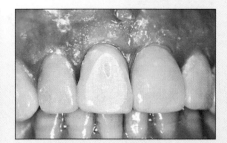 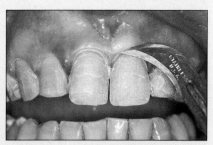

Fig 16-41a Initial removal of porcelain before tooth structure is reached.

Fig 16-41b Porcelain removed until the first area of enamel is visualized.

Fig 16-41c Exploring margins with a No. 12 scalpel blade to remove remaining resin composite and porcelain.

Veneer Removal

Removal of porcelain veneers is not only time-consuming but also difficult and technique sensitive, especially if the underlying tooth color is light. The veneer cannot be grooved with a bur and torqued in the same manner that a cemented gold crown is removed. The veneer must be removed with a diamond bur in the same way that enamel is removed during initial tooth preparation.

The dentist starts removing the porcelain in the midfacial area with a back-and-forth sweeping motion with a barrel diamond (Fig 16-41a). This must be done without water spray so that the operator can visualize the subtle color difference between the veneer and tooth structure as the interface is reached. Therefore, the dental assistant must cool the tooth with a constant stream of air. Once this interface is apparent (Fig 16-41b), the diamond bur is moved laterally away from the area of exposed enamel toward the periphery of the preparation. Care must be taken to remove as little enamel as possible during this step.

The procedure continues until only a small amount of porcelain remains at the margins. If there has been microleakage at the margins, the remaining marginal porcelain can be removed with a No. 12 scalpel blade. However, if the marginal seal is intact, the remainder of the porcelain must be cautiously removed with the diamond bur.

It is very important that the operator not lose orientation in relation to the porcelain-tooth interface. If this occurs, it is very easy to inadvertently remove all of the enamel. For this reason, one veneer should be completely removed before starting veneer removal on the next tooth.

After all porcelain veneers have been removed, gingival retraction cord is packed to clearly expose all margins. As the

final step of veneer removal, all margins are explored with a sharp No. 12 scalpel blade (Fig 16-41c), which commonly results in the removal of additional small areas of residual resin composite and porcelain.

Maintenance

The maintenance of the porcelain veneer restoration is similar to that of the porcelain crown. Devices such as an ultrasonic cleaner, air-abrasive polisher, and prophylaxis cup with pumice must be avoided. Surface stains may be removed from porcelain veneers with aluminum oxide polishing paste or diamond polishing paste on a felt wheel or rubber cup. Proximal stains may be removed with composite polishing strips. When scaling is performed around porcelain veneers, care must be taken not to chip the margins. If a fluoride preparation is needed by the patient, it should have a neutral pH; because of their ability to etch porcelain, neither acidulated phosphate fluoride nor stannous fluoride should be used.

The patient should be advised that foods and liquids with a high potential for staining, such as coffee and tea, increase the potential for marginal staining. The patient must also be made aware of the potential for the porcelain to fracture. Activities such as ice chewing and fingernail biting must be absolutely avoided. It is a good idea to make an occlusal guard appliance for all patients who have porcelain-veneer restorations. When porcelain-veneer restorations will oppose natural teeth or when the patient has a history of a parafunctional habit, a protective appliance should be fabricated to protect both the porcelain veneers and the opposing teeth.

Procedures for Insertion of Porcelain Veneers

Veneer Try-in

1. Check the veneers for fit on dies, and transilluminate to check for fracture lines.
2. Try in the veneers individually for fit, and then all together. Interproximal contact areas may need to be adjusted with a microfine diamond or disk. Do not make any other adjustments until veneers are bonded.
3. Clean the veneers with acetone and air dry. Place silane on the inner surface of each veneer and allow to air dry.
4. Choose a shade of resin composite or water-soluble try-in paste, place on the inside of the veneer, and try in.
5. If water-soluble try-in paste has been used, wash the veneer with water and air dry before loading with the unfilled resin and luting composite. If the shade is correct, skip steps 6 through 12, and proceed with step 13.
6. If the shade is incorrect, remove the try-in composite and select another shade, or customize the shade by adding tint to the luting composite.
7. If characterization (eg, blue in incisal areas, yellow at gingival areas) is required, tints and opaques should be placed only on the tooth and not on the inside of the veneer. The tints and opaques are brushed on the tooth in a thin layer and light cured for 30 seconds. All try-in composite must be removed from the tooth (facial, proximal, and lingual aspects) before curing the tints and opaques. Because the tooth was not etched, the cured tints and opaques can be scraped off easily with an explorer at the end of the try-in.
8. Once a combination of composite, tint, and/or opaque has been determined, make note of it so that it can be reproduced exactly for final luting.
9. Clean the try-in resin composite from the inside of the veneer with acetone using two different beakers. Clean the bulk of the resin composite with a brush dipped in the first beaker, then transfer the veneer to the second, clean beaker of acetone to remove the remaining resin composite.

Veneer Preparation

10. Place the veneers, etched side down, on a 2 × 2-inch gauze pad in a glass beaker of clean acetone, and place the beaker in an ultrasonic cleaner for 5 minutes.
11. Remove the veneers from the acetone and dry.
12. Place silane on the inner surface of the veneers and allow it to air dry.

Tooth Preparation

13. Place retraction cord in the sulcus of each prepared tooth (but not the mandibular incisors if the margins are more than 1.0 mm from the gingival crest).
14. Clean both central incisors with oil-free pumice paste. (This should be done for each tooth just before etching.)
15. Place clear plastic matrix or dead-soft metal matrix material on the distal aspects of both central incisors.
16. Etch both central incisors with 30% to 40% phosphoric acid for 20 seconds, wash for 3 seconds, and air dry to ensure adequate etch of the enamel.
17. Remoisten tooth surface.
18. If using a fourth-generation bonding agent, place several coats of primer and gently air dry until tooth surface is completely dry. Check for uniform shiny surface. If using a fifth- or sixth-generation bonding agent, place one to two coats and follow manufacturer's instructions for drying and curing.
19. If using a fourth-generation bonding agent, place the dentin adhesive on the tooth surface and the inner surface of the veneer. If using a fifth- or sixth-generation bonding agent, place the agent on the inner surface of the veneer.
20. If tints or opaques are necessary, place on the predetermined areas and light cure for 90 seconds.

Placement

21. Place bonding resin and light-cured resin composite into the veneer being bonded. Operatory light should be turned off at this time.
22. With shimstock (0.0005-inch thickness) between central incisors and clear plastic matrix strips or dead-soft metal matrix material on distal aspects of each central incisor, gently place veneers onto both central incisors and tease into place. Ensure that excess resin composite appears at all margins.
23. Remove excess resin composite from veneers with a small brush or explorer, depending on viscosity.
24. Visually inspect, standing in front of the patient to ensure that veneers are placed correctly. Ensure that mesial surfaces are in contact.
25. Lightly press facial surfaces of veneers and light cure from the lingual aspect for 30 seconds, then light cure from the facial aspect for 30 seconds.
26. Remove the excess resin composite only on the distal surfaces of the central incisors with a No. 12 scalpel blade to ensure that the veneers on lateral incisors will fit.
27. Visually inspect for voids and repair if possible.
28. Try in the left lateral incisor veneer to ensure correct fit.
29. Repeat steps 14 to 28 for each veneer being placed.

(continued)

Procedures for Insertion of Porcelain Veneers *(continued)*

Finishing

30. Remove minimal gingival flash of resin composite with a No. 12 scalpel blade. Move blade from veneer gingivally to avoid chipping the veneer's margin. Ensure that all excess resin composite is removed on the facial and proximal surfaces. Finishing of the margins with a rotary instrument should be avoided, as it will damage the root and remove the glaze from the veneer. This will cause an increase in plaque retention and elicit a gingival reaction.[15]

31. Remove excess resin composite from lingual surfaces with an egg-shaped, 12-fluted carbide bur.

32. Smooth lingual surfaces with composite polishing points or disks.

33. Check and adjust the occlusion in maximum intercuspation position and in excursions (with special attention to the distal incisal edges of maxillary lateral incisors).

34. Reshape incisal edges and contours while standing in front of the patient.

35. Reshape and contour incisal embrasures with a finishing diamond or thin separating disk.

36. Gingival margins should be smooth and require no finishing. If gingival margins are rough, smooth them with a finishing diamond or 12-fluted carbide bur. Be careful not to scar the cementum.

37. Polish all roughened porcelain using an abrasive-impregnated rubber porcelain polishing system (Brasseler or Shofu).

38. Finish the proximal areas with finishing and polishing strips.

39. Any visible porcelain that has been finished and smoothed with a rubber point should be polished with diamond polishing paste on a wet felt wheel and prophylaxis cup at the gingival margin. Be careful not to polish the cementum.

40. With the retraction cord still in place, re-etch and rebond (with rebonding or surface-sealing resin) all margins.

41. Remove the retraction cord.

42. Have the patient return in 1 week to inspect for excess composite and rough areas. At this time, final esthetic reshaping may be accomplished.

References

1. Fradeani M. Six-year follow-up with Empress veneers. Int J Periodontics Restorative Dent 1998;18:217–225.

2. Kihn PW, Barnes DM. The clinical longevity of porcelain veneers. J Am Dent Assoc 1998;129:747–752.

3. Kreulen CM, Creugers NHJ, Meijering AC. Meta-analysis of anterior veneer restorations in clinical studies. J Dent 1998;26:345–353.

4. Peumans M, Van Meerbeek B, Lambrechts P, Vuylsteke-Wauters M, Vanherle G. Five-year clinical performance of porcelain veneers. Quintessence Int 1998;29:211–221.

5. Shaini FJ, Shortall ACC, Marquis PM. Clinical performance of porcelain laminate veneers. A retrospective evaluation over a period of 6.5 years. J Oral Rehabil 1997;24:553–559.

6. Strassler HE, Weiner S. Long term clinical evaluation of etched porcelain veneer [abstract 1017]. J Dent Res 1998;77:233.

7. Van Gogswaardt DC, Van Thoor W, Lampert F. Clinical assessment of adhesively placed ceramic veneers after 9 years [abstract 1178]. J Dent Res 1998;77:779.

8. Peumans M, De Munck J, Fieuws S, Lambrechts P, Vanherle G, Van Meerbeek B. A prospective ten-year clinical trial of porcelain veneers. J Adhes Dent 2004;6:65–76.

9. Edelhoff D, Sorensen JA. Tooth structure removal associated with various preparation designs for anterior teeth. J Prosthet Dent 2002;87:503–509.

10. Levinson N. Psychological facets of esthetic dental health care: A developmental perspective. J Prosthet Dent 1990;64:486–491.

11. Hahn P, Gustav M, Hellwig E. An in vitro assessment of the strength of porcelain veneers dependent on tooth preparation. J Oral Rehab 2000;27:1024–1029.

12. Highton R, Caputo AA, Matyas J. A photoelastic study of stresses on porcelain laminate preparations. J Prosthet Dent 1987;58:157–161.

13. Schneider PM, Messer LB, Douglas WH. The effect of enamel surface reduction in vitro on the bonding of composite resin to permanent human enamel. J Dent Res 1981;60:895–900.

14. Troedson M, Derand T. Shear stresses in the adhesive layer under porcelain veneers—A finite analysis study. Acta Odontol Scand 1998;56:257–262.

15. Peumans M, Van Meerbeek B, Lambrechts P, Vanherle G. Porcelain veneers: A review of the literature. J Dent 2000;28:163–177.

16. Seymour KG, Cherukara GP, Samarawickrama DYD. Stresses within porcelain veneers and the composite lute using different preparation designs. J Prosthodont 2001;10:16–21.

17. Friedman MJ. A 15-year review of porcelain veneer failure—A clinician's observations. Compend Contin Educ Dent 1998;19:625–628, 630, 632 passim.

18. Crispin B. Esthetic moieties. J Esthet Dent 1993;5:37.

19. Rouse J, McGowan S. Restoration of the anterior maxilla with ultra-conservative veneers: Clinical and laboratory considerations. Pract Periodontics Aesthet Dent 1999;11:333–339.

20. Walls AWG, Steele JG, Wassell RW. Crowns and other extra-coronal restorations: Porcelain laminate veneers. Br Dent J 2002;193:73–82.

21. Cherukara GP, Seymour KG, Zou L, Samarawickrama DYD. Geographic distribution of porcelain veneer preparation depth with various clinical techniques. J Prosthet Dent 2003;89:544–550.

22. Cherukara GP, Seymour KG, Samarawickrama DY, Zou L. A study into the variations in the labial reduction of teeth prepared to receive porcelain veneers—A comparison of three clinical techniques. Br Dent J 2002;192:401–404.

23. Rouse JS. Full veneer versus traditional veneer preparation: A discussion of interproximal extension. J Prosthet Dent 1997;6:545–549.

24. Wylie SG, Tan HK, Brooke K. Restoring the vertical dimension of mandibular incisors with bonded ceramic restorations. Aust Dent J 2000;45:91–96.

25. Magne P, Douglas WH. Design optimization and evolution of bonded ceramics for the anterior dentition: A finite-element analysis. Quintessence Int 1999;30:661–672.

26. Castelnuovo J, Tjan AHL, Phillips K, et al. Fracture strength and failure mode for different ceramic veneer designs [abstract 1373]. J Dent Res 1998;77:803.

27. Kois JC. The restorative-periodontal interface: Biological parameters. Periodontol 2000 1996;11:29–38.

28. Andreason FM, Flugge E, Daugaard-Jensen J, Munksgaard EC. Treatment of crown fractured incisors with laminate veneer restorations. An experimental study. Endod Dent Traumatol 1992;8:30–35.

29. Bayne SC, Heymann HO, Wilder AD, et al. One-year clinical study of sclerotic vs. non-sclerotic dentin bonding [abstract 1221]. J Dent Res 1995;74:164.

30. Heymann HO, Bayne SC. Current concepts in dentin bonding: Focusing on dentinal adhesion factors. J Am Dent Assoc 1993;124:27–36.

31. Allen EP. Use of mucogingival surgical procedures to enhance esthetics. Dent Clin North Am 1988;32:307–330.

32. Rouse JS. Facial shell temporary veneers: Reducing chances for misunderstanding. J Prosthet Dent 1996;76:641–643.

33. Robbins J. Color management of the porcelain veneer. Esthet Dent Update 1992;3:132–135.

34. Barceleiro Mde O, De Miranda MS, Dias KR, Sekito T Jr. Shear bond strength of porcelain laminate veneer bonded with flowable composite. Oper Dent 2003;28:423–428.

35. Friedman M. Multiple potential of etched porcelain laminate veneers. J Am Dent Assoc 1987;122(special issue):83E–87E.

36. Linden JJ, Swift EJ, Boyer DB, Davis BK. Photo-activation of resin cements through porcelain veneers. J Dent Res 1991;70:154–157.

37. Reid JS. Tooth color modification and porcelain veneers. Quintessence Int 1988;19:477–481.

38. Robbins J. Color characterization of porcelain veneers. Quintessence Int 1991;22:853–856.

39. Seghi R, Gritz MD, Kim J. Colorimetric changes in composite resins due to visible light polymerization [abstract 892]. J Dent Res 1988;67:224.

40. Rotstein I, Mor C, Friedman S. Prognosis of intracoronal bleaching with sodium perborate preparation in vitro: 1-year study. J Endod 1993;19:10–12.

41. Haywood VB. Nightguard vital bleaching: Current concepts and research. J Am Dent Assoc 1997;128(suppl):19S–25S.

42. Torneck C, Titley K, Smith D, Adibfar A. The influence of time of hydrogen peroxide exposure on the adhesion of composite resin to bleached bovine enamel. J Endod 1990;16:123–128.

43. Godwin JM, Barghi N, Berry TG, et al. Time duration for dissipation of bleaching effects before enamel bonding [abstract 590]. J Dent Res 1992;71:179.

44. Magne P, Douglas W. Porcelain veneers: Dentin bonding optimization and biomimetic recovery of the crown. Int J Prosthodont 1999;12:111–121.

45. Hsu CS, Stangel I, Nathanson D. Shear bond strength of resin to etched porcelain [abstract 1095]. J Dent Res 1985;64:296.

Anterior Ceramic Crowns

17

Jeffrey S. Rouse

The provision of anterior ceramic crowns can be the most valuable and difficult service in dentistry. Protecting the natural dentition and providing an illusion of reality requires the practitioner to choose the correct ceramic system and prepare the site for success. This chapter discusses a systematic approach for selection of the proper ceramic system[1] and development of a foundation for the restoration that enables predictable results.

Decision-Making Factors

There are two common myths pertaining to anterior ceramics: *(1)* strength is the most important decision-making factor, and *(2)* all-ceramic crowns are always more esthetic.

Strength should not be the overriding factor in choosing an anterior ceramic crown system. While it is true that metal-ceramic crowns are stronger than all-ceramic systems, the real question is how much strength is required. The answer is that the crown must be able to resist fracture under load. Normal incisal bite force averages between 130 and 230 N.[2,3] The weakest ceramic choice, a nonadhesively cemented porcelain jacket crown, has an adequate load value (545 N) for the anterior region. Bonded ceramic crowns and IPS Empress (Ivoclar Vivadent; 2,180 N) have load values an order of magnitude greater than those generated during normal function.[3] In addition, the ultimate strengths for axial and oblique loads on anterior ceramic systems exceed the maximum normal bite-force peaks.[3] Normal functional loads, therefore, should not damage all-ceramic crowns (Table 17-1).

All-ceramic systems are not always more esthetic. In the hands of an average laboratory technician, all-ceramic systems will be repeatably more esthetic simply because of the lack of a metal core[4] (Fig 17-1). However, given proper preparation depths, skilled technicians can mimic natural teeth using a metal-ceramic system (Fig 17-2).

Metal-ceramic crowns are more appropriate for some patients than others. Teeth that are opaque or have high chroma and high value may be easier to match with metal-ceramic systems than with all-ceramic systems. A patient with a low lip line is a good candidate for metal ceramics, because the esthetic weakness of metal ceramics is most pronounced in the gingival third, where the opacity influences the brightness. The highly reflective opaque ceramic coating used to mask the metal is difficult to disguise when matching teeth with low color saturation or brightness (Fig 17-3). In the anterior region, many patients demand a perfect match of crown, tooth, and gingiva. This can be challenging for metal-core crowns. In an attempt to eliminate the gingival opacity, some ceramists stop the extension of the metal substructure up to 2 mm away from the shoulder.[5] This removes the highly reflective opacity in the gingival third, decreasing reflection and allowing light penetration into the cervical tooth structure, without

Table 17-1 | Comparison of all-ceramic restorative systems

Product	Flexural strength	Abrasiveness vs natural tooth	Special equipment	Other characteristics
Traditional feldspathic porcelain	110–150 MPa	Varies; higher leucite content yields higher wear	Special refractory die	No core material; uniform translucency and shade throughout; etchable for bonding to tooth
Pressable ceramics				
IPS Empress (Ivoclar Vivadent)	160–182 MPa	Comparable to natural tooth except when layered with conventional feldspathic porcelain	Special oven, die material, and molding process	Etchable for bonding to tooth; core material shaded and translucent
Optimal Pressable Ceramic	165 MPa	Same as for IPS Empress	Same as for IPS Empress	Same as for IPS Empress
Empress 2 (Ivoclar Vivadent)	350 MPa	Less wear than natural tooth	Same as for IPS Empress	Crown can be cemented or etched to bond; possible to do three-unit fixed partial denture for anterior teeth
Infiltrated ceramics				
In-Ceram (Vident)	450 MPa	Same as for conventional feldspathic porcelain	Special die material; high-temperature oven	Core material is more opaque; not etchable, must be cemented
In-Ceram Spinell (Vident)	350 MPa	Same as for In-Ceram	Same as for In-Ceram	Core material 20% more translucent than In-Ceram; not etchable, must be cemented
Milled ceramics				
Procera (Nobel Biocare)	600 MPa	Same as for In-Ceram	Special die scanner; computer with modem; CAD/CAM machine	Dense translucent core; not etchable, must be cemented
Zirconium oxide core ceramics	1,000 MPa	Same as for In-Ceram	Special CAD/CAM machine or dry pressed	Dense opaque core with limited dentin shades; not etchable, must be cemented, may be used for limited fixed partial dentures

Adapted from Rosenblum and Schulman.[4]

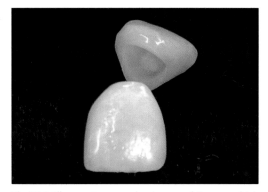

Fig 17-1 All-ceramic crowns have a porcelain core, which facilitates an esthetic match. These crowns provide adequate strength to resist functional loads.

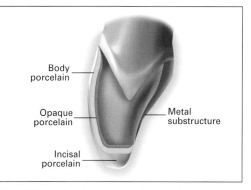

Body porcelain

Opaque porcelain

Metal substructure

Incisal porcelain

Fig 17-2 Porcelain layered over the metal substructure. (Illustrations for chapter 17 by John Bonfardeci, Studio Giovanni.)

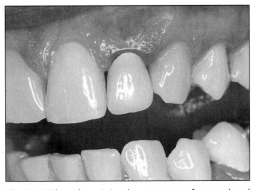

Fig 17-3 When there is inadequate space for metal and porcelain, the opaque porcelain may cause unnatural opacity (maxillary lateral incisor).

decreasing the strength of the crown.[6] Light transmission illuminates the gingiva and eliminates the dark gingival shadow sometimes found around metal-ceramic crowns.[6]

If practitioners should not make decisions based solely on the strength of metal-ceramic restorations or the esthetics of all-ceramic systems, then what criteria are appropriate? When esthetic demands are high, an enamel-bonded veneer is the first choice. Adequate enamel must be present, and the patient should have no more than moderate parafunctional habits. It is commonly agreed that enamel-bonded veneers are the most predictable, most esthetic, and strongest restorations for anterior teeth (see chapter 16). However, veneers are contraindicated when less than 50% of the prepared tooth is in enamel; a sound bonding surface is critical to the strength and success of porcelain restorations. In addition, veneers are not recommended when there is more than 2 mm of unsupported incisal porcelain in bruxers or more than 3 mm of unsupported incisal porcelain in nonbruxers.[1]

When veneers are contraindicated, choosing the correct anterior ceramic crown system is critical. The choice involves a hierarchy based on the esthetic goals of the patient, the preoperative condition of the tooth, and the load that the tooth will receive. The questions to be asked when deciding on the correct ceramic crown system are: (1) What are the esthetic demands, especially in the gingival third? (2) What is the quality of the bonding surface? and (3) Does the patient have parafunctional habits? If so, what is the severity?

Esthetic Demands

An evaluation of esthetics and a diagnosis should be conducted following the guidelines established in chapter 3. Patient expectations should be addressed before treatment begins. If there are limitations in the treatment, they should be discussed in advance. Diagnostic waxups or computer imaging may help determine what can be achieved with the restorations and aid in patient communication. Elements that affect the esthetic choice of materials include the color of the underlying structures (eg, post and core, discolored dentin) and the importance of the esthetic match in the gingival third.

Veneers bonded to enamel provide some of the most beautiful and dependable restorations for anterior teeth. The thin laminate of porcelain provides an optical refractive index similar to that of translucent enamel, allowing the natural tooth to act as the color substrate. Therefore, when the tooth substrate is an ideal color, a veneer restoration can be placed that is almost imperceptible (Figs 17-4a and 17-4b).

A ceramic crown can be thought of as a veneer of "enamel" porcelain over a "dentin" ceramic core (Fig 17-5). This "dentin" core material can be feldspathic porcelain, castable glass, heat-pressed leucite-reinforced ceramic, infiltrated alumina, lithium disilicate, or zirconium oxide.[7-11] All cores can be laminated with veneering porcelain or stain. The type of core material used in a particular patient depends on the underlying tooth structure (Table 17-2).

Because the core material has a perceptible effect on crown color,[13] the ideal core material should match the natural optical properties of dentin and mask any discoloration present.[12] Today, the feldspathic porcelains most closely mimic the opalescent and fluorescent properties of natural teeth. They are translucent, color stable, brilliant, and natural. Therefore, if the underlying tooth color is acceptable, full feldspathic crowns produce the most natural result, because they allow the underlying tooth color to show.[14]

If the "dentin" core color must be altered, the ceramic core selection changes (Fig 17-6). IPS Empress, Optimal Pressable Ceramic (OPC; Pentron), and Finesse All-Ceramic (Dentsply Ceramco) allow broader choices of substrate color with intermediate translucency. In-Ceram Alumina (Vident), Procera (Nobel Biocare), and In-Ceram Zirconia (Vident) provide a high-strength core that is relatively opaque. In-Ceram Alumina, for example, creates a core that is roughly 50% as translucent as dentin.[15] The influence of the core material is most noticeable in the gingival third. The more translucent the core, the more gray it appears as the darkness of the oral cavity shows through. This is most evident with translucent Optimal Pressed Ceramic and IPS Empress. A higher value or brightness is produced by the more opaque, reflective cores found in In-Ceram Alumina, In-Ceram Zirconia, and metal-ceramic crowns.[11]

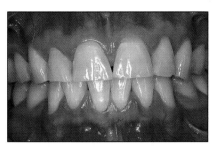

Fig 17-4a An increase in length and alteration of shape is required esthetically. The tooth color is acceptable, there are no restorations, and there is adequate enamel for bonding. Enamel-bonded veneers are the restorations of choice.

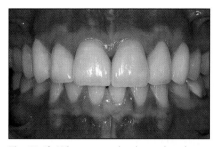

Fig 17-4b When properly planned and constructed, enamel-bonded veneers are almost imperceptible.

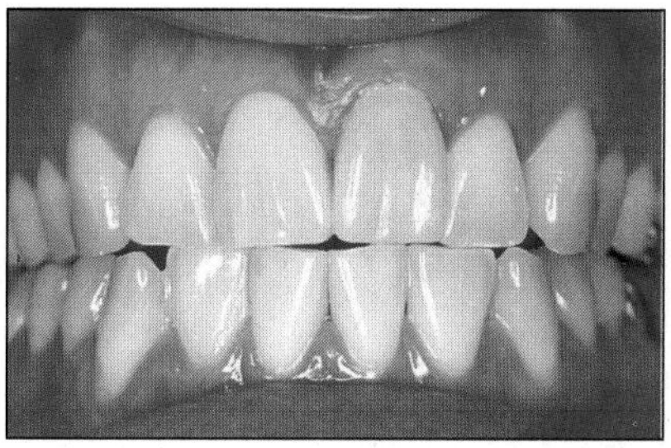

Fig 17-5 Unlike metal-ceramic crowns, cemented all-ceramic restorations are significantly influenced by the underlying color. In this case, an amalgam buildup shows through an all-ceramic crown on the maxillary left central incisor, making it too gray.

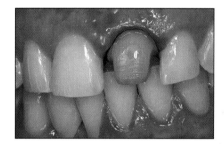

Fig 17-6 Dark prepared teeth are an esthetic challenge for all-ceramic restorations. The correct ceramic core must be chosen to minimize the effect of the discoloration.

Table 17-2	Selection criteria for anterior ceramic crown materials[12]										
Shade and appearance of natural teeth	Conventional feldspathic	Veneered Optimal	Colored Optimal	Veneered Empress	Colored Empress	Empress 2	In-Ceram	In-Ceram Spinell	Procera	Zirconium oxide	Metal-ceramic
Vita A-1 to A-2; Low color content, opaceous, high brightness	X							X	X	X	X
Vita A-3; Moderate color content, translucent body, opaque body	X	X	X	X	X	X	X	X	X	X	X
Vita A-3.5 to A-4; High color content, translucent or opaque	X	X	X	X	X	X	X	X	X	X	X
Altering shade from high color to low color			X		X	X	X	X	X	X	X
Translucent, low brightness, high color		X	X	X	X	X					
Translucent, grayish teeth		X		X							
Translucent, moderately bright teeth	X		X	X	X	X					

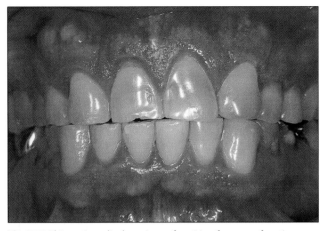

Fig 17-7 This patient displays signs of attrition from parafunction, erosion from chewing aspirin and swishing acidic juices, and cervical notching from abrasion and abfraction.

Quality of the Bonding Surface

Anterior crowns can be fixed to the tooth by traditional cementation or by bonding. Traditional cementation utilizes a cement such as glass ionomer or resin-modified glass-ionomer cement. Bonding uses a luting resin or a resin composite and resin adhesive. (In this chapter, the terms *cement* and *cementation* will be used, for the most part, to discuss insertion with traditional cements. The terms *resin cement*, *luting resin*, *bonding resin*, and *bonding* will be used in reference to resin bonding of restorations.) A traditional cement occupies the space between the restoration and the tooth surfaces but does not provide adhesion between them. In most cases, bonding provides adhesion to both surfaces. Because of this, a bonded crown may not have the same requirements for tooth preparation as a cemented crown. In addition, bonding acts to transfer force from the ceramic material to the underlying tooth structure and strengthens an all-ceramic restoration that would be relatively weak if cemented.

When most all-ceramic crowns are bonded, the ceramic is etched to create micromechanical retention for the resin cement. Bonding procedures, such as those described in chapter 8, are performed on the tooth. When the resin cement is polymerized, it forms a rigid union between the restoration and the tooth. Under function, the dentin bond allows the resin to transfer load to underlying tooth structure.[16] Properly bonded crowns have fracture strengths far greater than human bite force,[17–19] but functional and para-

functional forces and the hydrodynamic nature of dentin may decrease bond strength with time. If the dentin bond is compromised, the porcelain becomes more susceptible to fracture. A study by Neiva et al[19] comparing the fracture strength of three ceramic materials reported that bonded IPS Empress had a higher mean fracture strength than In-Ceram Alumina or Procera. However, with a compromised bond, IPS Empress was significantly weaker than the other systems.

The nature of the dentin surface significantly impacts the strength of the tooth-resin interface (Fig 17-7). The risk of debonding and fracture is magnified when the underlying dentin is less than optimal. Clinicians must recognize differences in dentin composition before planning restorations that depend on long-term dentin bonding.[20] Clinical evidence suggests that loss of cervical bonded restorations is more prevalent in older patients with more sclerotic dentin. Changes in the microstructure of dentin associated with aging have been hypothesized as the cause. Sclerotic dentin has been classified.[21] If no sclerosis is present, the dentin will appear light yellow and opaque (category 1). If there is significant sclerosis, the dentin will have a dark yellow or discolored appearance and will be glossy or translucent (category 4). These category 4 lesions are typically found in older individuals. When the long-term retention of cervical restorations was compared in sclerotic vs nonsclerotic lesions, dentin bond failures were 33% more frequent in category 4 sclerotic dentin than in other categories after 1 year.[21] Acid degradation of the dentin (due to bulimia and gastrointestinal reflux) yields an accelerated sclerosing of the dentin and poor bond strengths. Deep dentin can also significantly affect strength at the dentin-resin interface. The density of the dentinal tubules is greatest near the pulp. Tubules represent 28% volume of the dentin along the pulpal wall, compared to 4% volume at the dentinoenamel junction.[21] Adhesive bond strengths in deep dentin are generally lower because there is less intertubular dentin space for bonding and greater moisture flow that may interfere with bonding.

In addition to a compromised dentin surface, bending forces beyond the ceramic limits are a contraindication to bonded ceramics. Flexural fatigue, or abfraction, is the pathologic loss of hard tooth substance by biomechanical loading forces (see Fig 17-7). This loss is thought to be due to flexure and ultimate fatigue of enamel and/or dentin at some location distant from the actual point of loading. Cuspal deflection has been well documented.[22] Eccentric forces can generate cervical flexure, resulting in stress concentrations in a bonded crown.[23] Cervical restoration failure occurs more commonly in mandibular incisors than in maxillary incisors.[21] Tooth flexure can cause porcelain fracture or less obvious failure due to marginal leakage.

Carious or noncarious lesions or previous restorations may require a crown margin to be placed far apical to the gingival crest. Adhesion is affected by dentin moisture or other contaminants (blood, sulcular fluid, or saliva).[21] The inability to isolate subgingival margins prevents predictable dentin bonding and is therefore a contraindication to bonded-ceramic crowns.[21]

Strength is not a key criterion for a ceramic crown when the dentin bonding is maximized. When the ultimate bond is compromised, however, a bonded ceramic crown may not be the restoration of choice.

Parafunction

Parafunction is a physiologically normal activation of voluntary skeletal muscles to produce behaviors that lack functional purpose and are potentially injurious. It occurs cyclically, and because it is mediated by the limbic system, it is harder to control and change.[24] Human bite force on anterior teeth rarely exceeds 200 N, well within the tolerances of most ceramic systems. Forces are greater than normal during parafunctional episodes; the normal bite strength in some bruxers/clenchers can be as much as six times that of the non-bruxer.[25] Therefore, severe parafunction is damaging to all-ceramic systems because of forces generated beyond the dentin-resin bond strength and the ceramic force tolerance. This can result in sudden, catastrophic failure.

A more gradual failure of an all-ceramic system comes from fatigue failure. Testing confirms that cyclic loading is much more damaging than static loading, given the same total time and maximum load.[26] Cyclic loading decreases mean flexural strength of an all-ceramic system by an average of 15% to 60% of the corresponding static values.[27] Three modes of cyclic fracture can occur in an all-ceramic crown near the area of contact with an opposing tooth: (1) brittle-mode tensile cracks beginning on the occluding surface; (2) quasi-plastic mode microfractures within the ceramic material in a "yield" zone; and (3) radial cracking (under-surface tension flexes the core/ceramic veneer interface).[28] It has been postulated that these inner-surface cracks are the most likely cause of failure of cemented all-ceramic systems.[29] All of the fatigue modes of failure can occur with repeated functional loads. However, severe loading during parafunctional episodes magnifies the damage by coalescence of microcracks into a macroflaw, accelerating the loss of strength and reducing the lifespan of the ceramic restoration. A thorough evaluation of the patient's parafunctional history is required in choosing an anterior ceramic system.

Hierarchical Approach

Once practitioners have answered questions regarding esthetics, bonding substrate, and parafunction, a hierarchical approach can be used to select the best anterior ceramic restoration for each patient. The choices begin with veneer crowns and conclude with metal-ceramic crowns. The type of ceramic crown is chosen when a tooth meets all the indications for that level. Refinement within the hierarchy is then made by meeting additional criteria.

Veneer Crowns

Indications
1. Esthetics of primary importance
2. Mixed enamel and dentinal substrate
3. Minimal or no parafunction

Enamel-bonded porcelain laminate veneers are the most dependable and esthetic anterior ceramic restorations. A veneer allows the passage of light into the tooth, and the underlying tooth color provides a natural effect. A veneer crown is simply a veneer that covers the entire tooth. It is to be used only in selected cases, because transitions from thin to thicker porcelain make fabrication difficult. The preparation preserves remaining enamel and uses a conservative preparation design. The most common indication is for a peg-shaped lateral incisor. Another indication is a tooth with good enamel support, large proximal restorations, and endodontic access (Fig 17-8a). The enamel is reduced by 0.5 mm, the proximal restorations are removed, and the margins are finished with a light chamfer (Figs 17-8b and 17-8c).

Bonded All-Ceramic Crowns

Indications
1. High esthetic demands, especially in the gingival third
2. Dentin bonding substrate acceptable
3. Moderate to no parafunction

Key to bonded all-ceramic restorations is the ability to provide predictable dentin adhesion. Without a sound dentin-crown unit after bonding, all-ceramic bonded crowns are extremely weak and prone to fracture.[16-18] This class of ceramics includes feldspathic porcelain (on a refractory die), castable glass, and injection-molded ceramics. These systems provide the finest esthetics of the anterior ceramic crown categories because they most closely match the translucency, brilliance,

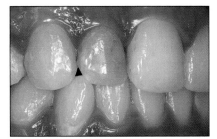

Fig 17-8a This lateral incisor had a large area of enamel available for bonding after preparation, but the interproximal restoration and lingual endodontic access made it an ideal candidate for a veneer crown.

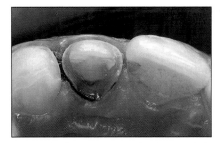

Fig 17-8b The preparation displays a subtle transition from 0.5 mm of facial reduction to 1.0 mm of lingual reduction.

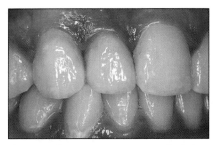

Fig 17-8c The veneer crown is in esthetic harmony with the natural central incisor and veneered canine.

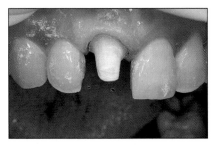

Fig 17-9a When the tooth substrate is acceptable for bonding and color, a bonded, feldspathic all-ceramic crown is indicated.

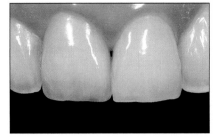

Fig 17-9b The bonded feldspathic crown provides functional predictability and natural esthetics.

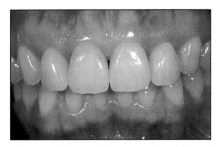

Fig 17-10 The maxillary central and lateral incisors are restored with IPS Empress crowns. When the tooth color is poor but a reliable bond is available, IPS Empress is a good choice because several core colors are available.

and qualities of natural tooth substrates. The difference between the systems is the varying degree of translucency in the core materials. Choices within this category should be based on which substrate most closely mimics that of the natural teeth. If the prepared tooth color is normal (Fig 17-9a), full feldspathic crowns produce the most natural core (Fig 17-9b).[11] However, when the crown substrate requires alteration of translucency or opacity, the core choice should be made accordingly.

IPS Empress and OPC are heat-processed, high-leucite pressed ceramics. They provide ceramists with multiple dentin shades and translucencies, which can be used to mask defects or match adjacent dentition. Once the proper dentin shade, or stump, is chosen, the core is fabricated using a lost-wax technique. The ceramist decides whether the crown will be cast in its entirety and then colored with surface stains or a cast coping will be layered with feldspathic porcelain. Surface staining involves placing heavily pigmented characterization colors on the crown, which is then covered with a glazing powder and fired. The layering technique is the recommended method for anterior ceramics (Fig 17-10). The preparation

depth must allow a core reduction such that the substructure resembles a veneer preparation. Enamel and incisal feldspathic porcelains are then veneered on the core. Both techniques provide very promising clinical results.[30,31] IPS Empress and OPC have comparable flexural strength.[32–35] The in vitro margin fit of IPS Empress has been reported to provide a mean marginal opening of 63 μm, with facial and lingual marginal openings being larger than mesial and distal marginal openings.[36] A survival rate for anterior crowns of greater than 95% has been reported through 11 years of observation.[37] Heat-pressed ceramics offer the benefit of wear values comparable to those of enamel, whereas most ceramic materials cause accelerated enamel wear.[38–41]

Cemented All-Ceramic Crowns

Indications
1. Moderate to high esthetic demands, especially in the gingival third
2. Poor-quality dentin bonding substrate
3. Moderate to no parafunction

Cemented all-ceramic crowns are used where esthetics is an overriding concern but the dentinal substrate does not provide for proper bonding. Because the core material is very strong, bonding to the underlying tooth structure is not necessary. Cementation requires fewer steps, is less technique sensitive, and has less opportunity for mishaps than do bonding procedures. Because the crown is cemented, the preparation must meet the retention and resistance requirements of any cemented crown. Esthetics is compromised slightly because the ceramic core is less translucent than bonded ceramic restorations and is more opaque than many natural tooth substrates. Because of the high strength of these ceramic materials, cemented ceramic crowns can be placed in patients with moderate or controlled parafunction.

The difference between the ceramic materials that must be bonded versus those that can be used in cemented crowns is found in the composition and processing techniques for the core. For example, In-Ceram Alumina is an 85% alumina, glass-infiltrated core fabricated on a resin die.[9,10] In-Ceram Spinell (Vident) is a mixture of alumina and magnesia made on a resin die.[9,10] Procera crowns have a 99% alumina core fabricated on a die designed from digitized specifications made from the master die. Empress 2 (Ivoclar Vivadent) is a lithium disilicate–based glass ceramic. In-Ceram Zirconia is a slip cast or dry-pressed zirconium core.

The In-Ceram Alumina core is fabricated using a process known as slip casting. A special gypsum die is produced to which an alumina and water mixture or "slip" is applied and shaped. The core is sintered (baked at high temperature) in a furnace, creating an interconnected porous network. The core material is then returned to the porcelain oven, and a lanthanum aluminosilicate glass is infiltrated into the pores of the core to add strength. Aluminous porcelain is then layered over the core to produce the final tooth form. This lengthy process requires at least three separate firings in the porcelain oven. Flexural strengths from 300 to 600 MPa have been reported for In-Ceram.[9,42] A clinical study in a private practice of 223 units demonstrated a 3-year survival rate of 96%. Anterior crowns had a higher survival rate (98%) than premolars (94%). The data showed that core fractures and porcelain fractures occurred at a rate of approximately 0.6% and 0.3% per year, respectively.[43] Additional in vivo studies confirm In-Ceram Alumina's high success rate.[4,44,45] Marginal integrity has been shown to be within clinically acceptable standards.[46] In-Ceram Spinell is based on the conventional In-Ceram technique, but the core is fabricated from a magnesium-alumina or "spinell" powder. The Spinell core material is more translucent than the regular In-Ceram material, improving the esthetics in the gingival third, but it is not as strong as regular In-Ceram (flexural strength of about 350 MPa)[9,10] (Figs

17-11a and 17-11b). Reports on a 5-year history with 40 anterior In-Ceram Spinell crowns showed a 97.5% success rate.[47]

Procera is another system that uses an alumina core (Figs 17-12a and 17-12b). The master die is scanned into a computer, and the surface contour of the die is mapped with the use of more than 50,000 measured values. An alumina coping is designed on the computer, and the relief space for the cementing agent is established. The data are then transmitted via modem to a production station, where the coping is manufactured with advanced powder technology and a computer-aided design/computer-assisted manufacture (CAD/CAM) technique. The coping contains high-purity (99.9%) aluminum oxide powder, which is milled and sintered. A veneering porcelain that is compatible with the coping is layered to develop crown contours and esthetics. The flexural strength of the core is reported to be greater than 600 MPa, with a fracture toughness of 4.48 MPa.[7] The mean load to failure of the core/veneer porcelain system is clinically acceptable when the veneer porcelain is more than 0.4 mm thick. The veneering porcelain doubles in strength at 0.9 mm.[48] With a 0.6-mm-thick Procera core, a tooth reduction of 1.0 to 1.5 mm is required. In a laboratory study, mean gap dimensions for marginal openings, internal adaptation, and precision of fit for Procera crowns were less than 70 µm.[49] Data on the clinical fit of Procera crowns indicated a mean marginal gap width of 80 to 95 µm for anterior crowns and 90 to 145 µm for posterior crowns.[50] A 5-year clinical study of Procera reported that 94 of the 97 crowns (97%) were rated either excellent or acceptable. No failures were reported for the anterior crowns evaluated.[51]

The Empress 2 core material provides better mechanical properties than the original IPS Empress. This allows it to be cemented or bonded. The core pattern is waxed to full contour and invested. The Empress 2 glass-ceramic ingots are heat pressed in a 920°C furnace under pressure and vacuum. The glass ceramic becomes viscous and flows into the lost-wax mold of the core. The Empress 2 core is coated with a glass ceramic containing fluoroapatite. These apatite crystals are similar in structure to those found in natural teeth. Reportedly, they allow the porcelain to mimic the optical properties of translucency, brightness, and opalescence of a natural tooth.[52] The Empress 2 core has a flexural strength of 350 ± 50 MPa, a fracture toughness of 3.2 MPa, and a failure load of 771 to 1,115 N.[53,54] The restorations exhibit excellent marginal fit. In a 3-year clinical evaluation of 27 restorations placed on posterior teeth the survival rate was 100%.[55] Results from a study on the mean gap dimensions and marginal opening for incisor crowns showed that Empress 2 had the smallest and most homogeneous gap dimensions (46 ± 1

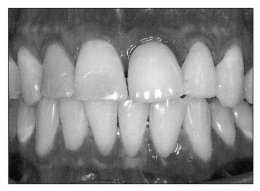

Fig 17-11a Preoperatively, the maxillary left central incisor had a large resin composite restoration. Because composite provides a poor substrate for bonding, a crown material that could be cemented was needed. In-Ceram Spinell was chosen because, unlike a metal-ceramic restoration, it could be made to match the adjacent teeth that were to be restored with porcelain veneers and bonded all-ceramic crowns.

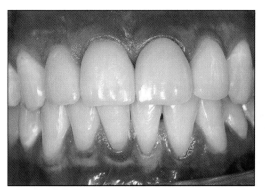

Fig 17-11b In-Ceram Spinell provided high-value, low-chroma restorations.

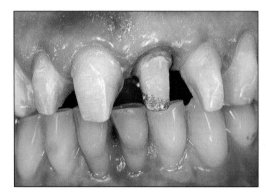

Fig 17-12a The post and core does not allow bonding. A cemented crown is an appropriate choice for the central incisor.

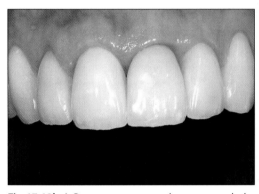

Fig 17-12b A Procera crown was chosen to mask the color of the post and core and to esthetically match the other all-ceramic restorations.

μm).[46] In addition, two studies reported no evidence of abrasion of the ceramic or the opposing teeth in vitro or in vivo.[40,41]

All-ceramic cementable crown cores may also be fabricated in zirconium oxide. It has outstanding mechanical properties and high biocompatibility. Zirconium oxide produces an extremely strong core (998 to 1,183N).[54,56,57] It is stronger than all other ceramic core materials.[58,59] In-Ceram Zirconia may be slip-cast like In-Ceram Alumina, dry-pressed, or milled from a solid die. In-Ceram Zirconia frameworks produced by a CAD/CAM system exhibited a mean marginal fit well below the clinically acceptable 100-μm limit.[60,61] A 3-year study of posterior fixed partial dentures produced from In-Ceram Zirconium showed no material failure.[62] The relative translucency of a zirconium oxide ceramic core is roughly equivalent to that of a metal core.[11] It is also extremely opaque with limited opportunity to alter the core color to match dentin shades.[63] While the core materials continue to improve in the strength and toughness, the weakness in the restorations continues to be the weaker veneering porcelains.[56,64]

Metal-Ceramic Crowns

Indications
1. Moderate esthetic demands
2. Poor-quality dentinal substrate
3. Severe to no parafunction

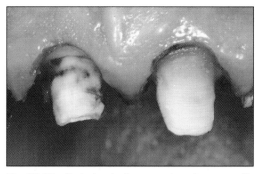

Fig 17-13a Endodontically treated and structurally compromised teeth are indications for metal-ceramic crowns.

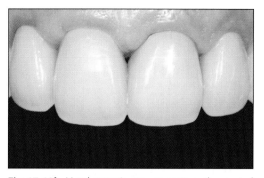

Fig 17-13b Metal-ceramic crowns restore the central and lateral incisors. A porcelain butt joint margin and 2 mm of metal reduction from the facial shoulder allow light to enter the tooth and illuminate the gingival third of the crown.

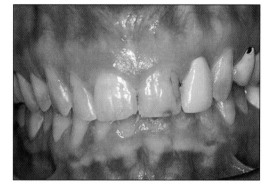

Fig 17-14a A careful consideration of the esthetic demands, bonding substrate, and any parafunction may lead to the use of multiple systems within the same patient.

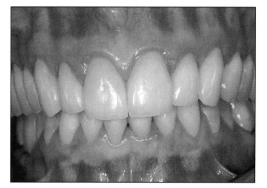

Fig 17-14b Veneers and bonded and cemented crowns were used to restore function and esthetics.

Porcelain-fused-to-metal crowns have a long history of success.[65] Introduced in the late 1940s, metal-ceramic crowns continue to be the most common complete-coverage anterior restoration. Porcelain margins were developed in the 1960s, and the technique later evolved with the introduction of shoulder porcelains.[6] Recent development of opalescent and fluorescent porcelains has dramatically improved esthetics of these restorations.[14]

The quality of the dentinal substrate does not play a role in the choice of metal-ceramic restorations since they are cemented, but resistance and retention requirements are of major importance. Patients with moderate to severe parafunction are best treated with porcelain-fused-to-metal crowns, which are inherently stronger than all-ceramic crowns.[66] Tooth contacts may be developed in metal rather than porcelain to decrease wear of the opposing dentition. Other indications for metal-ceramic crowns are a deep, tight incisor relationship and minimal dentin wall thickness after endodontic treatment. Neither allows sufficient reduction for

all-ceramic crowns. Preparations can be modified since metal surfaces as thin as 0.5 mm are usually adequate (Figs 17-13a and 17-13b). Metal ceramics are still preferred for fixed partial dentures.

Today clinicians have a plethora of anterior ceramic systems from which to choose. The decision should be based on esthetic goals, bonding requirements, and parafunctional habits rather than a favorite porcelain system. Dentists using a hierarchical approach to selecting anterior ceramic crowns will discover that several ceramic materials may be used within the same smile (Figs 17-14a and 17-14b).

Anterior Tooth Preparation

To provide a tooth preparation that meets the restorative and technical guidelines and provides predictable results, practitioners must understand and blend the biologic, mechanical, and esthetic components of tooth preparation.[67] All three

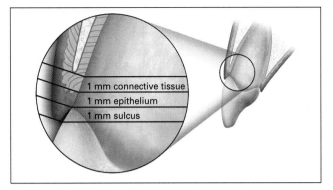

Fig 17-15a The biologic width comprises epithelial and connective tissue attachments. Crown preparations that impinge on the biologic width result in chronic inflammation.

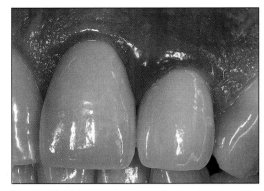

Fig 17-15b This crown's preparation impinged on biologic width interproximally. Inflammation had been present for 17 years.

categories are equally important. Biologic principles dictate finish-line position and pulpal preservation. Mechanical preparation principles include retention and resistance features, margin configuration, closure, and integrity. Principles of esthetics require that the tooth-restoration interface is not a visual focal point.

Biologic Principles

Margin location is the most important biologic parameter in predictably maintaining gingival health. The relationship between margin location and gingival health is well documented.[68–71] Even among patients receiving regular preventive dental care, subgingival margins are associated with increased probing depths and gingival inflammation.[68–70] The critical factor in maintaining healthy gingival tissue is the relationship between margin location and supracrestal fiber attachment.[72,73] If the restorative margins impinge on the supracrestal fiber attachment, chronic inflammation can result.[74–76] Practitioners must therefore balance the principles of periodontal health and the desire for concealed porcelain margins.[77] They must also be aware of the cervical limitations of crown preparations; a complete understanding of the dentogingival complex is paramount.

In 1921, Gottlieb[78] first described "an epithelial attachment of the gingiva to the hard tissues." Sicher[79] discussed the "dento-gingival junction" as the fibrous, connective tissue attachment of the gingiva and the epithelial attachment. The dimensions of this functional dentogingival unit were first reported by Gargiulo et al[80] (Fig 17-15a), who described the dentogingival junction as consisting of a sulcus, junctional epithelium, and gingival fiber attachment to cementum, coronal to the alveolar crest. The term biologic width was given to

this zone of connective tissue and epithelium by D. Walter Cohen (1962) in an unpublished presentation at Walter Reed Army Medical Center. This biologic zone was reintroduced to periodontics and restorative dentistry by Ingber et al[81] in 1977.

Gargiulo et al[80] provided an arithmetic outline for evaluating the tissue-tooth interface. The average for the connective tissue attachment, the least variable of the biologic components, is 1.07 mm. Connective tissue includes 10 different gingival fiber bundles, the periodontal ligament, cementum, and collagen fiber bundles embedded into the root surface; these embedded fiber bundles are called Sharpey's fibers. The connective tissue zone also contains the nerve and blood supply for the gingival tissues. The connective tissue attachment is the strongest part of the attachment and provides resistance that, under normal circumstances, prevents a periodontal probe or gingival retraction cord from penetrating to the bone. It includes the circumferential fibers that often produce facially evident inflammatory reactions to interproximal biologic width violations.[75,76]

Coronal to the connective tissue attachment is the epithelial attachment. The epithelial attachment has an average dimension of 0.97 mm.[80] The hemidesmosomal attachment of the epithelium provides a tight approximation of tissue to the tooth but is easily penetrated, especially in the presence of inflammation. The cells in this layer undergo a continual coronal migration with a complete turnover every 4 to 6 days. They attach to enamel, cementum, dentin, and even porcelain.

The term biologic width describes a vertical measurement of 2.04 mm, the combined width of the connective and epithelial attachments. If the margin of a restoration violates the 2-mm biologic width and impinges on the supracrestal fibers, substantial gingival inflammation often results[74–76] (Fig 17-15b).

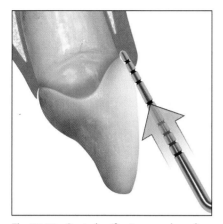

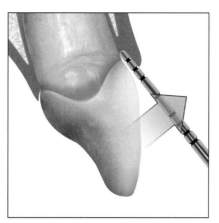

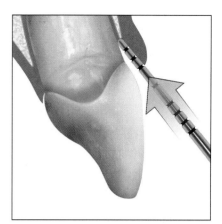

Fig 17-16a Crest classifications are based on the probing depths on the facial and interproximal surfaces from bone to free gingival margin. After the administration of local anesthesia, the probe is placed in the sulcus and pushed until it meets resistance.

Fig 17-16b The probe is angled to keep its tip on the root surface.

Fig 17-16c The probe is forced through the attachment apparatus until it engages bone. The depth is measured at the free gingival margin and the crest type classified.

The difficulty for practitioners is that Gargiulo's work presents a "contrived illusion of mathematical precision." The research suggests a vertical measurement of 0.69 mm for the sulcus.[80] This would make the total dentogingival complex, biologic width plus sulcus, approximately 3.00 mm. Yet, clinically, the dimensions vary greatly. Not every tooth has the average biologic width of 2 mm and a 1-mm sulcular depth.[81] Each tooth presents unique gingival measurements that must be assessed and used in treatment. Individual measurements of the total dentogingival complex must, therefore, be used in making restorative decisions.[82]

If the goal is to place a restorative margin in the sulcus without violating the biologic width, the base of the sulcus must be identified. However, this is extremely difficult. The periodontal literature indicates that the tip of the periodontal probe often penetrates the base of the sulcus and may extend into the connective tissue.[83] The depth of penetration depends on the level of inflammation, the diameter of the probe, and the pressure used on the probe. Because the sulcus depth can be identified only histologically, the distance from the free gingival margin to the crest of the alveolar bone is the only predictable measurement available to determine intracrevicular margin location. At the crown preparation appointment, the entire dentogingival complex is measured. After the administration of local anesthesia, a periodontal probe is pushed through the sulcus until resistance is felt (Fig 17-16a). The probe is then angled away from the clinical crown while the tip is still touching the root surface (Fig 17-16b) and is pushed completely to the osseous crest (Fig 17-16c). This

process is called *bone sounding*, and measurements are taken on the midfacial aspect of the tooth and at both facioproximal line angles. If the probe is not angled correctly there is a greater risk of the tip of the probe skipping past the thin facial plate of bone, resulting in an inaccurate measurement.

Measurements on anterior teeth can be categorized into three types of relationships between the free gingival margin and alveolar crest: normal, low, and high.[76,82] This relationship will influence margin placement, determine the stability of the attachment levels of the gingiva against the tooth, and influence the need for crown-lengthening surgery prior to restorative procedures. The critical factor in proper management of the soft tissues is accurate location of the alveolar crest, which allows the clinician to avoid impingement on the biologic width.

Normal Crest Relationship

In a normal crest relationship, the measurement from the free gingival margin to the osseous crest is 3 mm facially and 3 to 4.5 mm interproximally (Fig 17-17), which usually results in a gingival scallop of 3 to 4 mm and tissue levels that are stable in relation to the tooth. The normal crest is found on 85% of anterior teeth.[83] In the normal crest relationship, restorative margins can be placed 0.5 to 1.0 mm into the sulcus facially and 0.5 to 2.5 mm interproximally. The apical limit of the restorative margin is 2.5 mm coronal to the osseous crest. The retraction technique is not critical in this crest relationship because the gingival level is stable. Typically, a normal crest relationship should yield no recession and no loss of papilla height following routine intervention. Research indicates that

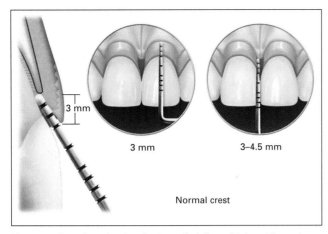

Fig 17-17 Sounding depths of 3.0 mm facially and 3.0 to 4.5 mm interproximally represent a normal crest relationship. The tissue should rebound completely after manipulation.

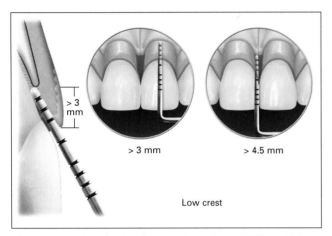

Fig 17-18 Sounding depths of greater than 3.0 mm facially and 4.5 mm interproximally represent a low crest relationship. Tissue response is not predictable after manipulation. Recession and "black triangles" are probable.

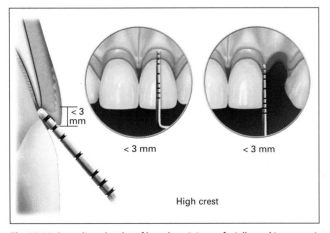

Fig 17-19 Sounding depths of less than 3.0 mm facially and interproximally represent a high-crest relationship. Intracrevicular preparation is difficult without biologic width violation.

a normal crest relationship will reestablish itself even if the tissue is completely denuded, although it may take up to 3 years to return to its normal form.[84,85]

Low Crest Relationship

A low crest relationship is the most difficult of all crest positions to manage and is found in 13% of anterior teeth.[83] The relationship of the free gingival margin to the osseous crest is greater than 3 mm facially and greater than 4.5 mm interproximally (Fig 17-18). The gingival scallop does not mimic the osseous crest. Patients with low crests are at high risk for facial recession and loss of papilla height because of the increased distance from the alveolar crest to the gingival margin. The position of the soft tissues on the tooth is not stable in teeth with a low crest relationship and can easily be altered unintentionally during treatment.

If maintenance of the tissue levels is critical during restorative procedures, practitioners have two options. One option is to correct the low crest surgically before tooth preparation, creating a normal crest relationship and thus achieving predictability. This can be accomplished by reducing the tissue height with an internally beveled gingivectomy so that the gingival crest is 3 mm coronal to the osseous crest. However, if the position of the cementoenamel junction, root anatomy, gingival architecture, osseous support, or esthetic demands prevent proactive treatment, the second option is to take great care to avoid damage to the attachment during preparation and impression making. The finish line of the preparation should be located at or coronal to the free gingival margin, and there should be minimal, if any, tissue retraction during impression making. The patient should be warned of the possible tissue changes before the preparation begins and have an understanding of the treatment options if tissue loss does occur. While not predictable, thicker tissue seems more resistant to recession following intervention.[86]

High Crest Relationship

Patients with high crests are the least common (2%) and pose the greatest risk for violation of biologic width.[84] Probing measurements are less than 3 mm facially or interproximally (Fig 17-19). The tissue levels are very stable, and the gingival scallop is flat, less than 3 mm. The high crest relationship sometimes occurs when excessive tissue covers the anatomic crown, such as in altered passive eruption,[87] or in patients with noncarious cervical lesions. However, it is most common adjacent to edentulous spaces where the gingival scallop has flattened. Margin location is determined by the demands of biologic width. High crest teeth, by definition, will only allow a restorative margin of less than 0.5 mm into the sulcus because of the short distance to the alveolar crest. These teeth are at high risk for biologic width impingement with intracrevicular margin placement. Gingival retraction for impressions should be minimal.

Pulpal Preservation

In one study, irreversible pulpitis occurred in 5.7% of cases in which crowns were placed on vital teeth.[88] Preoperative radiographs and pulp testing are important steps in determining pulp vitality prior to tooth preparation. Unfortunately, pulp testing cannot identify degrees of health. Separately or cumulatively, the effects of large restorations, leaking restorations, caries lesions, deep cracks, pins, etc increase the chances of pulpal necrosis after tooth preparation. Patients should be made aware of that risk preoperatively.

If the tooth preparation involves an increase of heat to the tooth, pulpal necrosis can occur. In one in vivo study in primates, pulpal injury occurred in 15% of teeth with a 5.5°C rise in temperature. An 11.1°C rise led to necrosis of the pulp in 60% of the teeth, and a 16.6°C rise caused necrosis of all the teeth tested.[89] Temperature changes have been monitored during complete-crown preparation. When an air/water spray coolant was used, a temperature decrease in the pulp chamber from 37°C to 25°C after 4 minutes of exposure occurred. However, when only air coolant was used, the pulpal temperature rose from 37°C to 48°C after 1 minute of continuous exposure.[90] Therefore, continuous air/water coolant is a critical factor in maintaining pulpal health.

Mechanical Principles

During tooth preparation, several mechanical principles must be followed. The preparations must incorporate retention and resistance form, structural durability, and marginal integrity.

Resistance and Retention

Retention is the feature of a crown preparation that resists dislodgment in a vertical direction or along the path of placement. In 1926, Ward[91] became the first practitioner to establish a standard for preparation taper. He prescribed 5% to 20% per inch or 3 to 12 degrees. Since then, recommendations have ranged from 3 to 5 degrees, to 6 degrees, to 10 to 14 degrees.[92] Jorgensen[93] indicated that there is a 50% reduction in retention when going from 5 to 10 degrees of taper. These tenets are heavily based on clinical empiricism and on two experiments in which crown and abutment analogs were pulled apart along their paths of insertion. The theoretical benefits of preparations with minimal convergence angles do not withstand scrutiny[94–96] and are difficult to produce in clinical practice. Divergence from parallel might have

to be as much as 12 degrees to be observed and produced clinically.[55,97] Routine preparations in practice have been measured at between 15 and 36 degrees without apparent detrimental effect to the longevity of the restorations.[98,99] For nonadhesively cemented restorations, the minimum convergence value required clinically is unknown, although total convergence up to 20 degrees has been shown to be acceptable.[96,100] Today, crowns with greater taper may be cemented with adhesive resin cements, minimizing the need to prepare the crowns to minimal convergence angles.[101]

Resistance is the feature of a tooth preparation that enhances the restoration's stability and resists dislodgment along an axis other than the path of placement.[102] Most retention studies utilize conventional pull-type tests to evaluate preparations and/or cements.[103,104] However, data on functional force vectors in the oral environment strongly suggest that these lift-off type forces are virtually nonexistent in the mouth.[105–107] During chewing, teeth are subjected to alternating combinations of buccolingual and occlusogingival forces.[108] These studies indicate that stresses that cause failure of an anterior restoration are repeated perpendicular or oblique forces.[95,107] Therefore, as Caputo and Standlee[109] concluded, "Resistance form is the most important factor that must be designed into any restoration if it is to succeed in function."

Resistance clinically is multifactoral. It is based on preparation taper, height, diameter, and cement type. Crowns generally loosen and fail by cleavage of the cement attachment without damaging the abutment or restoration.[96] The cement attachment fails when a portion of the abutment subjected to compressive and shear forces is unable to withstand load application. Attachment failure is a progressive phenomenon linked to increasing abutment taper. Increasing the preparation taper from 10 to 20 degrees creates a broader stress distribution and greater stress within the cement.[96] Clinically, a minimal preparation taper decreases the damaging effects of occlusal stress on the cement attachment, improving a crown's resistance.

The height and diameter of the final preparation are also related to resistance.[110] Resistance is increased by lengthening the axial walls of the preparation.[111] The minimum height for resistance is one half the diameter of the tooth.[112] This means that, on average, an anterior preparation must be 3.5 mm and a posterior preparation 4.0 mm in height. Of the total preparation height, the gingival 2 mm of the preparation must be on sound tooth structure to provide a proper ferrule,[113–116] and the other 1.5 mm or more can be in either tooth structure or buildup material (Fig 17-20). A ferrule is the marginal band of a crown which contacts tooth structure, providing protection from masticatory forces. In addition, the

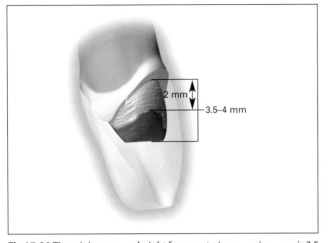

Fig 17-20 The minimum core height for an anterior ceramic crown is 3.5 mm. The cervical 2.0 mm of the facial and lingual aspects must be solid tooth structure for a proper ferrule.

ferrule requires a dentin thickness of 1 mm from the external surface of the crown preparation to the wall of any endodontic preparation.

Resistance is also affected by the mechanical properties of the cement.[96] The limiting threshold of each crown is the cement's resistance to fatigue in compression.[96] The more stress that will be placed on the cement, due to a severe taper and/or lack of preparation height, the more resistant the cement must be. Resin-modified glass-ionomer cements are more resistant than glass-ionomer cements, which are in turn more resistant than zinc phosphate cements. Most research on resistance and retention data is conducted on nonadhesively cemented crowns. Today, however, adhesive cements allow the placement of crowns that do not meet standard taper and length requirements. Yet, because the hydrodynamic nature of dentin bonding makes it unpredictable, it is suggested that all crown preparations meet minimum requirements.[20,21]

Structural Durability

Structural durability is the relationship between occlusal stress and material strength. It ensures that a restoration does not deform or fracture under load. In a metal-ceramic crown, the minimum metal thickness under porcelain is 0.4 to 0.5 mm for gold alloys and 0.2 mm for base-metal alloys. If the metal is too thin, it will flex under load, resulting in possible porcelain fracture. The minimum porcelain thickness over metal is 0.9 mm (0.2 mm for the opaque material and 0.7 mm for body porcelain). Ceramists prefer a 1.3- to 1.5-mm reduction for the axial surfaces of metal-ceramic crowns and a 2.0-mm reduction incisally/occlusally. The greater the reduction, the

easier it is to mask the opaque material in the gingival third of the crown with body porcelain. Most bonded all-ceramic crowns require a minimum thickness of 1.0 mm to provide esthetics and adequate strength. Cemented all-ceramic crowns require a circumferential tooth reduction of 1.5 mm for strength.

Marginal Integrity

A completely closed margin is unattainable clinically. Even the finest margins are not sufficiently closed to prevent bacterial ingress. To place it in perspective, the width of a human hair is 50 μm; bacteria responsible for caries are 4 to 5 μm in diameter. Because bacteria are constantly passing under restoration margins, patient resistance to disease is more important than the marginal opening of crowns. What, then, is an acceptable marginal opening? One study reported that when the margin of an inlay or onlay could not be visualized, a marginal discrepancy of 119 μm was found to be acceptable.[117] Bjorn and colleagues[118,119] reported that 83% of gold and 74% of porcelain crowns exhibited marginal defects; more than half were greater than 200 μm. Yet defective margins are to blame in only 10% of failed restorations. While all practitioners should strive for the finest margins possible, it is impossible to achieve a closed margin. The best possible margin enables the patient to floss and care for the restoration, minimizing cement dissolution and maximizing the patient's natural resistance factors. Because 100 μm is the smallest detectable ledge,[120] this can be used as a practical criterion for evaluating fit.

What margin design provides the best marginal integrity? The margin design selected does not have a significant effect on marginal seal.[121,122] Shoulder (Fig 17-21a), shoulder-bevel (Fig 17-21b), and chamfer (Fig 17-21c) finish line preparations all allow acceptable marginal fit when complete seating is achieved. The shoulder-bevel margin is the least esthetic choice. The bevel should be used only with metal-ceramic crowns and is suited for structurally compromised teeth where ferrule extension is important. If porcelain is placed on a bevel, the cementation process may cause porcelain breakage. In two studies, the geometry exhibiting the least marginal discrepancy after cementation was a shoulder preparation on a die-spaced casting, which was significantly better than that of a shoulder bevel or chamfer.[123,124] The shoulder finish line is thought to be better than the beveled shoulder because it allows the cement to escape more readily. The shoulder design exhibits less marginal distortion than a chamfer because of the crown's thickness adjacent to the margin. Stress analysis of various margin finish lines showed that chamfer and internally rounded shoulder preparations had the lowest stress concentration when loaded vertically, mini-

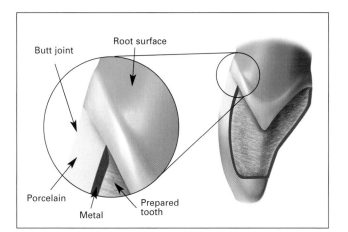

Fig 17-21a In the preferred substructure design for a porcelain facial margin, a uniform thickness of porcelain is carried to the finish line.

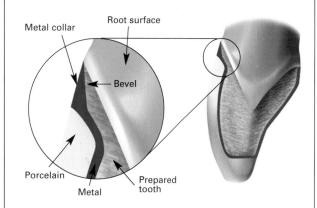

Fig 17-21b The preferred substructure design if a metal facial margin is desired. Metal covers the bevel and forms a butt joint with the porcelain.

mizing the risk of catastrophic ceramic failure under load.[125,126]

Esthetic Design

Porcelain margins must provide an esthetic transition from tooth to crown, preventing the margin from becoming the visual focal point. Such margins are easier to fabricate and more predictable when they are fabricated on a 90-degree shoulder preparation. This is true for metal-ceramic and most all-ceramic systems.[127–130] A chamfer requires minimal axial reduction and is appropriate for conservative all-ceramic restorations. It is the required finish line for the Procera scanner. It does not, however, provide an adequate reduction for metal-ceramic crowns. The opaque material used to mask the metal at the margin will show through the more translucent porcelain and will compromise the esthetics in the gingival third. A 90-degree shoulder between 1.0 and 1.5 mm in depth allows for a precise margin, maximum seating, and good esthetics. This preparation can be used for porcelain butt margins of metal-ceramic crowns or for all-ceramic crowns.

Functional Crown Preparation Technique

With a complete understanding of the key components of intracrevicular tooth preparation, practitioners can achieve predictability with a standardized, controlled, and functional crown preparation.[131] This preparation design works for any type of anterior ceramic crown. This technique also minimizes the number of burs, bur changes, and cost. Only four burs are used in the technique sequence described below.

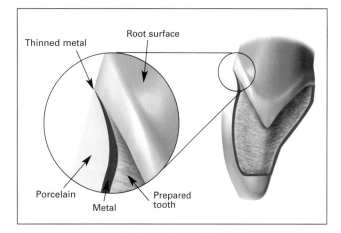

Fig 17-21c A 1.0 to 1.5 chamfer can be used for anterior ceramic restorations. It is the required finish line for the Procera scanner.

Bone Sounding

Before beginning any anterior crown preparation, a comprehensive evaluation of the underlying osseous structure is critical. Bone sounding to the osseous crest with a periodontal probe, as described in the Biologic Principles section of this chapter, should be performed to determine the dimension of the total dentinogingival complex. If the probing depth is 3.0 mm facially and 4.5 mm or less interproximally, the crest relationship is normal and tissue levels should remain stable. If, however, the probings are not normal, the patient must be made aware of the possible complications involved in the treatment, and the preparation and impression must be altered accordingly.

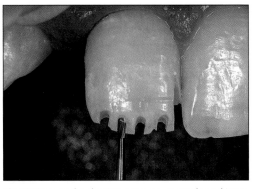

Fig 17-22 Incisal reduction grooves are made and inter-proximal contact is broken with a 330 carbide bur with a 2.0-mm cutting-head length.

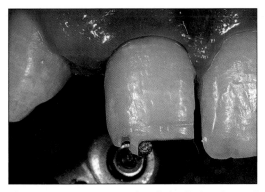

Fig 17-23 A 1.2-mm round-ended cylinder diamond completes the incisal reduction.

Incisal Reduction

The amount of incisal edge reduction is dictated by the planned final incisal edge position. There should be a 2.0-mm reduction from that point. This requires that a diagnostic waxup be completed before tooth preparation if the original incisal edge position is not acceptable. A 2.0-mm reduction allows the technician space to develop incisal translucency and halo effect without a loss of fracture strength of the porcelain.[132] Initial depth cuts are made with a No. 330 carbide bur that has a 2.0-mm cutting-head length (Fig 17-22); note that No. 330 burs from some manufacturers have a head length of less than 2.0 mm, so the head length should be measured. This same carbide bur can be used to open proximal contacts and is also excellent for use in occlusal reduction of posterior teeth. A 1.2-mm-diameter round-ended cylinder diamond is used to remove the remaining incisal-edge tooth structure to the level of the incisal depth cuts (Fig 17-23). This diamond is also used for facial and cervical reduction.

Facial Reduction

Viewed from the proximal aspect, anterior teeth have three facial planes: cervical, midfacial, and incisal. The incisal plane has been removed in the first step with a 1.2-mm-diameter round-ended cylinder diamond. The facial reduction focuses only on the midfacial plane, not the cervical. Depth cuts are prepared to the full depth of the diamond (Fig 17-24), which is aligned with the midfacial plane (Fig 17-25). The use of the 1.2-mm diamond as a depth gauge allows a more uniformly accurate preparation. Without the use of a device to help gauge reduction depth, teeth are routinely underprepared on

the facial aspect.[133] At this time, the cervical plane should receive almost no reduction. If the bur is angled to the cervical aspect, the facial plane would be severely underreduced. After two or three depth cuts, the same diamond is used for the remaining gross facial reduction.

Cervical Reduction

The cervical finish line is initially produced at the free gingival margin circumferentially (Fig 17-26). The tissue is not retracted prior to initial preparation. The primary cord can push the free gingival margin apically and flatten out the normal architecture up to 1.5 mm, which potentially increases the chances of biologic width violations at the line angles or interproximal areas (see Fig 17-15b). The 1.2-mm round-ended diamond is then used to create a finish line with a rounded internal line angle and slight lip rather than a flat shoulder. The recommended thickness is 1.0 to 1.5 mm depending on the type of crown chosen. Underreduction adjacent to the finish line will affect the emergence profile and facial contour of the restoration. This can predispose the restoration to technical and/or esthetic failure. Utilizing a 1.2-mm-diameter diamond allows the practitioner a guide for preparation depth adjacent to the finish line. This is critically important because studies indicate a large variation between recommended tooth reduction and that actually achieved (0.75 to 0.9 mm).[92]

Lingual Reduction

The finish line on the lingual is established at the free gingival margin with the same 1.2-mm-diameter diamond. Depending on the crown chosen, this finish line can be a light chamfer for metal using up to half of the diameter of the diamond

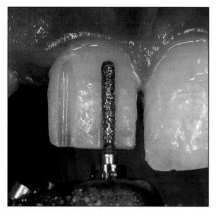

Fig 17-24 Multiple facial reduction grooves are made to the entire depth of the 1.2-mm-diameter diamond bur.

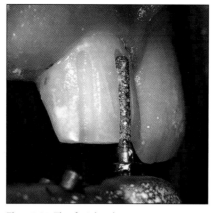

Fig 17-25 The facial reduction grooves must be oriented properly to ensure adequate mid-facial reduction. The gingival plane is not prepared at this point.

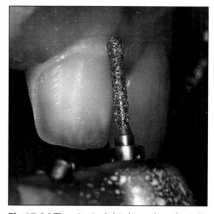

Fig 17-26 The gingival third is reduced axially by 1.2 mm to 0.5 mm apical to the free gingival crest. At this point, the shoulder should be rounded internally and a slight lip will be present at the outer edge of the finish line.

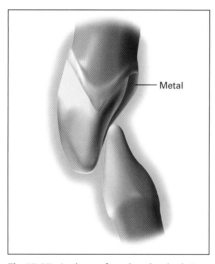

Fig 17-27a In the preferred occlusal relationship between a maxillary metal-ceramic crown and a natural mandibular incisor, the contact is on metal.

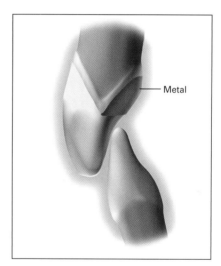

Fig 17-27b In a less desirable occlusal relationship, the opposing natural incisor contacts the restoration on porcelain. This is the recommended occlusal relationship when both maxillary and mandibular incisors are restored.

or a 1.2-mm shoulder for cemented all-ceramic systems if the bur is used to its full depth. The proper reduction on the lingual concavity is required to ensure functional anterior guidance, prevent interference with the envelope of function, and avoid development of contours that produce unacceptable phonetics. Without proper reduction, technicians are forced to overcontour the lingual aspect of the final restorations. This can move the condyle distally and produce joint discomfort.

In addition, a lisp after final restoration placement indicates an overcontoured lingual surface. Air flow becomes constricted, producing a whistle. A football-shaped diamond is designed to mimic the lingual concavity and provides the necessary reduction of 0.5 to 1.5 mm, depending on the choice of material used (Figs 17-27a and 17-27b). With the initial cervical reduction completed, a primary thin retraction cord is placed in the sulcus.

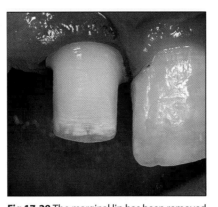

Fig 17-28 The marginal lip has been removed with a 1.6-mm round-ended diamond bur, leaving a 90-degree shoulder.

Preparation Completion

A 1.6-mm-diameter round-ended diamond bur with 3 degrees of taper is used to finish the preparation. The taper on the diamond is designed to create a minimum convergence angle. The large tip will remove the J-lip on the external surface produced by the 1.2-mm diamond and create a crisp shoulder or chamfer circumferentially. A round-ended diamond is chosen because of its versatility and ease of use. The rounded tip can simply cleave the J-lip and produce a shoulder. If the side of the bur is used, it will remove the lip at an angle, producing a deep chamfer. The round end is suggested over a flat-ended diamond for fabricating a shoulder finish line. With a round-ended diamond, the practitioner can lock his or her wrist and allow the bur to simply traverse along the J-lip, thus producing the shoulder finish line. A flat-ended diamond requires a much more deft touch because the angle of the end must be altered constantly to match the contours of the preparation. Most practitioners find that the flat-ended bur produces an irregular, inadequate finish line. The margin should be developed to the coronal aspect of the primary cord facially and level with the free gingival margin interproximally (Fig 17-28). This will ensure an intracrevicular margin location after normal gingival tissue rebound, which takes up to 3 months in patients with normal crests. In patients with low or high crests, margins should not extend apical to the gingival crest.

Impression Technique

An important factor in delivering high-quality restorations is providing the laboratory with an accurate impression. Practitioners must develop a technique that is reliable and repeatable.

Impression materials minimally displace gingival tissue, fluids, or debris, so successful retraction and isolation are mandatory. Various methods and techniques have been described in the literature for exposure of dry crown margins. They include mechanical, mechanical-chemical, rotary curettage, electrosurgery, and laser surgery (troughing). Regardless of the technique, four requirements must be satisfied for effective gingival retraction: (1) the tissue at the crown margins must be displaced horizontally to provide for an adequate bulk of impression material; (2) the tissue at the margin must be displaced vertically to expose the undercut apical to the finish line; (3) all gingival bleeding must be arrested; and (4) all hard and soft tissues must be dry.[134,135]

The mechanical-chemical technique, the most popular retraction technique today,[136,137] combines the mechanical displacement of the tissue with cord and the drying action of chemical agents. The retraction begins during crown margin preparation. The primary piece of dry cord (compression cord) is placed in the sulcus and cut so that the ends abut within the sulcus. After the final finish line preparation, aluminum sulfate gel is ejected around the sulcus. Aluminum sulfate is one of the least irritating of the retraction chemicals. It does not ionize readily, it retains its astringent qualities, and it is not toxic.[138] A larger, dry secondary cord (deflection cord) is packed through the aluminum sulfate, dragging the chemical into the sulcus. In studies by Laufer et al,[139,140] 50% to 90% of impressions of preparations with sulcular widths between 0.08 and 0.13 mm had defects. No detectable difference in distortion of impressions of preparations was found with sulcular widths of 0.2 mm or greater. This was confirmed by Aimjirakul et al[141] in a gingival sulcus simulation model that demonstrated that the viscoelastic behavior of elastomers depends on the width of the sulcus. The polyether materials showed greater sulcular penetration than other impression materials regardless of sulcular width. To achieve a crevicular width of 0.2 mm, the secondary cord optimally must remain in the gingival crevice for 4 minutes prior to making the impression.

Another difficult area for practitioners is managing the field. If the patient is involved in retracting the cheeks and lips and eliminating the parotid fluid flow, it frees the doctor and assistant to manage the tongue, saliva, sulcus, and impression. Absorbent parotid shields and cheek retractors are used to retract the lips and cheeks. The patient holds the retractors, leaving the operator's hands free (Fig 17-29). To achieve a crevicular width of 0.2 mm, a medium-sized cord should remain in the gingival sulcus for 4 minutes.[142] The double packing technique, in a patient with a normal crest, should produce no apical migration of the gingival crest.[143–145] The technique must be modified for low and high crest patients. Finish lines should be kept supragingival or equigingival to avoid recession and biologic width impingements. The impression technique on a low crest situation must use light packing pressure and smaller diameter cords to avoid trauma-induced recession. Rotary curettage, electrosurgery, and laser troughing are definitely contraindicated in low crest patients. A high crest case simply lacks the depth for the normal retraction cords, and smaller cords are recommended. The secondary cord should be removed wet to prevent renewed hemorrhage. The preparation is washed and dried to evaluate tissue displacement and hemorrhage control.

If the field is not dry, a 20% ferric sulfate solution can be used to cauterize the tissue. Ferric sulfate provides minimal tissue injury, and healing is more rapid than with aluminum chloride.[138] It must be placed directly against the cut tissues because it coagulates blood so quickly; if not, it is washed away by the extraneous blood, leaving a bleeding site. There have been reports of the tooth absorbing the ferric ion. In vitro tests, however, have failed to show corrosive effects or staining.[138] A disadvantage to the use of ferric compounds is that they inhibit the setting of polyether impression materials. If a dry field cannot be achieved rapidly, the sulcus width will decrease, increasing the risk of defects in the impression. Chemical agents and secondary cord should be replaced and the retraction attempted again.

Only after the field is acceptable is the impression material mixed. All impression materials are accurate enough to lead to production of well-fitting restorations.[146–148] Polyether and polyvinyl siloxane impression materials work well for multipurpose use and provide good soft and hard tissue detail.[149,150] Polyvinyl siloxane materials provide good elastic recovery; are dimensionally stable for indefinite periods; and are clean, odorless, and tasteless.[151] A disadvantage of polyvinyl siloxane is that because it is hydrophobic, it requires an absolutely dry field. Although many polyvinyl siloxane impression materials are advertised to be hydrophilic, research indicates that they are only reliable under dry conditions. In all situations, moisture leads to less detail reproduction compared to dry conditions.[152] Also, latex gloves may inhibit the set of polyvinyl siloxane. Even casual contact of the teeth or soft tissues with latex gloves can cause an inhibition of polymerization intraorally.[153–155]

Latex gloves do not affect polyether impressions. Polyether materials are inherently hydrophilic, so small amounts of blood or saliva do not affect accuracy.[152] Polyether is affected by ferric solutions and some disinfecting solutions. Because of its rigid set, it can be difficult to remove from the mouth, and it has a bad taste and smell.[146,147] Polyvinyl siloxane and poly-

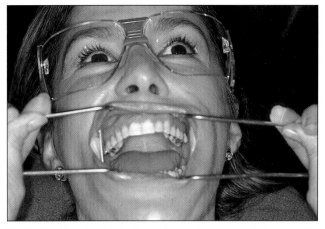

Fig 17-29 The patient helps in the impression process by holding the cheek retractors, keeping the dentist's and assistant's hands free to work.

ether materials can be used in a custom or stock tray, and studies have shown no difference in accuracy.[156,157] The working and setting times of the impression materials must be identified and followed precisely.

Shade

Success of an anterior ceramic crown depends on how well critical information is communicated between the dentist and laboratory. At least 75% of all remakes are caused by poor communication.[158] It is the dentist's challenge to predictably and accurately convey what is visualized in clear terms, allowing the technician to develop the "illusion of reality" in the ceramic material. The dentist must be able to perceive the color, understand and quantify the characteristics, and convey the information.

The experience of seeing color in teeth depends on six elements[159]:

1. *Light source:* Light is the basic necessity for vision. In order for a color to be seen, it must be present in the light source. For practitioners to perceive color, the operatory lighting should duplicate natural light as closely as possible. Full-spectrum lighting must emit the correct wavelengths, warmth, and intensity (150 to 250 foot candles) at the operating level. Eight 4-foot-long, full-spectrum light tubes should be positioned directly overhead. The spectral composition and warmth of the light can be measured with appropriate measuring devices.
2. *Amount of light:* As the amount of light decreases, the practitioner's ability to see color decreases.

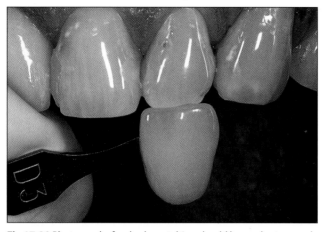

Fig 17-30 Photographs for shade matching should be made at an angle to avoid excess glare on the tooth surface. The shade tab should be held in line with the long axis of the tooth.

3. *Sensitivity of the eye:* Fourteen percent of males are color blind to one or more colors. Color blindness is rare in females. The condition increases progressively with age. Annual monitoring is appropriate for practitioners who need to perceive color predictably.

4. *The brain's interpretation of color:* Color must be perceived, not merely viewed. Any distortion of the stimulus by the receptor results in an error. Therefore, the light must be constant and controlled, viewing conditions standardized, and the eye and brain trained through repetition.

5. *Optical properties of the tooth:* Natural teeth are translucent; all of the light that enters is reflected or refracted. The amount of translucency depends on the structure and thickness of the enamel and dentin. The dentin is the primary source for color, and the enamel regulates the brightness.

6. *Condition of tooth and setting:* Factors that affect the interpretation include the color of the operatory walls, the patient's and dentist's clothes, the patient's napkin, and the patient's lipstick and skin tone. Once those factors are neutralized, the eye's ability to see yellow-orange improves color selection. Surrounding the tooth with a blue-colored material or looking at blue during shade selection is one way to increase the dentist's ability to detect small differences in the spectral composition of the tooth. With an understanding of color perception and tooth anatomy, practitioners can begin to describe tooth color composition.

A logical place to begin solving the shade-selection dilemma is with an understanding of the four dimensions of color. Artists describe color in terms of three dimensions: hue, chroma, and value. *Hue* is the basic color of an object. It is determined by the wavelength of the reflected light. Dentin is responsible for a tooth's hue. *Chroma* is a further refinement of the hue. It is a measurement of the dilution or saturation of the hue, from pale to intense. *Value* is a measure of the amount of light reflected by a tooth. It is also called *luminance* or *brightness*. It measures the gray scale from black (low value) to white. The thickness and character of enamel affect brightness. Teeth with thick enamel tend to be lower in value because the gray enamel masks the brighter dentin underneath. Teeth have a fourth dimension of color known as *maverick colors*. These are concentrated areas of color in the dentin of most teeth that differ from the overall color. They combine with the basic dentin color and project their resultant effect through the enamel. Maverick colors follow no set rules or pattern; they appear in different areas of the dentin and represent different color families in several degrees of concentration.

Once the four dimensions have been visualized, the components and perceptions must be translated into the language of dental ceramics.[158] Each individual dimension of color should be measured separately. A measuring device must be used to standardize the information provided to the technician. Commercial or customized tooth color guides incorporate much of the information required. Two guides should be used, one set up for value and the other for hue-chroma. The value can be selected first. Color should play no role in its selection. Practitioners should squint when choosing value. This will lower the amount of light entering the eye and decrease color perception. Next, hue-chroma is detected. All teeth are yellow; only the chroma varies. Chroma defines the color below the enamel. Commercial guides categorize hue-chroma as Vita A, B, C, and D families. The color family is determined by comparing the tooth to the fully saturated tab (A4, B4, C4, and D4). Second, the exact dilution within the family (1, 2, 3, 4) is measured. Custom shade guides can provide a more reliable means for measuring tooth color dimensions.[160] Each tab is a sample of what the ceramist is capable of producing with a given porcelain and technique. Maverick shades are the last to be selected. The family colors are narrow in spectrum (yellow, honey yellow, light and dark brown) but vary in concentration. The maverick guide is constructed of body modifiers and neutral porcelains.[157] Concentrations are determined as with chroma shades. After the dimensions are determined, the information is conveyed to the ceramist.

Communication between the dentist and laboratory can occur in three ways:

1. *Diagrams:* A representation of the tooth may be drawn. While this can be helpful for communicating difficult con-

tours and characteristics, it is difficult for the technician to interpret and very time-consuming.

2. *Custom stain tabs:* Painting colors on a shade tab can display chroma but cannot represent value. In addition, customizing is extremely time-consuming.
3. *Photographs:* Taking photographs of the teeth being restored along with matching shade guides is the most efficient and cost-effective method of shade selection (Fig 17-30).

Photographs must provide an accurate representation of nature. A 35-mm camera with neutral slide film (EPN 100, Kodak) maximizes the ceramist's ability to mimic reality. Digital photography has begun to replace film cameras. The ability to instantly view your results and the elimination of film processing are tremendous advantages. Electronic transfer to the laboratory allows improved communication. The disadvantage is the multiple errors that can occur in color reproduction. The camera and monitors must all be color-corrected to maximize results. Many operatory and laboratory shade matching systems have been introduced with varying success.

The more photographs that are taken, the more information the technician can obtain. If the anterior ceramic crown does not match at try-in, more photographs should be taken of the crown to allow the ceramist to modify it correctly. Personal contact between the ceramist and patient would be ideal, but this is often not possible.

Restoration Placement

The classification of anterior ceramic crowns is based on whether the prosthesis is adhesively retained or cemented. Veneers and bonded crowns rely on the formation of a resin bond between the tooth structure and porcelain. Cemented all-ceramic and metal-ceramic crowns are nonadhesively cemented with traditional cements rather than bonded to the preparation. Therefore, the placement protocol will vary significantly between the types of crowns.

Resin Bonding of All-Ceramic Crowns

The goal of adhesive bonding is to provide a marginal seal of the crown and adhesively retain it to the tooth. Resin bonding is technique sensitive and demands proper preparation of ceramic and tooth surfaces. It has been demonstrated that a strong, dependable bond between resin and porcelain can be achieved. The porcelain intaglio surface is etched with hydrofluoric acid to create micromechanical retention sites.[161] Silane

is added to the etched surface shortly before bonding and allowed to air dry. Silane coupling agents improve the resin bond to porcelain.[162]

The dentin-resin bond is less dependable than the resin-ceramic bond. Because hemorrhage and crevicular fluid flow may interfere with dentin bonding, teeth should be isolated with retraction cord before cementation. Preparations should be cleaned with pumice and/or antimicrobial solutions such as chlorhexidine. Because light polymerization decreases with increasing porcelain thickness[163] and because polymerization of the adhesive before cementation may result in resin pooling and incomplete seating, a chemically activated adhesive system should be applied according to the manufacturer's instructions.[164] This includes an etchant, primer, and dual-cure adhesive. A dual-cure resin cement is recommended for bonding of the crown for the same reason. Dual-cured resins have a slow, chemically activated autocure component and a light-activated component. The inside of the crown is painted with adhesive before addition of the luting resin. The crown is gently placed and excess cement removed with a brush. Then the crown is seated with additional pressure or lightly tapped to extrude excess luting resin at the margins. The luting resin is light cured through the facial and lingual aspects for 1 minute each. Excess resin is removed with a No. 12 scalpel blade. The occlusion is adjusted with diamond burs that have 15-μm diamond abrasive and 8-μm diamond abrasive under water spray. Finally, the porcelain is polished with a porcelain polishing kit.

Cementation of Nonbonded Crowns

The goals of nonadhesive cementation are complete seating of the crown and maximization of the physical properties of the cement. The preparation should be thoroughly cleaned with pumice and/or an antimicrobial solution. If the soft tissue interferes with complete seating, retraction cord should be placed. The cement should be mixed according to the manufacturer's instructions and loaded into the crown, and the crown should be seated. If the crown has metal margins, the patient should bite on an orangewood stick or cotton roll; the stick can be moved up and down and back and forth for a few seconds. This technique, called dynamic seating, results in more complete seating of the crown.[165] Every effort should be made to keep the crown dry during the initial setting phase, that is, the first 5 minutes after cementation.[166] The physical properties of most cements deteriorate if they become wet during setting. The final step is careful removal of the excess set cement with an explorer or scaler.

References

1. Spear FM, Winter RR. Esthetic alternatives for anterior teeth. Presented at the Annual Meeting of American Academy of Restorative Dentistry, Chicago, February 22, 1997.

2. Hagberg C. Assessment of bite force: A review. J Craniomandib Disord 1987;1:162–169.

3. Ludwig K. Studies on the ultimate strength of all-ceramic crowns. Dent Lab 1991;5:647–651.

4. Rosenblum MA, Schulman A. A review of all-ceramic restorations. J Am Dent Assoc 1997;128:297–307.

5. Lehner CR, Mannchen R, Scharer P. Variable reduced metal support for collarless metal-ceramic crowns: A new model for strength evaluation. Int J Prosthodont 1995;8:337–345.

6. Schaffner VB, Jones DW. Light transmission in shoulder porcelain of metal-ceramic restorations. Presented at the Annual Meeting of the Academy of Prosthodontics, Orlando, FL, May 17, 1994.

7. Andersson M, Razzoog ME, Oden A, Hegenbarth EA, Lang BR. Procera: A new way to achieve an all-ceramic crown. Quintessence Int 1998;29:285–296.

8. Bello A, Jarvis RH. A review of esthetic alternatives for the restoration of anterior teeth. J Prosthet Dent 1997;78:437–440.

9. Giordano RA. Dental ceramic restorative systems. Compend Contin Educ Dent 1996;17:779–794.

10. McLaren EA. All-ceramic alternatives to conventional metal-ceramic restorations. Compend Contin Educ Dent 1998;19:307–325.

11. Heffernan MJ, Aquilino SA, Diaz-Arnold AM, Haselton DR, Stanford CM, Vargas MA. Relative translucency of six all-ceramic systems. Part I: Core materials. J Prosthet Dent 2002;88:4–9.

12. Campbell SD. Clinical selection criteria for esthetic full crown restorations. Presented at the American Academy of Restorative Dentistry, Chicago, February 23, 1999.

13. Campbell SD, Tu SJ, Lund PS. Translucency of a new ceramic crown material [abstract 395]. J Dent Res 1997;76:63.

14. Rouse J, McGowan S. Restoration of the anterior maxilla with ultraconservative veneers: Clinical and laboratory considerations. Pract Periodont Aesthet Dent 1999;11:333–339.

15. Lund PS, Campbell SD, Giordano RA. Translucency of core and veneer materials for all-ceramic crowns [abstract 2135]. J Dent Res 1996;75:284.

16. Grossman DG. Photoelastic examination of bonded crown interfaces [abstract 719]. J Dent Res 1989;68:271.

17. Burke FJT. Fracture resistance of teeth restored with dentin-bonded crowns: The effect of increased tooth preparation. Quintessence Int 1996;27:115–121.

18. Burke FJT, Qualtrough AJE, Wilson NHF. A retrospective evaluation of a series of dentin-bonded ceramic crowns. Quintessence Int 1998;29:103–106.

19. Neiva G, Yaman P, Dennison JB, Razzoog ME, Lang BR. Resistance to fracture of three all-ceramic systems. J Esthet Dent 1998;10:60–66.

20. Marshall GW, Marshall SJ, Kinney JH, Balooch M. The dentin substrate: Structure and properties related to bonding. J Dent 1997; 25:441–458.

21. Heymann HO, Bayne SC. Current concepts in dentin bonding: Focusing on dentinal adhesion factors. J Am Dent Assoc 1993;124: 27–36.

22. Douglas WH. Clinical status of dentin bonding agents. J Dent 1989; 17:209–215.

23. Lee WC, Eakle WS. Possible role of tensile stress in the etiology of cervical erosive lesions of teeth. J Prosthet Dent 1984;52:374–380.

24. Gear RW. Neural control of oral behavior and its impact on occlusion. In: McNeill C (ed). Science and Practice of Occlusion. Chicago: Quintessence, 1997:59–60.

25. Gibbs CH, Mahan PE, Mauderli A, Lundeen HC, Walsh EK. Limits of human bite strength. J Prosthet Dent 1986;56:226–228.

26. Jung YG, Peterson IM, Kim DK, Lawn BR. Lifetime-limiting strength degradation from contact fatigue in dental ceramics. J Dent Res 2000;79:722–730.

27. Drummond JL, King TJ, Bapna MS, Koperski RD. Mechanical property evaluation of pressable restorative ceramics. Dent Mater 2000; 16:226–233.

28. Lawn BR, Deng Y, Lloyd IK, Janal MN, Rekow ED, Thompson VP. Materials design of ceramic-based layer structures for crowns. J Dent Res 2002;81:433–438.

29. Wakabayashi N, Anusavice KJ. Crack initiation modes in bilayered alumina/porcelain disks as a function of core/veneer thickness ratio and supporting substrate stiffness. J Dent Res 2000;79:1398–1404.

30. Lehner C, Studer S, Brodbeck U, Scharer P. Short-term results of IPS-Empress full-porcelain crowns. J Prosthodont 1997;6:20–30.

31. Lyzak WA, Campbell SD, Wen Z. Thermal cycling effects on the strength of Optimal Pressable Ceramic [abstract 2062]. J Dent Res 1997;76:271.

32. AbdelHalim T, Lyzak WA, Campbell SD, Wen Z. Effects of pressing programs on optimal pressable ceramic strength [abstract 2064]. J Dent Res 1997;76:271.

33. Burke FJT. Fracture resistance of dentin-bonded crowns constructed in a leucite-reinforced ceramic [abstract 1608]. J Dent Res 1999; 78:306.

34. Cattell MJ, Knowles JC, Clarke RL, Lynch E. The biaxial flexural strength of two pressable ceramic systems. J Dent 1999;27:183–196.

35. Gorman CM, McDevitt WE, Hill RG. Comparison of two heat-pressed all-ceramic dental materials. Dent Mater 2000;16:389–395.

36. Sulaiman F, Chai J, Jameson LM, Wozniak WT. A comparison of the marginal fit of In-Ceram, IPS Empress and Procera crowns. Int J Prosthodont 1997;10:478–484.

37. Fradeani M, Redemagni M. An 11-year clinical evaluation of leucite-reinforced glass-ceramic crowns: A retrospective study. Quintessence Int 2002;33:503–510.

38. Heinzmann JL, Krejci I, Lutz F. Wear and marginal adaptation of glass-ceramic inlays, amalgam and enamel [abstract 423]. J Dent Res 1990;69(special issue):161.

39. Imai Y, Suzuki S, Fukushima S. In vitro enamel wear of modified porcelains [abstract 50]. J Dent Res 1999;78:112.

40. Sorensen JA, Sultan E, Condon JR. Three-body in vitro wear of enamel against dental ceramics [abstract 909]. J Dent Res 1999;78:219.

41. Sorensen JA, Berge HX. In vivo measurement of antagonist tooth wear opposing ceramic bridges [abstract 2942]. J Dent Res 1999; 78:473.

42. Giordano R, Pelletier L, Campbell S, Pober R. Flexural strength of alumina and glass components of In-Ceram [abstract 1181]. J Dent Res 1992;71:253.

43. McLaren EA, White SN. Survival of In-Ceram crowns in a private practice: A prospective clinical trial. J Prosthet Dent 2000;83: 216–222.

44. Kappert HF, Altvater A. Field study on the accuracy of fit and the marginal seal of In-Ceram crowns and bridges [in German]. Dtsch Zahnarztl Z 1991;46:151–153.

45. Haselton DR, Diaz-Arnold AM, Hillis SL. Clinical assessment of high-strength all-ceramic crowns. J Prosthet Dent 2000;83:396–401.

46. Yeo IS, Yang JH, Lee JB. In vitro marginal fit of three all-ceramic crown systems. J Prosthet Dent 2003;90:459–464.

47. Fradeani M, Aquilano A, Corrado M. Clinical experience with In-Ceram Spinell crowns: 5-year follow up. Int J Periodontics Restorative Dent 2002;22:525–533.

48. Harrington Z, McDonald A, Knowles J. An in vitro study to investigate the load at fracture of Procera AllCeram crowns with various thickness of occlusal veneer porcelain. Int J Prosthodont 2003;16:54–58.

49. May KB, Russell MM, Razzoog ME, Lang BR. Precision of fit: The Procera AllCeram crown. J Prosthet Dent 1998;80:394–404.

50. Boening KW, Wolf BH, Schmidt AE, Kastner K, Walter MH. Clinical fit of Procera AllCeram crowns. J Prosthet Dent 2000;84:419–424.

51. Oden A, Andersson M, Krystek-Ondracek I, Magnusson D. Five-year clinical evaluation of Procera AllCeram crowns. J Prosthet Dent 1998;80:450–456.

52. Schweiger M, Holand W, Frank M, Rheinberger V. IPS Empress 2: A new pressable high-strength glass-ceramic for esthetic all-ceramic restorations. Quintessence Dent Technol 1999;22:143–151.

53. Seghi RR, Sorensen JA, Engelman MJ, et al. Flexural strength of new ceramic materials [abstract 1521]. J Dent Res 1990;89:299.

54. Pallis K, Griggs JA, Woody RD, Guillen GE, Miller AW. Fracture resistance of three all-ceramic restorative systems for posterior applications. J Prosthet Dent 2004;91:561–569.

55. Zimmer D, Gerds T, Strub JR. Survival rate of IPS-Empress 2 all-ceramic crowns and bridges Three year's results [in German]. Schweiz Monatsschr Zahnmed 2004;114:115–119.

56. Guazzato M, Albakry M, Ringer SP, Swain MV. Strength, fracture toughness and microstructure of a selection of all-ceramic materials. Part II. Zirconia-based dental ceramics. Dent Mater 2004;20:449–456.

57. Guazzato M, Albakry M, Ringer SP, Swain MV. Strength, fracture toughness and microstructure of a selection of all-ceramic materials. Part II. Zirconia-based dental ceramics. Dent Mater 2004;20:449–456.

58. Guazzato M, Proos K, Sara G, Swain MV. Strength, reliability and mode of fracture of bilayered porcelain/core ceramics. Int J Prosthodont 2004;17:142–149.

59. Chong KH, Cai J, Takahashi Y, Wozniak W. Flexural strength of In-Ceram alumina and In-Ceram zirconia. Int J Prosthodont 2002;5:183–188.

60. Tinschert J, Natt G, Mautsch W, Spiekermann H, Anusavice KJ. Marginal fit of alumina- and zirconia-based fixed partial dentures produced by a CAD/CAM system. Oper Dent 2001;26:367–374.

61. Coli P, Karlsson S. Fit of a new pressure-sintered zirconium dioxide coping. Int J Prosthodont 2004;17:59–64.

62. Suarez MJ, Lozano JF, Paz Salido M, Martinez F. Three-year clinical evaluation of In-Ceram Zirconia posterior FPDs. Int J Prosthodont 2004;17:35–38.

63. Heffernan MJ, Aquilino SA, Diaz-Arnold AM, Haselton DR, Stanford CM, Vargas MA. Relative translucency of six all-ceramic systems. Part II: Core and veneer materials. J Prosthet Dent 2002;88:10–15.

64. Al-Dohan HM, Yaman P, Dennison JB, Razzoog ME, Lang BR. Shear strength of core-veneer interface in bi-layered ceramics. J Prosthet Dent 2004;91:349–355.

65. Jones DW. Development of dental ceramics—A historical perspective. Dent Clin North Am 1985;29:621–644.

66. Campbell SD. A comparative strength study of metal-ceramic and all-ceramic materials: Modulus of rupture. J Prosthet Dent 1989;62:476–479.

67. Selby A. Fixed prosthodontic failure. A review and discussion of important aspects. Aust Dent J 1994;39:150–156.

68. Block PL. Restorative margins and periodontal health. J Prosthet Dent 1987;57:683–689.

69. Felton DA, Kanoy B, Bayne S, Wirthman G. Effect of in vivo crown margin discrepancies on periodontal health. J Prosthet Dent 1991;65:357–364.

70. Flores-de-Jacoby L, Zafiropoulus GG, Ciancio S. The effect of crown margin location on plaque and periodontal health. Int J Periodontics Restorative Dent 1989;9:197–205.

71. Sorensen JA, Torres TJ, Kang SK, Avera SP. Marginal fidelity of ceramic crowns with different margin designs [abstract 1365]. J Dent Res 1990;69(special issue):279.

72. Nevins M, Skurow HM. The intracrevicular restorative margin, the biologic width, and the maintenance of the gingival margin. Int J Periodontics Restorative Dent 1984;4(3):31–49.

73. Tarnow DP, Stahl SS, Magner A. Human gingival attachment response to subgingival crown placement. J Clin Periodontol 1986;13:563–569.

74. Kaiser DA, Newell DH. Technique to disguise the metal margin of the metal/ceramic crown. Am J Dent 1988;1:217–221.

75. Kois JC. The gingiva is red around my crowns: A differential diagnosis. Dent Econ 1993;4:101–105.

76. Kois JC. The restorative-periodontal interface: Biological parameters. Periodontol 2000 1996;11:1–10.

77. Hochman N, Yaffe A, Ehrlich J. Crown contour variations in gingival health. Compend Contin Educ Dent 1983;4:360–365.

78. Gottlieb B. Der epithelansatz am zahne. Dtsch Monatsschr Zahnheilkd 1921;39:142–148.

79. Sicher H. Changing concepts of the supporting dental structures. Oral Surg 1959;12:31–35.

80. Gargiulo AW, Wentz FM, Orban B. Dimensions and relations of the dentogingival junction in humans. J Periodontol 1961;32:261–267.

81. Ingber JS, Rose LF, Coslet JG. The "biologic width": A concept in periodontics and restorative dentistry. Alpha Omegan 1977;70:62–65.

82. Kois JC. Altering gingival levels: The restorative connection. Part I: Biologic variables. J Esthet Dent 1994;6(1):3–9.

83. Spray JR, Garnick JJ, Doles LR, Klawitter JJ. Microscopic demonstration of the position of periodontal probes. J Periodontol 1978;49:148–152.

84. Van Der Velden UJ. Regeneration of the interdental soft tissues following denudation procedures. Clin Periodontol 1982;9:455–459.

85. Pontoriero R, Carnevale G. Surgical crown lengthening: A 12-month clinical wound healing study. J Periodontol 2001;72:841–848.

86. Sanavi F, Wiesgold AS, Rose LF. Biologic width and its relation to periodontal biotypes. J Esthet Dent 1998;10:157–163.

87. Coslet JG, Vanarsdall R, Wiesgold A. Diagnosis and classification of delayed passive eruption of the dentogingival junction in the adult. Alpha Omegan 1977;10:24–28.

88. Jackson CR, Skidmore AE, Rice RT. Pulpal evaluation of teeth restored with fixed prostheses. J Prosthet Dent 1992;67:323–325.

89. Zach L, Cohen G. Pulpal response to externally applied heat. Oral Surg 1965;19:515–530.

90. Laforgia PD, Milano V, Morea C, Desiate A. Temperature change in the pulp chamber during complete crown preparation. J Prosthet Dent 1991;65:56–61.

91. Ward ML. The American Textbook of Operative Dentistry, ed 6. Philadelphia: Lea & Febiger, 1926:413.

92. Al-Omari WM, Al-Wahadni AM. Convergence angle, occlusal reduction, and finish line depth of full-crown preparations made by dental students. Quintessence Int 2004;35:287–293.

93. Jorgensen KD. The relationship between retention and convergence angles in cemented veneer crowns. Acta Odontol Scand 1955; 13:35–40.

94. Wiskott A, Nicholls JI, Belser UC. The effect of abutment length and diameter on resistance to fatigue loading. Int J Prosthodont 1997; 10:207–215.

95. Wiskott A, Nicholls JI, Belser UC. The relationship between convergence angle and resistance of cemented crowns to dynamic loading. Int J Prosthodont 1996;9:117–130.

96. Wiskott HWA, Krebs C, Scherrer SS, Botsis J, Belser UC. Compressive and tensile zones in the cement interface of full crowns: A technical note on the concept of resistance. J Prosthet Dent 1999;8:80–91.

97. Ohm E, Silness J. The convergence angle in teeth prepared for artificial crowns. J Oral Rehabil 1978;5:371–375.

98. Mack PJ. A theoretical and clinical investigation into the taper achieved on crown and inlay preparations. J Oral Rehabil 1980;7: 255–265.

99. Nordlander J, Weir D, Stoffer W, Ochi S. The taper of clinical preparations for fixed prosthodontics. J Prosthet Dent 1988;60:148–151.

100. Smith CT, Gary JJ, Conkin JE, Franks HL. Effective taper criterion for the full veneer crown preparation in preclinical prosthodontics. J Prosthodont 1999;8:196–200.

101. el-Mowafy OM, Fenton AH, Forrester N, Milenkovic M. Retention of metal ceramic crowns cemented with resin cements: Effect of preparation taper and height. J Prosthet Dent 1996;76:524–529.

102. Gilboe DB, Teteruck WR. Fundamentals of extracoronal tooth preparation. Part I. Retention and resistance form. J Prosthet Dent 1974;32:651–656.

103. Carter SM, Wilson PR. The effect of die spacing on crown retention. Int J Prosthodont 1996;9:21–29.

104. Wilson AH, Chan DC. The relationship between preparation convergence and retention of extracoronal retainers. J Prosthet Dent 1994;3:74–78.

105. Korioth TW, Waldron TW, Versluis A, Schulte JK. Forces and moments generated at the dental incisors during forceful biting in humans. J Biomech 1997;30:631–633.

106. Morikawa A. Investigation of occlusal force on lower first molar in function [in Japanese]. Kokubyo Gakkai Zasshi 1994;61:250–274.

107. Wiskott A, Belser U. A rationale for a simplified occlusal design in restorative dentistry: Historical review and clinical guidelines. J Prosthet Dent 1995;75:169–183.

108. Graf H, Geering AH. Rationale for clinical application of different occlusal philosophies. Oral Sci Rev 1977;10:1–10.

109. Caputo AA, Standlee JP. Biomechanics in Clinical Dentistry. Chicago: Quintessence, 1987:128.

110. Owen CP. Retention and resistance in preparations for extracoronal restorations. Part 2: Practical and clinical studies. J Prosthet Dent 1986;56:148–153.

111. Shillingburg HT, Hobo S, Whitsett LD. Fundamentals of Fixed Prosthodontics, ed 2. Chicago: Quintessence, 1981:79–96.

112. Zuckerman GR. Resistance form for the complete veneer crown: Principles of design and analysis. Int J Prosthodont 1988;1:302–307.

113. Eismann HF, Radke RA. Postendodontic restoration. In: Cohen S, Burns RC (eds). Pathways of the Pulp. St Louis: Mosby, 1987: 640–683.

114. Sorensen J, Engelman M. Ferrule design and fracture resistance of endodontically treated teeth. J Prosthet Dent 1990;63:529–536.

115. Trabert KC, Cooney JP. The endodontically treated tooth: Restorative concepts and techniques. Dent Clin North Am 1984;28:423–451.

116. Akkayan B. An in vitro study evaluating the effect of ferrule length on fracture resistance of endodontically treated teeth restored with fiber-reinforced and zirconia dowel systems. J Prosthet Dent 2004; 92:155–162.

117. Christensen GJ. Marginal fit of gold inlay castings. J Prosthet Dent 1966;16:297–305.

118. Bjorn AL, Bjorn H, Grkovic B. Marginal fit of restorations and its relation to periodontal bone level. I. Metal fillings. Odontol Revy 1969; 20:311–321.

119. Bjorn AL, Bjorn H, Grkovic B. Marginal fit of restorations and its relation to periodontal bone level. II. Crowns. Odontol Revy 1970;21:337–346.

120. Qualtrough AJE, Piddock V. Dental ceramics: What's new? Dent Update 2002;29:25–33.

121. Belser UC, MacEntee MI, Richter WA. Fit of three porcelain-fused-to-metal marginal designs in vivo: A scanning electron microscope study. J Prosthet Dent 1985;53:24–29.

122. Wright WE. Selection of proper margin configuration. J Calif Dent Assoc 1992;20:41–44.

123. Faucher RR, Nicholls JI. Distortion related to margin design in porcelain-fused-to-metal restorations. J Prosthet Dent 1980;43:149–155.

124. Pascoe DF. Analysis of the geometry of finish lines for full crown restorations. J Prosthet Dent 1978;40:157–162.

125. el-Ebrashi MK, Craig RG, Peyton FA. Experimental stress analysis of dental restorations. 3. The concept of the geometry of proximal margins. J Prosthet Dent 1969;22:333–345.

126. Gardner FM, Tillman-McCombs KW, Gaston ML, Runyan DA. In vitro failure load of metal-collar margins compared with porcelain facial margins of metal-ceramic crowns. J Prosthet Dent 1997; 78:1–4.

127. Abbate MF, Tjan AHL, Fox WM. Comparison of the marginal fit of various ceramic crown systems. J Prosthet Dent 1989;61:527–531.

128. Gavelis JR, Morency JD, Riley ED, Sozio RB. The effect of various finish line preparations on the marginal seal and occlusal seat of full crown preparations. J Prosthet Dent 1981;45:138–145.

129. Padilla MT, Bailed JH. Marginal configuration, die spacers, fitting of retainer/crowns, and soldering. Dent Clin North Am 1992;36: 743–765.

130. Vahidi F, Egloff ET, Panno FV. Evaluation of marginal adaptation of all-ceramic crowns and metal-ceramic crowns. J Prosthet Dent 1991;66:426–431.

131. Kois JC. New paradigms for anterior tooth preparation: Rationale and technique. Contemp Esthet Dent 1996;2(1):1–8.

132. Wall JC, Reisbick MH, Johnston WM. Incisal edge strength of porcelain laminate veneers restoring mandibular incisors. Int J Prosthodont 1992;5:441–446.

133. Aminian A, Brunton PA. A comparison of the depths produced using three different tooth preparation techniques. J Prosthet Dent 2003;89:19–22.

134. Chiche GJ, Harrison JD. Impression considerations in the maxillary anterior region. Compend Contin Educ Dent 1994;15:318–327.

135. Nemetz H, Donovan TE, Landesman H. Exposing the gingival margin: A systematic approach for the control of hemorrhage. J Prosthet Dent 1984;51:647–650.

136. Benson BW. Tissue displacement methods in fixed prosthodontics. J Prosthet Dent 1986;55:175–181.

137. Nementz E, Seibly W. The use of chemical agents in gingival retraction. Gen Dent 1990;3:104–108.

138. Donovan TE, Gandara BK, Nemetz H. Review and survey of medicaments used with gingival retraction cords. J Prosthet Dent 1985;53:525–531.

139. Laufer BZ, Baharav H, Ganor Y, Cardash HS. The effect of marginal thickness on the distortion of different impression materials. J Prosthet Dent 1996;76:466–471.

140. Laufer BZ, Baharav H, Cardash HS. The linear accuracy of impressions and stone dies as affected by the thickness of the impression margin. Int J Prosthodont 1994;7:247–252.

141. Aimjirakul P, Masuda T, Takahashi H, Miura H. Gingival sulcus simulation model for evaluating the penetration characteristics of elastomeric impression materials. Int J Prosthodont 2003;16:385–389.

142. Baharav H, Laufer BZ, Langer Y, Cardish HS. The effect of displacement time on gingival crevice width. Int J Prosthodont 1997;10:248–253.

143. Azzi R, Tsao TF, Carranza FA, Kenney EB. Comparative study of gingival retraction methods. J Prosthet Dent 1983;50:561–565.

144. Harrison JD. Effect of retraction materials on the gingival sulcus epithelium. J Prosthet Dent 1961;11:514–519.

145. Ruel J, Schuessler PJ, Malament K, Mori D. Effect of retraction procedures on the periodontium in humans. J Prosthet Dent 1980;44:508–515.

146. Ciesco JN, William MS, Sandrik JL, Mazur B. Comparison of elastic impression materials used in fixed prosthodontics. J Prosthet Dent 1981;45:89–94.

147. Dounis GS, Ziebert GJ, Dounis KS. A comparison of impression materials for complete-arch fixed partial dentures. J Prosthet Dent 1991;65:165–169.

148. Lin CC, Ziebert GJ, Donegan SJ, Dhuru VB. Accuracy of impression materials for complete-arch fixed partial dentures. J Prosthet Dent 1988;59:288–291.

149. Federick DR, Caputo A. Comparing the accuracy of reversible hydrocolloid and elastomeric impression materials. J Am Dent Assoc 1997;128:183–188.

150. Pratten DH, Novetsky M. Detail reproduction of soft tissue: A comparison of impression materials. J Prosthet Dent 1991;65:188–191.

151. Chee WWL, Donovan TE. Polyvinyl siloxane impression materials: A review of properties and techniques. J Prosthet Dent 1992;73:419–423.

152. Johnson GH, Lepe X, Aw TC. The effect of surface moisture on detail reproduction of elastomeric impressions. J Prosthet Dent 2003;90:228–234.

153. Chee WWL, Donovan TE, Kahn RL. Indirect inhibition of polymerization of a polyvinyl siloxane impression material: A case report. Quintessence Int 1991;22:133–135.

154. de Camargo LM, Chee WWL, Donovan TE. Inhibition of polymerization of polyvinyl siloxanes by medicaments used on gingival retraction cords. J Prosthet Dent 1993;70:114–117.

155. Kahn RL, Donovan TE. A pilot study of polymerization inhibition of poly (vinyl siloxane) materials by latex gloves. Int J Prosthodont 1989;2:128–130.

156. Gordon GE, Johnson GH, Drennon DG. The effect of tray selection on the accuracy of elastomeric impression materials. J Prosthet Dent 1990;63:12–15.

157. Rueda LJ, Sy-Munoz JT, Naylor WP, Goodacre CJ, Swartz ML. The effect of using custom or stock trays on the accuracy of gypsum casts. Int J Prosthodont 1996;9:367–373.

158. Muia P. Esthetic Restorations: Improved Dentist-Laboratory Communication. Chicago: Quintessence, 1993:81–95.

159. Zwimpfer M. Color, Light, Sight, Sense. Philadelphia: Schiffer Publishing, 1988:1–264.

160. Groh CL, O'Brien WJ, Boenke KM, Mora GP. Differences in color between fired porcelain and shade guides [abstract 813]. J Dent Res 1992;71:207.

161. Sorensen JA, Kang SK, Avera SA. Porcelain-composite interface microleakage with various porcelain surface treatments. Dent Mater 1991;7:118–121.

162. Stangel I, Nathanson D, Hsu CS. Shear strength of the composite bond to etched porcelain. J Dent Res 1987;66:1460–1465.

163. Boyer DB, Chan KC. Curing light activated composite cement through porcelain [abstract 1289]. J Dent Res 1989;68:476.

164. Bowen RL, Cobb EN. A method for bonding to dentin and enamel. J Am Dent Assoc 1983;107:734–736.

165. Rosenstiel SF, Gegauff AF. Improving cementation of complete cast crowns: A comparison of static and dynamic seating methods. J Am Dent Assoc 1988;117:845–848.

166. Curtis SR, Richards MW, Meiers JC. Early erosion of glass-ionomer cement at crown margins. Int J Prosthodont 1993;6:553–557.

Esthetic Inlays and Onlays

J. William Robbins
Dennis J. Fasbinder

There are several treatment options for esthetic Class 1 and Class 2 restorations, in addition to direct resin composite restorations. This chapter discusses tooth-colored inlays and onlays fabricated in resin composite and in ceramic materials. Restorations fabricated with computer-aided design/computer-assisted manufacture (CAD/CAM) technology will also be discussed.

Esthetic inlays and onlays have a number of characteristics in common, whether they are resin, ceramic, or fabricated with CAD/CAM technology.

General Considerations

Preparations

The preparations for ceramic and resin composite inlays and onlays are the same. Preparations for CAD/CAM inlays and onlays to be fabricated with the current CEREC (Sirona Dental) system do not differ from preparations for laboratory-fabricated inlays and onlays.

There is little research to support the efficacy of any preparation design over another.[1] However, based on knowledge of the materials and clinical experience, the divergent, relatively nonretentive preparation is most commonly advocated because of ease of placement (Fig 18-1). Resistance form may be incorporated with rounded proximal boxes, but grooves should not be used. Resistance and retention form for the restoration are provided primarily by adhesion to enamel and dentin. The walls and floors of the preparation should be smooth and even, and the internal angles should be rounded to enhance

adaptation of the restorative material (Fig 18-2). The occlusal reduction should be anatomic and, uniformly, a minimum of 2 mm for strength[2] (Fig 18-3).

There is no benefit to the placement of bevels at the occlusal or gingival margins; in fact, bevels should be avoided because thin margins of both resin composite and porcelain are susceptible to chipping during function.[3,4] A 90-degree butt joint minimizes the chipping problem but results in a visible demarcation between the tooth and the restoration. Therefore, when the esthetic blend of the restoration and the tooth is important, such as on the facial surface of a maxillary premolar, a long chamfer may be placed (see Fig 18-2).

Bases and Liners

The use of bases and liners is somewhat controversial. Initially, glass-ionomer bases were used for dentinal protection and to base the preparation to "ideal" form. However, it has been shown that it is not necessary to protect the dentin from the phosphoric acid etchant.[5] Therefore, glass-ionomer cement is recommended only for routine block-out of undercuts.

Provisional Restorations

Provisional restorations can be a challenge with esthetic inlays and, particularly, onlays because of the nonretentive design of the preparations. Provisional restorations can be made in the usual manner with acrylic resin or resin composite and cemented with temporary cement. It is commonly stated that a eugenol-containing cement should not be used with

Fig 18-1 Onlay preparation technique.

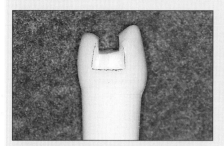

Fig 18-1a Simulation of amalgam preparation after removal of the amalgam.

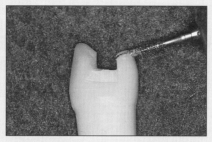

Fig 18-1b Use of a diamond of known diameter to make the first depth cut of 1 mm.

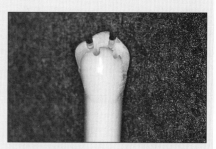

Fig 18-1c First depth cuts of 1 mm.

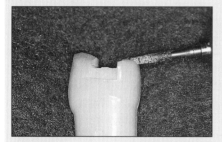

Fig 18-1d Use of a diamond of known diameter to make the second depth cuts of 1.0 mm.

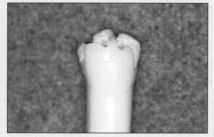

Fig 18-1e Second depth cuts of an additional 1 mm.

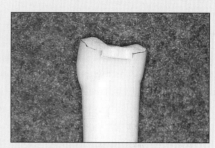

Fig 18-1f Occlusal reduction of 2 mm completed; however, sharp line angles remain in the box area.

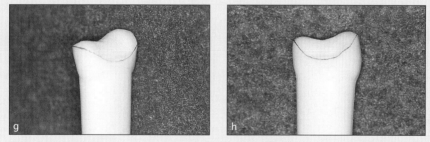

Figs 18-1g and 18-1h Completed smooth, flowing preparation without sharp angles.

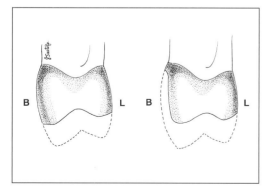

Fig 18-2 Standard onlay preparation *(left)* and modified onlay preparation *(right)* that includes coverage of facial surface to achieve a superior esthetic blend with the natural tooth color. B = buccal; L = lingual.

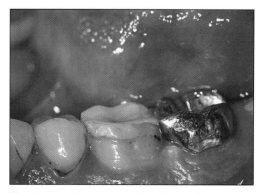

Fig 18-3 Inadequate occlusal reduction for porcelain onlay, resulting in fractured porcelain.

the provisional restoration when the final restoration will be bonded with a resin cement.[1,6] However, the literature is equivocal on the deleterious effect of eugenol. Some studies support the hypothesis that a eugenol-containing provisional cement inhibits the set of resin cements,[1,6,7] while others show that eugenol-containing provisional cements have no impact on bond strengths.[8–12] Because of the nonretentive design of the onlay preparation, the more retentive polycarboxylate cement is the temporary luting cement of choice. Small mechanical undercuts should be placed on the intaglio surface of the provisional restoration to aid in retention. If adjacent teeth are being restored, the provisional restorations can be connected to improve retention.

For inlay preparations, flexible light-cured materials, such as Fermit (Vivadent) or Barricade (Dentsply), may be used. To provide retention and to decrease sensitivity, a dentin primer can be placed in the preparation and air dried, or a small amount of resin-modified glass-ionomer cement liner can be placed on the pulpal floor and polymerized. The preparation is filled with the provisional material, and the patient is instructed to bite into maximum intercuspation to develop the occlusion. Excess material is removed with an explorer, and the provisional restoration is light cured. This technique is recommended only for short-term use in small preparations.[13]

Adhesive Cementation

Resin luting cement is the only material recommended for cementing this type of restoration because it bonds to enamel, dentin, and the restorative material. Luting resin cement limits microleakage and enhances the strength of the restoration.[14] It is commonly reported that indirect bonded restorations strengthen the prepared tooth[15,16]; however, this is not universally supported by the literature.[17] Dual-cured luting resin and dual-cured dentin bonding agents, which combine light-curing and chemical-curing components, should be used to bond all indirect posterior bonded restorations.[18,19] The light-curing component polymerizes rapidly on exposure to light of the proper wavelength, while the chemical-curing component undergoes a slow polymerization process in those areas to which the light does not penetrate. It is important that the curing light be applied to dual-cured resin for an adequate period of time, because the dual-cure process results in more complete polymerization than is achieved with chemical polymerization alone.[20,21] The shelf life of dual-cured resins is shorter than that of conventional light-cured resin composites. Therefore, a test batch of dual-cured luting resin should periodically be mixed and allowed to cure in a dark environment to ensure that it will polymerize in the absence of light. It should polymerize in the dark within 10 minutes.

Preparing the Restoration for Bonding

Adhesion is more reliably achieved to ceramic materials than to resin composite. Ceramics used in these restorations must be etched, creating durable micromechanical retention.[22] The ceramic inlay/onlay is prepared for bonding by etching the internal surface, usually with hydrofluoric acid. This is generally done at the laboratory but may be done chairside. Shortly before bonding, silane is applied to the etched surface to enhance wetting by the resin adhesive.[23,24]

Bonding to resin composite restorations is more difficult. The intaglio surface has no air-inhibited layer and relatively few unreacted methacrylate groups, so a reliable chemical bond does not form between the inlay and the resin cement.[25–27] Because the resin composite–cement interface may be the weak link, several procedures have been recommended to enhance the bond to resin. With hybrid resin composite, the intaglio surface should be carefully air abraded with 50-μm aluminum oxide (avoiding the margins)[28,29] and then cleaned with a steam cleaner or in an ultrasonic bath. The air abrasion provides a rough surface for frictional retention. The cleaned surface should be treated with an agent to allow better wetting by the cement. Silane is generally the preferred wetting agent.[26,30,31] Treatment with hydrofluoric acid has also been recommended to etch the glass particles in the hybrid resin composite, but laboratory research does not support the efficacy of this procedure.[25]

Bonding of microfilled resin composite restorations is even more problematic. Although not traditionally believed to be effective, air abrasion has been shown to enhance bond strength in one laboratory study.[29]

Preparing the Tooth for Bonding

The rubber dam is placed to ensure an isolated field (Fig 18-4a). Once the restoration is ready for bonding, a decision must be made regarding the type of dentin bonding agent. Fourth-generation light-cured adhesive systems should not be used under indirect posterior bonded restorations. The light-cured adhesive would need to be air thinned prior to polymerization to ensure absence of pooling of the adhesive, which would prevent complete seating of the restoration. However, it has been shown that air thinning of the light-cured adhesive resin significantly decreases the bond strength.[32] This leaves fourth-generation dual-cured systems, fifth-generation single-bottle systems, and sixth-generation self-etching systems. The technology continues to change rapidly, which makes the discussion of current dentin bonding agents difficult.

The technique with the most research support employs the dual-cured fourth-generation dentin bonding systems. The enamel and dentin are etched for 15 to 20 seconds, washed

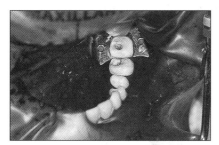

Fig 18-4a Rubber dam isolation for cementation of a quadrant of porcelain onlays.

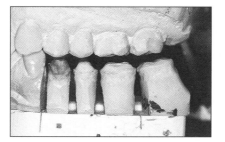

Fig 18-4b Master cast of a quadrant of porcelain onlay preparations. Note the amount of occlusal reduction.

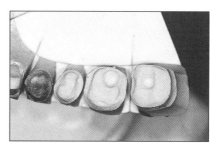

Fig 18-4c Occlusal view of onlay preparations.

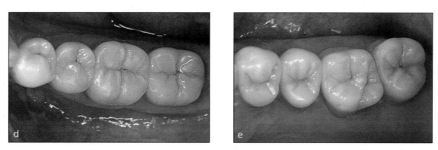

Figs 18-4d and 18-4e Porcelain onlays 2.5 years after placement. (Porcelain onlays created by Gilbert Young, CDT, GNS Dental Laboratory.)

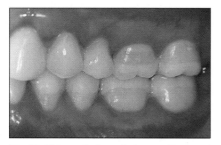

Fig 18-4f Lateral view of the maxillary and mandibular quadrants of porcelain onlays. The esthetic blend on the facial aspect of the maxillary premolars is better because the preparations were taken farther gingivally than on the molars.

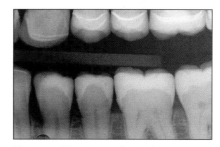

Fig 18-4g Bite-wing radiograph at 2.5 years showing porcelain onlays. Note different cement radiopacity in maxillary and mandibular restorations.

for 2 to 3 seconds, and air dried to enable visual inspection for an adequate enamel etch. The dentin is remoistened, and several coats of primer are applied. One laboratory study indicated that a 30-second application of primer with rubbing resulted in decreased microleakage compared to a 5-second priming.[33] The primer is completely air dried with gentle air pressure. The dual-cured adhesive is placed on the tooth and the intaglio surface of the restoration. The dual-cured luting resin is mixed and placed into the preparation and restoration, and the restoration is seated. Excess resin must be completely removed from the proximal-surface gingival margins with floss and interproximal instruments before polymerization of

the luting resin. Some clinicians recommend placement of a clear gel, such as glycerin, on the margins before polymerization in order to prevent the formation of an air-inhibited layer in the luting resin at the margin.[34] The margins may be finished with microfine diamonds or multifluted carbide finishing burs and a No. 12 scalpel blade, and they can be polished with disks, rubber points, or cups. After removal of the rubber dam, the occlusion is adjusted and the surface is polished to a high shine. The final step is rebonding, as described in chapter 10, with an unfilled or lightly filled resin (Figs 18-4b to 18-4g and Figs 18-5a to 18-5d).

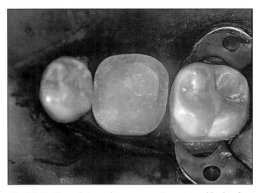

Fig 18-5a Porcelain onlay preparation, mandibular first molar.

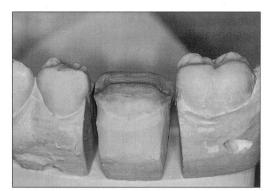

Fig 18-5b Master cast of prepared mandibular first molar for a porcelain onlay.

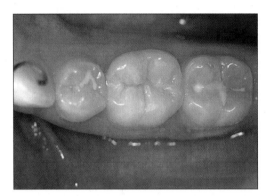

Fig 18-5c Completed porcelain onlay on mandibular first molar.

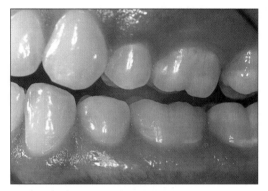

Fig 18-5d Buccal view of completed porcelain onlay on mandibular first molar. (Porcelain onlay created by Gilbert Young, CDT, GNS Dental Laboratory.)

The most commonly used bonding agents are in the fifth-generation group. These products generally require multiple coats for maximum bond strength.[21,35] The placement of multiple coats can potentially result in greater thickness of cured adhesive and areas of pooling, both of which can interfere with complete seating of the restoraton.[36] Also, many fifth- and sixth-generation products are incompatible with dual-cured and autocured luting composites. The clinician must ensure that the selected bonding agent and resin cement will polymerize together.

Maintenance

Maintenance is a very important factor in the longevity of esthetic inlays and onlays. As with all types of restorative dentistry, lack of preventive measures and the resulting caries can cause failure of the finest restoration. Use of devices such as ultrasonic scalers or air-abrasive polishers on these restorations must be avoided because they can cause surface and marginal damage. Calculus should be removed carefully with hand instruments. When scalers are used around a bonded inlay or onlay, care must be taken not to chip the margins. Surface stain may be removed from a restoration with aluminum oxide polishing paste or diamond polishing paste on a felt wheel or rubber cup. Because of their ability to etch porcelain, neither acidulated phosphate fluoride nor stannous fluoride solutions or gels should be used intraorally in patients with ceramic restorations. Only neutral sodium fluoride solutions should be used.

The patient should be advised that foods and liquids with a high potential for staining, such as coffee and tea, increase the potential for marginal staining. The patient must also be made aware of the potential for restoration fracture. Activities such as ice chewing and nail biting must be absolutely avoided. When a patient has a history of a parafunctional habit, a protective appliance should be fabricated to protect both the inlay or onlay and the opposing teeth.

Resin Composite Inlays and Onlays

Inlays and onlays made of resin composite are quite popular in Europe but have not gained wide acceptance in the United States. These restorations may be fabricated intraorally or on a cast. After polymerization, the restoration is bonded in place with a resin luting cement. Resin composite inlays can be highly esthetic and have certain advantages over direct resin composite and bonded ceramic restorations.

Advantages Over Direct Resin Composite Restorations

As discussed in chapter 10, inadequate proximal contours and open contacts can be common problems of direct resin composite restorations. These are less common problems with resin inlays, because contours and contacts can be developed outside of the mouth. If a contact is inadequate, it can easily be corrected prior to cementation.

Several problems associated with direct resin composite restorations are the result of polymerization shrinkage. During polymerization, resin composite shrinks on the order of 2% to 4%,[37] often causing a gap to form at the least retentive marginal interface, which is usually the gingival margin. Microleakage and bacterial ingress into the marginal gap may cause pulpal irritation and tooth sensitivity.[38] Current dentin adhesives have lessened, but not eliminated, the problem.[39,40] Polymerization shrinkage can also cause cuspal flexure, which is sometimes associated with craze lines in the enamel and postoperative sensitivity.[41]

In theory, polymerization shrinkage should be less of a problem with resin inlays because they are polymerized before cementation. The only polymerization shrinkage that occurs at the time of cementation is in the thin layer of resin cement. Resin inlays are reported to have less microleakage[42–44] and greater strength and·hardness[45–47] and to result in less postoperative sensitivity than direct resin composite restorations.[48]

While the in vitro data suggest that there are significant advantages to the resin inlay compared to the direct resin composite restoration, this is not corroborated by the in vivo data. In a 5-year clinical study[49] and another 11-year clinical study,[50] no statistically significant difference was found in the success rates for resin inlays compared to direct-placement resin composite restorations. Based on these data, and because of the increased cost of the resin inlay and the frequent need to remove more solid tooth structure for inlays, it is currently difficult to make a strong case in favor of the resin inlay over the direct resin composite restoration.

Secondary Polymerization

The superior physical properties of resin inlays are primarily due to more complete polymerization resulting from secondary polymerization procedures. Directly placed resin composites harden through a process of free-radical polymerization of methacrylate groups. In most cases, the polymerization reaction is initiated when a molecule within the resin composite (camphorquinone) forms free radicals when exposed to light of the appropriate wavelength (about 470 nm). The radicals react with a photoreducer (an aromatic or aliphatic amine) to initiate chain formation of the methacrylate groups. As polymerization progresses, the methacrylate chains grow and the material loses its fluidity. A hard surface forms and spreads progressively deeper into the resin composite. The reaction stops when the light is removed, the thickness is too great to allow adequate light penetration, or there are no more reactive molecules in close proximity to each other. Even with long curing times and powerful lights, incomplete polymerization occurs, particularly below the surface.[51]

Light-cured resin composite inlays undergo this initial polymerization but then are further polymerized with a combination of intense light, heat, and/or pressure. The postcure can be performed in a postcure unit specifically made for this purpose, in a toaster oven at approximately 250°F for 7 minutes,[45] or with a curing light or light box. Polymerization under pressure has been shown to increase both diametral tensile strength and stiffness of the restoration.[52] These secondary curing procedures are recommended with all indirect resin systems, although they may not be mentioned in all manufacturers' instructions.

Direct, Direct/Indirect, and Indirect Resin Composite Inlays and Onlays

Many resin composite inlay systems are available. For the purposes of this chapter, they are classified as direct (made on the tooth) or indirect (made on a cast).

Direct Resin Inlays

Inlays can be fabricated directly on the tooth (Fig 18-6). After preparation, a water-soluble separating medium and a matrix are placed on the tooth. The preparation is bulk filled with resin composite and light cured from all directions. The matrix is removed, and the inlay is teased out of the preparation. Because the resin composite shrinks during polymerization, the inlay is slightly smaller than the preparation and will come out easily if no undercuts are present. The inlay is then post-

Fig 18-6 Direct resin composite inlay technique.

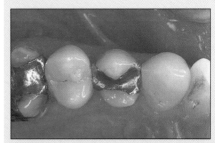

Fig 18-6a Preoperative view of a maxillary first premolar with an amalgam restoration that must be replaced.

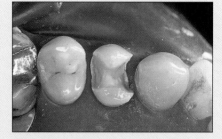

Fig 18-6b Preparation for a direct mesio-occlusodistal resin composite inlay.

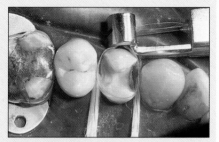

Fig 18-6c Placement of a matrix for a direct resin composite inlay.

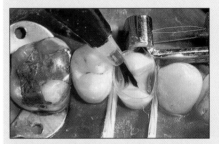

Fig 18-6d Placement of separating medium into the preparation.

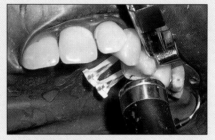

Fig 18-6e Light curing of the resin composite inlay, which was placed in bulk.

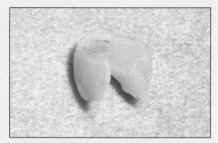

Fig 18-6f Resin composite inlay after it has been removed from the preparation.

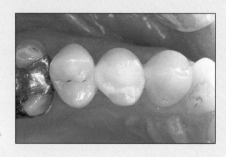

Fig 18-6g Two-year postoperative view of the direct mesio-occlusodistal resin composite inlay in the maxillary first premolar.

cured. Finally, it is tried in, adjusted, and bonded into the preparation (see the Direct Resin Inlay Technique box on p. 523).

Direct/Indirect Resin Inlays

When the direct/indirect method is used, an impression is made of the prepared tooth and a cast is poured (Figs 18-7a to 18-7o). Because this technique can be performed in one appointment, the master cast must be ready to use in a short period of time (5 minutes). Therefore, the products used must be compatible with the technique. The master die can be made from a silicone material (Mach 2, Parkell) or a master cast made from die stone (Snap-Stone, Whip Mix). The restoration is fabricated on the die and usually undergoes a primary (light-cured) and secondary (auxiliary curing unit) polymer-

ization. This process may be performed in the dental office or at a commercial laboratory.

Indirect Resin Inlays and Onlays

Resin inlays and onlays may also be fabricated by commercial laboratories. They can be constructed from either hybrid resin composite or microfilled resin composite. However, there is a newer generation of resin materials that has been termed *ceromer* or *ceramic-optimized polymer*.[48] These materials are reported to have greater durability, fracture toughness, wear resistance, esthetics, and repairability.[48] However, in one laboratory study, repaired ceromers were found to be 30% to 60% weaker than the parent material.[53]

Figs 18-7a to 18-7o Direct/indirect resin composite inlays using two different techniques.

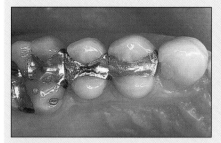

Fig 18-7a Preoperative view of the maxillary first and second premolars, which will be restored with direct/indirect resin composite inlays.

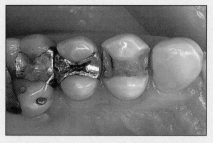

Fig 18-7b Preparation of the maxillary first premolar for a direct/indirect resin composite inlay.

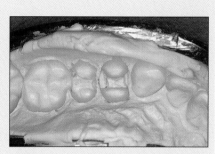

Fig 18-7c Impression of the inlay preparation.

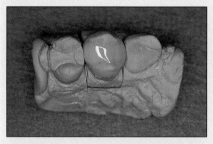

Fig 18-7d Indirect fabrication of the resin composite inlay on a silicone die that was made from the impression.

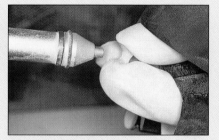

Fig 18-7e Air abrasion of the inner surface of the hybrid resin composite inlay with 50-μm aluminum oxide.

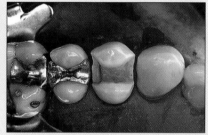

Fig 18-7f Preparation of the maxillary first premolar for cementation of the direct/indirect resin composite inlay.

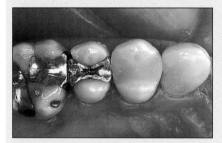

Fig 18-7g Direct/indirect resin composite inlay after cementation in the maxillary first premolar.

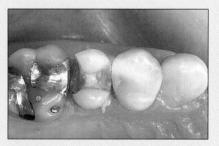

Fig 18-7h Preparation of the maxillary second premolar for direct/indirect resin composite inlay.

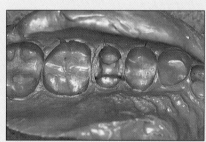

Fig 18-7i Impression of the maxillary second premolar for the resin composite inlay.

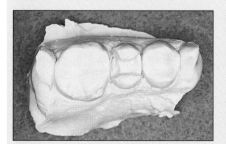

Fig 18-7j Stone die (Snap-Stone) of the inlay preparation.

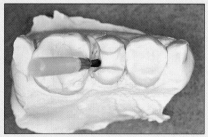

Fig 18-7k Painting the separator on the stone die prior to fabrication of the inlay.

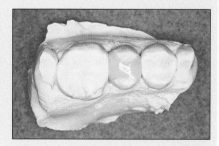

Fig 18-7l Fabrication of the direct/indirect resin composite inlay on the stone die.

Figs 18-7a to 18-7o *(continued)*

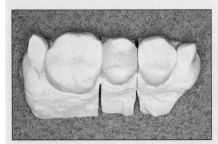

Fig 18-7m Stone die sawed and separated to allow for finishing of the inlay's margins.

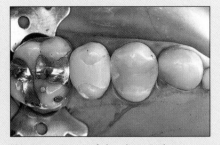

Fig 18-7n Try-in of the direct/indirect resin composite inlay in the maxillary second premolar.

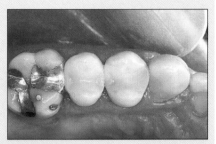

Fig 18-7o Direct/indirect resin composite inlays in the maxillary first and second premolars.

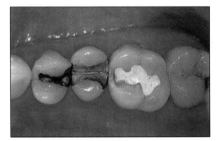

Fig 18-8a Preoperative view of maxillary premolars and first molar to be restored with ceromer restorations.

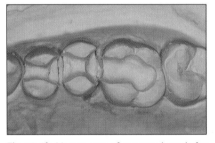

Fig 18-8b Master cast of prepared teeth for ceromer inlays.

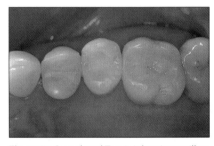

Fig 18-8c Completed Targis inlays in maxillary premolars and first molar.

There is minimal independent laboratory data available on the physical properties of the ceromer products. Ferracane[54] compared Artglass (Heraeus Kulzer) to the traditional hybrid composite, Charisma (Heraeus Kulzer). The fracture toughness of Artglass was higher than with Charisma; however, the flexural modulus and the hardness were higher with Charisma. Similarly, the physical properties were evaluated for Artglass, Targis (Ivoclar), and a traditional hybrid resin composite, Z100 (3M ESPE).[55] Targis demonstrated superior strength and Young's modulus compared to the other two products. The ceromer material may be combined with a fiber-reinforced material, which significantly increases fracture resistance.[56] However, flexural strength of fiber-reinforced ceromer has been shown to be significantly decreased after storage in water.[57] Ceromer restorations are bonded in the same manner as other indirect resin inlays/onlays (Figs 18-8a to 18-8c).

Posterior Bonded Porcelain Restorations

Ceramic inlays were introduced in 1913[58] but did not become popular because of difficulties in fabrication and a high failure rate.[1] In the 1980s, the development of compatible refractory materials made fabrication easier, and the development of adhesive resin cements greatly improved clinical success rates.[2]

The modern generation of bonded porcelain restorations was first described in 1983.[59] When it became clear that the technique had merit in anterior applications, interest developed in the use of bonded porcelain for posterior applications. In 1986, Redford and Jensen[60] described the strengthening effect of porcelain inlays on the fracture resistance of natural teeth. In 1988, Jensen[61] reported excellent clinical success in a 2-year in vivo study. The technique has since been refined to the point that porcelain inlays and onlays are now an accepted operative modality.

Direct Resin Inlay Technique

Fabrication

1. Select a shade prior to tooth dehydration.
2. Place the rubber dam to isolate the tooth to be restored.
3. Remove the existing restoration and/or carious tooth structure and make a preparation with 8 to 10 degrees of occlusal divergence. The preparation should be smooth, with rounded line angles and without margin bevels. Ensure that the gingival margin is on enamel; if not, choose an alternate restoration.
4. Coat the preparation with a thin layer of water-soluble lubricant.
5. Place the matrix band and wedge it.
6. Bulk load resin composite into the preparation and roughly form the occlusal anatomy.
7. Light cure for 40 seconds from the occlusal and proximal aspects.
8. Remove the wedge(s) and matrix band.
9. Remove the resin composite inlay with a spoon excavator or carver. If there are undercuts in the preparation or the composite bonds to the tooth, the inlay will have to be cut out and redone.
10. Postcure the inlay.

Placement

11. Return the inlay to the preparation and check interproximal contacts. Because of polymerization shrinkage, a three-surface inlay may not seat completely. When this occurs, lightly reduce the inner (axial) surfaces of both proximal boxes with a microfine diamond. Try the inlay in again, and repeat the process until the inlay seats completely. If interproximal contacts are open, roughen the surface, place a thin layer of unfilled resin, place a thin layer of resin composite, light cure, and readjust the contact(s).
12. Air abrade the inner surface of the inlay with 50-μm alumina.
13. Place silane on the intaglio surface of the restoration only and air dry.
14. Place a Tofflemire matrix on the prepared tooth to ensure that the etchant is not in contact with adjacent teeth.
15. Etch the preparation with 30% to 40% phosphoric acid etchant gel for 15 to 20 seconds, wash for 5 seconds, and air dry to ensure adequate enamel etch.
16. Remoisten the dentin and place several coats of dentin primer on damp dentin. Air dry the primer, gently at first, until the surface is completely dry, and confirm a uniform shiny surface.
17. Remove the Tofflemire matrix.
18. Mix and place a dual-cure adhesive, which is not light cured before restoration placement, on the walls of the preparation and on the inner surface of the restoration.
19. Mix dual-cure resin composite luting cement and place into the preparation and inner surface of the restoration with a syringe.
20. Gently place the restoration into the preparation and vibrate with a hand instrument to ensure that it is almost fully seated.
21. Remove excess composite luting cement with a brush both occlusally and interproximally.
22. Gently seat the restoration completely with an instrument on the occlusal surface, making sure that a bead of composite luting cement is expressed at all margins; confirm correct seating with an explorer at the margins.
23. While the assistant is holding the restoration in place, gently clean the interproximal margins with floss, an explorer, and a No. 12 scalpel blade, being careful not to cause bleeding. The interproximal margins must be completely finished before the resin composite luting cement polymerizes. Leave excess composite on the facial and lingual margins.
24. Cover all accessible interproximal margins with glycerin.
25. Complete polymerization by light curing for 90 seconds from the occlusal aspect and 30 seconds each from the facial and lingual aspects in interproximal areas.

Finishing

26. Finish all margins with 12-fluted carbide burs, finishing disks, and/or composite polishing points.
27. Remove the rubber dam and adjust the occlusion with articulating paper and a fine diamond (gross adjustment) and a 12-fluted, egg-shaped carbide bur (fine adjustment).
28. Complete polishing with composite polishing points and aluminum oxide polishing paste.
29. Etch with 30% to 40% phosphoric acid for 5 seconds, rinse, dry, apply rebonding (surface-sealing) resin, and polymerize.

Indications

The indications for posterior bonded porcelain restorations overlap those for direct and indirect posterior resin composite restorations, which have already been described. These restorations are indicated when there is an overriding desire for esthetics and all margins can be placed on enamel. Some clinicians recommend bonded porcelain rather than resin composite for larger restorations.[2]

Ceramic Inlay vs Resin Composite Inlay

Ceramic inlays are reported to leak less than resin composite inlays.[62–64] The marginal fidelity depends on technique and is laboratory dependent.[62] One laboratory study demonstrated better marginal fidelity with ceramic inlays,[64] while another study found better fit with resin inlays.[65] Pressed ceramic inlays have been shown to have an average marginal gap of less than 50 μm.[66] As previously described, adhesion of luting resin is more reliable and durable to etched porcelain material than to prepolymerized resin composite.

The main advantage of resin composite inlays is that they tend to be more user-friendly, both clinically and in the dental laboratory. The resin inlay can be placed into the preparation with moderate pressure to ensure complete seating without the fear of fracture. Also, if the interproximal contact is removed during the process of adjustment, it can easily be replaced with the addition of light-cured resin composite.

In contrast, the porcelain inlay is quite fragile and subject to fracture during the try-in phase. If the interproximal contact is inadvertently removed during adjustment, it can be replaced by the time-consuming procedure of adding low-fusing porcelain and refiring the inlay in a porcelain furnace.[67] Once it is removed from the porcelain furnace, the inlay must be re-etched with hydrofluoric acid. Alternatively, the contact can be replaced with resin composite after the proximal porcelain surface is etched with hydrofluoric acid and silanated.

One in vivo study[68] compared the clinical success of these two treatment modalities at 3 years and found that Class 2 ceramic inlays had a significantly higher breakage rate than indirect resin composite inlays. This finding was corroborated in a laboratory study[69] that found lower fracture resistance of porcelain inlays compared to resin inlays. Based on the limited data available, resin composite should be considered first for use in two- and three-surface inlay preparations of moderate width in premolar teeth.

Porcelain Onlay vs Resin Composite Onlay

The porcelain onlay has the same disadvantages as the porcelain inlay. Although some ceramic materials cause wear of opposing enamel,[70] they also provide long-term occlusal stability, which resin composite may not provide in a cuspal-coverage restoration.[71] The stronger bond of resin cement to porcelain is particularly important when cusps are covered. The stronger the bond, the more efficiently forces are transferred through the restoration and the cement and absorbed into the tooth.[14] For these reasons, when even one cusp of a posterior tooth is being covered with an esthetic bonded onlay, the porcelain onlay is preferred.

Porcelain onlays may be used routinely for the esthetic restoration of premolars. They may also be used as cuspal-coverage restorations for molars, although the occlusal forces will be greater in the molar region. Another indication for the porcelain onlay is in the restoration of a molar with a short occlusogingival dimension. In this circumstance, it is difficult to gain axial retention and resistance with a conventional crown preparation. However, the porcelain onlay preparation requires only 2 mm of occlusal reduction and no axial reduction for retention and resistance. The short molar, which would have previously required crown-lengthening surgery before placement of a complete-coverage crown, can now be restored more conservatively with the porcelain onlay.

Selection of appropriate patients is of paramount importance in the placement of posterior bonded porcelain restorations. For the greatest long-term predictable success, all margins should be on enamel. Also, the patient and the tooth to be restored should be amenable to rubber dam placement. Ideally, the patient should exhibit no signs of a parafunctional habit. In addition, the restoration should be fabricated so that it contacts in maximum intercuspation position of the mandible but has no contact on the porcelain in mandibular excursive movements.

Shade Selection

The shade used for a porcelain inlay or onlay is selected in the same way as for a metal-ceramic crown. Because of the thickness of the occlusal porcelain, the underlying tooth color and cement shade have a minimal effect on the shade of the final restoration except at the margins. As with porcelain veneers, use of a translucent resin cement is recommended to improve the esthetic blend at the margins.

Fabrication

The most common method of fabrication of porcelain inlays and onlays utilizes a refractory die. After a master die is poured in die stone, a refractory die is made by duplicating the master die or repouring the impression in a refractory material. The porcelain is baked on the refractory die, recovered, and fit to the master die. Variations in the fit of ceramic inlays and onlays are reported to be related more to the ability of the technician than to the type of ceramic material used.[62]

The newer generation of pressed ceramics is fabricated much differently. The restoration is waxed on a stone die in the traditional manner and invested in a special investment. The invested wax pattern is burned out as in the traditional lost-wax technique. An ingot of the pressed-ceramic material is heated and pressed into the lost-wax pattern space. After cooling, the investment is removed and the ceramic restoration is retrieved and finished in the same manner as a feldspathic porcelain restoration.

Porcelain Onlay Technique

Tooth Preparation

1. Select a shade prior to tooth dehydration.
2. Make a stent for fabrication of a provisional restoration.
3. Remove the existing restoration.
4. Ensure that the gingival margins are on enamel and that the tooth can be isolated with a rubber dam; if not, choose an alternate restoration.
5. After completion of the preparation, there should be room for at least a 2-mm thickness of porcelain. All internal line angles should be rounded and walls divergent occlusally. There should be no grooves or sharp angles.
6. Make an impression, using retraction cord if required.
7. Make a custom provisional restoration using the stent. Place undercuts in the intaglio surface of the provisional restoration.
8. Cement with a strong provisional cement; because the preparation has minimal resistance form, polycarboxylate cement is the cement of choice for luting the provisional restoration.

Restoration Placement

9. Check the restoration on the die for fit, and check for fracture lines with transillumination.
10. Place the rubber dam.
11. Remove the provisional restoration and clean cement from the preparation with an ultrasonic scaler or a slow-speed diamond and pumice with a brush.
12. Try in the porcelain restoration; adjust interproximal contacts with coarse Sof-Lex disks (3M), and polish with porcelain polishing points.
13. Clean the onlay with acetone and air dry.
14. Place silane on the etched internal surface of the onlay and air dry.
15. Place a Tofflemire matrix on the prepared tooth to ensure that the etchant does not contact adjacent teeth.
16. Etch the tooth with 30% to 40% phosphoric acid etchant gel for 20 seconds, wash for 5 seconds, and air dry to ensure adequate enamel etch.
17. Remoisten dentin and place several coats of dentin primer on damp dentin. Air dry the primer, gently at first, until the surface is completely dry, and confirm a uniform shiny surface.
18. Remove the Tofflemire matrix.
19. Mix and place a dual-cure adhesive, which should not be light cured before placement of the restoration; similarly, dual-cure adhesive must be placed on the inner surface of the restoration.
20. Mix dual-cure resin composite luting cement and place into the preparation and the inner surface of the restoration with a syringe.
21. Gently place the restoration into the preparation and vibrate with a hand instrument to ensure that it is almost fully seated.
22. Remove excess resin composite luting cement with a brush both occlusally and interproximally.
23. Gently seat the restoration completely with an instrument applied to the occlusal surface, making sure that a bead of composite is expressed at all margins. Confirm correct seating with an explorer at the margins.
24. While the assistant holds the restoration in place, gently clean interproximal margins with floss, an explorer, and a No. 12 blade, being careful not to cause bleeding. The interproximal margins must be completely finished before the resin composite polymerizes. Leave excess composite luting cement on facial and lingual margins.
25. Cover all accessible interproximal margins with glycerin.
26. Complete polymerization by light curing for 90 seconds from the occlusal aspect and 30 seconds each from the facial and lingual aspects in interproximal areas.

Finishing

27. Finish all margins with 12-fluted carbide burs or microfine diamonds, finishing disks, and/or composite polishing points.
28. Remove the rubber dam and adjust the occlusion with articulating paper and a microfine diamond.
29. Complete polishing with rubber porcelain polishing points.

Isolation

It is universally acknowledged that strict isolation is necessary for bonding posterior adhesive restorations. This is best accomplished with a well-placed rubber dam. If it is not possible to isolate the tooth with a rubber dam, an adhesive restoration should not be placed (see the Porcelain Onlay Technique box).

Resin Composite vs Porcelain

Wear

There are significant differences in the wear characteristics of resin composite and porcelain. Wear is not a significant factor in a porcelain restoration,[2] but traditional feldspathic porcelain is highly abrasive and can cause significant wear of the opposing dentition. A newer generation of low-fusing porcelains has been shown to cause significantly less wear of enamel than traditional feldspathic porcelain.[72,73] The new class of pressable ceramics, described previously, has become popular, in part because they are less abrasive to opposing teeth. These include Empress (Ivoclar Vivadent), Empress 2 (Ivoclar Vivadent), Optimal Pressed Ceramic (OPC, Jeneric/Pentron), and Finesse All-Ceramic (Dentsply). The first generation of Empress showed decreased wear of opposing enamel compared to traditional and low-fusing porcelains in vitro.[74] However, the newer generation, Empress 2, has shown almost no wear of opposing enamel, both in vitro[73] and in vivo at 6 months.[75] If long-term clinical studies confirm the low wear of opposing enamel, this will be a significant advance in ceramics.

The data concerning wear of resin composite materials have been somewhat contradictory.[76–78] Enamel is reported to wear at a rate of 30 μm/y in molars and 15 μm/y in premolars.[79] Most modern resin composite materials fall within that range.[54,78] Ferracane[54] reported that the wear of the traditional resin composite, Charisma, was lower than that of the ceromer, Artglass. Similarly, Reich et al[55] evaluated the wear of Artglass, Targis, and a traditional resin composite, Z100. Although Targis demonstrated superior physical properties, Z100 had the highest wear resistance. In another laboratory study,[80] the wear of three commercially available ceromer materials was compared to a cast-gold control. Targis demonstrated the greatest wear, followed by Artglass; Skulptur FibreKor (Jeneric/Pentron) demonstrated the least wear, which was approximately equal to that of gold. Similarly, the wear rates for Artglass and Targis were evaluated in a two-body wear test.[81] Targis demonstrated wear similar to that of enamel, and Artglass had significantly higher wear than enamel. Another laboratory study[82] reported that the wear resistance of indirect resin composites is similar to that of gold but is significantly more abrasive to antagonistic enamel.

Longevity

Results of short-term clinical studies of resin inlays are encouraging, but there is little long-term data. Bishop[83] reported one failure out of 92 resin inlays that had been in place for 7 months to 4 years. A Swedish study[84] reported that 29 of 30 resin inlays were excellent or acceptable at 17 months, while another study[85] reported good marginal integrity at 5 years. One American study[86] reported no failures among 60 resin inlays after 3 years, while another American study[68] reported that 10 of 145 resin inlays failed at 3 years. Another prospective clinical study[87] evaluated 64 indirect resin inlays/onlays over a period of 48 to 75 months with a mean time of 59

months. They reported three failures (5%) due to fractures (two) and caries (one). However, 18 of 64 restorations were rated as less than optimal, mostly due to the absence of interproximal contacts.

It is still not clear whether the resin inlay offers any advantages in terms of longevity over the direct-placement resin composite restoration. Two clinical studies reported no significant differences between resin inlays and direct resin composite restorations at 5 years[49] and at 11 years.[50]

There has been little clinical research on the longevity of the newer-generation ceromer restorations. One clinical study[88] of an experimental ceromer, now marketed as belleGlass (Kerr), reported 5-year results for 24 inlays and onlays. All restorations were performing satisfactorily, although 12% had interfacial staining and 58% had slight to moderate marginal degradation. Another clinical study[89] evaluated 99 ceromer inlays over a period of 6 to 53 months and reported a success rate of 98%.

Several clinical studies have evaluated the performance of ceramic inlays or onlays. The clinical success of traditional feldspathic inlays has been mixed. A 6-year retrospective study[90] reported a 25.8% failure rate among feldspathic porcelain onlays with and without metal reinforcement. One 4-year study[91] reported no failures in 50 inlays. Another study reported a 95% success rate with a mean evaluation period of 5.9 years.[92] Other clinical studies, however, have shown significantly higher failure rates. One study[93] reported that 21 of 145 inlays fractured at 3 years, while another study[94] reported 16% failure at 3 years. Still another study[95] reported a 20% failure rate at 8 years, while a similar study[96] reported an 84% success rate with a mean observation time of 6.3 years. If these high failure rates are confirmed by other clinical studies, the utility of the feldspathic porcelain inlay and onlay must be questioned.

Clinical results with the leucite-reinforced pressed ceramic restorations have been more promising. Several clinical studies[97–100] have shown excellent clinical success up to 7 years. However, a randomized 5-year clinical evaluation[101] of three ceramic inlay systems and gold inlays reported less promising results: 20% of the leucite-reinforced ceramic inlays failed, and 70% of all of the ceramic inlay systems demonstrated marginal ditching, while there were no failures among the gold inlays.

Failures

Two types of failure are most common with esthetic inlays and onlays: bulk fracture (see Fig 18-3) and marginal breakdown (Fig 18-9). Bulk fracture sometimes occurs in areas of cuspal coverage, particularly if the restorative material is less

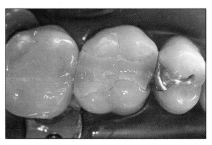

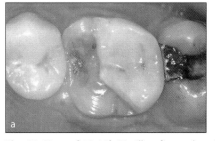

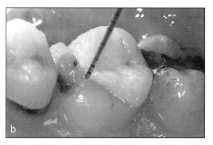

Fig 18-9 Maxillary first molar with a 7-year-old bonded Dicor (Dentsply) inlay demonstrating marginal ditching and a small fracture of the marginal ridge.

Figs 18-10a and 18-10b Maxillary first molar with 5-year-old bonded feldspathic porcelain onlay demonstrating bulk fracture.

than 2.0 mm thick (Fig 18-10a and 8-10b). It also occurs at the isthmus adjacent to a marginal ridge, where the porcelain is poorly supported by tooth structure.

Marginal ditching is a common finding in esthetic inlays and onlays.[88,101–104] Because resin cements tend not to be heavily filled, they wear more quickly than the adjacent restorations or tooth structure. This is particularly true if the marginal fit is poor.[105,106] Kawai and others[107] demonstrated a linear relationship between wear of resin cement and the horizontal marginal gap. They concluded that reduction of the marginal gap is an important clinical consideration in minimizing the wear of the resin cement. They also found hybrid resin cements to wear faster than microfilled resin cements. Isenberg and others[108] reported 3-year results of a clinical study of 121 CEREC inlay and onlay restorations. None of the restorations exhibited any evidence of interfacial staining, discoloration, or caries, but about 50% of the restorations exhibited gap dimensions large enough to be detected with an explorer. The rate of wear of the resin composite luting agent was linear over the first year, but no further vertical wear was noted over the course of the investigation. The depth-width ratio of the gap generally did not exceed 50%. However, Hayashi and others[109] recently reported results of an 8-year clinical study that evaluated marginal wear using an optical laser scanner. They found that marginal deterioration occurred in a sequential three-stage pattern. The initial stage of marginal deterioration occurred rapidly from initial placement to 21 months. In the second stage, the level of deterioration leveled off and progressed at a much slower rate. This stage ranged from 21 months to 72 months. During the third stage, the marginal deterioration again accelerated to a much faster rate during the sixth to the eighth year. If this data is confirmed in other clinical studies, indications for ceramic inlays may have to be reevaluated.

CAD/CAM Ceramic Restorations

CAD/CAM technology for the fabrication of ceramic restorations has been a significant development in dentistry. The vast majority of CAD/CAM systems have been designed for use in the dental laboratory. InLab (Sirona Dental), Procera (Nobel Biocare), LAVA (3M ESPE), and Cercon (Dentsply/Caulk) are but a few of the CAD/CAM systems dental laboratories are using in an effort to improve efficiency while utilizing modern ceramic materials.

The CEREC (CEramic REConstruction) system represents a unique CAD/CAM system that is used by dentists for chairside fabrication and delivery of ceramic restorations. It was developed by Dr Werner Mörmann, a dentist, and Marco Brandestini, an engineer, in 1980. Siemans initially marketed the CEREC 1 system in Europe in 1985, and the first clinical trials took place in 1987.[110] It was introduced in the United States in 1989. Since then, the system has evolved through a series of hardware and software upgrades to reach its present form, the CEREC 3D system.

The CEREC system allows the dentist to provide esthetic restorations in a single appointment.[111,112] The cavity preparation for an inlay, onlay, crown, or veneer is recorded to the computer using an optical imaging procedure via a camera. The 3D computer software program creates a three-dimensional virtual model of the preparation on which the restoration is designed. Once the restoration design is completed, the software program interprets the design data to direct-cutting diamonds to mill the final restoration from a prefabricated blank of restorative material. The final restoration is adhesively cemented to the tooth to complete the treatment.[110,113,114] This system offers a considerable time savings over conventional, laboratory-generated restorations that require multiple appointments.

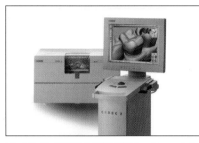

Fig 18-11 CEREC 3 CAD/CAM unit consisting of the acquisition unit and milling chamber.

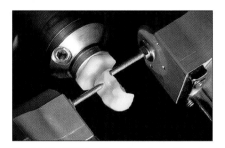

Fig 18-12 CEREC milling chamber with cylindrical diamond and tapered diamond.

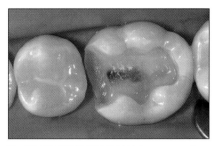

Fig 18-13 CEREC CAD/CAM inlay preparation.

Hardware and Software

The CEREC CAD/CAM system consists of an acquisition unit and a milling chamber or unit (Fig 18-11). The acquisition unit contains a computer with the three-dimensional design software, a liquid crystal display (LCD) monitor, and an intraoral camera for the optical imaging of the cavity preparation. The milling unit houses two motors. Each motor controls a cutting diamond for milling the final restoration from prefabricated blocks of restorative material (Fig 18-12). One motor has a cylindrical diamond that mills the entire internal surface of the restoration. It is available in 1.2- and 1.6-mm diameters. The other motor has a milling diamond that has a tapered cone shape and mills the entire external surface of the restoration. The milling unit also contains a water chamber for distilled water and lubricant additive that is used during the milling procedure to clean and lubricate the diamonds as they mill the restorative material. The acquisition and milling units communicate with each other via a radio transmitter.

The CEREC 3 camera has been redesigned with a detachable, protective cover that can be dry-heat sterilized. An additional hygienic feature is that the computer trackball used for computer graphic design can be removed and disinfected. The CEREC 3 monitor has been expanded in size and displays the tooth with 12 times magnification, compared to the CEREC 2 unit, which displayed the tooth at an 8 times magnification.

The introduction of the R1800 program by Sirona realized the goal of a three-dimensional CAD program for all single-tooth restorations. The capability to use a diagnostic waxup or pretreatment model to copy the desired contour and anatomy in the design of a new anterior or posterior crown has been a staple of the CEREC technique. The newly developed anterior veneer options provide the capability to replicate contralateral tooth contour to a veneer design. This significantly enhances the ability to replicate a patient's existing tooth contours with veneers.

Inlays/Onlays

How well the milled restoration fits depends, to a great extent, on the tooth preparation. Cavity preparations for CAD/CAM inlays and onlays are similar to those for conventional indirect ceramic inlays and onlays.[115,116] (Fig 18-13). The occlusal aspect of the preparation should be at least 2 mm deep to provide adequate strength for the ceramic restoration. All cavosurface margins should be well defined and have a 90-degree butt-joint configuration. This will allow the camera to record an accurate image of the cavosurface margin while providing strength to the restoration. Bevels and chamfer-style margins should not be used. The cavity walls of the proximal box should have at least 4 degrees of divergent taper.[117,118] All preparation floors should be smooth, but not necessarily flat. Concavities created by the removal of carious tooth structure or prior restorations may be blocked out with a liner or base, but this is not required to obtain an accurate fit of the restoration.

Veneers

Preparation designs for veneers are similar to those for other ceramic veneers, with the exception that the path of insertion of the veneer must be visible from the facial aspect of the tooth. Should an incisal- or proximal-wrap design be used, the angle of view of the camera must be from the incisal, and this requires the use of the crown program rather than the veneer program. This may lead to increased design editing and time to create the desired contours.

Figs 18-14a to 18-14d CEREC endo-crown. *(a)* Preparation facial view; *(b)* preparation occlusal view; *(c)* milled crown; *(d)* crown after adhesive cementation and adjustment. (Courtesy of Dr M. Shapiro.)

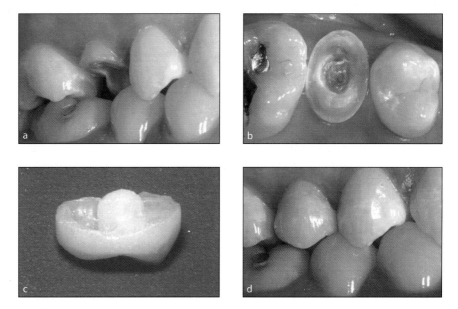

Crowns

The tooth preparation is the same as described for other all-ceramic crowns. There must be at least 2 mm of occlusal clearance and at least 1.2 mm of axial reduction. The computer graphic-design process is similar to that used for fabrication of an onlay; the milling process is somewhat longer. Many clinicians choose to characterize the monochromatic shade of the porcelain blocks with shade modifiers and a glaze prior to adhesive cementation.[117]

An additional preparation design has been suggested for CEREC crowns: the endodontic crown design. This design incorporates the core and short post into the crown as a single restoration (Figs 18-14a to 18-14d). This design significantly increases the surface area of the preparation available for adhesive cementation. It is particularly useful in teeth with short clinical crowns. This restoration has not been well evaluated clinically; however, preliminary reports from the University of Zurich, Switzerland, indicate that the cross-section area of the tooth may be a factor in retention and may be problematic for premolar teeth.

Computer-Aided Design

A dry field is necessary to ensure that the preparation is optically scanned with precision and accuracy. It is also critical to clearly isolate the gingival extent of the preparation from the adjacent soft tissues. For these reasons, the use of a rubber dam is essential. Following completion of the tooth preparation, an optical impression is recorded. The image is captured

by way of the intraoral camera, which reflects an infrared beam off of the surface of the tooth. Because enamel, dentin, bases, and soft tissues do not reflect the infrared beam equally well, the tooth must be coated with a uniform reflective material before imaging. The powder should also coat all adjacent structures that may be viewed in the optical scan (Fig 18-15). Several types of powder and devices are available for coating the preparation. Some manufacturers offer a titanium-dioxide powder that is applied with an aerosol spray can. A limitation of this technique is that the can must be held upright at all times to avoid the risk of spraying liquid into the powder container. A mechanical device is also marketed for applying the powder; the device is connected to an air line on the dental unit and is activated with a foot control. In addition, a liquid paint-on titanium-dioxide material is available.

The camera has a three-dimensional resolution that projects an image of the preparation on the monitor. To ensure accurate scanning of the preparation, the camera head is aligned in the long axis of the tooth, parallel to the planned path of insertion of the restoration, and an image is recorded. The image is viewed simultaneously on the video monitor. All portions of the preparation margins should be visible and distinct from adjacent structures. The camera head must be held motionless to record an accurate image without distortion of the preparation (Fig 18-16).

The design phase is initiated when the computer renders a virtual three-dimensional model of the cavity preparation from the recorded optical image (Fig 18-17). The three-dimensional capability of the software allows for the preparation model to be rotated in an infinite number of angles and

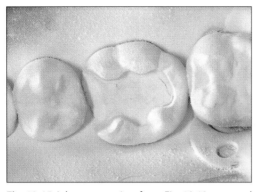

Fig 18-15 Inlay preparation from Fig 18-13 opaqued with titanium dioxide powder for the camera optical impression.

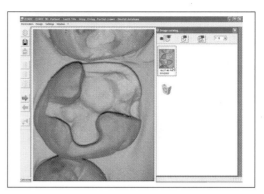

Fig 18-16 Optical impression of a powdered cavity preparation as viewed on the computer monitor.

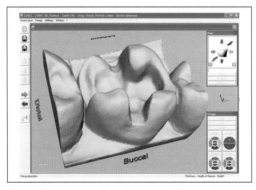

Fig 18-17 A preparation virtual model is calculated for the design of the restoration.

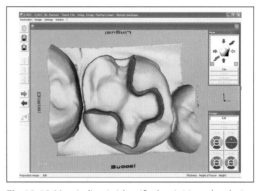

Fig 18-18 Margin line is identified to initiate the design of the restoration on the preparation virtual model.

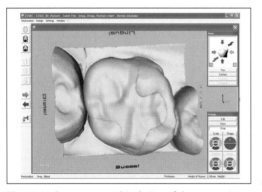

Fig 18-19 Computer graphic design of the restoration.

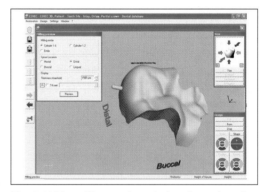

Fig 18-20 The milling preview window shows the calculated three-dimensional model of the restoration prior to milling.

views for design of the restoration. Following identification of the cavity margin by tracing the margin line (Fig 18-18), the restoration design is proposed on the monitor. A number of editing tools are available to customize the contours, anatomy, and occlusal relationship of the restoration (Fig 18-19).

Computer-Assisted Manufacture

When the milling function is activated, the software calculates a volume model of the restoration (Fig 18-20). Based on the calculated three-dimensional model of the restoration, the

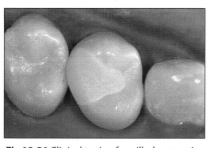

Fig 18-21 Clinical try-in of a milled restoration reveals an accurate margin adaptation. No try-in medium has been used, leading to the shade mismatch due to a dry field.

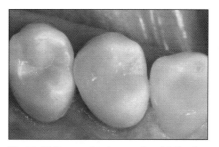

Fig 18-22 Restoration is completed following adhesive cementation and polishing.

computer then requests that the appropriately sized ceramic block be inserted in the milling chamber.

A number of ceramic materials are available for use in CEREC restorations.[119] To be used in the CEREC milling chamber, the restorative material is fabricated in a block form and mounted on a milling stub that can be inserted into the milling chamber. Vita Mark II blocks (Vident) are of a fine-grained, feldspathic porcelain that has a homogeneous structure. The fine grain of the Vita Mark II porcelain is reported to increase hardness of the material but decrease wear of the opposing dentition.[120] The material comes in nine Vita 3D master shades, as well as a bleach shade and an esthetic translucent line of shades. The Triluxe block, a tricolor block that simulates the variation in shade from cervical to incisal in a natural tooth, has also been introduced. Improvements in the software allow for restoration designs to be properly positioned within the tricolor block prior to milling. Al-Hiyasat and coworkers[121] reported that Vita Mark II ceramic material was less abrasive and more resistant to wear than conventional aluminous and bonded-ceramic materials.

ProCAD (Ivoclar Vivadent) was introduced in 1998 and is a leucite-reinforced ceramic similar to Empress 1 but with a finer particle size. The excellent clinical success with Empress 1 restorations is expected to be duplicated with the ProCAD material, as they are essentially the same restorations with different fabrication techniques. Both Vita Mark II and ProCAD materials can be characterized and glazed using stains applied chairside and a porcelain oven.

An innovative resin composite material that has been introduced for use with the CEREC system, Paradigm (3M ESPE) is a resin composite with the filler composed of zirconia silica.[122] The inorganic filler loading is 85% by weight, with an average particle size of 0.6 µm, and is radiopaque. A recent study has reported a randomized, longitudinal clinical trial comparing Paradigm inlays to Vita Mark II inlays over 3 years of clinical service.[123] The inlays were evaluated using modified US Public Health Service criteria on a yearly basis. The study determined that Paradigm inlays performed equally as well as Vita Mark II inlays at 3 years, with clinical advantages noted in inlay fracture resistance and color match.

Once the ceramic block has been locked in the milling chamber, the unit is ready to mill the restoration. The milling diamonds move in coordination with the movement of the metallic mounting of the ceramic block, which calibrates the position of the milling head. The ceramic block, rotating as it goes, is fed uniformly through the milling process. Milling time is a function of the size and complexity of the restoration and may range from 10 to 20 minutes on average.

Try-in and Cementation

Once the ceramic restoration is recovered from the milling chamber, the inlay is tried in (Fig 18-21). Adjustments to the proximal contacts may have to be made for the restoration to seat completely. The axiopulpal line angle and the gingival floor of the box are the places most likely to require adjustment.[124] Should the fit be unacceptable in some area, the design can be reloaded from the program disk and corrected, and a second restoration can be milled quickly.

The ceramic restoration should be etched and silanated prior to adhesive cementation. Use of a conventional adhesive cementation technique and a dual-cured resin cement is recommended. Contouring and refinement of anatomy can be accomplished after cementation with various microfine diamonds.[125] Finishing and polishing are completed with abrasive rubber points, disks, and cups or brushes with diamond polishing paste as for other ceramic restorations (Fig 18-22).

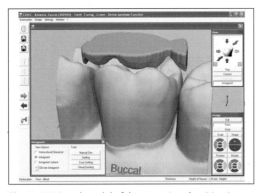

Fig 18-23 Virtual model of the opposing dentition is projected over the restoration design to evaluate the potential occlusal contacts.

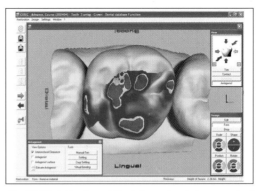

Fig 18-24 Activation of the interocclusal clearance tool indicates the location, size, and intensity of contact with opposing dentition.

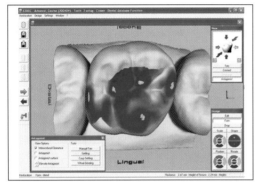

Fig 18-25 The application of editing tools has allowed for the refinement of the occlusal contacts in the restoration design prior to milling.

Advantages and Disadvantages

The main advantages of CAD/CAM technology are time savings, service to the patient, and utilization of optimal restorative material. The technique affords a dentist the opportunity to prepare, design, and fabricate a ceramic restoration in a single appointment, without the need for conventional impressions, provisional restorations, or dental laboratory support.

CAD/CAM technology offers excellent esthetics, durability, and at least short-term strengthening of the tooth. Roznowski et al[126] compared the fracture resistance of molars restored with various adhesive and nonadhesive restorations and reported that teeth restored with mesio-occlusodistal CEREC inlays were as strong as unprepared, unrestored teeth, while nonadhesive restorations weakened teeth.

The CAD/CAM systems are not without their disadvantages. Because the restoration is fabricated without the benefit of a die or articulated casts, development of occlusal relationships may be problematic. The software has several design options to overcome this apparent limitation. The correlation technique provides the opportunity to record the pretreatment occlusal anatomy, or that of a diagnostic waxup,

and copy it to the occlusal surface of the new restoration design. The existing occlusal relationships can be maintained in the new restoration. An alternative technique involves the use of the antagonist tool. A bite registration can be used to record the occlusal surface of the opposing dentition. The surface data is recorded to the software and superimposed over the design of the new restoration (Fig 18-23). This provides a degree of control in evaluating and developing occlusal relationships in the new restoration. It is not a "virtual articulator" in that it is a static recording and does not record interocclusal relationships in excursive mandibular movements. However, interocclusal relationships in maximum intercuspation position (centric occlusion) of the mandible can be determined and refined prior to milling (Figs 18-24 and 18-25). The milled restoration will require some adjustment after bonding to ensure absence of interferences in excursive mandibular movements.

A significant training period is required to achieve proficiency with the system. Participation in a 2-day initial training course is usually recommended, followed by laboratory practice on an additional 20 to 25 restorations. The initial cost of the system is also considerable; however, it is balanced against the minimal per-restoration cost of using the system as compared to laboratory-fabricated ceramic restorations. Generally, the actual cost of the CEREC restoration to the dentist is about 10% to 15% of the cost of a laboratory-fabricated ceramic restoration.

A major concern about CAD/CAM restorations has been their precementation marginal fit. Several studies have evaluated marginal openings in CAD/CAM restorations. Krejci and others[127] reported precementation marginal openings with CEREC 1 restorations to be in the range of 125 to 175 μm. However, after cementation, they found that more than 90% of enamel-ceramic interfaces had "continuous margins." They found that the quality of the marginal adaptation immediately after cementation does not seem to depend on precementation marginal fit.[127] Peters and Bieniek[128] reported results of a clinical study of 22 CEREC 1 inlays in which the average marginal fit was 121 μm with a range of 60 to 150 μm. Wilder[124] reported the average film thickness of resin cement at the occlusal cavosurface margin with CEREC 1 to be 89 ± 65 μm; the average thickness at the gingival margin was 105 ± 81 μm. By comparison, Christensen[129] reported that gold castings can be fabricated with marginal openings of less than 25 μm. Because of the relatively large precementation marginal gaps, the exposed resin cement was thought to be the weak link in the CEREC 1 restoration.

CEREC system hardware and software improvements have led to improvements in adaptation and marginal fit. Mörmann and Schug[130] evaluated the marginal fit of CAD/CAM inlays fabricated with the improved CEREC 2 unit using the COS 4.01 software program. They reported the overall mean interfacial margin width to be 56 ± 27 μm for CEREC 2 inlays and 84 ± 38 μm for CEREC 1 inlays. They also reported that the milling precision of the CEREC 2 unit was 2.4 times greater than that of the CEREC 1 unit. Benz and coworkers[131] also reported a mean occlusal interfacial width for CEREC 2 inlays of 48 ± 34 μm, a 35% improvement over the CEREC 1 inlays.

Ellingsen and Fasbinder[132] reported a study comparing the precementation fit of CEREC 2 crowns to CEREC 3 crowns. All areas of crown adaptation measured were significantly smaller for the CEREC 3 system compared to the CEREC 2 system except at the axial walls of the preparation. Cavosurface margin gaps of 47.5 ± 19.5 μm were reported for CEREC 3 crowns, and gaps of 97.0 ± 33.8 μm were reported for CEREC 2 crowns. The fit of CEREC 3 crowns is very nearly on par with that of gold castings.

Postoperative sensitivity following adhesive restorative procedures is not an uncommon problem. Although there are a number of reports documenting postoperative sensitivity for direct or indirect adhesive restorations, few of them deal directly with CEREC restorations. Sjogren and coworkers[133]

reported that 10 of 72 patients had postoperative sensitivity with Vita Mark I or II ceramic inlays. However, Heymann and colleagues[134] reported no postoperative sensitivity at any recall interval in their 4-year clinical trial of CEREC ceramic inlays. Fasbinder and coworkers[135] reported that 13% of 92 Vita Mark II onlays were rated slightly sensitive at 1 week and 4% at 2 weeks. All sensitivity was resolved by 1 month, and there was essentially no postoperative sensitivity throughout the remainder of the study. The CAD/CAM technique may play a role in minimizing postoperative sensitivity. The ability to deliver the restorations in a single appointment prevents the potential for dentin contamination during the temporization phase. Also, the use of manufactured blocks of porcelain and resin composite significantly restrict the influence of polymerization shrinkage since it is limited to the thickness of the resin cement.

Longevity/Clinical Studies

The failure rate of Vita Mark II porcelain inlays made with the CEREC technique has been reported to be very low. Sjogren and coworkers[136] reported four fractures among 66 Vita Mark II inlays over 5 years. Palleson and van Dijken[137] reported a single fractured Vita Mark II inlay among 16 pairs of CAD/CAM inlays over 8 years. Berg and Derand[138] reported 3 fractures among 115 Vita Mark II inlays over 5 years. Martin and Jedynakiewicz[139] performed a systematic review of clinical studies on intracoronal CEREC restorations. They reported a mean survival rate of 97.4% over a 4-year period. The primary reasons for failure were reported as fracture of the ceramic material, fracture of the supporting tooth, and postoperative sensitivity. Fracture of the ceramic material was generally a result of occlusal stress or insufficient material thickness. Otto and De Nisco[140] reported an 8% failure rate for ceramic inlays after 10 years of clinical service. Of the failures, 53% were caused by fractures of the ceramic material and 20% were due to tooth fracture. Hickel and Manhart[141] reviewed clinical studies in the dental literature during the 1990s and reported annual failure rates of posterior restorations in stress-bearing areas as 0% to 11.8% for laboratory-fabricated resin composite inlays, 0% to 7.5% for laboratory-fabricated ceramic inlays, and 0% to 4.4% for CAD/CAM ceramic restorations. They also reported bulk fracture as a frequent cause of failure for ceramic inlays.

The majority of clinical studies on CEREC restorations have been completed using the CEREC 1 and CEREC 2 units. The CEREC 3 unit was introduced in 2000, and results of long-term clinical studies are not yet available. However, a good clinical record has been established for CEREC restorations. Zuellig-Singer and Bryant[142] reported results of a 3-year clinical evaluation of CEREC inlays with four different luting agents. They reported one inlay fracture and that 94.6% of the restorations had continuous margins at 3 years. There was no significant difference in continuous-margin rates among the four luting materials. The authors also reported less wear with the microfilled luting resin as compared to that of the hybrid-composite and glass-ionomer luting materials. Heymann and coworkers,[134] in the previously mentioned clinical study of CEREC 1 inlays, reported no significant changes in the 50 CEREC inlays after 4 years of clinical service. There was no reported postoperative sensitivity, and there were no restoration fractures. Sjogren and coworkers[143] reported a 10-year clinical evaluation of 66 CEREC inlays. They reported an 11% failure rate after 10 years, with four inlay fractures, one tooth fracture, one restored tooth requiring endodontic treatment, and one inlay replaced due to postoperative symptoms. The survival rate at 10 years was estimated at 89%. They reported a significantly improved survival rate for CAD/CAM-fabricated inlays cemented with a chemically cured resin composite cement as compared to those cemented with a dual-cured resin cement. Otto and De Nisco[144] reported a 10-year prospective study of 200 CEREC 1 inlays and onlays. The primary failure mechanisms of the 15 failed restorations included restoration fracture (eight cases) and tooth fracture (three cases). Only three of the teeth that had failed restorations required crowns; the remaining restorations were repaired or the initial restoration replaced with another CEREC inlay or onlay. The Kaplan-Meier survival rate was 90.4% at 10 years.

Bindl and Mörmann[145] reported a study comparing CEREC crowns to reinforced ceramic-core crowns. Thirty-six anterior crowns in 24 patients were placed using equal numbers of CEREC crowns and In-Ceram Spinell crowns. The crowns were evaluated over a mean service time of 44.9 ± 10.3 months using modified US Public Health Service criteria. No significant difference in clinical performance between the two types of ceramic crowns was reported. Based on the studies cited above, the performance of the current generation of CEREC-fabricated restorations is expected to be excellent, and the use of this technology is predicted to grow steadily.

References

1. Banks RG. Conservative posterior ceramic restorations: A literature review. J Prosthet Dent 1990;63:619–626.
2. Burke FJT, Qualtrough AJE. Aesthetic inlays: Composite or ceramic? Br Dent J 1994;176:53–60.
3. Qualtrough AJ, Cramer A, Wilson NH, Roulet JF, Noack M. An in vitro evaluation of the marginal integrity of a porcelain inlay system. Int J Prosthodont 1991;4:517–523.
4. Wilson NHF, Wilson MA, Wastell DG, Smith GA. Performance of Occlusin in butt-joint and bevel-edged preparations: Five-year results. Dent Mater 1991;7:92–98.
5. Inokoshi S, Iwaku M, Fusayama T. Pulp response to a new adhesive restorative resin. J Dent Res 1982;61:1014–1019.
6. Nasedkin JN. Porcelain posterior resin-bonded restorations: Current perspectives on esthetic restorative dentistry. Part II. J Can Dent Assoc 1988;54:499–506.
7. Kelsey WP, Blankenau RJ, Latta MA. Resin bond strengths to dentin following placement of an adhere liner [abstract 986]. J Dent Res 1997;76:137.
8. Bocangel JS, Demarci FF, Turbino ML, et al. Influence of eugenol on the microleakage and bond strength of two bonding agents [abstract 421]. J Dent Res 1997;76:66.
9. Murdoch H, Scrabeck J, Dhuru J. The effect of eugenol on the shear bond strength of composite restorative materials [abstract 1012]. J Dent Res 1999;78:232.
10. Schwartz RS, Davis RD, Mayhew R. The effect of ZOE on the bond strength of resin to enamel. Am J Dent 1990;3:28–30.
11. Schwartz RS, Davis RD, Hilton TJ. Effect of temporary cements on the bond strength of a resin cement. Am J Dent 1992;5:147–150.
12. Sung E, Caputo A, Dail S. The effect of temporary cements on the composite resin bond strength [abstract 1320]. J Dent Res 1998;77:270.
13. Burgess JO, Haveman CW, Butzin C. Evaluation of resins for provisional restorations. Am J Dent 1992;5:137–139.
14. Derand T. Stress analysis of cemented or resin-bonded porcelain inlays. Dent Mater 1991;7:21–24.
15. Dalpino P, Francischone C, Ishikiriama A, France E. Fracture resistance of teeth directly and indirectly restored with composite resin and indirectly restored with ceramic materials. Am J Dent 2002; 15:389–394.
16. De Freitas C, Miranda M, de Andrade M, Flores V, Vaz L, Guimaraes C. Resistance to maxillary premolar fractures after restoration of Class II preparations with resin composite or ceromer. Quintessence Int 2002;33:589–594.
17. St-Georges AJ, Sturdevant JR, Swift EJ Jr, Thompson JY. Fracture resistance of prepared teeth restored with bonded inlay restorations. J Prosthet Dent 2003;89:551–557.
18. Jung H, Friedl KH, Haller A, Schmalz G. Curing efficiency of different polymerization methods through ceramic restorations. Clin Oral Investig 2001;5:156–161.
19. Ferrari M, Dagostin A, Fabianelli A. Marginal integrity of ceramic inlays luted with self-curing resin cements. Dent Mater 2003;19: 270–276.
20. Burquieres SH, Burgess JD, Ripps A. Bond strength of resin cement to the dentin varying curing modes and light intensity [abstract 2987]. J Dent Res 1999;78:479.
21. Hilton TJ, Schwartz RS, Ferracane JL. Fifth generation bonding agent application technique effects on bond strength [abstract 214]. J Dent Res 1998;77:132.
22. Bailey L, Bennett R. Two year bond results of Dicor ceramic/LA cement system [abstract 1734]. J Dent Res 1989;68:398.
23. Ozden AN, Akaltan F, Can G. Effect of surface treatments of porcelain in the shear bond strength of applied dual-cured cement. J Prosthet Dent 1994;72:85–88.
24. Thurmond JW, Barkmeler WW, Wilwerding TM. Effect of porcelain surface treatments on bond strengths of composite resin bonded to porcelain. J Prosthet Dent 1994;72:355–359.

25. Imamura GM, Reinhardt JW, Boyer DB, Swift EJ. Enhancement of resin bonding to heat-cured composite resin. Oper Dent 1996;21:249–256.

26. Lutz F. State of the art of tooth-colored restoratives. Oper Dent 1996;21:237–248.

27. Wendt SL. Microleakage and cusp fracture resistance of heat-treated resin composite inlays. Am J Dent 1991;4:10–14.

28. Latta M, Barkmeier W. Bond strength of a resin cement and a cured composite inlay material. J Prosthet Dent 1993;72:189–193.

29. Lucena-Martin C, Gonzalez-Lopez S, Navajas-Rodriguez de Mondelo JM. The effect of various surface treatments and bonding agents on the repaired strength of heat-treated composites. J Prosthet Dent 2001;86:481–488.

30. Ellakwa AE, Shortall AC, Burke FJ, Marquis PM. Effects of grit blasting and silanization on bond strengths of a resin luting cement to Belleglass HP indirect composite. Am J Dent 2003;16:53–57.

31. Tezvergil A, Lassila LV, Yli-Urpo A, Vallittu PK. Repair bond strength of restorative resin composite applied to fiber-reinforced composite substrate. Acta Odontol Scand 2004;62:51–60.

32. Hilton TJ, Schwartz RS. The effect of air thinning on dentin adhesive bond strength [abstract 243]. J Dent Res 1994;73:132.

33. Haws SM, Vargas MA, Guzman S, Cobb DS. Effect of primer application on microleakage of composite resins [abstract 403]. J Dent Res 1997;76:64.

34. Bergmann P, Noack MJ, Roulet JF. Marginal adaptation with glass ceramic inlays adhesively luted with glycerine gel. Quintessence Int 1991;22:739–744.

35. Bergeron C, Guzman S, Vargas MA. Bond strength of single-bottle adhesives: Multiple applications [abstract 213]. J Dent Res 1998;77:132.

36. Frankenberger R, Sindel J, Kramer N, Petschelt A. Dentin bond strength and marginal adaptation: Direct composite resins vs ceramic inlays. Oper Dent 1999;24:147–155.

37. Feilzer AJ, de Gee AJ, Davidson CL. Curing contraction of composites and glass ionomer cements. J Prosthet Dent 1988;59:297–300.

38. Brännström M. Infection beneath resin composite restorations: Can it be avoided? Oper Dent 1987;12:158–163.

39. Civelek A, Ersoy M, L'Hotelier E, Soyman M, Say EC. Polymerization shrinkage and microleakage in Class II cavities of various resin composites. Oper Dent 2003;28:635–641.

40. Loguercio A, Reis A, Ballester R. Polymerization shrinkage: Effects of constraint and filling technique in composite restorations. Dent Mater 2004;20:236–243.

41. van Dijken J, Horstedt P, Waern R. Directed polymerization shrinkage versus a horizontal incremental filling technique: Interfacial adaptation in vivo in Class II cavities. Am J Dent 1998;11:165–172.

42. Hasegawa EA, Boyer DB, Chan DCN. Microleakage of indirect composite inlays. Dent Mater 1989;5:388–391.

43. Robinson PB, Moore BK, Swartz ML. Comparison of micro-leakage in direct and indirect resin composite restorations in vitro. Oper Dent 1987;12:113–116.

44. Shorthall AC, Baylis RL, Baylis MA, Grundy JR. Marginal seal comparisons between resin bonded Class 2 porcelain inlays, posterior composite restorations and direct resin composite inlays. Int J Prosthodont 1989;2:217–223.

45. Kanca J. The effect of heat on the surface hardness of light-activated resin composites. Quintessence Int 1989;20:899–901.

46. Wendt SL. The effect of heat used as a secondary cure upon the physical properties of three resin composites. I. Diametral tensile strength, compressive strength and marginal dimensional stability. Quintessence Int 1987;18:265–271.

47. Wendt SL. The effect of heat used as a secondary cure upon the physical properties of three resin composites. II. Wear, hardness and color stability. Quintessence Int 1987;18:351–356.

48. Trushkowsky RD. Ceramic optimized polymer: The next generation of esthetic restorations—Part 1. Compend Cont Educ Dent 1997;18:1101–1112.

49. Wassell RW, Walls AWG, McCabe JF. Direct composite inlays versus conventional composite restorations: Five-year follow-up J Dent 2000;28:375–382.

50. Pallesen U, Qvist V. Composite resin fillings and inlays. An 11-year evaluation. Clin Oral Investig 2003;7:71–79.

51. Santos GC Jr, El-Mowafy O, Rubo JH, Santos MJ. Hardening of dual-cure resin cements and a resin cured with QTH and LED curing units. J Can Dent Assoc 2004;70:323–328.

52. Brosh T, Ferstand N, Cardash H, Baharav H. Effect of polymerization under pressure of indirect tensile mechanical properties of light-polymerized composites. J Prosthet Dent 2002;88:381–387.

53. Lyzak WA, Campbell SD, Wen Z. Flexural strength of repaired composite veneer materials for fixed prosthodontics [abstract 1333]. J Dent Res 1998;77:272.

54. Ferracane J. Evaluation of cure, properties, and wear resistance of Artglass dental composite. Am J Dent 1998;11:214–218.

55. Reich S, Sindel J, Morneburg TH. Wear of prosthetic composites dependent on mechanical matrix properties [abstract 2260]. J Dent Res 1998;77:914.

56. belleGlass Technical Data. Physical properties of indirect composite resins (reference 139AK74). Orange, CA: Kerr Laboratories, 1997.

57. Behr M, Rosentritt M, Lang R, Handel G. Flexural strength of fiber-reinforced bars after different types of loading [abstract 2305]. J Dent Res 1999;78:394.

58. Qualtrough AJE, Wilson NHF, Smith GA. The porcelain inlay: A historical review. Oper Dent 1990;15:61–70.

59. Horn HR. A new lamination: Porcelain bonded to enamel. N Y State Dent J 1983;49:401–403.

60. Redford DA, Jensen ME. Etched porcelain resin-bonded posterior restorations: Cuspal flexure, strength, and micro-leakage [abstract 1573]. J Dent Res 1986;65:334.

61. Jensen ME. A two-year clinical study of posterior etched-porcelain resin-bonded restorations. Am J Dent 1988;1:27–33.

62. Dietschi D, Maeder M, Holz J. In vitro evaluation of marginal fit and morphology of fired ceramic inlays. Quintessence Int 1992;23:271–278.

63. Karaagaclioglu L, Zaimoglu A, Akoren AC. Microleakage of indirect inlays placed on different kinds of glass ionomer cement linings. J Oral Rehabil 1992;19:457–469.

64. Thordrup M, Isidor F, Hørsted-Bindslev P. Comparison of marginal fit and microleakage of ceramic and composite inlays: An in vitro study. J Dent 1994;22:147–153.

65. Soares CJ, Martins LR, Fernandes Neto AJ, Giannini M. Marginal adaptation of indirect composites and ceramic inlay systems. Oper Dent 2003;28:689–694.

66. Audenino G, Bresciano ME, Bassi F, Carossa S. In vitro evaluation of fit of adhesively luted ceramic inlays. Int J Prosthodont 1999;12:342–347.

67. Scherer W, Futter H, Cooper H. Clinical technique for an in-office porcelain modification. J Esthet Dent 1991;3:23–26.

68. Hein DK, Christensen RP, Smith SL. 3 year breakage rate of class 2 tooth colored materials [abstract 1200]. J Dent Res 1997;76:163.

69. Soares CJ, Martins LR, Pfeifer JM, Giannini M. Fracture resistance of teeth restored with indirect-composite and ceramic inlays. Quintessence Int 2004;35:281–286.

70. Oh W, Delong R, Anusavice K. Factors affecting enamel and ceramic wear: A literature review. J Prosthet Dent 2002;87:451–459.

71. Magne P, Belser UC. Porcelain versus composite inlays/onlays: Effects of mechanical loads on stress distribution, adhesion, and crown flexure. Int J Periodontics Restorative Dent 2003;23:543–555.

72. Metzler KT, Woody RD, Miller AW, Miller BH. In vitro investigation of the wear of human enamel by dental porcelain. J Prosthet Dent 1999;81:356–364.

73. Sorensen JA, Sultan E, Condon JR. Three-body in vitro wear of enamel against dental ceramics [abstract 909]. J Dent Res 1999;78:219.

74. Imai, Y, Suzuki S, Fukushima S. In vitro enamel wear modified porcelains [abstract 50]. J Dent Res 1999;78:112.

75. Sorensen JA, Berge HX. In vitro measurement of antagonist tooth wear opposing ceramic bridges [abstract 2942]. J Dent Res 1999;78:473.

76. Burgoyne A, Nichols J, Brudvik J. In vitro two-body wear of inlay-onlay resin composite restorations. J Prosthet Dent 1991;65:206–214.

77. Gray W, Suzuki M, Jordan R, et al. Clinical evaluation of indirect composite restorations—3 year results [abstract 633]. J Dent Res 1991;70:344.

78. Walton JN. Esthetic alternatives for posterior teeth: Porcelain and laboratory-processed resin composites. J Can Dent Assoc 1992;58:820–823.

79. Lambrechts P, Braem M, Vuylsteke-Wauters M, Vanherle G. Quantitative in vivo wear of human enamel. J Dent Res 1989;68:1752–1754.

80. Suzuki S. In vitro wear of indirect resin composite restoratives [abstract 204]. J Dent Res 1998;77:657.

81. Kern M, Strub JR, Lu XY. Wear of composite resin veneering materials in a newly developed chewing simulator [abstract 2154]. J Dent Res 1998;77:901.

82. Suzuki S, Nagai E, Taira Y, Minesaki Y. In vitro wear of indirect composite restoratives. J Prosthet Dent 2002;88:431–436.

83. Bishop BM. A heat and pressure cured composite inlay system: A clinical evaluation. Aust Prosthodont J 1989;3:35–41.

84. Bessing C, Lundqvist P. A 1-year clinical examination of indirect resin composite inlays: A preliminary report. Quintessence Int 1991;22:153–157.

85. van Dijken JW, Horstedt P. Marginal breakdown of 5-year-old direct composite inlays. J Dent 1996;24:389–394.

86. Wendt SL, Leinfelder KF. Clinical evaluation of a heat treated composite inlay: 3-year results. Am J Dent 1992;5:258–262.

87. Leirskar J, Nordbo H, Thoresen NR, Henaug T, von der Fehr FR. A four to six years follow-up of indirect resin composite inlays/onlays. Acta Odontol Scand 2003;61:247–251 [erratum 2003;61:319].

88. O'Neal SJ, Givan DA, Suzuki S. Five year clinical performance of heat and pressure cured indirect composite [abstract 1628]. J Dent Res 1999;78:309.

89. Kukrer D, Gemalmaz D, Kuybulu E, Bozkurt F. A prospective clinical study of ceromer inlays: Results up to 53 months. Int J Prosthodont 2004;17:17–23.

90. Smales R, Etemadi S. Survival of ceramic onlays placed with and without metal reinforcement. J Prosthet Dent 2004;91:548–553.

91. Friedl KH, Schmalz G, Hiller KA, Bey B. In vitro evaluation of a feldspathic ceramic system: 4 year results. J Dent Res 1997;76:163.

92. Fuzzi M, Rappelli G. Ceramic inlays: Clinical assessment and survival rate. J Adhes Dent 1999;1:71–79.

93. Molin M, Karlsson S. A 3-year clinical follow-up study of a ceramic (OPTEC) inlay system. Acta Odontol Scand 1996;54:145–149.

94. Qualtrough AJE, Wilson NHF. A 3-year clinical evaluation of a porcelain onlay system. J Dent 1996;24:317–323.

95. Hayashi M, Tsuchitani Y, Kawamura Y, Miura M, Takeshige F, Ebisu S. Eight-year clinical evaluation of fired ceramic inlays. Oper Dent 2000;25:473–481.

96. Schulz P, Johansson A, Arvidson K. A retrospective study of Mirage ceramic inlays over up to 9 years. Int J Prosthodont 2003;16:510–514.

97. van Dijken JW, Hasselroth L, Ormin A, Olofsson AL. Clinical evaluation of extensive dentin enamel bonded all-ceramic onlays and onlay crowns [abstract 2713]. J Dent Res 1999;78:445.

98. Fradeani M, Aquilano A, Basseyi L. Longitudinal study of pressed glass ceramic inlays for four and a half years. J Prosthet Dent 1997;78:346–353.

99. Frankenberger R, Petschelt A, Kramer N. Leucite-reinforced ceramic inlays and onlays after six years: Clinical behavior. Oper Dent 2000;25:459–465.

100. Studer S, Lehner C, Scharer P. Seven year results of leucite-reinforced glass ceramic inlays and onlays [abstract 1375]. J Dent Res 1998;77:803.

101. Molin MK, Karlsson SL. A randomized 5-year clinical evaluation of 3 ceramic inlay systems. Int J Prosthodont 2000;13:194–200.

102. Krejci I, Lutz F, Reimer M. Wear of CAD/CAM ceramic inlays: Restorations, opposing cusps, luting cements. Quintessence Int 1994;25:199–207.

103. Krejci I, Guntert A, Lutz F. Scanning electron microscopic and clinical examination of resin composite inlays/onlays up to 12 months in situ. Quintessence Int 1994;25:403–409.

104. Van Meerbeek B, Inokoshi S, Willems G, et al. Marginal adaptation of four tooth-coloured inlay systems in vivo. J Dent 1992;20:18–26.

105. O'Neal SJ, Miracle RL, Leinfelder LF. Evaluating interfacial gaps for esthetic inlays. J Am Dent Assoc 1993;124:48–54.

106. Wilder AD. Clinical considerations of Cerec restorations. In: Mörmann WH (ed). Proceedings of an International Symposium on Computer Restorations. Chicago: Quintessence, 1991:141–149.

107. Kawai K, Isenberg B, Leinfelder KF. Effect of gap dimension on resin composite cement wear. Quintessence Int 1994;25:53–58.

108. Isenberg BP, Essig ME, Leinfelder KF. Three year clinical evaluation of CAD/CAM restorations. J Esthet Dent 1992;4:173–176.

109. Hayashi M, Tsubakimoto Y, Takeshige F, Ebisu S. Analysis of longitudinal marginal deterioration of ceramic inlays. Oper Dent 2004;29:386–391.

110. Mörmann WH, Gotsch T, Krejci I, Lutz F. Barbakow F. Clinical status of 94 CEREC ceramic inlays after 3 years in situ. In: Mörmann WH (ed). International Symposium on Computer Restorations. Chicago: Quintessence, 1991:355–363.

111. Mehl A, Hickel R. Current state of development and perspectives of machine-based production methods for dental restorations. Int J Comput Dent 1999;2:9–35.

112. Mörmann WH. Chairside computer-generated ceramic restorations: The CEREC third generation improvements. Pract Periodont Aesthet Dent 1992;4(7):9–16.

113. Mörmann WH, Brandestini M, Lutz F, Barbakow F. Chairside computer-aided direct ceramic inlays. Quintessence Int 1989;20: 329–339.

114. Mörmann WH. Symposium review. In: Mörmann WH (ed). Proceedings of an International Symposium on Computer Restorations. Chicago: Quintessence, 1991:17–21.

115. Fasbinder DJ. CEREC Operator's Manual. Charlotte, NC: Sirona Dental, 2004.

116. David SB, LoPresti JT. Tooth-colored posterior restorations using CEREC method CAD/CAM–generated ceramic inlays. Compend Cont Educ Dent 1994;15:802–810.

117. Burke FJT, Wilson NHF, Watts DC. The effect of cavity wall taper on fracture resistance of teeth restored with resin composite inlays. Oper Dent 1993;18:230–236.

118. Sato K, Matsumura H, Atsuta M. Relationship between cavity design and marginal adaptation in a machine-milled ceramic restorative system. J Oral Rehabil 2002;29:24–27.

119. Fasbinder DJ. Restorative material options for CAD/CAM restorations. Compend Contin Educ Dent 2002;23:911–922.

120. Krejci I. Wear of CEREC and other restorative materials. In: Mörmann WH (ed). Proceedings of an International Symposium on Computer Restorations. Chicago: Quintessence, 1991:245–251.

121. al-Hiyásat AS, Saunders WP, Sharkey SW, Smith G, Gilmour WH. Investigation of human enamel wear against four dental ceramics and gold. J Dent 1998;26:487–495.

122. Rusin RP. Properties and applications of a new composite block for CAD/CAM. Compend Contin Educ Dent 2001;22(6 suppl):35–41.

123. Fasbinder DJ, Dennison JB, Heys D, Lampe K. Clinical evaluation of CAD/CAM–generated composite inlays: 3 years [abstract 68]. J Dent Res 2003;82(special issue):B-21.

124. Wilder AD. Clinical considerations of CEREC restorations. In: Mörmann WH (ed). Proceedings of an International Symposium on Computer Restorations. Chicago: Quintessence, 1991:141–149.

125. Shearer AC, Kusy RP, Whitley JQ, Heymann HO, Wilson NHF. Finishing of MGC Dicor material. Int J Prosthodont 1994;7:167–173.

126. Roznowski M, Bremer B, Geurtsen W. Fracture resistance of human molars restored with various filling materials. In: Mörmann WH (ed). Proceedings of an International Symposium on Computer Restorations. Chicago: Quintessence, 1991:559–565.

127. Krejci I, Lutz F, Reimer M. Marginal adaptation and fit of adhesive ceramic inlays. J Dent 1993;21:39–46.

128. Peters A, Bieniek KW. SEM-examination of the marginal adaptation of computer machined ceramic restorations. In: Mörmann WH (ed). Proceedings of an International Symposium on Computer Restorations. Chicago: Quintessence, 1991:365–370.

129. Christensen GJ. Marginal fit of gold inlay castings. J Prosthet Dent 1966;16:297–305.

130. Mörmann WH, Schug J. Grinding precision and accuracy of fit of CEREC 2 CAD/CIM inlays. J Am Dent Assoc 1997;128:47–53.

131. Benz C, Benz B, El Mahdy K, Hickel R. Clinical evaluation of the CEREC II system in comparison to CEREC 1. In: Mörmann W (ed). CAD/CIM in Esthetic Dentistry. Chicago: Quintessence, 1996: 516–524.

132. Ellingsen LA, Fasbinder DJ. In vitro evaluation of CAD/CAM ceramic crowns [abstract 2640]. J Dent Res 2002;81(special issue):A-331.

133. Sjogren G, Bergman M, Molin M, Bessing C. A clinical examination of ceramic (CEREC) inlays. Acta Odontol Scand 1992;50:171–178.

134. Heymann HO, Bayne SC, Sturdevant JR, Wilder AD, Roberson TM. The clinical performance of CAD-CAM–generated ceramic inlays: A four-year study. J Am Dent Assoc 1996;127:1171–1181.

135. Fasbinder DJ, Lampe K, Dennison JB, Peters MC, Nematollahi K. Clinical performance of CAD/CIM generated ceramic onlays [abstract 2711]. J Dent Res 1999;78(special issue):444.

136. Sjogren G, Molin M, van Dijken JW. A 5-year clinical evaluation of ceramic inlays (CEREC) cemented with a dual-cured or chemically cured resin composite luting agent. Acta Odontol Scand 1998; 56:263–267.

137. Pallesen U, van Dijken JW. An 8-year evaluation of sintered ceramic and glass ceramic inlays processed by the CEREC CAD/CAM system. Eur J Oral Sci 2000;108:239–246.

138. Berg NG, Derand T. A 5-year evaluation of ceramic inlays (CEREC). Swed Dent J 1997;21:121–127.

139. Martin N, Jedynakiewicz NM. Clinical performance of CEREC ceramic inlays: A systematic review. Dent Mater 1999;15:54–61.

140. Otto T, De Nisco S. Computer-aided direct ceramic restorations: A 10-year prospective clinical study of CEREC CAD/CAM inlays and onlays. Int J Prosthodont 2002;15:122–128.

141. Hickel R, Manhart J. Longevity of restorations in posterior teeth and reasons for failure. J Adhes Dent 2001;3:45–64.

142. Zuellig-Singer R, Bryant RW. Three year evaluation of computer-machined ceramic inlays: Influence of luting agent. Quintessence Int 1998;29:573–582.

143. Sjogren G, Molin M, van Dijken JW. A 10-year prospective evaluation of CAD/CAM-manufactured (CEREC) ceramic inlays cemented with a chemically cured or dual-cured resin composite. Int J Prosthodont 2004;17:241–246.

144. Otto T, De Nisco S. Computer-aided direct ceramic restorations: A 10-year prospective clinical study of CEREC CAD/CAM inlays and onlays. Int J Prosthodont 2002;15:122–128.

145. Bindl A, Mörmann W. Survival rate of mono-ceramic and ceramic-core CAD/CAM–generated anterior crowns over 2–5 years. Eur J Oral Sci 2004;112:197–204.

537

Cast-Gold Restorations

Patrice P. Fan
Thomas G. Berry

The cast-gold restoration has lessened in popularity over the past 20 years because of the increased emphasis on esthetics, but it remains an excellent restoration with a long history of success. If used with care, gold alloy is considered to have the greatest longevity of any restorative material used in dentistry. This opinion is generally supported by longitudinal studies,[1–3] although it is disputed by other studies.[4–6] Cast gold may be used for intracoronal (inlays) or extracoronal (complete-coverage crowns) restorations, as well as for restorations that are a combination of both (onlays or partial-coverage crowns) (Figs 19-1a and 19-1b).

Gold castings present several advantages over direct restorative materials such as silver amalgam or resin composite. Because castings are fabricated using an indirect technique, it is possible to achieve nearly ideal contours and occlusion.[7] Gold alloy is a strong material that rarely fractures and, when used as an extracoronal restoration, can provide protection to the tooth.[8–10] Other materials such as titanium and nickel-chrome alloys have shown clinically acceptable results, but gold alloy remains the dental casting alloy of choice.[11] Gold wears at a rate similar to that of enamel, so it does not cause accelerated wear of the opposing teeth.[12] It casts easily and accurately, and, if a type II or type III gold is used, marginal adaptation can usually be improved after the restoration is cast.

Gold is also resistant to corrosion by virtue of its half cell potential, and it behaves as a cathode in the intraoral environment.[13] Gold shows better resistance to current at-home vital bleaching agents, such as 10% carbamide peroxide, compared to unpolished amalgam and nickel chrome.[14] However, galvanic corrosion has been shown to cause unpleasant, sometimes painful, transient effects when gold alloy is in direct contact with zinc-containing amalgam restorations. As passivation processes develop, naturally or by actively brushing the new amalgam restoration with tin oxide, side effects subside.[15–17]

The primary drawback to the use of cast gold rather than direct restorations is higher initial cost, because castings require at least two appointments for the patient and have associated laboratory costs. However, the long-term success of cast-gold restorations offsets this initial investment and decreases frequency of "remakes," preserving tooth structure, pulp vitality, and subsequent expense. For esthetic reasons, gold castings are usually used to restore posterior teeth that are not in the esthetic zone. Preparations for anterior teeth are usually designed so that the gold is hidden from direct observation (Figs 19-2a and 19-2b). Esthetics may also be preserved in maxillary posterior teeth when cast-gold restorations are used (Figs 19-3a and 19-3b). Postoperative tooth sensitivity following insertion of cast-gold restorations can usually be prevented with the proper use of sealers, liners, and bases.[18,19] This chapter addresses the indications, materials, and clinical steps for the fabrication of cast-gold restorations.

Indications

The indications for a cast-gold restoration range from a tooth with a relatively small caries lesion, restored with an inlay, to a severely weakened and/or malfunctioning tooth, restored with a complete-coverage crown. Cast-gold restorations may be used to restore teeth with caries lesions or to replace existing restorations. They are generally indicated for situations in

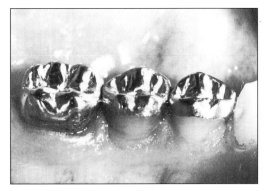

Fig 19-1a Partial- and complete-coverage cast restorations.

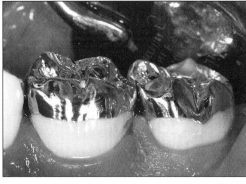

Fig 19-1b Partial-coverage cast (onlay) restorations.

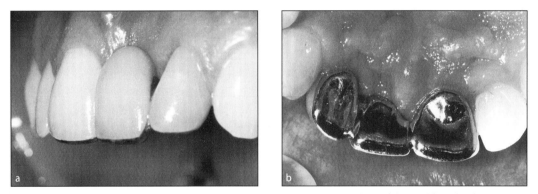

Figs 19-2a and 19-2b These anterior restorations are designed to display very little of the gold from the facial aspect. The incisal gold is angled so that light is not reflected directly back at the viewer.

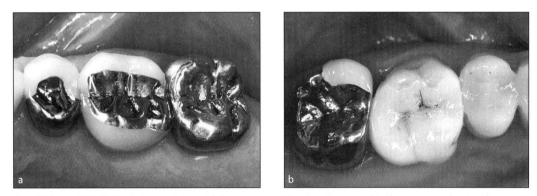

Figs 19-3a and 19-3b Posterior partial- and full-coverage gold restorations, used in the same quadrant with ceramic and ceramometal restorations, satisfy functional and esthetic demands.

which other, less expensive materials are not suitable for establishing proper proximal and/or occlusal contacts, creating appropriate axial contours, or protecting the remaining tooth structure. A cast-gold restoration may also be indicated when gold has been used to restore adjacent and/or opposing teeth, so that problems arising from use of dissimilar metals do not occur.[20,21] A cast-gold restoration may be specifically recommended for posterior areas and for alleviat-

ing the deleterious effects of bruxism. Reduction requirements for a full cast-gold crown are more conservative than for any other type of full-coverage restorations, and the wear properties of gold make it an ideal choice when there is opposing intact tooth structure.[12]

The morphology of posterior teeth, the number of carious surfaces, the number of restored surfaces, the width and depth of existing restorations,[22] and the occlusal relationships must be considered when the need for a cast restoration is determined. Non–working-side occlusal contacts can be especially important. Hiatt[23] has shown a significant increase in the number of vertical fractures in teeth with non–working-side contacts.

Basic Principles of Cast Restorations

While there are many acceptable techniques and designs for cast restorations, certain principles always apply.

Conservation of Tooth Structure

Preparations should be made as conservatively as possible to maximize the strength of the remaining tooth structure, lessen the likelihood of postoperative sensitivity and pulpal pathosis, and decrease the likelihood of tooth fracture. Tooth reduction should not exceed the amount that will allow adequate material thickness necessary to resist fracture, deformation, or wear during function. From an anatomic standpoint, nonfunctional cusps (buccal cusps of maxillary teeth, lingual cusps of mandibular teeth) of molars and functional cusps of maxillary premolars possess steep inclines. The enamel is also thinner on nonfunctional cusps. The clinician should keep these elements in mind during the treatment planning process.[24–27]

Tooth preservation involves more than simply minimizing the removal of tooth structure. Preparations must be designed to protect remaining tooth structure. This may involve additional reduction to remove weak tooth structure, or it may necessitate cuspal coverage. Studies have shown that as a cavity preparation gets wider[28,29] and deeper,[30] progressive weakening of the tooth occurs. When an inlay preparation exceeds one third of the intercuspal (buccal cusp tip to lingual cusp tip) width, an onlay or another extracoronal restoration should be considered to protect the cusps of the tooth. Indeed, a conservative three-surface (mesio-occlusodistal; MOD) restoration has proven to decrease tooth stiffness by 50% and a large three-surface restoration by as much as 78%. Gold onlays or full cast crowns provide greater resistance and a splinting effect to cusp movement. They virtually double the resistance to fracture when compared to an intact tooth.[31–33] This reinforcing effect is particularly significant in the maxillary premolars.

Two retrospective studies[34,35] concluded that a significant factor to prevent catastrophic failure of endodontically treated teeth was the presence of a full- or partial-coverage restoration. Another recent 9-year retrospective cohort study[36] demonstrated that endodontically treated teeth with intra-coronal restorations were six times more likely to fail catastrophically compared to teeth restored with full-coverage restorations.[34–36]

Because extracoronal restorations cover both facial and lingual surfaces, they protect remaining tooth structure and reduce the incidence of tooth fracture.[37]

Retention and Resistance Form

Retention and resistance form are two separate but related features of a preparation. Correctly incorporated, they resist unseating vertical, lateral, and oblique forces that are placed on the restoration during function or parafunction.[38] Retention form resists forces attempting to remove a restoration parallel to the path of insertion. Resistance form resists forces attempting to dislodge a restoration obliquely to the path of insertion. Retention form and resistance form are usually closely interrelated and may be difficult to distinguish clinically as separate features. However, they both are affected by four factors. The first is the resulting stress quantified by the ratio of applied force to surface area. The force itself varies in its magnitude, frequency, duration, and direction. The other three factors are the final tooth preparation geometry, the luting material type and thickness, and the tooth and crown surface texturing.[39–41]

Retention is gained when two or more walls oppose each other. These walls may be intracoronal, extracoronal, or a combination of the two (Figs 19-4a and 19-4b). The amount of retention created by these opposing walls is determined by several factors. The degree of convergence toward the occlusal (extracoronal walls) or divergence toward the occlusal (intracoronal walls) and the length of the walls are the most important factors. One long wall opposed by a short wall provides retention equivalent only to that imparted by the short wall. The longer[42] and more nearly parallel the walls, the greater the retention. The further apart the opposing walls and the greater the surface areas, the more retentive the restoration will be.[43] Certain implant internal connections have utilized these principles creating an effective self-locking morse taper configuration. In practice, the taper achieved bears little resemblance to those traditionally advocated in textbooks (a combined 6 to 12 degrees), and most teeth are prepared with a taper in excess of 12 degrees with clinical success.[44–46] Although a rapid loss of retention occurs as the taper progresses from 5 to 10 degrees for each wall,[47] a total convergence up to 16 degrees still provides adequate retention.[44,45]

At a constant taper, retention increases with increasing preparation length, surface area, and preparation diameter and also with the use of a resin-based cement combined with

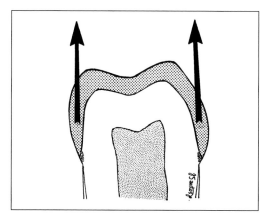

Fig 19-4a Complete-coverage, or full veneer, crowns rely on the opposing external walls to provide retention for the restoration. A slight taper of the walls in the occlusal direction provides a path of insertion.

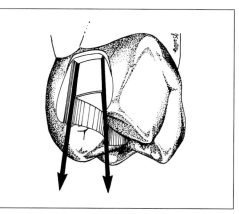

Fig 19-4b Inlays (pictured) and onlays rely on tapering opposing internal walls for retention.

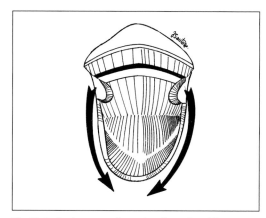

Fig 19-5a Resistance to lingual and rotational forces may be provided by proximal grooves.

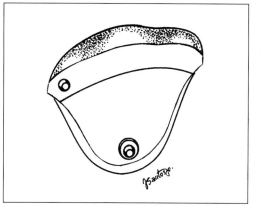

Fig 19-5b Pinholes also provide resistance to lingual displacement.

Fig 19-6 This maxillary molar preparation (a) shows the use of controlled taper, boxes, and a "pothole" to provide retention and resistance form for the full-coverage casting (b).

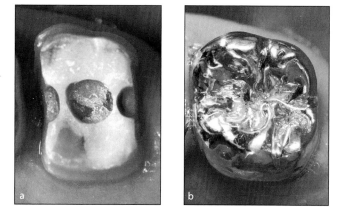

surface treatments.[39–41] It is important to note that the retention of a casting prior to cementation is not an indication of its retention postcementation.[48]

Addition of intracoronal features has different effects on retention and resistance. The addition of proximal boxes or pins improves both retention and resistance, whereas proximal grooves and potholes mostly enhance resistance form[49] (Figs 19-5 and 19-6). Posterior teeth that are short may present a problem despite their larger diameter. Short, wide preparations do not resist rotational forces well. Adding a groove or a pin will reduce this rotational radius and provide additional resistance.

In complete-coverage restorations, the addition of a circumferential groove in both the preparation and the crown has been shown to drastically improve retention.[50] A recent study[51] demonstrated that the positive influence of grooves or boxes is limited by the height, width, and taper of the existing preparation. The study showed that grooves and boxes seem to possess a limited effect on short, wide, and excessively tapered preparations. The most effective method to improve retention was to decrease the convergence of the preparation's 2.5-mm total height in the cervical 1.5 mm from 20 to 8 degrees.

Insufficient retention is a major cause of failure of fixed prostheses, exceeded only by failure due to dental caries and porcelain fracture.[6]

Recent developments in luting agents and techniques of metal conditioning allow bonding of cast restorations to the tooth. This greatly improves the resistance to displacement from the preparation. Although less often discussed, the cement's compression and shear strength as a function of film thickness along with the tooth-cement and cement-crown adhesive properties, appear to be essential parameters affecting retention and resistance. However, the long-term effectiveness of bonded castings is not yet known.

Resistance form is essential to providing long-term stability of cemented restorations. Taper has a limited influence. A variation of ±10% taper increases or decreases resistance by ±10%.[31,32] Indeed, the rationale for resistance form has evolved from a theoretical model[52,53] to a more clinically relevant idea.[31] The self-limiting taper concept, or "on-off" theory, has been challenged by the importance of the cement's properties, thickness, and mechanical behavior under compression.[41,53,54] Cement thickness should be kept at the minimum level compatible with seating of the restoration. Texturing the surface of the abutment and crown before cementation increases the resistance to dynamic lateral loading.[41]

Pulpal Considerations

Tooth preparation for any cast restoration involves dentin and, therefore, affects the pulp. Often in situations in which a restoration is indicated, the pulp has already been traumatized by caries and/or previous restorations. Prior to tooth preparation, the pulp should be tested for vitality, and radiographs should be taken. Tooth symptoms and restorative history should be noted. The additional trauma created by tooth preparation can be enough to cause necrosis of an unhealthy pulp. If the vitality of the pulp is questionable, a reevaluation of the pulpal vitality should be performed 4 to 6 months after the initial therapy. Endodontic therapy is easier and more predictable and economical for the patient if it is performed before the final restoration is placed. Endodontic therapy through an existing restoration is difficult and may lead to decreased crown retention, marginal leakage, and recurrent caries.[55] One study[56] determined that the cast-gold restoration presented the lowest rate of bacterial leakage when endodontic access openings were closed with either resin composite or amalgam, as compared to other types of full-coverage restorations. Hence, endodontic therapy should be performed prior to preparation.

Pulpal considerations for cast restorations are the same as those for direct restorations. The best pulpal protection is a thick layer of sound dentin. A thorough discussion of the subject can be found in chapter 5. The thinner the dentin, the more permeable and susceptible it is to penetration of bacteria and uncured monomers.[57,58] A pulpal reaction will be triggered if the remaining dentinal thickness (RDT) is less than 1 mm (see chapter 5). In situations in which the RDT is very thin, application of a sealer or liner is indicated, followed by an observation period to determine that the tooth remains symptom-free prior to seating the final restoration permanently.[59]

Certain anatomic considerations are critical to planning the preparation, especially in younger patients. The pulp horns may be large enough to be exposed during preparation. Examination of preoperative radiographs is imperative to identify potential problems. Because the pulp is narrower in the cervical region of the tooth, pulpal exposures are less likely to occur in this area.

Postcementation thermal sensitivity is sometimes a problem. Several methods to prevent or minimize this problem have been recommended. Some clinicians scrub the preparations with antimicrobial solutions to reduce bacterial contamination, a possible cause of postoperative sensitivity. Other factors affecting pulpal response include RDT and postoperative time.[59–61] Resin varnish should be avoided in favor of bonding or desensitizing systems. These have been shown to seal the dentin surface more effectively prior to cementation to prevent migration of bacteria into the tubules. Techniques vary depending on the cement used.[62]

Gingival Considerations

When a tooth is prepared for a cast restoration, finish lines (and therefore casting margins) can be placed supragingivally or intracrevicularly.[63] It is well established that supragingival crown margins are compatible with gingival health, but both configurations have their proponents.[64,65] However, there is general agreement that it is only at the completion of the initial periodontal therapy that the decision on the location of finish lines should be made.[66] Should crown lengthening be necessary, the waiting period before final tooth preparation should provide adequate time for healing and tissue stabilization.

Each margin location has its indications, as described below.

Supragingival margins present the following advantages:

- Preparation, impression, and temporization are facilitated.
- The restoration can be finished/cemented and cleaned with ease.
- Patient hygiene measures are more effective, and evaluation at recall is facilitated.
- Incidence of inflammation in adjacent tissues is reduced.

For partial-coverage restorations, the finish line should be kept in enamel that is supported by dentin wherever possible and should never be placed in areas of direct-contact occlusal function.

Intracrevicular margins may be warranted in the following situations:

- Existing restorations, caries lesions, or erosion require that the finish line be placed more apically.
- Refinement or modification of an existing finish line is needed.
- Additional retention or resistance form is needed.
- There is a long contact area on a proximal surface.
- The emergence profile requires modification.
- Root sensitivity is unresolved with conservative measures.

Note that esthetics is obviously not a criterion for margin placement in a cast-gold restoration.

From a restorative standpoint, subgingival margin placement increases the level of difficulty and reduces predictability. Periodontally, even a well-fitting margin may trigger a pathologic response.[67–70]

It is important to note that the term *subgingival* implies the placement of a restoration margin somewhere between the free gingival margin and the alveolar crest. *Intracrevicular* refers to the placement of a margin within the gingival sulcus and above the junctional epithelium or epithelial attachment (Fig 19-7). Ultimately, the fit, finish, and emergence profile at intracrevicular finish lines may be as significant to gingival health as the location of the finish line in relation to the free gingiva.[71,72]

One other controversial issue pertains to restoration margins impinging on the biologic width. Gargiulo's biologic concept and dimensions have been challenged.[73–75] Of the three

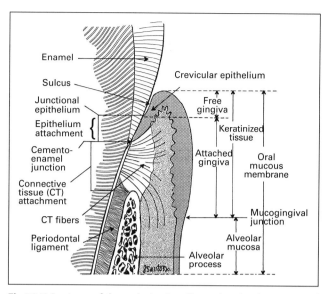

Fig 19-7 Anatomy of the periodontium illustrating the three zones of the dentogingival junction.[63]

components of the biologic width, only the connective tissue attachment seems to be relatively constant. Sulcular depth and epithelial attachment show wide variations. Histologically, the sulcus depth is at 0.5 mm, whereas clinically, it ranges from 1 to 4 mm and is affected by probing force, tooth position, and tissue health status. The dentogingival complex follows human biologic variability. The most predictable method to assess the patient's specific biologic width is to probe the osseous crest.[74]

Biologic width violation can result in an inflammatory response leading to attachment loss, pocket formation, and osseous resorption. Most studies were performed on animals, and there is actually very limited data on biologic width.[75]

The consequences of restoration margins impinging on the biologic width remain controversial. A recent 2-year prospective study failed to correlate the violation of biologic width with bone resorption or gingival recession. On the other hand, a statistically significant increase in probing depth and gingival inflammation was observed, but its clinical significance remains uncertain.[75]

It is important to remember that the bone scallop approximately parallels the cementoenamel junction (CEJ) circumferentially.[73–75] Frequently, a preparation finish line on an anterior tooth does not parallel this osseous scallop, thus inducing an interproximal violation of biologic width.

The interproximal bone in posterior areas has a flat architecture and adequate thickness, so a scallop pattern in the restoration finish line is not as necessary. However, a thin labial or buccal plate over a root prominence is not uncommon, so these areas are at risk.[76] A phenotype characterized by a slender tooth and thin gingival tissue may be prone to gingival recession following a biologically or mechanically aggressive procedure.[77] A minimum of 3 mm height of attached gingiva and free gingiva should be present prior to any restorative procedure in which the finish line approaches gingival tissue.[63]

If possible, finish lines should not be prepared deeper than 0.5 to 1.0 mm into the sulcus[78,79] or closer than 1.0 mm to the base of the sulcus.[63] A more complete discussion of this subject may be found in chapter 1.

Because gingival health may be adversely affected by intracrevicular finish lines,[66,69,80–83] finish lines should be placed supragingivally if the situation permits. When finish lines must be placed within the gingival crevice because of caries lesions, existing restorations, fractures, root sensitivity, or short clinical crowns,[84,85] care must be exercised to minimize the damage to gingival tissues. The fragile soft tissue may be reflected by careful placement of deflection cord (gingival retraction cord), prior to final preparation of the finish line, to avoid soft tissue damage.

Finish Lines

The term *finish line* refers to the border of the preparation where the prepared tooth structure meets the unprepared surface of the tooth. The type of finish line depends on the clinical situation. A smooth, well-defined finish line is beneficial, regardless of the design used, to facilitate laboratory procedures and finishing of the restoration. Selection of the type of finish line may be dictated by the shape of the tooth (bell shaped vs flat) (Fig 19-8), the desired location of the finish line, or operator preference. The most common types of finish lines for cast restorations are knife-edged, chamfer, and shoulder. Both the chamfer and the shoulder configurations may be beveled or unbeveled (Fig 19-9a).

According to a dental survey, there is no agreement on the ideal finish line.[86] The type of finish line and presence or absence of a bevel will depend upon tooth morphology, its location, and the type of restorative material used.

The Slip Joint vs the Butt Joint Theory

Despite a lack of consensus regarding the maximal allowable marginal gap, a gap between 39 and 120 µm may be considered acceptable.[87–90] It has long been held that the addition of bevels to cast-gold preparations helps to reduce marginal gaps.[91] However, this was based on mathematical models that did not take cement thickness into account. As explicitly demonstrated by Ostlund[92] and supported by others,[93,94] beveling beyond 45 degrees significantly increases the cement-filled opening (Fig 19-9b). Simply put, the steeper the bevel angle, the larger the vertical discrepancy (opening) between the edge of the casting and the finish line. This assumes that the casting is fully relieved, allowing minimum cement thickness. Another study[95] later demonstrated that crowns with shoulder finish line configuration had better marginal fit than did those with beveled finish line configuration. The study did not describe or quantify the amount of difference of internal fit of the castings. Factors such as existing taper, die relief spacer thickness, laboratory technique, cement material properties, finishing technique, and seating force play important roles in the ultimate finish line fit.[88,96] Research suggests that finish line form and cement do not significantly affect the fit of cemented crowns. However, marginal fit varies continuously around the tooth, making an evaluation subjective and arduous.[97–99]

Knife-edged Configuration

A knife-edged finish line requires the least amount of tooth reduction. It is sometimes used with a bell-shaped tooth because creation of a heavier margin would require excessive removal of tooth structure. Generally, a knife-edged finish line is not desirable because it is more difficult than other finish lines to discern on a die, and it tends to result in overcontoured restorations. These thin margins are more difficult to wax and cast accurately and are susceptible to distortion under occlusal forces. However, the configuration is commonly used on the mesial aspect of a mesially tipped molar, on the lingual aspects of mandibular molars, and on root surfaces of periodontally involved teeth. It should be noted that excellent results may be obtained with knife-edged finish lines in expert hands coupled with outstanding laboratory support when the gold finish lines are accessible for finishing and are in enamel.[100]

Chamfer Configuration

A chamfer is often the preferred finish line for cast-gold extracoronal restorations. It is more conservative than a shoulder finish line and generates less stress at the cement interface.[101] It creates a well-defined and easily identified margin that provides room for adequate thickness of gold without overcontouring the restoration. Care must be taken not to tilt the bur toward the tooth, because that will increase taper, or away from the tooth, because that will create undercuts.

Shoulder Configuration

The shoulder finish line is used primarily where a bulk of material is needed to strengthen the restoration at the margins, as for all-porcelain or metal-ceramic restorations. It is the least conservative of the finish line types for cast gold. It also has the most critical fit, since there is no bevel present on the

Fig 19-8 Flat proximal surfaces *(left)* allow the easy formation of a chamfered finish line, while bell-shaped anatomy *(right)* makes it difficult to create such a finish line without severe reduction of the proximal surface.

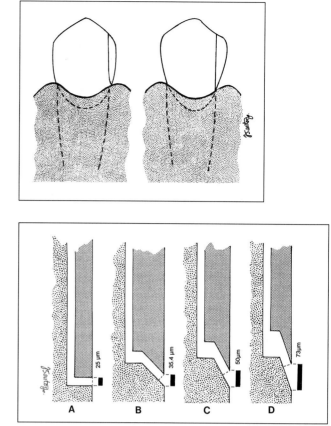

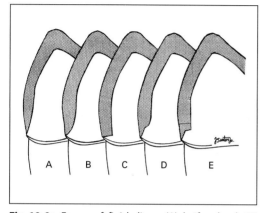

Fig 19-9a Forms of finish lines: (A) knife-edged; (B) chamfer; (C) shoulder; (D) beveled chamfer; (E) beveled shoulder.

Fig 19-9b Effect of the same cement film thickness on cervical marginal openings, comparing a shoulder marginal configuration with no bevel and beveled shoulders at varied bevel angles: (A) butt margin with 90-degree cavosurface angle; (B) shoulder margin with 45-degree bevel; (C) shoulder margin with 60-degree bevel; (D) shoulder margin with 70-degree bevel. The broken line represents the cement film thickness of 25 μm at the margin. As steepness of the bevel increases, the marginal opening increases.[94]

restoration that can be burnished against the preparation to reduce marginal opening.

Chamfer or Shoulder with a Bevel

This design is preferred by clinicians who believe that a beveled margin is easier to detect in an impression and that it makes the margins of the casting more burnishable. A bevel is recommended for proximal boxes. However, for full cast crowns, the bevel can increase the risk of encroachment on the epithelial attachment.

Contours

The establishment of proper contours of the restoration depends on proper tooth preparation. An overcontoured casting is often the result of an underprepared tooth. If

removal of tooth structure is insufficient, the crown has to be overcontoured to obtain sufficient thickness of metal. Overcontoured crowns encourage plaque retention, resulting in gingival inflammation[102,103] (Fig 19-10). Even with overcontoured crowns, however, gingival health can be maintained if the patient practices excellent oral hygiene measures.[104]

Whereas Wheeler[105] proposed that convexities be created in the gingival third of artificial crowns to deflect food away from the free gingiva. Herlands et al[106] however, showed that the maximum bulge in the natural crown at its greatest diameter is no more than 0.5 mm greater than at the CEJ and that the impaction mechanism of gingival injury does not occur. The biologic acceptability of undercontouring is often observed when a provisional crown is lost from a prepared tooth for an extended time without adverse effects on the surrounding gingiva.[104] A natural contour (ie, the exact

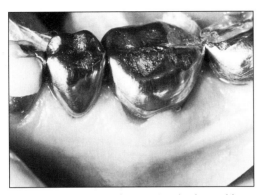

Fig 19-10 Overcontoured restorations lead to problems. Note the loss of normal gingival contours and the edematous appearance of the tissue.

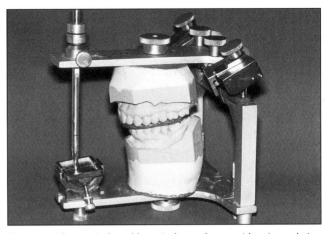

Fig 19-11 The semiadjustable articulator, shown with a jaw relation record in place, simulates mandibular movements more closely than the simple articulators.

replacement of the axial and proximal morphology) is the desired form for cast-gold restorations when the gingival crest is at a normal level.

When the free gingival margin is apical to the CEJ because of recession or surgery, a flattened contour best reproduces the contour of the root surface.[104] Flat contours are recommended occlusal to furcations to allow access for cleaning.

Stein[107] described the contour of a restoration adjacent to the gingiva as the emergence profile. He stated that the proximal emergence profiles of all natural teeth are either flat or concave. This natural contour provides an open gingival embrasure that promotes good oral hygiene.

Occlusion

No restoration, no matter how well crafted, will be successful if it does not function correctly. Satisfactory occlusion is required if the restoration is to achieve adequate function and patient comfort.

Establishing biologically acceptable occlusion starts with careful planning. The teeth opposing the one to be restored (whether in a natural or restored state) should be properly aligned and in the desired occlusal plane. Occlusal surfaces should be well formed. If these conditions do not exist, the opposing dentition should be recontoured or restored, if possible. Failure to do so may seriously compromise the occlusal relationships and, in turn, the future health and function of the involved teeth,[108] as well as the patient's comfort.[109,110]

Existing occlusal relationships should be identified with marking tape in maximum intercuspation position (centric occlusion), centric relation, and excursive movements. Tooth

fremitus, radiographic evidence of ligament widening, and wear patterns should be noted. It is essential to determine the precise etiology (eg, physiologic forces with compromised periodontal support or pathologic forces on a normal periodontium) of occlusal traumatism. A broken cusp may result from an overload in working or nonworking movements and is often associated with a large existing restoration. Malpositioned teeth, open contacts, and uneven marginal ridges may warrant additional therapy.[94,108,110]

Acceptable occlusion has several characteristics. Multiple contact points exist between opposing teeth that come into contact simultaneously during closure. The maximum closure position is referred to as *maximum intercuspation*. Ideally, the facial cusps of the mandibular posterior teeth and the lingual cusps of the maxillary posterior teeth contact the opposing teeth in a fossa or on a marginal ridge so that the occlusal contacts stabilize the teeth in both arches. In some cases, contact of mandibular and maxillary anterior teeth separates the posterior teeth during any eccentric movement of the jaw. This occlusal relationship is referred to as *anterior guidance* or *mutually protected occlusion*.[111,112] Another occlusal relationship, referred to as group function, sometimes exists or is created. In this relationship, several teeth on the functional side share equally in the contact during lateral movements of the mandible.[113]

A major benefit of indirect fabrication of a restoration is the ability to form the wax pattern to the desired occlusal relationships. The wax pattern (and ultimately the restoration) must contact its antagonist(s) in the prescribed contact areas at precisely the instant the other teeth contact. A premature contact or an interference in excursive movements may be

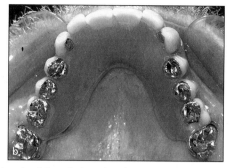

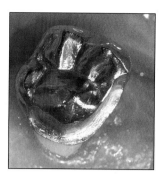

Figs 19-12a and 19-12b Gold occlusal onlays and canine inlays designed to decrease wear and preserve the occlusal scheme in this removable partial denture.

Fig 19-12c This type IV gold crown has been milled to provide optimum integration with the removable partial denture framework.

uncomfortable, produce loosening or accelerated wear of the restoration or its antagonist, and/or damage the health of the tooth and its supporting structures.[114,115]

Occlusion should be developed with mounted casts on an articulator. For single-unit castings, a simple hinge articulator may be adequate, although it allows accurate reproduction of maximum intercuspation only. Lateral or protrusive interferences must be adjusted in the mouth. In more complicated situations, as for multiple units, use of a more sophisticated semiadjustable articulator may be indicated (Fig 19-11). When casts are mounted on a semiadjustable articulator with a facebow, the lateral and protrusive movements of the mandible may be simulated with reasonable accuracy.[116]

To verify the accuracy of the relationship of the mounted casts, the patient's occlusal contacts should be checked intraorally with shimstock. If a small discrepancy exists between the patient's occlusal contacts and those on the mounted casts, the casts can be corrected with shimstock, thin articulating paper, and a carving instrument. If the discrepancy is great, it will be necessary to remount the casts. If the casts are mounted accurately and the casting is correctly fabricated, minimal adjustment will be necessary at the placement appointment.

Types of Cast Restorations

The variety of cast restorations ranges from inlays (small intracoronal restorations) to complete-coverage castings (restorations that cover the entire coronal surface of the tooth) (Figs 19-12a to 19-12c). Onlays and partial-coverage castings are hybrids that possess both intracoronal and extracoronal features. The design chosen should be the one that removes the least amount of sound tooth structure while restoring the

missing tooth structure and enabling the tooth to withstand functional and parafunctional forces.

Inlay

The gold inlay is a treatment option for small Class 2 caries lesions. Although used less frequently than in the past, the inlay has a long history of success. It is not uncommon to see a patient who has multiple inlays that are 30 years old and still clinically serviceable.[117]

Inlays are entirely intracoronal restorations, most commonly with occlusal and proximal extensions (Fig 19-13). Preparations should be as conservative as possible to maintain tooth strength. If the occlusal width of the preparation exceeds one third to one half the buccolingual intercuspal distance, a restoration offering more protection for the cusps, such as an onlay, should be planned.[29] The occlusal contacts should be entirely on gold or enamel, not on a margin of the restoration.

Occlusal Preparation

Initial entry is made in the central fossa with a tapered fissure bur to establish the pulpal floor (Fig 19-14). Theoretically, the ideal occlusal depth is 1 mm in dentin or 2.5 mm at the triangular ridges. Depth is ultimately determined by the extent of existing caries lesions or restorations or the need for additional retention. The occlusal outline is extended mesiodistally along the central groove and stopped just short of the marginal ridge. The bur is held vertically in the long axis of the tooth throughout the preparation. This position and the bur's taper provide the 3- to 5-degree divergence of the facial and lingual walls (total divergence of 6 to 10 degrees) toward the occlusal aspect of the tooth (Fig 19-15).

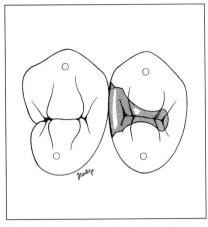

Fig 19-13 An inlay is an intracoronal restoration.

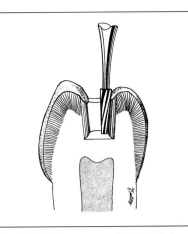

Fig 19-14 The correct pulpal depth for an inlay is established with a tapered fissure bur. It can be used to create the flat floors and well-defined internal angles.

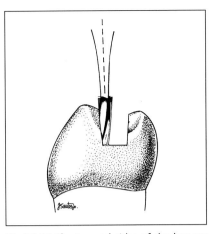

Fig 19-15 The tapered sides of the bur are used to help establish the desired occlusal divergence of the walls.

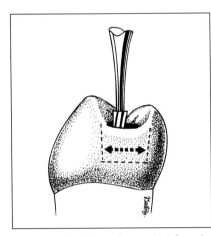

Fig 19-16 A thin layer of enamel is left on the proximal surface to protect the adjacent tooth while the proximal box is being prepared.

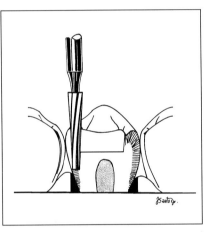

Fig 19-17 A flat gingival floor with an axial wall with slight convergence to the occlusal is created. The gingival floor is established occlusal to the gingival tissue, unless otherwise dictated.

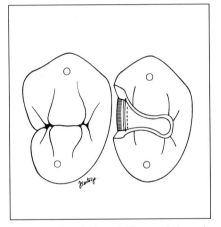

Fig 19-18 The gingivoaxial line angle is made an even depth into the tooth from the facial to the lingual wall, and the axial wall converges occlusally.

Proximal Boxes

The tapered fissure bur is used to create mesial and/or distal proximal boxes. A thin layer of proximal enamel is left to protect the adjacent tooth while the proximal box is formed (Fig 19-16). The faciolingual dimension is determined by any existing restoration or caries lesion and the relationship of the proximal surface to the adjacent tooth. The gingival floor of the box should have an axial depth of approximately 1.0 to 1.5 mm. Ideally, the gingival extension should be established occlusal to the height of the papilla (Fig 19-17). However, the presence of a caries lesion or an existing restoration, or the need for a longer wall to ensure adequate retention, may require extension to a subgingival location. The contour of the axial wall of the box should follow the faciolingual contour of the external surface of the tooth (Fig 19-18). The box should extend to the facial and lingual borders of the contact area, and the bevels should extend the preparation slightly beyond the box. This extension allows access to the gold margins facially and lingually for finishing with a disk.

Refinement

All of the preparation floors and walls should be smooth, all walls except the axial walls should be divergent occlusally, the axial walls should be convergent occlusally, and internal angles should be well defined (Figs 19-14 and 19-19). It is critical that no undercut area exists that could interfere with

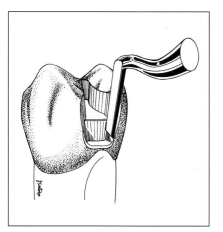

Fig 19-19 A hand instrument, such as an enamel hatchet, is helpful in smoothing the walls of the preparation.

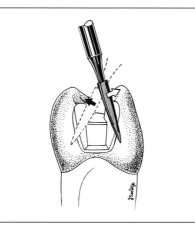

Fig 19-20 The facial and lingual proximal bevels or flares should be established slightly beyond the contact area and blended with the gingival bevel.

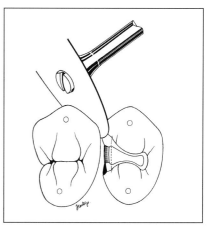

Fig 19-21 A rotary disk, placed at an angle of 45 degrees, can provide a smooth, flat bevel without undercuts.

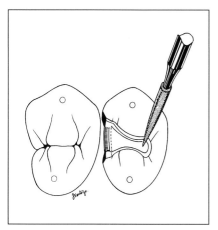

Fig 19-22a A thin, flame-shaped diamond or finishing bur is used to create a short but distinct bevel at the occlusal finish lines.

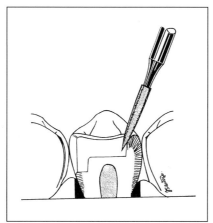

Fig 19-22b The bevel is extended across the entire occlusal margin and blended with the other bevels.

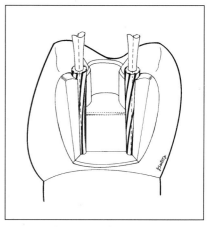

Fig 19-23 The tapered fissure bur (No. 169) is positioned at an angle to give an occlusal divergence for the retentive grooves. The grooves should be at a depth of half the diameter of the bur.

placement and withdrawal. All cavosurface margins must be distinctly defined (Figs 19-19 to 19-21).

Proximal Bevel

The proximal bevel or flare is established on the facial and lingual walls of the box with a garnet disk, a No. 7901 bur, or a thin, flame-shaped diamond bur (see Figs 19-20 and 19-21).ᐧ A finishing bur or diamond bur must be used carefully to avoid developing an undercut in the facial and lingual walls at the faciogingival or linguogingival line angle. An undercut is less likely to occur when a disk is used (see Fig 19-21). The walls of the preparation should diverge from the gingival floor in the occlusal direction. The proximal bevels should blend smoothly with the gingival and occlusal bevels.

Bevels of Horizontal Cavosurface Angles

A No. 7901 finishing bur or a thin, flame-shaped diamond bur is used to place 0.5-mm-wide occlusal, proximal, and gingival bevels along the entire cavosurface finish line (Figs 19-20, 19-22a, and 19-22b). A gingival margin trimmer may also be used to place the gingival bevels if access is too limited to use a bur. The bevels should be at an angle of approximately 45 degrees to the external surface of the tooth.

Retention Grooves

If retention grooves are needed to provide additional retention and resistance form, a No. 169 tapered fissue bur is used to place them to bisect the facioaxial and linguoaxial line angles of the box (Fig 19-23). The grooves must diverge

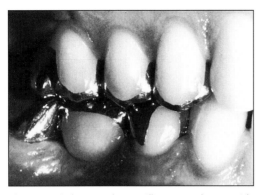

Fig 19-24 Onlays on the maxillary premolars provide protection to the facial cusps.

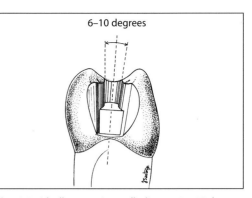

Fig 19-25 Ideally, opposing walls diverge 6 to 10 degrees for the inlay preparation.

toward the occlusal aspect in a facial and lingual direction, and the axial walls should converge occlusally.

Onlay

The onlay is essentially an inlay that covers one or more cusps. A complete onlay covers the entire occlusal surface; a partial onlay covers only a portion of the occlusal surface. The onlay incorporates the principles of both extracoronal and intracoronal restorations. Although it is generally more conservative than a partial- or complete-coverage crown, it provides the same protection of the remaining tooth structure (Fig 19-24).

There are several important features of the preparation. All finish lines are beveled. A bevel or flare creates a second plane designed to allow, with burnishing, close adaptation of the gold to the tooth. A beveled shoulder is used for the centric holding cusps (lingual cusps of maxillary posterior teeth and buccal cusps of mandibular posterior teeth) and a long bevel or chamfer is used for the noncentric cusps. The gingival margin and the facial and lingual walls of the proximal boxes are designed like those for the inlay, with their well-defined bevel or flare. These finish lines are blended to form an uninterrupted finish line around the entire preparation. The gingival floors of the proximal boxes are essentially beveled shoulders.

The width and depth of the occlusal portion of the preparation and of the proximal boxes are often dictated by the presence of an old restoration and/or a caries lesion. If additional resistance and retention form are needed, retention grooves may be placed at the axiofacial and axiolingual line angles.

A tapered fissure bur is recommended for preparing the outline form because its taper helps to establish the desired total occlusal divergence of 6 to 10 degrees for the internal facial and lingual walls. The axial walls of the proximal boxes converge toward the occlusal surface.

Occlusal Preparation

The initial entry is made in the central fossa to a depth of approximately 1.0 mm into dentin (total depth of approximately 2.5 mm in the tooth). In some cases, it may be necessary to extend some portions of the preparation to a greater depth because of carious dentin or a previous restoration or for additional retention. The occlusal outline form is extended by moving the bur laterally, cutting with the side of the bur. The occlusal outline form should be as conservative as the caries lesion or old restoration permits. The bur is kept in the long axis of the intended path of insertion so that the taper of the bur provides the desired 3- to 5-degree divergence for each internal cavity wall.

Proximal Boxes

The boxes are created on the proximal surfaces. The facial and lingual walls should exhibit a combined divergence occlusally of 6 to 10 degrees from each other as was provided in the occlusal area of the preparation (Fig 19-25). The faciolingual dimension is likely to be determined by the presence of a restoration, caries lesion, and/or the relationship of the proximal surface to the adjacent tooth (Fig 19-26). The bevels at the facial and lingual cavosurface angles will extend the preparation slightly beyond the proximal contact area so that the margins of the restoration will be accessible for finishing with a disk (Fig 19-27).

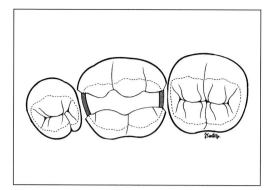

Fig 19-26 The proximal box is extended to or slightly beyond the contact area. Bevels will provide the desired proximal clearance.

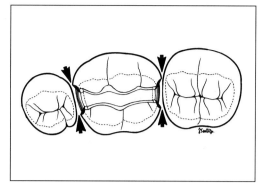

Fig 19-27 After the bevels are placed, there is access for completing the preparation's finish lines and the margins of the restoration.

Cuspal Reduction

A carbide or diamond bur is used to reduce the cusps. Depth cuts of 1.5 to 2.0 mm are made for the centric (vertical holding) cusp(s), and cuts of 1.0 to 1.5 mm are made for the noncentric cusp(s) (Fig 19-28). A bur with a measured diameter is used to gauge the depth of the cuts. The side of the bur is held parallel to the cuspal inclines to make the depth cuts. After the depth cuts are placed, a uniform reduction of the cusps that parallels the general anatomic contours of the occlusal surface is made. The cuspal heights are reduced to the full extent of the depth cuts (Figs 19-29 and 19-30). Reduction for the centric holding cusps is generally greater than that for the noncentric cusps because less thickness of the restoration is needed to withstand occlusal forces exerted against a noncentric cusp.

Shoulder Preparation

A shoulder is prepared on the external surface of the centric cusp to provide a band of metal (ferrule) to protect the tooth. The bur is held parallel to the external surface of the tooth to prepare a shoulder about 1.0 mm in height and 1.0 mm in axial depth. The finish line should extend gingivally at least 1.0 mm beyond any occlusal contacts. The occlusoaxial line angles are rounded (Fig 19-31). There must be adequate (1.0- to 1.5-mm) clearance in all eccentric mandibular movements.

Noncentric Cusp

A chamfer or long bevel may be used instead of a shoulder on the noncentric cusp(s). The bur is positioned at an angle of approximately 45 degrees to the axial surface (Fig 19-32). This provides a ferrule effect for additional protection of the cusp.

Gingival Bevel

A smooth and distinct bevel is established on the gingival margins with a No. 7901 finishing bur, a thin, flame-shaped diamond bur, or a gingival margin trimmer. This bevel should be approximately 0.5 mm in width and at an angle of approximately 45 degrees to the external surface of the tooth.

Shoulder Bevel

A 1.0-mm bevel is placed on the shoulder with a No. 7901 or fine diamond bur. This bevel is blended with the proximal bevels. Any corners or sharp angles at the junction of the various bevels and across the occlusoaxial line angles are eliminated (Fig 19-33).

Proximal Bevels

The proximal bevel or flare is established with a garnet disk, a fine, flame-shaped diamond bur, or a No. 7901 bur. Creation of an undercut during beveling at the faciogingival or linguogingival line angles must be avoided. Divergence is established from the gingival floor occlusally. The proximal bevels should blend smoothly with the gingival bevel and the buccal and lingual bevels.

Retention Grooves

If retention grooves are needed, they can be placed in both proximal boxes. A No. 169 bur is used to bisect the facioaxial and linguoaxial line angles. The grooves must diverge toward the occlusal aspect faciolingually and converge toward the occlusal aspect axially to be aligned with the internal path of insertion (Fig 19-34).

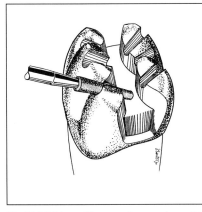

Fig 19-28 A bur of known diameter is used to establish depth cuts to guide the correct reduction of the cusps—1.5- to 2.0-mm-deep cuts on centric holding cusps and 1.0- to 1.5-mm-deep cuts in noncentric cusps.

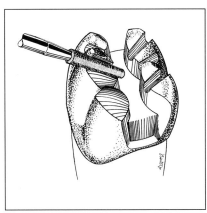

Fig 19-29 The buccal cusps are reduced in accordance with the occlusal anatomy of the tooth.

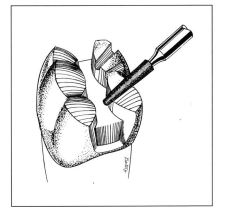

Fig 19-30 The lingual cusps of the mandibular teeth require less reduction because they are not holding cusps.

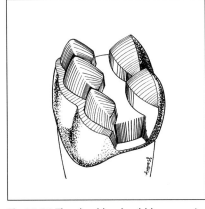

Fig 19-31 The shoulder should have precise line angles.

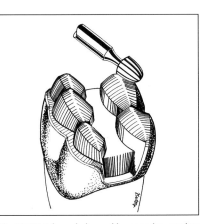

Fig 19-32 A barrel-shaped bur can be used to create the chamfer on the noncentric cusp(s).

Partial-Coverage Crown

The partial-coverage crown, or partial veneer crown, covers only a portion of the outer circumference or axial surfaces of the tooth and completely covers the occlusal surface. For instance, a three-quarter crown has three of the four axial surfaces covered by the restoration, usually leaving the facial axial surface unprepared, except at its occlusal extent; this is to preserve the facial surface for esthetics. A seven-eighths crown, usually used for maxillary molars, covers three and one-half of the four axial surfaces, usually leaving the mesiofacial half of the facial surface of the tooth unprepared. Leaving part of the external surface of the tooth uncovered offers several potential benefits. It conserves tooth structure and

avoids potential insult to the periodontium adjacent to the unrestored tooth surface.[82] Cementation is generally easier and seating is more complete than for a complete-coverage crown because escape of the excess cement is facilitated. The uncovered tooth surface allows for pulp testing.[115] Preservation of the facial surface eliminates the need to match the shade of the adjacent teeth with a ceramic material. Because it is not necessary to veneer the casting with a tooth-colored material, the laboratory procedures are simplified.[118]

Retention and resistance of the partial veneer crown are provided by a combination of extracoronal and intracoronal features. The extracoronal retention is created by opposing axial walls on the mesial and distal surfaces that have a combined convergence toward the occlusal of approximately 6 to

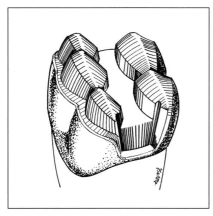

Fig 19-33 Finished onlay preparation. Internal angles are precise, occlusal line angles are rounded, the walls have the correct taper, the grooves are correctly positioned, and all the finish lines are smooth and continuous.

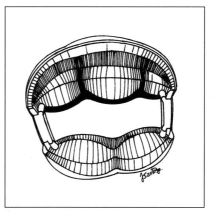

Fig 19-34 The retention grooves are placed at the linguoaxial and facioaxial line angles but do not undermine the enamel.

10 degrees. This is supplemented with grooves or boxes in the proximal walls that provide not only added retention but also resistance to lingual displacement. A slight overlay of the facial cusp protects it from fracture and provides some resistance form.

The extensions of the proximal and facial portions of the preparation can vary in design according to the specific needs. If the tooth is located so that the facial cusps are readily visible, esthetic concerns may dictate a modification of the standard design to conceal the gold. In such cases, the mesial proximal wall is extended toward the facial surface only far enough to barely break contact. Reduction of the mesial incline of the mesiofacial cusp of molars and the mesial incline of the facial cusp of premolars is limited. The distal incline is reduced more to provide protection and the ferrule effect. This more esthetic design is shown in Fig 19-35.

Because partial-coverage crowns are infrequently placed on anterior teeth, this section focuses on the posterior teeth.

Occlusal Reduction

Depth cuts are made by laying the side of the bur (of measured diameter) against the cuspal inclines (Fig 19-36) and reducing them to the desired depth (Fig 19-37). The total reduction of the centric cusp should be 1.5 to 2.0 mm, and that of the noncentric cusp should be 1.0 to 1.5 mm. The remaining occlusal surface is reduced, but the general anatomic contours are maintained (Fig 19-38). As previously mentioned, less reduction may be desirable in some areas for esthetic reasons. The placement of an occlusal channel and the facial bevel are discussed later.

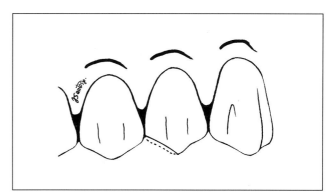

Fig 19-35 Limited reduction of the mesiofacial incline of the facial cusp and greater reduction of the distofacial incline of a maxillary tooth provide some protection to the cusp while limiting the display of gold in a partial-coverage restoration.

Lingual Reduction

The axial wall of the lingual surface is reduced with a round-ended tapered diamond bur. Close attention must be paid to the desired path of insertion to establish parallelism. A two-plane reduction of the tooth is needed to maintain natural contours. Because of the anatomic differences in the lingual contours of the maxillary and the mandibular teeth, the second plane on the lingual surface of a maxillary tooth will be more pronounced. The gingival portion of the lingual surface should have a 3- to 5-degree convergence occlusal to the path of insertion (Fig 19-39), and the second plane should be offset about 30 degrees.

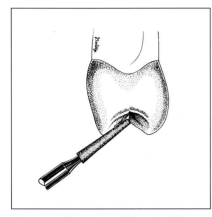

Fig 19-36 The diamond bur is held at the same angle as the natural slope of the cusp to create an even occlusal reduction for partial-coverage crowns.

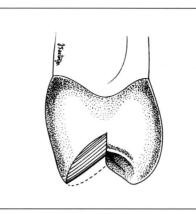

Fig 19-37 Removal of 1.0 to 1.5 mm of tooth structure from the noncentric cusp serves as a guide to reducing the rest of the occlusal surface.

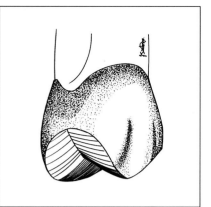

Fig 19-38 The occlusal reduction has followed the original contours of the occlusal surface.

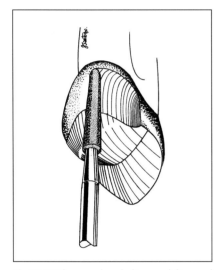

Fig 19-39 The round-ended tapered diamond bur is very effective in creating the proper taper and in creating a chamfer finish line.

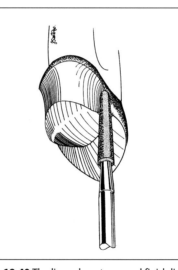

Fig 19-40 The lingual contours and finish line should be carried into the proximal surfaces. Lack of access may require use of a thinner diamond initially.

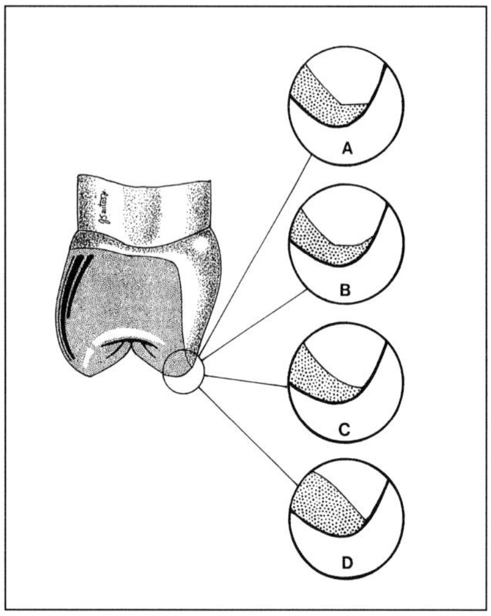

Fig 19-41 Variation in occlusobuccal finish lines for maxillary partial coverage crown—(A) flat bevel, (B) contrabevel, and (C) knife-edged—are acceptable finish lines. A bevel is not absolutely necessary with adequate enamel support; however, the finish line in (D) would compromise finish and resistance form with unsupported enamel, making a bevel necessary. (Redrawn from Shillingburg et al,[119] after Ingraham et al[120] and Richter and Ueno.[71])

Proximal Reduction

The proximal surfaces are reduced in one plane. A 3- to 5-degree taper is established from the finish line to the occlusoaxial line angle. Space limitations may require use of a thin tapered diamond initially until enough space has been created to use a round-ended tapered diamond bur. The round-ended diamond bur has a more appropriate shape to create a chamfer finish line (Fig 19-40).

Finish Lines

The junction of each proximal wall and the lingual wall is blended so that there is a smooth transition. This procedure is especially important at the finish line. The gingival finish lines are placed slightly coronal to the gingival tissue if possible. The presence of caries lesions or existing restorations may alter the level of finish line placement, but, regardless of where the finish line is located, the transition should be

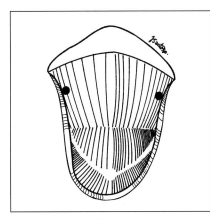

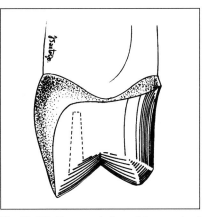

Fig 19-42a Before the proximal grooves are prepared, their desired location is marked with a pencil or an indentation made by a bur. This aids in obtaining the correct faciolingual location.

Fig 19-42b The angulation of the proximal groove is equally important, so visualization is critical.

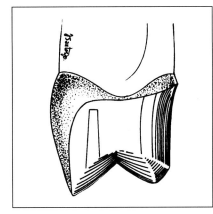

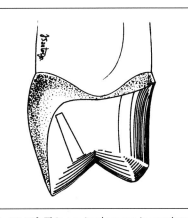

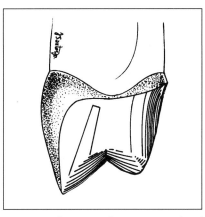

Fig 19-43a Alignment of the proximal groove with the long axis of the tooth provides the best compatibility with the rest of the preparation design.

Fig 19-43b This proximal groove is angulated too much toward the lingual surface and will not provide adequate resistance to lingual rotation.

Fig 19-43c This proximal groove is angulated too much toward the facial surface, creating an undercut in relation to the lingual surface of the preparation, thus interfering with the path of insertion.

smooth and well defined. For the buccal finish line of partial-coverage crowns for maxillary teeth, several different configurations may be used, balancing the need for resistance form and for facial esthetics (Fig 19-41).

Proximal Grooves

The grooves are initiated in the proximal areas with a No. 170 bur (or a No. 169 bur for a small tooth). The grooves are located as far facially as possible without undermining the facial enamel. It may be helpful to mark the proposed location of the grooves before they are prepared (Figs 19-42a and 19-42b). Because the grooves must have a path of draw compatible with each other and with the axial walls, their angulation must be carefully planned before they are begun. As a general rule for posterior teeth, the grooves should be

parallel to the long axis of the tooth (Fig 19-43a). The axial walls of the two grooves should converge occlusally. Failure to align the grooves correctly will result in a preparation that does not have an acceptable path of insertion (Figs 19-43b and 19-43c).

The axial depth of each groove is made equal to or slightly greater than the diameter of the No. 170 bur. After the first proximal groove is cut, the groove on the opposite side of the preparation is cut in the same fashion so that it aligns with the first groove and with the axial walls (Fig 19-44). The grooves may be enlarged, and the internal walls may be left rounded or more acutely refined to form boxes. In many cases, a box form is present after the removal of an existing restoration. Existing boxes may be modified and incorporated in the preparation in lieu of grooves (Fig 19-45).

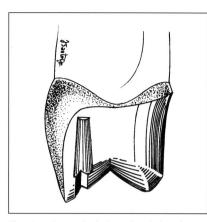

Fig 19-44 Properly designed and placed proximal groove.

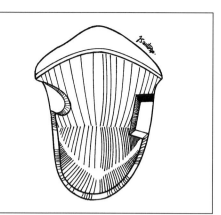

Fig 19-45 A groove is located on one proximal surface and a box on the other. Both meet the requirements for occlusal divergence of the facial and lingual walls and convergence of the axial wall toward the opposite proximal wall. The groove has a lingual "lip" to enhance resistance to lingual displacement.

Occlusal Channel

The resistance form and strength of the restoration can be enhanced by preparation of an occlusal channel. A channel may already exist if an occlusal restoration has been removed. If not, it may be prepared. A flat-ended tapered carbide or diamond bur is used to cut the channel or to remove undercuts in an existing channel. The channel allows the space for a "staple" of thicker metal in the restoration that resists lingual displacement and helps the restoration resist deformation under pressure (Fig 19-46).

Facial Bevel

Placement of the facial finish line differs in the maxillary teeth and the mandibular teeth. Because the maxillary facial cusp is usually the noncentric cusp, only a 1.0-mm layer of metal and a short bevel are required to protect the cusp (Fig 19-47). Placement of a shoulder and a bevel are recommended for the facial cusp in mandibular teeth to help restorations withstand the forces on centric cusps. A shoulder extending 1.0 mm long occlusogingivally and 1.0 mm deep axially is placed into the facial surface across the facial cusp with a straight fissure bur held parallel to the external surface of the tooth (Fig 19-48). A 0.5- to 1.0-mm-wide bevel is placed with a fine diamond or a finishing bur. The finish line should be placed gingival to any occlusal contacts.

Final Refinement

All the sharp external angles of the preparation are rounded. Sharp angles make it more difficult to pour the stone into the impression without bubbles. Even if the die is poured without

bubbles, it has fragile edges that are easily abraded during laboratory procedures. After all the angles of the preparation are rounded, the surfaces are smoothed with a fine-grit diamond bur. Figure 19-49 illustrates some completed preparations.

Complete-Coverage Gold Castings

As its name implies, the complete-coverage, or full veneer, casting includes coverage of the entire coronal portion of the tooth. Extensive loss of tooth structure is the most common indication for complete coverage. For esthetic reasons, this restoration tends to be limited to molars. Because the restoration involves the entire circumference of the tooth, control of occlusal and proximal relationships allows improvements in occlusion and proximal contacts. Correction of tooth positioning is sometimes possible.

Retention is provided primarily or entirely by the extracoronal walls. A complete-coverage crown is the most retentive of the casting designs.[121,122] One or more grooves or boxes can be added to the preparation if additional retention and resistance form are needed.

Proximal Reduction

A thin, tapered carbide or diamond bur is placed at either the facial or lingual embrasure and used to cut proximal tooth structure toward the opposite embrasure (Figs 19-50a and 19-50b). The bur should be extended cervically to the desired location of the gingival finish line. Unless a caries lesion or an old restoration dictates otherwise, the gingival finish line

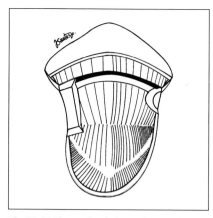

Fig 19-46 The occlusal channel generally parallels the contour of the facial surface rather than cutting straight across the tooth to the opposite wall. Note the inadequate proximal groove, which provides little resistance to lingual displacement.

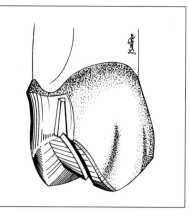

Fig 19-47 Note the shape of the occlusal channel as it comes across the occlusal surface to connect to the proximal groove. Also note the small facial bevel.

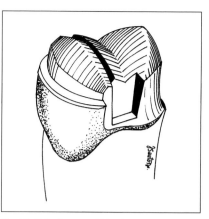

Fig 19-48 In the mandible, the centric holding cusp requires a facial design similar to that of the onlay preparation.

Fig 19-49 *Preparations for partial-coverage crowns require the same refinement of walls, floors, and bevels as are needed for inlay and onlay preparations.*

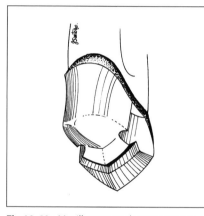

Fig 19-49a Maxillary premolar preparation.

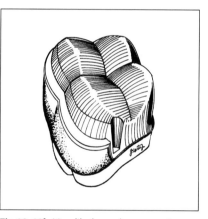

Fig 19-49b Mandibular molar preparation.

should be established at least 0.5 mm supragingivally. The reduction must be at the expense of the tooth being prepared to avoid damage to the enamel of the adjacent tooth. The reduction, when completed, should taper occlusally 3 to 5 degrees toward the opposing proximal wall. The opposing wall is prepared in the same manner. Once enough space has been created to permit access, a round-ended tapered diamond is used to complete the proximal reduction and place a gingival chamfer.

Occlusal Reduction

A series of depth cuts is made on the occlusal surface with a diamond or a fissure bur. Both the facial and lingual cuspal inclines are cut to a depth of at least 1.5 mm to allow an adequate thickness of metal for strength and wear. An even reduction that follows the original anatomic contours allows the development of the appropriate occlusal anatomy in the restoration. The corrugated effect of this occlusal reduction adds strength to the crown.

Facial and Lingual Reduction

The facial and lingual surfaces are each reduced in two planes to allow reproduction of normal contours in the restoration. The first plane, extending occlusally from the gingival finish line, should have a 3- to 5-degree taper to the path of insertion (Fig 19-51). The second plane should be angled at 30 to

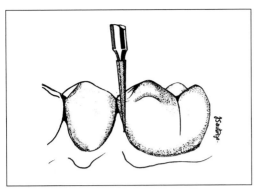

Fig 19-50a Use of a thin, flame-shaped diamond bur is recommended to initiate the proximal reduction of the preparation for a complete-coverage restoration.

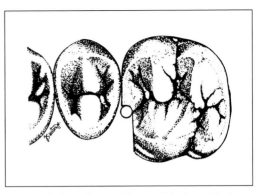

Fig 19-50b The reduction is kept within the original contours of the tooth so that abrasion of the adjacent tooth is avoided.

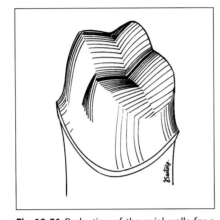

Fig 19-51 Reduction of the axial walls for a complete-coverage restoration is identical to that for the partial-coverage crowns, except the facial wall is also included. At this stage, the facial and lingual walls are each in one plane.

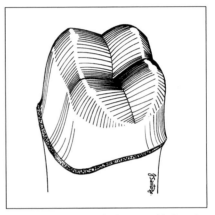

Fig 19-52 The second plane is added to the facial and lingual walls. The second plane should be at a 30- to 45-degree angle to the long axis and involves the occlusal third of the centric holding cusp and the occlusal fourth of the noncentric cusp.

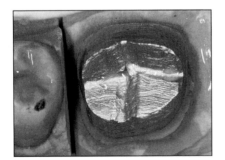

Fig 19-53a Die of full crown preparation, mandibular left first molar, occlusal view.

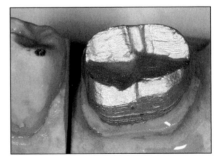

Fig 19-53b Facial view of preparation showing the second plane of reduction.

45 degrees to the first plane to allow desired facial and lingual contours to be reestablished (Figs 19-52 and 19-53). This second plane should begin at the occlusal third of the wall for the centric cusp and the occlusal fourth for the noncentric cusp. A round-ended, tapered diamond is used to make these reductions. A modified conservative full-coverage preparation, involving supragingival margins on both lingual and buccal aspects, has shown excellent long-term results.[100]

Refinement

The parts of the preparation are blended to eliminate indefinite areas along the finish line, irregularities in the walls, and sharp corners. A finish line that is distinct around the whole preparation must be established. The facioproximal and linguoproximal line angles often need to be rounded and distinctly defined. All of the sharp corners of the preparation, such as the occlusoaxial line angles, are rounded. The surfaces of the preparation should be relatively smooth. The preparation is viewed carefully from more than one angle to ensure that there are no undercuts within any wall, between the walls, or in relationship to an adjacent tooth.

Try-In

Before the casting is fitted to the prepared tooth, it should be adjusted to fit the master die. The intaglio surface of the casting is inspected under magnification for bubbles or other imperfections,[123,124] which can be removed with a small round bur. The die is checked for defects or abraded areas. The casting should not be forced onto the die. If the casting does not seat easily, the die should be sprayed with a disclosing medium and the crown should then be gently reseated. The disclosing medium should mark areas that are binding on the inside of the casting. These areas can be relieved with a bur (No. 2 or No. 4 round bur). This process is repeated until the casting is fully seated.

Once the casting is fully seated on the die, the interproximal contacts are checked and necessary adjustments made. This is best accomplished on a solid cast, especially if there are multiple castings. The occlusion in maximum intercuspation (MI) is adjusted until the restoration holds shimstock equally as well as the adjacent natural teeth. The location and size of the occlusal contacts are marked with articulating paper. A finishing bur, stone, or abrasive disk is used to make any modifications needed. After MI contacts on the restoration are similar to MI contacts on other teeth in the quadrant or arch, if the type of cast articulation is fairly accurate, contacts in excursive movements are marked and adjusted to remove excursive interferences. The internal surface of the casting

may be carefully air abraded with aluminum oxide, avoiding the margins, in preparation for the clinical try-in. Air abrasion provides a dull, matte finish. Any area that binds during intraoral seating of the casting creates a bright, burnished mark. If these steps are accomplished with precision before the patient arrives, minimal chair time should be required for adjustments.

Once adjustments have been made on the cast, the casting is tried on the prepared tooth to determine the fit. Adjustments to the proximal contacts are made if needed. The internal surface is inspected for shiny spots. The shiny spots are adjusted, and the casting is reseated. The casting is removed and reinspected for new shiny spots. This process may need to be repeated several times until the casting is fully seated.

An alternative method to seat castings employs disclosing media. Disclosing media include chloroform and rouge, disclosing pastes or waxes[125] and impression materials.[126] Whatever the choice, the medium is placed on the internal surface of the casting, and it is then seated. The casting is removed and inspected for abrasion of the disclosing medium that allows the gold to show through. These areas are adjusted as needed, more disclosing medium is placed, and the casting is reseated. This process is continued until the casting is fully seated.

The fitting process is completed when the margins are flush against the finish lines of the preparation and there is no binding when the restoration is seated. The casting should fit passively in place. A tight fit usually means the casting is not fully seated. Use of a die spacer medium, painted onto the die to within 0.5 to 1.0 mm of the finish line prior to wax pattern fabrication, will usually simplify the process of fitting the casting.[126]

Marginal Finishing

Marginal finishing is done prior to cementation to adapt and polish margins that have already been determined to be satisfactory. The goal is to develop a margin that is adapted to the preparation finish line, extends to, but not beyond, the finish line, and blends with the contours of the tooth.[127] The casting must be fully seated before an attempt can be made to adapt and finish the margins.

Margin location determines whether margin finishing can be done on the tooth. Subgingival and/or interproximal margins are very difficult to reach without damaging the soft tissue, bone, or the tooth itself. For these margins, all finishing must be done on the die. Easily accessible margins can be finished while the casting is seated on the tooth (Fig 19-54). If the margin is tightly adapted but slightly overcontoured or undercontoured, a white stone or abrasive disk can be used

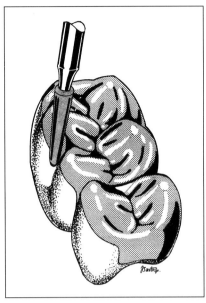

Fig 19-54 A fine diamond bur or finishing stone is held perpendicular to the margin and moved parallel to the margin to reduce small discrepancies in the marginal area.

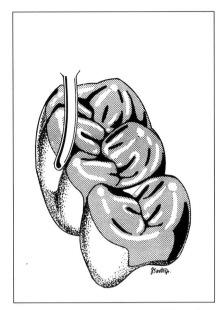

Fig 19-55a Pressure is applied with the side or tip of the burnisher, moved parallel to the marginal area to adapt it more tightly to the tooth.

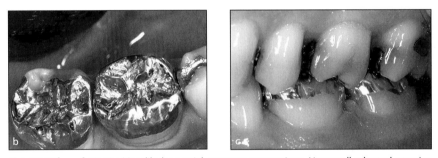

Figs 19-55b and 19-55c Mandibular partial-coverage restorations. Note well-adapted margins that have been burnished.

in a low-speed handpiece to reduce the protruding surface, whether it is gold or enamel. When finished, the gold margin should be flush with the tooth structure, and adjacent contours of the restoration should be continuous with natural tooth contours. The stone or disk should be rotated from the metal to the tooth or parallel to the margin, but never from tooth to gold. Rubber points or fine-grit abrasive disks may be used to produce a high luster if access permits. Care must be exercised to avoid damage to the soft tissue or abrasion of the tooth surface.

Marginal adaptation can sometimes be improved by hand burnishing, both on the die and on the tooth prior to cementation. Well-controlled pressure is applied with a beavertail or ball burnisher, held adjacent to, and moved parallel to, the

gold margin (Figs 19-55a to 19-55c). The burnisher should not be placed directly on the margin. Pressure should be applied with a back-and-forth motion (parallel to the margin) that moves slowly closer to the margin. Because a small area of the burnisher is contacting the gold, a great deal of pressure (force per unit area) is applied. The casting is stabilized during the burnishing process to ensure that it does not change position. It is also critical to have good finger rests to ensure that the burnisher does not slip off the tooth and injure the soft tissue or the tooth itself if the burnishing is done in the mouth. Some additional benefit may be achieved by burnishing the margins of the casting on the tooth during the cementing procedure, before the cement sets.

Cementation

The final step in the process is luting or cementation of the casting. Cement failure has been shown to be the second[128] or third[129] most important factor in the failure of cast restorations. A thin layer of the luting agent (cement) is placed in the casting and on the walls of the preparation, and the casting is then seated on or in the tooth. The cement hardens within a few minutes, and the excess is removed. The luting agent fills the gap between the casting and tooth to provide retention and to minimize leakage at the margin. Some luting agents, such as zinc phosphate cement, provide retention entirely from frictional resistance to displacement. Others, such as the adhesive resin cements, bond to the tooth and/or the casting to provide adhesion in addition to frictional resistance. It appears that resin cements or resin-modified glass-ionomer cements provide superior retention and have better physical properties. However, it is essential to understand that no cement will compensate for inadequate preparation resistance and retention form in the long term. Therefore, when sound preparation design principles can be used, the choice of cement is of little clinical relevance.[130,131] But clinical situations often vary from the ideal, so cement selection can be of real importance. An understanding of the advantages and limitations of each type of cement is relevant.

Selection of a Luting Agent

The most commonly used luting agents today are zinc phosphate, glass-ionomer, polycarboxylate, resin, and resin-modified glass-ionomer cements.[132] A survey[133] of 10,000 dentists conducted in 1990 revealed that glass-ionomer cements were used most frequently for cementation of crowns (42%), followed by polycarboxylate (33%), zinc phosphate (22%), resin cement (2%), and zinc oxide–eugenol (1%) cements. Since that time, resin cements and resin-modified glass-ionomer cements have gained popularity, with much of the current research in the area of cements focused on these two materials. The type of cement used does not seem to influence the final margin adaptation, so the ease of manipulation and strict adherence to the protocol for each specific luting agent have a more significant impact on the ultimate strength and solubility properties that, in turn, affect the clinical performance of the final restoration.[130,134] Because the indications and procedures for each luting agent are different, they are discussed separately.

Zinc Phosphate Cement

Zinc phosphate cement consists of a powder containing 90% zinc oxide and 10% magnesium oxide that is incorporated into a liquid containing approximately 67% phosphoric acid.[20] Among the many luting agents available, zinc phosphate has the longest record (more than 100 years) of successful use.[135] It has good compressive strength and low film thickness, and it is relatively easy to manipulate.[20] Excess cement is easily removed after it has set. Relatively high compressive and tensile strengths make it a good choice for long-span fixed partial dentures.[136] In a study of zinc phosphate cement samples taken from castings that had been in service for up to 48 years, the cement was found to have maintained a stable chemical structure.[137]

Zinc phosphate cement is slightly soluble in oral fluids, allows relatively high levels of microleakage,[138] and is sometimes associated with postoperative sensitivity.[139,140] Despite these drawbacks, it is not unusual to see patients with gold castings that were cemented more than 30 years ago with zinc phosphate cement. In a study of eight restorations that had been in service for 22 years despite positive microleakage tests, no evidence of carious tooth structure, sensitivity, or pulpal degeneration was observed.[141]

Zinc phosphate cement should be mixed on a glass slab that has been chilled, preferably to just above the dew point to avoid water condensation that could contaminate the mix and weaken the set cement. Powder should be mixed into the liquid in small increments over a large area of the glass slab. This method dissipates the heat released during the exothermic setting reaction and provides a longer working time. The slower the mix and cooler the glass slab, the longer the working time. A cool glass slab also allows more powder to be incorporated into the liquid, resulting in improved physical properties.[142] From a practical standpoint, refrigerated glass slabs (4° to 8°C) always induce water condensation, but the coldness of the slab still allows the incorporation of more powder to the mix, which compensates for the water contamination and leads to improved compressive strength.[143]

Powder is added until the mixed material adheres to the spatula to form a 1-inch string when the spatula is lifted from the glass slab. The mixing should be completed within 90 seconds after initiation. If the mixing is prolonged beyond approximately 90 seconds, the hardening of the cement caused by the setting reaction may be confused with having achieved the proper powder-liquid ratio.[144] Its relatively long working time makes zinc phosphate cement a good choice when multiple castings are luted at the same time.

Glass-Ionomer Cement

Traditional glass-ionomer luting cement is a modification of the glass-ionomer restorative material. It consists of a powder containing aluminum fluorosilicate glass particles that are incorporated into a liquid containing polyalkenoic acids. In some products, these acids are freeze-dried and included in the powder that is mixed with water.[145] It bonds to tooth structure by formation of ionic bonds to hydroxyapatite crystals in enamel and dentin.[145] It is speculated that glass ionomers have the potential to inhibit caries because of fluoride release, but the critical level of fluoride release over time to prevent caries is well beyond the release rate of current glass-ionomer luting cements.[146,147] Glass-ionomer luting cement has a low film thickness (20 to 25 μm) and better physical properties than zinc phosphate cement.[20,148,149] However, a glass ionomer may take a significant amount of time before reaching ultimate strength.[150,151] Glass-ionomer cements may be hand-mixed but are also available in preweighed capsules that allow mixing in an amalgamator. Persistent reports of excessive postoperative sensitivity associated with glass-ionomer luting agents have not been borne out in clinical studies.[152–155] Glass-ionomer cements appear to be more technique sensitive than zinc phosphate cements because the surface of the preparation needs to remain moist before cementation and the cement at the margin of the restoration must be isolated from moisture but not desiccated after cementation.[130]

Glass-ionomer cement is very sensitive to early moisture contamination. If exposed to external moisture during the setting reaction (usually 5 minutes), the reaction is interrupted, resulting in a cement with high solubility and poor physical properties.[156] Therefore, glass-ionomer cement should not be used until contamination can be prevented. As with glass-ionomer restorative materials, dehydration is also a problem.[157] Excess cement should not be removed from the margins for at least 5 minutes after the crown is seated. Leaving a bead of excess cement in place protects the underlying layers of cement from moisture contamination.[158] Because glass-ionomer cement bonds to the tooth surface, excess cement is somewhat difficult to remove once set, particularly in the interproximal areas.

When glass-ionomer cement is mixed by hand, the premeasured powder is incorporated into the premeasured liquid in bulk as quickly as possible. A chilled slab has been shown to increase the working time significantly for glass-ionomer cements, as it has for zinc phosphate cements.[159] Most manufacturers now offer an encapsulated form of glass-ionomer luting cement; this results in properly proportioned cement that is thoroughly mixed in a few seconds. Glass-ionomer cement has a relatively short working time, so a single mix should be limited to luting no more than two or three units. If additional units have to be luted, a new mix of cement should be used.

Resin-Modified Glass-Ionomer Cements

Like the resin cements and traditional glass-ionomer cements, the resin-modified glass-ionomer cements are modified restorative materials. The combination of resin and glass-ionomer chemistries overcomes some of the problems with moisture contamination and dehydration experienced with glass-ionomer cements[160] and eliminates many of the steps necessary for resin cements.[132] In addition, they release fluoride, providing potential anticaries activity.[161] Resin-modified glass-ionomer cements have physical properties between those of conventional glass-ionomer and resin cements.[149] Their adhesive properties to tooth structure are similar to those of traditional glass ionomers,[162] and they have adequately low film thicknesses.[163,164] They absorb fluids during and after setting, causing a net expansion.[165,166] One anecdotal clinical report and two in vitro studies[167–169] have linked early resin-modified glass-ionomer formulations with all-ceramic crown fractures. The current generation of resin-modified glass-ionomer cements has apparently overcome this deficiency.[170,171]

Resin Luting Cements

Adhesive cements, and especially resin cements, present additional challenges. First, they are significantly more technique sensitive than traditional luting agents. Most require multiple time-consuming steps and strict moisture control. In addition, resin cements are very difficult to remove from crown margins once they are completely set. Removal of cement flash is made difficult by the relative inaccessibility of crown margins, irregular root topography, and the clear or tooth-colored nature of many resin cements. For these reasons, many clinicians do not use resin cements routinely for posterior applications. However, some circumstances dictate the use of resin cement. Due to their adhesive properties, a resin cement is the material of choice when luting a crown with minimal retention and resistance features. In addition, resin cements must be used when bonding all-ceramic noncore crowns. As is the case with most dental materials, a clear understanding of the advantages and disadvantages, as well as clinical indications, is essential when making a material selection for a given circumstance.

The resin cements are especially designed for use with bonded ceramic restorations, but they may also be used with cast restorations. They are generally supplied as a dual-paste system in which the two parts are mixed just prior to the cementation process. Polymerization may be initiated by a chemical catalyst or by a combination of a chemical catalyst and a light-activated catalyst, but for cast restorations, chemically cured cements are indicated. Resin cements differ from resin composite restorative materials primarily in their reduced filler content[172]; reduction of the filler content leads to better flow and reduced film thickness, which are desirable properties for a luting cement.[173] Some resin cements contain fillers that are capable of providing fluoride release,[174] although there is questionable therapeutic effect due to the low levels and short duration of fluoride release.[175]

Resin cements have the best physical properties of all of the cements.[149,176,177] They are virtually insoluble in oral fluids and have the highest compressive and tensile strengths of all the cements. They also exhibit less microleakage[178] than other luting agents. If used in combination with a dentin adhesive system, they bond to tooth structure and to some metals.[142] For this reason, as previously stated, they are often recommended for less retentive preparations.[179–181]

There are several potential problems associated with resin cements. There is great variation in the physical properties and handling characteristics among resin cements,[163] which can cause confusion for clinicians. The film thickness tends to be greater than that of other cements,[163,182,183] so incomplete seating of the casting could be a problem. This is especially true when a dentin adhesive is used, because without due care, it can pool in the internal angles of the preparation. Resin cements require the most clinical steps if used with an adhesive system, so there is more chance for an error in technique to occur. There are no long-term clinical studies to determine if the high retention values and low microleakage are long lasting in castings cemented with resin cements.

Polycarboxylate and Zinc Oxide–Eugenol Cements

Polycarboxylate and zinc oxide–eugenol cements are no longer widely used with cast restorations. Their properties are generally inferior to those of the cements previously discussed. Historically, some clinicians have used them if a tooth has had a history of sensitivity. They have also been used as temporary luting agents and with stainless steel crowns.

Preparing the Tooth for Cementation

Although some materials are more adversely affected by the presence of contaminants than others, no material fares well if used in the presence of oils, debris, saliva, blood, or other significant contamination. It is important to ensure that the area is cleaned, free of excess moisture, and well isolated. Bleeding and other significant sources of contamination must be well controlled. Temporary cements leave a layer of debris on the dentin surface[184] that should be removed before

cementation. This may be accomplished with pumice, detergents, and/or cleaning agents.

Some clinicians recommend the additional step of disinfecting the preparation with chlorhexidine, EDTA, or benzalkonium. The rationale is that bacteria are a primary cause of postoperative sensitivity,[60,61] so disinfection of the dentin surface will lower the number of microbes and thus reduce one cause of sensitivity. Another approach is to use desensitizing agents, usually including HEMA or a potassium oxalate–based salt. These agents can be applied immediately before final impression and/or after etching if a bonded resin system is used. They essentially disinfect the dentin and seal the tubules. Their use seems not to interfere with crown retention regardless the type of luting cement used.[185–187]

In addition to cleaning and isolating the preparation, specific additional steps are recommended to prepare the tooth to receive certain cements. Preparation surface texturing obtained either by rotary instruments or sandblasting with 50-μm aluminum oxide has been shown to increase crown retention significantly, regardless of the choice of cement.[172,188,189]

Zinc Phosphate Cement

Because zinc phosphate cement exhibits the most microleakage of any cement[163] and has been associated with postcementation sensitivity, several methods have been recommended to prevent sensitivity by "sealing" the dentin prior to cementation. Copal varnish has a long history of use for this purpose, with anecdotal reports of success. However, copal varnish doesn't disinfect the dentin, and its effectiveness has limited duration.[190] More recently, use of dentin primers and adhesives to seal the dentin before cementation has resulted in reports of decreased sensitivity. However, a recent study has noted a marked (42%) decrease in retention with the application of a resin-based sealer prior to cementation. Conversely, an increase in retention was noticeable with glass-ionomer and resin-modified glass-ionomer cements.[191]

Glass-Ionomer Cements

For glass-ionomer cements, the tooth should be clean and slightly moist.[152] No cavity varnish should be placed that might prevent bonding of this luting agent to the tooth surface. The area should be well isolated to prevent moisture contamination during the luting process and for several minutes following the seating of the restoration.

Resin Cements

Most resin cements have corresponding dentin adhesive systems that are applied immediately before cementation. In most cases, the preparation is etched and a primer and adhesive are placed. Each adhesive system has specific instructions for its use that must be followed precisely to obtain the best results. Failure to follow the specific directions for both the adhesive and the luting resin can mean the difference between success and failure. It must be emphasized that excellent isolation is a necessity when a resin cement is used.

A small amount of the cement should be mixed and observed before cementation procedures are started to confirm that the cement will set. Some autocuring resin cements have short shelf lives and lose their ability to polymerize.

Resin-Modified Glass-Ionomer Cements

One of the advantages of resin-modified glass-ionomer cements is that the cementation procedure is fairly simple. Multiple bonding steps are not necessary, and no special preparation of the tooth surface is performed, other than to make it clean and slightly moist. Removal of excess cement is relatively easy.

Preparing the Casting for Cementation

After adjustments have been made and the external surface of the casting has been polished, the internal surface of the casting should be air abraded with aluminum oxide to produce a uniform, slightly roughened finish. Margins must be avoided or protected when the internal surface is air abraded. The casting should then be cleaned to remove any contaminants, such as polishing compounds. Ammonia, detergents, or various other cleaning solutions may be used in an ultrasonic bath, or the casting can be cleaned with a steam cleaner.

If an adhesive resin cement is used, additional retention can be obtained by tin-plating the inside of the casting.[192,193] A number of inexpensive tin-plating systems that can be used to deposit a thin layer of tin on the surface of the gold alloy are commercially available. This simple process can be done in the laboratory or operatory in a few minutes.[192] A newer generation of metal surface treatments, the Rocatec[194] (3M ESPE) and Silicoater[195] (Kulzer) systems, both produce a coating that has been shown to significantly increase bond strength of resin to metal. Yet another alternative that has shown promising results is the use of an adhesive system that has an alloy primer.[196]

Seating the Casting

With zinc phosphate and glass-ionomer cements, the cement is mixed and placed in the casting. Some clinicians also like to place a layer of the cement on the walls of the preparation for intracoronal restorations. The casting should be half filled,

and all of the margins should be covered. Once the casting is seated with finger pressure, the patient is instructed to bite on an orangewood stick or other seating instrument. The instrument is moved up and down and then side to side. This technique, called *dynamic seating*, results in more complete seating of the casting.[197] The margins are checked with an explorer to determine that complete seating has been accomplished.

The excess cement must be removed with proper timing and care. If removal is attempted before the cement is set, thin strands of cement may be dragged from under the margins, thus creating voids. The bead of extruded cement has been shown to protect the cement at the margin from moisture contamination.[158] Therefore, it is important to check the cement to ensure that it has set before the excess is removed. Excess cement may be removed with an explorer or curette and floss or yarn. The gingival crevice should be flushed with water frequently to remove any loose particles. As a final step, an assistant should supply a continuous stream of air to each margin while the clinician gently reflects the free gingiva with an explorer to check for any remaining cement. Cement left subgingivally can cause tissue inflammation. A knot is tied in the floss and then the floss is pulled back and forth through the gingival embrasure to remove loose pieces from the interproximal areas.

As discussed previously, there are some distinct advantages of adhesive resin luting cements in certain situations, but their use requires different seating procedures than those used for zinc phosphate and glass-ionomer cements. For each resin-based cement, manufacturer's instructions should be followed closely. The internal surface of the casting should be air abraded, tin-plated, or both, to increase retention. Procedure guides accompanying the resin cement should be adhered to. Removal of excess adhesive resin cement from exposed areas of the tooth and adjacent teeth can be a bit difficult, so a large amount of excess cement should be avoided. The adhesive and luting materials are mixed and applied according to the manufacturer's instructions, and the casting is seated using procedures similar to those used for other cements. Setting times for these materials vary, and the time to remove excess cement is critical, so, again, instructions must be followed closely.

The occlusion is reevaluated and final adjustments are made, if necessary. The patient is informed of the possibility of postcementation sensitivity and that a minor additional adjustment of the occlusion may be necessary. The patient is instructed in proper oral hygiene measures to ensure prevention of caries and periodontal problems.

References

1. Bentley C, Drake EW. Longevity of restorations in dental school clinic. J Dent Educ 1986;50:594–600.

2. Marynuik GA. In search of treatment longevity—A 30 year perspective. J Am Dent Assoc 1984;109:739–744.

3. Mjör IA. Placement and replacement of restorations. Oper Dent 1981;6:49–54.

4. Minker JS. Simplified full coverage preparations. Dent Clin North Am 1965;9:355–372.

5. Mjör IA, Jokstad A, Qvist V. Longevity of posterior restorations. Int Dent J 1990;40:11–17.

6. Vanderhaug J. A 15-year clinical evaluation of fixed prosthodontics. Acta Odontol Scand 1991;49:35–40.

7. Shillingburg HT, Jacobi R, Brackett SE. Fundamentals of Tooth Preparation. Chicago: Quintessence, 1987:112.

8. Salis SG, Good J, Stokes A, Kirk E. Patterns of indirect fracture in intact and restored human premolar teeth. Endod Dent Traumatol 1987;3:10–14.

9. Sorensen JA, Martinoff JT. Intracoronal reinforcement and coronal coverage: A study of endodontically treated teeth. J Prosthet Dent 1984;51:780–784.

10. Oden A, Tullberg M. Cracks in gold cemented on amalgam restorations. Acta Odontol Scand 1985;43:15–17

11. Stoll R, Fisher C, Springer M, Stachniss V. Margin adaptation of partial crowns cast in pure titanium and in a gold alloy—An in vitro study. J Oral Rehabil 2002;29:1–6.

12. Delong R, Pintado MR, Douglas WH. The wear of enamel opposing shaded ceramic restorative materials: An in vitro study. J Prosthet Dent 1992;68:42–48.

13. Enderle J, Blanchard S, Bronzino J. Introduction to Biomedical Engineering. San Diego, CA: Academic Press, 2000: 554–557.

14. Canay S, Cehreli MC, Bilgic S. In vitro evaluation of the effect of a current bleaching agent on the electrochemical corrosion of dental alloys. J Oral Rehabil 2002;29:1014–1019.

15. Walker RS, Wade AG, Iazzetti G, Sarkar NK. Galvanic interaction between gold and amalgam: Effect of zinc, time and surface treatments. J Am Dent Assoc 2003;134:1463–1467.

16. Meyer RD, Meyer J, Taloumis LJ. Intraoral galvanic corrosion: Literature review and case report. J Prosthet Dent 1993;69:141–143.

17. Willershausen-Zonnchen B, Gross E, Dermann K, Sonnabend E. In vitro study on the corrosion behavior of two amalgams in direct contact to different cast metal alloys [in German]. Dtsch Zahnarztl Z 1991;46:290–292.

18. Johnson GH, Lepe X. Crown retention with the use of a 5% glutaraldehyde sealer on prepared dentin. J Prosthet Dent 1998;79:671–676.

19. Felton DA, Bergenholtz G, Kanoy BE. Evaluation of the desensitizing effect of Gluma dentin bond on teeth prepared for complete coverage restorations. Int J Prosthodont 1991;4:292–298.

20. Craig RG. Restorative Dental Materials, ed 6. St Louis: Mosby, 1980:57.

21. Phillips RW. Skinner's Science of Dental Materials, ed 9. Philadelphia: Saunders, 1991:296.

22. Lagouvardos P, Sourai P, Douvitsas G. Coronal fractures in posterior teeth. Oper Dent 1989;14:28–32.

23. Hiatt WH. Incomplete crown–root fracture in pulpal periodontal disease. J Periodontol 1973;44:369–379.

24. Eakle WS, Maxwell EH, Braly BV. Fractures of posterior teeth in adults. J Am Dent Assoc 1986;112:215–218.

25. Cavel WT, Kelsey WP, Blankenau RJ. An in vitro study of cuspal fracture. J Prosthet Dent 1985;53:38–42.

26. Cameron CE. Cracked tooth syndrome. J Am Dent Assoc 1976;93:971–975.

27. Gher ME, Dunlap RH, Anderson MH, Kuhl LV. Clinical survey of fractured teeth. J Am Dent Assoc 1987;114:174–177.

28. Larson TD, Douglas WH, Geistfeld RE. Effects of prepared cavities on the strength of teeth. Oper Dent 1981;6:2–5.

29. Vale WA. Cavity preparation. Ir Dent Rev 1956;2:33–41.

30. Blazer PK, Land MR, Cochran RA. Effects of designs of Class 2 preparations on resistance of teeth to fracture. Oper Dent 1983;8:6–10.

31. Morin DL, Douglas WH, Cross M, Delong R. Biophysical stress analysis of restored teeth: Experimental strain measurement. Dent Mater 1988;4:41–48.

32. Hood JAA. Methods to improve fracture resistance of teeth. In: Vanherle G, Smith, DC (eds). International Symposium on Posterior Composite Resin Dental Restorative Materials. St Paul, MN: 3M, 1985:443–450.

33. Reeh ES, Douglas WH, Messer HH. Stiffness of endodontically treated teeth related to restoration technique. J Dent Res 1989;68:1540–1544.

34. Sorensen JA, Martinoff JT. Intracoronal reinforcement and coronal coverage: A study of endodontically treated teeth. J Prosthet Dent 1984;51:780–784.

35. Cheung GS, Chan TK. Long-term survival of primary root canal treatment carried out in a dental teaching hospital. Int Endod J 2003;36:117–128.

36. Aquilino SA, Caplan DJ. Relationship between crown placement and the survival of endodontically treated teeth. J Prosthet Dent 2002;87:256–263.

37. Salis SG, Hood JA, Stokes AN, Kirk EE. Patterns of indirect fracture in intact and restored human premolar teeth. Endod Dent Traumatol 1987;3:10–14.

38. Graf H, Geering AH. Rationale for clinical application of different occlusal philosophies. Oral Sci Rev 1977;10:1–10.

39. Wiskott HWA, Nicholls JI, Belser UC. The relationship between abutment taper and resistance of cemented crowns to dynamic loading. Int J Prosthodont 1996;9:117–130.

40. Wiskott HWA, Nicholls JI, Belser UC. The effect of tooth preparation height and diameter on the resistance of complete crowns to fatigue loading. Int J Prosthodont 1997;10:207–215.

41. Wiskott HWA, Belser UC, Scherrer SS. The effect of film thickness and surface texture on the resistance of cemented extracoronal restorations to lateral fatigue loading. Int J Prosthodont 1999;12:255–262.

42. Gilboe DB, Teteruck WR. Fundamentals of extracoronal tooth preparation. Retention and resistance form. J Prosthet Dent 1974;32:651–656.

43. Jorgensen KD. The relationship between retention and convergence angle in cemented veneer crowns. Acta Odontol Scand 1955;13:35–40.

44. Owen CP. Retention and resistance in preparations for extracoronal restorations. Part II: Practical and clinical studies. J Prosthet Dent 1986;56:148–153.

45. Ohm E, Silness J. The convergence angle in teeth prepared for artificial crowns. J Oral Rehabil 1978;5:371–375.

46. Mack PJ. A theoretical investigation into the taper achieved on crown and inlay preparations. J Oral Rehabil 1980;7:255–265.

47. Dodge WR, Weed RM, Baez RJ, Buchanan RN. The effect of convergence angle on retention and resistance form. Quintessence Int 1985;16:191–197.

48. Guyer SE. Multiple preparations for fixed prosthodontics. J Prosthet Dent 1970;32:529–553.

49. Weed RM. Determining adequate crown convergence. Tex Dent J 1980;98:14–16.

50. Chan KC, Hormati AA, Boyer DB. Auxiliary retention for complete crowns provide by cement keys. J Prosthet Dent 1981;45:152–157.

51. Proussaefs P, Campagni W, Bernal G, Goodacre C, Kim J. The effectiveness of auxiliary features on a tooth preparation with inadequate resistance form. J Prosthet Dent 2004;91:33–41.

52. Parker MH, Gunderson RB, Gardner FM, Calverley MJ. Quantitative determination of taper adequate to provide resistance form: Concept of limiting taper. J Prosthet Dent 1988;59:281–288.

53. Zukermann GR. Factors that influence the mechanical retention of complete crown. Int J Prosthodont 1988;1:196–200.

54. McMullen AF 3rd, Himel VT, Sarkar NK. An in vitro study of the effect endodontic access preparation has upon the retention of porcelain fused to metal crowns of maxillary central incisors. J Endod 1989;15:154–156.

55. Mulvay PG, Abbott PV. The effect of endodontic access cavity preparation and subsequent restorative procedures on molar crown retention. Aust Dent J 1996;41:134–139.

56. Trautmann G, Gutmann JL, Nunn ME, Witherspoon DE, Berry WC, Romero GG. Restoring teeth that are endodontically treated through existing crowns. Part III: Material usage and prevention of bacterial leakage. Quintessence Int 2001;32:27–32.

57. Hamid A, Hume WR. The effect of dentin thickness on diffusion of resin monomers. J Oral Rehabil 1997;24:20–25.

58. Camps J, Tardieu C, Dejou J, Franquin JC, Ladaique P, Rieu R. In vitro cytotoxicity of dental adhesive systems under simulated pulpal pressure. Dent Mater 1997;13:34–42.

59. Camps J, Dejou J, Remusat M, About I. Factors influencing pulpal response to cavity restorations. Dent Mater 2000;16:432–440.

60. Brännström M, Vojinovic O. Response of the dental pulp to invasion of bacteria around three filling materials. J Dent Child 1976;43:83–89.

61. Cox CF, Suzuki S. Re-evaluating pulp protection: Calcium hydroxide liners vs. cohesive hybridization. J Am Dent Assoc 1994;125:823–831.

62. Chang JC, Chan JT, Chheda HN, Iglesias A. Microleakage of a 4-methacryloxyethyl trimellitate anhydride bonding agent with amalgams. J Prosthet Dent 1996;75:495–498.

63. Wilson RD, Maynard JG. Intracrevicular restorative dentistry. Int J Periodontics Restorative Dent 1981;1:35–49.

64. Valderhaug J. Periodontal considerations and carious lesions following the insertion of fixed prosthesis: A 10-year follow-up study. Int Dent J 1980;30:296–304.

65. Koth DL. Full crown restoration and gingival inflammation in a controlled population. J Prosthet Dent 1982;48:681–685.

66. Waerhaug J. Histologic considerations which govern where the margins of restorations should be located in relation to the gingival. Dent Clin North Am 1960;5:161–176.

67. Renggli HH, Regolati B. Gingival inflammation and plaque accumulation by well-adapted supragingival and subgingival proximal restorations. Helv Odontol Acta 1972;16:99–101.

68. Mormann W, Regolati B, Renggli HH. Gingival reaction to well-fitted subgingival proximal gold inlays. J Clin Periodontol 1974;1:120–125.

69. Newcomb GM. The relationship between the location of subgingival crown margins and gingival inflammation. J Periodontol 1974;45:151–154.

70. Ericsson I, Lindhe J. Recession in sites with inadequate width of keratinized gingiva. An experimental study in the dog. J Clin Periodontol 1984;11:95–103.

71. Richter WA, Ueno H. Relationship of crown margin placement to gingival inflammation. J Prosthet Dent 1973;30:156–161.

72. Ackerman MB. The full coverage restoration in relation to the gingival sulcus. Compend Contin Educ Dent 1997;18:1131–1138, 1140.

73. Gargiulo AW, Wentz FM, Orban BJ. Dimensions and relations of the dentogingival junction in humans. J Periodontol 1961;32:261–267.

74. Kois JC. Altering gingival levels: The restorative connection. Part I: Biologic variables. J Esthet Dent 1994;6:3–9.

75. Gunay H, Seeger A, Tschernitschek H, Geurtsen W. Placement of the preparation line and periodontal health—A prospective 2-year clinical study. Int J Periodontics Restorative Dent 2000;20:173–181.

76. Ruben MP, Smukler H, Schulman S, Kon S, Bloom AA. Healing of periodontal surgical wounds. In: Goldman HM, Cohen DW (eds). Periodontal Therapy, ed 6. St Louis: Mosby, 1980:640–754.

77. Koke U, Sander C, Heinecke A, Muller HP. A possible influence of gingival dimensions on attachment loss and gingival recession following placement of artificial crowns. Int J Periodontics Restorative Dent 2003;23:439–445.

78. Dragoo JR, Williams GB. Periodontal tissue reactions to restorative procedures. Int J Periodontics Restorative Dent 1981;1(1):9–23.

79. Mount GJ. Crown and the gingival tissues. Aust Dent J 1970;15:253–258.

80. Jameson LM. Comparison of the volume of crevicular fluid from restored and nonrestored teeth. J Prosthet Dent 1979;41:209–214.

81. Silness J. Periodontal conditions in patients treated with dental bridges. II. The influence of full and partial crowns on plaque accumulation, development of gingivitis and pocket formation. J Periodont Res 1970;5:219–230.

82. Silness J. Periodontal conditions in patients treated with dental bridges. Part III. The relationship between the location of the crown and margin and the periodontal condition. J Periodont Res 1970;5:225–229.

83. Reitemeier B, Hansel K, Walter MH, Kastner C, Toutenburg H. Effect of posterior crown margin placement on gingival health. J Prosthet Dent 2002;87:167–172.

84. Kay HB. Esthetic considerations in the definitive periodontal prosthetic management of the maxillary anterior segment. Int J Periodontics Restorative Dent 1982;2(3):45–59.

85. Nevins M, Skurow HM. The intracrevicular restorative margin, the biologic width, and the maintenance of the gingival margin. Int J Periodontics Restorative Dent 1984;4(3):31–49.

86. Butel Em, Campbell JC, DiFiore PM. Crown margin design: A dental school survey. J Prosthet Dent 1991;65:303–305.

87. Byrne G, Goodacre CJ, Dykema RW, Moore BK. Casting accuracy of high-palladium alloys. J Prosthet Dent 1986;55:297–302.

88. Teteruck WR, Mumford G. The fit of certain dental casting alloys using different investing materials and techniques. J Prosthet Dent 1966;16:910–927.

89. Christensen GJ. Marginal fit of gold onlays. J Prosthet Dent 1966;16:297–305.

90. McLean JW, von Fraunhofer JA. The estimation of film thickness by an in vivo technique. Br Dent J 1971;131:107–111.

91. Rosner D. Function, placement and reproduction of bevels for gold casting. J Prosthet Dent 1963;13:1160–1166.

92. Ostlund LE. Cavity design and mathematics: Their effect on gaps at the margins of cast restorations. Oper Dent 1985;10:122–137.

93. Grieve AR. A study of dental cements. Br Dent J 1969;127:405–410.

94. Panno FV, Vahidi F, Gulker I, Ghalili KM. Evaluation of the 45-degree labial bevel with a shoulder preparation. J Prosthet Dent 1986;56:655–661.

95. Pascoe DF. Analysis of the geometry of finish lines for full crown restorations. J Prosthet Dent 1978;40:157–162.

96. Fusayama T, Ide K, Hosoda H. Relief of resistance of cement of full cast crowns. J Prosthet Dent 1964;14:95–105.

97. Byrne G. Influence of finish-line form on crown cementation. Int J Prosthodont 1992;5:137–144.

98. Piemjai M. Effect of seating force, margin design, and cement on marginal seal and retention of cast metal crowns. Int J Prosthodont 2001;14:412–416.

99. Mitchell CA, Pintado MR, Douglas WH. Nondestructive, in vitro qualification of crown margins. J Prosthet Dent 2001;85:575–584.

100. Tucker RV. The full gold crown: An overview. Oper Dent 2000;25:130–133.

101. el-Ebrashi MK, Craig RG, Peyton FA. Experimental stress analysis of dental restorations. 3. The concept of the geometry of proximal margins. J Prosthet Dent 1969;22:333–338.

102. Morris ML. Artificial crown contours and gingival health. J Prosthet Dent 1962;12:1146–1156.

103. Parkinson CF. Excessive crown contours facilitate endemic plaque niches. J Prosthet Dent 1976;35:424–429.

104. Youdelis RA, Weaver JD, Sapkos S. Facial and lingual contours of artificial complete crown restorations and their effect on periodontium. J Prosthet Dent 1973;29:61–66.

105. Wheeler RC. Complete crown form and the periodontium. J Prosthet Dent 1961;11:722–734.

106. Herlands RE, Lucca JJ, Morris HL. Forms, contours, and extensions of full coverage restorations in occlusal reconstruction. Dent Clin North Am 1962;6:147–162.

107. Stein RS. Periodontal dictates for esthetic ceramometal crowns. J Am Dent Assoc 1987;Dec(special issue):63E–75E.

108. Krough-Paulsen WG, Olsson A. Occlusal disharmonies and dysfunction of the stomatognathic system. Dent Clin North Am 1966;10:627–635.

109. Bell WE. Temporomandibular Disorders: Classification/Diagnosis/Management, ed 2. Chicago: Year Book, 1986:219.

110. Schluger S, Yuodelis R, Page RC, Johnson RH. Periodontal Diseases, ed 2. Philadelphia: Lea & Febiger, 1990:125–137.

111. D'Amico A. Functional occlusion of the natural teeth of man. J Prosthet Dent 1961;11:899–915.

112. Ogawa T, Ogimoto T, Koyano K. Pattern of occlusal contacts in lateral positions: Canine protection and group function validity in classifying guidance patterns. J Prosthet Dent 1998;80:67–74.

113. Schuyler CH. Considerations of occlusion in fixed partial dentures. Dent Clin North Am 1959;3:175–185.

114. Kaiser DA, Becker CM, Malone WFP. Designs for cast metal restorations. Am J Dent 1998;11:199–201.

115. Kahn AE. Partial versus full coverage. J Prosthet Dent 1960;10:167–172.

116. Gibbs CH, Lundeen HL. Advances in Occlusion. Littleton, MA: PSG, 1982:2–32.

117. Donovan T, Simonson RJ, Guentin CT, Tucker RV. Retrospective clinical evaluation of 1,314 cast gold restorations in service from 1 to 52 years. J Esthet Restor Dent 2004;16:194–204.

118. Shillingburg HT. Cast gold restorations. In: Clark JW (ed). Clinical Dentistry. New York: Harper & Row, 1976.

119. Shillingburg HT, Hobo S, Whitsett LD, Jacobi R, Brackett SE. Fundamentals of Fixed Prosthodontics, ed 3. Chicago: Quintessence, 1997:132.

120. Ingraham R, Bassett RW, Koser JR. An Atlas of Cast Gold Procedures, ed 2. Buena Park, CA: Uni-Tro College Press, 1969:34.

121. Lorey RE, Myers GE. The retentive qualities of bridge retainers. J Am Dent Assoc 1968;76:568–572.

122. Potts RG, Shillingburg HT, Duncanson MG. Retention and resistance of preparations for cast restorations. J Prosthet Dent 1980;43:303–308.

123. Gerhardt DE. Seating the cast gold restoration. Gen Dent 1987;35:479–480.

124. Ostlund LE. Improving the marginal fit of the cast restorations. J Am Acad Gold Foil Oper 1974;17:56–60.

125. Kaiser DA, Wise HB. Fitting cast gold restorations with the aid of disclosing wax. J Prosthet Dent 1980;43:227–228.

126. Van Nortwick WG, Gettlemen L. Effect of internal relief, vibration and venting on the vertical seating of cemented crowns. J Prosthet Dent 1981;45:395–399.

127. Kaiser DA. Anatomy of the cast gold margin. J Prosthet Dent 1983;50:437–440.

128. Schwartz NL, Whitsett LD, Berry TG, Stewart JL. Unserviceable crowns and fixed partial dentures: Life-span and causes for loss of serviceability. J Am Dent Assoc 1970;81:1395–1401.

129. Walton JN, Gardner FM, Agar JR. A survey of crown and fixed partial denture failures: Length of service and reasons for replacement. J Prosthet Dent 1986;56:416–421.

130. Donovan TE, Cho GC. Contemporary evaluation of dental cements. Compend Contin Educ Dent 1999;20:197–179, 202–208, 210 passim.

131. Zidan O, Ferguson GC. The retention of complete crowns prepared with three different tapers and luted with four different cements. J Prosthet Dent 2003;89:565–571.

132. Diaz-Arnold AM, Vargas MA, Haselton DR. Current status of luting agents for fixed prosthodontics. J Prosthet Dent 1999;81:135–141.

133. Christensen GJ, Christensen R. Use Survey—1990. Clin Res Assoc Newsletter 1990;14:1–3.

134. White SN, Yu Z, Tom J, Sangsurasak S. In vivo marginal adaptation of cast crowns luted with different cements. J Prosthet Dent 1995;74:25–32.

135. Ames WB. A new oxyphosphate for crown seating. Dent Cosmos 1892;34:392–393.

136. Shillingburg HT, Hobo S, Whitsett LD. Fundamentals of Fixed Prosthodontics. Chicago: Quintessence, 1981:376–377.

137. Margerit J, Cluzel B, Leloup JM, et al. Chemical characterization of in vivo aged zinc phosphate dental cements. J Mater Sci Mater Med 1996;7:623–628.

138. White SN, Yu Z, Tom JF, Sangsurasak S. In vivo microleakage of luting cements for cast crowns. J Prosthet Dent 1994;71:333–338.

139. Norman RD, Swartz ML, Phillips RW, Vermani RV. A comparison of the intraoral disintegration of three dental cements. J Am Dent Assoc 1969;78:777–782.

140. White SN, Sorensen JA, Kang SK, Caputo AA. Microleakage of new crown and fixed partial denture luting agents. J Prosthet Dent 1992;67:156–161.

141. Kydd WL, Nicholls JI, Harrington G. Marginal leakage of cast gold crowns luted with zinc phosphate cement: An in vivo study. J Prosthet Dent 1996;75:9–13.

142. Smith DC. Dental cements. Current status and future prospects. Dent Clin North Am 1983;6:763–792.

143. Jost-Brinkmann PG, Rabe H, Miethke RR. Materials properties of zinc phosphate cements after delayed setting on refrigerated slabs [in German]. Fortschr Kieferorthop 1989;50:1–11.

144. Osborne JW, Wolff MS, Berry JC. Variance in powder-liquid ratio in zinc phosphate cement for luting castings [abstract 468]. J Dent Res 1986;65:778.

145. Katsuyama S, Ishikawa T, Fujii B (eds). Glass Ionomer Dental Cement: The Materials and Their Clinical Use. Diehnelt DE (trans). St Louis: Ishiyaku EuroAmerica, 1993.

146. Staninec M, Giles WS, Saiku JM, Hattori M. Caries penetration and cement thickness of three luting agents. Int J Prosthodont 1988;1:259–263.

147. Musa A, Pearson GJ, Gelbier M. In vitro investigation of fluoride ion release from four resin modified glass polyalkenoate cements. Biomaterials 1996;17:1019–1023.

148. White SN, Furuichi R, Kyomen SM. Microleakage through dentin after crown cementation. J Endod 1995;21:9–12.

149. White SN, Yu Z. Compressive and diametral tensile strengths of current adhesive luting agents. J Prosthet Dent 1993;69:568–572.

150. Mojon P, Hawbolt EB, McEntee MI, Ma PH. Early bond strength of luting cements to precious alloy. J Dent Res 1992;71:633–639.

151. Matsuya S, Maeda T, Ohta M. IR and NMR analyses of hardening and maturation of glass ionomer cement. J Dent Res 1996;75:1920–1927.

152. Johnson GH, Powell LV, DeRouen TA. Evaluation and control of post-cementation pulpal sensitivity: Zinc phosphate and glass ionomer cements. J Am Dent Assoc 1993;124:38–46.

153. Jokstad A, Mjor IA. Ten years' clinical evaluation of three luting agents. J Dent 1996;24:309–315.

154. Kern M, Kleimeier B, Schaller HG, Strub JR. Clinical comparison of post-operative sensitivity for a glass ionomer and a zinc phosphate luting cement. J Prosthet Dent 1996;75:159–162.

155. Pameijer CH, Nilner K. Long term clinical evaluation of three luting materials. Swed Dent J 1994;18:59–67.

156. Um CM, Oilo G. The effect of early water contact on glass-ionomer cements. Quintessence Int 1992;23:209–214.

157. Hornsby PR. Dimensional stability of glass-ionomer cements. J Chem Tech Biotechnol 1980;30:595–601.

158. Curtis SR, Richards MW, Dhuru VB, Meiers JC. Early erosion of glass-ionomer cement at crown margins. Int J Prosthodont 1993;6:553–557.

159. Fricker J, Hirota K, Tamiya Y. The effects of temperature on the setting of glass ionomer (polyalkenoate) cements. Aust Dent J 1991;36:240–242.

160. Wilson AD, Prosser JK, Powis DM. Mechanism of adhesion of polyelectrolyte cements to hydroxyapatite. J Dent Res 1983;62:590–592.

161. Wilson AD. Resin-modified glass-ionomer materials. Int J Prosthodont 1990;3:425–429.

162. Sidhu SK, Watson TF. Resin-modified glass-ionomer materials. Part 1: Properties. Dent Update 1995;22:429–431.

163. White SN, Yu Z. Film thickness of new adhesive luting agents. J Prosthet Dent 1992;67:782–785.

164. White SN, Yu Z, Tom JF, Sangsurasak S. In vivo marginal adaptation of cast crowns luted with different cements. J Prosthet Dent 1995;74:25–32.

165. Kanchanavasita W, Pearson S, Pearson GJ. Water sorption characteristics of resin-modified glass-ionomer cements. Biomaterials 1997;18:343–349.

166. Yap AU. Resin-modified glass ionomer cements: A comparison of water sorption characteristics. Biomaterials 1996;17:1897–1900.

167. Miller MB. The reality of nonscience-based newsletters. Quintessence Int 1996;27:655–656.

168. Sindel J, Frankenberger R, Kramer N, Petschelt A. Crack formation of all-ceramic crowns dependent on different core build-up and luting materials. J Dent 1999;27:175–181.

169. Leevailoj C, Platt JA, Cochran MA, Moore BK. In vitro study of fracture incidence and compressive fracture load of all-ceramic crowns cemented with resin-modified glass ionomer and other luting agents. J Prosthet Dent 1998;80:699–707.

170. Duncan JP, Pameijer CH. Retention of parallel-sided titanium posts cemented with six luting agents: An in vitro study. J Prosthet Dent 1998;80:423–428.

171. Snyder MD, Lang BR, Razzoog ME. The efficacy of luting all ceramic crowns with resin-modified glass ionomer cement. J Am Dent Assoc 2003;134:609–612.

172. Jacobson PH, Rees JS. Luting agents for ceramic and polymeric inlays and onlays. Int Dent J 1992;42:145–149.

173. Aquilino SA, Diaz-Arnold AM, Piotrowski TJ. Tensile fatigue limits of prosthodontic adhesives. J Dent Res 1991;70:208–210.

174. Burgess JO, Norling BK, Cardenas HL. Fluoride release and flexural strength of five fluoride releasing luting agents. J Dent Res 1996;75(special issue):70.

175. McMillen K, Kerby RE, Thakur A, Johnson WM. Fluoride release of resin-based luting agents. J Dent Res 1996;75:68.

176. Shinkai K, Suzuki S, Leinfelder KF, Katch Y. Effect of gap dimensions on wear resistance of luting agents. Am J Dent 1995;8:149–151.

177. White SN, Yu Z. Physical properties of fixed prosthodontic resin composite luting agents. Int J Prosthodont 1993;6:384–389.

178. Blair KF, Koeppen RG, Schwartz RS, Davis RD. Microleakage associated with resin composite–cemented, cast glass ceramic restoration. Int J Prosthodont 1993;6:579–584.

179. Hunsaker JK, Christensen GJ, Christensen RP, et al. Retentive characteristics of dental cementation materials. Gen Dent 1993;44:464–467.

180. Krabbendam CA, Ten Harkel HC, Duijesters PPE, Davidson CL. Shear bond strength determinations on various kinds of luting cements with tooth structure and cast alloys using a new testing device. J Dent 1987;15:77–81.

181. O'Sullivan BP, Johnson PF, Blosser RL, et al. Bond strength of a luting composite to dentin with different bonding systems. J Prosthet Dent 1987;58:171–175.

182. Levine WA. An evaluation of the film thickness of resin luting agents. J Prosthet Dent 1989;62:175–181.

183. Staninec M, Giles WS, Saiku JM, Hattori M. Caries penetration and cement thickness of three luting agents. Int J Prosthodont 1988;1:259–265.

184. Schwartz RS, Davis RD, Hilton TJ. Effect of temporary cements on the bond strength of a resin cement. Am J Dent 1992;5:147–150.

185. Cobb DS, Reinhardt JW, Vargas MA. Effect of HEMA-containing dentin desensitizers on shear bond strength of a resin cement. Am J Dent 1997;10:62–65.

186. Reinhardt JW, Krell KV. Effect of desensitizers and bonding agents on radicular dentin permeability [abstract 1332]. J Dent Res 1997;76:180.

187. Swift EJ, Lloyd AH, Felton DA. The effect of resin desensitizing agents on crown retention. J Am Dent Assoc 1997;128:195–200.

188. Ayad MF, Rosenstiel SF, Salama M. Influence of tooth surface roughness and type of cement on retention of complete cast crowns. J Prosthet Dent 1997;77:116–121.

189. Tjan AHL, Tjan AH, Greive JH. Effects of various cementation methods on the retention of prefabricated posts. J Prosthet Dent 1987; 58:309–313.

190. Tarim B, Suzuki S, Suzuki S, Cox CF. Marginal integrity of bonded amalgam restorations. Am J Dent 1996;9:72–76.

191. Johnson GH, Hazelton LR, Bales DJ, Lepe X. The effect of a resin-based sealer on crown retention for three types of cement. J Prosthet Dent 2004;91:428–435.

192. Imbery TA, Davis RD. Evaluation of tin plating systems for a high-noble alloy. Int J Prosthodont 1993;6:55–59.

193. Olin PS, Hill EME. Tensile strength of air abraded vs tin plated metals luted with three cements [abstract 188]. J Dent Res 1991;70:387.

194. Robin C, Scherrer S, Wiskott H, de Rijk W, Belser U. Weibull parameters of composite resin bond strength to porcelain and noble alloy using Rocatec System. Dent Mater 2002;18:389–395.

195. Vojvodic D, Jerolimov V, Celebic A, Catovic A. Bond strengths of silicoated and acrylic resin bonding systems to metal. J Prosthet Dent 1999;81:1–6.

196. Yamada Y, Tsubota Y, Fukushima S. Effect of restoration method on fracture resistance of endodontically treated maxillary premolars. Int J Prosthodont 2004;17:94–98.

197. Rosenstiel SF, Gegauff AF. Improving cementation of complete cast crowns: A comparison of static and dynamic seating methods. J Am Dent Assoc 1988;117:845–848.

Restoration of Endodontically Treated Teeth

J. William Robbins

A great deal of research has been published on the restoration of endodontically treated teeth.[1] Despite the large number of in vitro and in vivo investigations, there is still much confusion regarding ideal treatment. Scurria et al[2] followed up the restorative outcome of 1,199 endodontically treated teeth through an insurance claims system and reported that the percentage of noncrown restorations placed during the subsequent 2 years after endodontic therapy was 67% in the anterior tooth group, 54% in the premolar group, and 50% in the molar group. Based on these data, it seems clear that there continues to be significant confusion regarding the restoration of endodontically treated teeth. It is the purpose of this chapter to analyze the research and present a logical approach to this subject.

When faced with the challenge of restoring an endodontically treated tooth, the dentist must decide, first, whether a post is required and, second, the type of restoration that is indicated. In the past, a post was thought to strengthen the root of an endodontically treated tooth. This philosophy pervaded dental education until laboratory research began to cast doubts on this assumption. It is widely held today that the primary purpose of post placement is to retain the core buildup material or to reinforce the remaining coronal tooth structure.

The longevity of endodontically treated teeth is difficult to evaluate because of the many mitigating factors. Perhaps the most important factor that is not reported in clinical studies is the amount of remaining coronal tooth structure before the final restoration. This factor is much more important than others that are reported, such as post material and design, ce-

ment, and core material. Mentink and others[3] reported an 82% success rate in post-restored teeth after 10 years. Torbjorner and others[4] reported a 2.1% failure rate per year. Finally, Nanayakkara and others[5] reported the median survival rate to be 17.4 years.

The long-term clinical success of an endodontically treated tooth is dependent on many factors. It has been reported that the majority of failures are due to inadequate restorative therapy, followed by tooth loss due to periodontal reasons. Relatively few endodontically treated teeth are lost because of failed endodontic therapy.[6] When endodontic therapy fails, the most common reason is inadequate cleaning and obturation of the canal system.[7] However, it has been reported that the clinician is a key element in the success of endodontically treated teeth. Success rates for specialists in endodontics have been reported to be between 70% and 95%,[8] while success for generalists has been reported to be 64% and 75%.[9] In recent years, it has become obvious that another important failure mechanism is orthograde contamination, that is, contamination via leakage of oral fluids apically within the root.[10–12] This can be due to the loss of or leakage around a provisional restoration or marginal leakage around a definitive restoration. Coronal sealing of the root canal system should be accomplished as soon as possible after completion of the root canal therapy.[13]

The decision to place a post is based on several parameters. These include the position of the tooth in the arch, occlusion, function of the restored tooth, amount of remaining tooth structure, and canal configuration. Each of these considerations will be discussed in detail.

Indications for Placement of Posts

Anterior Teeth

Anterior and posterior teeth function much differently; therefore, they must be evaluated separately. The anterior tooth receives predominantly shear forces, which act on both the clinical crown and the root. Although some laboratory studies[14,15] have indicated that a post strengthens an intact anterior endodontically treated tooth, the majority of studies[16–18] have suggested that the fracture resistance of these teeth is not affected by, or is decreased with, placement of a post. Therefore, when a complete-coverage restoration is not required for esthetic or functional reasons (eg, to serve as an abutment for a fixed or removable partial denture), a post is not indicated. However, if a complete-coverage restoration is indicated in an endodontically treated anterior tooth for esthetics or function, a post may be indicated.[19] This is especially true for maxillary lateral incisors and mandibular incisors.

With maxillary central incisors and canines, the decision to place a post should be based on the amount of remaining coronal tooth structure, as well as the occlusion and function of the tooth. If there is a significant amount of remaining coronal tooth structure, the crown preparation should be accomplished before the decision regarding post placement is made. Once the axial preparation is completed and the access preparation is cleaned, the dentist can make the decision as to whether the remaining coronal tooth structure needs the reinforcement of a post. If the decision is made, based on the functional requirements of the tooth, that the remaining coronal tooth structure is adequate to support the crown, resin composite can be bonded into the access preparation. However, if there is doubt regarding the adequacy of the resistance form of the coronal portion of the tooth, then a post or post and core is indicated.

Posterior Teeth

For the posterior tooth, the decisions are more clear-cut. The forces on posterior teeth are predominately vertical. Therefore, reinforcement of coronal tooth structure is not commonly needed, as it is in anterior teeth. Because of the morbidity associated with post placement (Fig 20-1), a post is indicated in a posterior tooth only when other more conservative retention and resistance features cannot be used for the core. These features include chamber retention, amalgam pins, and threaded pins, all of which have been shown to be exceedingly effective (see chapter 11).[20]

In 1980, Nayyar and Walton[21] described the amalcore, or coronal-radicular, restoration. Rather than placing a post, the pulp chamber and coronal 2.0 to 3.0 mm of each canal are used for retention of the buildup material (Figs 20-2a to 20-2c). Subsequently, several authors reported laboratory data on the fracture resistance of the amalcore. Kern and others[22] and Christian and others[23] reported that the placement of a post in the distal canal of a mandibular molar increases the fracture resistance of the amalcore. However, in these studies the specimens were stressed in compression at 60 and 90 degrees, respectively. This angle of force does not reproduce the vertical forces that molars receive in vivo. In a similar study, Plasmans and others[24] found no statistically significant difference between the amalcore alone and the amalcore with a post when stressed at 45 degrees. Kane and Burgess[25] reported that the placement of two horizontal threaded pins in the buccal and lingual walls of the amalcore restoration provides a significant increase in fracture resistance. In a retrospective clinical study of more than 400 coronal-radicular restorations, Nayyar and Walton[21] reported no failures that could be attributed to the core buildup. The coronal-radicular buildup has proven to be a predictable and cost-effective restorative modality for posterior endodontically treated teeth.

It has been commonly stated that threaded pins should not be placed in endodontically treated teeth because they will cause the teeth to crack. However, no clinical data are available to support this belief. In fact, current data indicate that there is very little difference between the dentin of endodontically treated teeth and vital dentin.[26,27] There is also a move to completely discard traditional retention and resistance features in deference to the adhesively retained core buildup. With regard to core retention, Tjan and others[28] reported that dentin adhesive performed better than mechanical retention with resin composite, while threaded pins performed better with amalgam in vitro. One 6-year clinical study supports the effectiveness of the adhesively retained complex amalgam without auxiliary retention.[29] However, sufficient long-term clinical data are not available to support the efficacy of using a dentin bonding agent as the sole means of core retention. Therefore, until the efficacy of the adhesively retained buildup can be demonstrated in long-term clinical studies, it would be prudent to use adhesive materials in conjunction with traditional retention and resistance features.

Although a post is not commonly required to retain the core in a posterior tooth, a post may be indicated when the tooth is to serve as an abutment for a removable partial denture.[30] In this circumstance, the forces that play on the tooth are not physiologic, and coronal reinforcement may be necessary (Fig 20-3). In maxillary molars, a post is generally placed only in the palatal canal, and in mandibular molars, in the distal canal.

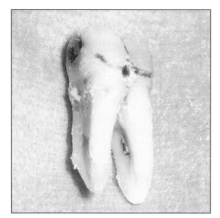

Fig 20-1 Mandibular molar with post perforation in the mesial concavity of the distal root.

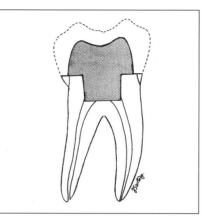

Fig 20-2a Amalcore with adequate chamber retention.

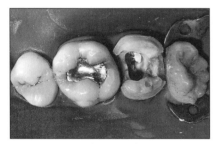

Fig 20-2b Amalcore preparation in a maxillary second molar.

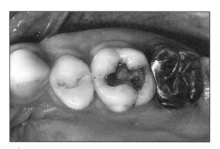

Fig 20-2c Definitive amalcore restoration in the maxillary second molar.

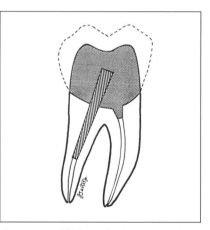

Fig 20-3 Mandibular molar that does not have a large enough pulp chamber for chamber retention of the core buildup. A post is used for retention of the core.

Fig 20-4 (a) Preoperative view of an endodontically treated maxillary second premolar. (b) Maxillary second premolar after restoration with a tapered prefabricated post and amalgam core. The canal was not enlarged for post placement.

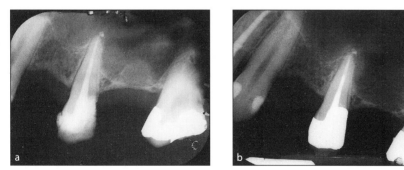

Maxillary premolars are a unique subset of posterior endodontically treated teeth. Because these teeth are subjected to a mixture of shear and compressive forces, the need for a post and core in a maxillary premolar is not as clear. If the remaining coronal tooth structure is inadequate, if the clinical crown is tall in relation to its diameter at the point where it enters the alveolar bone, or if the tooth receives significant lateral stress, a post may be indicated (Fig 20-4). In addition, if the premolar serves as an abutment for a removable partial denture, a post and core may be indicated.[30] Conversely, if the coronal portion of the tooth is relatively short and functions more like a molar, a post is not usually indicated.

When the decision is made to place a post, the delicate morphologic structure of the maxillary premolar root must be considered during preparation of the post space.[31,32] Posts that necessitate minimal canal enlargement should be chosen for maxillary premolars. Ideally, after completion of the endodontic obturation, the canal should not be further enlarged. Rather, the post should be modified to fit the canal. This philosophy would commonly dictate the placement of a conservative tapered post in the maxillary premolar (see Fig 20-4).

Considerations in Post Design

Prior to choosing a post system, the dentist must have a clear understanding of the effect of several variables on the post-tooth combination. These variables include post design (Fig 20-5), post length, post diameter, venting, surface roughness, canal preparation, method of cementation, and luting medium.

Post Design

In general, it has been reported that the active threaded post has the greatest retention, followed by the parallel post; the tapered post has the least retention.[33–35] Therefore, the post should be chosen, in part, by the amount of post retention that the clinical situation requires. If the canal length is adequate, usually considered to be 7.0 to 8.0 mm, and the canal configuration is normal, either the tapered or parallel post may be selected. However, if the length of post space available is minimal or the canal space is funnel shaped, an active post may be required because of the difficulty in gaining adequate axial retention.

Post Length

Increased post length results in increased retention.[34,35] However, a minimum of 4.0 mm of gutta-percha should be left in the apical portion of the canal space to minimize the risk of apical leakage.[36,37] A passive post should usually be as long as possible without encroaching on the remaining gutta-percha or causing perforation in a curved canal.[38]

Post Diameter

It is commonly stated that endodontically treated teeth are more susceptible to fracture because they exhibit increased brittleness.[39,40] However, more current research questions the validity of this assumption.[26,27] Regardless of the effect of endodontic therapy on the brittleness of a tooth, the dentist has no control over this variable. It is known that the fracture resistance of a restored endodontically treated tooth decreases as the amount of dentin removed increases.[41] Increased post diameter produces minimal, if any, increase in post retention[42,43] and significantly increases internal stresses within the tooth.[44,45] Therefore, increasing the diameter of the post is not the preferred method of increasing its retention. The diameter of the post should be as small as possible while retaining the necessary rigidity.

Venting

Because of the intraradicular hydrostatic pressure created during cementation of the post,[46] a means for cement to escape must always be provided. Because virtually all prefabricated posts have a venting mechanism incorporated in their design, this factor is most important with the custom cast post. A vent may be incorporated in the pattern before casting or cut into the post with a bur prior to cementation.

Surface Preparation

Surface roughening, such as air abrading or notching, of the post increases post retention.[47–51] Surface texture is usually incorporated in prefabricated posts; however, this feature must be added to the custom cast post and core. Composite core retention to titanium posts has been shown to increase significantly utilizing the Silicoater (Kulzer), Rocatec[52] (3M ESPE), or Cojet (3M ESPE) surface treatments.[53]

Canal Preparation

Several methods of preparing the post space and their effect on apical seal have been investigated. These include use of rotary instruments, heated instruments, and solvents.[36,54–57] The literature is equivocal on preparation of the post space; no method has been shown to be consistently superior. When a rotary instrument is used, care must be taken to ensure that only the gutta-percha is removed. The canal space should not be routinely enlarged. It has also been shown that post space preparation with a rotary instrument can generate large temperature increases on the root surface.[58] Therefore, caution must be exercised during canal space preparation. Immediate preparation (immediately after the endodontic filling) of the post space has been compared to delayed preparation (waiting at least 24 hours).[54,56,59–61] Again, neither method has been consistently shown to be superior.

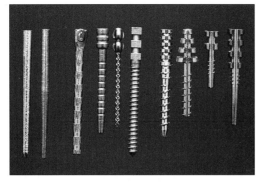

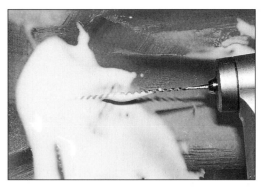

Fig 20-5 Prefabricated posts. *(left to right)* Passive tapered: Endowel (Star), Filpost (Ivoclar Vivadent); passive parallel: Parapost Plus (Coltène Whaledent), BCH (3M), Unity (Coltène Whaledent), Boston Post (Roydent); active: Flexipost (Essential Dental Systems), V-Lock (Brasseler), Radix (Caulk), Cytco (Maillefer).

Fig 20-6 Lentulo spiral used to place cement into the canal space.

Cementation of Posts

The actual method of post cementation has been investigated,[62,63] including placement of the cement on the post, and/or placement of the cement in the canal with a lentulo spiral, a paper point, or an endodontic explorer. The lentulo spiral is the superior instrument for cement placement (Fig 20-6). The cement may also be placed in the canal with a needle tube, as long as the tip of the tube is inserted to the bottom of the canal space and the cement is extruded from the tip as it is slowly removed from the canal. After the cement is placed in the canal, the post is coated with the cement and inserted. When zinc phosphate cement is used, it has been shown that the placement of an organic solvent (Cavidry, Parkell) in the canal before cementation of the post increases retention.[64]

Luting Cements

Cements for posts and post-and-core restorations have been investigated extensively.[35,65–70] These include zinc phosphate, polycarboxylate, glass ionomer, and filled and unfilled resin composites. Both zinc phosphate and glass ionomer are commonly used because of their ease of use and their history of clinical success. In recent years, resin cements as well as resin-modified glass-ionomer cements have become popular luting agents. The data are not clear regarding the superiority of one cement over another. Schwartz and others[71] reported increased retention with zinc phosphate cement over resin cement regardless of whether a eugenol-containing sealer had been used. Duncan and Pameijer[72] reported that a resin-modified glass-ionomer cement coupled with a dentin bonding agent had greater retention than resin composite cement,

glass-ionomer cement, or zinc phosphate cement. Some laboratory studies[73–75] have shown a significant increase in post retention with resin cements, but other studies[71,76,77] have not confirmed this finding. There are two problems with the use of resin composite cements. First, resin cement is technique sensitive because of its short working time. Second, it is difficult to remove all of the gutta-percha and eugenol-containing endodontic sealer from the prepared canal without removing excess tooth structure. This residue in the surface irregularities of the prepared canal prevents adequate conditioning of the dentin[78] and inhibits the set of the polymer.[66,76,77,79,80] However, one laboratory study indicated that the use of eugenol-containing sealer has no impact on resin bond strength in the canal.[81]

With traditional resin cements, a dentin bonding agent must first be placed in the canal. The choice of bonding agent is very important. Current available dentin bonding agents are fourth generation (separate primer and adhesive), fifth generation (one-bottle systems), and sixth generation (self-etching systems). Because of their low pH, many fifth- and sixth-generation dentin bonding agents are not compatible with autocure and/or dual-cure resin composites. A scanning electron microscope (SEM) study[82] confirmed the superiority of a fourth-generation compared to a fifth-generation bonding agent. With the advent of a newer generation of self-etching resin cements that do not require bonding agents, it appears that this group of luting agents will become the material of choice. Each cement has distinct advantages and should be chosen based on these advantages in a given situation. However, the choice of luting agent is clearly not the key factor in the longevity of a post-restored tooth. No cement can overcome the inadequacies of a poorly designed post.

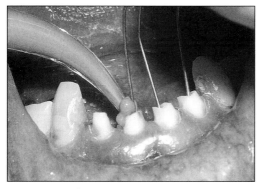

Fig 20-7a Use of 25-gauge needles to allow air to escape from canals during the impression making to ensure a complete impression of the canal spaces.

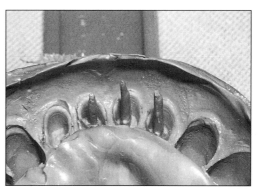

Fig 20-7b Final impression of canal spaces for laboratory fabrication of custom cast posts.

Types of Posts

Custom Cast Post

The custom cast post and core has a long history of success in restorative dentistry. However, laboratory studies[83–86] have consistently shown that the fracture resistance of teeth restored with custom cast posts is lower than that of teeth restored with many different prefabricated posts. In addition, retrospective clinical studies[4,87] have shown prefabricated parallel posts to have greater clinical success than custom cast posts. This, coupled with the added expense and extra appointment required to fabricate the custom cast post, makes its routine use questionable.

There are several circumstances in which the custom cast post is the post of choice:

1. When multiple post-and-core restorations are planned in the same arch, the laboratory-fabricated custom cast post is the most time- and cost-efficient method. The teeth are prepared for the posts, and the final crown preparations are completed so that all crown margins are on tooth structure. It is important that the crown preparation be completed before the impression for the post and core is made so that the axial contours of the core can be fabricated correctly.

   An impression is made with an elastomeric impression material used in an injection technique, which allows the impression material to flow into the total length of the prepared canal space (Figs 20-7a and 20-7b). This can be best accomplished using one of the following techniques. A 25-gauge needle is placed into the canal before the impres-

sion is made. The syringe material is then injected into the canal until it begins to flow out the top of the orifice. While the syringe material is being injected, the needle is slowly removed from the canal. The needle serves as an escape channel for the trapped air and allows the elastomeric impression material to reproduce the entire length of the canal space. Alternatively, the syringe material may be placed directly into the canal with a needle tube, which is attached to the syringe. The tip of the needle tube must be long enough to extend to the entire length of the prepared canal space. The elastomeric material is injected as the needle tube is slowly removed from the canal. No reinforcement of the impression material in the canal space is required with the newer impression materials. The impression is poured, and the custom posts are fabricated in the laboratory. At a subsequent appointment, the posts are cemented and the final impression for the restorations is made without further tooth preparation.

2. When a small tooth, such as a mandibular incisor, requires a post and core, a prefabricated post may be difficult to use. Commonly, there is minimal space around the post for the core buildup material. In this situation, the custom cast post serves well.

3. Occasionally, the angle of the core in relation to the root must be altered. It is not advisable to bend prefabricated posts; therefore, the custom cast post and core most successfully fulfills this need (Figs 20-8a and 20-8b).

4. When an all-ceramic noncore (without opaque substructure, such as zirconia) restoration is placed, it is necessary to have a core buildup that approximates the color of natural tooth structure. Because resin composite is not the core material of choice in high-stress situations, porcelain

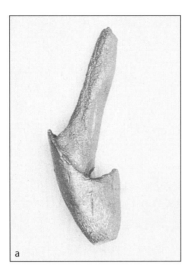

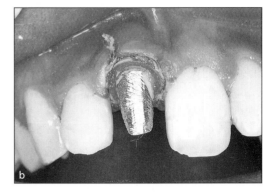

Figs 20-8a and 20-8b Custom cast post to allow a change in the angle of the core in relation to the post.

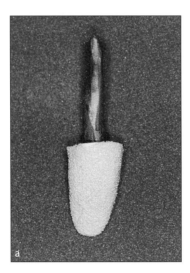

Fig 20-9 *(a)* Custom cast post with porcelain fired to the core for improved esthetics. *(b)* Maxillary central incisor with a custom cast post ready to receive an all-ceramic crown.

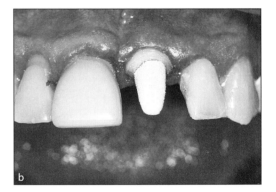

may be fired to the surface of the core of a custom cast post to simulate natural tooth color. The porcelain on the core can be etched, and the all-ceramic crown can be adhesively bonded (Fig 20-9).

Prefabricated Posts

In recent years, there has been a significant increase in the number of post systems available. Traditional prefabricated posts may be divided into three major groups: passive tapered, passive parallel, and active.

Passive Tapered Post

A goal of all post systems should be minimal removal of tooth structure before post placement. Therefore, the ideal post

system requires no further preparation after removal of the gutta-percha. Because the natural shape of the canal is tapered, the passive tapered post best fulfills this criterion (see Fig 20-5). The major advantage of the passive tapered post is that the post can be modified to fit the tapered canal rather than the canal having to be enlarged to fit the post.

The major disadvantage is that the tapered post provides the least retention. This means that the retention must be gained through increased post length. When the root is not long enough to allow for adequate post length (7.0 to 8.0 mm), a more retentive post is indicated. A second commonly stated disadvantage of the tapered post is the alleged wedging effect, which results in increased stress[88] and root fracture. This effect has been demonstrated in laboratory studies[83,85] with custom cast tapered post–and-core restorations. Howev-

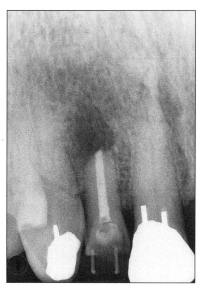

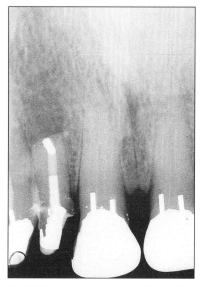

Fig 20-10a Preoperative view of a maxillary lateral incisor with a short canal space.

Fig 20-10b Tooth after restoration with a Brasseler V-Lock active post and amalgam core.

er, this theoretical wedging effect does not appear to be valid when a passive tapered post is used in conjunction with an acceptable core material and a crown.[49]

The primary indication for the passive tapered post is in teeth with small canals and thin, fragile roots, such as maxillary premolars (see Fig 20-4). However, it may be used routinely in teeth with normal canal configuration and sufficient canal length to provide the necessary retention.

Passive Parallel Post

The prefabricated post by which all other posts are measured has traditionally been the Parapost (Coltène Whaledent) (see Fig 20-5). The success of this post style has been demonstrated clinically,[4,87] as well as in the laboratory.[33–35,89] Compared to other post designs, the parallel post has been shown to provide the most favorable stress distribution.[88] The passive parallel post has greater retention than the passive tapered post.[90] However, a biologic price must be paid for this increased retention. The naturally tapered canal space must be enlarged to accommodate a parallel post. Enlargement of this canal space is not consistent with the ideal of maintaining as much tooth structure as possible. For this reason, use of the passive parallel post is recommended when increased retention is needed and the parallel canal preparation will not jeopardize the integrity of the root.

Active Post

An active post is one that engages (screws into) the dentin in the canal space. There are several styles of active posts, including those requiring a tap, self-tapping posts, split-shank posts, and hybrid posts, which contain both active and passive features (see Fig 20-5). It is difficult to generalize about active posts because of their design differences. However, the V-Lock (Brasseler) and the Flexipost (Essential Dental Systems) have performed well in the laboratory,[66] and it has been the author's experience that they perform well in clinical use.

Traditionally, the major concern about active posts has been the potential for vertical fracture of the tooth during placement of the post.[43,91] However, many laboratory studies support the use of the newer generation of active posts.[92–97] It has been shown that the active post should not be "bottomed out" when it is inserted.[96] After complete seating of an active post, it should be unscrewed one fourth of a turn. This results in decreased residual stress in the root. It has also been shown that, at shorter lengths, the active post produces less stress than other styles of prefabricated posts.[43] Therefore, active posts are indicated when the canal length is insufficient to gain adequate retention with a passive post (eg, in a short canal space or partially occluded canal due to a broken instrument or post) (Figs 20-10a and 20-10b).

Nonmetallic Post Systems

Carbon Fiber Posts

In recent years, a new generation of nonmetallic posts has been developed and marketed as a major advance in technology (Figs 20-11a and 20-11b). The post that has received the most attention is the carbon fiber–reinforced post. The proposed advantages are that the post can be bonded to the tooth with resin cement and that carbon fiber has a modulus of elasticity (rigidity) similar to that of dentin, resulting in greater post flexibility. The major disadvantages of the carbon fiber post are its dark color and radiolucent appearance in a radiograph (see Fig 20-11b).

There have been several laboratory investigations of the carbon fiber post; unfortunately, the results are equivocal. These posts are advertised to have a similar modulus to dentin and a much lower modulus than traditional stainless steel. One study supports this claim,[98] while another does not.[99] The carbon fiber post was also found to have a 15% decrease in strength and stiffness after soaking in water for 30 weeks.[100] Several in vitro studies investigated the fracture resistance of teeth restored with the carbon fiber post compared to teeth restored with stainless steel or titanium posts. One group of studies found that the teeth restored with the carbon fiber post fractured with significantly less force than those restored with metal posts.[101–104] Other studies found the fracture strength of the carbon fiber post–restored teeth to be equal to or greater than that of teeth restored with metal posts.[105–107] In these fracture resistance studies, there was a significant discussion regarding the nature of the root fractures that occurred at failure. Most studies found the fractures to be more favorable with the carbon fiber post,[102,103,105–107] while one study found root fractures to be more favorable with the metal posts.[108]

In vitro retention of the carbon fiber post has also been evaluated. One study found its retention to be greater than that of metal posts when cemented with either resin cement or glass-ionomer cement.[108] Another study found the retention of the carbon fiber post and the metal posts to be equal using a resin cement,[109] while another study found the stainless steel post to be approximately 45% more retentive than the carbon fiber post bonded with resin cement.[98] Similarly, the retention of the resin composite core to the post head has been evaluated in vitro. Two studies found the retention of the core material to metal posts to be superior to that of carbon fiber post.[99,110] Additionally, one study found the retention of resin composite to a carbon fiber post to be significantly enhanced when the post is first air abraded.[111]

Because the laboratory data do not lead to a clear conclusion regarding the clinical utility of the carbon fiber post, a decision must be made based on an understanding of the tooth-post-core-crown combination. The idea that the post should have the same rigidity as the tooth, resulting in less stress, is appealing for the root. However, this idea disregards the effect of flexibility on the core with a cemented or bonded crown on top of the core. It would seem that a flexible core would ultimately result in marginal breakdown at the crown-tooth interface. In a study utilizing two-dimensional finite element analysis, stresses related to both stainless steel and carbon fiber posts were evaluated.[112] It was found that the use of the carbon fiber post reduced the stresses within the canal but increased the stresses at the restoration margins.

Ultimately, the effectiveness of the carbon fiber post must be confirmed with long-term clinical data. Most of the reported data are retrospective clinical studies. King and Setchell[113] reported a 25% failure rate of the carbon fiber post at 7 years compared to less than a 10% failure rate with metal posts. The failures occurred at the resin cement–post interface. However, the study sample was small (n = 27), and a gold core was cast to the carbon fiber post. Fredriksson and others[114] reported no failures due to dislodgment or root fracture in a retrospective clinical study of 236 teeth restored with the carbon fiber post for a mean duration of 32 months. Ferrari and others[115] compared the carbon fiber post with the custom cast post over 4 years. They reported no failures in the carbon fiber post group due to the post, while 11% of the cast post group failed due to root fracture and crown dislodgment. In another retrospective study, Ferrari and others[116] reported on the clinical success at 6 years of three types of carbon fiber posts placed in 1,304 teeth. They reported a failure rate of only 3.2%. Finally, in a prospective clinical study, Mannocci and others[117] reported 3-year results comparing the carbon fiber post with the custom cast post. Only one carbon fiber post out of 226 placed failed; this was due to post dislodgment. In contrast, 10 of 194 of the custom cast posts failed, all due to root fracture.

Tooth-Colored Posts

A major obstacle to the esthetic restoration of an endodontically treated anterior tooth that requires a post is the dark color of the post, which casts a shadow at the tooth-gingiva interface. This is true for both the black carbon fiber post and the all-metal post. In an attempt to overcome this problem, several other tooth reinforcement methods have been advocated, including zirconium-coated carbon fiber posts, all-zirconium posts, prefabricated fiber-reinforced resin posts

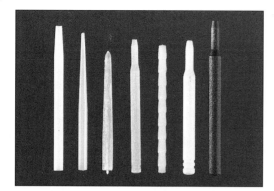

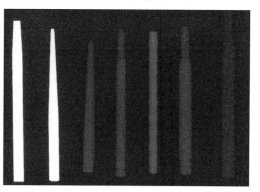

Fig 20-11a Nonmetallic posts. *(left to right)* Cosmopost (Ivoclar Vivadent), Cerapost (Brasseler), Luscent Anchor (Dentatus), Light-post (Bisco), FibreKor Post (Jeneric/Pentron), Aestheti-Plus (Bisco), and C-Post (Bisco).

Fig 20-11b Radiograph of nonmetallic posts in Fig 20-11a.

(see Figs 20-11a and 20-11b), and direct resin composites reinforced with fiber. To conceal the color of the carbon fiber post, one manufacturer has coated the carbon fiber post with white zirconium (AesthetiPlus, Bisco). One laboratory study found the physical properties of this post to be similar to those of the uncoated carbon fiber post.[101] Many of the tooth-colored posts are not radiopaque, rendering them invisible on a radiograph. A recent laboratory study[118] found that only three of seven composite fiber posts evaluated were radiopaque.

The all-zirconium posts, Cosmopost (Ivoclar Vivadent) and Cerapost (Brasseler), are white, biocompatible,[119] and radiopaque (see Figs 20-11a and 20-11b). They are reported to have a higher modulus of elasticity than stainless steel.[120,121] When used in conjunction with a resin composite core material, a very esthetic post and core can be fabricated (Figs 20-12a and 20-12b). However, it has been reported that zirconium posts are manufactured with a wide range of defects, resulting in some posts with very low fracture resistance.[122] In addition, it has been shown that the zirconium post is not etchable with hydrofluoric acid.[121,123] This means that neither the resin cement nor the resin composite core material will predictably bond to the post.[81,124] This lack of bond between the post and the resin composite results in decreased retention of the core as well as greater coronal microleakage with the zirconia post.[125] Because of the inability to get a strong bond between the zirconia post and the resin composite core and/or resin luting cement, there is a temptation to notch the post to enhance the retention. However, it has been shown that notching the post significantly decreases the fracture resistance and should be avoided.[126]

Additionally, Dietschi and others[127] reported a decreased bond between zirconium and composite after fatigue testing. However, it has been shown that the bond strength to resin composite can be improved by Cojet (3M ESPE) treatment as well as with air abrasion and silane application.[53] One method used to overcome the problem of bonding resin composite core material to the zirconium post has been described.[128] A leucite-reinforced ceramic (Empress, Ivoclar Vivadent) is pressed to the prefabricated zirconium post (Figs 20-13a and 20-13b). This reportedly provides an adequate bond between the post and core and provides an excellent substrate for bonding of the final all-ceramic crown.

Stresses surrounding the zirconium post were evaluated in a photoelastic study.[129] The zirconium post demonstrated higher stresses at the occlusal emergence location than those recorded for metal posts. Additionally, it was shown in a laboratory study that more catastrophic root fractures occurred with zirconia posts compared to metal and carbon fiber posts.[130] Koutayas and Kern[128] recently described the current options for all-ceramic post-and-core systems; however, other than two short-term clinical studies[120,131] and a few case reports,[132–135] little useful information is available.

Recently, prefabricated fiber-reinforced composite posts, FibreKor Post (Jeneric/Pentron), Luscent Anchor (Dentatus), Light-Post (Bisco), D. T. Light-Post (Rechurches Tecniques Dentaires RTD), and Fiber White (Coltène/Whaledent) have become available (see Figs 20-11a and 20-11b). One study found the fiber-reinforced resin post to be as strong as the carbon fiber post and approximately twice as rigid.[111] However, it has been shown in laboratory studies that the bond strength of resin composite core material to resin dowels is

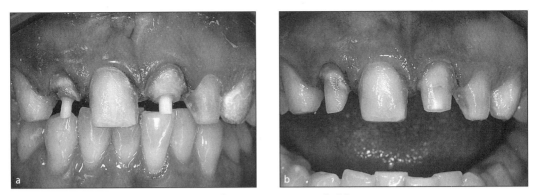

Figs 20-12a and 20-12b All-zirconium posts with resin composite core buildups.

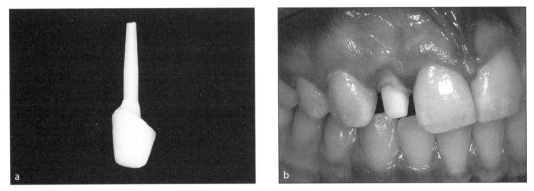

Fig 20-13a and 20-13b Cerapost with leucite-reinforced pressed ceramic core (Empress).

significantly less compared to the mechanical retention to titanium posts.[124,136]

Finally, a technique has been advocated to directly build a post and core in the tooth using composite and a woven polyester bondable ribbon.[137] A laboratory study found the fracture resistance of teeth restored in this manner to be significantly less than that of those restored with carbon fiber posts or metal posts.[101] One laboratory study[138] compared the fracture strength of teeth restored with several of these tooth-colored post systems. It was found that the Empress post and core was the weakest, followed by the zirconium Cosmopost with a ceramic core (see Figs 20-13a and 20-13b). The Vectris (Ivoclar Vivadent) post and resin composite core was significantly stronger than the all-ceramic post and core but significantly weaker than a prefabricated titanium post with a composite core, which was the strongest.

Removal of this newer generation of bonded nonmetallic posts, in comparison to metallic posts, is reported to be easier with the carbon fiber posts and fiber-reinforced composite posts, and more difficult with the zirconium posts.

At present, the laboratory data regarding the nonmetallic post systems are equivocal. Additionally, few clinical data sup-

port the use of any of the tooth-colored post systems. However, there is a growing body of clinical research literature to support the use of the carbon fiber post. Caution in the use of all of the nonmetallic post systems is advised when minimal coronal tooth structure remains and high core strength is required.

Intraradicular Reinforcement of Structurally Compromised Roots

Clinicians are occasionally faced with the difficult task of restoring an endodontically treated tooth in which much of the internal canal dentin has been lost (Fig 20-14). Traditionally, the custom cast post and core has been used in this situation. However, an alternative method of restoring flared canals has been described.[139] The missing internal tooth structure is replaced with bonded resin composite, and a traditional metal post is bonded into the newly created canal space (Figs 20-15a to 20-15c). A laboratory study[140] compared the fracture resistance of teeth restored with the custom cast post to the resin composite–metal post technique. The missing internal tooth structure was replaced with bond-

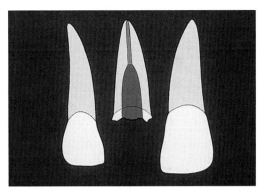

Fig 20-14 Structurally compromised root due to loss of internal radicular tooth structure.

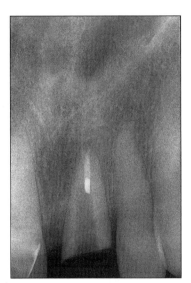

Fig 20-15a Radiograph of a structurally compromised root due to the iatrogenic removal of a broken post.

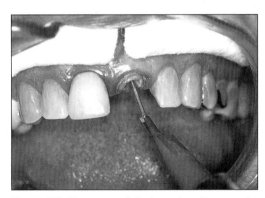

Fig 20-15b Placement of dual-cured resin composite core material into the prepared canal with a needle tube.

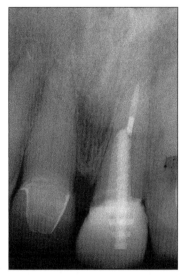

Fig 20-15c Radiograph of the structurally compromised root restored with bonded resin composite and a prefabricated metal post (V-Lock).

ed resin composite and cured using a light-conducting plastic post, temporarily inserted during light curing. The resin composite–metal post technique resulted in significantly greater fracture resistance than that seen in the custom cast post group. It is postulated that the intimate fit of the custom cast post to the weakened dentin walls results in lower fracture resistance. In a similar but simpler technique, the canal can be prepared for bonding and an autopolymerizing resin composite can be placed in the canal immediately before the insertion of a prefabricated metal post.

The Retention Triad

The real difficulty in restoring an endodontically treated tooth occurs when minimal coronal tooth structure remains. In this circumstance, the dentist must consider both retention of the post and core and resistance of the post-core-crown combination.

Retention is defined as the force that resists a tensile or pulling force. Retention of a post can be gained in three ways (Fig 20-16). The first method to gain retention is through adequate post length in the canal.[34,35] To gain this axial retention, it is imperative that the canal space not be overenlarged iatrogenically or by caries. In an anterior tooth, adequate length is commonly considered to be in the range of 7.0 to 8.0 mm, plus 4.0 mm of gutta-percha that should be left undisturbed at the apex.[37]

The design of the post may be either tapered or parallel. The tapered post requires less removal of tooth structure during preparation of the post space but exhibits poorer retention than does the parallel post. However, when the parallel

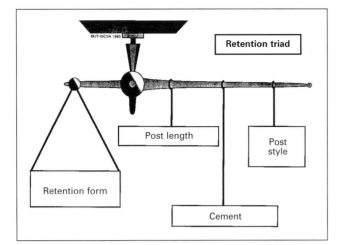

Fig 20-16 Retention triad.

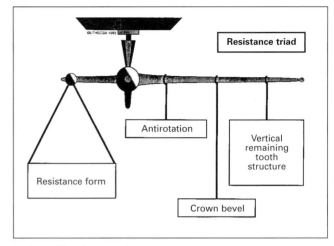

Fig 20-17 Resistance triad.

post is employed, more tooth structure must be removed, especially at the apical end of the post space. Both of these post designs are acceptable, and the decision should be based on the canal and root configurations, available post space, and the amount of retention required.

The second factor affecting retention is post style. When the decision is made that the canal length is inadequate to retain a passive post, an active post should be selected. This can occur with short clinical roots or because of obstructions in the canal space. An active post can also serve effectively when the canal space has been overenlarged. The active post can actively engage the dentin in its terminal 2 to 3 mm to gain retention. The weakened coronal portion of the canal space is not engaged, possibly resulting in less stress.

The third part of the retention triad is the luting agent used to cement the post. The idea of bonding a post into the canal with resin cement to increase retention is theoretically appealing. However, the gutta-percha and zinc oxide–eugenol cement smeared in the canal irregularities make the bonded post a dream more than a reality. When technology enables the removal of canal contaminants noninvasively, resin cement will probably be the luting agent of choice. However, until that time, no available cement can overcome the problems created by a poorly engineered post.

The Resistance Triad

The second and most important consideration in the design of the post restoration is the resistance of the tooth-post-crown combination. If the resistance requirements are not met, the probability of failure is high, regardless of the retentiveness of the post.[141] Three parameters of resistance must be considered (Fig 20-17). The resistance triad consists of the crown bevel, vertical remaining coronal tooth structure, and antirotation feature(s). These features work in combination; if one of the features is minimal or nonexistent, one or both of the remaining features must be increased.

The first feature of the resistance triad is the *crown bevel* (Fig 20-18). The bevel is that part of the crown margin that extends past the post-and-core margin onto the natural tooth structure. To be effective, it must encircle the tooth (360 degrees) and ideally extend at least 2.0 mm onto tooth structure below the post-and-core margin.[142,143] It is not always possible to develop a bevel in every crown preparation. Because all-ceramic crowns and crowns with porcelain labial margins cannot be constructed with a metal collar, it is not possible to use a bevel with these types of crowns. It may also be difficult to prepare a bevel when the remaining coronal tooth structure is minimal. If tooth structure has been lost to fracture or caries, it is sometimes not possible to gain the necessary bevel because of impingement of the crown margin on the biologic width.

The second feature of the resistance triad is *vertical remaining tooth structure* (Fig 20-19). Traditionally, it was taught that the face of a root should be flattened prior to construction of the post and core (Fig 20-20). However, it has been shown that leaving as much natural vertical remaining tooth structure as possible will significantly increase the resistance of the final restoration (Figs 20-21a and 20-21b).[144–146] Unfortunately, because of caries, trauma, or iatrogenic removal, vertical remaining tooth structure is not always available.

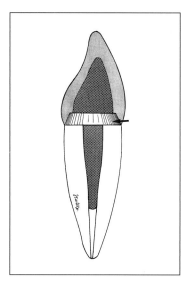

Fig 20-18 Crown bevel around periphery of root surface to increase resistance form.

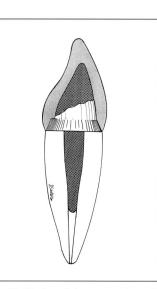

Fig 20-19 Remaining coronal tooth structure should be left to strengthen the post-core-crown combination.

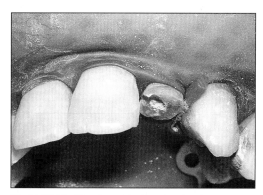

Fig 20-20 Maxillary lateral incisor that has been unnecessarily flattened prior to placement of the post and core.

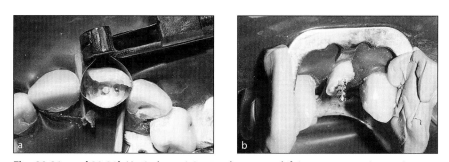

Figs 20-21a and 20-21b Vertical remaining tooth structure left in core preparations to increase resistance form.

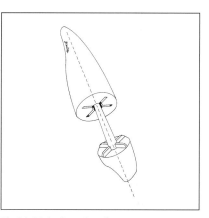

Fig 20-22 Antirotation slots.

The third feature of the resistance triad is *antirotation*. Every post and core must have an antirotation feature incorporated in the preparation.[50,86] An elongated or oblong canal orifice can provide the antirotation effect for the post and core. However, as the canal becomes more round, the need for incorporation of antirotation features becomes more important. This is especially true for anterior teeth. Auxiliary pins and keyways, prepared in the face of the root before construction of the post, are the most common antirotation devices (Fig 20-22).

The three features of the resistance triad are generally easy to incorporate in the preparations of posterior teeth. If there is not enough tooth structure to allow the placement of a bevel, a simple crown-lengthening procedure will generally expose enough tooth structure to allow for bevel placement after healing. It is also easier to incorporate antirotation features in posterior teeth because of their larger size.

However, the features of the resistance triad are generally more difficult to incorporate into the preparations of anterior teeth. Commonly, not as much vertical tooth structure remains, and it is more difficult to incorporate antirotation features because of the smaller tooth size. If, for reasons related to the biologic width or, more commonly, for esthetic reasons, it is not possible to place a substantial metal margin, a very important part of the resistance triad is absent. If there is also minimal vertical remaining tooth structure, the prognosis for the tooth is guarded unless more vertical tooth structure can be incorporated in the preparation. Because anterior crown lengthening generally results in an esthetically unacceptable gingival discontinuity, the treatment of choice, prior to placement of the restoration, is orthodontic eruption.[147] After forced eruption, there is then sufficient remaining vertical tooth structure to significantly improve both the resistance form and the prognosis.

Buildup Materials

With the increased use of prefabricated posts in recent years, the choice of core material has received much interest. Unfortunately, no material possesses all of the ideal characteristics (see box). In selecting a core buildup material, the dentist must consider both the functional requirements of the core and the amount of remaining natural tooth structure. There are currently five widely used core materials: glass ionomer, resin composite, resin-modified glass ionomer, amalgam, and cast metal.

Conventional glass-ionomer materials have the advantages of fluoride release, ease of manipulation, natural color, biocompatibility, corrosion resistance, and dimensional stability in a wet environment.[148] However, they have the major disadvantage of low fracture toughness, which means that the material is susceptible to propagation of cracks. Unfortunately, the fracture toughness is not improved with the addition of silver reinforcement.[149] Therefore, conventional and silver-reinforced glass ionomers can be recommended only for use in posterior teeth in which at least 50% of natural coronal tooth structure remains.

In recent years, resin-modified glass-ionomer materials have gained popularity as core materials. An initial laboratory study[150] indicated that, in addition to the aforementioned advantages of glass-ionomer cement, resin-modified glass-ionomer cements have physical properties similar to those of resin composite. However, another laboratory study found one resin-modified glass ionomer inferior to resin composite in strength.[151] Until their success can be confirmed with clinical studies, resin-modified glass-ionomer cements should be used cautiously in high-stress situations.

Resin composite is the most popular core material because it is easy to use. It is available in light-cure, dual-cure, and autocure formulations. It is provided as both a tooth-colored material to be used as a core material under anterior all-ceramic restorations and as a color-contrast material to be used under metallic restorations. Adequate compressive strength[83,85] and fracture toughness[149] have been confirmed by static load testing. However, resin composite has not performed as successfully when tested with dynamic repeated load tests.[152,153] This type of laboratory test is used to simulate the small, repeated loads of function and parafunction in the oral cavity. It appears that resin composite undergoes plastic deformation under a small repeated load, which may lead to core failure. Another disadvantage of resin composite is that it is not dimensionally stable in a wet environment.[154] As it absorbs water, the buildup expands. This is clinically relevant if a provisional restoration over a resin composite core is lost after the impression has been made for the crown. At delivery, the crown will not fit accurately because of the dimensional expansion of the core.

Resin composite is an adequate buildup material when some vertical tooth structure remains to help support the core buildup. However, it is not recommended for situations in which the entire coronal portion of the tooth is to be replaced with the core material.

Amalgam, as a core buildup material, has several disadvantages. Its early strength is low, necessitating a 15- to 20-minute wait, even when fast-setting spherical alloy is used, until the buildup can be prepared for the crown. It is messy to prepare and can result in irreversible staining of the marginal gingiva during preparation. However, its strength has been confirmed in laboratory studies under both static and dynamic loads.[83,152,153] Therefore, in a high-stress situation in which most of the coronal portion is replaced with the core, either amalgam or custom cast metal is the material of choice (Figs 20-23a and 20-23b).

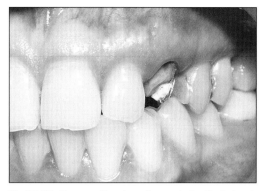

Fig 20-23a Preoperative view of an endodontically treated maxillary canine.

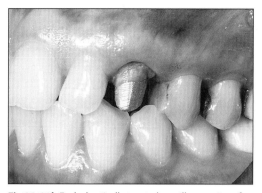

Fig 20-23b Endodontically treated maxillary canine after restoration with a prefabricated post and amalgam core.

Definitive Restorations

Multiple materials and techniques are available for the definitive restoration of the endodontically treated tooth. Because the functional requirements are significantly different for anterior and posterior teeth, they are discussed separately.

Anterior Teeth

It has been demonstrated in the laboratory that the endodontically treated anterior tooth has a fracture resistance approximately equal to that of a vital tooth.[16,18,84] Therefore, when a significant amount of coronal tooth structure remains, there is no need to place a post, and a conventional resin composite restoration in the access preparation is the treatment of choice (Fig 20-24). When a moderate amount of coronal tooth structure is missing but approximately 50% of the coronal enamel remains, the bonded porcelain veneer may be the restoration of choice (Figs 20-25a to 20-25d). Again, there is no need for post placement with the porcelain veneer.

When the decision is made to fabricate a crown for an anterior endodontically treated tooth, a post is commonly indicated. This is especially true for maxillary lateral incisors and mandibular incisors. The decision to place a post is based on the amount of remaining coronal tooth structure after completion of the crown preparation and the functional occlusal requirements. Therefore, the tooth should first be prepared for the crown; then the decision is made regarding the need for a post based on the strength of the remaining natural coronal tooth structure. If a post is required, the canal space is prepared, the post cemented, and the core buildup completed.

Posterior Teeth

In posterior teeth, the forces on the occlusal surfaces are more vertical. Laboratory data indicate that the access preparation has a minimal effect on the fracture resistance of posterior endodontically treated teeth.[155] Based on these data, some authors question the need for cuspal-coverage restorations in these posterior teeth. It has also been demonstrated in the laboratory that teeth with mesio-occlusodistal (MOD) preparations can be strengthened to match the values achieved by unprepared teeth if bonded restorations are placed.[156–161] In a retrospective clinical study, Kanca[162] reported a high clinical success rate in restoring endodontically treated posterior teeth with resin composite restorations. Other laboratory studies, however, have indicated that MOD resin composite restorations in maxillary premolars have no more strengthening effect than similar MOD unbonded amalgam restorations.[163–165] In a retrospective clinical study, Hansen[166] compared the long-term efficacy of resin composite and amalgam in the restoration of endodontically treated premolars. During the first 3 years, teeth restored with amalgam had a greater incidence of cuspal fracture. However, in years 3 through 10, fractures occurred with approximately the same frequency in both groups.

In the face of confusing and contradictory data, it is difficult for the practitioner to develop a treatment philosophy with a sound scientific basis. It seems clear that in wider preparations the strengthening effect of the bonded resin composite restoration is real. However, it has been shown that the strengthening effect diminishes significantly with both thermal cycling[167] and functional loading[168] of the restoration. Because both of these phenomena occur in the

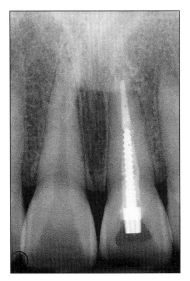

Fig 20-24 Endodontically treated maxillary central incisor that received an unnecessary post.

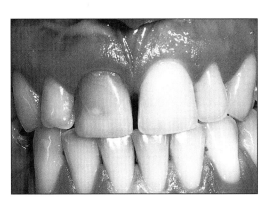

Fig 20-25a Preoperative view of a maxillary right central incisor.

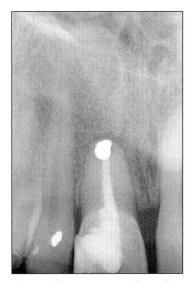

Fig 20-25b Preoperative radiograph.

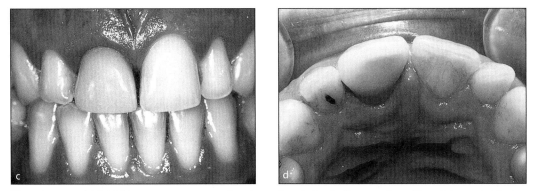

Figs 20-25c and 20-25d Seven-year postoperative views of endodontically treated maxillary right central incisor restored with a porcelain veneer.

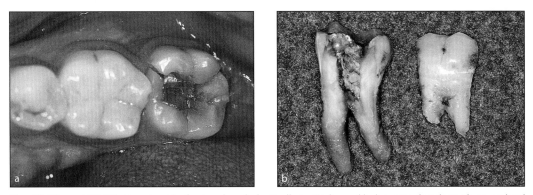

Figs 20-26a and 20-26b Unrestorable, fractured, endodontically treated mandibular second molar with an occlusal amalgam restoration.

oral environment, the long-term strengthening effect of the intracoronal bonded restoration must be questioned. It has also been proposed that a portion of the sensory feedback mechanism is lost when the neurovascular tissue has been removed from the tooth in the course of endodontic therapy, an effect confirmed in an in vivo study.[169] Clinically, this means the patient can inadvertently bite with more force on an endodontically treated tooth than on a vital tooth due to the impaired sensory feedback mechanism (Figs 20-26a and 20-26b).

Both clinical[87] and laboratory[170] studies have demonstrated that the key element in the successful restoration of endodontically treated posterior teeth is the placement of a cuspal-coverage restoration. Although the intracoronal bonded restoration is appealing, based on the current data, the most prudent course of action is to place a restoration that covers all cusps when restoring the endodontically treated posterior tooth. This can be one of a wide variety of restorations, including metal or ceramometal crowns and metal or ceramic onlays.

References

1. Robbins JW. Restoration of the endodontically treated tooth. Dent Clin North Am 2002;46:367–384.
2. Scurria MS, Shugars DA, Hayden WJ, Felton DA. General dentist's patterns of restoring endodontically treated teeth. J Am Dent Assoc 1995;126:775–779.
3. Mentink AGB, Meeuwissen R, Kayser AF, Mulder J. Survival rate and failure characteristics of the all metal post and core restoration. J Oral Rehabil 1993;20:455–461.
4. Torbjorner A, Karlsson S, Odman P. Survival rate and failure characteristics for two post designs. J Prosthet Dent 1995;73:439–444.
5. Nanayakkara L, McDonald A, Setchell DJ. Retrospective analysis of factors affecting the longevity of post crowns [abstract 932]. J Dent Res 1999;78:222.
6. Vire DE. Failure of endodontically treated teeth: Classification and evaluation. J Endod 1991;17:338–342.
7. Weine FS. Endodontic Therapy, ed 5. St Louis: Mosby, 1996:14.
8. Weiger R, Axmann-Kremar K, Lost C. Prognosis of conventional root canal treatment reconsidered. Endod Dent Traumatol 1998;14:1–9.
9. Eriksen HM. Endodontology—Epidemiologic considerations. Endod Dent Traumatol 1991;7:189–195.
10. Barrieshi KM, Walton RE, Johnson WT, Drake DR. Coronal leakage of mixed anaerobic bacteria after obturation and post space preparation. Oral Surg Oral Med Oral Pathol Oral Radiol Endod 1997;84:310–314.
11. Fox K, Gutteridge DL. An in vitro study of coronal microleakage in root canal–treated teeth restored by the post and core technique. Int Endod J 1997;30:361–368.
12. Alves J, Walton R, Drake D. Coronal leakage: Endotoxin penetration from mixed bacterial communities through obturated, post-repaired root canals. J Endod 1998;24:587–591.
13. Helling I, Gorfil C, Slutzky H, Kopolovic K, Zalkind M, Slutzky-Goldberg I. Endodontic failure caused by inadequate restorative procedures: Review and treatment recommendations. J Prosthet Dent 2002;87:674–678.
14. Kantor ME, Pines MS. A comparative study of restorative techniques for pulpless teeth. J Prosthet Dent 1977;38:405–412.
15. Trabert KC, Caputo AA, Abou-Rass M. Tooth fracture—A comparison of endodontic and restorative treatments. J Endod 1978;4:341–345.
16. Guzy GE, Nichols JI. In vitro comparison of intact endodontically treated teeth with and without endo-post reinforcement. J Prosthet Dent 1979;42:39–44.
17. Robbins JW, Earnest L, Schumann S. Fracture resistance of endodontically treated cuspids: An in vitro study. Am J Dent 1993;6:159–161.
18. Trope M, Maltz DO, Tronstad L. Resistance to fracture of restored endodontically treated teeth. Endod Dent Traumatol 1985;1:108–111.
19. Zakhary SY, Nasr HH. In vitro assessment of intact endodontically treated anterior teeth with different restorative procedures. Egypt Dent J 1986;32:221–239.
20. Robbins JW, Burgess JO, Summitt JB. Retention and resistance features for complex amalgam restorations. J Am Dent Assoc 1989;118:437–442.
21. Nayyar A, Walton RE. An amalgam coronal radicular dowel and core technique for endodontically treated posterior teeth. J Prosthet Dent 1980;44:511–515.
22. Kern SB, von Fraunhofer JA, Mueninghoff LA. An in vitro comparison of two dowel and core techniques for endodontically treated molars. J Prosthet Dent 1984;51:509–514.
23. Christian GW, Button GL, Moon PC, England MC, Douglas HB. Post core restoration in endodontically treated posterior teeth. J Endod 1981;7:182–185.
24. Plasmans PJ, Visseren LG, Vrijhoef MM, Kayser FA. In vitro comparison of dowel and core techniques for endodontically treated molars. J Endod 1986;12:382–387.
25. Kane J, Burgess JO. Modification of the resistance form of amalgam coronal-radicular restorations. J Prosthet Dent 1991;65:470–474.
26. Huang TG, Schilder H, Nathanson D. Effects of moisture content and endodontic treatment on some mechanical properties of human dentin. J Endod 1992;18:209–215.
27. Sedgley CM, Messer HH. Are endodontically treated teeth more brittle? J Endod 1992;18:332–335.
28. Tjan AHL, Munoz-Viveros CA, Valencia-Rave GM. Tensile dislodgment of composite/amalgam cores: Dentin adhesives versus mechanical retention [abstract 1355]. J Dent Res 1997;76:183.
29. Summitt JB, Burgess JO, Berry TG, et al. Six-year clinical evaluation of bonded and pin-retained complex amalgam restorations. Oper Dent 2004;29:269–276.
30. Sorensen JA, Martinoff JT. Endodontically treated teeth as abutments. J Prosthet Dent 1985;53:631–636.
31. Yaman P, Zillich R. Restoring the endodontically treated bi-rooted premolar—The effect of endodontic post preparation on width of root dentin. J Mich Dent Assoc 1986;68:79–81.
32. Zillich R, Yaman P. Effect of root curvature on post length in restoration of endodontically treated premolars. Endod Dent Traumatol 1985;1:135–137.
33. Cooney JP, Caputo AA, Trabert KC. Retention and stress distribution of tapered-end endodontic posts. J Prosthet Dent 1986;55:540–546.
34. Johnson JK, Sakamura JS. Dowel form and tensile force. J Prosthet Dent 1978;40:645–649.
35. Standlee JP, Caputo AA, Hanson EC. Retention of endodontic dowels: Effects of cement, dowel length, diameter, and design. J Prosthet Dent 1978;39:401–405.
36. Mattison GD, Delivanis PD, Thacker RW, Hassell KT. Effect of post preparation on the apical seal. J Prosthet Dent 1984;51:785–789.
37. Neagley RL. The effect of dowel preparation on apical seal of endodontically treated teeth. Oral Surg Oral Med Oral Pathol 1969;28:739–745.
38. Sorensen JA, Martinoff JT. Clinically significant factors in dowel design. J Prosthet Dent 1984;52:28–35.

39. Carter JM, Sorensen SE, Johnson RR, Teitelbaum RL, Levine MS. Punch shear testing of extracted vital and endodontically treated teeth. J Biomech 1983;16:841–848.

40. Helfer AR, Melnick S, Schilder H. Determination of moisture content of vital and pulpless teeth. Oral Surg Oral Med Oral Pathol 1972; 34:661–670.

41. Deutsch AS, Musikant BL, Cavallari J, et al. Root fracture during insertion of prefabricated posts related to root size. J Prosthet Dent 1985;53:782–789.

42. Assif D, Bliecher S. Retention of serrated endodontic posts with a composite luting agent: Effect of cement thickness. J Prosthet Dent 1986;56:689–691.

43. Standlee JP, Caputo AA, Collard EW, Pollack MH. Analysis of stress distribution by endodontic posts. Oral Surg Oral Med Oral Pathol 1972;33:952–960.

44. Mattison GD. Photoelastic stress analysis of cast-gold endodontic posts. J Prosthet Dent 1982;48:407–411.

45. Mattison GD, von Fraunhofer JA. Angulation loading effects on cast-gold endodontic posts: A photoelastic stress analysis. J Prosthet Dent 1983;49:636–638.

46. Gross MJ, Turner CH. Intra-radicular hydrostatic pressure changes during the cementation of post-retained crowns. J Oral Rehabil 1983;10:237–249.

47. Colley IT, Hampson EL, Lehman ML. Retention of post crowns. Br Dent J 1968;124:63–69.

48. Maniatopolous C, Pilliar RM, Smith DC. Evaluation of shear strength at the cement endodontic post interface. J Prosthet Dent 1988; 59:662–669.

49. Richer JB, Lautenschlager EP, Greener EH. Mechanical properties of post and core systems. Dent Mater 1986;2:63–66.

50. Ruemping DR, Lund MR, Schnell RJ. Retention of dowels subjected to tensile and torsional forces. J Prosthet Dent 1979;41:159–162.

51. Tjan AHL, Whang SB. Retentive properties of some simplified dowel-core systems to cast gold dowel and core. J Prosthet Dent 1983;50:203–206.

52. Akisli I, Ozcan M, Nergiz I. Effect of surface conditioning techniques on the resistance of resin composite core materials on titanium posts. Quintessence Int 2003;34:766–771.

53. Sahafi A, Peutzfeld A, Asmussen E, Gotfredsen K. Effect of surface treatment of prefabricated posts on bonding of resin cement. Oper Dent 2004;29:60–68.

54. Dickey DJ, Harris GZ, Lemon RR, Luebke RG. Effect of post space preparation on apical seal using solvent techniques and Peeso reamers. J Endod 1982;8:351–354.

55. Kwan EH, Harrington GW. The effect of immediate post preparation on apical seal. J Endod 1981;7:325–329.

56. Madison S, Zakariasen KL. Linear and volumetric analysis of apical leakage in teeth prepared for posts. J Endod 1984;10:422–427.

57. Suchina JA, Ludington JR. Dowel space preparation and the apical seal. J Endod 1985;11:11–17.

58. Hussey DL, Biagioni PA, McCullagh JJP, Lamey PJ. Thermographic assessment of heat generated on the root surface during post space preparation. Int Endod J 1997;30:187–190.

59. Bourgeois RS, Lemon RR. Dowel space preparation and apical leakage. J Endod 1981;7:66–69.

60. Portell FR, Bernier WE, Lorton L, Peters DD. The effect of immediate versus delayed dowel space preparation on the integrity of the apical seal. J Endod 1982;8:154–160.

61. Schnell FJ. Effect of immediate dowel space preparation on the apical seal of endodontically filled teeth. Oral Surg Oral Med Oral Pathol 1978;45:470–474.

62. Goldman M, DeVitre R, Tenca J. Cement distribution and bond strength in cemented posts. J Dent Res 1984;63:1392–1395.

63. Goldstein GR, Hudis SI, Weintraub DE. Comparison of four techniques for cementation of posts. J Prosthet Dent 1986;55:209–211.

64. Maryniuk GA, Shen C, Young HM. Effects of canal lubrication on retention of cemented posts. J Am Dent Assoc 1984;109:430–433.

65. Brown JD, Mitchem JC. Retentive properties of dowel post systems. Oper Dent 1987;12:15–19.

66. Burgess JO, Summitt JB, Robbins JW. The resistance to tensile, compression, and torsional forces provided by four post systems. J Prosthet Dent 1992;68:899–903.

67. Chapman KK, Worley JL, von Fraunhofer JA. Retention of prefabricated posts by cements and resins. J Prosthet Dent 1985;54:649–652.

68. Krupp JD, Caputo AA, Trabert KC, Standlee JP. Dowel retention with glass ionomer cement. J Prosthet Dent 1979;41:163–166.

69. Radke RA, Barkhordar RA, Podesta RE. Retention of cast endodontic posts: Comparison of cementing agents. J Prosthet Dent 1988; 59:318–320.

70. Young HM, Shen C, Maryniuk GA. Retention of cast posts relative to cement selection. Quintessence Int 1985;16:357–360.

71. Schwartz RS, Murchison DF, Walker WH. Effects of eugenol and non-eugenol endodontic sealer cements on post retention. J Endodont 1998;24:564–567.

72. Duncan JP, Pameijer CH. Retention of parallel-sided titanium posts cemented with six luting agents: An in vitro study. J Prosthet Dent 1998;80:423–428.

73. Goldman M, De Vitre R, White R, Nathanson D. An SEM study of posts cemented with an unfilled resin. J Dent Res 1984;63: 1003–1005.

74. Nathanson D. New views on restoring the endodontically treated tooth. Dent Econ 1993;83:48–50.

75. Wong B, Utter JD, Miller BH, et al. Retention of prefabricated posts using three different cementing procedures [abstract 1360]. J Dent Res 1995;74:181.

76. Nourian L, Burgess JO. Tensile load to remove cemented posts cemented with different surface treatments [abstract 1788]. J Dent Res 1994;73:325.

77. Paschal JE, Burgess JO. Tensile load to remove posts cemented with different cements [abstract 1362]. J Dent Res 1995;74:182.

78. Serafino C, Gallina G, Cumbo E, Ferrari M. Surface debris of canal walls after post space preparation in endodontically treated teeth: A scanning electron microscope study. Oral Surg Oral Med Oral Pathol Oral Radiol Endod 2004;97:381–387.

79. Burgess JO, Re GJ, Nunez A. Effect of sealer type on post retention [abstract 1356]. J Dent Res 1997;76:183.

80. Millstein P, Robison B, Rankin C. Effects of EDTA/NaOCL and resin cement on post tooth retention [abstract 1527]. J Dent Res 1999; 78:296.

81. Kurtz JS, Perdigao J, Geraldeli S, Hodges JS, Bowles WR. Bond strengths of tooth-colored posts, effect of sealer, dentin adhesive, and root region. Am J Dent 2003;16(spec no.):31A–36A.

82. Vichi A, Grandini S, Davidson C, Ferrari M. An SEM evaluation of several adhesive systems used for bonding fiber posts under clinical conditions. Dent Mater 2002;18:495–502.

83. Chan RW, Bryant RW. Post-core foundations for endodontically treated posterior teeth. J Prosthet Dent 1982;48:401–406.

84. Lovdahl PE, Nicholls JI. Pin-retained amalgam cores vs. cast-gold dowel cores. J Prosthet Dent 1977;38:507–514.

85. Moll JFP, Howe DF, Svare CW. Cast gold post and core and pin-retained composite resin bases: A comparative study in strength. J Prosthet Dent 1978;40:642–644.

86. Newburg RE, Pameijer CH. Retentive properties of post and core systems. J Prosthet Dent 1976;36:636–643.

87. Sorensen JA, Martinoff JT. Intracoronal reinforcement and coronal coverage: A study of endodontically treated teeth. J Prosthet Dent 1984;51:780–784.

88. Hong-so Yang, Lang L, Molina A, Felton D. The effects of dowel design and load direction on dowel-and-core restorations. J Prosthet Dent 2001;85:558–567.

89. Isador F, Brondum K. Intermittent loading of teeth with tapered individually cast or prefabricated, parallel-sided posts. Int J Prosthodont 1992;5:257–261.

90. Qualtrough A, Chandler M, Purton D. A comparison of the retention of tooth-colored posts. Quintessence Int 2003;34:199–201.

91. Burns DA, Krause WR, Douglas HB, Burns DR. Stress distribution surrounding endodontic posts. J Prosthet Dent 1990;64:412–418.

92. Boyarsky H, Davis R. Root fracture with dentin-retained posts. Am J Dent 1992;5:11–14.

93. Caputo AA, Hokama SN. Stress and retention properties of a new threaded endodontic post. Quintessence Int 1987;18:431–435.

94. Felton DA, Webb EL, Kanoy BE, Dugoni J. Threaded endodontic dowels: Effects of post design on incidence of root fracture. J Prosthet Dent 1991;65:179–187.

95. Greenfeld RS, Roydhouse RH, Marshall FJ, Schoner B. A comparison of two post systems under applied compressive shear loads. J Prosthet Dent 1989;61:17–24.

96. Ross RS, Nicholls JI, Harrington GW. A comparison of strains generated during placement of five endodontic posts. J Endod 1991;17:450–456.

97. Thorsteinsson TS, Yaman P, Craig RG. Stress analyses of four prefabricated posts. J Prosthet Dent 1992;67:30–33.

98. Purton DG, Love RM. Rigidity and retention of carbon fibre versus stainless steel canal posts. Int Endod J 1996;29:262–265.

99. Purton DG, Payne JA. Comparison of carbon fiber and stainless steel root canal posts. Quintessence Int 1996;27:93–97.

100. Narva KK, Lassila LVJ, Vallittu PK. Comparison of mechanical properties of commercial carbon graphite fiber root canal posts [abstract 418]. J Dent Res 1999;78:158.

101. Hollis RA, Christensen GJ, Christensen W, et al. Comparison of strength for seven different post materials [abstract 3421]. J Dent Res 1999;78:533.

102. Martinez-Insua A, Da Silva L, Rilo B, Santana U. Comparison of the fracture resistances of pulpless teeth restored with a cast post and core or carbon-fiber post with a composite core. J Prosthet Dent 1998;80:527–532.

103. Sidoli GE, King PA, Setchell DJ. An in vitro evaluation of a carbon fiber-based post and core system. J Prosthet Dent 1997;78:5–9.

104. Wong EJ, Ruse ND, Greenfield RS, Coil JM. Initial failure of post/core systems under compressive shear loads [abstract 2269]. J Dent Res 1999;78:389.

105. Dean JP, Jeansonne BG, Sarkan N. In vitro evaluation of a carbon fiber post. J Endod 1998;24:807–810.

106. Isador F, Odman P, Brondum K. Intermittent loading of teeth restored using prefabricated carbon fiber posts. Int J Prosthodont 1996;9:131–136.

107. King PA, Setchell DJ. An in vitro evaluation of a prototype CFRC prefabricated post developed for the restoration of pulpless teeth. J Oral Rehabil 1990;17:599–609.

108. Stockton L, Williams P. Retention and shear bond strength of 2 post systems. Oper Dent 1999;24:210–216.

109. Drummond JL, Toepke TR, King TJ. Pullout strength of thermal and loaded cycled carbon and stainless steel posts [abstract 3393]. J Dent Res 1999;78:530.

110. Millstein P, Maya A, Freeman Y, O'Leary J. Comparing post and core retention with post head diameter [abstract 1528]. J Dent Res 1999;78:296.

111. Triolo PT, Trajtenberg C, Powers JM. Flexural properties and bond strength of an esthetic post [abstract 3538]. J Dent Res 1999;78:548.

112. Holmgren EP, Mante FK, Shokoufeh E, Afsharzand Z. Stresses in post and core build-up materials [abstract 934]. J Dent Res 1999;78:222.

113. King PA, Setchell DJ. 7 year clinical evaluation of a prototype CFRC endodontic post. [abstract 2235]. J Dent Res 1997;76:293.

114. Fredriksson M, Astback J, Pamenius M, Arvidson K. A retrospective study of 236 patients with teeth restored by carbon fiber-reinforced epoxy resin posts. J Prosthet Dent 1998;80:151–157.

115. Ferrari M, Vichi A, Garcia-Godoy F. A retrospective study of fiber-reinforced epoxy resin posts vs. cast posts and cores: A four year recall. Am J Dent (in press).

116. Ferrari M, Mason PN, Mannocci F, Vichi A. Retrospective study of clinical behavior of several types of fiber posts. Am J Dent (in press).

117. Mannocci F, Vichi A, Ferrari M, et al. Carbon fiber posts, clinical and laboratory studies. The esthetical endodontic posts. In: Proceedings from the Second International Symposium. Reconstruction with Carbon Fiber Posts. Milan, Italy: Hippocrates Edizioni Medico-Scientifiche, 1998:18–19.

118. Finger W, Ahlstrand W, Fritz U. Radiopacity of fiber-reinforced resin posts. Am J Dent 2002;15:81–84.

119. Ichikawa Y, Akagawa Y, Nikai H, Tsuru H. Tissue compatibility and stability of a new zirconia ceramic in vivo. J Prosthet Dent 1992;68:322–326.

120. Meyerberg KH, Kuthy H, Scharer P. Zirconia posts: A new all-ceramic concept for nonvital abutment teeth. J Esthet Dent 1995;7:73–80.

121. Rovatti L, Mason ON, Dallare EA. The esthetical endodontic posts. In: Proceedings from the Second International Symposium. Reconstructions with Carbon Fiber Posts. Milan, Italy: Hippocrates Edizioni Medico-Scientifiche, 1998:12.

122. Fischer H, Rentzsch W, Marx R. Elimination of low-quality ceramic posts by proof testing. Dent Mater 2002;18:570–575.

123. Sahafi A, Peutzfeldt, Asmussen E, Gotfredsen K. Bond strength of resin cement to dentin and to surface-treated posts of titanium alloy, glass fiber, and zirconia. J Adhes Dent 2003;5:153–162.

124. Al-harbi F, Nathanson D. In vitro assessment of retention of four esthetic dowels to resin core foundation and teeth. J Prosthet Dent 2003;90:547–555.

125. Usumez A, Cobankara F, Ozturk N, Eskitascioglu G, Belli S. Microleakage of endodontically treated teeth with different dowel systems. J Prosthet Dent 2004;92:163–169.

126. Oblak C, Jevnikar P, Kosmac T, Funduk N, Marion L. Fracture resistance and reliability of new zirconia posts. J Prosthet Dent 2004;91:342–348.

127. Dietschi D, Romelli M, Goretti A. Adaptation of adhesive posts and cores to dentin after fatigue testing. Int J Prosthodont 1997;10:498–507.

128. Koutayas SO, Kern M. All-ceramic posts and cores: The state of the art. Quintessence Int 1999;30:383–392.

129. Snyder TC, Caputo AA. Retention and load transfer characteristics of zirconium dioxide endodontic dowels [abstract 1529]. J Dent Res 1999;78:297.

130. Hu YH, Pang LC, Hsu CC, Lau YH. Fracture resistance of endodontically treated anterior teeth restored with four post-and-core systems. Quintessence Int 2003;34:349–353.

131. Kern M, Simon MHP, Strub JR. Clinical evaluation of all ceramic zirconia posts: A pilot study [abstract 2234]. J Dent Res 1997;76:293.

132. Ahmad I. Yttrium–partially stabilized zirconium dioxide posts: An approach to restoring coronally compromised nonvital teeth. Int J Periodontics Restorative Dent 1998;18:455–465.

133. Ahmad I. Zirconium oxide post and core system for the restoration of an endodontically treated incisor. Pract Periodont Aesthet Dent 1999;11:197–204.

134. Zalkind M, Hochman N. Direct core buildup using a preformed crown and a prefabricated zirconium oxide post. J Prosthet Dent 1998;80:730–732.

135. Zalkind M, Hochman N. Esthetic considerations in restoring endodontically treated teeth with posts and cores. J Prosthet Dent 1998;79:702–705.

136. Coelho Santos G Jr, El-Mowafy O, Hernique Rubo J. Diametral tensile strength of a resin composite core with non-metallic prefabricated posts: An in vitro study. J Prosthet Dent 2004;91:335–341.

137. Karna JC. A fiber composite laminate endodontic post and core. Am J Dent 1996;9:230–232.

138. Furer C, Rosentritt M, Behr M, Handel G. Fracture strength of all-ceramic, metal, and fiber reinforced posts and cores [abstract 1489]. J Dent Res 1998;77:818.

139. Lui JL. Composite resin reinforcement of flared canals using light-transmitting plastic posts. Quintessence Int 1994;25:313–319.

140. Saupe WA, Gluskin AH, Radke RA. A comparative study of fracture resistance between morphologic dowel and cores and a resin-reinforced dowel system in the intraradicular restoration of structurally compromised roots. Quintessence Int 1996;27:483–491.

141. Isador F, Brondum K, Ravnholt G. The influence of post length and crown ferrule length on the resistance to cyclic loading of bovine teeth with prefabricated titanium posts. Int J Prosthodont 1999;12:78–82.

142. Libman W, Nicholls J. Load fatigue of teeth restored with cast posts and cores and complete crowns. Int J Prosth 1995;2:155–161.

143. Akkayan B. An in vitro study evaluating the effect of ferrule length on fracture resistance of endodontically treated teeth restored with fiber-reinforced and zirconia dowel systems. J Prosthet Dent 2004;92:155–162.

144. Sorensen JA, Engelman MJ, Mito WT. Effect of ferrule design on fracture resistance of pulpless teeth [abstract 142]. J Dent Res 1988;67:130.

145. Pierrisnard L, Bohin F, Renault P, Barquins M. Corono-radicular reconstructions of pulpless teeth: A mechanical study using finite element analysis. J Prosthet Dent 2002;88:442–448.

146. Zhi-Yue L, Yu-xing Z. Effects of post-core design and ferrule on fracture resistance of endodontically treated maxillary central incisors. J Prosthet Dent 2003;89:368–373.

147. Starr C. Management of periodontal tissues for restorative dentistry. J Esthet Dent 1991;3:195–208.

148. Cooley R, Robbins J, Barnwell S. Stability of glass ionomer used as a core material. J Prosthet Dent 1990;64:651–653.

149. Lloyd CH, Adamson M. The development of fracture toughness and fracture strength in posterior restorative materials. Dent Mater 1987;3:225–231.

150. Lattner ML. Fracture Resistance of Five Core Materials for Cast Crowns [thesis]. San Antonio, TX: University of Texas, 1994.

151. Levartovsky S, Goldstein GR, Georgescu M. Shear bond strength of several new core materials. J Prosthet Dent 1996;75:154–158.

152. Huysmans MC, Van Der Varst PG, Schafer R, Peters MC, Plasschaert AJ, Soltesz U. Fatigue behavior of direct post and core restored premolars. J Dent Res 1992;71:1145–1150.

153. Kovarik RE, Breeding LC, Caughman WF. Fatigue life of three core materials under simulated chewing conditions. J Prosthet Dent 1992;68:584–590.

154. Oliva RA, Lowe JA. Dimensional stability of silver amalgam and composite used as core materials. J Prosthet Dent 1987;57:554–559.

155. Reeh ES. Reduction in tooth stiffness as a result of endodontic restorative procedures. J Endod 1989;15:512–516.

156. Jensen ME, Redford DA, Williams BT, Gardner F. Posterior etched-porcelain restorations: An in vitro study. Compend Contin Educ Dent 1987;8:615–622.

157. Landy NA, Simonsen RJ. Cusp fracture strength in Class 2 composite resin restorations [abstract 39]. J Dent Res 1984;63:175.

158. Morin D, DeLong R, Douglas WH. Cusp reinforcement by the acid-etch technique. J Dent Res 1984;63:1075–1078.

159. Reeh ES, Douglas WH, Messer HH. Stiffness of endodontically treated teeth related to restoration technique [abstract 1510]. J Dent Res 1988;67:301.

160. Share J, Mishell Y, Nathanson S. Effect of restorative material on resistance to fracture of tooth structure in vitro [abstract 622]. J Dent Res 1982;61:247.

161. Wendt SL, Harris BM, Hunt TE. Resistance to cusp fracture in endodontically treated teeth. Dent Mater 1987;3:232–235.

162. Kanca J. Conservative resin restoration of endodontically treated teeth. Quintessence Int 1988;19:25–28.

163. Joynt RB, Wieczkowski G, Klockowoski R, Davis EL. Effects of composite restorations on resistance to cuspal fracture in posterior teeth. J Prosthet Dent 1987;57:431–435.

164. Joynt RB, Davis EL, Wieczkowski GJ, Williams DA. Fracture resistance of posterior teeth restored with glass ionomer–composite resin systems. J Prosthet Dent 1989;62:28–31.

165. Stampalia LL, Nicholls, JI, Brudvik JS. Fracture resistance of teeth with resin-bonded restorations. J Prosthet Dent 1986;55:694–698.

166. Hansen EK. In vivo cusp fracture of endodontically treated premolars restored with MOD amalgam or MOD resin fillings. Dent Mater 1988;4:169–173.

167. Eakle WS. Effect of thermal cycling on fracture strength and microleakage in teeth restored with a bonded composite resin. Dent Mater 1986;2:114–117.

168. Fissore B, Nicholls JI, Yuodelis RA. Load fatigue of teeth restored by a dentin bonding agent and a posterior composite resin. J Prosthet Dent 1991;65:80–85.

169. Randow K, Glantz P. On cantilever loading of vital and non-vital teeth. Acta Odontol Scand 1986;44:271–277.

170. Hoag EP, Dwyer TG. A comparative evaluation of three post and core techniques. J Prosthet Dent 1982;47:177–181.

Index